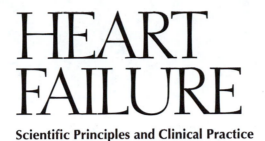

HEART FAILURE

Scientific Principles and Clinical Practice

HEART FAILURE

Scientific Principles and Clinical Practice

Edited by

Philip A. Poole-Wilson, M.D., F.R.C.P., F.A.C.C., F.E.S.C.

Professor of Cardiology, Department of Cardiac Medicine, National Heart and Lung Institute, Imperial College of Science, Technology and Medicine, London, England

Wilson S. Colucci, M.D., F.A.C.C.

Professor of Medicine and Physiology, Boston University School of Medicine; Associate Chief of Cardiology and Director, Cardiomyopathy Program, Boston Medical Center; Chief of Cardiology, Veterans Affairs Medical Center, Boston, Massachusetts

Barry M. Massie, M.D.

Professor of Medicine and Associate Staff, Cardiovascular Research Institute, University of California, San Francisco, School of Medicine; Director, Coronary Care Unit, and Chief, Hypertension Clinic, Veterans Affairs Medical Center, San Francisco, California

Kanu Chatterjee, M.B., F.R.C.P.

Professor of Medicine, Lucie Stern Professor of Cardiology, Vilensky Research Professor of Cardiology, and Associate Chief, Division of Cardiology, Department of Medicine, University of California, San Francisco, School of Medicine, San Francisco, California

Andrew J. S. Coats, D.M., F.R.C.P., F.R.A.C.P., F.E.S.C., F.A.C.C.

Viscount Royston Professor of Cardiology, Department of Cardiac Medicine, National Heart and Lung Institute, Imperial College of Science, Technology and Medicine; Director of Cardiology, Royal Brompton Hospital, London, England

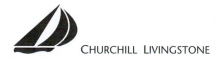

CHURCHILL LIVINGSTONE

New York, Edinburgh, London, Madrid, Melbourne, San Francisco, Tokyo

Library of Congress Cataloging-in-Publication Data

Distributed in the United Kingdom by Churchill Livingstone, Robert Stevenson House, 1–3 Baxter's Place, Leith Walk, Edinburgh EH1 3AF, and by associated companies, branches, and representatives throughout the world.

Medical knowledge is constantly changing. As new information becomes available, changes in treatment, procedures, equipment and the use of drugs become necessary. The editors/authors/contributors and the publishers have, as far as it is possible, taken care to ensure that the information given in this text is accurate and up to date. However, readers are strongly advised to confirm that the information, especially with regard to drug usage, complies with the latest legislation and standards of practice.

The Publishers have made every effort to trace the copyright holders for borrowed material. If they have inadvertently overlooked any, they will be pleased to make the necessary arrangements at the first opportunity.

Acquisitions Editor: *Allan Ross*
Assistant Editor: *Jennifer Hardy*
Production Editor: *Donna C. Balopole*
Production Supervisor: *Sharon Tuder*
Cover Design: *Jeannette Jacobs*

Production services provided by Bermedica Production, Ltd.

Printed in the United States of America

First published in 1997   7   6   5   4   3   2   1

To our families, mentors, and students

Contributors

William T. Abraham, M.D.

Assistant Professor of Medicine, Division of Cardiology, Department of Medicine, University of Colorado School of Medicine; Director, Health Failure Program, University of Colorado Health Sciences Center, Denver, Colorado

Inder S. Anand, M.D., F.R.C.P., D.Phil. (Oxon)

Professor of Medicine, Cardiovascular Division, Department of Medicine, University of Minnesota Medical School; Staff Cardiologist, Veterans Affairs Medical Center, Minneapolis, Minnesota

Bert Andersson, M.D., Ph.D.

Senior Consultant in Cardiology, Division of Cardiology, Department of Heart and Lung Diseases, Sahgrenska University Hospital, and Wallenberg Laboratory for Cardiovascular Research, Göteborg University, Göteborg, Sweden

Stefan D. Anker, M.D.

Research Registrar, Department of Cardiac Medicine, National Heart and Lung Institute, Imperial College of Science, Technology and Medicine; Honorary Registrar, Royal Brompton Hospital, London, England

Stephen G. Ball, M.A., Ph.D., F.R.C.P.

Professor of Cardiology and Chairman of Institute for Cardiovascular Research, University of Leeds Medical School; Consultant Cardiologist, Leeds General Infirmary, Leeds, England

Yochai Birnbaum, M.D.

Research Fellow in Cardiology, Heart Institute, Good Samaritan Hospital, Los Angeles, California

Arie Blitz, M.D.

Chief Resident, Division of Cardiothoracic Surgery, Department of General Surgery, University of California, Los Angeles, UCLA School of Medicine, Los Angeles, California

Gisèle Bonne, Ph.D.

Researcher, Unité de Recherche INSERM 153, Institut de Myologie, Groupe Hospitalier Pitié-Salpêtrière, Paris, France

Elias H. Botvinick, M.D.

Professor of Medicine and Radiology, University of California, San Francisco, School of Medicine; Co-Director, Adult Noninvasive Cardiac Laboratory, UCSF Hospitals, San Francisco, California

Roland R. Brandt, M.D.

Instructor of Medicine, Mayo Medical School; Research Fellow, Cardiorenal Research Laboratory, Division of Cardiovascular Diseases, Department of Internal Medicine, Mayo Clinic and Mayo Foundation, Rochester, Minnesota

Michael R. Bristow, M.D., Ph.D.

Professor of Medicine and Head, Division of Cardiology, Department of Medicine, University of Colorado School of Medicine; Director, Temple Hoynes Buell Heart Center, University of Colorado Health Sciences Center, Denver, Colorado

John C. Burnett, Jr., M.D.

Professor of Medicine and Physiology, Mayo Medical School; Director, Cardiorenal Research Laboratory, Division of Cardiovascular Diseases, Department of Internal Medicine, Mayo Clinic and Mayo Foundation, Rochester, Minnesota

A. John Camm, M.D.

Professor of Clinical Cardiology, Cardiological Sciences, St. George's Hospital Medical School; Honorary Consultant Cardiologist, St. George's Hospital, London, England

Lucie Carrier, Ph.D.

Researcher, Unité de Recherche INSERM 153, Institut de Myologie, Groupe Hospitalier Pitié-Salpêtrière, Paris, France

Bianca Maria Cattaneo, M.D.

Research Fellow in Cardiology, Department of Medicine, San Gerardo University Hospital, Monza, Milan, Italy; Centro Auxologico Italiano, Milan, Italy

Kanu Chatterjee, M.B., F.R.C.P.

Professor of Medicine, Lucie Stern Professor of Cardiology, Vilensky Research Professor of Cardiology, and Associate Chief, Division of Cardiology, Department of Medicine, University of California, San Francisco, School of Medicine, San Francisco, California

Tony M. Chou, M.D.

Assistant Clinical Professor of Medicine, Division of Cardiology, Department of Medicine, University of California, San Francisco, School of Medicine, San Francisco, California

John G. F. Cleland, M.D., F.R.C.P., F.E.S.C., F.A.C.C.

British Heart Foundation Senior Research Fellow and Honorary Consultant Cardiologist, Medical Research Council Clinical Research Initiative in Heart Failure, University of Glasgow, Glasgow, Scotland

Andrew J. S. Coats, D.M., F.R.C.P., F.R.A.C.P., F.E.S.C., F.A.C.C

Viscount Royston Professor of Cardiology, Department of Cardiac Medicine, National Heart and Lung Institute, Imperial College of Science, Technology and Medicine; Director of Cardiology, Royal Brompton Hospital, London, England

Robert J. Cody, M.D.

The James H. and Ruth J. Wilson Professor of Medicine, Division of Cardiology, Ohio State University Medical Center, Columbus, Ohio

Wilson S. Colucci, M.D., F.A.C.C.

Professor of Medicine and Physiology, Boston University School of Medicine; Associate Chief of Cardiology and Director, Cardiomyopathy Program, Boston Medical Center; Chief of Cardiology, Veterans Affairs Medical Center, Boston, Massachusetts

Aman S. Coonar, B.Sc. (Hons), M.B.B.S., M.R.C.P.

British Heart Foundation Junior Research Fellow, Department of Cardiological Sciences, St. George's Hospital Medical School, London, England

Martin R. Cowie, M.B., ChB., B.Med.Biol., M.R.C.P.

Research Fellow in Clinical Epidemiology, Department of Cardiac Medicine, National Heart and Lung Institute, Imperial College of Science, Technology and Medicine, London, England

Michael W. Dae, M.D.

Professor of Radiology and Medicine, University of California, San Francisco, California

Henry J. Dargie, F.R.C.P., F.E.S.C.

Co-Director, Clinical Research Initiative in Heart Failure, University of Glasgow; Consultant Cardiologist, West Glasgow Hospitals University NHS Trust, Glasgow, Scotland

Teresa De Marco, M.D., F.A.C.C.

Associate Professor of Medicine, Medical Director, Heart Transplantation, and Co-Director, Heart Failure Evaluation and Treatment Program, Division of Cardiology, Department of Medicine, University of California, San Francisco, School of Medicine, San Francisco, California

Helmut Drexler, M.D.

Professor of Medicine and Chief, Department of Cardiology, Medizinische Hochschule Hannover, Hannover, Germany

Uri Elkayam, M.D.

Professor of Medicine, Division of Cardiology, Department of Medicine, University of Southern California School of Medicine; Director, Heart Failure Program, University of Sourthern California University Hospital, Los Angeles, California

Arthur M. Feldman, M.D., Ph.D.

Harry S. Tack Professor of Medicine and Chief, Division of Cardiology, University of Pittsburgh Medical Center, Pittsburgh, Pennsylvania

Gary S. Francis, M.D.

Professor, Department of Medicine, University of Minnesota Medical School; Director, Acute Cardiac Care, University of Minnesota Hospital and Clinics, Minneapolis, Minnesota

William Frishman, M.D.

Professor and Associate Chairman, Department of Medicine, Albert Einstein College of Medicine of Yeshiva University/Montefiore Medical Center, Bronx, New York

Stephen J. Fuller, M.A., D.Phil.

British Heart Foundation Lecturer in Basic Science, Department of Cardiac Medicine, National Heart and Lung Institute, Imperial College of Science, Technology and Medicine, London, England

Derek Gibson, M.A., M.B., F.R.C.P.

Consultant Cardiologist, Royal Brompton Hospital, London, England

Thomas D. Giles, M.D.

Professor, Department of Medicine, Louisiana State University School of Medicine in New Orleans; Director, Program in Heart Failure and Hypertension, Louisiana State University Medical Center, New Orleans, Louisiana

Jaswinder S. Gill, M.A., M.D., M.R.C.P., F.A.C.C.

Consultant Cardiologist, Department of Cardiology, Guy's Hospital; Honorary Senior Lecturer, UMDS, Guy's and St. Thomas's Medical and Dental Schools, University of London, London, England

Guido Grassi, M.D.

Assistant Professor, Department of Medicine, San Gerardo University Hospital, Monza, Milan, Italy; University of Milan, Centro di Fisiologia Clinica e Ipertensione, Maggiore Hospital, Milan, Italy

Barry H. Greenberg, M.D.

Professor of Medicine and Director, Heart Failure/ Transplant Cardiology Program, Division of Cardiovascular Medicine, Department of Medicine, University of California, San Diego, School of Medicine, San Diego, California

Garrie J. Haas, M.D.

Director of the Heart Failure Special Care Unit, Cleveland Clinic Foundation, Cleveland, Ohio

Derek Harrington, B.Sc., M.R.C.P.

Robert Luft Research Fellow in Cardiology, Department of Cardiac Medicine, National Heart and Lung Institute, Imperial College of Science, Technology and Medicine, London, England

Mary H. Hawthorne, Ph.D., R.N.

Associate Professor and Director of the Adult Nurse Practitioner Program, Duke University School of Nursing, Durham, North Carolina

Denise D. Hermann, M.D.

Assistant Clinical Professor of Medicine, Heart Failure/Transplant Cardiology Program, Division of Cardiovascular Medicine, Department of Medicine, University of California, San Diego, School of Medicine, San Diego, California

Stuart J. Hutchison, M.D.

Clinical Instructor in Cardiology, Division of Cardiology, Department of Medicine, University of California, San Francisco, School of Medicine, San Francisco, California; Assistant Professor, Department of Medicine, University of Toronto Faculty of Medicine, St. Michael's Hospital, Toronto, Canada

Joanne S. Ingwall, Ph.D.

Professor of Medicine (Physiology) and Senior Biochemist, NMR Laboratory for Physiological Chemistry, Cardiovascular Division, Department of Medicine, Brigham and Women's Hospital and Harvard Medical School, Boston, Massachusetts

William B. Kannel, M.D., M.P.H.

Professor of Medicine and Public Health, Department of Medicine, Section of Preventive Medicine and Epidemiology, Boston University School of Medicine/Framingham Heart Study, Framingham, Massachusetts

David A. Kass, M.D.

Associate Professor, Departments of Medicine and Biomedical Engineering, Johns Hopkins University School of Medicine, Baltimore, Maryland

David M. Kaye, M.B.B.S., Ph.D., F.R.A.C.P., F.A.C.C.

Postdoctoral Research Fellow, Cardiovascular Division, and Department of Medicine, Harvard Medical School, Brigham and Women's Hospital, Boston, Massachusetts

Ralph A. Kelly, M.D.

Assistant Professor of Medicine, Harvard Medical School; Associate Physician, Brigham and Women's Hospital, Boston, Massachusetts

Robert A. Kloner, M.D., Ph.D.

Professor of Medicine, Division of Cardiology, Department of Medicine, University of Southern California School of Medicine; Director of Research, Heart Institute, Good Samaritan Hospital, Los Angeles, California

Uwe Kühl, Ph.D.

Department of Cardiology, Freie Universität Berlin; Medical Clinic of Internal Medicine, Benjamin Franklin Hospital, Berlin, Germany

Hillel Laks, M.D.

Professor and Chief, Division of Cardiothoracic Surgery, Department of General Surgery, University of California, Los Angeles, UCLA School of Medicine, Los Angeles, California

Carl V. Leier, M.D.

Overstreet Professor of Medicine and Pharmacology, Director, Division of Cardiology, and Cardiology Director of Heart Transplantation, The Ohio State University College of Medicine, Columbus, Ohio

Thierry H. LeJemtel, M.D.

Professor, Division of Cardiology, Department of Medicine, Albert Einstein College of Medicine of Yeshiva University, Bronx, New York

Jonathan Leor, M.D.

Director of Coronary Care Unit and Assistant Director, Cardiology Division, Soroka Medical Center; Senior Lecturer, Faculty of Health Sciences, Ben Gurion University, Beer Sheva, Israel

Giuseppe Mancia, M.D.

Professor of Medicine, Department of Internal Medicine, University of Milan, Milan, Italy; Head, First Division of Internal Medicine, San Gerardo University Hospital, Monza, Milan, Italy

Barry M. Massie, M.D.

Professor of Medicine and Associate Staff, Cardiovascular Research Institute, University of California, San Francisco, School of Medicine; Director, Coronary Care Unit, and Chief, Hypertension Unit, Veterans Affairs Medical Center, San Francisco, California

Theresa A. McDonagh, B.Sc., M.B., Ch.B., M.R.C.P.

Clinical Lecturer, Clinical Research Initiative in Heart Failure, University of Glasgow; Honorary Senior Registrar, Department of Cardiology, West Glasgow Hospitals University NHS Trust, Glasgow, Scotland

Robert S. McKelvie, M.D., Ph.D., F.R.C.P.(C)

Associate Professor of Medicine, Division of Cardiology, McMaster University Faculty of Health Sciences; Consultant in Cardiology, Hamilton Civic Hospitals-General Division, Hamilton, Ontario, Canada

William J. McKenna, B.A., M.D., F.A.C.C., F.E.S.C., F.R.C.P.

Professor of Cardiac Medicine, Department of Cardiological Sciences, St. George's Hospital Medical School, London, England

James P. Morgan, M.D., Ph.D.

Associate Professor of Medicine, Harvard Medical School; Chief, Cardiovascular Division, Beth Israel Hospital, Boston, Massachusetts

Celia M. Oakley, M.D., F.R.C.P., F.A.C.C., F.E.S.C.

Professor of Clinical Cardiology, Department of Medicine, Royal Postgraduate Medical School, Hammersmith Hospital, London, England

Paul J. Oldershaw, M.A., M.D., F.R.C.P.

Consultant Cardiologist, Royal Brompton Hospital, London, England

Milton Packer, M.D.

Dickinson W. Richards Professor of Medicine and Professor of Pharmacology, Columbia University College of Physicians and Surgeons; Chief, Division of Circulatory Physiology, and Director, Center for Heart Failure Research, Columbia-Presbyterian Medical Center, New York, New York

Ted Plappert, C.V.T.

Echocardiography Technician, Cardiovascular Division, Hospital of the University of Pennsylvania (HUP), Philadelphia, Pennsylvania

Philip A. Poole-Wilson, M.D., F.R.C.P., F.A.C.C., F.E.S.C.

Professor of Cardiology, Department of Cardiac Medicine, National Heart and Lung Institute, Imperial College of Science, Technology and Medicine, London, England

J. David Port, Ph.D.

Assistant Professor of Medicine, Division of Cardiology, Department of Medicine, and Assistant Professor, Department of Pharmacology, University of Colorado School of Medicine, Denver, Colorado

Andrew N. Redington, M.D., F.R.C.P.

Professor of Congenital Heart Disease, Department of Paediatric Cardiology, National Heart and Lung Institute–Royal Brompton Hospital Trust, Imperial College of Science, Technology and Medicine, London, England

Peter J. Richardson, M.D., F.R.C.P.

Consultant Cardiologist, Cardiac Department, King's College Hospital, London, England

Heinrich R. Schelbert, M.D.

Profesor of Pharmacology and Radiological Sciences, Vice Chair, Department of Molecular and Medical Pharmacology, Chief, Nuclear Medicine Service, University of California, Los Angeles, UCLA School of Medicine, Los Angeles, California

Frank Scholl, M.D.

Resident, Division of Cardiothoracic Surgery, Department of General Surgery, University of California, Los Angeles, UCLA School of Medicine, Los Angeles, California

Heinz-Peter Schultheiss, M.D.

Professor of Medicine and Chief, Department of Cardiology, Freie Universität Berlin; Medical Clinic of Internal Medicine, Benjamin Franklin Hospital, Berlin, Germany

Ketty Schwartz, Ph.D.

Director of Research, Unité de Recherche INSERM 153, Institut de Myologie, Groupe Hospitalier Pitié-Salpêtrière, Paris, France

Bodo Schwartzkopff, M.D.

Assistant Professor, Medical Clinic and Policlinic B, Division of Cardiology, Pneumology and Angiology, Department of Internal Medicine, Heinrich-Heine University, Düsseldorf, Germany

Thomas W. Smith, M.D.

Professor of Medicine, Harvard Medical School; Chief, Cardiovascular Division, Brigham and Women's Hospital, Boston, Massachusetts

Martin G. St. John Sutton, F.R.C.P., F.A.C.C., F.E.S.C.

Professor of Medicine, University of Pennsylvania School of Medicine; Director, Cardiovascular Imaging Program, Hospital of the University of Pennsylvania (HUP), Philadelphia, Pennsylvania

Rodney H. Stables, M.A., M.R.C.P.

Senior Registrar in Cardiology, Royal Brompton Hospital, London, England

Randall C. Starling, M.D., M.P.H.

Associate Professor of Internal Medicine, Section of Heart Failure and Cardiac Transplant Medicine, Department of Cardiology, Cleveland Clinic Foundation, Cleveland, Ohio

Lynne Warner Stevenson, M.D.

Associate Professor of Medicine, Harvard Medical School; Clinical Director, Cardiomyopathy and Heart Failure Service, Brigham and Women's Hospital, Boston, Massachusetts

Bodo E. Strauer, M.D.

Professor and Director, Medical Clinic and Policlinic B, Division of Cardiology, Pneumology and Angiology, Department of Internal Medicine, Heinrich-Heine University, Düusseldorf, Germany

Peter H. Sugden, M.A., D.Phil.

Reader in Biochemistry, Department of Cardiac Medicine, National Heart and Lung Institute, Imperial College of Science, Technology and Medicine, London, England

Martin J. Sullivan, M.D.

Associate Professor, Division of Cardiology, Department of Medicine, Duke University Medical Center, Durham, North Carolina

George C. Sutton, M.D., F.R.C.P., F.A.C.C.

Consultant Cardiologist, The Hillingdon Hospital, Uxbridge, Middlesex, England; Senior Lecturer, National Heart and Lung Institute, Imperial Colloege of Science, Technology, and Medicine, London, England

Karl Swedberg, M.D., Ph.D.

Chief, Department of Medicine, Östra University Hospital, Göteborg, Sweden

Bernard Swynghedauw, Ph.D., M.D., F.E.S.C.

Director of Research, Institut National de la Santé et de la Recherche Médicale, U172-INSERM, Hopital Lariboisière, Paris, France

Lip-Bun Tan, B.Sc.(Hons), M.B.B.Chir., D.Phil, F.R.C.P., F.E.S.C.

Mautner Stroke BHS Senior Lecturer, Institute of Cardiovascular Research, University of Leeds Medical School; Consultant Cardiologist, Killingback Hospital and St. James's University Hospital, Leeds, England

John R. Teerlink, M.D.

Howard Hughes Medical Institute Postdoctoral Research Fellow, Cardiovascular Research Unit, University of California, San Francisco, School of Medicine, and Section of Cardiology Research, Northern California Institute for Research and Education, Veterans Affairs Medical Center, San Francisco, California

Konstantinos Vlachonassios, M.D.
Fellow, Division of Cardiology, Department of Medicine, University of Southern California School of Medicine, Los Angeles, California

Peter D. Wagner, M.D.
Professor of Medicine and Bioengineering, Department of Medicine, University of California, San Diego, School of Medicine, San Diego, California

Karl T. Weber, M.D.
Professor of Medicine, Division of Cardiology, Department of Internal Medicine, University of Missouri Health Sciences Center, Columbia, Missouri

Susan E. Wiegers, M.D.
Assistant Professor of Medicine, Cardiovascular Division, Department of Medicine, University of Pennsylvania School of Medicine; Director, HUP Cardiac Clinic, and Associate Director, Noninvasive Imaging, Cardiovascular Division, Hospital of the University of Pennsylvania (HUP), Philadelphia, Pennsylvania

Mohamad H. Yamani, M.D.
Cardiology Fellow, University of Michigan Medical School, Ann Arbor, Michigan

James B. Young, M.D.
Head, Section of Heart Failure and Cardiac Transplant Medicine, Department of Cardiology, Cleveland Clinic Foundation, Cleveland, Ohio

Salim Yusuf, D. Phil., F.R.C.P.(C)
Professor of Medicine, and Director, Division of Cardiology, McMaster University Faculty of Health Sciences; Director, Preventive Cardiology and Therapeutics Research Program, Hamilton Civic Hospital Research Center, Hamilton, Ontario, Canada

Irving H. Zucker, Ph.D.
Professor and Chairman, Department of Physiology and Biophysics, University of Nebraska College of Medicine, Omaha, Nebraska

Preface

Heart failure to some is a clinical syndrome or a medical condition detected and treated by physicians. To others heart failure is an abbreviation for a fundamental physiopathologic state in which the organ responsible for delivering blood to the pulmonary and systemic circulations becomes limited in its capacity to act as a pump with inevitable consequences for the body as a whole. Heart failure is then seen as the end state of all diseases of the heart and is a condition that will threaten the survival of the organism as a whole. Sir Thomas Lewis put it well in 1933 when he wrote "the very essence of cardiovascular medicine is recognition of early heart failure."

Heart failure is a common disease occurring in approximately 1 percent of the total population and in up to 10 percent of the elderly population. The prognosis is in general poor. Carefully undertaken and properly designed studies have shown that new treatments have a favorable effect on both symptoms and the duration of life. In almost no other branch of clinical medicine has evidence been assessed so critically with regard to efficacy and outcome. Heart failure fulfills the three simple criteria for identifying diseases that should have a high priority and be the focus of healthcare programs; it is common, it can be detected, and treatment is effective.

The last two decades have seen a transformation in knowledge about heart failure, the ability of physicians to diagnose heart failure, and the development of new and effective treatments. This has been a consequence of basic research, the availability of new technology such as echocardiography, the introduction of numerous new drugs, and of human endeavor.

Many research workers were attracted to the subject by the interest, excitement, and enthusiasm that emanated from the many opportunities arising from the introduction of heart transplantation and from research programs directed toward creating, as yet unsuccessfully, a long-term artificial heart.

Heart Failure: Scientific Principles and Clinical Practice brings together much of the current knowledge about heart failure. The topic has become so large and diverse that a multiauthored book, utilizing experts in each field, is essential if the most current and comprehensive information is to be presented. Because overlap is inevitable in this context, differences in approaches and interpretations are to be anticipated. Additionally, this book provides both basic and practical clinical backgrounds that are necessary for the understanding of the physiologic mechanisms of heart failure and its diagnosis and management.

Heart Failure is intended for the interested reader, to be dipped into by practicing physicians, and to be used as a source of information and reference by cardiologists and those specializing in heart failure. Our aim is to facilitate the dissemination of information on current thinking with regard to heart failure and thus to make a small contribution to the benefit of patients with this condition.

Philip A. Poole-Wilson, M.D., F.R.C.P., F.E.S.C.
Wilson S. Colucci, M.D., F.A.C.C.
Barry M. Massie, M.D.
Kanu Chatterjee, M.B., F.R.C.P.
Andrew J. S. Coats, D.M.

Acknowledgments

Producing a major reference work that covers a broad and rapidly evolving subject such as heart failure requires a tremendous effort from a large number of individuals. The most important, of course, are the contributing authors. Each chapter has been authored by one or more experts in a specific area, and, as such, we recognize that our authors have numerous, and at many times, overwhelming, clinical, scientific, and teaching responsibilities. We are honored that they agreed to participate in this endeavor and delighted that they have done so in such an outstanding manner.

Others have made less obvious, but no less vital, contributions. We also gratefully acknowledge the work and the tolerance of our administrative and secretarial staffs and the assistance of the personnel at Churchill Livingstone.

Finally, we must express our gratitude to our colleagues, trainees, and students. Our daily interactions with them are what makes the science and medicine of heart failure continually stimulating and provides the impetus for undertaking a project such as this.

Contents

Color plates appear following page 18.

Cellular Physiology of Myocyte Contraction

James P. Morgan

This chapter focuses on the cellular mechanisms that modulate contraction/relaxation cycles of the mammalian myocyte. Normal contraction and relaxation of the heart require synchronous interaction of numerous subcellular processes; abnormalities at any of these sites can potentially produce significant systolic or diastolic dysfunction (or both). The initial sections of this chapter focus on normal cellular processes and the latter on how these processes may function abnormally in the presence of cardiac hypertrophy and heart failure.

EXCITATION-CONTRACTION AND REPOLARIZATION-RELAXATION COUPLING PROCESSES

The central part played by the calcium ion (Ca^{2+}) in regulating contraction/relaxation cycles of the heart is illustrated in Figure 1-1.[1,2] For the purposes of discussion, four major cellular sites participate in the regulation of cardiac excitation-contraction and repolarization-relaxation coupling via effects on intracellular Ca^{2+} availability or cellular responsiveness: sarcolemma, sarcoplasmic reticulum, troponin–tropomyosin regulatory complex, and actin and myosin filaments. The intracellular availability of calcium is regulated primarily by the sarcolemma and sarcoplasmic reticulum; and calcium responsiveness is controlled by the regulatory troponin–tropomyosin complex of the myofilaments. Therefore as a broad general scheme, one can consider two major calcium-dependent processes that regulate the contraction and relaxation of the myocyte: (1) those that alter the availability of free myoplasmic Ca^{2+} for activation and maintenance of contraction; and (2) those that alter the responsiveness of the myofilaments to Ca^{2+} activation (Fig. 1-1).[3]

One of the seminal observations that focused attention on the vital role of Ca^{2+} in the heart was by Stanley Ringer in 1883, when he noted that the calcium ion was necessary to maintain contractile function in isolated myocardial preparations.[4] During the years since Ringer's finding, a general consensus has developed concerning the cellular processes involved, with the major advances occurring only since the 1960s. Although a number of specific issues remain to be resolved, the generally accepted scheme is as follows (Fig. 1-1): Excitation-contraction coupling is initiated when depolarization allows trigger Ca^{2+} to enter the myoplasm through calcium channels located in the sarcolemma. This trigger calcium releases a much larger quantity of activator Ca^{2+} from intracellular stores in the sarcoplasmic reticulum. The released Ca^{2+} diffuses toward the myofilaments, where some of it is bound by troponin C of the myofilament regulatory complex. The interaction of Ca^{2+} with troponin C initiates contraction; repolarization-relaxation coupling begins when Ca^{2+} dissociates from troponin C and is resequestered by the sarcoplasmic reticulum, followed by repolarization of the cell. Intracellular Ca^{2+} homeostasis is maintained by sarcolemmal mechanisms that extrude Ca^{2+} from the myocyte. Such mechanisms include the sodium-calcium exchanger and an adenosine triphosphate (ATP)-dependent calcium pump. Synchronous function of each of these multiple processes permits the heart to maintain a 10,000-fold concentration gradient for Ca^{2+} across the sarcolemma.

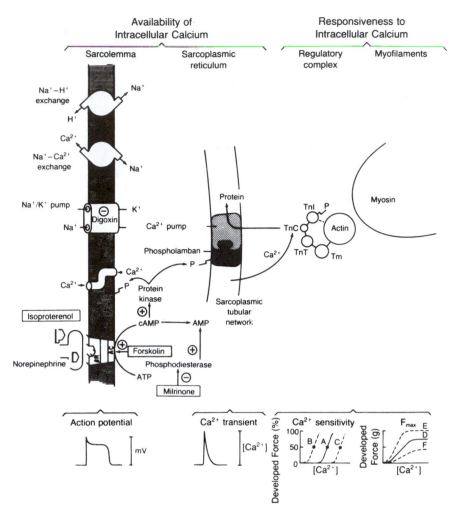

Fig. 1-1. Four major cellular sites for the regulation of excitation-contraction coupling in the mammalian heart: sarcolemma, sarcoplasmic reticulum, regulatory complex, and myofilaments. Cardiac contractility may be altered by changing either the availability of intracellular calcium for activation or the responsiveness of the myofilaments to intracellular calcium. Calcium availability is regulated predominantly by sites in the sarcolemma and sarcoplasmic reticulum that can be functionally monitored by means of the action potential and calcium transient, respectively. Responsiveness to intracellular calcium is regulated predominantly by the troponin–tropomyosin complex, attached to actin, and the myofilaments actin and myosin. These components can be functionally assessed by the calcium sensitivity and maximal calcium-activated force (F_{max}) of fibers rendered hyperpermeable to calcium. See the text for details. The Ca^{2+} transient is the depolarization-induced increase and decrease in the intracellular calcium concentration: $[Ca^{2+}]$; Ca^{2+} sensitivity is the relation between the intracellular calcium concentration and cardiac activation, expressed as a percentage of peak developed force. Curves A and D are baseline values of the sensitivity of myofilaments to calcium and F_{max}, respectively. Ca^{2+} sensitivity and F_{max} can change independently of each other. Curves B and E show enhancement, and curves C and F depression, of sensitivity and F_{max}, respectively. Tnl, troponin l; TnC, troponin C; TnT, troponin T; Tm, tropomyosin; βR, beta-adrenergic receptor; AC, adenylate cyclase; cAMP, cyclic AMP; P, phosphorylation. (From Morgan,[1] with permission.)

Second Messengers

In addition to calcium, other second messenger systems exist in the myocyte that play important roles with regard to modulation of cellular Ca^{2+} levels, among the most important of which are cyclic adeno-sine monophosphate (cAMP) inositol triphosphate, and diacylglycerol.[5,6] cAMP modulates intracellular Ca^{2+} through the activation of a protein kinase (cA kinase).[7] cAMP activates cA kinase by binding to the regulatory subunit of the enzyme, triggering a conformational change that allows its catalytic subunit to dissociate and phosphorylate protein substrates. In the heart, phosphorylation of sites on the sarcolemma, sarcoplasmic reticulum, and troponin–tropomyosin regulatory complex have profound effects on both systolic and diastolic Ca^{2+} concentrations. Phosphorylation of the L-type, voltage-dependent calcium channels of sarcolemma increases the influx of Ca^{2+} during depolarization and thereby not only triggers the release of a proportionately larger quantity of this ion from the sarcoplasmic reticulum but provides a larger amount available to load cellular stores for release during subsequent action potentials.[8] Both effects increase the force of systolic contraction. Simultaneously, cA kinase phosphorylates phospholamban, the regulatory subunit of the calcium pump of the sarcoplasmic reticulum, and so enhances the rate of Ca^{2+} resequestration.[9] Phosphorylation of the troponin–tropomyosin complex at the TnI site decreases the affinity of troponin C for Ca^{2+} and facilitates dissociation of the Ca^{2+}–troponin C complex.[10] The phosphorylation of phospholamban and of troponin I enhances the rate of diastolic relaxation of the heart. The cA kinase activity is sensitive to small changes in cAMP concentrations within the physiologic range.[11] The cA kinase activity ratio fluctuates from beat to beat, with maximum activity occurring during systole[12]; exposure of myocardium to agents that elevate intracellular cAMP levels, such as β-agonists, have been demonstrated to increase the cA kinase activity ratio. The interesting hypothesis has been proposed, but not yet proved, that cAMP, cA kinase, or both are compartmentalized in the heart and become accessible to each other in response to selected stimuli.[7,13]

By a G protein-mediated process after receptor binding, several cardiotonic agents, including α-adrenergic agonists and endothelin, have been reported to activate phospholipase C-mediated hydrolysis of phosphoinositol-4,5-biphosphate (PIP_2) in the cardiac sarcolemma.[5,14] The product of this reaction is 1,2-diacylglycerol (DAG) and inositol-1,4,5-triphosphate (IP_3). Both components act as second messengers in the heart. IP_3 has been reported to act directly on the sarcoplasmic reticulum, inducing the release of a sensitive Ca^{2+} pool, perhaps by actions on a specific IP_3-gated Ca^{2+} release channel. This mechanism appears to account partially for the positive inotropic effects of α-agonists and endothelin in some species. Elevated cellular Ca^{2+} levels may in turn enhance relaxation by activating Ca^{2+} calmodulin-dependent protein kinase II (CaM kinase II), which can phosphorylate phospholamban and increase activity of the sarcoplasmic reticular Ca^{2+} pump.[15] DAG activates a Ca^{2+}- and phospholipid-dependent kinase, protein kinase C, and promotes its translocation to the sarcolemma. Protein kinase C appears to have

long-term effects on the expression of a number of gene products involved with cell growth and may also modulate the action of IP_3. Moreover, under some circumstances, such as with endothelin or cytokine stimulation, it may mediate a negative inotropic effect.[16,17] Despite a growing awareness of the potential importance of the IP_3/DAG second messenger pathways in the cellular physiology of the heart, many important details remain to be elucidated.

Sarcolemma

As demonstrated in Figure 1-1, the cardiac sarcolemma contains the multiple channels, exchangers, and pumps necessary for maintaining intracellular Ca^{2+} homeostasis.[1,18] Multiple agonist receptors are present that couple sarcolemmal signals to various intracellular second messenger pathways, including cAMP (β_1, β_2, histamine, and glucagon receptors), cyclic guanosine monophosphate (cGMP) (cholinergic, adenosine receptors), and IP_3/DAG (α-adrenergic, endothelin, and angiotensin receptors). These systems are discussed in more detail in subsequent chapters.

The intracellular Na^+ concentration, because of its effect on Na^+/Ca^{2+} exchange, is an important determinant of cellular Ca^{2+} levels.[19] The Na^+/Ca^{2+} exchanger of the sarcolemma operates down the concentration gradient for sodium, exchanging three Na^+ for one Ca^{2+}; therefore when the exchanger operates in the outward direction to extrude Na^+, a negative potential is generated within the cell.[20] Processes that increase intracellular Na^+ concentrations, such as inhibition of Na^+/K^+-ATPase with digoxin, increase Ca^{2+} entry via this exchange mechanism. Experimental evidence suggests that the exchanger may operate in both inward and outward directions for Ca^{2+} during the cardiac cycle.[19] Along with the Na^+/H^+ exchanger,[21,22] the Na^+/Ca^{2+} exchanger plays an important role in governing calcium homeostasis in the mammalian heart. As discussed below, alterations in the function of these exchangers may markedly alter intracellular Ca^{2+} modulation under the influence of drugs (i.e., endothelin) and in the setting of several disease states, including heart failure. The Na^+/K^+-ATPase (sodium pump) also plays an important role in maintaining Ca^{2+} homeostasis. Inhibition of this ATPase by agents such as digoxin leads to increased intracellular Na^+ concentrations, enhanced Na^+/Ca^{2+} exchange, and elevated levels of intracellular Ca^{2+}.[23] The slow inward calcium current (I_{si}) plays an essential role in excitation-contraction coupling in the heart both as a trigger for the release of Ca^{2+} from the sarcoplasmic reticulum and as a source of Ca^{2+}

to load stores for release during subsequent action potentials. Two types of calcium channel contribute to the inward Ca^{2+} current in myocardium: (1) low threshold T-type calcium channels that are activated by small depolarizations from resting membrane potential; and (2) high threshold L-type channels.[18] The L-type channels activate and inactivate at potentials significantly more positive than T-type channels, are sensitive to dihydropyridine-type Ca^{2+} blockers, and appear to be responsible for conducting most of the inward Ca^{2+} current. In addition, the L-type calcium channels are voltage- and calcium-dependent and may be inactivated by depolarization or increased intracellular Ca^{2+} concentrations. Calcium ions entering via I_{si} may contribute some of the Ca^{2+} that activates contraction, but most of the Ca^{2+} activity appears to originate from the sarcoplasmic reticulum.[18,24,25]

Sarcoplasmic Reticulum

The sarcoplasmic reticulum is the most important Ca^{2+} store within the heart.[26] It is useful to view this organelle as consisting of two functionally important parts: the subsarcolemmal cisternae, which are located in close proximity to the sarcolemma; and the sarcotubular network, which closely invests the contractile apparatus.[27] Based on studies in skeletal muscle where the large cells facilitate visualization of sarcoplasmic reticular Ca^{2+} handling, the subsarcolemmal cisternae can be considered the sites of Ca^{2+} release and the sarcotubular network the site of Ca^{2+} reuptake.[26] Although separation of the sarcoplasmic reticulum into these two functionally distinct sites is undoubtedly an oversimplification, it allows Ca^{2+} restitution to be viewed in part as the process responsible for Ca^{2+} transport within the sarcoplasmic reticulum from reuptake to release sites. This scheme has utility in terms of considering phenomena such as frequency-response relations and treppe as well as the mechanism of postextrasystolic potentiation.[18] As discussed above, the rate at which Ca^{2+} is resequestered is under the modulatory control of phospholamban. Phosphorylation of phospholamban by cA kinase or CaM kinase II can markedly enhance the rate of Ca^{2+} reuptake and enhance diastolic relaxation.

Contractile Elements

The contractile proteins actin and myosin plus ATP undergo a sequence of interactions that result in cell shortening, as described in Figure 1-2.[27,28] During diastole, the troponin–tropomyosin complex prevents actin and myosin from interacting. The binding of Ca^{2+} to troponin C (Fig. 1-1) induces a conformational change in the complex that permits crossbridges to form and sarcomere shortening to develop. Relaxation of the myocyte occurs when Ca^{2+} diffuses away from its binding sites on troponin C and the troponin–tropomyosin complex again assumes an inhibitory conformation. This sequence of events is repeated during every contraction/relaxation cycle.

Phosphorylation of troponin I (Fig. 1-1), one of the regulatory subunits, has the effect of decreasing the affinity of troponin C for Ca^{2+}. As a result, Ca^{2+} dissociates from troponin C at a faster rate, enhancing relaxation. There is evidence that drugs and disease states can affect contractile element interactions (see below).

Mitochondria

The mitochondria are the primary suppliers of ATP for the cardiac myocyte. ATP is required to fuel the ion pumps (including the sarcolemmal and sarcoplasmic reticular ATPases) that remove Ca^{2+} from the cytosol during diastole. ATP is also necessary for normal function of the sarcolemmal Na^+ pumps. In addition, ATP interaction with the high-affinity binding site of myosin is required for normal relaxation of the myocyte. Normally, intracellular levels of ATP, in the micromolar range, are adequate to keep the myosin energized, prevent formation of rigor bonds, and maintain normal dissociation of crossbridges to permit relaxation.[29]

CELLULAR ALTERATIONS WITH CARDIAC HYPERTROPHY AND FAILURE

Systolic Versus Diastolic Heart Failure

Patients with heart failure can be divided into two major categories depending on whether their predominant functional problems are caused by decreased contractility (systolic failure) or impaired relaxation (diastolic failure). Approximately one-third of patients with symptomatic heart failure have a normal ejection fraction and symptoms that are entirely or in large measure a result of diastolic dysfunction.[29] A negative lusitropic (i.e., impaired relaxant) state may be caused by structural changes in the heart, including hypertrophy, fibrosis, or infiltrative processes; however, subcellular abnormalities in re-

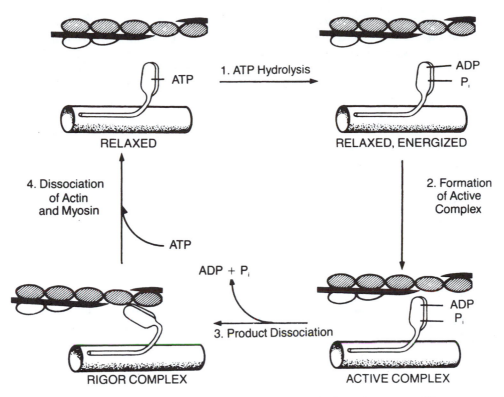

Fig. 1-2. Reaction mechanism for actomyosin ATPase (simplified) in four steps. The sequence begins at the upper left, where ATP binding to myosin has dissociated the thick and thin filaments, causing the muscle to relax. Hydrolysis of myosin-bound ATP (step 1) transfers the energy of the nucleotide to the cross-bridge in a relaxed, energized state (upper right). Interaction of the cross-bridge with actin in the thin filament (step 2) leads to formulation of the active complex (lower right) in which the energy derived from ATP is still associated with the cross-bridge. Dissociation of ADP and P_i, the products of ATP hydrolysis (step 3), leads to the formation of a rigor bond, in which the chemical energy has been expended to perform mechanical work: the motion of the cross-bridge. The cycle ends and the muscle returns to its resting state when ATP binding to the rigor complex (step 4) dissociates the cross-bridge from the thin filament. (From Katz,[27] with permission.)

polarization-relaxation coupling appear to be present in many cases.[1,5,29–31] Factors that (1) slow the detachment of cross-bridges (e.g., intracellular alkalosis), which in turn increases the affinity of troponin C for Ca^{2+}, (2) impair resequestration of Ca^{2+} by the sarcoplasmic reticulum (e.g., decreased level of phosphorylation of calmodulin due to a decreased degree of cAMP-mediated cA kinase activation), or (3) cause a diminished rate of Ca^{2+} extrusion via the Na^+/Ca^{2+} exchanger (e.g., due to a relative increase in cellular Na^+ levels, brought about by Na^+/K^+-ATPase inhibition with digoxin) may also delay the rate of diastolic relaxation. Positively inotropic agents may have (1) positive lusitropic effects (i.e., isoproterenol and other agonists that increase cellular cAMP levels through phosphorylation of phospholamban and troponin I, as well as the L-type Ca^{2+} channels); (2) negative lusitropic effects (i.e., endothelin and other agonists that activate protein kinase C, which affects Na^+/H^+ exchange to produce cytoplasmic alkaliniza-

tion), or (3) no lusitropic effect, with no change in the lusitropic state (i.e., increases in extracellular Ca^{2+}).[1] These concepts are important because most patients with chronic heart failure have some degree of diastolic dysfunction combined with systolic dysfunction, and an intervention with negatively lusitropic actions can potentially exacerbate contractile abnormalities.[32–34]

Human Heart Failure

Abnormalities of electrophysiologic properties, sarcoplasmic reticular function, energy utilization and supply, and contractile element interaction have been identified in experimental studies in animals and patients with heart failure.[35] The findings suggest that intracellular Ca^{2+} modulation may be abnormal in the failing heart. The initiation worldwide of active cardiac transplantation programs has made available for investigational use both control and myopathic human cardiac tissue. Myopathic tissue is obtained from the hearts of patients undergoing transplantation who demonstrate in vivo the signs, symptoms, and hemodynamic values of end-stage failure. Control tissue is obtained from surgical waste tissue or donor hearts not suitable for transplantation.

Several groups have used calcium indicators to study intracellular Ca^{2+} modulation in tissue from control and myopathic human hearts and have found marked differences with regard to the configuration of the Ca^{2+} transient, action potential, and duration of isometric or isotonic contraction and relaxation.[36,37] Figure 1-3 shows the Ca^{2+} transients recorded with the bioluminescent protein aequorin, isometric twitches, and action potentials in tissue from representative patients with (1) no known cardiac disease, (2) end-stage dilated cardiomyopathy, and (3) end-stage hypertrophic cardiomyopathy.[39] Note that the aequorin signal recorded from the control muscle in Figure 1-3 consists of a single component that rises to a peak and then declines toward baseline before peak tension is reached. Similar mo-

nophasic calcium signals have been recorded with aequorin from nonfailing human atrial and ventricular muscle, and they appear to be typical of both animal and human working myocardium.[36] In normal mammalian working myocardium, the aequorin signal seems to reflect predominantly the release and reuptake of Ca^{2+} by the sarcoplasmic reticulum.[34,35,37] In contrast, the calcium transients recorded from myopathic muscles were not only prolonged compared to these of the controls but consisted of two temporally distinct components, labeled L_1 and L_2 in Figure 1-3. Note that the plateau phase of the cardiac action potential was prolonged in myopathic muscle compared to that in the controls. These data indicate that the prolonged contraction of myopathic muscle in vitro appears to correlate with changes in $[Ca^{2+}]_i$. Moreover, these results, if extrapolated to the failing human heart in vivo, may explain the myocardial relaxation abnormalities seen in patients with dilated cardiomyopathy.[37]

To test if myopathic muscle has a diminished capacity to handle increases in cytoplasmic Ca^{2+}, calcium concentration–response curves were obtained

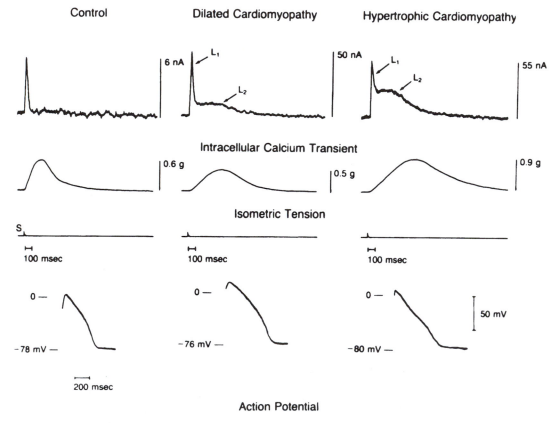

Fig. 1-3. Recordings representing, from top to bottom, aequorin light tracing (i.e., $[Ca^{2+}]_i$), isometric tension, stimulus(s) artifact, and action potentials from control and myopathic human trabeculae carneae maintained in vitro. Light is expressed in nanoamperes (nA) of anode current; tension in grams (g), action potentials in millivolts (mV). L_1 and L_2, two components in $[Ca^{2+}]_i$ transient. (From Morgan,[39] with permission.)

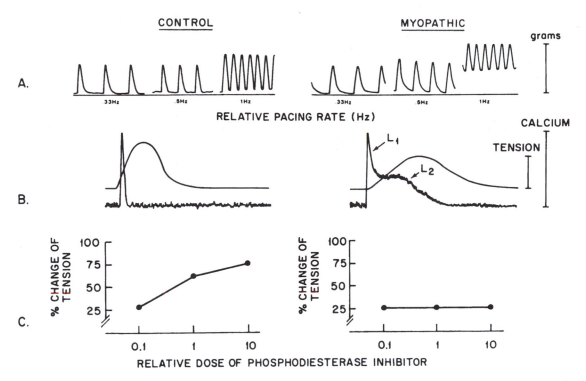

CONTROL   MYOPATHIC

RELATIVE PACING RATE (Hz)

Fig. 1-4. Tracings showing signatures of heart failure in isolated human myocardium. **(A)** Reversal of the force–frequency relation from positive to negative staircase going from lower to higher pacing frequencies. **(B)** Prolonged $[Ca^{2+}]_i$ transient and twitch; two components (L_1 and L_2) in the $[Ca^{2+}]_1$ transient. **(C)** Markedly diminished response to phosphodiesterase inhibitors, such as milrinone. (From Perreault,[37] with permission.)

for the two types of muscle shown in Figure 1-4.[37] In control and myopathic muscle, increases in extracellular Ca^{2+} produced a concentration-dependent positive inotropic effect that was associated with a corresponding increase in the amplitude of the calcium transient. In contrast, in the myopathic muscles, increasing concentrations of extracellular calcium ($[Ca^{2+}]_o$) produced a progressive rise in the amplitude of the abnormal second component of the light signal (L_2) relative to the first component. This change in the Ca^{2+} transient was associated with a prolonged isometric contraction. In contrast, the time course of contraction in control muscle was not significantly changed by concentrations of $[Ca^{2+}]_o$ up to four times normal values. Moreover, higher concentrations of $[Ca^{2+}]_o$ produced increased end-diastolic levels of $[Ca^{2+}]_i$ and incomplete relaxation before initiation of the next twitch. These data are consistent with the hypothesis that the myopathic muscle has diminished capacity to maintain Ca^{2+} hemostasis in the presence of normal and increased transsarcolemmal gradients.

Additional studies with the pharmacologic agents ryanodine (an alkaloid that blocks release of Ca^{2+} by the sarcoplasmic reticulum) and verapamil (a calcium-channel blocking agent) suggested that the ab-

normal L_2 component of the calcium transient in myopathic muscle reflects dysfunction of both the sarcolemma and the sarcoplasmic reticulum.[34] The former may cause increased Ca^{2+} entry, possibly via voltage-dependent channels, and increased Na^+/Ca^{2+} exchanger; the latter may cause slowed restoration of low resting tone during diastole owing to a decreased rate of Ca^{2+} resequestration.

The inability of myopathic muscle to maintain Ca^{2+} homeostasis seems to be a primary cause of systolic and diastolic dysfunction.[1,34] This point is well illustrated by the frequency–response relation in myopathic muscle, as shown in Figure 1-5. In most mammalian species when the frequency of pacing is increased, a positive inotropic effect occurs (i.e., the positive treppe effect). This phenomenon has been demonstrated for normal human and animal myocardium.[18] Figure 1-5 shows that a negative treppe effect occurs in myopathic myocardium.[40] As the frequency of contraction is increased from 0.33 to 1.00Hz, fusion of the Ca^{2+} transients and twitches occurred with incomplete relaxation and elevation of the end-diastolic tension and Ca^{2+}. At higher pacing frequencies, these changes were associated with a decrease in active tension generation, although the total tension that developed was increased. Although

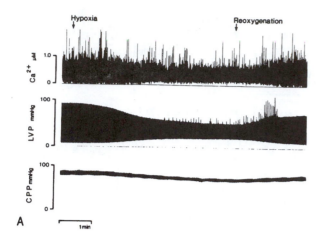

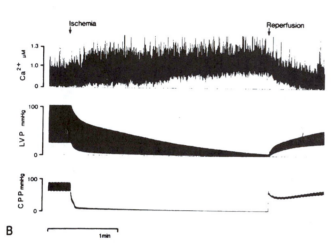

Fig. 1-5. Recordings from isolated buffer-perfused ferret heart at 30°C paced at 125–130 beats per minute. Simultaneous recording of $[Ca^{2+}]_i$ transients (top), isovolumic left ventricular pressures (LVP) (middle), and coronary perfusion pressures (bottom) during 5 minutes of hypoxia followed by reoxygenation **(A)** or 3 minutes of global ischemia followed by reperfusion **(B)**. Note that $[Ca^{2+}]_i$ and LVP correlate in the presence of hypoxia but seem to be uncoupled in the presence of ischemia. CPP, coronary perfusion pressure. (From Kihara,[40] with permission.)

these abnormalities may have been exacerbated by the relatively hypothermic connections of these experiments, the results provide a clear example of a situation in which abnormal Ca^{2+} handling can lead to both diastolic and systolic dysfunction.

Changes in Cellular Ca^{2+} Modulation with Heart Failure

Heart failure has been associated with a variety of structural and biochemical abnormalities that affect Ca^{2+} modulation and may explain the systolic and diastolic alterations that occur.[1,36] At the level of the sarcolemma, changes have been reported in the numbers or coupling of adrenergic receptors and in L-type calcium channels. The density of Ca^{2+} ATPase uptake sites on the sarcoplasmic reticulum appears to be decreased, and the mechanisms that regulate calcium release are impaired. The structure of the contractile apparatus and regulatory subunits is reportedly altered in some types of failing animal and human hearts. The energy-supplying capacity of the mitochondria may also be impaired in the failing heart. Therefore a variety of abnormalities may be present with the potential to affect multiple steps in the excitation-contraction and repolarization-relaxation pathways.

There is pharmacologic evidence that abnormalities in second messenger pathways other than the Ca^{2+} pathway may contribute to cellular changes during heart failure.[32] The inotropic effectiveness of phosphodiesterase inhibitors, such as milrinone, are markedly reduced in muscles from patients with heart failure. In contrast, the effectiveness of inotropic stimulation with the adenylate cyclase activator forskolin are preserved. After a minimally effective concentration of forskolin was given to elevate cAMP levels, the inotropic responses of muscle from failing hearts to phosphodiesterase inhibitors was markedly potentiated. Taken together, these results indicate that an abnormality in the production of cAMP may be a fundamental defect in patients with end-stage heart failure, thereby affecting each of the steps in the excitation-contraction and repolarization-relaxation-contraction coupling under its modulatory control. Direct measurements of total cellular cAMP have provided conflicting results, perhaps because of localization of this cyclic nucleotide into distinct, compartmentalized subcellular pools.

Changes in Myofilament Ca^{2+} Responsiveness

Changes in the responsiveness of the myofilaments to Ca^{2+} can have an important effect on cardiac contraction and relaxation.[1] The relations between Ca^{2+} binding to troponin C and the degree of activation of the myofilaments may be substantially altered by drug and disease states. As shown in Figure 1-1, a change in calcium responsiveness may manifest as altered Ca^{2+} sensitivity (generally defined as the amount producing 50 percent maximal activation) or maximal calcium-activated force. In Figure 1-1, the basal level of sensitivity of the myofilaments to Ca^{2+} is indicated by curve A and the maximal calcium-activated force at baseline by curve D. Curves B and E show enhancement and curves C and F depression of sensitivity and maximal calcium-activated force, respectively. Common clinical conditions, such as ischemia, depress the generation of maximal force, probably through development of acidosis and accumulation of inorganic phosphate as intracellular stores of ATP are consumed.[40–43] With ischemia, a marked increase in intracellular Ca^{2+} occurs that is not translated into improved systolic or diastolic performance, reflecting the predominance of mechanisms acting downstream from the site at which Ca^{2+} combines with troponin C (Fig. 1-5). In contrast, hypoxia appears to be a commonly occurring example of acute heart failure in which contractile performance remains coupled to intracellular Ca^{2+} (Fig. 1-5), apparently because the desensitizing effects of inorganic phosphate and H^+ ions are washed away by continued coronary perfusion (Fig. 1-5).

The myocardial stunning that occurs after brief periods of myocardial ischemia are associated with normal cellular Ca^{2+} levels at a time when the generation of systolic pressure is depressed.[44–46] The mechanism of this response may include altered Ca^{2+} affinity of troponin C, phosphorylation of myosin light chains, phosphorylation of C protein, or changes in the lattice structure of the myofilaments. In general, studies of myopathic animal and human myocardium have failed to reveal substantial alterations in calcium responsiveness as a cause of contractile dysfunction.[47–49] However, pharmacologic agents may differentially affect the responsiveness of myofilaments to Ca^{2+} in myopathic myocardium compared with normal, raising the intriguing possibility of the development of therapeutic agents that selectively enhance the contractility or relaxant properties of the failing heart. In summary, altering the responsiveness of the myofilaments to Ca^{2+} is an important approach to the control of cardiac contractile function that may have therapeutic utility in clinical medicine.

Hypertrophy and Heart Failure

Most failing hearts demonstrate a significant degree of myocyte hypertrophy due to preexisting pressure or volume-overload states or as a compensatory response to contractile dysfunction and myocyte dropout. Therefore an important question is whether the abnormalities in excitation-contraction and repolarization-relaxation coupling described above are pathognomonic of heart failure or merely a reflection of the degree of cardiac hypertrophy that is present.

Several lines of evidence indicate that hypertrophy may be responsible for these changes. First, cardiac muscles from animals and patients with heart failure of multiple causes have substantial degrees of compensatory hypertrophy.[35] Patients with end-stage heart failure often have more than a 75 percent increase in mean fiber diameter. Second, the abnormalities in Ca^{2+} modulation found in myopathic myocardium are also present in muscle from patients with hypertrophic cardiomyopathy and hyperdynamic systolic function.[35] Third, the severity of at least some of the abnormalities in cellular Ca^{2+} modulation described above can be correlated with the degree of myocyte hypertrophy that is present. Fourth, many of the structural changes reported in the failing heart have also been reported with compensated hypertrophy, including decreased sarcoplasmic reticular Ca^{2+}-ATPase messenger RNA (mRNA) and isoform shifts in the regulatory subunits of the troponin–tropomyosin complex. Taken together, these observations suggest that changes in intracellular Ca^{2+} modulation may be initially compensatory but when more fully developed may ultimately lead to decompensation of cardiac function. Elevated intracellular levels of Ca^{2+} may provide a signal for the synthesis of proteins responsible for the hypertrophic process. It remains to be determined how these presumably compensatory mechanisms contribute to the development of cardiac decompensation and failure.

Future Directions

Although many important details remain to be determined, it is clear that changes in intracellular Ca^{2+} play a central role in the regulation of contraction and relaxation of cardiac muscle. It must be kept in mind, though, that there are other important second messengers that play major roles in these processes including cAMP and perhaps IP_3 and DAG, which may exacerbate or produce abnormal intracellular Ca^{2+} modulation. Moreover, changes in the steps distal to contractile proteins may play crucial roles in mediating the contraction and relaxation of cardiac muscle under normal and pathophysiologic conditions. An understanding of the basic mechanisms of excitation-contraction and repolarization-relaxation coupling and the ways in which they are affected by the development of pathophysiologic states is essential for developing rational preventive and therapeutic approaches to heart failure.[50] It remains to be determined whether molecular or pharmacologic interventions designed to directly affect the processes that control intracellular Ca^{2+} availability or myofilament Ca^{2+} responsiveness can improve survival or the quality of life for patients with heart failure. Logic suggests that it should be possible to develop appropriate approaches, but to date cardiotonic drugs have yet to be developed that can match even the modest successes of angiotensin-converting enzyme inhibition and vasodilator therapy for management of clinical heart failure.

REFERENCES

1. Morgan JP: Mechanisms of disease. Abnormal intracellular modulation of calcium as a major cause of cardiac contractile dysfunction. N Engl J Med 1991;325:625

2. Rasmussen H: The calcium messenger system. N Engl J Med 1986;314:1094, 1164

3. Blinks JR, Endoh M: Modification of myofibrillar responsiveness to Ca^{++} as an inotropic mechanism. Circulation, suppl. III 1986;73:85

4. Ringer S: A further contribution regarding the influence of the different constituents of the blood on the contraction of the heart. J Physiol (Lond) 1883;4:29–42

5. Katz AM: Interplay between inotropic and lusitropic effects of cyclic adenosine monophosphate on the myocardial cell. Circulation 1990;82:17

6. Williamson JR, Monch JR: Second messengers of inositol lipid metabolism and Ca^{2+} signaling. pp. 1729–1744. In Fozzard HA, Haber E, Jennings RB, Katz AM, Morgan HE (eds): The Heart and Cardiovascular System. Lippincott-Raven, Philadelphia, 1992

7. Shabb JB, Corbin JD: Protein phosphorylation in the heart. pp. 1539–1562. In Fozzard HA, Haber E, Jennings RB, Katz AM, Morgan HE (eds): The Heart and Cardiovascular System. Lippincott-Raven, Philadelphia, 1992

8. Sperelakis N, Wahler GM: Regulation of Ca^{2+} influx in myocardial cells by beta adrenergic receptors, cyclic nucleotides, and phosphorylation. Mol Cell Biochem 1988;82:19–28

9. Tada M, Kirchberger MA, Katz AM: Phosphorylation of a 22,000-dalton component of the cardiac sarcoplasmic reticulum by adenosine 3':5'-monophosphate-dependent protein kinase. J Biol Chem 1975;250:2640–2647

10. Katz AM: Cyclic adenosine monophosphate effects on the myocardium. A man who blows hot and cold with one breath. J Am Coll Cardiol 1983; 2:143–9

11. Ogreid D, Doskeland SO: Activation of protein kinase isoenzymes under near physiological conditions. Evidence that both types (A and B) of cAMP binding sites are involved in the activation of protein kinase by cAMP and 8-N_3-cAMP. FEBS Lett 1982;150:161–166

12. Krause E-G, Bartel S, Beyerdorfer I et al: Transient changes in cyclic AMP and in the enzymic activity of protein kinase and phosphorylase during the cardiac cycle in the canine myocardium and the effect of propranolol. Mol Cell Biochem 1989;89:181–186

13. Bode DC, Brunton LL: Post-receptor modulation of the effects of cyclic AMP in isolated cardiac myocytes. Mol Cell Biochem 1988;82:13–18

14. Berridge MJ: Inositol triphosphate and diacylglycerol. Two interacting second messengers. Annu Rev Biochem 1987;56:159–193

15. Katz S, Remtulla MA: Phosphodiesterase protein activator stimulates calcium transport in cardiac microsomal preparations enriched in sarcoplasmic reticulum. Biochem Biophys Res Commun 1978;83:1373–1379

16. Rozanski GJ, Witt RC: Interleukin-1 enhances beta-responsiveness of cardiac L-type calcium current suppressed by acidosis. Am J Physiol 1994;267:H1361–1367

17. Kramer BK, Smith TW, Kelly RA: Endothelin and increased contractility in adult rat ventricular myocytes. Role of intracellular alkalosis induced by activation of the protein kinase C-dependent Na^+-H^+ exchanger. Circ Res 1991;68:269–279

18. Gibbons WR, Zygmunt AC: Excitation-contraction coupling in heart. pp. 1249–1279. In Fozzard HA, Haber E, Jennings RB, Katz AM, Morgan HE (eds): The Heart and Cardiovascular System. Lippincott-Raven, New York, 1992

19. Sheu S-S, Blaustein MP: Sodium/calcium exchange and control of cell calcium and contractility in cardiac and vascular smooth muscles. pp. 903–943. In Fozzard HA, Haber E, Jennings RB, Katz AM, Morgan HE (eds): The Heart and Cardiovascular System. Lippincott-Raven, New York, 1992

20. Mullins LJ: Ion Transport in Heart. Lippincott-Raven, New York, 1981

21. Seiler SM, Cragoe EJ, Jones LR: Demonstration of a Na^+/H^+ exchange activity in purified canine cardiac sarcolemmal vesicles. J Biol Chem 1985;260:4869–4876

22. Periyasamy SM, Kakar S, Garbid KD, Askari A: Ion specificity of cardiac sarcolemmal Na^+/H^+ antiporter. J Biol Chem 1990;265:6035–6041

23. Eisner DA, Smith TW: The Na-K pump and its effectors in cardiac muscle. pp. 863–902. In Fozzard HA, Haber E, Jennings RB, Katz AM, Morgan HE (eds): The Heart and Cardiovascular System. Lippincott-Raven, New York, 1992

24. Fabiato A: Myoplasmic free calcium concentrations reached during the twitch of an intact isolated cardiac cell and during calcium-induced release of calcium from the sarcoplasmic reticulum of a skinned cardiac cell from the adult rat or rabbit ventricle. J Gen Physiol 1981;78:457–497

25. Fabiato A, Fabiato F: Calcium-induced release of calcium from the sarcoplasmic reticulum of skinned cells from adult human, dog, cat, rabbit, rat, and frog hearts and from fetal and new-born rat ventricles. Ann NY Acad Sci 1978;307:491–522

26. Lytton J, MacLennan DH: Sarcoplasmic reticulum. In Fozzard HA, Haber E, Jennings RB, Katz AM, Morgan HE (eds): The Heart and Cardiovascular System. pp. 1203–1222. Lippincott-Raven, New York, 1992

27. Katz AM: Physiology of the Heart. 2nd Ed. Lippincott-Raven, New York, 1992

28. Taylor EW: Mechanism and energetics of actomyosin ATPase. pp. 1281–1294. In Fozzard HA, Haber E, Jennings RB, Katz AM, Morgan HE (eds): The Heart and Cardiovascular System. Lippincott-Raven, New York, 1992

29. Apstein CA, Morgan JP: Cellular mechanisms underlying left ventricular diastolic dysfunction. pp. 3–24. In Gaasch WH, Le Winter MM (eds): Left Ventricular Diastolic Dysfunction and Heart Failure. Lea & Febiger, Philadelphia, 1994

30. Katz AM: Cardiomyopathy of overload: a major determinant of prognosis in congestive heart failure. N Engl J Med 1990;322:100

31. Katz AM: Requirements of contraction and relaxation. Implications for inotropic stimulation of the failing heart. Basic Res Cardiol 1989;84:47

32. Feldman MD, Copelas L, Gwathmey JK et al: Deficient production of cyclic AMP. Pharmacologic evidence of an important cause of contractile dysfunction in patients with end-stage heart failure. Circulation 1987; 75:331

33. Erdmann E: The effectiveness of inotropic agents in isolated cardiac preparations from the human heart. Klin Wochenschr 1988;66:1

34. Gwathmey JK, Copelas L, MacKinnon R et al: Abnormal intracellular calcium handling in myocardium from patients with end-stage heart failure. Circ Res 1987;61:70

35. Gwathmey JK, Warren SE, Briggs GM et al: Diastolic dysfunction in hypertrophic cardiomyopathy. Effect on active force generation during systole. J Clin Invest 1991;87:1023

36. Hasenfuss G, Holubarsch C, Just H, Alpert NR (eds): Cellular and Molecular Alterations in the Failing Human Heart. Springer-Verlag, New York, 1992

37. Perreault CL, Williams CP, Morgan JP: Cytoplasmic calcium modulation and systolic versus diastolic dysfunction in myocardial hypertrophy and failure. Circ 1993;87:VII-31–VII-37

38. Phillips PJ, Gwathmey JK, Feldman MD et al: Post-extrasystolic potentiation and the force-frequency relationship. Differential augmentation of myocardial contractility in working myocardium from patients with end-stage heart failure. J Mol Cell Cardiol 1990; 22:99–110

39. Morgan JP, Erny RE, Allen PD, Grossman W, Gwathmey JK: Abnormal intracellular calcium handling. A major cause of systolic and diastolic dysfunction in ventricular myocardium from patients with heart failure. Circulation, suppl. III 1990;81:21–32

40. Kihara Y, Grossman W, Morgan JP: Direct measurement of changes in intracellular calcium transients during hypoxia, ischemia, and reperfusion of the intact mammalian heart. Circ Res 1989;65:1029

41. Steenbergen C, Murphy E, Levy L, London RE: Elevation in cytosolic free calcium concentration early in myocardial ischemia in perfused rat heart. Circ Res 1987;60:700

42. Marban E, Kitkaze M, Kusuoka H et al: Intracellular free calcium concentration measured with ^{19}F NMR spectroscopy in intact ferret hearts. Proc Natl Acad Sci USA 1987;84:6005

43. Mohabir R, Lee HC, Kurz RW, Clusin WT: Effects of ischemia and hypercarbia acidosis on myocyte calcium transients, contraction, and pH{-i} in perfused rabbit hearts. Circ Res 1991;69:1525

44. Carrozza JP, Bentivegna LA, Williams CP et al: Decreased myofilament responsiveness in myocardial stunning follows transient calcium overload during ischemia and reperfusion. Circ Res 1992;71:6

45. Krause SM, Jacobus WE, Becker LC: Alterations in cardiac sarcoplasmic reticulum calcium transport in the postischemic "stunned" myocardium. Circ Res 1989;65:526–530

46. Kusuoka H, Koretsune Y, Chacko VP, Weisfeldt ML, Marban E: Excitation-contraction coupling in postischemic myocardium. Does failure of activator Ca^{2+} transients underlie stunning? Circ Res 1990;66: 1268–1276

47. Hajjar RJ, Gwathmey JK, Briggs GM, Morgan JP: Differential effect of DP1 201–106 on the sensitivity of myofilaments to Ca^{2+} in intact and skinned trabeculae from control and myopathic human hearts. J Clin Invest 1988;82:1578

48. Wankerl M, Bohm M, Morano I et al: Calcium sensitivity and myosin light chain pattern of atrial and ventricular skinned cardiac fibers from patients with various kinds of cardiac diseases. J Mol Cell Cardiol 1990; 22:1425

49. Perreault CL, Brozovich FV, Ransil BJ, Morgan JP: Effects of MCI-154 on Ca^{2+} activation of skinned human myocardium. Eur J Pharmacol 1989;165:305

50. Francis GS, McDonald K, Chu C, Cohn JN: Pathophysiologic aspects of end-stage heart failure. Am J Cardiol 1995;75:11A–16A

2 | Cardiac Interstitium

Karl T. Weber

Former axioms, presumed truths, require revision as the body of knowledge advances.

- *Axiom 1*: When the myocardium falters as a muscular pump, cardiac myocytes must be faulty. Not so. Perfectly normal giant mastodons, trapped in tar, were unable to function or indeed survive their unfavorable environment, which can likewise be the case for cardiac myocytes.
- *Axiom 2*: Relative to myocytes, the interstitial space and its structural proteins are unimportant to the diseased heart if for no other reason than the turnover of these proteins is too slow to be of any relevance. Not so. Structural proteins turnover is a dynamic process.[1] Myocardial collagen remodeling is an integral feature of many disease states and an abnormal interstitium can represent an adverse environment for cardiac myocytes. Fibrillar type I collagen surrounds myocytes; it courses between them, connects them to one another, and has the tensile strength of steel.[2] Fibrillar collagen is a major determinant of tissue stiffness, myocyte length, and contraction.

Concepts of cardiac muscle mechanics, set forth more than three decades ago,[3] emphasize the importance of elastic elements positioned in series and in parallel with a contractile element represented by myocytes. Interest in myocardial contractility, a biochemical property of cardiac muscle, emphasized the role of contractile proteins and sarcoplasmic reticulum handling of calcium. Short-changed were the elastic elements and their anatomic correlates; consequently, the importance of the structural composition of tissue was overlooked. This experience serves to remind us that we are what we know based on what we believe to be true at the time.

Scanning electron microscopy drew attention to the extensive fibrillar collagen network in the heart.[4] Such morphologic studies paved the way for investigations that have explored the functional significance of fibrillar collagen and drew attention to the interstitium in general. Not surprisingly, fibrillar collagen proved to be a major determinant of tissue stiffness.[5] For those clinging to previous axioms, further investigation was still necessary. For others, who acknowledged a role for the interstitium in the diseased heart, regulation of collagen turnover was a next logical target. The latter studies created more of a balance between the importance of elastic and contractile components in governing the mechanical behavior of the normal and failing myocardium. Moreover, they drew attention to the progressive nature of collagen remodeling found throughout the right and left ventricles in various disease states. They further emphasized that highly specialized parenchymal cells can be innocent bystanders to iterations in their stromal environment. The importance of stroma, relative to parenchyma, is now a recognized feature of various diseases that affect the kidney, liver, lung, and pancreas.

The cardiac interstitium is the focus of this chapter. A major component of this extracellular space, in terms of tissue stiffness and structural remodeling, are type I and III fibrillar collagens. All impor-

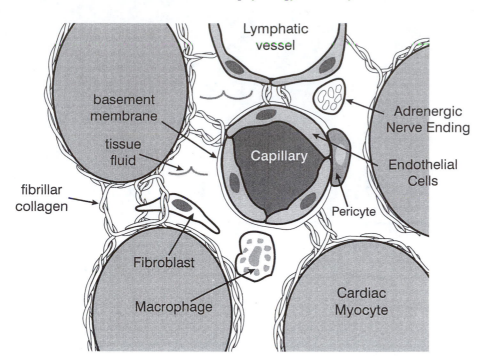

Fig. 2-1. Cardiac interstitium situated between cardiac myocytes.

tant to matrix and tissue remodeling is the regulation of collagen turnover, based on the behavior of fibroblasts and fibroblast-like cells, governed by signals derived locally or from the circulation. Material presented herein builds on previous reviews of the cardiac interstitium[6,7] and addresses current information regarding the dynamic behavior of cells residing in fibrous tissue.

INTERSTITIAL SPACE: BRIEF OVERVIEW

The cardiac interstitium is composed of structures and cells depicted in Figure 2-1. The normal interstitium includes: (1) type I and III collagens, the major fibrillar collagens; (2) lesser quantities of type IV, V, and VI collagens, found in cell membranes or the pericellular space; (3) a small amount of elastin; (4) glycosaminoglycans and glycoproteins associated with these structural proteins; (5) adrenergic nerve endings; (6) blood and lymph-containing vessels; (7) cells of mesenchymal origin that include fibroblasts, pericytes, valvlar interstitial cells, and macrophages; and (8) tissue fluid, formed as an ultrafiltrate of plasma and containing signals that arise from parenchymal and mesenchymal cells and nerve endings to regulate the behavior and growth of fibroblasts or fibroblast-like cells.

Phenotypically transformed fibroblasts appear in the interstitium during wound healing to orchestrate fibrogenesis and subsequent matrix remodeling. Inflammatory cells gain access to the interstitium from the circulation and contribute to tissue repair. The type of inflammatory cell involved is influenced by the nature of the chemical signal(s) that has been activated and is expressed as regulatory polypeptides (e.g., cytokines and growth factors).

Like skeletal muscle, the normal fibrillar collagen network of the myocardium is divided into epimysium, perimysium, and endomysium.[7] Each serves various functions, reviewed elsewhere.[6,7] Contiguous with the internalized collagen network of the myocardium is its exteriorized segment found in chordae tendineae and heart valve leaflets.[8] Valve leaflets, a site of high collagen turnover, offer a unique opportunity to study the regulation of collagen turnover by valvlar interstitial cells.

MATRIX AND TISSUE STIFFNESS: BRIEF OVERVIEW

Myocardial tissue exhibits a resistance to stretch (i.e., stiffness) during diastole. It includes postcontraction relengthening of tissue during the isovolumic relaxation period and stretching of tissue during rapid filling and following atrial contraction. Furthermore, dynamic elastance of tissue is present during contraction.[9,10] Concepts of cardiac tissue mechanics were developed years ago for the intact heart[11] and excised cardiac tissue.[12] As depicted in Figure 2-2, these concepts included a contractile element (represented by cardiac myocytes) and elastic

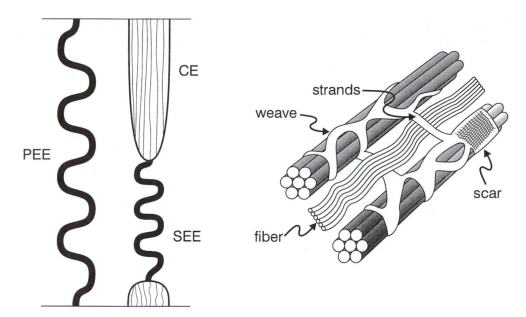

Fig. 2-2. Concepts of cardiac mechanics include a contractile element (CE) and elastic elements placed either in series with (SEE) or in parallel to (PEE) the CE. Anatomic correlates of SEE and PEE include various components of the fibrillar collagen network and replacement fibrosis (or scarring).

elements (positioned either in series with the contractile elements or in parallel with the contractile element and in series with the elastic elements). Anatomic correlates of in-series elastic elements are now recognized to include structural proteins that connect myocytes and their intracellular cytoskeletal proteins to one another and muscle bundles to one another. Scar tissue replacing necrotic myocytes likewise represents an in-series elastic element. Collagen fibers that form a weave of connective tissue that ensheathes muscle bundles as well as myocytes, and that course between myocytes and bundles represent in-parallel elastic elements. Specific characteristics of fibrillar collagens that determine tissue stiffness include not only their overall concentration but also fiber thickness and configuration, fiber alignment relative to myocytes and their distribution within tissue, the percentage of stiff type I collagen relative to more resilient type III collagen, and the degree of collagen cross-linking.

Various clinical and experimental studies[13–19] have demonstrated the importance of disproportionate fibrillar collagen accumulation, or fibrosis, on tissue stiffness. As reviewed elsewhere,[5] these studies addressed (1) the presence of fibrosis in the hypertrophied ventricle with abnormal stiffness; (2) the importance of fibrosis to abnormal myocardial stiffness, with or without cardiac myocyte hypertrophy; (3) the prevention of fibrosis to preserve normal tissue stiffness; and (4) regression of fibrosis, which would normalize tissue stiffness in either hypertrophied or nonhypertrophied ventricles.

Using a simple expression of collagen network remodeling (i.e., the percent of tissue occupied by collagen or its collagen volume fraction), the following broad statements can be made: (1) A two- to threefold increase in tissue collagen adversely influences diastolic stiffness whereas systolic stiffness is preserved. (2) A four-fold or more rise in collagen volume fraction is associated with a further rise in diastolic stiffness and a decline in systolic stiffness (or systolic dysfunction), expressed as a decline in ejection fraction and percent shortening.

REGULATION OF COLLAGEN TURNOVER

Normal Myocardium

Collagen concentrations of the right and left ventricles (RVs and LVs) are equivalent in the 28-day-old heart of the rabbit fetus.[20] At 7 days after birth the RV and LV collagen concentrations have increased beyond that found in utero but remain equivalent.[20] A fall in pulmonary vascular resistance (and so in RV systolic wall stress) occurs at birth with a regression in RV myocyte size during the neonatal period. Accordingly, collagen concentration in the RV 28 days after birth is now greater than in the LV. This natural remodeling of the RV after birth demonstrates that ventricular loading is a determinant of myocyte size but not collagen turnover. Given its larger mass, LV collagen content (concentration × mass) is greater than that in the adult RV.

Collagen turnover in the adult heart is normally a dynamic process. Daily fractional collagen synthesis of 5 percent has been observed,[1] with nearly 60 percent of newly synthesized collagen degraded rapidly within the lysosomes and endoplasmic reticulum of interstitial fibroblasts, hereafter referred to as *cardiac fibroblasts*. Extracellular degradation is mediated by various neutral proteases, including collagenase, produced by fibroblasts. Interstitial collagenase exists largely in latent form.[21,22] A 60 to 80 percent increase in collagenase activity appears after activation of matrix metalloproteinases. Myocardial collagenase is activated by trypsin, plasmin, and neutrophil elastase. The molecular weight of this metalloproteinase is estimated to be 52 kDa.

Are hemodynamic factors or locally produced substances responsible for collagen turnover? Several observations address this question. First, the collagen concentration of atrial tissue with its minimal loading is severalfold greater than that in ventricular tissue. Second, collagen concentration of minimally loaded RV is nearly twice that of the LV. These findings suggest that hemodynamic load is not a major determinant of collagen synthesis. Third, collagen formation was not altered in young rabbits treated with propranolol or practolol, β-adrenergic receptor antagonists that reduce myocardial work.[23] Contrariwise, after 5 weeks of treatment of young rats with an angiotensin-converting enzyme (ACE) inhibitor, enalapril, which did not alter arterial pressure, the collagen content of the RV, LV, aorta, and superior mesenteric artery were each less than that found in age- and gender-matched, untreated, normotensive controls.[24] Collectively, these observations support a role for locally produced angiotensin II in regulating collagen turnover. A role for angiotensin II is further supported by studies of collagen turnover in cultured cardiac fibroblasts, where collagen synthesis is increased, and the collagenolytic activity of culture medium was decreased by this peptide.[25,26] Additionally, inhibition of ACE may increase local concentrations of bradykinin, which in turn promotes the formation of such substances as prostaglandins (PG), and nitric oxide. In cultured fibroblasts these substances inhibit collagen synthesis and increase collagen degradation.[27,28]

Normal Valve Leaflets

Valve leaflets provide a unique site when considering a role for ventricular loading versus local or circulating substances in regulating collagen turnover. After surgically induced unilateral renal ischemia and activation of the secondary renin-angiotensin-aldosterone system (RAAS), mRNA expression of type I and III collagens and their proteins in the rat myocardium[29] is increased. It was expressed as perivascular fibrosis of intramyocardial coronary arteries in both the pressure-overloaded, hypertrophied LV and the normotensive, nonhypertrophied RV.[30] In this same model, increased expression of these transcripts and proteins were found in mitral and aortic valve leaflets of the hypertensive LV and in the tricuspid valve of the normotensive RV.[31] These in vivo findings implicate an association between a circulating substance (e.g., angiotensin II) and collagen accumulation and demonstrate that hypertension, or ventricular loading, is responsible for myocyte hypertrophy, not fibrous tissue formation.

Valvular interstitial cells (VICs), responsible for collagen turnover at this site of high collagen turnover, were studied, given that quantitative in vitro autoradiographic studies can localize intact valve leaflets as a site of high-density ACE[32-34] and AT$_1$ receptor binding.[34] Monoclonal ACE antibody immunolabeling identified the VIC as the cell expressing this ectoenzyme.[35] Morphologically, VICs resemble pericytes, fibroblast-like cells residing in vascular adventitia, another site of high collagen turnover. Both VICs and pericytes contain α-smooth muscle actin microfilaments, and accordingly both are contractile. Angiotensin II induces contraction of both VICs and pericytes.[35-37] Does angiotensin II influence VIC collagen turnover, and is it produced by VICs? To address these questions, Katwa et al.[35] isolated VICs from adult rat heart valve leaflets and maintained them in culture, a procedure that eliminated hemodynamic factors as a confounding variable. Whether VICs have components requisite for generating angiotensin II was addressed first.

Cultured VICs from each valve and their cell membranes demonstrated high-density ACE binding by in vitro autoradiography. Intact VICs likewise expressed ACE, as detected by monoclonal ACE immunolabeling. The reverse transcriptase polymerase chain reaction revealed that cultured VICs contain ACE transcript. ACE substrate utilization in cultured VICs was found to include angiotensin I, bradykinin, substance P, and enkephalins. Therefore ACE bound to VICs has both angiotensin I-converting and kininase II activities. AT$_1$ receptors were identified in VIC membranes by competitive binding and Western immunoblot assays; AT$_2$ receptors were not found. Preliminary studies[38] indicated that intact VICs have the transcript for angiotensinogen, the requisite precursor for angiotensin peptides, and that they also have a nonrenin aspartyl protease

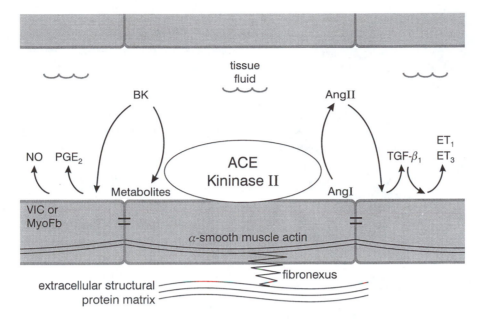

Fig. 2-3. Autocrine/paracrine responses of valvar interstitial cells (VIC) or myofibroblasts (MyoFb) to locally produced angiotensin II (AngII). This process may include elaboration of transforming growth factor β_1 and subsequent production of endothelins (ET$_1$ and ET$_3$). Angiotensin I (AngI) produced by these cells arises from hydrolysis of angiotensinogen (Ao) by an aspartyl protease. It may occur intra- or extracellularly. Membrane-bound ectoenzyme, angiotensin-converting enzyme (ACE), converts AngI to AngII. ACE also functions as a kininase II involved in the degradation of bradykinin (BK), as well as substance P and enkephalins (not shown). Both VIC and MyoFb contain α-smooth muscle actin microfilaments and are attached to matrix proteins by a fibronexus. Each of these cells is connected to neighboring cells by gap junctions (=).

(likely cathepsin D) for converting angiotensinogen to angiotensin I, thereby eliminating any absolute dependence on renin. Tissue stores of renin are derived from the circulation[39] and are not sustained in anephric animals or in cultured VICs. Cultured VICs were shown to generate angiotensins I and II. Whether angiotensin I formation occurs intra- or extracellularly requires further study. Locally produced angiotensin II could serve to regulate VIC collagen synthesis and degradation and VIC contraction in an autocrine/paracrine manner. This point requires further study. What is known about these issues is presented below.

In situ hybridization demonstrated that cultured VICs contain type I collagen mRNA, and that collagen synthesis and type I collagen mRNA expression are each increased when these cells, maintained in serum-deprived conditions, are incubated with angiotensin II. Whether this presumptive transcriptional event is a direct or indirect response to angiotensin II must be addressed. Angiotensin II, as depicted in Figure 2-3, enhances expression of transforming growth factor β_1 (TGFβ_1) and endothelins, each of which can augment cardiac fibroblast collagen synthesis and reduce collagenase activity.[40,41] As is the case in other (noncardiac) fibroblasts and vas-

cular smooth muscle cells, other locally produced substances, such as bradykinins, prostaglandins, and nitric oxide, inhibit collagen synthesis and promote collagen degradation.[27,42] Thus there exists the potential for a paradigm of local reciprocal regulation (Figure 2-4) of collagen turnover.

Diseased Heart and Related Structures

The heart's wound healing response can be used to gauge the regulation of collagen accumulation in the diseased myocardium. Various experimental models (Table 2-1) have been used for this purpose, including models associated with parenchymal cell death (i.e., cardiac myocyte necrosis) due to ischemic injury (coronary ligation). Models of cell loss following administration of a catecholamine, infusion of angiotensin II, or potassium depletion secondary to chronic aldosterone or deoxycorticosterone treatment (uninephrectomized rats on a high sodium diet) have also been used. Models where myocyte necrosis is not a requisite include those with fibrosis of visceral pericardium following pericardiotomy, endocardial fibrosis remote to myocardial infarction, foreign-body fi-

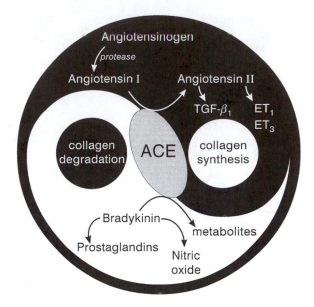

Fig. 2-4. Paradigm of reciprocal regulation to collagen turnover in cardiovascular tissue may exist. Stimulators of fibrosis include angiotensin II, transforming growth factor β_1 and endothelins 1 and 3. Inhibitors of fibrosis include bradykinin, prostaglandins, and nitric oxide. Stimulators would increase collagen synthesis and reduce collagenase activity. Inhibitors would behave just the opposite.

brosis associated with placement of a silk ligature around a coronary artery without subsequent infarction, or perivascular fibrosis of intramural coronary arterioles that appears either remote to the infarction or in association with chronic angiotensin II or aldosterone treatment.

Table 2-1. Sites of High-Density ACE Binding in Normal and Diseased Heart

Normal heart
   Heart valves
   Adventitia of intramyocardial coronary arteries
Diseased heart
   Scar in infarcted RV or LV
   Endocardial fibrosis remote to MI
   Perivascular fibrosis and microscopic scars remote to MI
   Foreign-body fibrosis surrounding silk ligature
   Pericardial fibrosis after pericardiotomy
   Endomyocardial fibrosis after isoproterenol administration
   Perivascular fibrosis of RV and LV with chronic AngII or ALDO administration
   Microscopic scars of RV and LV with chronic AngII or ALDO administration

   Abbreviations: MI, myocardial infarction; RV and LV, right and left ventricles; AngII, angiotensin II; ALDO, aldosterone.

Regardless of whether myocyte necrosis has occurred, fibroblasts are pivotal to healing. In adult tissues fibroblasts retain pluripotentiality and, accordingly, exhibit marked diversity in their functions, a trait presumptively related to distinct phenotypic subtypes.[43-45] For different tissues or within a given tissue, fibroblasts demonstrate extensive clonal heterogeneity. Several days after myocyte loss—due to coronary ligation or freeze-thaw injury—fibroblast-like cells appear at the site of repair.[46,47] Larger than cardiac fibroblasts, these cells have a prominent, wrinkled nucleus and endoplasmic reticulum. In addition, they have α-smooth muscle actin microfilaments that may have been acquired during phenotypic transformation or may have persisted in pericytes that now assume the role of the wound healing fibroblast. These actin filaments contribute to the ability of these cells to contract[48] and to their wrinkled nucleus, which is indicative of contractile activity. Various mediators of inflammation, including angiotensin II and prostaglandins, induce contraction; papaverine promotes relaxation.[48] These contractile, fibroblast-like cells are central to tissue repair and are termed *myofibroblasts*.[49] The contraction of granulation tissue is mediated by myofibroblasts and their contractile behavior. Mandatory components of tissue contraction includes myofibroblasts having cell-to-cell and cell-to-stroma connections. Such remodeling of granulation tissue appears weeks after its formation and accounts for a reduction in the volume of infarcted myocardium, infarct thickness, and retraction of scar tissue.[50-52] Signals responsible for the appearance of myofibroblasts in the heart, albeit presently unknown, may be derived from the circulation, cardiac fibroblasts, neighboring endothelial cells, platelets, or invading inflammatory cells. This subject requires further study. In other tissues $TGF\beta_1$ has been implicated in evoking this response.[53-57]

Using immunohistochemical labeling, Sun et al.[47] found α-smooth muscle actin-containing fibroblasts located in granulation that formed at the site of infarct repair; they also found that these cells expressed ACE. Myofibroblasts are therefore largely responsible for high-density ACE binding seen by in vitro autoradiography (Plate 2-1) at this site.[47] Other cells expressing ACE at the site of infarction include endothelial cells and macrophages. The appearance of ACE in myofibroblasts likely serves to regulate local concentrations of angiotensin II, bradykinin, and related peptides that contribute to the healing response. Myofibroblasts at the site of infarction express type I collagen mRNA,[47] the major fibrillar collagen found in scar tissue.[58-60] The number of myofibroblasts at the site of a myocardial infarction (MI)

Color Insert

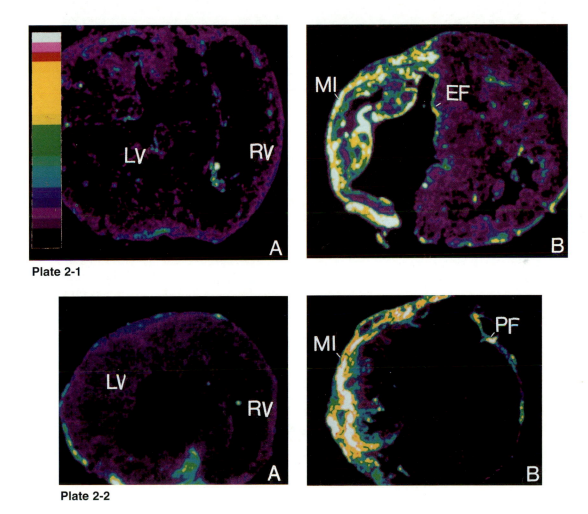

Plate 2-1

Plate 2-2

Plate 2-1. Autoradiographic detection of angiotensin-converting enzyme (ACE) binding density in (**A**) the normal rat myocardium and (**B**) 8 weeks after myocardial infarction. ACE binding density is low throughout the normal myocardium. Marked ACE binding appears at sites of fibrous tissue formation, including the site of infarction (MI), endocardial fibrosis of the interventricular septum (EF), and remote to the infarct in the right ventricle (RV).

Plate 2-2. Autoradiographic detection of angiotensin II receptor binding in myocardium of (**A**) sham-operated rat and (**B**) 8 weeks after infarction. Angiotensin II receptor binding is normally low throughout the myocardium but becomes marked at sites of fibrosis, including placement of silk ligature (**A,** lower center), infarct scar (MI), and pericardial fibrosis (PF) seen in Fig. B and also left side of Fig. A. By competitive binding, only AT_1 receptors have been identified in the normal and fibrosed myocardium. (From Sun Y and Weber KT: Angiotensin II receptor binding following myocardial infarction in the rat. Cardiovasc Res 1994;28:1623, with permission.)

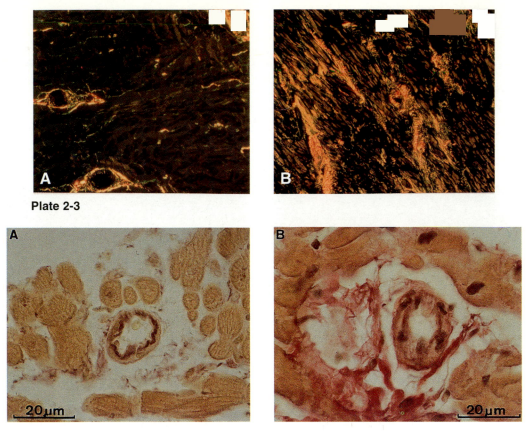

Plate 2-3

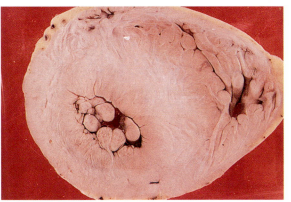

Plate 24-1

20 µm

20 µm

Plate 27-1

Plate 2-3. Human hypertensive heart disease is associated with an extensive remodeling of the myocardium by fibrous tissue, which includes a perivascular/interstitial fibrosis. In the picrosirius-polarization technique, fibrillar collagen appears yellow or light green and myocytes dark brown. **(A)** Normal human left ventricle; **(B)** hypertrophied human left ventricle demonstrating the extensive perivascular fibrosis of intramyocardial coronary arteries with extensions into the contiguous interstitial space. (From Weber KT and Brilla CG: Pathological hypertrophy and cardiac interstitium: Fibrosis and renin-angiotensin-aldosterone system. Circulation 1991;83:1849, with permission.)

Plate 24-1. Media hypertrophy of intramyocardial arteriole surrounded by collagen (reddish stained by EvG) in arterial hypertension **(B)** compared with normotensive subject **(A).** (From Schwartzkopff B, Motz W, Frenzel H, et al. Structural and functional alterations of the intramyocardial coronary arterioles in patients with arterial hypertension. Circulation 1993;88:993, with permission.)

Plate 27-1. Cross-section of the heart in hypertrophic cardiomyopathy. Severe asymmetric hypertrophy, papillary muscle hypertrophy, and obliteration of ventricular cavity.

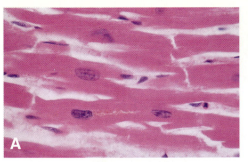

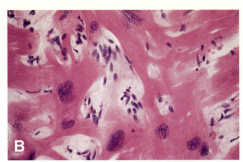

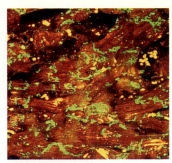

Plate 27-2

Plate 27-3

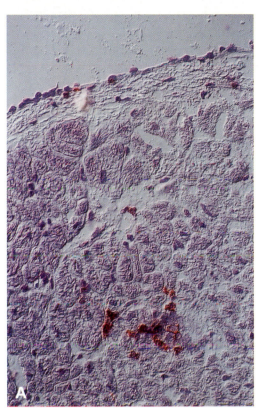

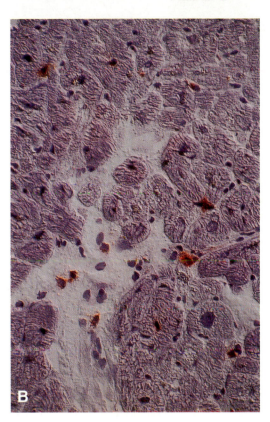

Plate 29-1

Plate 27-2. (A) Microscopy of normal heart section reveals ordered myocytes. **(B)** Microscopic section of hypertrophic cardiomyopathy heart section demonstrates severe myocyte architectural disarray.

Plate 27-3. Altered patterns of gap junction distribution in areas of myofiber disarray in hypertrophic cardiomyopathy. Gap junction immunostaining (green) shows a random dispersion on the myocyte surface instead of being confined to well-defined intercalated disc areas. Confocal laser scanning image, anti-connexin 43 immunostaining (×200). (From Sepp R, Severs NJ, and Gourdie RG: Altered patterns of cardiac intercellular junction distribution in hypertrophic cardiomyopathy. Heart, 1996, in press, with permission.)

Plate 29-1. Immunohistochemical staining of inflammatory cells. **(A)** Focal and **(B)** diffuse chronic lymphocytic infiltration stained with anti-CD3 antibodies (A&B, ×400). *(Plate continues.)*

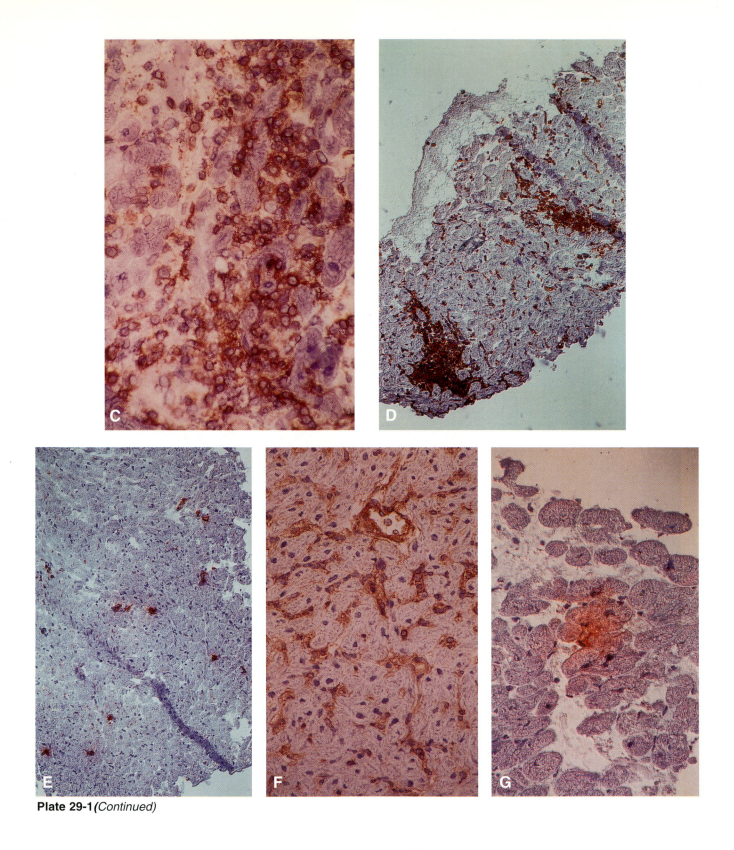

Plate 29-1. (*Continued*). **(C&D)** Acute myocarditis stained 1 week after onset of symptoms (C, ×400; D, ×100). **(E)** Activated macrophages (antibody 27E10, ×100). HLA-DR expression in **(F)** inflamed myocardium. **(G)** Interferon-γ released from an activated macrophage (F&G, ×400).

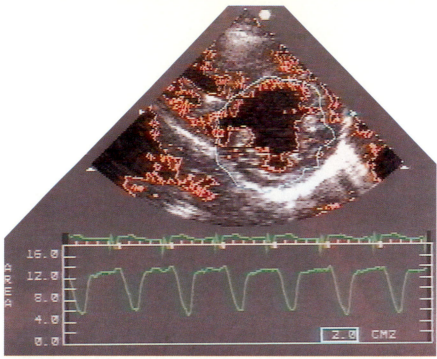

Plate 32-1

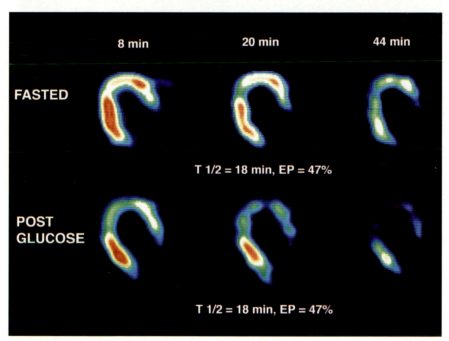

Plate 35-1

Plate 32-1. Automated border detection applied to a parasternal short axis view from a heart transplant recipient with normal systolic function. The area change over time has been calculated on line by the system and is displayed in graph form below the two-dimensional image.

Plate 35-1. Selected serial ^{11}C palmitate images obtained in a patient with nonischemic cardiomyopathy in the fasted state and after glucose loading. The images on the left were acquired at 8 minutes after ^{11}C palmitate administration, in the center at 20 minutes, and on the right at 44 minutes. Note the heterogeneous clearance of ^{11}C palmitate from the left ventricular myocardium in the fasted state. Glucose loading, as seen in the lower panel, markedly accentuates this heterogeneity. The figure further indicates the more rapid clearance of ^{11}C palmitate from the anterior wall. (From Sochor H, Schelbert H, Schwaiger M et al: Studies of fatty acid metabolism with positron emission tomography in patients with cardiomyopathy. Eur J Nucl Med 1986;12:S66–S69, with permission.)

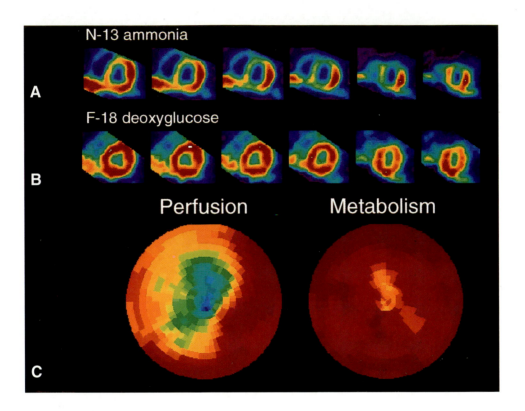

Plate 35-2. Quantitative assessment of a blood flow metabolism mismatch in a patient with ischemic cardiomyopathy. **(A)** Contiguous short axis cuts of the myocardial ^{13}N ammonia and **(B)** the myocardial [18]F 2-deoxyglucose uptake are shown. **(C)** The polar map of myocardial perfusion indicates an extensive flow defect involving the anterior wall and the interventricular septum. This is consistent with the reduced ^{13}N ammonia uptake in the anterior wall and the interventricular septum as seen on the short axis cuts. In contrast, [18]F 2-deoxyglucose uptake is relatively homogeneous demonstrating a rather extensive blood flow metabolism mismatch. (Courtesy of Marcelo Di Carli, M.D., UCLA School of Medicine, Los Angeles, CA.)

are gradually reduced in number, but residual cells persist for prolonged periods.[46,47,61]

ACE-positive myofibroblasts are likewise found at sites of fibrosis that appear remote to LV infarction.[47] Macrophages and endothelial cells are not found at these sites. Considered a reactive fibrosis, they include the endocardial fibrosis of the interventricular septum, the perivascular fibrosis of intramural vessels found in the RV, the pericardial fibrosis that follows pericardiotomy (without infarction), and the foreign-body fibrosis that surrounds silk ligatures around the left coronary artery (without infarction). At each of the aforementioned sites, myofibroblasts would be shown to express type I collagen mRNA by in situ hybridization.[47] Thus myofibroblasts are the dominant cell involved in stromal formation irrespective of the location or nature of the inciting stimulus to connective tissue formation in the heart and its related structures.

Wound healing is normally confined to injured tissue and must therefore be regulated by locally generated signals. Cytokine expression, for example, is confined to sites of injury. What regulates cytokine expression is less well understood. Parenchymal cell necrosis may be important,[62] but it is not a requisite to fibrous tissue reactions as evidenced from the above findings. Even as late as 12 weeks after left coronary artery ligation with infarction, increased ACE mRNA expression and activity were observed in tissue homogenates obtained from the RV. It was not the case, however, for systemic organs.[63] In this infarct model, plasma renin and ACE activity are not increased. In keeping with the presence of myofibroblasts ACE activity, ACE binding density is increased 8 weeks after an MI at both the site of injury and remote sites of fibrous tissue formation (Plate 2-1).[47] The appearance of ACE in fibrous tissue, expressed in myofibroblasts, is independent of circulating angiotensin II. This situation contrasts to endothelial cell ACE.[64] Myofibroblasts appear to have an intrinsic ability (i.e., protease and ACE activities) that is required to generate their own signals (e.g., angiotensins I and II), which directly or indirectly (e.g., $TGF\beta_1$, bradykinin, PGE_2), regulate collagen turnover in an autocrine/paracrine manner.

In support of the indirect (paracrine) regulation of collagen turnover is the finding that angiotensin II induces cultured neonatal rat cardiac fibroblasts to express $TGF\beta_1$ mRNA.[65] Fibroblasts produce PGE_2 in response to bradykinin stimulation.[28,66] Kinins and prostanoids are endogenous hormones whose role as chemical mediators of inflammation is well recognized. Their involvement in wound healing in the heart has not been systematically examined. Bradykinin, PGI_2, and PGE_2 have each been de-

tected in coronary sinus drainage. During myocardial ischemia and following infarction, the bradykinin concentration in sinus effluent rises severalfold.[67–71] A similar response is observed for sinus concentrations of angiotensin II and PGE_2.[66,71] Whether the early release of bradykinin after infarction arises from the coronary vasculature or other cells is presently unknown. Nevertheless, the release of bradykinin after infarction may be an integral feature of the heart's inflammatory response. Bradykinin-induced coronary vascular hyperpermeability and subsequent interstitial edema can adversely influence LV diastolic and systolic function.[70] Early potentiation of bradykinin release by ACE inhibitor administration after infarction could impair ventricular function.

Several days after acute infarction, the release of PGE_2 is markedly increased by administration of bradykinin, suggesting that inflammatory cells may be involved.[66] Various mesenchymal cells, including squamous epithelial cells of visceral and parietal pericardium, pleura, and peritoneum,[72–74] fibroblasts of various organs,[75–77] and cultured mesothelial cells of pericardium[78] are able to synthesize prostanoids. Whether these nonendothelial cells release bradykinin, a stimulus to prostaglandin synthesis,[75] is yet uncertain. Both bradykinin and PGE_2 alter cultured cardiac fibroblast collagen turnover.[75,79] Fibroblast-like cells, isolated on day 7 from the site of infarction, demonstrate increased cyclooxygenase activity and increased prostanoid production, including PGE_2.[80] Bradykinin-induced release of PGE_2 from the heart remains increased 30 days after MI.[66] Microsomes prepared from infarcted myocardium at 3 weeks and as late as 3 months after coronary ligation demonstrate increased prostaglandin synthesis. The persistence of PGE_2 production well beyond the inflammatory phase of tissue repair suggests that nonvascular, noninflammatory cells may be involved. Whether angiotensin peptides, bradykinin, and PGE_2 are released by myofibroblasts has not yet been assessed.

If locally generated angiotensin II is to influence fibrogenesis, receptor–ligand binding in myofibroblasts is a requisite. Using in vitro quantitative autoradiography [(^{125}I-Sar^1, Ile^8)-angiotensin II], Sun and Weber[81] found high-density angiotensin II receptor binding at each of the fibrous tissue sites noted earlier for the rat infarct model (Plate 2-2).[81] The angiotensin II receptor subtype involved, determined by displacement with an AT_1 (Dup 753, losartan) or AT_2 (PD 123177) receptor antagonist, indicated AT_1 not AT_2, receptor binding. AT_1 receptor binding density was marked at the site of the MI and remote sites involving the RV and septum. In sham-operated rats, the fibrosed visceral pericardium and foreign-body fibrosis were also sites of high AT_1 receptor binding. Cells that express AT_1 receptors at these sites remain to be elucidated, but myofibroblasts are likely candidates. Nonetheless, the anatomic association between ACE and AT_1 receptors at sites of fibrous tissue formation support the proposition that local concentrations of angiotensin II contribute to tissue repair.

Further evidence in support of the putative role of angiotensin II in regulating fibrous connective tissue formation is derived from in vivo studies that used either an ACE inhibitor or AT_1 receptor antagonist. In dogs with anterior infarction, captopril[82] and enalapril[83] were each found to influence wound healing at the site of cell loss, including the appearance of flatter infarct scars and less collagen in the infarct zone. In 4-week-old spontaneously hypertensive rats (SHRs), quinapril, given in a dose that did not prevent hypertension, was found to attenuate the expected rise in aortic collagen volume fraction that appeared at 30 weeks of age.[84] Circulating RAAS is not activated in SHRs and therefore does not account for these findings. After infarction, another model without circulating RAAS activation, perindopril, attenuated the endomyocardial fibrosis that appeared in the nonnecrotic rat LV.[85] Similarly, captopril prevented the expected proliferation of fibroblast-like cells and fibrosis in the noninfarcted rat RV and septum following LV infarction.[86] On the other hand, an AT_1 receptor antagonist, losartan, prevented fibrosis but not fibroblast proliferation at these remote sites.[87] Lisinopril prevents pericardial fibrosis following pericardiotomy, without infarction.[81] Despite the presence of myocyte injury associated with angiotensin II administration lisinopril attenuates microscopic scarring.[88] The cardioprotective effect of ACE inhibitors in models of wound healing that are independent of circulating angiotensin II implicate local production of angiotensin II as contributing to fibrous tissue formation. The importance of a local accumulation of bradykinin, PGE_2, and nitric oxide cannot be discounted as contributing to this altered wound healing response.

Circulating Hormones and Reactive Fibrosis

When local mediators of wound healing (e.g., angiotensin II) gain access to the circulation and are not neutralized, they can promote a wound healing response at distant sites. This reaction represents a wound healing response gone awry. It would explain the reactive fibrosis that appears in systemic and coronary arterioles in association with chronic eleva-

tions in circulating angiotensin II. A role for aldosterone cannot be discounted (*vide infra*). Numerous experimental models (Table 2-2) have been used to address the relative contribution of these hormones. The aforementioned perivascular/interstitial fibrosis appears in the hypertensive, hypertrophied LV after surgically induced unilateral renal ischemia, where endogenous plasma angiotensin II and aldosterone are each increased.[15,89–92] The normotensive, nonhypertrophied RV is also involved,[90] further implicating a role for these circulating effector hormones of the RAAS. Treatment of these animals with captopril prevented this remodeling.[93] Increased collagen found in the nonhypertrophied LV and the hypertrophied RV after pulmonary artery banding in cats[94] further implicates these hormones. This classic model of RAAS activation is accompanied by the appearance of pleural effusions and ascites that follows angiotensin II- and aldosterone-induced urinary sodium retention.[95] Bilateral renal ischemia follows placement of a band (suprarenal) on the ascending, thoracic, or subdiaphragmatic abdominal aorta and is accompanied by an increase in myocardial collagen synthesis,[96,97] which can be prevented by digitoxin.[98]

Other in vivo studies demonstrated that the pathologic accumulation of fibrous tissue appears with neither the pressure-overload hypertrophy induced by infrarenal aortic banding[90] nor the volume-overload hypertrophy associated with uninephrectomy and a high sodium diet,[90] a compensated arteriovenous fistula,[91,99] chronic anemia,[100] atrial septal defect,[101] or the hypertrophy induced by chronic thyroxine administration.[100,102] In each of these circumstances

---

Table 2-2. Experimental Models That Address the Importance of Hemodynamic Versus Hormonal Factors Contributing to Hypertrophy With or Without Fibrosis

Hypertrophy with fibrosis
    Unilateral renal ischemia
    Aldosterone (uninephrectomy, high Na^+ diet)
    Deoxycorticosterone acetate (uninephrectomy, high Na^+ diet)
    Angiotensin II administration
    Suprarenal aortic banding
    Pulmonary artery banding

Hypertrophy without fibrosis
    Anemia
    Arteriovenous fistula
    Atrial septal defect
    Thyroxine administration
    Infrarenal aortic band
    Uninephrectomy plus high Na^+ diet
    Aldosterone plus low-dose spironolactone

the circulating RAAS is not activated so long as renal perfusion is sustained.

A perivascular fibrosis of intramural vessels of the RV and LV, as well as systemic arterioles, has been observed in rats receiving angiotensin II by implanted osmotic minipump and in uninephrectomized rats on a high sodium diet that received either d-aldosterone[90,103] or deoxycorticosterone acetate (DOCA).[104] With exogenous administration of angiotensin II, the plasma angiotensin II and aldosterone levels increase; whereas with aldosterone treatment, plasma renin activity and angiotensin II are suppressed.[90,105] Chronic DOCA treatment suppresses plasma renin activity and circulating levels of angiotensin II and aldosterone.[106] The reactive perivascular fibrosis of intramyocardial coronary arterioles of the RV and LV that accompanies chronic mineralocorticoid excess[64,90,103,104] has been confirmed.[107,108] The latter studies further demonstrated that this reactive fibrosis was accompanied by increased expression of types I and III collagen transcripts in the nonhypertrophied RV and the hypertrophied LV, whereas atrial natriuretic peptide mRNA was expressed only in the hypertrophied LV.[108] Type I corticoid receptor binding in the heart by either aldosterone or DOCA, a nonclassic site of action for these mineralocorticoids, is responsible for this adverse remodeling as evidenced by the protective effect of a corticoid receptor antagonist.

In rats receiving aldosterone pretreatment and continued treatment with an aldosterone receptor antagonist (spironolactone) prevented both perivascular fibrosis and scarring of the myocardium. It was true for both a small dose of spironolactone, which did not prevent hypertension or LV hypertrophy (LVH), and a large dose, which achieved these endpoints.[109] To further address the role of arterial pressure, captopril was used to prevent hypertension in rats receiving aldosterone for 8 weeks; given the independent source of aldosterone, captopril did not interfere with the effects of this hormone; and as a result, it did not prevent reactive myocardial fibrosis. Further evidence in support of a role for circulating mineralocorticoids in hypertrophy and remodeling comes from other studies.[110] Rats with an intracerebroventricular infusion of aldosterone, which produced comparable arterial hypertension via central mechanisms, were compared to rats that received this steroid by subcutaneous administration. Central administration did not lead to LVH or remodeling. These findings further implicate a direct role for circulating aldosterone in promoting myocardial remodeling. Finally, aldosterone administration to uninephrectomized rats on a low sodium diet was associated with a marked elevation in plasma aldosterone but not reactive fibrosis. The results of the various in vivo studies suggest a clear association between chronic inappropriate (relative to sodium intake) elevations in circulating angiotensin II or aldosterone and the reactive fibrous tissue response. Fibrogenic mechanism(s) remain uncertain and may indeed be distinct for each hormone. Various other chronic mineralocorticoid excess states, in both humans and rats, have been related to adverse vascular remodeling (Table 2-3).[111]

To address the pathophysiologic basis for myocardial fibrosis in rats receiving angiotensin II or aldosterone in promoting myocardial fibrosis, each hormone was administered separately by implanted minipump to previously normal rats.[64] Hearts were examined at 2, 4, and 6 weeks of hormone treatment. Important differences in the temporal appearance of myocardial fibrosis were induced by each hormone, emphasizing the likelihood that responsible mechanisms differ for the hormones. Within 2 weeks of angiotensin II treatment, a perivascular fibrosis of intramural coronary vessels was present in both the RV and LV and became more extensive over the 6-weeks course of treatment.

Perivascular fibrosis is a nonspecific histopathologic finding that often accompanies abnormal coronary vascular permeability. Macromolecular escape to angiotensin II infusion was examined using cardiac lymph in dogs and an antibody to plasma fibronectin in rats. In dogs, where a filtration-independent model was used, intravenous angiotensin II for 90 minutes increased cardiac lymph protein concentration (relative to plasma protein). To address a role for increased arterial (coronary perfusion) pressure, an equipotent dose of methoxamine was compared to angiotensin II. Despite comparable increments in arterial pressure, there was no escape of protein in the methoxamine-treated animals,[112] suggesting that angiotensin II has a specific effect on the coronary vasculature that was independent of arterial pressure. Subsequent studies, comparing a pressor to a nonpressor dose of angiotensin II, demonstrated that the escape of plasma protein into cardiac lymph was related to the release of nitric oxide and could be prevented by co-administration of a nitric oxide synthase inhibitor (L-NAME). It was not the case for a cyclooxygenase inhibitor.[113]

The sequence of events leading to perivascular fibrosis was next examined in rats. Within 48 hours of angiotensin II treatment, localized deposits of plasma fibronectin were evident within the media and adventitia of intramyocardial coronary arterioles with extensions into the adjacent interstitial space. Immunolabeling of large intramural arteries or veins was not detected. A cellular response was

Table 2-3. Vascular Remodeling of Systemic and Coronary Arterioles in Chronic Mineralocorticoid Excess States (Inappropriate Relative to Dietary Sodium)

Mineralocorticoid	Human condition	Experimental model
Aldosterone	Primary hyperaldosteronism	
	Adrenal adenoma	ALDO infusion (1K; high Na$^+$)^a
	Secondary hyperaldosteronism	
	Bartter syndrome	AngII infusion
	Renal ischemia	Renal ischemia
	Heart failure	Rapid pacing
Deoxycorticosterone	11β-Hydroxylase deficiency	
	Congenital	DOCA administration
	Acquired (anabolic steroids)	Androgen administration
Apparent mineralocorticoid excess	11β-HSD inhibition	Glycyrrhizic acid
	Carbenoxolone	administration

Abbreviations: ALDO, aldosterone; AngII, angiotensin II; DOCA, deoxycorticosterone acetate; 11β-HSD, 11β-hydroxysteroid dehydrogenase; 1K = uninephrectomy; high Na$^+$ = high sodium diet.

^{a}Remodeling was not seen with aldosterone infusion and low-sodium diet or with uninephrectomy and high-sodium diet alone. (From Weber et al.,[111] with permission.)

also now evident within the adventitia of these vessels and appeared to involve fibroblasts and macrophages. On day 4, plasma fibronectin staining of the media and adventitia of arterioles was more extensive and widespread than that noted earlier, as was the case for its extension into the interstitial space. On day 7 of angiotensin II, the walls of the intramyocardial coronary arterioles had become thicker, with diffuse fibronectin labeling evident in the media, adventitia, and neighboring interstitial space. The increased cellularity of the adventitia remained evident in involved vessels on days 4 and 7. Although fibroblasts and macrophages were still apparent, by day 7 no polymorphonuclear neutrophils (PMNs) were found. By day 10 and 14 of the infusion, widespread involvement of intramyocardial coronary arterioles was evident, and plasma fibronectin labeling was present in the media and adventitia of these vessels. Again, the large intramural arteries and veins were not involved. The presence of an increased number of cells, presumably fibroblasts and macrophages, was still evident, and a perivascular fibrosis of arterioles, represented by an increased accumulation of fibrillar collagen, was present on day 14. Type I collagen mRNA-producing cells were seen only in the myocardium of angiotensin II-infused animals (vis-a-vis age-matched, untreated controls). They appeared in both ventricles on days 4 and 7 of the infusion. Grains were abundant in these cells, which were located in the adventitia and perivascular space of many, but not all, coronary arterioles. Within the interstitial space there were also cells that expressed type I collagen mRNA. Based on their morphologic features, which included an elongated fusiform shape with elongated nuclei and prominent nucleoli, these cells appeared to be fibroblasts or had a fibroblast-like phenotype. These cells were not seen in control animals.

In uninephrectomized rats on a high sodium diet receiving aldosterone, reactive or reparative fibrosis was not evident until 4 weeks, when it appeared in both ventricles, becoming more extensive at 6 weeks. It was not until 4 weeks or more that arterial pressure began to rise in these animals. Pathophysiologic events associated with the perivascular fibrosis that accompanies aldosterone treatment remains to be examined. Thus although fibrosis was seen in both ventricles with each model, a combined elevation in circulating angiotensin II and aldosterone led to more rapid appearance of the fibrous tissue response than the elevation in plasma aldosterone alone. Mechanisms involved in promoting fibrogenesis require further investigation.

Circulating Hormones and Reparative Fibrosis

Chronic activation of the RAAS is also associated with cardiac myocyte necrosis and subsequent reparative fibrosis that presents as microscopic scarring. Myocyte necrosis accompanies inappropriate elevations in plasma angiotensin II in the absence of hypertension.[105,114] Anti-cardiac myosin or anti-fibronectin antibodies have been used as a sensitive means to detect the myocyte injury[105,115] that accompanies administration of a small dose of angiotensin II and that does not elevate arterial pressure until day 5. In angiotensin II-infused animals, both ventricles were found to contain multifocal areas of cardiac myocyte injury on day 1, associated with scattered PMNs and clusters of macrophages. On day 7 these areas of injured myocytes and wound healing contained fibroblasts. Microscopic scars were evident on day 14. Necrosis was prevented by adrenergic receptor antagonists, not other antihypertensive drug regimens.[116] The role of angiotensin II-induced release of catecholamines from the adrenal medulla was therefore considered. Bilateral adrenal medullectomy prevented the loss of parenchymal cells that appeared in response to angiotensin II. Total adrenalectomy likewise provided a similar outcome, whereas spironolactone, given to rats with intact adrenals, was not cardioprotective.[115] Thus myocyte necrosis is not a direct toxic effect of angiotensin II or aldosterone but, instead, an indirect response to angiotensin II-induced release of catecholamines from the adrenal medulla.

Myocyte necrosis and scarring is also evident after mineralocorticoid excess created by aldosterone[103,117] or DOCA[104,118] in previously uninephrectomized rats receiving a high sodium diet. More than 3 weeks of mineralocorticoid treatment is required, however. Spironolactone and amiloride, with their potassium-sparing effects (albeit through different mechanisms of action), were found to prevent microscopic scarring in the RV and LV of rats treated with aldosterone for 8 weeks.[117,119] Dietary KCl supplementation has a similar protective effect in rats receiving DOCA.[118] On the other hand, spironolactone, but not amiloride, prevents perivascular fibrosis,[109,117] indicating that potassium loss is not responsible for this reactive fibrosis. Thus myocardial potassium depletion in the setting of chronic mineralocorticoid excess contributes to myocyte necrosis and reparative fibrosis. This phenomenon would explain the microscopic scarring of the myocardium reported in a patient with Bartter syndrome,[120] a weightlifter taking anabolic steroids,[121] and in cases where androgens create a chronic excess of deoxycorticosterone (DOC) by 11β-hydroxylase inhibition.[122]

These various in vivo and in vitro studies of collagen regulation indicate the following: (1) ventricular hypertrophy, expressed as an increment in parenchymal mass based on cardiac myocyte growth, is regulated by myocyte work determined by either ventricular systolic pressure or filling volume; (2) chronic infusions of angiotensin II or aldosterone did not lead to RV hypertrophy; (3) fibrous tissue formation at normal or pathologic sites is related to local concentrations of angiotensin II (and perhaps bradykinin and PGE_2); (4) perivascular fibrosis is associated with chronic inappropriate elevations in circulating angiotensin II and appears in response to enhanced vascular permeability, not altered ventricular loading; (5) scarring, or reparative fibrosis, follows myocyte necrosis of diverse cause and is associated with catecholamine release by angiotensin II[105,114] and myocardial potassium depletion due to chronic mineralocorticoid excess[118]; and (6) separate regulatory controls[123,124] determine myocyte growth and stromal structure and, accordingly, determine whether myocardial tissue remains normal or becomes pathologic in appearance.[125,126]

INTERSTITIUM AND THE FAILING HEART

The definition of heart failure must be addressed before proceeding with this discussion. From the perspective of the heart, a physiologic definition of heart failure is the inability of the heart to serve its purpose as a muscular pump. Such inability is due an abnormality within the myocardium and is therefore referred to as *cardiac failure*. This situation is in contrast to lesions within the valvar structures or pericardium or to reduced circulating blood volume or hemoglobin, which cause *circulatory failure*.[127] Cardiac (or myocardial) failure may manifest only during diastole, where it is referred to as *primary diastolic dysfunction*. The latter typically occurs because myocardial stiffness has been impaired by an infiltrative process (e.g., amyloid deposition) or adverse accumulation of fibrillar collagen. The LV fails to accommodate pulmonary venous return and left atrial emptying without an abnormal rise in its filling pressure. Secondarily, pulmonary venous pressure rises. Resting systolic function is preserved in this setting, but it too falters when the heart rate rises. Tachycardia associated with exercise, for example, shortens the diastolic filling period and compromises ventricular filling. As a result, forward blood flow falters during physical activity. *Primary systolic dysfunction* is present when the heart fails to provide metabolizing tissues with oxygen at a rate that is in keeping with their requirements. With advanced, severe failure this situation can occur at rest; with less severe failure it appears only with heightened levels of oxygen requirement and can be gauged according to the maximal oxygen uptake attained during exercise and by the appearance of the exercise anaerobic threshold.[128] Diastolic and systolic dysfunction can coexist.

Congestive heart failure (CHF) refers to a clinical syndrome comprising a constellation of symptoms and signs that arise because of congested organs and underperfused tissues. Renal perfusion is central to the evolution of this syndrome. CHF is not a specific disease entity per se, given the many etiologic forms of heart disease that can lead to its appearance. Once perfusion is impaired, kidneys elaborate renin and activate the circulating RAAS, which leads to sodium and water retention. This response is not compensatory, given that intravascular volume and sodium intake are normal. Instead, it is inappropriate. At first, the intravascular volume expands, manifesting clinically as neck vein distension. Subsequently, the extravascular volume rises and can present as pleural or pericardial effusion, ascites, or peripheral edema. In patients and experimental animals, it has been clearly shown that such signs and symptoms of CHF are associated with circulating RAAS activation. Whether it accompanies various causes of circulatory failure, such as pulmonary artery banding in cats, suprarenal aortic banding in rats, or supravalvlar aortic stenosis in dogs, myocardial failure following infarction or idiopathic cardiomyopathy in humans is irrelevant to the kidneys. They are underperfused and dictate that sodium and water be retained. The terms *compensated* and *decompensated* are frequently used to indicate the absence or presence of CHF, respectively. By implication, these terms infer the absence or presence of sodium avidity.

What is the contribution of the cardiac interstitium to myocardial failure? In humans the major etiologic factors associated with chronic cardiac failure are ischemic heart disease (with previous MI) and hypertensive heart disease. The interstitial space, site of an adverse accumulation of fibrillar collagen, is central to impaired ventricular function with each entity. In the explanted human heart, examined microscopically after heart transplantation in patients with advanced symptomatic failure secondary to ischemic heart disease, extensive remodeling of the RV and LV was found.[129] As seen in Figure 2-5, it included a reparative and interstitial fibrosis that was severalfold greater than the macroscopic scar(s) that followed previous infarction(s). This adverse fibrous tissue response was held responsible for cardiac failure. With human hypertensive heart disease there is a similar pattern of reparative and reactive fibrous tissue responses involving both the hypertrophied LV and the nonhypertrophied RV. The extensive microscopic scarring and perivascular/interstitial fibrosis of the LV is shown in Plate 2-3, contrasted to the normal human LV. Such remodeling has been found

in humans and rats with chronic mineralocorticoid excess (inappropriate for dietary sodium intake), as indicated in Table 2-3. Circulating effector hormones of the RAAS and DOC have been associated with myocardial fibrosis.

In rats with unilateral renal ischemia having persistent activation of the circulating RAAS, which is based first on the viability of the "endocrine" (ischemic) kidney and subsequently on the viability of the contralateral kidney, a progressive adverse accumulation of fibrillar collagen appears in the hypertensive, hypertrophied LV and the normotensive, nonhypertrophied RV. This perivascular/interstitial fibrosis leads to a rise in collagen volume fraction of each ventricle. Initially, a two- to threefold rise in collagen is expressed as abnormal myocardial stiffness (primary diastolic dysfunction), whereas systolic stiffness and ejection fraction are preserved. This picture is the pathophysiologic setting found at 8 weeks in this model. At 32 weeks, the continued accumulation of collagen has created a fourfold or more rise in the collagen volume fraction. At this juncture, there is LV dilatation plus impaired contractility, reduced cardiac output, and combined diastolic and systolic dysfunction.[17,130]

One study addressed the transition from compensated to decompensated failure in SHRs.[19,131,132] Throughout much of its adult life the SHRs model of arterial hypertension and LVH without circulating RAAS activation. The appearance of CHF in this model, expressed as tachypnea, labored breathing, and pleural effusion, was accompanied by a fourfold rise in the LV collagen volume fraction and abnormal diastolic stress-strain relation of LV tissue (Fig. 2-6). At this time, RV hypertrophy had also appeared likely secondary to chronic pulmonary venous hypertension created by the failing LV. The appearance of CHF in the SHR model was also heralded by the increased expression of extracellular matrix gene transcripts for fibronectin, type I and III fibrillar collagens, and TGF/β_1. This change occurred in both the hypertrophied LV and RV and was not found in age-matched, compensated SHRs or normotensive, age-matched genetic controls. Transcripts for β-myosin or sarcoplasmic reticulum ATPase were not altered in either ventricle of compensated or decompensated animals. These findings further emphasize the importance of an adverse accumulation of fibrillar collagen to myocardial diastolic and systolic failure.

An inadequate fibrillar collagen network, characterized by degradation of collagen fibers and likely mediated by enhanced collagenolytic and gelatinolytic activity, leads to muscle fiber slippage, wall thinning, and LV spherization.[6] This has been observed early in the course of rapid pacing-induced

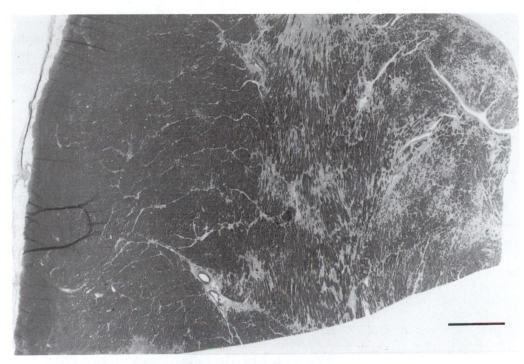

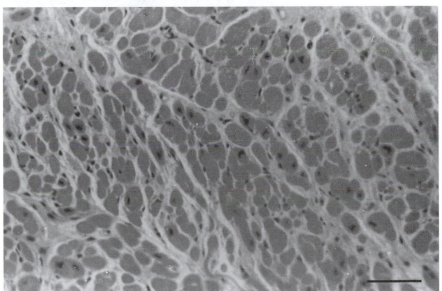

Fig. 2-5. Myocardial fibrosis is a major component of the adverse remodeling found in the explanted human heart with chronic ischemic heart disease. (**Upper**) Extensive replacement and interstitial fibrosis are seen in noninfarcted left ventricular tissue of such a heart at low magnification. (**Lower**) Higher magnification demonstrating interstitial fibrosis and variability of cardiac myocyte size seen remote to the infarct site. (From Beltrami et al.,[129] with permission.)

heart failure in dogs.[125,133–135] Only later, and with prolonged activation of the circulating RAAS,[136] does fibrosis appear.[99]

Enhanced proteinase activity and morphologic evidence of fibrillar collagen degradation has been found within the segment of myocardium that is ischemic[137] or is ischemic followed by reperfusion.[138] The thinning and impaired contractility of the is-

chemic segment seen in this setting may be explained by the loss of collagen that normally preserves ventricular architecture and muscle fiber alignment.

Collagen degradation is also an early component of tissue repair. Matrix metalloproteinases (MMPs) reside in the myocardium in a latent or inactive form.[21,22] Once activated, MMP-1 (interstitial colla-

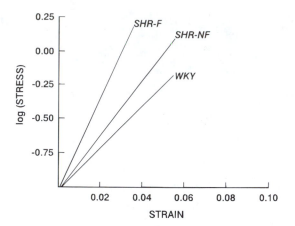

Fig. 2-6. Log stress-strain relation for cardiac tissue obtained from the left ventricle of spontaneously hypertensive rats (SHR). Animals with decompensated heart failure (SHR-F) and those without failure (SHR-NF) are compared to normotensive, nonfailing genetic controls (WKY). Examples were obtained from individual preparations. An increase in tissue stiffness is seen in SHR-F. (Adapted from Conrad et al.,[19] with permission.)

genase) degrades fibrillar collagen into characteristic one- and three-quarter fragments; MMP-2 and MMP-9 are gelatinases that degrade these smaller fragments. Hence cellular production of MMP-1 is not needed to initiate collagen degradation. A transient increase in collagenase activity appears in the infarcted LV on day 2, peaks at day 7, and declines thereafter, accompanied by a concomitant increase and contribution in collagenolytic activity of gelatinases.[139] This collagenase activity arises from the latent pool, as an increase in collagenase (MMP-1) mRNA expression does not appear until day 7 in the infarcted LV. Changes in MMP-1 activity or mRNA expression are not observed at sites remote to the infarct. Tissue inhibitors (TIMP) neutralize collagenolytic activity. Transcription of TIMP mRNA occurs at 6 hours in the infarcted LV, peaks on day 2, and slowly declines thereafter. No change in TIMP mRNA expression is observed at remote sites. Fibroblast-like cells are responsible for the transcription of MMP-1 and TIMP mRNAs.

Hence at the site of infarction, posttranslational

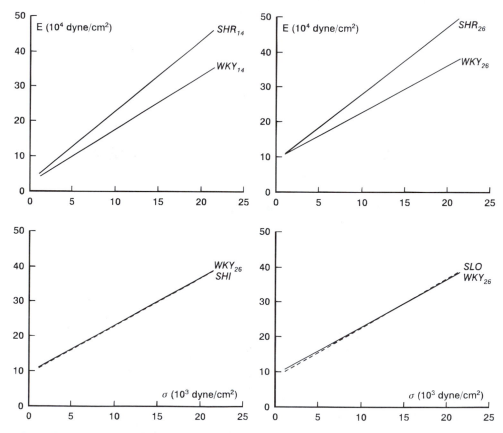

Fig. 2-7. Tangent elastic modulus (E) and end-diastolic wall stress (σ) obtained in intact isovolumetrically contracting left ventricle of adult SHRs at 14 weeks of age (SHR$_{14}$) and after 12 weeks of low- or high-dose lisinopril (SLO or SHI) compared to 26-week-old, untreated SHR (SHR$_{26}$) and age-matched nonfailing genetic controls (WKY). Low-dose lisinopril did not normalize arterial pressure or cause hypertrophy to regress, whereas high-dose treatment achieved these endpoints. In either case, regression of fibrosis normalized the ventricular stiffness. (Adapted from Brilla et al.,[30] with permission.)

activation of latent collagenase (MMP-1) plays a dominant role in tissue repair. Transcription of collagenase mRNA occurs when latent extracellular MMP-1 is reduced through activation of the latent pool of collagenase and gelatinases. In turn, TIMP mRNA synthesis is regulated by activation of MMPs. The balance between collagenase activation and TIMP inhibition therefore determines collagenolysis in infarcted tissue. Fibroblasts and fibroblast-like cells, and their synthesis and degradation of collagen, are essential to fibrogenesis and subsequent remodeling of fibrous tissue.

REGRESSION OF INTERSTITIAL FIBROSIS

The regression of myocardial fibrosis—the structural basis for impaired tissue stiffness—is based on restoring the balance between parenchyma and stroma and normalizing stiffness. It may or may not also require regression of cardiac myocyte size depending on the presence or absence of ventricular hypertrophy. Normalized structure of the interstitial compartment would translate into normalized function of the organ. Over the years many clinical and experimental studies have addressed the regression in LV mass without consideration of normalizing the abnormal tissue structure.

The regression of fibrosis must be based on recognition that the myocardial remodeling process is not simply an outcome of ventricular loading. Reversal of perivascular/interstitial fibrosis, for example, depends on neutralizing stimulatory factors that promote fibrous tissue formation as well as regressing stroma, which likely require proteolytic digestion. The latter must occur in a tissue-specific manner without inducing lathyrism. Experimental studies suggest that it can be accomplished.

Using a treatment trial format in adult 14-week-old SHRs where myocardial fibrosis is an established component of the hypertrophied myocardium, the animals were given lisinopril for 12 weeks. It was recognized that myocyte and stromal compartments are under separate controls, so two doses of lisinopril were used.[30] A small dose that did not significantly normalize arterial pressure and therefore did not cause the LV hypertrophy to regress was compared to a large dose, which normalized arterial pressure and did cause hypertrophic regression. In each case, regression of the fibrosis was observed; and in each case abnormal diastolic stiffness, evident at 14 and 26 weeks of age in untreated SHRs, was normalized (Fig. 2-7). This study not only demonstrated the feasibility of regressing fibrosis but that structural re-

modeling of the hypertrophied myocardium was the major determinant of abnormal tissue stiffness. It also raises the prospect of reversible heart failure in patients with primary diastolic dysfunction.

ACKNOWLEDGMENT

This work was supported in part by NIH grant ROI-HL-31701.

REFERENCES

1. Laurent GJ: Dynamic state of collagen. Pathways of collagen degradation in vivo and their possible role in regulation of collagen mass. Am J Physiol 1987; 252:C1
2. Burton AC: Relation of structure to function of the tissues of the wall of blood vessels. Physiol Rev 1954; 34:619
3. Abbott BC, Mommaerts WFHM: A study of inotropic mechanisms in the papillary muscle preparation. J Gen Physiol 1959;42:533
4. Caulfield JB: Alterations in cardiac collagen with hypertrophy. p. 49. In Tarazi RC, Dunbar JB (eds): Perspectives in Cardiovascular Research. Vol. 8. Cardiac Hypertrophy in Hypertension. Lippincott-Raven, New York, 1983
5. Weber KT, Brilla CG, Janicki JS: Myocardial fibrosis. Functional significance and regulatory factors. Cardiovasc Res 1993;27:341
6. Weber KT: Cardiac interstitium in health and disease. The fibrillar collagen network. J Am Coll Cardiol 1989;13:1637
7. Weber KT: Cardiac interstitium. Extracellular space of the myocardium. p. 1465. In Fozzard HA, Haber E, Jennings RB, Katz AM, Morgan HE (eds): The Heart and Cardiovascular System. 2nd Ed. Lippincott-Raven, New York, 1991
8. Robinson TF, Geraci MA, Sonnenblick EH, Factor SM: Coiled perimysial fibers of papillary muscle in rat heart. Morphology, distribution, and changes in configuration. Circ Res 1988;63:577
9. Sagawa K, Suga H, Shoukas AA, Bakalar KM: End-systolic pressure/volume ratio. A new index of ventricular contractility. Am J Cardiol 1977;40:748
10. Shroff SG, Janicki JS, Weber KT: Mechanical and energetic behavior of the intact left ventricle. p. 129. In Fozzard HA, Haber E, Jennings RB, Katz AM, Morgan HE (eds): The Heart and Cardiovascular System. 2nd Ed. Lippincott-Raven, New York, 1991
11. Fry DL, Griggs DM, Greenfield JC: Myocardial mechanics. Tension-velocity-length relationships of heart muscle. Circ Res 1964;14:73
12. Hefner LL, Bowen TE: Elastic components of cat papillary muscle. Am J Physiol 1967;212:1221
13. Hess OM, Schneider J, Koch R et al: Diastolic function and myocardial structure in patients with myocardial hypertrophy. Special reference to normalized viscoelastic data. Circulation 1981;63:360
14. Villari B, Campbell SE, Hess OM et al: Influence of collagen network on left ventricular systolic and dia-

stolic function in aortic valve disease. J Am Coll Cardiol 1993;22:1477

15. Doering CW, Jalil JE, Janicki JS et al: Collagen network remodeling and diastolic stiffness of the rat left ventricle with pressure overload hypertrophy. Cardiovasc Res 1988;22:686

16. Jalil JE, Doering CW, Janicki JS et al: Fibrillar collagen and myocardial stiffness in the intact hypertrophied rat left ventricle. Circ Res 1989;64:1041

17. Weber KT, Janicki JS, Pick R, Capasso J, Anversa P: Myocardial fibrosis and pathologic hypertrophy in the rat with renovascular hypertension. Am J Cardiol 1990;65:1G

18. Bing OHL, Fanburg BL, Brooks WW, Matsushita S: The effect of the lathyrogen β-amino proprionitrile (BAPN) on the mechanical properties of experimentally hypertrophied rat cardiac muscle. Circ Res 1978;43:632

19. Conrad CH, Brooks WW, Hayes JA et al: Myocardial fibrosis and stiffness with hypertrophy and heart failure in the spontaneously hypertensive rat. Circulation 1995;91:161

20. Caspari PG, Gibson K, Harris P: Changes in myocardial collagen in normal development and after β blockade. p. 99. In Harris P, Bing RJ, Fleckenstein A (eds): Recent Advances in Studies on Cardiac Structure and Metabolism. Vol. 7. Biochemistry and Pharmacology of Myocardial Hypertrophy, Hypoxia, and Infarction. University Park Press, Baltimore, 1976

21. Tyagi SC, Matsubara L, Weber KT: Direct extraction and estimation of collagenase(s) activity by zymography in microquantities of rat myocardium and uterus. Clin Biochem 1993;26:191

22. Tyagi SC, Ratajska A, Weber KT: Myocardial matrix metalloproteinase(s): localization and activation. Mol Cell Biochem 1993;126:49

23. Caspari PG, Newcomb M, Gibson K, Harris P: Collagen in the normal and hypertrophied human ventricle. Cardiovasc Res 1977;11:554

24. Keeley FW, Elmoselhi A, Leenen FHH: Enalapril suppresses normal accumulation of elastin and collagen in cardiovascular tissues of growing rats. Am J Physiol 1992;262:H1013

25. Villarreal FJ, Kim NN, Ungab GD, Printz MP, Dillman WH: Identification of functional angiotensin II receptors on rat cardiac fibroblasts. Circulation 1993; 88:2849

26. Brilla CG, Zhou G, Matsubara L, Weber KT: Collagen metabolism in cultured adult rat cardiac fibroblasts. Response to angiotensin II and aldosterone. J Mol Cell Cardiol 1994;26:809

27. Dayer J-M, Roelke MS, Krane SM: Effects of prostaglandin E_2, indomethacin, trifluoperazine and drugs affecting the cytoskeleton on collagenase production by cultured adherent rheumatoid synovial cells. Biochem Pharmacol 1984;33:2893

28. Diaz A, Munoz E, Johnston R, Korn JH, Jimenez SA: Regulation of human lung fibroblast α1 (I) procollagen gene expression by tumor necrosis factor α, interleukin-1β, and prostaglandin E_2. J Biol Chem 1993;268:10364

29. Chapman D, Eghbali M: Expression of fibrillar types I and III and basement membrane collagen type IV genes in myocardium of tight skin mouse. Cardiovasc Res 1990;24:578

30. Brilla CG, Janicki JS, Weber KT: Impaired diastolic function and coronary reserve in genetic hypertension. Role of interstitial fibrosis and medial thickening of intramyocardial coronary arteries. Circ Res 1991;69:107

31. Willems IEMG, Havenith MG, Smits JFM, Daemen MJAP: Structural alterations in heart valves during left ventricular pressure overload in the rat. Lab Invest 1994;71:127

32. Pinto JE, Viglione P, Saavedra JM: Autoradiographic localization and quantification of rat heart angiotensin converting enzyme. Am J Hypertens 1991;4:321

33. Yamada H, Fabris B, Allen AM et al: Localization of angiotensin converting enzyme in rat heart. Circ Res 1991;68:141

34. Sun Y, Diaz-Arias AA, Weber KT: Angiotensin-converting enzyme, bradykinin and angiotensin II receptor binding in rat skin, tendon and heart valves. An in vitro quantitative autoradiographic study. J Lab Clin Med 1994;123:372

35. Katwa LC, Ratajska A, Cleutjens JPM et al: Angiotensin converting enzyme and kininase-II-like activities in cultured valvular interstitial cells of the rat heart. Cardiovasc Res 1995;29:57

36. Filip DA, Radu A, Simionescu M: Interstitial cells of the heart valves possess characteristics similar to smooth muscle cells. Circ Res 1986;59:310

37. Sims DE: The pericyte—a review. Tissue Cell 1986; 18:153

38. Katwa LC, Ratajska A, Cleutjens JPM et al: Valvular interstitial cells. Implications for a local angiotensin system and collagen turnover [abstract]. Circulation, suppl. I 1994;90:1

39. Danser AHJ, van Katz JP, Admiraal PJJ et al: Cardiac renin and angiotensins. Uptake from plasma versus in situ synthesis. Hypertension 1994;24:37

40. Guarda E, Katwa LC, Myers PR, Tyagi SC, Weber KT: Effects of endothelins on collagen turnover in cardiac fibroblasts. Cardiovasc Res 1993;27:2130

41. Katwa LC, Guarda E, Weber KT: Endothelin receptors in cultured adult rat cardiac fibroblasts. Cardiovasc Res 1993;27:2125

42. Kolpakov V, Gordon D, Kulik TJ: Nitric oxide-generating compounds inhibit total protein and collagen synthesis in cultured vascular smooth muscle cells. Circ Res 1995;76:305

43. Schor SL, Schor AM: Clonal heterogeneity in fibroblast phenotype. Implications for the control of epithelial-mesenchymal interactions. Bioessays 1987;7: 200

44. McCulloch CAG, Bordin S: Role of fibroblast subpopulations in periodontal physiology and pathology. J Periodont Res 1991;26:144

45. Sappino AP, Schürch W, Gabbiani G: Differentiation repertoire of fibroblastic cells. Expression of cytoskeletal proteins as marker of phenotypic modulations. Lab Invest 1990;63:144

46. Vracko R, Thorning D: Contractile cells in rat myocardial scar tissue. Lab Invest 1991;65:214

47. Sun Y, Cleutjens JPM, Diaz-Arias AA, Weber KT: Cardiac angiotensin converting enzyme and myocardial fibrosis in the rat. Cardiovasc Res 1994;28:1423

48. Gabbiani G, Hirschel BJ, Ryan GB, Statkov PR, Majno G: Granulation tissue as a contractile organ. A study of structure and function. J Exp Med 1972; 135:719

49. Gabbiani G: The myofibroblast. A key cell for wound healing and fibrocontractive diseases. p. 183. In Deyl Z, Adam M (eds): Connective Tissue Research. Chemistry, Biology, and Physiology. Alan R Liss, New York, 1981

50. Fishbein MC, Maclean D, Maroko PR: Experimental myocardial infarction in the rat. Am J Pathol 1978; 90:57

51. Jugdutt BI, Amy RWM: Healing after myocardial infarction in the dog. Changes in infarct hydroxyproline and topography. J Am Coll Cardiol 1986;7:91

52. Jugdutt BI: Left ventricular rupture threshold during the healing phase after myocardial infarction in the dog. Can J Physiol Pharmacol 1987;65:307

53. Desmouliere A, Geinoz A, Gabbiani F, Gabbiani G: Transforming growth factor-β1 induces α-smooth muscle actin expression in granulation tissue myofibroblasts and in quiescent and growing cultured fibroblasts. J Cell Biol 1993;122:103

54. Bruijn JA, Roos A, de Geus B, de Heer E: Transforming growth factor-β and the glomerular extracellular matrix in renal pathology. J Lab Clin Med 1994;123:34

55. Ronnov-Jessen L, Petersen OW: Induction of α-smooth muscle actin by transforming growth factor-β1 in quiescent human breast gland fibroblasts. Implications for myofibroblast generation in breast neoplasia. Lab Invest 1993;68:696

56. Vyalov SL, Gabbiani G, Kapanci Y: Rat alveolar myofibroblasts acquire α-smooth muscle actin expression during bleomycin-induced pulmonary fibrosis. Am J Pathol 1993;143:1754

57. Bennett NT, Schultz GS: Growth factors and wound healing. Biochemical properties of growth factors and their receptors. Am J Surg 1993;165:728

58. Bishop J, Greenbaum J, Gibson D, Yacoub M, Laurent GJ: Enhanced deposition of predominantly type I collagen in myocardial disease. J Mol Cell Cardiol 1990;22:1157

59. Weber KT, Janicki JS, Shroff SG et al: Collagen remodeling of the pressure-overloaded, hypertrophied nonhuman primate myocardium. Circ Res 1988;62:757

60. Mukherjee D, Sen S: Collagen phenotypes during development and regression of myocardial hypertrophy in spontaneously hypertensive rats. Circ Res 1990;67:1474

61. Willems IEMG, Havenith MG, De Mey JGR, Daemen MJAP: The α-smooth muscle actin-positive cells in healing human myocardial scars. Am J Pathol 1994;145:868

62. Thompson NL, Bazoberry F, Speir EH et al: Transforming growth factor beta-1 in acute myocardial infarction in rats. Growth Factors 1988;1:91

63. Hirsch AT, Talsness CE, Schunkert H, Paul M, Dzau VJ: Tissue-specific activation of cardiac angiotensin converting enzyme in experimental heart failure. Circ Res 1991;69:475

64. Sun Y, Ratajska A, Zhou G, Weber KT: Angiotensin converting enzyme and myocardial fibrosis in the rat receiving angiotensin II or aldosterone. J Lab Clin Med 1993;122:395

65. Sadoshima J, Izumo S: Molecular characterization of angiotensin II-induced hypertrophy of cardiac myocytes and hyperplasia of cardiac fibroblasts. Critical role of the AT$_1$ receptor subtype. Circ Res 1993;73:413

66. Evers AS, Murphree S, Saffitz JE, Jakschik BA, Needleman P: Effects of endogenously produced leukotrienes, thromboxane, and prostaglandins on coronary vascular resistance in rabbit myocardial infarction. J Clin Invest 1985;75:992

67. Baumgarten CR, Linz W, Kunkel G, Schölkens BA, Wiemer G: Ramaprilat increases bradykinin outflow from isolated hearts of rat. Br J Pharmacol 1993;108:293

68. Kimura B, Sumners C, Phillips MI: Changes in skin angiotensin II receptors in rats during wound healing. Biochem Biophys Res Commun 1992;187:1083

69. Kimura E, Hashimoto K, Furukawa S, Hayakawa H: Changes in bradykinin level in coronary sinus blood after the experimental occlusion of a coronary artery. Am Heart J 1973;85:635

70. Hashimoto K, Hirose M, Furukawa K, Hayakawa H, Kimura E: Changes in hemodynamics and bradykinin concentration in coronary sinus blood in experimental coronary artery occlusion. Jpn Heart J 1977;18:679

71. Noda K, Sasaguri M, Ideishi M, Ikeda M, Arakawa K: Role of locally formed angiotensin II and bradykinin in the reduction of myocardial infarct size in dogs. Cardiovasc Res 1993;27:334

72. Herman AG, Claeys M, Moncada S, Vane JR: Biosynthesis of prostacyclin (PGI$_2$) and 12L-hydroxy-5, 8, 10, 14-eicosatetraenoic acid (HETE) by pericardium, pleura, peritoneum and aorta of the rabbit. Prostaglandins 1979;18:439

73. Dusting GJ, Nolan RD: Stimulation of prostacyclin release from the epicardium of anaesthetized dogs. Br J Pharmacol 1981;74:553

74. Nolan RD, Dusting GJ, Jakubowski J, Martin TJ: The pericardium as a source of prostacyclin in the dog, ox and rat. Prostaglandins 1982;24:887

75. Goldstein RH, Polgar P: The effect and interaction of bradykinin and prostaglandins on protein and collagen production by lung fibroblasts. J Biol Chem 1982;257:8630

76. Bareis DL, Manganiello VC, Hirata F, Vaughan M, Axelrod J: Bradykinin stimulates phospholipid methylation, calcium influx, prostaglandin formation, and cAMP accumulation in human fibroblasts. Biochemistry 1983;80:2514

77. Ahumada GG, Sobel BE, Needleman P: Synthesis of prostaglandins by cultured rat heart myocytes and cardiac mesenchymal cells. J Mol Cell Cardiol 1980;12:685

78. Satoh K, Prescott SM: Culture of mesothelial cells from bovine pericardium and characterization of the arachidonate metabolism. Biochim Biophys Acta 1980;930:283

79. Baum BJ, Moss J, Breul SD, Crystal RC: Association in normal human fibroblasts of elevated levels of adenosine 3':5'-monophosphate with a selective decrease in collagen production. J Biol Chem 1978;253:3391

80. Weber DR, Stroud ED, Prescott SM: Arachidonate metabolism in cultured fibroblasts derived from normal and infarcted canine heart. Circ Res 1989;65:671

81. Sun Y, Weber KT: Angiotensin II receptor binding

following myocardial infarction in the rat. Cardiovasc Res 1994;28:1623

82. Jugdutt BI, Humen DP, Khan MI, Schwarz-Michorowski BL: Effect of left ventricular unloading with captopril on remodeling and function during healing of anterior transmural myocardial infarction in the dog. Can J Cardiol 1992;8:151

83. Jugdutt BI, Khan MI, Jugdutt SJ, Blinston GE: Effect of enalapril on ventricular remodeling and function during healing after anterior myocardial infarction in the dog. Circulation 1995;91:802

84. Albaladejo P, Bouaziz H, Duriez M et al: Angiotensin converting enzyme inhibition prevents the increase in aortic collagen in rats. Hypertension 1994;23:74

85. Michel J-B, Lattion A-L, Salzmann J-L et al: Hormonal and cardiac effects of converting enzyme inhibition in rat myocardial infarction. Circ Res 1988;62:641

86. Van Krimpen C, Smits JFM, Cleutjens JPM et al: DNA synthesis in the non-infarcted cardiac interstitium after left coronary artery ligation in the rat heart. Effects of captopril. J Mol Cell Cardiol 1991;23:1245

87. Smits JFM, van Krimpen C, Schoemaker RG, Cleutjens JPM, Daemen MJAP: Angiotensin II receptor blockade after myocardial infarction in rats. Effects on hemodynamics, myocardial DNA synthesis, and interstitial collagen content. J Cardiovasc Pharmacol 1992;20:772

88. Sun Y, Ratajska A, Weber KT: Inhibition of angiotensin converting enzyme and attenuation of myocardial fibrosis by lisinopril in rats receiving angiotensin II. J Lab Clin Med 1996

89. Jalil JE, Doering CW, Janicki JS et al: Structural vs. contractile protein remodeling and myocardial stiffness in hypertrophied rat left ventricle. J Mol Cell Cardiol 1988;20:1179

90. Brilla CG, Pick R, Tan LB, Janicki JS, Weber KT: Remodeling of the rat right and left ventricle in experimental hypertension. Circ Res 1990;67:1355

91. Michel JB, Salzmann JL, Ossondo Nlom M et al: Morphometric analysis of collagen network and plasma perfused capillary bed in the myocardium of rats during evolution of cardiac hypertrophy. Basic Res Cardiol 1986;81:142

92. Thiedemann KU, Holubarsch C, Medugorac I, Jacob R: Connective tissue content and myocardial stiffness in pressure overload hypertrophy. A combined study of morphologic, morphometric, biochemical and mechanical parameters. Basic Res Cardiol 1983;78:140

93. Jalil JE, Janicki JS, Pick R, Weber KT: Coronary vascular remodeling and myocardial fibrosis in the rat with renovascular hypertension. Response to captopril. Am J Hypertens 1991;4:51

94. Buccino RA, Harris E, Spann JF, Sonnenblick EH: Response of myocardial connective tissue to development of experimental hypertrophy. Am J Physiol 1969;216:425

95. Davis JO, Howell DS, Southworth JL: Mechanisms of fluid and electrolyte retention in experimental preparations in dogs. III. Effect of adrenalectomy and subsequent desoxycorticosterone acetate administration on ascites formation. Circ Res 1953;1:260

96. Lindy S, Turto H, Uitto J: Protocollagen proline hydroxylase activity in rat heart during experimental cardiac hypertrophy. Circ Res 1972;30:205

97. Grove D, Zak R, Nair KG, Aschenbrenner V: Biochemical correlates of cardiac hypertrophy. IV. Observations on the cellular organization of growth during myocardial hypertrophy in the rat. Circ Res 1969;25:473

98. Turto H: Collagen metabolism in experimental cardiac hypertrophy in the rat and effect of digitoxin treatment. Cardiovasc Res 1977;11:358

99. Weber KT, Pick R, Silver MA et al: Fibrillar collagen and the remodeling of the dilated canine left ventricle. Circulation 1990;82:1387

100. Bartosova D, Chvapil M, Korecky B et al: The growth of the muscular and collagenous parts of the rat heart in various forms of cardiomegaly. J Physiol (Lond) 1969;200:285

101. Marino TA, Kent RL, Uboh CE et al: Structural analysis of pressure versus volume overload hypertrophy of cat right ventricle. Am J Physiol 1985;18:H371

102. Holubarsch C, Holubarsch T, Jacob R, Medugorac I, Thiedemann K: Passive elastic properties of myocardium in different models and stages of hypertrophy. A study comparing mechanical, chemical and morphometric parameters. p. 323. In Alpert NR (ed): Perspectives in Cardiovascular Research. Vol. 7. Myocardial Hypertrophy and Failure. Lippincott-Raven, New York, 1983

103. Hall CE, Hall O: Hypertension and hypersalimentation. I. Aldosterone hypertension. Lab Invest 1965;14:285

104. Selye H: The general adaptation syndrome and the diseases of adaptation. J Clin Endocrinol 1946;14:285

105. Tan LB, Jalil JE, Pick R, Janicki JS, Weber KT: Cardiac myocyte necrosis induced by angiotensin II. Circ Res 1991;69:1185

106. Brilla CG, Weber KT: Mineralocorticoid excess, dietary sodium and myocardial fibrosis. J Lab Clin Med 1992;120:893

107. Young M, Fullerton M, Dilley R, Funder J: Mineralocorticoids, hypertension, and cardiac fibrosis. J Clin Invest 1994;93:2578

108. Robert V, Van Thiem N, Cheav SL et al: Increased cardiac types I and III collagen mRNAs in aldosterone-salt hypertension. Hypertension 1994;24:30

109. Brilla CG, Matsubara LS, Weber KT: Anti-aldosterone treatment and the prevention of myocardial fibrosis in primary and secondary hyperaldosteronism. J Mol Cell Cardiol 1993;25:563

110. Gòmez Sànchez EP: Mineralocorticoid modulation of central control of blood pressure. Steroids 1995;60:69

111. Weber KT, Sun Y, Campbell SE et al: Chronic mineralocorticoid excess and cardiovascular remodeling. Steroids 1995;60:125

112. Reddy HK, Campbell SE, Janicki JS, Zhou G, Weber KT: Coronary microvascular fluid flux and permeability. Influence of angiotensin II, aldosterone and acute arterial hypertension. J Lab Clin Med 1993;121:510

113. Sigusch HH, Ou R, Campbell SE, Katwa LC, Weber KT: Angiotensin II and coronary vascular hyperpermeability. Role of hypertension vs. nitric oxide and prostaglandin E2 [abstract]. Circulation, suppl. I 1994;90:1

114. Ratajska A, Campbell SE, Weber KT: Fibronectin and collagen accumulation within cardiac myocytes.

Remodeling found in spontaneously hypertensive rats [abstract]. J Mol Cell Cardiol, suppl. III 1993; 25:S39

115. Ratajska A, Campbell SE, Sun Y, Weber KT: Angiotenin II associated cardiac myocyte necrosis. Role of adrenal catecholamines. Cardiovasc Res 1994;28:684

116. Bhan RD, Giacomelli F, Wiener J: Adrenoreceptor blockade in angiotensin-induced hypertension. Effect on rat coronary arteries and myocardium. Am J Pathol 1982;108:60

117. Brilla CG, Weber KT: Reactive and reparative myocardial fibrosis in arterial hypertension in the rat. Cardiovasc Res 1992;26:671

118. Darrow DC, Miller HC: The production of cardiac lesions by repeated injections of desoxycorticosterone acetate. J Clin Invest 1942;21:601

119. Campbell SE, Janicki JS, Matsubara BB, Weber KT: Myocardial fibrosis in the rat with mineralocorticoid excess. Prevention of scarring by amiloride. Am J Hypertens 1993;6:487

120. Potts JL, Dalakos TG, Streeten DHP, Jones D: Cardiomyopathy in an adult with Bartter's syndrome. Hemodynamic, angiographic, and metabolic studies. Am J Cardiol 1977;40:995

121. Campbell SE, Farb A, Weber KT: Pathologic remodeling of the myocardium in a weightlifter taking anabolic steroids. Blood Press 1993;2:213

122. Fink CS, Gallant S, Brownie AC: Peripheral serum corticosteroid concentrations in relation to the rat adrenal cortical circadian rhythm in androgen-induced hypertension. Hypertension 1980;2:617

123. Lund DD, Twietmeyer TA, Schmid PG, Tomanek RJ: Independent changes in cardiac muscle fibres and connective tissue in rats with spontaneous hypertension, aortic constriction and hypoxia. Cardiovasc Res 1979;13:39

124. Kozlovskis PL, Fieber LA, Pruitt DK et al: Myocardial changes during the progression of left ventricular pressure-overload by renal hypertension or aortic constriction. Myosin, myosin ATPase and collagen. J Mol Cell Cardiol 1987;19:105

125. Weber KT, Brilla CG: Pathological hypertrophy and cardiac interstitium. Fibrosis and renin-angiotensin-aldosterone system. Circulation 1991;83:1849

126. Bing OHL, Sen S, Conrad CH, Brooks WW: Myocardial function structure and collagen in the spontaneously hypertensive rat. Progression from compensated hypertrophy to haemodynamic impairment. Eur Heart J, suppl. F 1984;5:43

127. Katz LN, Feinberg H, Shaffer AB: Hemodynamic aspects of congestive heart failure. Circulation 1960; 21:95

128. Weber KT, Kinasewitz GT, Janicki JS, Fishman AP: Oxygen utilization and ventilation during exercise in patients with chronic cardiac failure. Circulation 1982;65:1213

129. Beltrami CA, Finato N, Rocco M et al: Structural basis of end-stage failure in ischemic cardiomyopathy in humans. Circulation 1994;89:151

130. Capasso JM, Palackal T, Olivetti G, Anversa P: Left ventricular failure-induced by long term hypertension in rats. Circ Res 1990;66:1400

131. Conrad CH, Boluyt MO, Brooks WW et al: Effect of captopril on TGF-β_1 gene expression, myocardial stiffness, and fibrosis in the spontaneously hypertensive rat [abstract]. Circulation, suppl. I 1994;90:1

132. Boluyt MO, O'Neill L, Meredith AL et al: Alterations in cardiac gene expression during the transition from stable hypertrophy to heart failure. Marked upregulation of genes encoding extracellular matrix components. Circ Res 1991;69:1058

133. Spinale FG, Zellner JL, Tomita M, Crawford FA, Zile MR: Relation between ventricular and myocyte remodeling with the development and regression of supraventricular tachycardia-induced cardiomyopathy. Circ Res 1991;69:1058

134. Armstrong PW, Stopps TP, Ford SE, DeBold AJ: Rapid ventricular pacing in the dog. Pathophysiologic studies of heart failure. Circulation 1986;74:1075

135. Armstrong PW, Moe GW, Howard RJ, Grima EA, Cruz TF: Structural remodeling in heart failure. Gelatinase induction. Can J Cardiol 1994;10:214

136. Riegger GAJ, Liebau G, Holzschuh M et al: Role of the renin-angiotensin system in the development of congestive heart failure in the dog as assessed by chronic converting-enzyme blockade. Am J Cardiol 1984;53:614

137. Sato S, Ashraf M, Millard RW, Fujiwara H, Schwartz A: Connective tissue changes in early ischemia of porcine myocardium. An ultrastructural study. J Mol Cell Cardiol 1983;15:261

138. Zhao M, Zhang H, Robinson TF et al: Profound structural alterations of the extracellular collagen matrix in postischemic dysfunctional ("stunned") but viable myocardium. J Am Coll Cardiol 1987;10:1322

139. Cleutjens JP, Guarda E, Weber KT: Transcriptional and post-transcriptional regulation of interstitial collagenase after myocardial infarction in the rat heart [abstract]. Circulation, suppl. I 1993;88:1

3 Biologic Determinants of Myocardial Function

Bernard Swynghedauw

Cardiac hypertrophy and failure are interesting meeting points between clinicians and basic researchers. Cardiac hypertrophy is not a disease per se but the physiologic adaptation of the heart to a mechanical overload, which in turn is a consequence of a disease. Cardiac hypertrophy is in fact one of the numerous examples of the general phenomenon termed "biologic adaptation." The *expression* of the gene (i.e., the phenotype), in terms of protein and mRNA and physiologic function, is modified. The *structure* of the gene (i.e., the genotype[1]) is unchanged, and the modifications observed in genetic diseases are in fact causal and not consequential.

Cardiac failure and cardiac hypertrophy are accompanied by peripheral phenomena that reflect the adaptation of the peripheral circulation to hemodynamic changes due to the fall in cardiac output or the causal loading conditions themselves. These phenomena include plasma hormone or peptide modifications and phenotypic changes at the level of the vessels.

Biologic adaptation is a daily necessity and results in a new, improved thermodynamic status. Without adaptation the organ or organism simply cannot survive, and there is consequently no adaptation. There is no finalism in this basic process; the finalism is in fact defined a posteriori. The new genetic program is mainly fetal, simply because it is the only new program available for the cell (Fig. 3-1). The same rationale applies in sociology to studies on the adaptation of a given social group or population. The comparison with sociologic adaptation is also valid in terms of economy. *Economy* is the ratio between the energy utilized and the energy produced, which means force relative to energy or heat produced during mechanical engineering or muscle mechanics. The science called economy is also the science of energy utilization: The economy of a country is indeed said to be in bad shape when the country spends more goods than it produces.[2,3] Cardiac failure indicates the limits of this mechanical adaptation and is aggravated by two additional factors: senescence and fibrosis.

SARCOMERE CHANGES

In humans, changes in the expression of genes encoding contractile proteins explain the enhanced contractility of the atria. The contractility compensates for the depressed early ventricular filling and, but only in part, the modifications of both ventricular contractility and active relaxation.

Isomyosin Shift to V3

The myosin molecule is composed of a pair of heavy chains (MHC) and two pairs of light chains (MLC1 and MPLC2; P means phosphorylatable). In the rat heart, which is our model, there are three isomyosins (V1, V2, V3), all of which possess the same pairs of MLC, MLC1v, and MPLC2v but differ by their MHC composition: $\alpha\alpha$ in V1, $\alpha\beta$ in V2, and $\beta\beta$ in V3. The fast skeletal myosin is composed of a different pair of MHC and MLC molecules. The slow skeletal isomyosin is similar to V3, as it is composed of the same MHC molecules ($\beta\beta$) and MLC1 molecule (MLC1v,

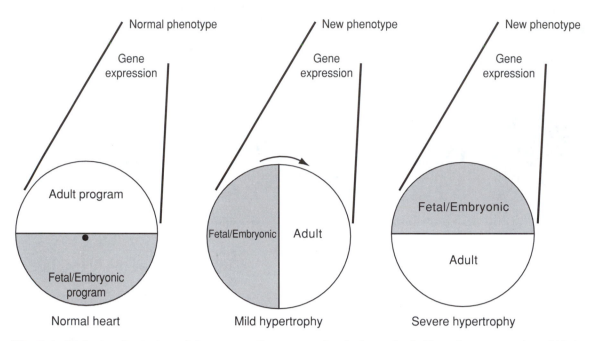

Fig. 3-1. Biologic adaptation of the myocardium to mechanical overload. Note the progressive shift in genetic expression to the fetal program. This working hypothesis takes into account various modifications in genetic expression, including the overall increase in gene expression responsible for hypertrophy, noninduction of various genes (e.g., the Ca^{2+}-ATPase of SR and the β_1-adrenergic and muscarinic receptors), and several shifts in isogene expression (e.g., those occurring with the isomyosins or the isosubunit α of the Na^+/K^+-ATPase).

or s) but differs from V3 by a specific MPL2s molecule. The myosin ATPase active site is located on the MHC head and depends on the structure of these subunits; $\alpha\alpha$-isoMHC has the highest ATPase activity, whereas $\beta\beta$-isoMHC has low enzymatic activity. Moreover, in phylogeny, when muscles from various species are compared, a good correlation has been found between myosin ATPase (i.e., the type of MHC isoform) and the maximum shortening velocity (Vmax).[2,3]

In response to chronic mechanical overload, myocyte genes from various striated muscles respond in the same way whatever the muscle type (i.e., atrial, ventricular, or fast skeletal muscle). The responses are (1) inhibition of the expression of those genes coding for fast MHC, which differ in the heart (α-MHC) and skeletal muscle (MHCf); and (2) activation of a unique gene (β-MHC) in all three muscles.[2] At the same time there are no major specific modulations for expression of the MLC genes. Such harmonious and complex regulations require a common mechanism for the two muscles and for the three genes α-MHC, MHCf, and β-MHC. The regulation is mostly, if not only, transcriptional. After experimental aortic stenosis, the increase in the amount of β-MHC mRNA precedes by 1 day the phenotypic protein changes, which demonstrates that the level of

the regulation is not translational.[4,5] By days 2–3 after banding the aorta, β-MHC mRNA was hardly detectable and was mainly restricted to the inner part of the left ventricle and around the coronary arteries of both ventricles, suggesting that the signal originates from the hemodynamic changes.[6] Transcriptional regulation was directly demonstrated during the development, using a technique called run-on, which consists in directly measuring the production of mRNA in isolated nuclei, which eliminates the effects of the translational processes.[7]

In the heart, the changes in isomyosin depend on the species and the type of muscle (atrium or ventricle). In every mammalian species so far studied, normal atrium shortens faster than ventricle. Accordingly, the atrial content in the $\alpha\alpha$-MHC chain isoform is always much higher than that of the $\beta\beta$-isoform. The maximum shortening velocity and myosin composition of the ventricles vary from one species to another: In the rat the $\alpha\alpha$-isoform is predominant, whereas normal human ventricle is entirely composed of the slow MHC $\beta\beta$-isoform. In the rat ventricle, cardiac overload rapidly induces (within 2 hours in an isolated heart[8]) a shift from the $\alpha\alpha$-isoform to $\beta\beta$-MHC. In humans and in some other mammalian species, the shift does not occur and cannot occur, as the human ventricle is already composed of $\beta\beta$-MHC. The shift occurs in the atria, including in humans. Atrial overload is indeed accompanied by a fall in the content in $\alpha\alpha$-MHC, parallels the echocardiographically determined atrial size.[2,9]

Measurements of the maximum shortening velocity of a totally unloaded myocardium can only be made in vitro using the papillary muscle and the quick-release technique. By so doing, it has been demonstrated that the slowing of Vmax is a fundamental process linked to mechanical overload, which allows the heart to adapt to the new environmental requirements and which occurs in every species so far studied, including humans.[2,3] The isomyosin shift is apparently insensitive to overload in the ventricles of humans, cats, pigs, dogs, and guinea pigs. Several studies suggest that in these species the slowing of the calcium transient and the phenotypic changes in membrane proteins are predominantly involved as determinants in the decrease in Vmax.

An excellent argument comes from analysis of the mechanical properties of detergent-treated skinned fibers from pressure-overloaded hearts. Contraction was triggered directly by adenosine triphosphate (ATP), as there are no membranes. In such a preparation, the time constant in milliseconds for tension recovery after a quick stretch reflects the rate of cross-bridge cycling. This time constant was significantly lengthened by the process of overload in rats but not in guinea pigs, a species in which sarcomere composition is not modified as in humans, suggesting that in guinea pigs the adaptational process does not involve the sarcomere, as in the rat.[10]

In humans the subject is still controversial. The above argument applies to the guinea pig, but the same experiments measuring the time constant have not been performed on human strips.

Other Myosin Changes

In the heart the maximum velocity of shortening Vmax is obtained by extrapolation from the force–velocity curve, a complex function with many variables. Vmax is in fact sensitive to both the rate of cross-bridge cycling and the number of active bridges; and a new mechanism of regulation located at the level of the cross-bridge cycling and different from the isomyosin shift has been proposed. The cyclic adenosine monophosphate (cAMP)-induced inotropic response, which is known to involve activation of the calcium channels, also has a direct effect on a given isomyosin. Mechanical overload may also directly influence cross-bridge cycling through an isomyosin-specific

mechanism analogous to that described for cAMP, providing an interesting new possibility to explain why in species such as humans the Vmax is depressed while the isomyosin profile remains unchanged. It has been suggested, but not demonstrated, that the signal responsible for this direct effect on the myosin molecule originates from the endothelium.[11,12]

Other Sarcomere Proteins

Sarcomere proteins are reputedly not modified during chronic overload, although there are few reports, if any, dealing with this question. One of the reasons this question is still open is the repeated finding of diminished ATPase activity in crude myofibrils from failing hearts, at least in human hearts during New York Heart Association (NYHA) stage IV.[13,14] This enzymatic change is not accompanied by any isomyosin shift as previously described, and a likely hypothesis to explain it is suggested by a role for troponin T, which belongs to a highly polymorphic family.[15]

Sarcomere sensitivity to calcium is usually explored on skinned fibers by drawing the pCa-active force curve. The sensitivity to calcium in the overloaded ventricle in rat, rabbit, and guinea pig is unchanged.[10] Different findings were obtained in human atria from patients having valvar disease. In these patients the pCa curve was shifted to the right, indicating diminished sensitivity to the cation, which has constituted a rationale for developing a new family of inotropic drugs that could enhance the sensitivity of the sarcomere to calcium.[16]

ENERGETICS

It is now possible to accurately quantitate mechanical properties and economy on isolated fibers from human hearts, as in the rabbit, by using cardioplegic solutions that have a reversible effect, such as 2,3-butanedione monoxime (BDM), to store the myocardial strips and protect them from dissection injury and microthermopiles to measure heat production.[14,17]

Using this technique, it is possible to demonstrate a fall in the peak isometric tension and maximum tension rise in pressure-overloaded rabbits and humans, even those with congestive heart failure, which indicates the existence of a deficit at the level of the myofiber. In addition, the contraction is more economical and the heat produced at the same moment is more reduced than the tension.

During each cross-bridge cycle, only one high energy bond (one ATP molecule) is hydrolyzed and produces heat; therefore heat production represents the number of cross-bridges that are active during the contraction. The average force developed by an individual myosin cross-bridge can then be calculated by dividing the average force–time integral measured by a force gauge on the whole muscle fiber by the heat liberated. The force–time integral of each myosin cross-bridge is increased in experimental compensatory hypertrophy and in the failing human heart, which means that cross-bridges cycle more economically.[17]

The important conclusion was that the general process of adaptation previously described for compensatory hypertrophy in rats or rabbits also applies to humans. In other words, from a thermodynamic point of view, the cardiac myofiber isolated from a failing human myocardium contracts more economically.

We can ask the same question for humans as for the rat model: What are the biologic determinants of such a basic phenomenon? It is indeed possible to partition this heat into a tension-dependent heat, which is the heat produced by the mechanical phenomena (i.e., the cross-bridge movement), and a tension-independent heat, which is the heat produced by calcium movement. Both are improved in experimental models in which we know that there is a shift in isomyosin and changes in membrane proteins, as well as in the human ventricle.

MEMBRANE PROTEINS

Changes in genetic expression during compensatory hypertrophy occur at the membrane level and are complex (Table 3-1). They involve (1) shifts in isogenes expression; (2) overexpression of certain genes in parallel with cardiac growth (therefore the concentration of the corresponding proteins remains unchanged although there is more protein per heart and; (3) some genes not activated by mechanical overload and whose products (i.e., the corresponding mRNA and proteins) are diluted in the already hypertrophied myocyte or myocardium (the concentration of these proteins thus falls).

Calcium Movements and Their Determinants

The calcium transient is studied using markers of free intracellular calcium (e.g., aequorin). In cardiac compensatory hypertrophy in the ferret,[50] the peak

of the transient was unchanged, but its duration was significantly augmented. In cardiac failure in humans[51] the transient is also prolonged and consists of fast and slow components.

Converging reports on both the Ca^{2+}-ATPase of the sarcoplasmic reticulum (SR) and on the dihydropyridine binding sites and slow inward current of Ca^{2+} have repeatedly reached the same conclusion using nearly identical models. During chronic overload the SR is less capable of pumping Ca^{2+} against the SR–cytoplasmic calcium gradient because the density of the Ca^{2+}-ATPase is lower. de la Bastie et al., in our laboratory,[34] studied in parallel the Ca-ATPase mRNA and protein and its function in chronically pressure-overloaded rat hearts. They also found diminished mRNA content of SR Ca^{2+}-ATPase relative to the content of ribosomal RNA; and for total Ca^{2+}-ATPase protein, they found a decrease in the active phosphorylated protein densities. More important was the finding that Ca^{2+} uptake relative to milligrams of SR was decreased, although it was normal relative to the amount of Ca^{2+}-ATPase, which was determined immunologically. Similar findings have been reported in humans by our group[36] and more recently by the group of Drexler[33]; that is, there is a fall in the density of Ca^{2+}-ATPase per cell or per surface area of SR, which explains the diminution of Ca^{2+} uptake.

The situation for the ryanodine channels, which are in fact calcium channels in charge of calcium release from the SR, is more confused. These receptors are bulky proteins that are activated in the myocardium by an autocatalytic phenomenon termed calcium-induced calcium release. This mode of regulation is specific for the heart and differs for skeletal or smooth muscle. The number of ryanodine receptors in cardiac hypertrophy is likely to be different according to the animal species. With mild cardiac hypertrophy in the guinea pig and ferret, there is a significant diminution in the density of ryanodine receptors that parallels the fall of Ca^{2+}-ATPase. The changes are less pronounced in rats, and the diminution in ryanodine receptor density is significant only when the degree of hypertrophy reaches +60 percent.[44] The situation is entirely different in humans. With human cardiomyopathies there is a twofold increase in the ryanodine-binding capacity; nevertheless the number of active calcium release channels, as quantitated by measuring the calcium release from microsomal preparations in vitro with an ultrarapid filtration technique, is unmodified.[45]

Assuming that the adult rat heart contains 46 million myocytes, the total number of calcium channels has been estimated at around 9000 fmol/mg protein

Table 3-1. Myocardial Phenotypic Changes in Ventricular Hypertrophy and Failure in Animal Models and Humans[a]

	Rat	Human	References
Sarcomere proteins			
Myofibrillar ATPase	↓	↓	13, 14
Cross-bridge cycling	Imp.	Imp.	14, 17, 18
Isomyosin shift to V3	+	0	2, 4, 9
Fetal MLC reexpressed	0	+	19, 20
IsoTNT shift to TNT2	??	+	15
Tropomyosin, TNI, C	=	=	21
Membrane receptors			
β1-AR	↓	↓	22, 23
β2-AR	=	=	22, 23
M2-R	↓	=	22, 23
Gαi2	=	↑	24
Gαs	=	=	25
Adenylate cyclase	↓	↓	22, 23
Adenosine R	??	=	26
Angio II R			
Type 1	↓	↓	27, 28
Type 2	↑	↓	27, 28
Membrane enzymes and exchangers			
Na^+/K^+-ATPase	=	↓	29, 30, 31
shift to α3-subunit	+	0	29, 30, 31
Na^+/Ca^{2+} exchanger	↓	↑	32, 33
Na^+/H^+ exchanger	??	??	
Ca^{2+}-ATPase of SR	↓	↓	33, 34, 35, 36
Phospholamban	↓	??	33, 34, 35
Calsequestrine	??	=	35
Ionic channels (current density)			
Ca^{2+} channel, L type	=	= or	37, 38, 39
Na^+ channel	↑	??	40, 41
K^+ channels			
I_{t0}	↓	??	41, 42
I_k	±↓	??	42
I_{k1}	↑	??	42
I_{ACh}, I_{ATP}	??	??	42
Na^+/Ca^{2+} exchange, $I_{(Na-Ca)}$	↑	?	32, 33, 42, 43
Ryanodine receptor	↓	↑	44, 45
Energetics			
Isocreatine kinase shift	+	+ +	46, 47
IsoLDH shift	+	+	48, 49

Abbreviations: ?, controversial; ??, unknown; MLC, myosin light chain; AR, adrenergic receptors; R, receptor; LDH, lactate dehydrogenase; Imp, improved.

[a]Animal models are generally compensatory hypertrophy; studies in humans are mostly dealing with failing hearts.

or 12×10^4 calcium channels per myocyte (or 15 sites/mm^2) using a radioactive dihydropyridine ligand and a one-site model. In rats at 45 weeks after aortic coarctation, the number of channels per myocyte increases to 20×10^4, which results in an unchanged density. Nevertheless, no more than 2–10 percent of these sites are likely to be functional. Several groups have measured the slow inward current of calcium (I_{Ca}) in compensatory hypertrophy on isolated cells by the whole cell patch clamp technique in the presence of agents such as cesium chloride, which allows one to eliminate overlapping outward currents. Their results were similar: The peak magnitude of the calcium current was unchanged when expressed in nanoamperes normalized per membrane surface area.[37–39]

In the heart, which is a tissue in which the Ca^{2+}-ATPase of the plasma membrane is poorly active (compared to vascular tissue, for example), the Na^+/Ca^{2+} exchanger is mainly responsible for calcium release from the cell; as such, it plays a major role in reestablishing calcium homeostasis during diastole. This exchanger is electrogenic and creates a current called $I_{(Na-Ca)}$. It does not directly utilize energy but is active at low intracellular concentration of sodium, which in turn depends on the activity of the energy-consuming Na^+/K^+-ATPase, the so-called sodium pump. Clearly, both the Na^+/Ca^{2+} exchanger and Na^+/K^+-ATPase are two systems that are functionally linked.

The modifications of such a duo are species-specific. Such species specificity is not surprising if we remember the species specificity of ventricular calcium metabolism, which is highly dominated by the activity of SR in such species as rats and is more dependent on plasma membrane exchanges.

Na^+/K^+-ATPase, located in the plasma membrane, is composed of two subunits, α and β, each being polymorphic. It is specifically inhibited by glycosides, and its main function is to pump three Na^+ out of the cell in exchange for two K^+. This enzyme is quite expensive for the cell in terms of ATP consumption. Kinetic studies of the enzyme and binding studies of ouabain showed two affinity sites in a normal rat heart that correspond in adults to two isoforms, $\alpha1$ and $\alpha2$. A third isoform, $\alpha3$, is mainly embryonic. In normal rat hearts, $\alpha1$ and $\alpha2$ are approximately equal in proportion; $\alpha2$, which has the highest affinity for ouabain, has the lowest affinity for Na^+ and is mainly responsible for the therapeutic effect; whereas $\alpha1$, the low affinity form, is responsible for toxicity.

Kinetic studies of the enzymes and glycoside binding studies have shown a rather complex pattern of changes in the presence of compensatory hypertrophy in rats: diminution in the number of low affinity sites for ouabain, increased density in the high affinity sites, and slowing of the dissociation rate constant for ouabain (k-1) at both sites. Physiologic studies, in full agreement with these findings, showed slowing of the recovery for a normal contraction after short infusion of the drug, which is the physiologic counterpart of lengthening of the dissociation constant for ouabain and diminished toxicity of the glycoside. Molecular biologic techniques have confirmed these data. In the rat there is a shift from the $\alpha2$ subunit isoform (with low affinity for ouabain and high affinity to sodium) to $\alpha3$, which is the fetal isoform (high affinity for ouabain and low affinity for sodium), which in turn enhances intracellular sodium concentration and influences the activity of the Na^+/Ca^{2+} exchanger. The latter is modified in the hypertrophied rat heart. In isolated sarcolemmal vesicles the Na^+-dependent $^{45}Ca^{2+}$ influx and efflux were both depressed, suggesting diminished density of the exchanger.[29-31]

In guinea pigs the specific activity of Na^+/K^+-ATPase is depressed. In humans with end-stage heart failure, the situation is still different. Even in normal heart the isoforms of Na^+/K^+-ATPase have affinities for sodium different from those in the rat. In addition, they are unchanged in the presence of hypertrophy. The trabeculae isolated from human failing hearts are more sensitive to ouabain, which may be at least partly due to a mean reduction of 42 percent in the concentration of Na^+/K^+-ATPase but not in an alteration in its catalytic properties.[31] By contrast, both the Na^+/Ca^{2+} exchanger mRNA and protein levels were increased.[33]

Calcium Homeostasis of Hypertrophy: Physiologic Consequences

There are, in any cell, two levels of control for calcium homeostasis: (1) the cytoplasm and (2) the endoplasmic or sarcoplasmic reticulum. It is difficult for the moment to propose even a scheme for compensatory hypertrophy in humans. Nevertheless, we have enough information on one species, the rat, to outline a few important points concerning calcium metabolism in the hypertrophied myocyte.

Free calcium transient in cytoplasm is normal during diastole in compensatory hypertrophy. In addition, both diastolic pressure and resting tension are unchanged, which would be impossible if the intracellular calcium were elevated. The well documented decrease in calcium transport at the level of Ca^{2+}-ATPase in SR is compensated by diminution of the ryanodine receptors, suggesting that at least in this species calcium release and uptake are in equilibrium at the level of the SR. By contrast, we know that the inward current for calcium is unchanged or even enhanced, and the activity of the two proteins that release calcium in the external space (i.e., Na^+/Ca^{2+} exchange and Na^+/K^+-ATPase) is deeply modified, suggesting that calcium homeostasis could not be maintained at the level of the plasma membrane.

How do these changes explain the modifications of cardiac function in the failing heart? Calcium homeostasis in the hypertrophied cardiocyte thus appears fragile, as the calcium uptake through the sarcolemma is normal in contrast to the processes that pump calcium out of the cytoplasm. Such an equilibrium appears unstable and may render the cell highly sensitive to any abnormal influx of calcium. It has indeed been clearly demonstrated in cardiac hypertrophy that both the anoxia-induced increase in myocardial stiffness and the calcium-induced arrhythmias are exaggerated.[52,53]

Such a hypothesis explains why the arrythmogenicity of the hypertrophied heart is equally linked to the degree of hypertrophy and the degree of fibrosis[54] and why the hypertrophied heart is more easily excitable. The fall in Ca^{2+}-ATPase of SR correlates well with the relaxation parameters and is usually considered the biologic explanation of the alterations of active relaxation that occur during cardiac hypertrophy. Finally, prolongation of the calcium transient is a rational, but incomplete, explanation of the slowing of Vmax. It is also interesting to note that the drop in Ca^{2+}-ATPase correlates with the isomyosin changes in rats, as does the relaxation and the shortening velocities.[55] In compensatory hypertrophy, contraction and active relaxation are nondissociable parameters.

Action Potential and QT Duration

In mammalian hearts, mechanical overload and senescence constantly result in lengthening of the action potential duration. The prolongation of the action potential explains the inversion of the T wave and the increase of the QT interval. Both clinical studies and experiments on hypertrophied isolated myocytes have demonstrated that lengthening of the QT interval, which is the electrocardiographic equivalent of the duration of the action potential, has prognostic significance.[56] The action potential duration depends on several ionic currents (Table 3-1): (1) The slow inward current of calcium (I_{Ca}) contributes to the plateau phase and is probably not involved, at least in the rat, because its density is unchanged. (2) The potassium currents are outward currents that accelerate repolarization. There are three main voltage-dependent potassium channels. A major defect has been reported in rat cardiac hypertrophy: 80 percent depression of the early transient outward current (I_{to}), which is likely to constitute the main explanation for prolongation of the action potential at least in this species.[42] The delayed rectifier outward current (I_k) is reduced in feline models of hypertrophy, whereas the background inward rectifier current (I_{k1}) is likely to be increased. (3) The Na^+/Ca^{2+} exchange creates an inward depolarization current. Its activation could create a long-lasting slow inward current and participate to the lengthening of the action potential. This point is still debatable.[41]

Autonomic Nervous System

During cardiac failure several levels of the autonomic nervous system (ANS) are modified: The plasma catecholamine level is elevated and consti-tutes a major risk factor; the sensitivity to isoproterenol, in terms of both inotropic and chronotropic effects, is hampered; the heart rate variability (HRV) is hampered and such a change is a major risk factor[57]; and most of the reflexes of the ANS are abnormal,[58] including the baroreflexes, for example. In addition, in response to the elevated plasma catecholamine level, homologous regulation of the transduction system occurs; the myocardial β-receptor density is down-regulated and the $G\alpha i2$ cardiac content up-regulated. Muscarinic receptors are unchanged.[22–25]

During the compensatory phase of cardiac hypertrophy in rats, despite normal plasma catecholamine content, the β_1-adrenergic and muscarinic receptors are equally down-regulated; moreover, their density on the cell membrane and the density of the corresponding mRNAs are decreased by 30 percent, suggesting that the corresponding genes, as the gene encoding the Ca^{2+}-ATPase of SR, belong to a family of genes that are not activated by mechanical overload and that the expressed proteins are diluted in the hypertrophied heart (Table 3-1).[22] Such a mechanism may protect the heart against acute stress. Therefore the β-adrenergic receptor down-regulation during heart failure is likely to have a double origin: It is a homologous down-regulation in response to the elevated plasma catecholamine content and an adaptational consequence of mechanical overload, exactly as the other phenotypic changes above described. Unexplained is the fact that phosphodiesterase inhibitors, including amrinone, glucagon, and, at least during the compensatory phase, forskolin, an activator of the cyclase itself, have a reduced inotropic effect on hypertrophied hearts.[59]

CARDIAC HORMONES

The heart is also an endocrine gland and is able to produce at least one hormone, atrial natriuretic factor (ANF), which is specifically secreted by the atria in response to a mechanical stress, such as an enhanced plasma volume. This small peptide has a strong natriuretic effect, which may compensate for a volume overload, and plays an important physiologic role. Cardiac mechanical overload is associated with an enhanced ANF mRNA content, which not only is located in the atrial but concerns the overloaded ventricle.[60]

The same situation occurs for the renin-angiotensin system (RAS). The plasma level of angiotensin II is unchanged by chronic mechanical overload but is elevated in renovascular hypertension and when

Table 3-2. Renin-Angiotensin System During Senescence and in Cardiac Hypertrophy and Failure

RAS	Senescence	Hypertrophy	Failure
Circulating	Down-regulated	Normal	Activated
Myocardial	Activated (left ventricle only)	Activated	Activated

(Data from Kawaguchi and Kitabatake,[61] and Heymes et al.[62])

failure occurs. The myocardial RAS is normally poorly active and may even be (in the rat, for example) nearly absent in the ventricle. Nevertheless, it is highly inducible by mechanical stress, and the mRNAs of the various components of the myocardial RAS are overexpressed during mechanical overload. The same is also true for the two angiotensin II receptor subtypes[27,28] (Tables 3-1 and 3-2).

FIBROSIS

The passive compliance of the left ventricular chamber depends on both chamber dilatation and intrinsic myocardial stiffness (as assessed by the diastolic stress–strain relation). The main determinant of myocardial (and arterial) stiffness is fibrosis (i.e., collagen concentration).

Fibrosis is not inevitably linked to mechanical overload, and there are several experimental and clinical models of mechanically overloaded hearts with unchanged myocardial stiffness and collagen content, including volume overload, and infrarenal aortic constriction (Table 3-3). With chronic cardiac overload, the left ventricle collagen concentration is

likely to be a factor independent of mechanics and whose determinants are senescence, myocardial ischemia, inflammatory processes, and, as recently demonstrated, angiotensin II, catecholamines, and aldosterone plasma levels. These hormonal factors play a role independently; for example, aldosterone alone creates fibrosis with no intervention by angiotensin II.[62–65]

Fibrosis is likely to play a major role during transition from the compensatory stage to the stage of cardiac failure. In a study on spontaneously hypertensive rats, it has been demonstrated that the major biologic marker for this transition is an increase in the collagen mRNA concentration (Table 3-4).[67–69] Morphologic quantitation of myocardial fibrosis in humans has also shown a good correlation between myocardial function and the degree of fibrosis.[66]

Table 3-3. Origins of Ventricular Fibrosis

Senescence: compensatory fibrosis + ????
Ischemia: reparative fibrosis
Inflamatory processes: Chagas disease, myocarditis
Hormones
    Angiotensin II
    Aldosterone
    Catecholamines
    Serotonin
Note: There are no arguments in favor of a direct involvement of mechanical overload in fibrogenesis. No fibrosis is seen after aortic insufficiency, aortocaval fistulas, infrarenal aortic stenosis.

(Data from Besse et al.,[55] Weber and Brilla,[63] Weber et al.,[64] Robert et al.,[65] and Schaper and Speiser.[66])

Table 3-4. Transition to Failure

Anatomic data
  ↑ RV and liver weights
Contractile proteins
  ↓ α-Myosin heavy chain; α-skeletal actin
  = β-Myosin heavy chain; myosin light chain 2; α-cardiac actin
RAS and ANF
  Activation of the RAS
  ANF expressed in the LV and RV
Ca^{2+}-ATPase of the SR
  ↓ in the RV
  = in the LV (but ?)
Extracellular matrix
  ↑ Fibronectin (mainly EIIIA), collagen, and TGFβ in RV and LV

Abbreviations: SHRs, spontaneously hypertensive rats; RV, LV, right and left ventricles; SR, sarcoplasmic reticulum; RAS, renin-angiotensin system; ANF, atrial natriuretic factor; TGFβ, transforming growth factor β.

The results are based on a comparison of nonfailing (13–14 months old) SHRs and failing SHRs (18–19 months old).

(Data from Bolyut et al.[67])

SENESCENCE

Studies on cardiovascular senescence are far from being academic, as epidemiologic studies have shown that diseases of the heart comprise one of the major causes of mortality among the overall population and the main cause in people over 65 years of age. The senescent heart, in the absence of any cardiovascular disease, is mainly though not solely an overloaded heart. The overload results from enhanced impedance of the large vessels, which is the basic characteristic of the senescent vessels.[70]

Clinical and experimental studies revealed that in the aging heart a loss of myocytes and fibrosis are associated with myocyte hypertrophy, which is more significant in the left ventricle than the right ventricle. Histochemical studies have shown an abnormal accumulation of fibrillar collagen around the vessels and within the interstitium. The concentrations of the two main components of fibrosis, collagen I and fibronectin, increase during aging. By contrast, type I and type III procollagen mRNA levels were reduced in the senescent rat heart, showing that changes in myocardial collagen mRNA and protein were not synchronous, suggesting that during senescence collagen concentration is not transcriptionally regulated.[69] Fibrosis is the major determinant of arrhythmias and impaired ventricular filling, both of which characterize senescent myocardial function.

In experimental models of senescence, sarcomere proteins, contractility parameters and relaxation velocity, action potential duration, and myoplasmic calcium transient are altered as during mechanical overload. The papillary muscles of aged rats contracts also more economically than that of young rats.[55] Compared to young animals, the ventricles of 24-month-old rats contains more slow isomyosin, less SR Ca^{2+}-ATPase,[55] fewer β_1-adrenergic and muscarinic receptors,[71,72] and a less active Na^+/Ca^{2+} exchanger.[70]

Aging, as mechanical overload, is accompanied by several modifications of the autonomous myocardial system that are likely to be located "down the road"; it explains the well documented depression of heart rate variability and the fact that elderly people, during exercise, maintain their maximal cardiac output by increased utilization of the Frank-Starling mechanism with only slight tachycardia or no increase in the heart rate at all.[73]

The phenotypes of the senescent and the mechanically overloaded rat hearts resemble one another on a large number of parameters, including mechanical data and several changes in membrane proteins. They mainly differ on three points: fibrosis and arrhythmias, which are much more abundant and frequent during senescence, and adaptation to exercising, which proceeds differently in the two conditions.

Plasma ANF levels are elevated in healthy elderly people and old rats, compared to the levels in young individuals. In vitro the basal ANF secretory rate was greater in atria from aged animals. In addition, the relative levels of mRNA coding for ANF showed a strong activation in the left, but not the right, ventricle. Aging is also associated with low plasma levels of angiotensin I, renin activity, and angiotensinogen, and high expression of the myocardial angiotensinogen and angiotensin-converting enzyme (ACE) mRNAs.[62] Cardiac failure is mainly a disease of the elderly; the average age of the patients of most of the clinical trials, including the CONSENSUS study on ACE inhibitors (ACEI) is around 65 years. Obviously most of the patients in the ACEI study have a low level of plasma angiotensin I, and the question is how ACEI works in the elderly. The answer is most likely to be found in the various tissue renin-angiotensin systems, at least the one located in the myocardium.

The modifications in protein synthesis and degradation and mRNA content that occur with aging suggest that the senescent heart may be unable to adapt to an increased load and would be unable to hypertrophy further in response to mechanical stress. This question is of crucial interest, as cardiac failure is more frequent after age 65 years than before. Several experimental investigators have tried to answer this question, and the general opinion is that the senescent heart responds more slowly to mechanical overload than the young hearts, but that the final result is the same in terms of myocardial mass.[55]

CONCLUSION

The biologic determinants of myocardial dysfunction in cardiac hypertrophy and failure are the following.

1. Systolic dysfunction.
   a. Isomyosin shift and prolonged calcium transient are responsible for the depressed Vmax and improved economy.
   b. Diminished cardiac output depends on the same determinants as Vmax; fibrosis and the limits of peripheral adaptation play a crucial role.
2. Diastolic dysfunction.
   a. Slow, active relaxation depends on numerous factors; nevertheless, the densities of Ca^{2+}-ATPase in the SR and phospholamban seem to be determinant.
   b. Depressed early ventricular filling is a direct function of ventricular fibrosis.

c. Increased atrial contribution is made possible by the isomyosin shift in atria.

d. Anoxia-induced myocardial stiffness is exaggerated in the presence of hypertrophy due to the poor buffering capacity of the hypertrophied myocyte in terms of calcium homeostasis.

3. Heart rate and arrhythmias.
   a. High incidence of severe arrhythmias leading to sudden death depends on the degree of fibrosis and the degree of prolonged action potential and calcium transient.
   b. Main determinants of the action potential and QT duration are K currents (mainly I_{to}, at least in rats). The QT length dispersion depends on fibrosis. QT length variability depends on K currents, adrenergic and vagal systems, and fibrosis.

4. Heart rate variability. This measurement is a noninvasive technique to evaluate the activity of the autonomous nervous system. The variability depends on the central nervous system, baroreflexes, and myocardial adrenergic/muscarinic receptor balance.

Finally, the major determinants for transition between compensatory hypertrophy and cardiac failure are (1) the limits and imperfections of the general process of biologic adaptation at the levels of the myocardium and the periphery; and (2) fibrosis (Table 3-4), which in turn depends on various hormones, ischemia, and above all senescence (Table 3-3).

REFERENCES

1. Swynghedauw B: Molecular Cardiology for the Cardiologists. Kluwer, Boston, 1995
2. Swynghedauw B: Developmental and functional adaptation of contractile proteins in cardiac and skeletal muscle. Physiol Rev 1986;66:710
3. Swynghedauw B: Cardiac Hypertrophy and Failure. INSERM–Libbey, Paris, 1990
4. Lompré AM, Schwartz K, d'Albis A et al: Myosin isozymes redistribution in chronic heart overloading. Nature 1979;282:105
5. Lompré AM, Nadal-Ginard B, Mahdavi V: Expression of the cardiac ventricular α and β myosin heavy-chain genes is developmentally and hormonally regulated. J Biol Chem 1984;255:6437
6. Schiaffino S, Samuel JL, Sassoon D et al: Nonsynchronous accumulation of α-skeletal actin and β myosin heavy chain mRNAs during early stages of pressure overload-induced cardiac hypertrophy demonstrated by in situ hybridization. Circ Res 1989;64:937
7. Boheler KR, Chassagne C, Martin X et al: Cardiac expressions of α and β myosin heavy chains and sarcomeric alpha actins are regulated through transcriptional mechanisms. Results from nuclear run-on assays in isolated rat cardiac nuclei. J Biol Chem 1992;267:12979
8. Delcayre C, Klug D, Van Thiem N et al: Aortic perfusion pressure as early determinant of β-isomyosin expression in perfused hearts. Am J Physiol 1992;263:H1537
9. Mercadier JJ, de la Bastie D, Ménasché P et al: Alphamyosin heavy chain isoform and atrial size in patients with various types of mitral valve dysfunction. A quantitative study. J Am Coll Cardiol 1987;9:1024
10. Clapier-Ventura R, Mekhfi H, Oliviero P et al: Pressure overload changes cardiac skinned fibers mechanics in rats, not in guinea pigs. Am J Physiol 1988;254:H517
11. Winegrad S, Weisberg A: Isozyme specific modification of myosin ATPase by cAMP in rat heart. Circ Res 1987;60:384
12. Hoh JFY, Rossmanith GH, Kwan LJ et al: Adrenaline increases the rate of cycling of crossbridges in rat cardiac muscle as measured by pseudo-random binary noise-modulated perturbation analysis. Circ Res 1988;62:452
13. Leclercq JF, Swynghedauw B: Myofibrillar ATPase, DNA and hydroxyproline content of human hypertrophied heart. Eur J Clin Invest 1976;6:27
14. Alpert NR, Mulieri LA, Hasenfuss G: Myocardial chemomechanical energy transduction. p. 111. In Fozzard HA, Haber E, Jennings RB, Katz AM, Morgan HE (eds): The heart and Cardiovascular System. Lippincott-Raven, Philadelphia, 1992
15. Anderson PAW, Malouf NN, Oakeley AF et al: Troponin T isoform expression in humans. A comparison among normal and failing heart, fetal heart and adult and fetal skeletal muscle. Circ Res 1991;69:1226
16. Rüegg JC: Calcium in Muscle Contraction. Springer-Verlag, Berlin, 1992
17. Hasenfuss G, Holubarsch, C, Just H, Alpert NR: Cellular and Molecular Alterations in the Failing Human Heart. Steinkopff Verlag, Darmstadt, 1992
18. Alpert NR, Mulieri LA: Increased myothermal economy of isometric force generation in compensated cardiac hypertrophy induced by pulmonary artery constriction in the rabbit. Circ Res 1982;491:50
19. Cummins P: Transitions in human atrial and ventricular myosin light-chain isoenzymes in response to cardiac-pressure-overload-induced hypertrophy. Biochem J 1982;205:195
20. Hirzel H, Tuchsmid C, Sneider J et al: Relationship between myosin isoenzyme composition, hemodynamics and myocardial structure in various forms of human cardiac hypertrophy. Circ Res 1985;57:729
21. Rüegg JC, Solaro RJ: Calcium-sensitizing positive inotropic drugs. p. 457. In Gwathmey JK (ed): Heart Failure. Basic Science and Clinical Aspects. Marcel Dekker, New York, 1993
22. Mansier P, Chevalier B, Barnett DB et al: Beta adrenergic and muscarinic receptors in compensatory cardiac hypertrophy of the adult rat. Pflugers Arch 1993;424:354
23. Brodde OE: The functional importance of beta 1 and beta 2 adrenoceptor in the human heart. Am J Cardiol 1988;62:24C
24. Eschenhagen T, Mende U, Nose M et al: Isoprenaline-induced increase in mRNA levels of inhibitory G-pro-

tein α subunit in rat heart. Arch Pharmacol 1991;341:609

25. Moalic JM, Bourgeois F, Mansier P et al: β_1-Adrenergic receptor and Gas mRNAs in rat heart as a function of mechanical load and thyroxine intoxication. Cardiovasc Res 1993;27:231

26. Hershberger RE, Feldman AM, Bristow MR. A1-adenosine receptor inhibition of adenylate cyclase in failing and non-failing ventricular myocardium. Circulation 1991;83:1343

27. Lopez JJ, Lorell BH, Ingelfinger JR et al: Distribution and function of cardiac angiotensin AT_1- and AT_2-receptor subtypes in hypertrophied rat hearts. Am J Physiol 1994;267:H844

28. Regitz-Zagrosek V, Friedel N, Heymann A et al: Regulation, chamber localization, and subtype distribution of angiotensin II receptors in human hearts. Circulation 1995;91:1461

29. Charlemagne D, Maixent JM, Preteseille M et al: Ouabain binding sites and (Na^+,K^+)-ATPase activity in rat cardiac hypertrophy. Expression of the neonatal forms. J Biol Chem 1986;261:185

30. Charlemagne D, Orlowski J, Oliviero P et al: Alteration of Na,K-ATPase subunit mRNA and protein levels in hypertrophied heart. J Biol Chem 1994;269:1541

31. Shamraj OI, Grupp IL, Grupp G et al: Characterization of Na/K-ATPase, its isoforms, and the inotropic response to ouabain in isolated failing human hearts. Cardiovasc Res 1993;27:2229

32. Hanf R, Drubaix I, Lelièvre L: Rat cardiac hypertrophy. Altered sodium-calcium exchange activity in sarcolemmal vesicles. FEBS Lett 1988;236:145

33. Studer R, Reinecke H, Bilger J et al: Gene expression of the cardiac Na^+-Ca^{2+} exchanger in end-stage human heart failure. Circ Res 1994;75:443

34. De la Bastie D, Levitsky D, Rappaport L et al: Function of the sarcoplasmic reticulum and expression of its Ca^{2+} ATPase gene in pressure overload-induced cardiac hypertrophy in the rat. Circ Res 1990;554:66

35. Arai M, Matsui H, Periasamy M: Sarcoplasmic reticulum gene expression in cardiac hypertrophy and heart failure. Circ Res 1994;74:555

36. Mercadier JJ, Lompré AM, Duc P et al: Altered sarcoplasmic reticulum Ca^{2+}-ATPase gene expression in the human ventricle during end-stage heart failure. J Clin Invest 1990;85:305

37. Mayoux E, Callens F, Swynghedauw B et al: Adaptional process of the cardiac Ca^{2+} channels to pressure overload. Biochemical and physiological properties of the dihydropyridine receptors in normal and hypertrophied rat hearts. J Cardiovasc Pharmacol 1988;12:390

38. Scamps F, Mayoux E, Charlemagne D et al: Ca current in single isolated cells from normal and hypertrophied rat heart. Effect of β adrenergic stimulation. Circ Res 1990;67:199

39. Gwathmey JK: Heart Failure. Basic Science and Clinical Aspects. Marcel Dekker, New York, 1993

40. Barrington PL, Harvey RD, Mogui DJ et al: Na current (I_{Na}) and inward rectifying K current (I_{K1}) in cardiocytes from normal and hypertrophied right ventricles of cat [abstract]. Biophys J 1988;53:426

41. Swynghedauw B, Coraboeuf E: Basic aspects of myocardial function, growth, and development. Cardiac hypertrophy and failure. p. 771. In Willerson JT, Cohn JN (eds): Cardiovascular Medicine Churchill Livingstone, New York, 1994

42. Coulombe A, Montaza A, Richer P et al: Reduction of calcium-independent transient outward current density in DOCA-salt hypertrophied rat ventricular myocytes. Pflugers Arch 1994;427:47

43. Hatem SN, Sham JKS, Morad M: Enhanced Na-Ca exchange activity in cardiomyopathic Syrian hamster heart. Circulation 1994;74:253

44. Rannou F, Sainte-Beuve C, Oliviero P et al: Adaptation to haemodynamic overload of dihydropyridine and ryanodine receptors in rat, ferret and guinea pig hearts. Implications for excitation-contraction coupling. J Mol Cell Cardiol 1995;27:1225

45. Rannou F, Dambrin G, Marty I et al: Expression of the cardiac ryanodine receptor mRNA in the hypertrophied rat heart. Cardiovax Res (in press)

46. Younes A, Schneider JM, Bercovici J, Swynghedauw B: Creatine kinase isoenzymes redistribution in chronically overloaded myocardium. Cardiovasc Res 1985;19:15

47. Ingwall J, Fossel E: Dynamics of energy metabolism in hypertrophied myocardium, the transition to failure. p. 601. In Alpert NR (ed): Myocardial Hypertrophy and Failure. Lippincott-Raven, Philadelphia, 1983

48. Revis NW, Cameron ASV: The relationship between fibrosis and lactate dehydrogenase isozymes in experimental hypertrophic heart of rabbits. Cardiovasc Res 1978;12:348

49. Revis NW, Thomson RY, Cameron ASV: Lactate dehydrogenase isozymes in the human hypertrophic heart. Cardiovasc Res 1977;11:172

50. Gwathmey JK, Morgan JP: Altered calcium handling in experimental pressure-overload hypertrophy in the ferret. Circ Res 1985;57:836

51. Gwathmey JK, Copelas L, MacKinnon R et al: Abnormal intracellular calcium handling in myocardium from patients with end-stage heart failure. Circ Res 1987;61:70

52. Callens-ElAmrani F, Snoeckx L, Swynghedauw B: Anoxia-induced changes in ventricular diastolic compliance in two models of hypertension in rats. J Hypertens 1992;10:229

53. Pye MP, Cobbe SM: Mechanism of ventricular arrhythmias in cardiac hypertrophy and failure. Cardiovasc Res 1992;26:740

54. Chevalier B, Heudes D, Heymes C et al: Trandolapril decreases prevalence of ventricular ectopic activity in middle-aged SHR. Circulation 1995;92:1947

55. Besse S, Assayag P, Delcayre C et al: Normal and hypertrophied senescent rat heart. Mechanical and molecular characteristics. Am J Physiol 1993;265:H183

56. Algra A, Tijssen JGP, Roelandt JRTC et al: QT interval variables from 24 hour electrocardiography and the two year risk of sudden death. Br Heart J 1993;70:43

57. Bigger JT, Fleiss JL, Rolzitzky LM et al: Frequency domain measures of heart period variability to assess risk late after myocardial infarction. J Am Coll Cardiol 1993;21:729

58. Carré F, Maison-Blanche P, Mansier P et al: Phenotypic determinants of heart rate variability in cardiac hypertrophy and failure. Eur Heart J, suppl. D 1994;15:58

59. Eschenhagen T: G proteins and the heart. Cell Biol Int 1993;17:723

60. Mercadier JJ, Samuel JL, Michel JB et al: Atrial natri-

uretic factor gene expression in rat ventricle during experimental hypertension. Am J Physiol 1989;257: H979

61. Kawaguchi H, Kitabatake A: Renin-angiotensin system in failing heart. J Mol Cell Cardiol 1995;27:201
62. Heymes C, Swynghedauw B, Chevalier B: Activation of angiotensinogen and angiotensin converting enzyme gene expression in the left ventricle of senescent rats. Circulation 1994;90:1328
63. Weber KT, Brilla CG: Pathological hypertrophy and cardiac interstitium. Fibrosis and renin-angiotensin-aldosterone system. Circulation 1991;83:1849
64. Weber KT, Brilla CG, Janicki JS: Myocardial fibrosis. Its functional significance and regulatory factors. Cardiovasc Res 1993;27:341
65. Robert V, Thiem NV, Cheav SL et al: Increased cardiac types I and III collagen mRNAs in aldosterone-salt hypertension. Hypertension 1994;24:30
66. Schaper J, Speiser B: The extracellular matrix in the failing human heart. p. 303. In Hasenfuss G, Holubarsch, C, Just H, Alpert NR (eds): Cellular and Molecular Alterations in the Failing Human Heart. Steinkopff Verlag, Darmstadt, 1992
67. Bolyut MO, O'Neill L, Meredith AL et al: Alterations in cardiac gene expression during transition from stable hypertrophy to heart failure. Circ Res 1994;75:23
68. Conrad CH, Brooks WW, Hayes JA et al: Myocardial fibrosis and stiffness with hypertrophy and heart failure in the SHR. Circulation 1995;91:161
69. Besse S, Robert V, Assayag P et al: Non-synchronous changes in myocardial collagen mRNA and protein during aging. Effect of DOCA-salt hypertension. Am J Physiol 1994;267:H2237
70. Besse S, Delcayre C, Chevalier B et al: Is the senescent heart overloaded and already failing? A review. Cardiovasc Drugs Ther 1994;8:581
71. Chevalier B, Mansier P, Teiger E, et al: Alterations in β adrenergic and muscarinic receptors in aged rat heart. Effects of chronic administration of propranolol and atropine. Mech Ageing Dev 1991;60:215
72. Hardouin S, Bourgeois F, Besse S, et al: Decreased accumulation of β_1-adrenergic receptors, Gαs and total myosin heavy chain messenger RNAs in the left ventricle of senescent rat heart. Mech Ageing 1993;71:169
73. Lakatta E: Cardiovascular regulatory mechanisms in advanced age. Physiol Rev 1993;73:413

Cellular and Molecular Biology of the Myocardium: Growth and Hypertrophy

4

Peter H. Sugden
Stephen J. Fuller

The growth of normal mammalian cardiac myocytes can be divided into two distinct phases.[1] Prenatally they proliferate rapidly, with mitosis slowing toward birth and completely ceasing early in the neonatal period. Thereafter the myocyte increases in size, accreting myofibrils, subcellular organelles, and so on (myocyte eutrophy) in order to fulfill the obligatory requirement for increased contractile capacity during maturational growth. Myocytic growth contributes significantly to the overall growth of the heart, although other elements (blood vessels, connective, nervous tissues) are also involved. The adult cardiac myocyte is thus an example of a terminally differentiated cell, and only in extreme circumstances has any recurrence of myocyte division been well documented biochemically and then only in the less-differentiated atrial myocyte.[2]

In addition, the adult cardiac myocyte grows adaptively to any externally imposed requirement for increased contractile work, which can arise under a variety of physiologic and pathologic conditions. [Unlike skeletal muscle, the heart does not possess satellite cells (quiescent adult myoblasts) that proliferate and are recruited to form myotubes when suitably stimulated.] This reaction is the hypertrophic response, which can be defined as an increase in myocyte size in excess of that predicted (e.g., based on age), in response to a stimulus. Although hypertrophy shares some common features with eutrophy (e.g., accumulation of myofibrils), it is in many ways distinct, with the principal differences apparent at the level of gene expression. Myocyte hypertrophy is

an important contributor to the loosely termed clinical entity "cardiac hypertrophy" (principally ventricular hypertrophy), which occurs when increased contractile power is needed. Thus classically, if the heart must eject blood against increased pressure (as in hypertensive or stenotic states) or must increase its net cardiac output (as with valvular regurgitation), it adapts by increasing its myocyte mass. These pressure and volume overloads give rise to characteristic patterns of cardiac hypertrophy.[3] Pressure overload causes gross thickening of the ventricular wall in the absence of chamber enlargement (concentric hypertrophy). The myocyte cross-sectional area increases to a greater extent than the cell length,[4-6] suggesting parallel deposition of sarcomeres. Epicardial myocytes enlarge more than mid- or endocardial myocytes, with smaller myocytes enlarging more than the larger cells.[6] Volume overload causes chamber enlargement with a limited increase in wall thickness (eccentric hypertrophy). Here myocyte length increases more than the cross-sectional area, suggesting deposition of sarcomeres in series.[7] How the two forms of hemodynamic overload lead to differential deposition of sarcomeres is not understood. More complex patterns of hypertrophy have been described.[8] Although ventricular hypertrophy is undoubtedly a physiologically important response during its initial stages (because it maintains or increases cardiac output), in its later stages it is an independent risk factor in humans for sudden cardiac death and other events of a cardiac origin.[9] The form of cardiac hypertrophy encountered most frequently in the clinical context is the more localized reactive hypertrophy that follows myocardial infarction. It has been estimated that the heart can lose up to 25 percent of its myocyte population, with the surviving myocytes adapting by hypertrophy to substitute for those lost. Here the hypertrophy prolongs survival.

CELL CYCLE IN SKELETAL AND CARDIAC MUSCLE

Cell Cycle Regulation in Skeletal Muscle

The reasons the cardiac myocyte withdraws from the cell cycle are unclear. By analogy with skeletal muscle, the involvement of homodimeric DNA binding proteins of the basic helix-loop-helix (bHLH) class has been suggested. In skeletal muscle the transition between proliferating myoblasts and nondividing myotubes is determined in part by the expression of so-called muscle determination genes encoding bHLH proteins of the MyoD class (MyoD, myogenin, MRF4, myf-5).[10] In addition, bHLH proteins of the Id class (inhibitor of DNA binding) prevent binding of MyoD class proteins to DNA. Id proteins are MyoD-like proteins that lack the DNA binding domain. They are thought to form heterodimeric complexes with MyoD that are unable to bind to DNA because two DNA binding domains are required for productive binding. Id proteins thus promote proliferation rather than differentiation.

As in other cell types, the reentry of skeletal myoblasts, which are arrested at the G_0–G_1 stage into the cell cycle, is dependent on phosphorylation of the Rb protein, the product of the retinoblastoma gene, by cell cycle protein kinases.[11,12] Current evidence suggests that, in addition to the DNA binding activity of the MyoD homodimer, MyoD interacts with unphosphorylated or hypophosphorylated Rb and prevents its phosphorylation.[13] This interaction locks Rb in its hypophosphorylated form and is responsible for cell cycle arrest and induction of muscle-specific gene expression during myogenesis.[13]

Cell Cycle Regulation in the Cardiac Myocyte

Although the analogy with skeletal muscle is useful, cell cycle control in cardiac myocytes may be somewhat different. Thus whereas cell division and expression of muscle-specific genes are mutually exclusive in skeletal muscle,[14] both being under the control of the MyoD-like proteins, cell division in the heart is not dependent on the absence of the contractile apparatus.[15] Furthermore, MyoD-like proteins are not found in the heart; and despite intensive efforts, no cardiac equivalents of these regulatory proteins have been identified.[15] The most recent data suggest that tumor-suppressor genes in addition to Rb, such as p53 and the Rb-like protein p107, may play a role in the terminal differentiation of cardiac muscle cells.[1,16] In contrast to MyoD, Id mRNA is present in ventricular myocytes during the early postnatal proliferative phase and declines in the adult heart.[17]

Division of the Cardiac Myocyte: Reinducible?

Controlled reentry of the cardiac myocyte into the cell cycle could be of considerable clinical significance. Because the mechanisms controlling the cell cycle in these myocytes are poorly understood, success has been limited. A general strategy in other cells is to elicit cell-restricted overexpression of an oncogene. The oncogenic capacity of the SV40 large tumor antigen (T-Ag) has been attributed to its binding tumor suppressor proteins (e.g., Rb) preventing them from inhibiting entry into the cell cycle.[18] Thus although Rb interacts with both MyoD and large T-Ag, the end results are diametrically opposed. In myotubes the effect of large T-Ag is dominant over MyoD.[13] In an attempt to produce a spermatid-specific tumor in transgenic mice with a transgene in which large T-Ag is fused to the 5′ and 3′ flanking regions of the mouse protamine 1 gene, the presence of right atrial tumors was detected.[19] These cells proliferated in culture, and some displayed a degree of spontaneous beating for up to 5 months. However, most did not beat, and none of the clonal lines selected had a myosin-positive phenotype. Using a more direct approach, large T-Ag was introduced into primary cultures of neonatal myocytes by recombinant adenoviral infection, with mitosis resuming within 72 hours.[20] Expression of the ventricular myosin light chain-2 (vMLC-2) gene, a ventricular-specific marker, was retained; and the cells could be passaged for a limited time. However, no continuous cell lines were forthcoming.

Cardiospecific expression of large T-Ag has been a more productive approach. Atrial-specific expression of large T-Ag in transgenic mice by fusion with the promoter region of the atrial natriuretic factor (ANF) gene resulted in the development of large right atrial tumors.[21] Myocyte-like cells could be propagated as transplantable tumor lines in syngeneic animals.[22]

Cells could be obtained from these tumors that retained many of the characteristics of atrial myocytes, and they proliferated in culture.[22,23] However, even these cells cannot be passaged indefinitely. Myocytes in transgenic mice expressing an α-myosin heavy chain (α-MHC) promoter/large T-Ag fusion gene were hyperplastic in both atria and ventricles.[24] Both types of myocyte could be passaged and maintained many features of the differentiated phenotypes, though T tubules and an extensive sarcoplasmic reticulum were conspicuously absent. The extent to which these cells can be passaged remains to be assessed.

Another approach has been to prepare transgenic mice in which the heart selectively overexpresses the c-*myc* proto-oncogene during development. These hearts are enlarged and contain a greater number of myocytes than those from normal mice (indicating increased hyperplasia).[25–27] However, the myocytes are smaller than normal, and their responses to hypertrophic agonists differ. Ca^{2+} may be involved in the regulation of cell growth, and cardiospecific overexpression of a calmodulin transgene (calmodulin is a small Ca^{2+}-binding regulatory protein) in mice led to myocyte hyperplasia,[28,29] principally involving the atria. (The ANF promoter region was utilized to ensure cardiospecificity, which may explain the greater atrial involvement.) Adult rat ventricular cells have been transformed by growth in conditioned media from a rat thyroid cell line.[30] This RCVC cell line had a doubling time of 20 hours, displayed contact inhibition, and possessed slow inward currents typical of the L-type Ca^{2+} channel (blocked by nifedipine).

The overall conclusion is that until the basic mechanisms that lead to withdrawal of the cardiac myocyte from the cell cycle are better understood, it is not possible to induce controlled reentry into the cell cycle. Furthermore, the absence of a differentiated cardiac myocyte cell line and the poor viability of isolated adult myocytes or perfused hearts means that study of the relatively protracted hypertrophic response must rely on the use of primary cultures of myocytes from neonatal (rat) or embryonic (chick) hearts.

EXPERIMENTAL MODELS FOR THE STUDY OF MYOCYTE HYPERTROPHY

Although cardiac hypertrophy can be induced experimentally in vivo with relative ease, the recent rapid advances in the understanding of myocyte hypertrophy are attributable to the development of a suitable model system, namely primary cultures of ventricular myocytes from neonatal rat heart.[31–34] Although some success in culturing adult mammalian ventricular myocytes has been reported,[35,36] the rat cells certainly undergo rapid phenotypic adaptation despite maintaining a rod-shaped morphology.[37] Clinically, cardiac hypertrophy is primarily an adult disease, and the question of the broader applicability of the neonatal model must be considered. The hypertrophic response in the neonatal myocyte probably simulates adequately the situation in the adult myocyte in vivo,[38] particularly with respect to the signaling pathways utilized (because of their universality) and the transcriptional changes observed. Some differences do exist. The fibroblast growth factor (FGF) receptor is expressed in the neonatal myocyte,[39] and FGF is hypertrophic.[40] However, the FGF receptor is not readily detected in the adult myocyte.[39] Equally, the applicability of the rat model to human cardiac hypertrophy should be considered, and again there are some differences. For example, α-MHC is constitutively expressed in the adult rat myocyte, where a transcriptional transition leads to expression of β-MHC during hypertrophy. In the human, β-MHC is constitutively expressed,[41] but even so its expression must be up-regulated in the presence of hypertrophy. In the future the use of transgenic mice and ventricular myocytes isolated from these animals is likely to increase, examples of which are already appearing in the literature.

TRANSCRIPTIONAL ALTERATIONS IN THE HYPERTROPHIED MYOCYTE

Hypertrophy of the ventricular myocyte is characterized in vivo and in cell culture models by a range of morphologic and biochemical changes.[38,42] The myocyte enlarges, and the complement of myofibrils is increased (Fig. 4-1). These changes can be simulated in vitro. Although changes in morphology also occur during maturational growth, specific transitions in gene expression distinguish hypertrophy from maturation (Table 4-1). Both up-regulation and down-regulation are observed. In ventricular myocytes from rats, immediate early genes (IEGs), such as genes encoding transcription factors (e.g., c-*fos* and *Egr*-1), are rapidly (within minutes) but transiently expressed in response to hypertrophic stimuli.[34] In addition to its transience, expression of IEGs is characterized by the absence of a requirement for de novo protein synthesis during their transcriptional induction, showing that the protein factors necessary for

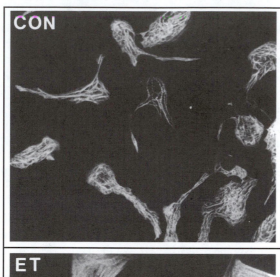

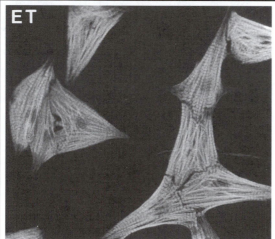

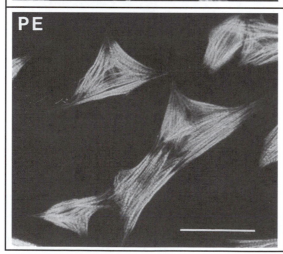

Fig. 4-1. Exposure of cultured ventricular myocytes to endothelin 1 or phenylephrine causes their hypertrophy. Cells were cultured in the absence of agonist (CON) or in the presence of 100 nM endothelin 1 (ET) OR 50 μM phenylephrine (PE) for 24 hours. They were fixed, permeabilized, and incubated with an antibody against β-myosin heavy chain (β-MHC), then with a biotinylated secondary antibody, and finally with steptavidin-Texas Red. The bar on the micrographs is 50 μm. The control myocytes are small, and myofibrils containing β-MHC are sparse and poorly organized. For cells exposed to ET or PE, the cell profile is increased, as is expression of β-MHC. The myofibrils are well organized and are clearly cross-striated. (Micrographs prepared by Dr. Angela Clerk, Department of Cardiac Medicine, National Heart and Lung Institute.)

their induction are present constitutively.[43] Other proteins involved in the regulation of gene expression (Id) are reexpressed in adult ventricular myocytes by hypertrophic agonism.[17]

In the medium term, the myocyte reverts to a pattern of gene expression more akin to that in the fetal heart with reexpression of ANF, β-MHC, and skeletal muscle (SkM) α-actin. In the longer term, expression of a number of constitutively expressed genes [e.g., vMLC-2, cardiac muscle (CM) α-actin] is upregulated, whereas the expression of others (e.g., the cardiac fast Na^+ channel) is unaltered. Increased expression of vMLC-2 and CM α-actin proteins increases sarcomerogenesis. These transcriptional changes are also seen in rat models of hypertrophy in vivo.[38] Additionally, the expression of certain genes is down-regulated in the presence of hypertrophy in vivo. Examples include the sarcoplasmic reticulum (SR) Ca^{2+}-release channel (the ryanodine receptor) and SR Ca^{2+}-ATPase-2 (SERCA-2),[44] which are responsible for cycling Ca^{2+} out of and into the SR. Down-regulation of gene expression has not been studied extensively in cell culture models. The characterization of transcriptional changes is incomplete, and many more probably remain to be added to this list. A recent addition is brain natriuretic factor (BNF). BNF is expressed at an early stage during the hypertrophic response in the cultured myocyte, and, unlike IEGs, expression is maintained.[45] Although it is clearly difficult to study the transient changes (e.g., IEG expression) in humans, certain of the alterations in gene expression described in rat models have been detected in association with human cardiac hypertrophy (e.g., reexpression of ANF[46–48]).

The overall effect of the longer-term changes in gene expression in the adult animal may be to return the cardiac myocyte to a less well differentiated phenotype that is closer to the fetal cell. The physiologic functions of the longer-term phenotypic alterations are becoming clearer. The expression of β-MHC may allow greater energy efficiency in terms of contraction,[49] whereas the expression of SkM α-actin may increase contractility.[50] The increased expression of

Table 4-1. Gene Transcription During Cardiac Hypertrophy

Gene	Induction, Up-regulation, or Reexpression	Time Scale (hours)
c-*fos*	Induction	< 1
c-*jun*	Induction	< 1
Egr-1	Induction	< 1
Atrial natriuretic factor	Reexpression	12–24
Skeletal muscle α-actin	Reexpression	12–24
β-Myosin heavy chain	Reexpression	12–24
Ventricular myosin light chain 2	Up-regulation	24–48
Cardiac muscle α-actin	Up-regulation	24–48
Brain natriuretic factor	?	< 1–48

ANF may be a homeostatic response to reduce blood pressure in the presence of hypertension.[38]

HYPERTROPHIC AGONISM

Numerous agonists and interventions induce hypertrophy in cultured ventricular myocytes[38,42] (Table 4-2). Naturally occurring agonists include vasoactive peptides (e.g., the potent vasoconstrictors ET-1[51–54] and angiotensin II[55–60]), physiologic or synthetic sympathoadrenal agonists acting principally through the α_1-adrenergic receptor (AdR) (e.g., norepinephrine and phenylephrine),[32–34,61–64] peptide growth factors [e.g., FGF,[40,65] transforming growth factor β,[40,65] insulin-like growth factor-1 (IGF-1)[66–68] and IGF-2[69]], and mechanical interventions.[70–72] β-Adrenergic agonism has been more tenuously linked to the hypertrophic response, and the effect may be indirect.[35,36,73,74] A variety of hypertrophic factors have been described, including a circulating factor (myotrophin) present in the plasma of hypertensive rats[75] and a factor secreted by the nonmyocytic cells in the heart.[76] Most recently a factor (cardiotrophin 1) present in the conditioned medium from differentiated embryoid bodies has been cloned and shown to be a member of a cytokine family.[77] It is not clear to what extent each of these agonists contributes to myocyte hypertrophy in vivo. The etiology of the response is likely to be multifactorial, and inputs from individual agonists may be separable on a temporal basis. Some interventions (e.g., stretch) may act indirectly through autocrine, paracrine, juxtacrine, or intracrine loops.[76,78–80] It is also difficult to assess the importance of local versus systemic changes in neurohumoral tone.

Table 4-2. Hypertrophic Agonists in Cardiac Myocytes

Agonist	Receptor Subtype	Receptor Coupling Mechanism
Endothelin-1	ET_A	$Gq/PtdInsP_2$ hydrolysis
α_1-Adrenergic agonists	Pharmacologically defined α_{1A} and cloned α_{1B}?	$Gq/PtdInsP_2$ hydrolysis
Angiotensin II	AT-1	$Gq/PtdInsP_2$ hydrolysis
Fibroblast growth factors	Not defined	Receptor protein tyrosine kinase
Insulin-like growth factor 1	No known subtype	Receptor protein tyrosine kinase
Transforming growth factor β	Not known	Receptor protein serine/threonine kinase
Insulin-like growth factor 2	No known subtype	Not known
Stretch	Not known	Endogenous angiotensin II production

Abbreviations: ET, endothelin; Ptd Ins P_2, phosphatidylinositol-4,5-bisphosphate; AT, angiotensin.

RECEPTOR COUPLING

Receptor-Coupled Hydrolysis of Membrane Phosphatidylinositols

Many established hypertrophic agonists (Table 4-2) activate at Gq-coupled receptors (Fig. 4-2). The potential importance of the αq-coupled pathway has been emphasized by the finding that a plasmid encoding a constitutively active αq is hypertrophic when transfected into myocytes.[81] For sympathoadrenal agonists and ET-1, the α_1-AdrR or the ET_A-receptor subtype is involved. Ligand-binding to these heptahelical transmembrane receptors results in the exchange of guanosine triphosphate (GTP) for guanosine diphosphate (GDP) in the heterotrimeric G protein Gq [α(GDP)·$\beta\gamma$] with the concomitant dissociation of Gq [α(GTP)·$\beta\gamma$] into α(GTP) and $\beta\gamma$ in the plane of the membrane. $Gq_{\alpha(GTP)}$ then activates the membrane-bound enzyme phospholipase Cβ(PLCβ), resulting in hydrolysis of the membrane phospholipid phosphatidylinositol-4,5-bisphosphate (PtdInsP$_2$) into the dual second messengers diacylglycerol (DAG) and inositol-1,4,5-trisphosphate (IP$_3$). Although IP$_3$ is important in the regulation of intracellular Ca^{2+} movements in many cell types, it does not appear to have an important function in this regard in cardiac myocytes. Thus although the IP$_3$ receptor Ca^{2+} release channel is present in the cardiac myocyte, it is located in the intercalated disc region and is more likely to be involved in cell–cell signaling than control of intracellular Ca^{2+} release.[82]

The second product of PtdInsP$_2$ hydrolysis, DAG, is the physiologic activator of the phospholipid-dependent protein kinase protein kinase C (PKC). Protein kinases are enzymes that phosphorylate other proteins by transferring the γ-phosphate group from adenosine triphosphate (ATP) to hydroxyl groups within their protein substrates, thereby altering their functions (e.g., their enzymatic activity). Two major classes exist in eukaryotes: those that phosphorylate seryl or threonyl residues (protein Ser/Thr kinases) and those that phosphorylate tyrosyl residues (protein Tyr kinases). The susceptibility of Ser/Thr or Tyr residues to phosphorylation is determined largely by the neighboring primary amino sequence[83] and their steric availability to the kinases. PKC is a protein Ser/Thr kinase that, as described below, is thought to play a major role in the hypertrophic response mediated through Gq-coupled receptors.

Mechanically stretching myocytes activates multiple signaling pathways,[78] including PtdInsP$_2$ hydrolysis, PKC, phospholipase A$_2$, and tyrosine kinases. The current theory is that it is mediated by local re-

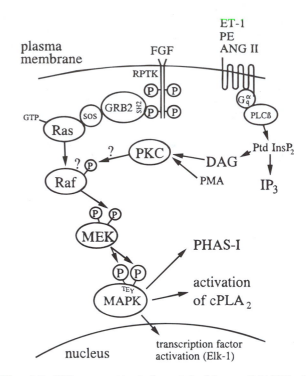

Fig. 4-2. Mitogen-activated protein kinase (MAPK) signaling cascade. Binding of extracellular growth factors, such as fibroblast growth factor (FGF), to their membrane-bound monomeric receptor protein tyrosine kinases (RPTKs) promotes RPTK dimerization followed by trans-autophosphorylation on Tyr residues in RPTKs. Through its Src homology 2 (SH2) domains, the adapter protein GRB2 translocates the guanine nucleotide exchange factor sos to the membrane where it promotes the GTP-loading of Ras. Rasl·GTP binds the protein Ser/Thr kinase Raf, thereby translocating it to the membrane. Here other poorly understood additional reactions lead to full activation of Raf. Raf phosphorylates and activates the protein Thr/Tyr kinase MEK [MAPK kinase], which in turn activates MAPK by phosphorylating it on both a Thr and a Tyr residue. MAPK phosphorylates cytoplasmic proteins, such as cytoplasmic phospholipase A$_2$ (cPLA$_2$) and PHAS-I (which is involved in the regulation of protein synthesis). Phosphorylation and activation of transcription factors (e.g., Elk-1) may involve the translocation of MAPK into the nucleus. Binding of endothelin 1 (ET-1) and α_1-adrenergic agonists such as phenylephrine (PE) and angiotensin II (ANG II) to their individual heptahelical receptors promotes GTP loading of the α-subunit of the heterotrimeric ($\alpha\beta\gamma$) G protein Gq. Gq(α·GTP) activates phospholipase Cβ (PLCβ), stimulating hydrolysis of phosphatidylinositol-2, 5-bisphosphate (PtdInsP$_2$) to diacylglycerol (DAG) and inositol-1, 4, 5-trisphosphate (IP$_3$). DAG is the physiologic activator of the "classic" and "novel" protein kinase C (PKC) subfamilies. The tumor-promoting phorbol ester PMA also directly activates these PKCs. Activation of PKC leads to activation of the MAPK cascade by mechanisms that are still ill-defined (but that may involve direct phosphorylation of Raf).

lease of angiotensin II,[79] which then couples to a Gq-linked receptor in the heart.[84,85] If this pathway is correct, the in vivo significance is considerable.

Receptor Protein Tyrosine Kinases

A second pathway for hypertrophy is coupled to receptor protein tyrosine kinases (RPTKs). After ligand binding, monomeric receptors (e.g., those of the FGF receptor family) dimerize. Receptors such as the IGF-1 receptor heterotetramer already exist as a functional dimer (two $\alpha\beta$ units). These receptors then undergo transautophosphorylation on Tyr residues, which triggers a series of responses[86] outlined below. In common with Gq-coupled receptors, one end result is stimulation of the mitogen-activated protein kinase (MAPK) cascade,[87] which is discussed later. Parenthetically and with regard to the hypertrophy seen in the insulin resistance (or plurimetabolic) syndrome characterized by hypertension, hyperinsulinemia, and insulin resistance,[88,89] we believe that there is no convincing evidence that insulin (which acts through an RPTK similar to the IGF-1 receptor) is a direct-acting hypertrophic agonist.

α_1-Adrenoceptor Subtypes

The α_1-AdrR subtype responsible for the hypertrophic response is of considerable pharmacologic interest. As shown by molecular cloning, a number of α_1-AdrR subtypes (α_{1A}-, α_{1B}-, α_{1C}-, and α_{1D}-AdrRs) are expressed in mammalian cells.[90] Using a pharmacologic approach with subtype-selective antagonists, two AdrR populations (α_{1A}- and α_{1B}-AdrRs) have been identified.[91] Both are linked to the stimulation of PtdIns hydrolysis.[92] In agreement with the proportions of receptor subtypes defined by ligand binding data, the α_{1A}-subtype contributes about 20 percent and the α_{1B}-subtype contributes the remainder of the input to PtdInsP$_2$ hydrolysis in the adult rat myocyte.[92] It has been difficult to unify the classification of subtypes as defined by the pharmacologic and molecular cloning approaches. It is agreed that the α_{1B}-AdrRs, defined by either approach, are identical. The pharmacologic α_{1A}-AdrR is now thought to be the cloned α_{1C}-AdrR.[90] Although originally thought to be absent from rat heart, the α_{1C}-AdrR has now been detected in cardiac myocytes by RNase protection assays[93] along with the α_{1B}- and α_{1D}-AdrRs.[94] Whether a specific receptor subtype is responsible for the hypertrophic response is difficult to assess, the problem being that the principal method of investigation has involved the use of subtype-selective antagonists.

Using the α_{1A}-AdrR selective antagonist 5-methylurapidil, Knowlton et al.[95] concluded that α_1-AdrR-mediated hypertrophy was pharmacologically an α_{1A}-AdrR (not α_{1B}-AdrR) response. In contrast, mice carrying a constitutively active α_{1B}-AdrR transgene that is expressed in a cardiospecific manner developed hypertrophy.[96]

IMPORTANCE OF PROTEIN KINASE C

As described above, a number of hypertrophic agonists (e.g., ET-1 and α_1-adrenergic agonists) promote the hydrolysis of PtdInsP$_2$ to produce DAG and InsP$_3$.[51,92,97,98] Evidence supports a role for DAG, the physiologic activator of PKC, in the mediation of Gq-coupled hypertrophy. PKC is a family of protein Ser/Thr kinases that has been divided on the basis of structural and regulatory properties into three subfamilies: classic, novel, and atypical.[99–101] All require phospholipid (e.g., phosphatidylserine) for activity, but the requirements for other regulatory molecules differ.[99] Only the cPKCs are Ca^{2+}-dependent. cPKCs and nPKCs are activated by DAG from agonist-stimulated hydrolysis of phospholipids (PtdInsP$_2$[102] and possibly phosphatidylcholine[103–105]). PKC is a major intracellular binding protein (although there may be others) for tumor-promoting phorbol esters such as phorbol 12-myristate-13-acetate (PMA), which can substitute for DAG.[106] These compounds have been particularly useful for implicating PKC in the regulation of cellular processes.

Several lines of evidence suggest involvement of PKC in the regulation of the hypertrophic response. First, ET-1 and phenylephrine (both powerful hypertrophic agonists) activate the isoforms of PKC predominating in ventricular myocytes (i.e., nPKC-δ and nPKC-ϵ)[107–110] There may be preferential activation of one of these isoforms. In our hands, nPKC-ϵ requires lower concentrations of agonists for activation than nPKC-δ.[110] Second, PMA (or its homologs) induces hypertrophy in cultured myocytes.[111–115] Third, transfection of myocytes with PKC constitutively activated by large N-terminal deletions stimulates promoter activity for β-MHC,[116] ANF,[114] and vMLC-2,[114] markers of the hypertrophic response. Although these experiments can be criticized because such large deletions remove regulatory sequences, thereby creating nonspecific protein kinases, transfection of ventricular myocytes with PKC isoforms constitutively activated by point mutations or small deletions in their inhibitory pseudosubstrate sites[100,101,117] also activates the ANF promoter.[118] Interestingly, cPKC-α, nPKC-ϵ, and aPKC-ζ produce comparable degrees of activation, implying that if there is any specificity of PKC, it must reside elsewhere (e.g., tissue-specific expression of isoforms,[108] preferential activation by agonists[110]). Finally, a PKC construct in which catalytic domain residues had been deleted acts in a dominant-negative manner to down-regulate the phenylephrine stimulation of β-MHC promoter activity.[119] This action presumably involves sequestration of DAG or protein substrates by the mutant PKC.

REGULATION OF THE MITOGEN-ACTIVATED PROTEIN KINASE CASCADE

MAPK (also known as the extracellular signal-regulated kinase, ERK) is thought to play a central role in cell growth and differentiation[120,121] (Fig. 4-2). It was first identified[122,123] as a highly conserved protein Ser/Thr kinase activated in a number of cell lines in response to peptide growth factors (fibroblast, nerve, platelet-derived, epidermal) acting through RPTKs.[86] Binding of ligands to these RPTKs stimulates their dimerization and their transautophosphorylation on Tyr residues. This reaction promotes association of proteins containing Src homology 2 (SH2) domains with specific phospho-Tyr residues in the RPTKs.[124] SH2 domain proteins include (1) GRB2, an adapter protein that bridges binding of the guanine nucleotide exchange factor (GEF) Sos to RPTKs[125-131]; (2) PtdIns 3-kinase (PI-3K) (not shown), which catalyzes synthesis of the putative signaling molecule PtdInsP$_3$ by phosphorylation of PtdInsP$_2$[132]; and (3) PLCγ (not shown), which hydrolyzes PtdInsP$_2$ to DAG and InsP$_3$.[133,134] These pathways have not yet been characterized in the cardiac myocyte.

The following pathway couples ligand-binding at RPTKs to activation of MAPK.[120,135,136] The binding of GRB2 to phosphorylated RPTKs through its SH2 domains and to Pro-rich sequences in Sos through its SH3 domains translocates Sos to the membrane, where it interacts with the small G protein Ras,[125,130,137] which is analogous to the α-subunit of the heterotrimeric G proteins. The GEF activity of Sos exchanges GDP bound to Ras for GTP.[138] Ras•GTP, the active form of Ras, is instrumental in the activation of the protein Ser/Thr kinase, Raf, by translocating it to the membrane.[139] However, binding of Ras•GTP to Raf is not sufficient to activate fully the protein kinase activity of Raf, and it is presumed that further modifications of Raf (possibly involving its phosphorylation) supercede in the membrane fraction. A major function of Raf is its role as a MAPK kinase kinase and thus to phosphorylate and activate MAPK kinase [MAPKK or MEK, for MAPK (or ERK) kinase].[139,140] Full activation of MEK1 by Raf requires the phosphorylation of two Ser residues.[141-143] MEK activates MAPK by phosphorylating a Tyr and a Thr residue within a conserved Thr-Glu-Tyr (TEY) sequence.[135] Activated MAPK then phosphorylates its own substrates. There is good evidence that activation of this pathway is hypertrophic in myocytes. Transfection of myocytes with constitutively active Ras[81,144] or Raf[145] induces the transcriptional changes typical of the hypertrophic response; Ras also induces the morphologic changes. Furthermore, dominant negative MAPK down-regulates the transcriptional changes in response to α-adrenergic agonism.[146]

The RPTK-coupled pathway of MAPK activation may be of less significance in the heart than the Gq-coupled pathway (through which the stretch-activated pathway may also act[71,78]) (Fig. 4-2). Although increased tyrosine phosphorylation of proteins in addition to MAPK is a characteristic of the hypertrophic response,[78,147] they are not necessarily RPTKs. MEK and MAPK are rapidly and transiently activated in heart by the powerfully hypertrophic agonists ET-1, α_1-adrenergic agonists, and PMA,[87,110,148,149] implicating Gq, PLCβ, PtdInsP$_2$ hydrolysis, and PKC. PKC is further implicated by the finding that chronic exposure of myocytes to PMA, which results in the loss of cPKCs and nPKCs from myocytes, down-regulates the activation of MAPK in response to PMA, ET-1, or α-adrenergic stimulation.[87] The pathway from PKC to MEK is poorly characterized,[120] although there may be elements in common with the RPTK → MAPK pathway. Work in other systems has suggested that PKC can directly phosphorylate and activate Raf,[150] but it is too early to say if it occurs in the heart. Heterotrimeric G proteins of the Gi class also activate the MAPK cascade in a Ras/Raf-dependent manner.[151,152] Activation of the Gi-coupled events is sensitive to pertussis toxin, which adenosine diphosphate (ADP)-ribosylates Gi$_\alpha$. Thus although some of the effects of ET-1 are Gi-dependent,[153,154] the activation of MAPK by ET-1 is not inhibited by pertussis toxin in myocytes.[155]

CONSEQUENCES OF MAPK ACTIVATION

MAPK phosphorylates a large number of proteins with intracellular signaling functions (preferentially at a Pro-X-Ser/Thr-Pro consensus sequence

156–158), which leads to altered functions/activities of the substrate proteins.[158] The substrates for MAPK in the heart remain poorly characterized. Substrates well characterized in other cell types include cytoplasmic phospholipase A_2 (cPLA$_2$)[159] and the transcription factor Elk-1.[160] Phosphorylation of cPLA$_2$ stimulates arachidonate release and the formation of lysophospholipids from membrane phospholipids.[159] Arachidonate release occurs during stretch-induced hypertrophy,[78] although it is not clear if cPLA$_2$ is responsible. Phosphorylation of Elk-1 and its interaction with the serum response factor (SRF) allows transactivation of genes containing the cis serum response element (SRE) in their promoter regions.[160] Transcription of the IEG proto-oncogene c-fos is regulated in this manner.[160] A novel molecular mechanism for the stimulation of protein synthesis translation has been identified. It involves MAPK-catalyzed phosphorylation[161] of PHAS-I (phosphorylated heat- and acid-stable protein regulated by insulin) in the rat[162] or 4E-BPI protein in humans[163] that releases initiation from a restraint caused by the sequestration of initiation factor eIF-4E. Although it is not known if it occurs in myocytes, PMA,[164] α_1-adrenergic agonism,[165] and ET-1[98] acutely activate protein synthesis and protein accretion (Fig. 4-1) in these cells. Other proteins phosphorylated by MAPK include structural proteins (e.g., microtubule-associated proteins, myelin basic protein, lamins, talins). "Retrophosphorylation" of Sos, Raf, and MEK by MAPK has also been detected[166–170] and may be important for the operation of negative feedback loops that lead to inactivation of the cascade.[168,169,171]

Although there is relatively good evidence that activation of the MAPK cascade is involved in the development of the hypertrophic phenotype, it may not be sufficient to induce the full response. Thus Raf and MAPK do not seem to be involved in the changes in myofibrillar organization observed with hypertrophy but are involved in the transcriptional alterations.[145,146] In contrast, activated Ras is able to induce the full response.[81,144] In a variety of nonmyocyte cell types, interaction of the actin cytoskeleton with myosin is involved in the cytokinesis associated with the end-stage of mitosis and is controlled by small G proteins of the Rho family,[172] which are related to Ras. It is not clear which second messengers are involved in the regulation of Rho•GTP loading. In nonmuscle cells, α-actinin (which is also a component of the Z-band in the myofibrils of striated muscle) interacts with PI 3-K[173] and its substrate PtdInsP$_2$.[174] These interactions may be involved in cytoskeletal reorganization. In muscle cells regulation of the protein–pro-

tein (e.g., actin, myosin, tropomyosin, troponins, α-actinin) interactions involved in myofibrillar assembly is still poorly understood, and it is not known if small G proteins are involved.

REGULATION OF TRANSCRIPTION

cis and trans Sites

As described above, the transcriptional changes seen with hypertrophy distinguish it from maturational growth. Transcription is controlled, at least in part, by the binding of trans-acting protein transcription factors to cis-regulatory sequences present in the noncoding regions of the genome. These oligonucleotide sequences have consensus motifs that are recognized by transcription factors; and they are frequently present in the promoter regions that lie upstream (i.e., on the 5' side) from the transcriptional initiation site and the coding region (Fig. 4-3).

Activator Protein-1 Sites

One of the better understood mechanisms of transcriptional activation is mediated at the activator protein-1 (AP-1) site present in the promoter regions in various genes.[43,175–177] AP-1 sites possess a TGAGTCAG octanucleotide consensus motif and were originally recognized as being involved in the transactivation of transcription by PMA. (The alternative nomenclature for PMA is 12-O-Tetradecanolyphorbol-13-acetate, or TPA. Hence the alternative nomenclature for the AP-1 site is the TPA-responsive element, or TRE.) AP-1 was subsequently recognized as being a c-Jun/c-Fos transcription factor heterodimer that binds to and transactivates at the TGAGTCAG sequence. Other transcription factors related to c-Jun (Jun B, Jun D) or c-Fos (Fos B, Fra 1, Fra 2) have been cloned. The dimerization process involves the leucine zipper motifs (a single leucine residue every seventh residue repeated four times in an α-helix) present in both factors, and the DNA binding involves an adjacent region rich in basic amino acids [hence the term basic leucine zipper (bZIP) proteins]. Although c-Jun can form homodimers that weakly transactivate, c-Fos is unable to homodimerize.

The transactivating ability of the c-Jun/c-Fos heterodimer is increased by the phosphorylation of Ser-63 and Ser-73 in the c-Jun amino-terminal transacti-

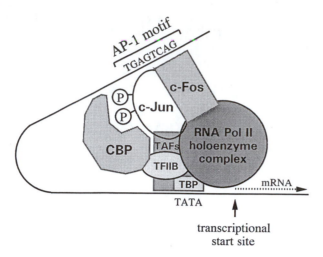

Fig. 4-3. Scheme of the protein–DNA and protein–protein interactions at the transcriptional initiation site of a gene containing AP-1 regulatory sequences in its promoter region. The site for initiation of transcription by the enzyme responsible for mRNA synthesis [RNA polymerase (pol) II] is frequently a TATA tetranucleotide consensus sequence (the TATA box) that lies about 30 bp upstream from the transcriptional start site. Various proteins factors [the TATA binding protein (TBP), a variety of TBP-associated factors (TAFs)] are constitutively associated with the TATA box. In a pathway thought to be common for both the AP-1 and the CRE transcription factors, phosphorylation of c-Jun in the c-Jun/c-Fos dimer bound by JNKS at AP-1 sites or phosphorylation of the CRE binding protein (CREB) by cAMP-dependent protein kinase at CREs promotes binding of the adapter protein CBP (CREB binding protein).[204] CBP also binds to the basal transcription factor TFIIB through its activation domain. TFIIB in turn binds to TBP and is involved in pol II recruitment. The assembly of this polymeric protein complex at the promoter region of a gene allows initiation of transcription.

vation domain, which by promoting association of co-activators and RNA polymerase II at the transcriptional initiation site stimulates transcription of AP-1 regulated genes (see Figure 4-3 for the interactions involved). Although it might be anticipated that phosphorylation of these residues would be increased by PMA, PMA seems to be relatively ineffective and in fact promotes dephosphorylation of Ser residues closer to the carboxyl-terminus in the c-Jun DNA binding domain.[178] Phosphorylation of Ser-63 and Ser-73 is catalyzed by a family of protein Ser/Thr kinases, the Jun N-terminal kinases (JNKs)[179] in human cell lines. JNKs show considerable homology with MAPKs but, in contrast to MAPK, are poorly activated by growth factors or PMA. They are activated by cell stress (e.g., ultraviolet light). The analogous enzymes in the rat are hence also known as stress-activated protein kinases (SAPKs). It is not yet known if JNKs/SAPKs are present in heart.

Regulation of *c-fos* Expression Through the Serum Response Element

The IEG c-*fos* is expressed in ventricular myocytes in response to hypertrophic stimuli[38] and has been used as a marker of the hypertrophic response.[78] The role of the translated c-Fos protein in activation at AP-1 sites is described above. The c-*fos* promoter region contains a *cis* SRE, an AP-1 site of unknown significance, and a site that may be principally involved in signaling from RPTKs (the sis-inducible element, SIE).[160] One pathway for stimulation of c-*fos* expression involves the formation of a ternary complex between a 62-kDa ternary complex factor (p62-TCF), a ubiquitously expressed SRF, and the SRE. p62-TCF is homologous with the transcription factor Elk-1[180] and is a member of the Ets group of transcription factors.[181] Although Elk-1 can bind to *cis* Ets sequences autonomously, the sequence specificity is broadened by interaction with SRF, which is capable of binding to a consensus (CArG) sequence in the SRE adjacent to the Ets site. The stimulation of c-*fos* expression may be at least partly attributable to a MAPK-catalyzed phosphorylation of sites in the C-terminal regulatory domain of Elk-1.[160,182,183] It is not clear if this regulatory pathway applies to other TCF homologs, although sequence studies predict that it should.

Expression of *Egr*-1

Expression of *Egr*-1 IEG is co-regulated with c-*fos* expression[184] and is enhanced by exposure of ventricular myocytes to hypertrophic agonists.[34,185] *Egr*-1 expression may be a better IEG marker of the hypertrophic response than c-*fos*, as its pattern of expression is more specifically correlated with development of the appropriate phenotype.[34] Down-regulation of *Egr*-1 expression using antisense oligodeoxynucleotide methodology down-regulated some aspects of the hypertrophic response on exposure of myocytes to ET-1.[186] The *Egr*-1 promoter region contains several SREs, which are responsible for its induction by vasopressin in mesangial cells.[187] Preliminary evidence indicates that phosphorylated Egr-1 binds to its *cis* consensus sequence more efficiently than the dephosphorylated species.[188] Thus transcription factor activation may generally involve phosphorylation.

IDENTIFICATION OF *cis*-ACTING REGULATORY MOTIFS RESPONSIBLE FOR UP-REGULATION OF GENES DURING HYPERTROPHY

ANF Promoter Region

Up-regulation of the transcription of ANF, vMLC-2, β-MHC, and c-*fos* has been used as a marker of the hypertrophic response.[38] To identify the *cis*-acting elements, the general approach is to sequence the 5′-flanking region of a gene and then prepare a series of nested deletions or mutations in this sequence. A fusion gene construct is then prepared in which the regulatory 5′-flanking regions are coupled to a reporter gene that encodes a protein that is both easy to assay and not expressed in normal mammalian cells (e.g., bacterial chloramphenicol acetyltransferase, firefly luciferase). The constructs are then transfected into cultured ventricular myocytes, and reporter gene expression in response to hypertrophic agonism is examined. Thus phenylephrine inducibility was unaffected by deletion of the −3003 to −638 basepair (bp) region (Fig. 4-4).[64] However, deletion of the −638 to −323 bp region decreased inducibility by 60 percent, implying that this region contains elements that control inducibility. The −638 to −323 bp region contains a number of consensus sequences for binding for transcription factors, including AP-1, CArG/SRE, and Egr-1 sites as well as an activator protein 2 (AP-2) site and a cyclic adenosine monophosphate (AMP)-responsive element (CRE).[64] In the atrial myocyte, PMA or overexpression of c-*fos* or c-*jun* activated ANF expression, implying the importance of the AP-1 site,[189] although the effects of c-*fos* overexpression on ANF promoter activity may not be simple.[189]

To study ANF promoter function in vivo during pressure-overload hypertrophy, Rockman et al.[190] used transgenic mice in which the −500 to 0 bp 5′-flanking region of the human ANF gene was fused with an SV40 large T-antigen (T-Ag) reporter. The −500 to 0 bp region was sufficient to confer atrial-specific expression on the reporter. Following aortic constriction, left ventricular expression of endogenous ANF was induced, but reporter expression was not up-regulated. This experiment shows that at least some of the elements controlling atrial-specific expression of ANF lie in the −500 to 0 bp region, but that those controlling pressure-overload specific expression probably do not.

vMLC-2 Promoter Region

A similar approach has established that cardiac-specific expression and α_1-adrenergic inducibility of the vMLC-2 gene declines hand-in-hand on progressive deletion from the −250 bp region through to the transcriptional initiation site, although there is evidence that the −2700 to −800 bp region may also contain elements that regulate specificity and inducibility.[64] The −250 bp upstream region contains three regions (HF-1, HF-2, HF-3) conserved between rat and chick, implying a regulatory function.[191] Whole site[191] or double point[192] mutations combined with transient transfection have shown that HF-1 and to a lesser extent HF-2 bestow cardiac specificity and inducibility on vMLC-2 expression, whereas HF-3 and a consensus E-box site (which binds muscle-specific transcription factors) immediately upstream of HF-1 were superfluous. Furthermore, the 28 bp HF-1 element conferred cardiac specificity and inducible expression on a neutral (thymidine kinase) promoter. In subsequent studies, a ubiquitous factor,

Fig. 4-4. Inducibility of ANF gene promoter activity by phenylephrine (PE). Fusion genes were prepared in which various lengths of the atrial natriuretic factor (ANF) gene promoter region that lies 5′ upstream from the transcriptional initiation site (0 bp) were linked to a luciferase reporter. Cardiac myocytes were transfected with plasmids containing these constructs, and the ability of PE to induce ANF promoter activity (as measured by luciferase activity) was assessed. Loss of the −638 to −323 bp noncoding promoter region caused a large decrease in PE inducibility, implying that this region contains elements important in this response. (Data from Knowlton et al.[64])

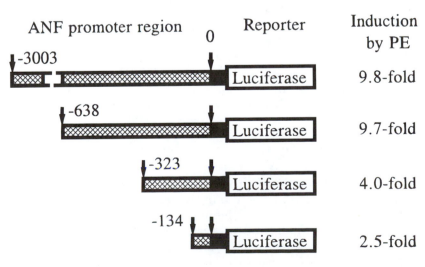

TF•HF-1a, and a muscle-specific factor, TF•HF-1b/MEF-2, which bound to HF-1, were identified in nuclear extracts of cardiac myocytes.[192] Expression cloning subsequently identified a novel HF-1b transcription factor that is restricted to terminally differentiated tissues.[193] Using in vivo footprinting to identify sites occupied by cardiac nuclear factors, another element, termed MLE-1, was discovered. This site contains an upstream stimulating factor (USF)-binding site, which is required for maximal activity of the vMLC-2 promoter in transient expression assays.[194] Studies in transgenic mice harboring vMLC-2/luciferase constructs with mutations in the putative promoter elements have confirmed the importance of the HF-1a and HF-1b sites.[195,196] Mutation of the HF-2 element had little effect on transgene expression, whereas mutation of the HF-3 site and to a lesser extent the E-box increased expression in muscle.[196] These studies suggest that the HF-3 and E-box elements may serve as negative regulatory elements to maintain ventricular-specific expression.

β-MHC Promoter Region

Studies on the β-MHC promoter region have identified a proximal "enhancer core" consensus sequence (originally identified in viral enhancers) between −215 and −196 bp that binds the mammalian transcriptional enhancer factor-1 (TEF-1).[197] The proximal enhancer core also contains a 7 bp M-CAT motif that is known to be responsible for expression of cardiac troponin T and other genes.[198] TEF-1 and the M-CAT binding factor may be closely related.[199] Promoter mapping showed that α_1-adrenergic- or cPKC-β-inducibility of β-MHC also maps to this region.[200] The implication is that a PKC-dependent phosphorylation event in some way increases the transactivating activity of TEF-1 and mediates α_1-adrenergic inducibility. In this regard, the closely related factor C/EBP is phosphorylated by PKC in vitro, which leads to an increase in transactivating activity.[201] Thus there may be sites additional to AP-1/TRE sequences that confer inducibility by phorbol esters and PKC.

Other Promoter Regions

Analogous promoter mapping studies have shown that TEF-1 may also be involved in the regulation of the SkM α-actin promoter, although its full expression may require binding of transcription factors to the SREs that are present,[202] and the gene is also regulated by AP-1.[203] Equally, promoter mapping

has shown that the c-*fos* promoter SRE is important in the activation of c-*fos* expression by stretch in cultured cardiac myocytes.[78]

CONCLUSIONS

Although understanding the cellular and molecular biology of cardiac myocyte growth has rapidly advanced, there is still much to be learned. The factors underlying cell cycle arrest seen in the adult cardiac myocyte must be clarified. The signaling pathways involved in the hypertrophic response and regulation of the concomitant changes in gene expression need to be elucidated. In the longer term, the mechanisms of myofibrillar assembly must be unraveled and the signals responsible for the differing patterns of myofibrillar assembly seen in the various anatomic patterns of hypertrophy clarified.

REFERENCES

1. Claycomb WC: Control of cardiac muscle cell division. Trends Cardiovasc Med 1992;2:231
2. Rumyantsev PP: DNA synthesis in atrial myocytes of rats with aortic stenosis. Adv Myocardiol 1983;4:147
3. Grossman WM, Jones D, McLaurin LP: Wall stress and patterns of hypertrophy in the human left ventricle. J Clin Invest 1975;56:56
4. Smith SH, Bishop SP: Regional myocyte size in compensated right ventricular hypertrophy in the ferret. J Mol Cell Cardiol 1985;17:1005
5. Campbell SE, Rakusan K, Gerdes AM: Change in cardiac myocyte size distribution in aortic-constricted neonatal rats. Basic Res Cardiol 1989;84:247
6. Campbell SE, Korecky B, Rakusan K: Remodeling of myocyte dimensions in hypertrophic and atrophic rat hearts. Circ Res 1991;68:984
7. Gerdes AM, Campbell SE, Hilbelink DR: Structural remodeling of cardiac myocytes in rats with arteriovenous fistulas. Lab Invest 1988;57:708
8. Ganau A, Devereux RB, Roman MJ et al: Patterns of left ventricular hypertrophy and geometric remodeling in essential hypertension. J Am Coll Cardiol 1992;19:1550
9. Levy D, Garrison RJ, Savage DD, Kannel WB, Castelli WP: Prognostic implications of echocardiographically determined left ventricular mass in the Framingham Heart Study. N Engl J Med 1990;322:1561
10. Weintraub H, Davis R, Tapscott S et al: The myoD gene family. Nodal point during specification of the muscle cell lineage. Science 1991;251:761
11. Wiman KG: The retinoblastoma gene. Role in cell cycle control and differentiation. FASEB J 1993;7:841
12. Hamel PA, Phillips RA, Muncaster M, Gallie BL: Speculations on the roles of *RB1* in tissue-specific

differentiation, tumor initiation, and tumor progression. FASEB J 1993;7:846

13. Gu W, Schneider JW, Condorelli G et al: Interaction of myogenic factors and the retinoblastoma protein mediates muscle cell commitment and differentiation. Cell 1993;72:309

14. Nadal-Ginard B: Commitment, fusion and biochemical differentiation of a myogenic cell line in the absence of DNA synthesis. Cell 1978;15:855

15. Olson EN: Regulation of muscle transcription by the MyoD family. The heart of the matter. Circ Res 1993;72:1

16. Kim KK, Soonpaa MH, Daud AI et al: Tumor suppressor gene expression during normal and pathological myocardial growth. J Biol Chem 1994;269:22607

17. Springhorn JP, Ellingsen O, Berger HJ, Kelly RA, Smith TW: Transcriptional regulation in cardiac muscle. Coordinate expression of Id with a neonatal phenotype during development and following a hypertrophic stimulus in adult rat ventricular myocytes in vitro. J Biol Chem 1992;267:14360

18. Ludlow JW: Interactions between SV40 large-tumor antigen and the growth suppressor proteins pRB and p53. FASEB J 1993;7:866

19. Behringer RR, Peschon JJ, Messing A et al: Heart and bone tumors in transgenic mice. Proc Natl Acad Sci USA 1988;85:2648

20. Sen A, Dunnmon P, Henderson SA, Gerard RD, Chien KR: Terminally differentiated neonatal rat myocardial cells proliferate and maintain specific differentiated functions following expression of SV40 large T antigen. J Biol Chem 1988;263:19132

21. Field LJ: Atrial natriuretic factor-SV40 T antigen transgenes produce tumors and cardiac arrhythmias in mice. Science 1988;239:1029

22. Steinhelper ME, Lanson NA Jr, Dresdner KP et al: Proliferation in vivo and in culture of differentiated adult atrial cardiomyocytes from transgenic mice. Am J Physiol 1990;259:H1826

23. Delcarpio JB, Lanson NA Jr, Field LJ, Claycomb WC: Morphological characterization of cardiomyocytes isolated from a transplantable cardiac tumor derived from transgenic mouse atria (AT-1 cells). Circ Res 1991;69:1591

24. Katz EB, Steinhelper ME, Delcarpio JB et al: Cardiomyocyte proliferation in mice expressing alpha-cardiac myosin heavy chain-SV40 T-antigen transgenes. Am J Physiol 1992;262:H1867

25. Jackson T, Allard MF, Sreenan CM et al: Transgenic animals as a tool for studying the effect of the c-myc proto-oncogene on cardiac development. Mol Cell Biochem 1991;104:15

26. Robbins RJ, Swain JL: C-myc protooncogene modulates cardiac hypertrophic growth in transgenic mice. Am J Physiol 1992;262:H590

27. Matiuck NV, Swain JL: Proto-oncogenes and cardiac development. Trends Cardiovasc Med 1992;2:61

28. Gruver CL, George SE, Means AR: Cardiomyocyte growth regulation by Ca^{2+}-calmodulin. Trends Cardiovasc Med 1992;2:226

29. Gruver CL, DeMayo F, Goldstein MA, Means AR: Targeted developmental overexpression of calmodulin induces proliferative and hypertrophic growth of cardiomyocytes in transgenic mice. Endocrinology 1993;133:376

30. Caviedes P, Olivares E, Salas K, Caviedes R, Jaimov-

ich E: Calcium fluxes, ion currents and dihydrophyridine receptors in a new immortal cell line from rat heart muscle. J Mol Cell Cardiol 1993;25:829

31. Simpson P, Savion S: Differentiation of rat myocytes in single cell cultures with and without proliferating nonmyocardial cells. Cross-striations, ultrastructure, and chronotropic response to isoproterenol. Circ Res 1982;50:101

32. Simpson P, McGrath A, Savion S: Myocyte hypertrophy in neonatal rat heart cell cultures and its regulation by serum and by catecholamines. Circ Res 1982; 51:787

33. Simpson P: Stimulation of hypertrophy of cultured neonatal rat heart cells through an α_1-adrenergic receptor and induction of beating through an α_1- and β_1-adrenergic receptor interaction. Evidence for independent regulation of growth and beating. Circ Res 1985;56:884

34. Iwaki K, Sukhatme VP, Shubeita HE, Chien KR: α- and β-Adrenergic stimulation induces distinct patterns of immediate early gene expression in neonatal rat myocardial cells. fos/jun Expression is associated with sarcomere assembly; Egr-1 induction is primarily an α_1-mediated response. J Biol Chem 1990;265: 13809

35. Clark WA, Rudnick SJ, LaPres JJ, Lesch M, Decker RS: Hypertrophy of isolated adult feline heart cells following β-adrenergic-induced beating. Am J Physiol 1991;261:C530

36. Clark WA, Rudnick SJ, LaPres JJ, Andersen LC, LaPointe MC: Regulation of hypertrophy and atrophy in cultured adult heart cells. Circ Res 1993;73:1163

37. Ellingsen O, Davidoff AJ, Prasad SK et al: Adult rat ventricular myocytes cultured in defined medium. Phenotype and electromechanical function. Am J Physiol 1993;265:H747

38. Chien KR, Knowlton KU, Zhu H, Chien S: Regulation of cardiac gene expression during myocardial growth and hypertrophy. Molecular studies of an adaptive physiologic response. FASEB J 1991;5:3037

39. Engelmann GL, Dionne CA, Jaye MC: Acidic fibroblast growth factor and heart development. Role in myocyte proliferation and capillary angiogenesis. Circ Res 1993;72:7

40. Parker TG, Packer SE, Schneider MD: Peptide growth factors can provoke "fetal" contractile protein gene expression in rat cardiac myocytes. J Clin Invest 1990;85:507

41. Cummins P: Contractile protein transitions in human cardiac overload. Reality and limitations. Eur Heart J, suppl. F 1986;5:119

42. Komuro I, Yazaki Y: Control of cardiac gene expression by mechanical stress. Annu Rev Physiol 1993; 55:55

43. McMahon SB, Monroe JG: Role of primary response genes in generating cellular responses to growth factors. FASEB J 1992;6:2707

44. Arai M, Matsui H, Periasamy M: Sarcoplasmic reticulum gene expression in cardiac hypertrophy and heart failure. Circ Res 1994;74:555

45. Hanford DS, Thuerauf DJ, Murray SF, Glembotski CC: Brain natriuretic peptide is induced by α_1-adrenergic agonists as a primary response gene in cultured rat cardiac myocytes. J Biol Chem 1994;269:26227

46. Edwards BS, Ackermann DM, Lee ME et al: Identification of atrial natriuretic factor with ventricular tis-

sue in hamsters and humans with congestive heart failure. J Clin Invest 1988;81:82

47. Day M, Schwartz D, Wiegand RC et al: Ventricular atriopeptin. Unmasking of messenger RNA and peptide synthesis by hypertrophy or dexamethasone. Hypertension 1987;9:485

48. Gardner DG: Molecular biology of natriuretic peptides. Trends Cardiovasc Med 1994;4:159

49. Moalic JM, Charlemagne D, Mansier P, Chevalier B, Swynghedauw B: Cardiac hypertrophy and failure—a disease of adaptation. Circulation, suppl. IV 1993;87:21

50. Hewett TE, Grupp IL, Grupp G, Robbins J: α-Skeletal muscle actin is associated with increased contractility in the mouse heart. Circ Res 1994;74:740

51. Shubeita HE, McDonough PM, Harris AN et al: Endothelin induction of inositol phospholipid hydrolysis, sarcomere assembly, and cardiac gene expression in ventricular myocytes. A paracrine mechanism for myocardial cell hypertrophy. J Biol Chem 1990;265:20555

52. Suzuki T, Hoshi H, Mitsui Y: Endothelin stimulates hypertrophy and contractility of neonatal rat cardiac myocytes in a serum-free medium. FEBS Lett 1990;268:149

53. Gardner DG, Newman ED, Nakamura KK, Nguyen KP: Endothelin increases the synthesis and secretion of atrial natriuretic peptide in neonatal rat cardiocytes. Am J Physiol 1991;261:E177

54. Ito H, Hirata Y, Hiroe M et al: Endothelin-1 induces hypertrophy with enhanced expression of muscle-specific genes in cultured neonatal rat cardiomyocytes. Circ Res 1991;69:209

55. Aceto JF, Baker KM: [Sar 1]angiotensin II receptor-mediated stimulation of protein synthesis in chick heart cells. Am J Physiol 1990;258:H806

56. Baker KM, Aceto JF: Angiotensin II stimulation of protein synthesis and cell growth in chick heart cells. Am J Physiol 1990;259:H610

57. Baker KM, Chernin MI, Wixson SK, Aceto JF: Renin-angiotensin system involvement in pressure-overload cardiac hypertrophy in rats. Am J Physiol 1990;259:H324

58. Baker KM, Aceto JF: Angiotensin II stimulation of protein synthesis and cell growth in chick heart cells. Am J Physiol 1990;259:H610

59. Sadoshima J, Izumo S: Molecular characterization of angiotensin II-induced hypertrophy of cardiac myocytes and hyperplasia of cardiac fibroblasts. Critical role of the AT_1 receptor subtype. Circ Res 1993;73:413

60. Sadoshima J, Izumo S: Signal transduction pathways of angiotensin II-induced c-fos gene expression in cardiac myocytes in vitro. Circ Res 1993;73:424

61. Meidell RS, Sen A, Henderson SA, Slahetka MF, Chien KR: α_1-Adrenergic stimulation of rat myocardial cells increases protein synthesis. Am J Physiol 1986;251:H1076

62. Lee HR, Henderson SA, Reynolds R et al: α_1-Adrenergic stimulation of cardiac gene transcription in neonatal rat myocardial cells. Effects on myosin light chain-2 gene expression. J Biol Chem 1988;263:7352

63. Ikeda U, Tsuruya Y, Yaginuma T: α_1-Adrenergic stimulation is coupled to cardiac myocyte hypertrophy. Am J Physiol 1991;260:H953

64. Knowlton KU, Baracchini E, Ross RS et al: Co-regulation of the atrial natriuretic factor and cardiac myosin light chain-2 genes during α-adrenergic stimulation of neonatal rat ventricular cells. Identification of cis sequences within an embryonic and a constitutive contractile protein gene which mediate inducible expression. J Biol Chem 1991;266:7759

65. Parker TG, Schneider MD: Growth factors, proto-oncogenes, and plasticity of the cardiac phenotype. Annu Rev Physiol 1991;53:179

66. Ito H, Hiroe M, Hirata Y et al: Insulin-like growth factor-1 induces hypertrophy with enhanced expression of muscle specific genes in cultured rat cardiomyocytes. Circulation 1993;87:1715

67. Donohue TJ, Dworkin LD, Lango MN et al: Induction of myocardial insulin-like growth factor-I gene expression in left ventricular hypertrophy. Circulation 1994;89:799

68. Duerr RL, Huang S, Miraliakbar HR et al: Insulin-like growth factor 1 enhances ventricular hypertrophy and function during the onset of experimental cardiac failure. J Clin Invest 1995;95:619

69. Adachi S, Ito H, Akimoto H et al: Insulin-like growth factor-II induces hypertrophy with increased expression of muscle specific genes in cultured rat cardiomyocytes. J Mol Cell Cardiol 1994;26:789

70. Komuro I, Kaida T, Shibazaki Y et al: Stretching cardiac myocytes stimulates protooncogene expression. J Biol Chem 1990;265:3595

71. Komuro I, Katoh Y, Kaida T et al: Mechanical loading stimulates cell hypertrophy and specific gene expression in cultured rat cardiac myocytes. Possible role of protein kinase C activation. J Biol Chem 1991;266:1265

72. Sadoshima J, Jahn L, Takahashi T, Kulik TJ, Izumo S: Molecular characterization of stretch-induced adaptation of cultured cardiac cells. An in vitro model of load induced cardiac hypertrophy. J Biol Chem 1992;267:10551

73. Bishopric NH, Kedes L: Adrenergic regulation of the skeletal α-actin gene promoter during myocardial cell hypertrophy. Proc Natl Acad Sci USA 1991;88:2132

74. Bishopric NH, Sato B, Webster KA: β-Adrenergic regulation of a myocardial actin gene via a cyclic AMP-independent pathway. J Biol Chem 1992;267:20932

75. Sen S, Kundu G, Mekhail N et al: Myotrophin. Purification of a novel peptide from spontaneously hypertensive rat heart that influences myocardial growth. J Biol Chem 1990;265:16635

76. Long CS, Henrich CJ, Simpson PC: A growth factor for cardiac myocytes is produced by cardiac nonmyocytes. Cell Regul 1991;2:1081

77. Pennica D, King KL, Shaw et al: Expression cloning of cardiotrophin 1, a cytokine that induces cardiac myocyte hypertrophy. Proc Natl Acad Sci USA 1995;92:1142

78. Sadoshima J, Izumo S: Mechanical stretch rapidly activates multiple signal transduction pathways in cardiac myocytes. Potential involvement of an autocrine/paracrine mechanism. EMBO J 1993;12:1681

79. Sadoshima J, Xu Y, Slayter HS, Izumo S: Autocrine release of angiotensin II mediates stretch-induced hypertrophy of cardiac myocytes in vitro. Cell 1993;75:977

80. Ito H, Hiroe M, Hirata Y et al: Endothelin ET_A recep-

tor antagonist blocks cardiac hypertrophy provoked by hemodynamic overload. Circulation 1994;89:2198

81. LaMorte VJ, Thorburn J, Absher D et al: G$_q$- and Ras-dependent pathways mediate hypertrophy of neonatal rat ventricular myocytes following α_1-adrenergic stimulation. J Biol Chem 1994;269:13490

82. Kijima Y, Saito A, Jetton TL, Magnuson MA, Fleischer S: Differential intracellular location of inositol 1, 4, 5-trisphosphate and ryanodine receptors in cardiomyocytes. J Biol Chem 1993;268:3499

83. Kemp BE, Pearson RB: Protein kinase recognition sequence motifs. Trends Biochem Sci 1990;15:342

84. Allen IS, Cohen NM, Dhallan RS et al: Angiotensin II increases spontaneous contractile frequency and stimulates calcium current in cultured neonatal rat heart myocytes. Insights into the underlying biochemical mechanisms. Circ Res 1988;62:524

85. Baker KM, Singer HA: Identification and characterization of guinea pig angiotensin II receptor. Coupling to inositol phosphate production. Circ Res 1988;62:896

86. Fantl WJ, Johnson DE, Williams LT: Signalling by receptor tyrosine kinases. Annu Rev Biochem 1993;62:453

87. Bogoyevitch MA, Glennon PE, Andersson MB et al: Endothelin-1 and fibroblast growth factors stimulate the mitogen-activated protein kinase signaling cascade in cardiac myocytes. The potential role of the cascade in the integration of two signaling pathways leading to myocyte hypertrophy. J Biol Chem 1994;269:1110

88. Reaven GM: Role of insulin resistance in human disease (syndrome X). An expanded definition. Annu Rev Med 1993;44:121

89. Reaven GM, Laws A: Insulin resistance, compensatory hyperinsulinaemia, and coronary heart disease. Diabetologia 1994;37:948

90. Ford APDW, Williams TJ, Blue DR, Clarke DE: α_1-Adrenoreceptor classification. Sharpening Occam's razor. Trends Pharmacol Sci 1994;15:167

91. Minneman KP: α_1-Adrenergic subtypes, inositol phosphates and sources of cell Ca^{2+}. Pharmacol Rev 1988;40:87

92. Lazou A, Fuller SJ, Bogoyevitch MA, Orfali KA, Sugden PH: Characterization of the stimulation of phosphoinositide hydrolysis by α_1-adrenergic agonists in adult rat heart. Am J Physiol 1994;267:H970

93. Rokosh DG, Bailey BA, Stewart AFR et al: Distribution of α1c-adrenergic receptor mRNA in adult rat tissues by RNase protection assay and comparison with α1b and α1d. Biochem Biophys Res Commun 1994;200:1177

94. Stewart AF, Rokosh DG, Bailey BA et al: Cloning of the rat α_{1C}-adrenergic receptor from cardiac myocytes. α_{1C} α_{1B} α_{1D} mRNAs are present in cardiac myocytes but not cardiac fibroblasts. Circ Res 1994;75:796

95. Knowlton KU, Michel MC, Itani M et al: The α_{1A}-adrenergic receptor subtype mediates biochemical, molecular, and morphological features of cultured myocardial cell hypertrophy. J Biol Chem 1993;268:15374

96. Milano CA, Dolber PC, Rockman HA et al: Myocardial expression of a constitutively active α_{1B}-adrenergic receptor in transgenic mice induces cardiac hypertrophy. Proc Natl Acad Sci USA 1994;91:10109

97. Brown JH, Buxton IL, Brunton LL: α_1-Adrenergic and muscarinic cholinergic stimulation of phosphoinositide hydrolysis in adult rat cardiomyocytes. Circ Res 1985;57:532

98. Sugden PH, Fuller SJ, Mynett JR et al: Stimulation of adult rat vetricular myocyte protein synthesis and phosphoinositide hydrolysis by the endothelins. Biochim Biophys Acta 1993;1175:327

99. Nishizuka Y: Intracellular signalling by hydrolysis of phospholipids and activation of protein kinase C. Science 1992;258:607

100. Hug H, Sarre TF: Protein kinase C isozymes. Divergence in signal transduction. Biochem J 1993;291:329

101. Dekker LV, Parker PJ: Protein kinase C—a question specificity. Trends Biochem Sci 1994;19:73

102. Berridge MJ: Inositol trisphosphate and calcium signalling. Nature 1993;361:315

103. Exton JH: Signaling through phosphatidylcholine breakdown. J Biol Chem 1990;265:1

104. Billah MM, Anthes JC: The regulation and cellular functions of phosphatidylcholine hydrolysis. Biochem J 1990;269:281

105. Dennis EA, Rhee SG, Billah MM, Hannun YA: Role of phospholipase in generating lipid second messengers in signal trasduction. FASEB J 1991;5:2068

106. Castagna M, Takai Y, Kaibuchi K et al: Direct activation of calcium-activated, phospholipid-dependent protein kinase by tumor-promoting phorbol esters. J Biol Chem 1982;257:7847

107. Bogoyevitch MA, Parker PJ, Sugden PH: Characterization of protein kinase C isotype expression in adult rat heart. Protein kinase C-ϵ is a major isotype present, and it is activated by phorbol esters, epinephrine and endothelin. Circ Res 1993;72:757

108. Rybin VO, Steinberg SF: Protein kinase C isoform expression and regulation in the developing heart. Circ Res 1994;74:299

109. Pucéat M, Hilal-Dandan R, Strulovici B, Brunton LL, Brown JH: Differential regulation of protein kinase C isoforms in isolated neonatal and adult rat cardiomyocytes. J Biol Chem 1994;269:16938

110. Clerk A, Bogoyevitch MA, Andersson MB, Sugden PH: Differential activation of protein kinase C isoforms by endothelin-1 and phenylephrine, and subsequent stimulation of p42- and p44mitogen-activated protein kinases in ventricular myocytes cultured from neonatal rat hearts. J Biol Chem 1994;269:32848

111. Henrich CJ, Simpson PC: Differential acute and chronic response of protein kinase C in cultured neonatal rat heart myocytes to α_1 adrenergic and phorbol ester stimulation. J Mol Cell Cardiol 1988;20:1081

112. Dunnmon PM, Iwaki K, Henderson SA, Sen A, Chien KR: Phorbol esters induce immediate-early genes and activate cardiac gene transcription in neonatal rat myocardial cells. J Mol Cell Cardiol 1990;22:901

113. Allo SN, McDermott PJ, Carl LL, Morgan HE: Phorbol ester stimulation of protein kinase C activity and ribosomal DNA transcription. J Biol Chem 1991;266:22003

114. Subeita HE, Martinson EA, van Bilsen M, Chien KR, Brown JH: Transcriptional activation of the cardiac myosin light chain 2 and atrial natriuretic factor genes by protein kinase C in neonatal rat ventricular myocytes. Proc Natl Acad Sci USA 1992;89:1305

115. Allo SN, Carl LL, Morgan HE: Acceleration of growth of cultured cardiomyocytes and translocation of protein kinase C. Am J Physiol 1992;263:C319

116. Kariya K, Karns LR, Simpson PC: Expression of a constitutively activated mutant of the β-isozyme of protein kinase C in cardiac myocytes stimulates the promoter of the β-myosin heavy chain isogene. J Biol Chem 1991;266:10023

117. Kemp BE, Parker MW, Hu S, Tiganis T, House C: Substrate and pseudosubstrate interactions with protein kinases. Determinants of specificity. Trends Biochem Sci 1994;19:440

118. Decock JBJ, Gillespie-Brown J, Parker PJ, Sugden PH, Fuller SJ: Classical, nover and atypical isoforms of PKC stimulate ANF- and TRE/AP-1-regulated-promoter activity in ventricular cardiomyocytes. FEBS Lett 1994;356:275

119. Houser SR, Karns LR, Kariya K, Simpson PC: A dominant negative protein kinase C mutant inhibits α_1-adrenergic induction of the β-myosin heavy chain promoter. Circulation, suppl. I 1993;88:I333

120. Marshall CJ: MAP kinase kinase kinase, MAP kinase kinase and MAP kinase. Curr Opin Gen Dev 1994;4:82

121. Robbins DJ, Zhen E, Cheng M et al: MAP kinases ERK1 and ERK2. Pleiotropic enzymes in a ubiquitous signaling network. Adv Cancer Res 1994;63:93

122. Sturgill TW, Ray LB, Erikson E, Maller JL: Insulin-stimulated MAP-2 kinase phosphorylates and activates ribosomal protein S6 kinase II. Nature 1988;334:715

123. Boulton TG, Nye SH, Robbins DJ et al: ERKs. A family of protein-serine/threonine kinases that are activated and tyrosine phosphorylated in response to insulin and NGF. Cell 1991;65:663

124. Zhou S, Shoelson SE, Chaudhuri M et al: SH2 domains recognize specific phosphopeptide sequences. Cell 1993;72:767

125. Lowenstein EJ, Daly RJ, Batzer AG et al: The SH2 and SH3 domain-containing protein GRB2 links receptor tyrosine kinases to ras signaling. Cell 1992;70:431

126. Egan SE, Giddings BW, Brooks MW et al: Association of Sos Ras exchange protein with Grb2 is implicated in tyrosine signal transduction and transformation. Nature 1993;363:45

127. Gale NW, Kaplan S, Lowenstein EJ, Schlessinger J, Bar-Sagi D: Grb2 mediates the EGF-dependent activation of guanine nucleotide exchange on Ras. Nature 1993;363:88

128. Li N, Batzer A, Daly R et al: Guanine-nucleotide-releasing factor hSos1 binds to Grb2 and links receptor tyrosine kinases to Ras signalling. Nature 1993;363:85

129. Reif K, Buday L, Downward J, Cantrell DA: SH3 domains of the adapter molecule Grb2 complex with two proteins in T cells. The guanine nucleotide exchange protein Sos and a 75-kDa protein that is a substrate for T cell antigen receptor-activated tyrosine kinases. J Biol Chem 1994;269:14081

130. Skolnik EY, Batzer A, Li N et al: The function of GRB2 in linking the insulin receptors to Ras signaling pathways. Science 1993;260:1953

131. Rozakis-Adcock M, Fernley R, Wade J, Pawson T, Bowtell D: The SH2 and SH3 domains of mammalian Grb2 couple the EGF receptor to the Ras activator mSos1. Nature 1993;363:83

132. Fry MJ: Structure, regulation and function of phosphoinositide 3-kinase. Biochim Biophys Acta 1994;1226:237

133. Cockcroft S, Thomas GMH: Inositol-lipid-specific phospholipase C isoenzymes and their differential regulation by receptors. Biochem J 1992;288:1

134. Rhee SG, Choi KD: Regulation of inositol phospholipid-specific phospholipase C isoenzymes. J Biol Chem 1992;267:12393

135. Nishida E, Gotoh Y: The MAP kinase cascade is essential for diverse signal transduction pathways. Trends Biochem Sci 1993;18:128

136. Blumer KJ, Johnson GL: Diversity in function and regulation of MAP kinase pathways. Trends Biochem Sci 1994;19:236

137. McCormick F: How receptors turn Ras on. Nature 1993;363:15

138. Feig LA: Guanine-nucleotide exchange factors. A family of positive regulators of Ras and related GTPases. Curr Opin Cell Biol 1994;6:204

139. Daum G, Eisenmann-Tappe I, Fries H-W, Troppmair J, Rapp UR: The ins and outs of Raf kinases. Trends Biochem Sci 1994;19:474

140. Kyriakis JM, App H, Zhang X. P. et al: Raf-1 activates MAP kinase kinase. Nature 1992;358:417

141. Huang W, Alessandini A, Crews CM, Erikson RL: Raf-1 forms a stable complex with Mek1 and activates Mek1 by serine phosphorylation. Proc Natl Acad Sci USA 1993;90:10947

142. Alessi DR, Saito Y, Campbell DG et al: Identification of the sites in MAP kinase kinase-1 phosphorylated by p74raf-1. EMBO J 1994;13:1610

143. Zheng C-F, Guan K-L: Activation of MEK family kinase requires phosphorylation of two conserved Ser/Thr residues. EMBO J 1994;13:1123

144. Thorburn A, Thorburn J, Chen S-Y et al: HRas-dependent pathways can activate morphological and genetic markers of cardiac muscle cell hypertrophy. J Biol Chem 1993;268:2244

145. Thorburn J, McMahon M, Thorburn A: Raf-1 kinase activity is necessary and sufficient for gene expression changes but not sufficient for cellular morphology changes associated with cardiac myocyte hypertrophy. J Biol Chem 1994;269:30580

146. Thorburn J, Frost JA, Thorburn A: Mitogen-activated protein kinases mediate changes in gene expression, but not cytoskeletal oganization associated with cardiac muscle hypertrophy. J Cell Biol 1994;126:1565

147. Sadoshima J, Qiu Z, Morgan JP, Izumo S: Angiotensin II and other hypertrophic stimuli mediated by G protein-coupled receptors activate tyrosine kinase, mitogen-activated protein kinase, and 90-kD S6 kinase on cardiac myocytes. The critical role of Ca^{2+}-dependent signaling. Circ Res 1995;76:1

148. Bogoyevitch MA, Glennon PE, Sugden PH: Endothelin-1, phorbol esters and phenylephrine stimulate MAP kinase activities in ventricular cardiomyocytes. FEBS Lett 1993;317:271

149. Lazou A, Bogoyevitch MA, Clerk A et al: Regulation of mitogen-activated protein kinase cascade in adult rat heart preparations in vitro. Circ Res 1994;75:932

150. Kolch W, Heidecker G, Kochs G et al: Protein kinase

C α activates RAF-1 by direct phosphorylation. Nature 1993;364:249

151. Howe LR, Marshall CJ: Lysophosphatidic acid stimulates mitogen-activated protein kinase activation via a G-protein-coupled pathway requiring p21^{ras} and p74^{raf-1}. J Biol Chem 1993;268:20717

152. Johnson GL, Gardner AM, Lange-Carter C et al: How does the G protein, G$_{i2}$, transduce mitogenic signals. J Cell Biochem 1994;54:415

153. Hilal-Dandan R, Urasawa K, Brunton LL: Endothelin inhibits adenyl cyclase and stimulates phosphoinositide hydrolysis in adult cardiac myocytes. J Biol Chem 1992;267:10620

154. Hilal-Dandan R, Merck DT, Lujan JP, Brunton LL: Coupling of the type A endothelin receptor to multiple responses in adult rat cardiac myocytes. Mol Pharmacol 1994;45:1183

155. Bogoyevitch MA, Clerk A, Sugden PH: Activation of the mitogen-activated protein kinase cascade by pertussis toxin-sensitive and -insensitive pathways in cultured ventricular cardiomyocytes. Biochem J 1995;309:437

156. Alvarez E, Northwood IC, Gonzalez RA et al: Pro-Leu-Ser/Thr-Pro is a consensus primary sequence for substrate protein phosphorylation. J Biol Chem 1991;266:15277

157. Gonzalez FA, Raden DL, Davis RJ: Identification of substrate recognition determinants for human ERK1 and ERK2 protein kinases. J Biol Chem 1991;266:22159

158. Davis RJ: The mitogen-activated protein kinase signal transduction pathway. J Biol Chem 1993;268:14553

159. Lin LL, Wartmann M, Lin AY et al: cPLA2 is phosphorylated and activated by MAP kinase. Cell 1993;72:269

160. Treisman R: Ternary complex factors. Growth factor regulated transcriptional activators. Curr Opin Gen Dev 1994;4:96

161. Haystead TAJ, Haystead CMM, Hu C, Lin T-A, Lawrence JC Jr: Phosphorylation of PHAS-I by mitogen-activated protein (MAP) kinase. Identification of a site phosphorylated by MAP kinase in vitro and in response to insulin in rat adipocytes. J Biol Chem 1994;269:23185

162. Hu C, Pang S, Kong X, Velleca M, Lawrence JC: Molecular cloning and tissue distribution of PHAS-I, an intracellular target for insulin and growth factors. Proc Natl Acad Sci USA 1994;91:3730

163. Pause A, Belsham GJ, Gingras A-C et al: Insulin-dependent stimulation of protein synthesis by phosphorylation of a regulator of 5'-cap function. Nature 1994;371:762

164. Fuller SJ, Sugden PH: Protein synthesis in rat cardiac myocytes is stimulated at the level of translation by phorbol esters. FEBS Lett 1989;247:209

165. Fuller SJ, Gaitanaki CJ, Sugden PH: Effects catecholamines on protein synthesis in cardiac myocytes and perfused hearts isolated from adult rats. Stimulation of translation is mediated through the α_1-adrenoceptor. Biochem J 1990;266:727

166. Anderson NG, Li P, Marsden LA et al: Raf-1 is a potential substrate for mitogen-activated protein kinase. Biochem J 1991;277:573

167. Matsuda S, Gotoh Y, Nishida E: Phosphorylation of Xenopus mitogen-activated protein (MAP) kinase kinase by MAP kinase kinase kinase and MAP kinase. J Biol Chem 1993;268:3277

168. Ueki K, Matsuda S, Tobe K et al: Feedback regulation of mitogen-activated protein kinase kinase kinase activity of c-Raf-1 by insulin and phorbol ester stimulation. J Biol Chem 1994;269:15756

169. Cheniack AD, Klarlund JK, Czech MP: Phosphorylation of the Ras nucleotide exchange factor Son of Sevenless by mitogen-activated protein kinase. J Biol Chem 1994;269:4717

170. Saito Y, Gomez N, Campbell DG et al: The threonine residues in MAP kinase kinase 1 phosphorylated by MAP kinase in vitro are also phosphorylated in nerve growth factor-stimulated phaeochromocytoma (PC12) cells. FEBS Lett 1994;341:119

171. Brunet A, Pagès G, Pouysségur J: Growth factor-stimulated MAP kinase induces rapid retrophosphorylation and inhibition of MAP kinase kinase (MEK1). FEBS Lett 1994;346:299

172. Hall A: Small GTP-binding proteins and the regulation of the actin cytoskeleton. Annu Rev Cell Biol 1994;10:31

173. Shibasaki F, Fukami K, Fukui Y, Takenawa T: Phosphatidylinositol 3-kinase binds to α-actinin through the p85 subunit. Biochem J 1994;302:551

174. Fukami K, Endo T, Imamura M, Takenawa T: α-Actinin and vinculin are PIP$_2$-binding proteins involved in signaling by tyrosine kinase. J Biol Chem 1994;269:1518

175. Karin, M: The AP-1 complex and its role in transcriptional control by protein kinase C. p. 235. In Cohen P, Foulkes JG (eds): The Hormonal Control of Gene Transcription. Elsevier, Amsterdam, 1991

176. Hunter T, Karin M: The regulation of transcription by phosphorylation. Cell 1992;70:375

177. Karin M: Signal transduction from cell surface to the nucleus through phosphorylation of transcription factors. Curr Opin Cell Biol 1994;6:415

178. Boyle WJ, Smeal T, Defize LHK et al: Activation of protein kinase C decreases phosphorylation of c-*Jun* at sites that negatively regulate its DNA binding activity. Cell 1991;64:573

179. Davis RJ: MAPKs. New JNK expands the group. Trends Biochem Sci 1994;19:470

180. Hipskind RA, Rao VN, Mueller CGF, Reddy ESP, Nordheim A: Ets-related protein Elk-1 is homologous to the c-*fos* regulatory factor p62^{TCF}. Nature 1991;354:531

181. Wasylyk B, Han SL, Giovane A: The Ets family of transcription factors. Eur J Biochem 1993;211:7

182. Gille H, Sharrocks AD, Shaw PE: Phosphorylation of transcription factor p62TCF by MAP kinase stimulates ternary complex formation at c-*fos* promoter. Nature 1992;358:414

183. Marais R, Wynne J, Treisman R: The SRF accessory protein Elk-1 contains a growth factor-regulated transcriptional activation domain. Cell 1993;73:381

184. Sukhatme VP, Cao X, Chang LC et al: A zinc finger-encoding gene coregulated with c-*fos* during growth and differentiation, and after cellular depolarization. Cell 1988;53:37

185. Neyses L, Nouskas J, Luyken J et al: Induction of immediate-early genes by angiotensin II and endothelin-1 in adult rat cardiomyocytes. J Hypertens 1993;11:927

186. Neyses L, Nouskas J, Vetter H: Inhibition of endothe-

lin-1 induced myocardial protein synthesis by an antisense oligonucleotide against the early growth response gene-1. Biochem Biophys Res Commun 1991; 181:22

187. Rupprecht HD, Sukhatme VP, Rupprecht AP, Sterzel RB, Coleman DL: Serum response elements mediate protein kinase C dependent transcriptional induction of early growth response gene-1 by arginine vasopressin in rat mesangial cells. J Cell Physiol 1994;159: 311

188. Huang R-P, Adamson ED: The phosphorylated forms of the transcription factor, Egr- 1, bind to DNA more efficiently than non-phosphorylated. Biochem Biophys Res Commun 1994;200:1271

189. Kovacic-Milivojevic B, Gardner DG: Divergent regulation of the human atrial natriuretic peptide gene by c-*jun* and c-*fos*. Mol Cell Biol 1992;12:292

190. Rockman HA, Ross RS, Harris AN et al: Segregation of atrial-specific and inducible expression of an atrial natriuretic factor transgene in an in vivo murine model of cardiac hypertrophy. Proc Natl Acad Sci USA 1991;88:8277

191. Zhu H, Garcia AV, Ross RS, Evans SM, Chien KR: A conserved 28-base-pair element (HF-1) in the rat cardiac myosin light-chain-2 gene confers cardiac-specific and α-adrenergic-inducible expression in cultured neonatal rat myocardial cells. Mol Cell Biol 1991;11:2273

192. Navankasattusas S, Zhu H, Garcia AV, Evans SM, Chien KR: A ubiquitous factor (HF-1a) and a distinct muscle factor (HF-1b/MEF-2) form an E-box-independent pathway for cardiac muscle gene expression. Mol Cell Biol 1992;12:1469

193. Zhu H, Nguyen VT, Brown AB et al: A novel, tissue-restricted zinc finger protein (HF-1b) binds to the cardiac regulatory element (HF-1b/MEF-2) in the rat myosin light-chain 2 gene. Mol Cell Biol 1993;13:4432

194. Navankasattusas S, Sawadogo M, van Bilsen M, Dang CV, Chien KR: The basic helix-loop-helix protein upstream stimulating factor regulates the cardiac ventricular myosin light-chain 2 gene via independent cis regulatory elements. Mol Cell Biol 1994; 14:7331

195. Lee KJ, Ross RS, Rockman HA et al: Myosin light chain-2 luciferase transgenic mice reveal distinct regulatory programs for cardiac and skeletal muscle-specific expression of a single contractile protein gene. J Biol Chem 1992;267:15875

196. Lee KJ, Hickey R, Zhu H, Chien KR: Positive regulatory elements (HF-1a and HF-1b) and novel negative regulatory element (HF-3) mediate ventricular muscle-specific expression of myosin light-chain 2-luciferase fusion genes in transgenic mice. Mol Cell Biol 1994;14:1220

197. Kariya K, Farrance IKG, Simpson PC: Transcriptional enhancer factor-1 in cardiac myocytes interacts with an α_1-adrenergic and β-protein kinase C-inducible element in the rat β-myosin heavy chain promoter. J Biol Chem 1993;268:26658

198. Ordahl CP: Developmental regulation of sarcomeric gene expression. Curr Top Dev Biol 1992;26:145

199. Farrance IK, Mar JH, Ordahl CP: M-CAT binding factor is related to the SV40 enhancer binding factor, TEF-1. J Biol Chem 1992;267:17234

200. Kariya K, Karns LR, Simpson PC: An enhancer core element mediates stimulation of the rat β-myosin heavy chain promoter by an α_1-adrenergic agonist and activated β-protein kinase C in hypertrophy of cardiac myocytes. J Biol Chem 1994;269:3775

201. Mahoney CW, Shuman J, McKnight SL, Chen HC, Huang KP: Phosphorylation of the CCAAT-enhancer binding protein by protein kinase C attenuates site-selective DNA binding. J Biol Chem 1992;267:19396

202. MacLellan WR, Lee T-C, Schwartz RJ, Schneider MD: Transforming growth factor-β response elements of the skeletal α-actin gene. Combinatorial action of serum response factor YY1, and the SV40 enhancer-binding protein, TEF-1. J Biol Chem 1994; 269:16754

203. Bishopric NH, Jayasena V, Webster KA: Positive regulation of the skeletal α-actin gene by Fos and Jun in cardiac myocytes. J Biol Chem 1992;267:25535

204. Nordheim A: CREB takes CBP to tango. Nature 1994; 370:177

5 Molecular Genetics of Cardiomyopathies

Gisèle Bonne
Lucie Carrier
Ketty Schwartz

Cardiomyopathies represent a variety of myocardial diseases that are an important cause of morbidity and mortality throughout the world and whose classification has evolved since the middle of this century. Currently, they are defined as "heart muscle diseases of unknown etiology" and are classified as dilated, hypertrophic, or restrictive, depending on the type of functional impairment.[1] Although apparently clear, this clinical classification presents major limitations, and over the past few years new and unexpected insights into the pathogenesis and classification of cardiomyopathies has emerged from the localization and identification of disease genes of several inherited forms. This chapter focuses on the inherited forms of hypertrophic cardiomyopathy (HCM) and dilated cardiomyopathy (DCM) for which an abnormal gene or defective protein has been identified. Particular emphasis is placed on the principles of reverse genetics or positional cloning, the striking genetic heterogeneity of these inherited cardiomyopathies, and the functional consequences and clinical implications of the identified mutations.

HISTORICAL PERSPECTIVE OF MOLECULAR GENETICS

The fundamental discovery during the 1950s and 1960s of the structure and organization of the DNA molecule and the implication that DNA was passing on genetic information to subsequent generations were made in prokaryotes. Until the 1970s it was technically impossible to isolate and analyze a gene from eukaryotes, mainly because of the disproportion between the estimated mean size of individual genes and that of the whole genome. Each gene represents about one millionth of the DNA molecule; and although there is enough DNA to form about 10 million genes, less than 1 percent of DNA is used to code for proteins. The difficulty was thus to isolate a sequence of 1 pg from 1 μg of DNA and to prepare it in sufficient amounts. Major progress was made during the 1970s with the development of techniques that finally led to modern molecular biology and genetics.

The basic principles of in vitro transcription made it possible to generate complementary DNA (cDNA) from messenger RNA (mRNA)[2,3] and to digest DNA by specific restriction endonucleases, which allowed cutting the DNA into fragments of different sizes.[4,5] These processes opened the route for cloning and thus for obtaining any DNA sequence in large quantities in an appropriate host.[6] Rapid nucleic sequencing followed,[7,8] as did the discovery by Southern that after separation of DNA fragments by electrophoresis on agarose or polyacrylamide gel the DNA can be transferred from the gel through capillary action to a nitrocellulose buffer.[9] The fears raised by these new genetic manipulations, which led to the moratorium of P. Berg and to the Asilomar Conference in 1975,[10] slowed the pace of advancement. Important discoveries rapidly followed, however, that were pivotal to the widespread development of recombinant DNA techniques. Examination of DNA from several individuals revealed sequence variations that are known to involve one nucleotide every 200 to 500 bp of homologous genes.[11] Some of these DNA changes involve restriction endonuclease cleavage sites, which are either created or abolished; these changes were called restriction fragment length polymorphisms (RFLPs). The process of disease gene identification was thus started followed by the concept of linkage analysis in 1980.[12]

Linkage analysis—the first step of reverse genetic or positional cloning—determines in a given pedigree the co-segregation of a distinct allele of a genetic locus with the disease trait transmitted in a mendellian fashion. The likelihood for linkage (Lod scores) is analyzed with statistical computer programs.[13,14] Positive Lod scores indicate close linkage between the disease gene and the analyzed locus and permit estimation of the genetic distance that separates them. RFLP are biallelic by definition. It became rapidly evident that in the absence of large kindreds they are poorly informative markers, as the expected frequency of heterozygosity at a locus is directly related to the number of common alleles in a population. The discovery of hypervariable loci due to repeat polymorphisms, which occur secondary to variations in the number of tandem repeats, was based on the development of polymorphic genetic markers (see Nakamura et al.[15] for review). These short interspersed tandem repeats or microsatellites are widely distributed in the genome and can be readily isolated from genomic libraries. There has been an impressive increase in the list of microsatellite markers: More than 800 had been reported at the end of 1992,[16] and more than 6,000 are now available (see Weber[17] for review). They constitute an almost continuous set of highly informative markers covering the genome and now have a dramatic impact on disease gene identification. Various polymerase chain reaction (PCR)-based techniques have been reported to detect them: (1) phosphorus 32 (^{32}P)-5′-end-labeled oligonucleotides; (2) ^{32}P incorporated during PCR amplification reaction; (3) ^{32}P-3′-end-tailed probes; (4) nonradioactive probes to hybridize the amplification product transferred onto a membrane after electrophoresis; and (5) a technique using a fluorescence-based automated DNA fragment analyzer which has been applied to large-scale genetic mapping (see Dausse et al.[18] for review). More recently, we have developed a method based on the use of ^{33}P and the β-imager (Biospace, Paris, France), which is a highly sensitive gaseous detector[19] that has several advantages over the tradi-

tional approaches, including its time-saving and efficiency.[18]

The final steps of positional cloning—disease gene isolation and validation—are particularly laborious and time-consuming.

1. When a new disease locus is specifically assigned on the genome, it may be possible to "query" that chromosomal region in a computer database and have a list of genes and expressed sequence tags (ESTs) assigned to the same region. These genes and ESTs are then considered candidates for that particular disease. The features of the genes are compared to the features of the disease to find the gene that is the strongest candidate for that particular disease. If no such genes are found, the second approach consists in gene cloning from libraries as cosmids or yeast artificial chromosomes.

2. Subsequently and finally, intragenic abnormalities of that gene are sought in affected individuals using procedures for mutation detection to discover if the candidate gene is the disease gene. Several useful mutation detection techniques have evolved with the advent of PCR. The various methods have complementary strengths, and a suitable procedure for virtually any experimental situation is now available (see Grompe[20] for review). Large gene alterations can be detected by cytogenetic techniques, Southern blot hybridization, or PCR-based techniques. The detection of single base changes (the most common type of mutation at most loci) can be carried out by several techniques, such as denaturing gradient gel electrophoresis (DGGE),[21] single-strand conformation polymorphisms (SSCP),[22] heteroduplex analysis or double-strand conformation polymorphisms (DSCP),[23,24] RNase A cleavage,[25] chemical mismatch cleavage,[26] or direct sequencing.[7,8] All of these methods can be applied to genomic DNA or cDNA reverse-transcribed from RNA purified from lymphoblastoid cell lines.

HYPERTROPHIC CARDIOMYOPATHY

Clinical Symptoms and Prevalence

Although various teams have systematically described the unique features of HCM since the mid 1950s, isolated observations of myocardial diseases that can usually be interpreted as HCM were reported earlier. The first was in France by Vulpian[27] followed by one in Germany by Schmincke, who proposed that primary subaortic stenosis was the cause of progressive hypertrophy.[28] HCM is now defined by the presence of unexplained left ventricular hypertrophy that is usually predominant in the interventricular septum and may or may not be associated with right ventricular hypertrophy. This particular phenotype can change with time and so may lead to confusion. Hypertrophy that is recognized on echocardiography develops during the adolescent growth phase and usually persists throughout adult life. In some patients, however, the septum later thins, and the left ventricle becomes more like that seen with DCM. In most patients significant cellular disorganization (myocardial disarray) is present in the interventricular septum and the free wall. Within the myocyte, the myofibrillar arrangement itself may also be abnormal with loss of the usual parallel arrays. The disease is associated with diastolic dysfunction, myocardial ischemia, and life-threatening arrhythmias that can result in sudden death. The clinical features of HCM are heterogeneous. There is considerable variability in the morphologic manifestations of ventricular hypertrophy[29,30] and the prognosis of affected individuals.[31–33] This variation is often most apparent between unrelated families, but intrafamilial heterogeneity may also be pronounced. The prevalence of HCM is reported to be 17.9 per 100,000 individuals.[34]

Familial Forms

The fact that HCM is sometimes familial has been known for a long time. The first genetic study of familial hypertrophic cardiomyopathy (FHC) was performed more than 30 years ago by Hollman et al., who described a kindred with asymmetric cardiac hypertrophy inherited as an autosomal dominant trait.[35] Studies carried out before the development of echocardiography underestimated the familial incidence of HCM. Two large family studies performed with two-dimensional echocardiography showed that HCM is familial in 50 to 60 percent of cases.[36,37] This number is probably underestimated and will certainly increase in the future, as genetic data have indicated that some apparent sporadic forms of the disease are in fact related to de novo and inherited mutations. In most instances the mode of inheritance is autosomal dominant.[36–38]

Physiopathologic Hypotheses

Although HCM is a cardiac disease of unknown etiology, five main hypotheses have been suggested for the primary defect that causes HCM[39]: (1) abnormal myocardial calcium kinetics, which could explain the diastolic dysfunction; (2) abnormal sympathetic stimulation because of heightened responsiveness of the heart to or excessive production of circulating catecholamines or reduced neuronal uptake of cardiac norepinephrines; (3) abnormally thickened coronary arteries that do not dilate normally and so lead to myocardial ischemia with resultant fibrosis and abnormal compensatory hypertrophy; (4) subendocardial ischemia, which depletes the energy stores essential for the uptake of calcium during diastole, increasing diastolic stiffness; and (5) structural abnormalities, such as catenoid configuration of the septum, that lead to myocardial cell hypertrophy and disarray. As is shown in the rest of this chapter, one striking result of the genetic analyses is that none of these hypotheses has been validated as a primary cause of familial HCM.

Genetic Analyses of Familial HCM

Because FHC is inherited as an autosomal dominant trait, all affected members of a given family must have an identical genetic defect. In unrelated families with HCM, the defect need not to be the same; that is, either a distinct mutation in the same gene (allelic or intragenic heterogeneity) or a mutation in different genes (nonallelic or intergenic heterogeneity) can lead to the same phenotype. This situation is indeed what has been found.

CMH1 AND β-MHC GENE MUTATIONS

The first locus for FHC (CMH1) was identified on chromosome 14q11–q12 (Fig. 5-1).[40,41] The genes coding for the two cardiac myosin heavy chain (MHC) isoforms (α and β) are located in tandem on this locus and were therefore unexpected candidate genes. With the use of refined genetic mapping and DNA analysis, the β-MHC gene was subsequently identified as the morbid gene carrying a point mutation[42] that resulted in substitution of a single amino acid in the myosin molecule. After this initial description, several other families have shown evidence of linkage to CMH1.[43–46] At the present time, 29 published missense mutations have been found in the β-MHC gene (see Schwartz et al.[41] for review). All are localized to either the head region or the junction of the head/rod domains. Almost simultaneously, our team and a group from South Africa found that arginine 403 is a hot spot for mutations, suggesting a major role of this residue in the maintenance of normal function of the MHC molecule.[47,48] In one family, a deletion involving the carboxyl-terminal region of the β-MHC has also been found,[49] but it is not clear if it is the cause of the disease in this family.

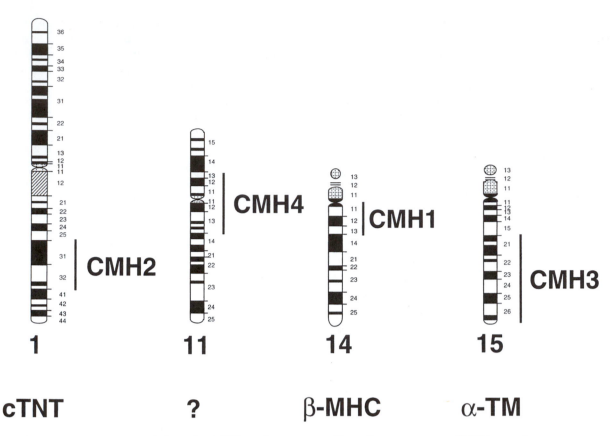

Fig. 5-1. Chromosomal loci for FHC and corresponding disease genes: CMH1 on chromosome 14q11–q12, CMH2 on chromosome 1q3, CMH3 on chromosome 15q2, and CMH4 on chromosome 11p13–q13. cTNT, cardiac troponin T gene; β-MHC, β-myosin heavy chain gene; α-TM, α-tropomyosin gene. (From Schwartz et al.,[41] with permission.)

Intergenic Heterogeneity of FHC

It is well known that FHC is phenotypically heterogeneous according to clinical and echocardiographic analysis and pathologic findings (see Maron et al.[50] for review). It was a surprise to discover in 1990 that FHC was also genetically heterogeneous, as in two of four families no linkage to CMH1 was found.[51] The next major problem with the genetic analysis was to obtain access to large informative pedigrees (more than 50 members). To circumvent this problem and to analyze small or medium-size families, we have used two highly informative microsatellite markers contained in the β-MHC gene, which we named MYOI and MYOII.[52–55] Analysis of these microsatellites enabled us to exclude linkage to CMH1 in eight unrelated medium-size families.[54] Almost simultaneously, other families in which the disease gene was not linked to CMH1 were identified.[44,46,55–58] This hypothesized genetic heterogeneity was subsequently confirmed by our team (and by others) by the discovery of three other loci, on chromosomes 1q3 (CMH2),[59] 15q2 (CMH3),[60] and 11p13–q13 (CMH4).[61] We have evidence that a fifth locus ex-

ists,[62] and it has been reported that a new disease locus on chromosome 7q3 associates FHC with the Wolff-Parkinson-White syndrome.[63]

The proportion of FHC that can be attributed to each CMH loci is not yet known. We have screened 28 unrelated French families by haplotype analysis; 14 families were not informative, showing linkage to more than one locus. Among the other 14 families, five were linked to CMH1, two to CMH2, none to CMH3, and three to CMH4; four appeared unmapped to any of the known loci (L. Carrier et al., unpublished data). This distribution among French families is in agreement with that found by Watkins et al. in families of various origins[64] and suggests that each locus makes only a small contribution to the total disease prevalence.

CMH2 and CMH3: Cardiac Troponin T and α-Tropomyosin Gene Mutations

By synteny with the murine genome and precise genetic analysis, the disease genes for the CMH2 and CMH3 loci have been identified (Fig. 5-1). They encode for two proteins of the thin filament of the sarcomere: cardiac troponin T (cTNT) on CMH2 and α-tropomyosin (α-TM) on CMH3.[65] Two missense mutations were found in the α-TM gene in exon 5.[64,65] As for the cTNT gene, a total of eight sequence changes were identified that exhibited the features expected of disease-causing mutations.[64,65] Six were missense mutations, which alter the encoded amino acid; one is a deletion of three nucleotides, which does not cause a frameshift; and the last is a point mutation in the 5' splice donor site of intron 15, which results in truncated mRNAs. The missense mutations affect nucleotides encoding a region involved in calcium-insensitive binding to α-tropomyosin, and the mutation at the donor site produces markedly aberrant cardiac troponin T mRNA transcripts, which alter the carboxyl-terminus of troponin T, a region contributing to calcium-dependent binding to tropomyosin. These observations that α-tropomyosin and cardiac troponin T, which along with β-MHC have central roles in the structure and function of the sarcomere in striated muscle, suggest that one of the pathophysiologic mechanisms of FHC could be impaired function of the contractile apparatus.

CMH4: SEARCHING FOR THE DISEASE GENE

The finding that FHC is, at least for some families, a disease of the sarcomere suggests that mutations in other contractile protein genes from either the thick or the thin filament, or in any protein implicated in filament assembly, may account for FHC at other loci including CMH4 on chromosome 11p13–q13. At the present time only one family has been reported as showing linkage to CMH4,[61] but we have evidence that at least two other families are linked to this single locus as well. Enlargement of the first family, identification of two others, and analysis of 14 other new informative microsatellite markers has allowed us to identify new recombinant individuals and to reduce the candidate interval from 23 centimorgan (cM) to 9 cM.[66] From the 60 genes already located in this interval, none encodes for another sarcomeric protein. The cardiac troponin C gene, which is one of the thin component of the thin filament, was not mapped to the genome, and we tried to locate it. The analysis of DNA isolated from hybrid cell lines containing specifically human chromosome 11 did not allow us to map the cardiac troponin C gene on CMH4 (data not shown). Subsequently, we tested another hypothesis of an energetic defect, and the gene encoding subunit VIII of the cytochrome c oxidase complex was located in the interval. No major alterations and no point mutations

were found in this gene, indicating that it was not the disease gene of the CMH4 locus.[67] It is clear that much more work is needed to identify this disease gene.

Functional Consequences of β-Myosin Heavy-Chain Gene Mutations

None of the previous physiopathologic hypotheses of FHC would have led us to suspect that one of the molecular bases could be a defect in the contractile apparatus; nevertheless, certain forms of the disease involve mutations in sarcomeric protein genes. Of course, neither linkage analyses nor the identification of point mutations is sufficient to prove that the mutations are the origin of FHC. Some clues have nevertheless been provided for β-MHC gene mutations.

First, all of the mutations present the characteristics of disease-causing mutations. They co-segregate with the disease in the proband's pedigrees and are never found in unaffected individuals, and the amino acid substitutions they produce occur at residues that have been conserved throughout vertebrate evolution, implying particular functional or structural importance.

Second, the tertiary structure of the head region of the myosin polypeptide[68,69] allows identification of the location of each of the β-MHC mutations relative to the functional domains and prediction of conformational changes in polypeptide folding and shape in response to particular amino acid substitutions. One striking finding is that all of the 29 mutations described to date are within functional regions of the molecule: the ATP-binding site, actin-binding site, or head–rod junction region (Table 5-1). This finding was not predicted from the primary structure of the molecule and suggests that the mutations could have a deleterious effect on the various functions of the myosin molecule. Indeed, for the Asn232Ser mutation that we found,[70] a modified function of the myosin has been predicted because an increase in actin-activated ATPase activity of the myosin has been observed with a monoclonal antibody directed against the region containing residues 215 to 248.[71]

Third, some β-MHC mutations were found to be expressed at mRNA and protein levels in both the myocardial and skeletal muscle of affected individuals. The Arg403Gln mutation was found to be expressed in mRNA of both the myocardial and biceps muscle of the same proband,[72,73] and the mutant Arg719Trp β-MHC protein was found to be present

Table 5-1. Predicted Localization of the β-MHC Mutations in the Three-Dimensional Model of the Molecule

Localization in the molecule	Amino acid substitution	Exon	Nucleotide substitution
ATP binding site	Thr 124 Ile	5	C → T
	Arg 143 Gln	5	G → A
	Tyr 162 Cys	5	A → G
	Gln 222 Lys	8	C → A
	Asn 232 Ser	8	A → G
	Arg 249 Gln	9	G → A
	Gly 256 Glu	9	G → A
Actin binding site	Arg 403 Gln	13	G → A
	Arg 403 Leu	13	G → T
	Arg 403 Trp	13	C → T
	Phe 513 Cys	15	T → G
	Gly 584 Arg	16	G → C
	Val 606 Met	16	G → A
	Lys 615 Asn	16	G → C
"Cleft" region	Arg 453 Cys	14	C → T
"Reactive cysteines" region	Gly 716 Arg	19	G → A
	Arg 719 Trp	19	C → T
	Arg 719 Gln	19	G → A
	Arg 723 Cys	20	C → T
	Pro 731 Leu	20	C → T
	Gly 741 Arg	20	G → C
	Gly 741 Arg	20	G → A
Interaction with essential light chains	Asp 778 Gly	21	A → G
Head–rod junction	Arg 870 His	22	G → A
	Leu 908 Val	23	C → G
	Glu 924 Lys	23	G → A
	Glu 930 Lys	23	G → A
	Glu 935 Lys	23	G → A
	Glu 949 Lys	23	G → A

(From Dufour C: Hétérogénéité Génétique de la Cardiomyopathie Hypertrophique. Doctoral thesis, University of Paris, Paris, 1995, with permission.)

in the myocardium and skeletal muscle of two unrelated patients.[74–76] It is not known if the other types of β-MHC mutant alleles are transcribed into the corresponding proteins.

Fourth, de novo myosin mutations have been found in patients with sporadic hypertrophic cardiomyopathy whose parents were clinically and genetically unaffected, and one of these mutations was transmitted to an affected child.[77,78]

Fifth, myofibrillar organization appears to be intact in a patient with the Arg403Gln mutation,[76] and protein stability does not seem to be markedly affected in mammalian nonmuscle cells transfected with expression constructs encoding seven different FHC mutants.[79] However, the ability to form filaments seems to be impaired, as up to one-third of the transfected cells fail to form filamentous structures.[79] It should be pointed out, however, that the latter studies were carried out in nonmuscle cell types. It is thus not completely clear if the mutant MHC proteins are indeed abnormally assembled in the muscle context, and it is equally unclear if this arrangement would explain myofibrillar disarray in FHC.

Sixth, although the basal ATPase activities of an Arg403Gln mutant truncated myosin produced in baculovirus are similar to the wild type, the actin-activated ATPase activity is markedly depressed, as is the in vitro motility of the actin filaments across myosin fragments on a nitrocellulose substrate.[80] The same conclusion was drawn by Cuda et al.[75] with an Arg403Gln mutated myosin isolated directly from a fresh biopsy of skeletal muscle of a patient.

Seventh, in vitro studies have analyzed the contractile properties of single slow-twitch muscle fibers from patients with various β-MHC gene mutations.[81] Fibers containing either Gly741Arg or Arg403Gln mutations displayed abnormal contractile properties (i.e., abnormal force–velocity relations and reduced power output). If these results, observed in skeletal slow-twitch muscle fibers, could be translated to the cardiac muscle context, one can predict that the above β-MHC mutations would result in alteration of the force velocity and thus in alteration of the pressure velocity of the cardiac muscle. The authors suggested that, at a given pressure, a heart containing a mutant myosin would produce less power than a normal heart of the same size. Hence, one way for the heart to compensate for this aberration would be to undergo hypertrophy, which would decrease the load on the individual myosin cross-bridge. It should be pointed out that fibers with Gly256Glu mutation did not present any impaired contractile properties,[81] indicating that more complete analysis is required before a general view of the pathogenesis of FHC can be offered.

Phenotype–Genotype Relations

Phenotype/genotype analyses carried out to date for β-MHC gene mutations are preliminary but so far have not shown a clear relation between a given mutation and the clinical features or prognosis of FHC (see Schwartz et al.[41] for review). Three aspects have been analyzed and can be highlighted.

1. The degree and the pattern of hypertrophy may be different in unrelated families carrying the same mutation or even in relatives of the same family, but the number of affected individuals in a given family is in many instances too small to provide conclusive evidence.[41] For instance, it was observed that the Val606Met mutation is associated with various degrees of hypertrophy in three unrelated families, but this finding did not influence the outcome.[82]

2. There were important differences in the survival of affected individuals from one mutation to another. Kaplan-Meier analyses, showing the survival of affected members of a family,[82] at first suggested that a mutation that produced no change in the charge of the β-MHC molecule would be more benign than other mutations. This view was challenged by Fananapazir et al.,[83] who found the same so-called benign mutations in another kindred where there was a low survival rate at 50 years of age and a high incidence of sudden death and disease-related deaths.

3. There is much evidence that many of the point mutations in the β-MHC gene are associated with low penetrance. For example, in our pedigrees with Arg403Leu, Arg403Trp, and Asn232Ser mutations, there are 28 gene carriers; and as many as eight of them, aged 21 to 51 years, are healthy and do not present any electro- or echocardiographic features of HCM.[47,70] These findings emphasize the role of other factors, including environmental differences, acquired traits (e.g., differences in life style, risk factors, exercise), or modifier genes that could modulate the phenotypic expression of the disease.

Phenotype/genotype analyses of other affected genes, including the α-TM gene on chromosome 15 and the cTNT gene on chromosome 1, are at an early stage and do not allow any definite conclusions to be made. Preliminary studies suggest differences in phenotypes and prognosis according to the type of mutation.[59,60,64,65]

DILATED CARDIOMYOPATHY

Clinical Symptoms and Prevalence

Dilated cardiomyopathies (DCMs) are characterized by a large ventricular dilation, impaired systolic function, development of progressive refractory congestive heart failure, and a poor prognosis. DCMs are the most common forms of cardiomyopathy, their prevalence in the US population being estimated at 36.5 per 100,000 persons.[34]

Familial Forms

Although it was generally considered to be a multifactorial disease related to various toxic environmental factors, there is, as in HCM, a strong genetic component in DCM, estimated to be present in approximately 20 percent of cases.[84] In the present study, segregation analysis of the pedigrees supported the evidence for a single dominant locus with incomplete penetrance. In most cases, however, the size of the family and the number of affected individuals do not allow an accurate analysis of the mode of inheritance. Autosomal dominant transmission was nevertheless most frequently observed,[85–87] and autosomal-recessive,[85–87] and X-linked[85,88] inheritances have been found. The apparent heterogeneity in the mode of transmission raises the possibility of numerous genetic factors being involved or the intervention of both genetic and multifactorial factors in degrees varying from one individual to another.[87]

Disease Genes

Two reports of particular interest have begun to reveal the genetic origin of this pathology. In three pedigrees with X-linked DCM, defects in the dystrophin genes and low abundance of cardiac dystrophin but not skeletal muscle dystrophin were found. The authors demonstrated that this disease is associated with deletion of the muscle-promoter region and the first exon of the gene.[89,90] A reduced dystrophin content was also found in the BIO 14.6 hamster, which is a widely recognized animal model of DCM.[91] The pathogenetic hypothesis for this type of DCM is disruption of the membrane cytoskeleton of the myocyte due to reduced dystrophin content. This hypothesis has been reinforced by finding a deficiency of a dystrophin-associated glycoprotein in this same strain of hamster.[92] Because Duchenne and Becker muscular dystrophies are due to dystrophin gene abnormalities and there are some reports of Becker dystrophy with predominant or even exclusive cardiac involvement,[93,94] the possibility was raised that some patients with DCM are in fact carriers of a dystrophin gene defect. In a series of patients with familial and nonfamilial DCM, screening for dystrophin gene defects did not reveal any known deletions observed for Duchenne and Becker muscular dystrophies.[95] It should be pointed out that only 14 exons were studied, and the promoter region of the gene was not analyzed. It is possible that the proportion of cases of DCM related to the dystrophin gene in individuals with DCM should be limited to cases of X-linked cardiomyopathy and cardiomyopathy with muscle abnormalities.

Most recently, a morbid gene that causes both an atrioventricular conduction defect and DCM in a large kindred with autosomal dominant transmission has been mapped to chromosome 1p1–q1.[96] The gene has not yet been found, but the authors speculate that the gap protein connexin 40 is a candidate gene for this particular phenotype of DCM.

CONCLUSIONS

The development of molecular genetics has brought completely new insights to the understanding of HCM and DCM, which were previously known as idiopathic diseases. This development has marked the dawn of a new era—genetic cardiology—and the HCMs have opened this fascinating route.

Genetic analyses of HCM are revealing a more complex picture than might have been expected from clinical studies. Three disease genes have been identified, indicating a high intergenic heterogeneity; and within these genes many mutations have been found, reflecting an intragenic or allelic heterogeneity. All of these mutations lead to the same overall phenotype. The genes encode components of the sarcomere—β-MHC, cTNT, and α-TM—which suggests that certain forms of FHC are diseases of the sarcomere. Other unidentified disease genes for FHC exist that could encode other components of the contractile apparatus or could be implicated in regulation of the contraction-relaxation cycle. It is clear that much more work is needed to identify these disease genes and to analyze the functional consequences of all the identified mutations before we are in a position to propose a general and unifying hypothesis for the pathogenesis of this disease. Finally, from the functional in vitro analyses, as well as from the in vivo analyses with transgenic animals and the crystallographic structural studies, major repercussions in the comprehension of normal sarcomere function and indeed of regulation of the cardiac contraction can be predicted.

REFERENCES

1. Report of the WHO/IFSC task force on the definition and classification of cardiomyopathies. Br Heart J 1980;44:672–673
2. Baltimore D: Viral RNA-dependent DNA polymerase. Nature 1970;226:1209–1211
3. Temin HM, Mizutani S: Viral RNA-dependent DNA polymerase. Nature 1970;225:1211–1213
4. Kelly TJJ, Smith HO: A restriction enzyme from Haemophilus influenzae. II. Base sequence of the recognition site. J Mol Biol 1970;51:393–409
5. Smith HO, Wilcox KW: A restriction enzyme from Haemophilus influenzae. I. Purification and general properties. J Mol Biol 1970;51:379–391
6. Cohen S, Chang A, Boyer H, Helling R: Construction of biological functional plasmids in vitro. Proc Natl Acad Sci USA 1973;70:3240–3244
7. Maxam AM, Gilbert W: A new method for sequencing DNA. Proc Natl Acad Sci USA 1977;74:560–564
8. Sanger F, Couison AR: A rapid method for determining sequences in DNA by primed synthesis and DNA polymerase. J Mol Biol 1975;94:444–448
9. Southern EM: Detection of specific sequences among DNA fragments separated by gel electrophoresis. J Mol Biol 1975;98:503–512
10. Watson JD, Tooze J: The DNA Story. A Documentary History of Gene Cloning. WH Freeman, San Francisco, 1981
11. Kan YW, Dozy AM: Polymorphism of DNA sequence adjacent to human β-globin structural gene. Relationship to sickle mutation. Proc Natl Acad Sci USA 1978; 75:5631–5635
12. Botstein D, White RL, Kolnick M, Davis RW: Construction of a genetic linkage map using restriction fragment length polymorphisms. Am J Hum Genet 1980;32:314–331
13. Ott J: Linkage analysis and family classification under heterogeneity. Ann Hum Genet 1983;47:311–320
14. Lathrop GM, Lalouel JM: Easy calculations of Lod scores and genetic risks on small computers. Am J Hum Genet 1984;36:460–465
15. Nakamura Y, Leppert M, O'Connell P et al: Variable

number of tandem repeat (VNTR) markers for human gene mapping. Science 1987;235:1616–1621

16. Weissenbach J, Gyapay G, Dib C et al: A second generation linkage map of the human genome. Nature 1992; 359:794–801

17. Weber JL: Know thy genome. Nature Genet 1994;7: 343–344

18. Dausse E, Quemener E, Schwartz K: [33]P and B-imager. Application for genotyping of microsatellite markers. Biotechniques 1995;18:426–430

19. Charpak G, Dominik W, Zaganidis N: Optical imaging of the spatial distribution of β-particles emerged from surfaces. Proc Natl Acad Sci USA 1989;86:1741–1745

20. Grompe M: The rapid detection of unknown mutations in nucleic acids. Nature Genet 1993;5:111–117

21. Myers RM, Fischer SG, Maniatis T et al: Modifications of the melting properties of duplex DNA by attachment of a GC-rich DNA sequence as determined by denaturing gradient gel electrophoresis. Nucleic Acids Res 1985;13:3110–3129

22. Orita M, Suzuki Y, Sekiya T, Hayashi K: Rapid and sensitive detection of point mutations and DNA polymorphisms using the polymerase chain reaction. Genomics 1990;5:874–879

23. Nagamine CM, Chan K, Lau YFC: A PCR artifact. Generation of heteroduplexes. Am J Hum Genet 1989; 45:337–339

24. White MB, Carvalho M, Derse D et al: Detecting single base substitutions as heteroduplex polymorphisms. Genomics 1992;12:301–306

25. Myers RM, Larin Z, Maniatis T: Detection of single base substitutions by ribonuclease A cleavage. Science 1985;230:303–305

26. Cotton RGH, Rodrigues NR, Campbell RD: Reactivity of cytosine and thymine in single-base-pair mismatches with hydroxylamine and osmium tetroxide and its application to the study of mutations. Proc Natl Acad Sci USA 1988;85:4397–4401

27. Vulpian A: Contribution à l'étude des rétrécissements de l'orifice ventricolo-aortique. Arch Physiol 1868;3: 220–222

28. Schmincke A: Ueber linkseitige muskulose Conus-stenosen. Dtsch Med Wochenschr 1907;33:1–8

29. Shapiro LM, McKenna WJ: Distribution of left ventricular hypertrophy in hypertrophic cardiomyopathy. A two-dimensional echocardiographic study. J Am Coll Cardiol 1983;2:437–444

30. Maron BJ, Gottdiener JS, Epstein S: Patterns and significance of distribution of left ventricular hypertrophy in hypertrophic cardiomyopathy. A wide angle, two dimensional echocardiographic study of 125 patients. J Am Cardiol 1981;48:418–428

31. Maron BJ, Lipson LC, Roberts WC et al: "Malignant" hypertrophic cardiomyopathy. Identification of a subgroup of families with unusual frequent premature death. Am J Cardiol 1978;41:1133–1140

32. Mckenna W, Deanfield J, Faruqui A et al: Prognosis in hypertrophic cardiomyopathy. Role of age and clinical, electrocardiographic and hemodynamic features. Am J Cardiol 1981;47:532–538

33. Spirito P, Chiarella F, Carratino L et al: Clinical course and prognosis of hypertrophic cardiomyopathy in an outpatient population. N Engl J Med 1989;320: 749–755

34. Codd MB, Sugrue DD, Gersh BJ, Melton LJ: Epidemiology of idiopathic dilated and hypertrophic cardiomyopathy. Circulation 1989;80:564–572

35. Hollman A, Goodwin JF, Teare D, Renwick JW: A family with obstructive cardiomyopathy (asymmetrical hypertrophy). Br Heart J 1960;22:449–456

36. Maron BJ, Nichols PF, Pickle LW et al: Patterns of inheritance in hypertrophic cardiomyopathy. Assessment by M-mode and two-dimensional echocardiography. Am J Cardiol 1984;53:1087–1094

37. Greaves SC, Roche AHG, Neutze JM et al: Inheritance of hypertrophic cardiomyopathy. A cross sectional and M mode echocardiographic study of 50 families. Br Heart J 1987;58:259–266

38. Clark CE, Henry WL, Epstein SE: Familial prevalence and genetic transmission of idiopathic subaortic stenosis. N Engl J Med 1973;289:709–714

39. Wynne J, Brauwald E: The cardiomyopathies and myocarditis. Toxic, chemical, and physical damage to the heart. pp. 1394–1450. In Braunwald E (ed): Heart Disease. A Textbook of Cardiovascular Medicine. WB Saunders, Philadelphia, 1992

40. Jarcho JA, McKenna W, Pare JAP et al: Mapping a gene for familial hypertrophic cardiomyopathy to chromosome 14ql. N Engl J Med 1989;321:1372–1378

41. Schwartz K, Carrier L, Guicheney P, Komajda M: The molecular basis of cardiomyopathies. Circulation 1995;91:532–540

42. Geisterfer-Lowrance AAT, Kass S, Tanigawa G et al: A molecular basis for familial hypertrophic cardiomyopathy. A β cardiac myosin heavy chain gene missense mutation. Cell 1990;62:999–1006

43. Solomon SD, Geisterfer-Lowrance AAT, Vosberg HP et al: A locus for familial hypertrophic cardiomyopathy is closely linked to the cardiac myosin heavy chain genes, CRI-L436, an CRI-L329 on chromosome 14 at q11–q12. Am J Hum Genet 1990;47:389–394

44. Hejtmancik JF, Brink PA, Hill R et al: Localization of gene for familial hypertrophic cardiomyopathy to chromosome 14ql in a diverse US population. Circulation 1991;83:1592–1597

45. Epstein ND, Cohn GM, Cyran F, Fananapazir L: Differences in clinical expression of hypertrophic cardiomyopathy associated with two distinct mutations in the β-myosin heavy chain gene. A 908 Leu → Val mutation and a 403 Arg → Gln mutation. Circulation 1992; 86:345–352

46. Dausse E, Schwartz K: Genetic heterogeneity of familial hypertrophic cardiomyopathy. Neuromuscul Disord 1993;3:483–486

47. Dausse E, Komajda M, Dubourg O et al: Familial hypertrophic cardiomyopathy. Microsatellite haplotyping and identification of a hot-spot for mutations in the β-myosin heavy chain gene. J Clin Invest 1993;92: 2807–2813

48. Moolman JC, Brink PA, Corfield VA: Identification of a new missense mutation at Arg403, a CpG mutation hotspot, in exon 13 of the β-myosin heavy chain gene in hypertrophic cardiomyopathy. Hum Mol Genet 1993;2:1731–1732

49. Marian AJ, Yu QT, Mares A et al: Detection of a new mutation in the β-myosin heavy chain gene in an individual with hypertrophic cardiomyopathy. J Clin Invest 1992;90:2156–2165

50. Maron BJ, Bonow RO, Cannon RO et al: Hypertrophic cardiomyopathy. Interrelations of clinical manifesta-

tions, pathophysiology, and therapy. N Engl J Med 1987;316:780–789, 844–852

51. Solomon SD, Jarcho JA, McKenna WJ et al: Familial hypertrophic cardiomyopathy is a genetically heterogeneous disease. J Clin Invest 1990;86:993–999

52. Polymeropoulos MH, Xiao H, Rath DS, Merril CR: Dinucleotide repeat polymorphism at the human cardiac beta-myosin gene. Nucleic Acids Res 1991;19:4019

53. Fougerousse F, Dufour C, Roudaut C, Beckmann JS: Dinucleotide repeat polymorphism at the human gene for cardiac beta-myosin heavy chain (MYH7). Hum Mol Genet 1992;1:64

54. Schwartz K, Dufour C, Fougerousse F et al: Exclusion of myosin heavy chain and cardiac actin gene involvement in hypertrophic cardiomyopathies of several French families. Circ Res 1992;71:3–8

55. Epstein ND, Fananapazir L, Lin HJ et al: Evidence of genetic heterogeneity in five kindreds with familial hypertrophic cardiomyopathy. Circulation 1992;85:635–647

56. Harada H, Kimura A, Nishi H et al: Genetic analysis of hypertrophic cardiomyopathy. Circulation, suppl. I 1992;86:591

57. Hirschfield W, Hunter J, Corfield V et al: Chromosome 14 linkage studies in South African families with hypertrophic cardiomyopathy. Eur Heart J 1992;13:32–37

58. Ko YL, Lien WP, Chen JJ et al: No evidence for linkage of familial hypertrophic cardiomyopathy and chromosome 14ql locus D14S26 in a Chinese family. Evidence for genetic heterogeneity. Hum Genet 1992;89:597–601

59. Watkins H, MacRae C, Thierfelder L et al: A disease locus for familial hypertrophic cardiomyopathy maps to chromosome 1q3. Nature Genet 1993;3:333–337

60. Thierfelder L, MacRae C, Watkins H et al: A familial hypertrophic cardiomyopathy locus maps to chromosome 15q2. Proc Natl Acad Sci USA 1993;90:6270–6274

61. Carrier L, Hengstenberg C, Beckmann JS et al: Mapping of a novel gene for familial hypertrophic cardiomyopathy to chromosome 11. Nature Genet 1993;4:311–313

62. Hengstenberg C, Charron P, Isnard R et al: Mise en évidence d'un cinquième locus impliqué dans les cardiomyopathies hypertrophiques familiales. Arch Mal Coeur 1994;87:1655–1662

63. MacRae C, Ghaisas N, Kass S et al: Familial hypertrophic cardiomyopathy with Wolff-Parkinson-White syndrome maps to a locus on chromosome 7q3. J Clin Invest 1995;96:1216–1220

64. Watkins H, McKenna WJ, Thierfelder L et al: Mutations in the genes for cardiac troponin T and α-tropomyosin in hypertrophic cardiomyopathy. N Engl J Med 1995;332:1058–1064

65. Thierfelder L, Watkins H, MacRae C et al: α-Tropomyosin and cardiac troponin T mutations cause familial hypertrophic cardiomyopathy. A disease of the sarcomere. Cell 1994;77:701–712

66. Carrier L, Bercovici J, Bonne G et al: Reduction of the CMH4 locus in familial hypertrophic cardiomyopathy by fine haplotype analysis. Presented to the XV World Congress of the International Society for Heart Research, Prague, July 1995

67. Bonne G, Carrier L, Komajda M, Schwartz K: The COX8 gene is not the disease gene of the CMH4 locus in familial hypertrophic cardiomyopathy. J Med Genet (in press)

68. Rayment I, Rypniewski WR, Schmidt-Bäse K et al: Three-dimensional structure of myosin subfragment-1. A molecular motor. Science 1993;261:50–56

69. Rayment I, Holden HM, Whittaker M et al: Structure of the actin-myosin complex and its implication for muscle contraction. Science 1993;261:58–65

70. Dufour C, Dausse E, Fetler L et al: Identification of a mutation near a functional site of the β cardiac myosin heavy chain gene in a family with hypertrophic cardiomyopathy. J Mol Cell Cardiol 1994;9:1241–1247

71. Eldin P, Cathiard AM, Léger J et al: Probing functional regions in cardiac isomyosins with monoclonal antibodies. Biochemistry 1993;32:2542–2547

72. Perryman MG, Yu QY, Marian AJ et al: Expression of a missense mutation in myocardial tissue in hypertrophic cardiomyopathy. J Clin Invest 1992;90:271–277

73. Yu QT, Ifegwu J, Marian AJ et al: Hypertrophic cardiomyopathy mutation is expressed in messenger RNA of skeletal as well as cardiac muscle. Circulation 1993;87:406–412

74. Greve G, Friedman D, Roberts R: A missense mutation in β-myosin heavy chain gene is expressed on the mRNA and protein level in cardiac tissue from an individual with hypertrophic cardiomyopathy. Eur Heart J, suppl. 1994;15:554

75. Cuda G, Fananapazir L, Zhu WS et al: Skeletal muscle expression and abnormal function of β-myosin in hypertrophic cardiomyopathy. J Clin Invest 1993;91:2861–2865

76. Vybiral T, Roberts R, Epstein H: Accumulation and assembly of myosin in hypertrophic cardiomyopathy with the 403 Arg to Gln β-myosin heavy chain mutations. Circ Res 1992;71:1404–1409

77. Watkins H, Thierfelder L, Hwang DS et al: Sporadic hypertrophic cardiomyopathy due to de novo myosin mutations. J Clin Invest 1992;90:1666–1671

78. Greve G, Mares A, Bachinski L, Roberts R: A sporadic mutation in the β-myosin heavy chain gene transmits hypertrophic cardiomyopathy to the offspring of two generations. [abstract]. Circulation 1993;88:I-572

79. Straceski AJ, Geisterfer-Lowrance A, Seidman CE et al: Functional analysis of myosin missense mutations in familial hypertrophic cardiomyopathy. Proc Natl Acad Sci USA 1994;91:589–593

80. Sweeney HL, Straceski AJ, Leinwand LA et al: Heterologous expression of a cardiomyopathic myosin that is defective in its actin interaction. J Biol Chem 1994;269:1603–1605

81. Lankford E, Epstein ND, Fananapazir L, Sweeney HL: Abnormal contractile properties of muscle fibers expressing β-myosin heavy chain gene mutations in patients with hypertrophic cardiomyopathy. J Clin Invest 1995;95:1409–1414

82. Watkins H, Rosenzweig T, Hwang DS et al: Characteristic and prognostic implications of myosin missense mutations in familial hypertrophic cardiomyopathy. N Engl J Med 1992;326:1106–1114

83. Fananapazir L, Epstein ND: Genotype-phenotype correlations in hypertrophic cardiomyopathy. Insights provided by comparisons of kindreds with distinct and identical β-myosin heavy chain mutations. Circulation 1994;89:22–32

84. Michels VV, Moll PP, Miller FA et al: The frequency of

familial dilated cardiomyopathy in a series of patients with idiopathic dilated cardiomyopathy. N Engl J Med 1992;326:77–82

85. Mestroni L, Miani D, Di Lenarda A et al: Clinical and pathologic study of familial dilated cardiomyopathy. Am J Cardiol 1990;65:1449–1453

86. Zimmerman E, Chwojnik A, Lerman J: Idiopathic dilated cardiomyopathy with or without mild dilation of the cardiac ventricles in multiple family members. Am J Cardiol 1992;69:972–973

87. Zachara E, Caforio ALP, Carboni GP et al: Familial aggregation of idiopathic dilated cardiomyopathy. Clinical features and pedigree analysis in 14 families. Br Heart J 1993;69:129–135

88. Berko BA, Swift M: X-linked dilated cardiomyopathy. N Engl J Med 1987;316:1186–1191

89. Muntoni F, Cau M, Ganau A et al: Brief report. Deletion of the dystrophin muscle-promoter region associated with X-linked dilated cardiomyopathy. N Engl J Med 1993;329:924–925

90. Towbin JA, Hejtmancik JF, Brink P et al: X-linked dilated cardiomyopathy. Molecular genetic evidence of linkage to the Duchenne muscular dystrophy (dys-trophin) gene at Xp21 locus. Circulation 1993;87:1854–1865

91. Iwata Y, Nakamura H, Fujiwara K, Shigekawa M: Altered membrane-dystrophin association in the cardiomyopathic hamster heart muscle. Biochem Biophys Res Commun 1993;190:589–595

92. Roberds SL, Ervasti JM, Anderson RD et al: Disruption of the dystrophin-glycoprotein complex in the cardiomyopathic hamster. J Biol Chem 1993;268:11496–11499

93. Casazza F, Brambilla G, Salvato A et al: Cardiac transplantation in Becker muscular dystrophy. J Neurol 1988;235:496–498

94. Kamakura K, Kawai M, Arahata K et al: A manifesting carrier of Duchenne muscular dystrophy with severe myocardial symptoms. J Neurol 1990;237:483–485

95. Michels VV: Genetics of idiopathic dilated cardiomyopathy. Heart Failure 1993;10:87–94

96. Kass S, MacRae C, Graber HL et al: A gene defect that causes conduction system disease and dilated cardiomyopathy maps to chromosome 1p1–1q1. Nature Genet 1994;7:546–551

6 ATP Synthesis in the Normal and Failing Heart

Joanne S. Ingwall

Adenosine triphosphate (ATP) is the high energy phosphate-containing compound directly used for excitation and contraction in muscle cells. Cleavage of the terminal phosphate (the phosphoryl bond) by ATPases releases chemical energy that is converted into the work of contraction (myosin ATPase), ion movements (Na^+/K^+- and Ca^{2+}-ATPases), and macromolecular synthesis. The reaction is:

$$MgATP + H_2O \leftrightarrow MgADP + Pi + H^+$$

Chemical energy that can be used to do work is called free energy. Although the free energy of ATP hydrolysis is high (-7.3 kcal/mol) compared to other high-energy phosphate-containing compounds, the concentration of ATP in the cytosol of cardiac myocytes is low. Adult mammalian ventricular tissue contains approximately 5 μmol/g wet weight, which is equivalent to 10 mmol/L (millimolar) of intracellular water or 30 to 35 μmol/g cardiac protein. This amount of ATP is sufficient to maintain pump function for only about 50 beats. Thus the cell must continually resynthesize ATP to maintain normal pump function and cellular viability. The metabolic pathways that produce ATP in the heart are described in this chapter. What is known (and not known) about how these pathways for ATP synthesis change during heart failure is also discussed.

REGULATION OF ATP CONCENTRATION

The distinction between the amount or concentration of ATP versus its turnover rate is central to our understanding of bioenergetics and the control of metabolism. In the normal heart the ATP concentration remains constant, but its rate of synthesis and degradation (turnover rate) varies. The energetics of changing cardiac work illustrates this principle. As the workload of the heart increases, oxygen consumption (a good index of the ATP synthesis rate) proportionately increases; yet ATP content is essentially unchanged. Thus the ATP turnover rate but not its concentration increases. This example also illustrates the important principle that the ATP synthesis rate matches the ATP utilization rate.

Another important principle essential to understanding bioenergetics is that the chemical reactions that use ATP are "driven" by high ATP/adenosine diphosphate (ADP) ratios, whereas ATP synthesis reactions are inhibited by high ATP/ADP ratios. The principle of feedback control of ATP synthesis pathways by ATP itself is central for understanding the regulation of intermediary metabolism.

One expression that defines the energy state of the cell is the adenylate energy charge. It is defined as ATP + 0.5 ADP/ATP + ADP + adenosine monophosphate (AMP) and distinguishes between utilizable ATP (the numerator) and total adenine nucleotide pool (the denominator). In well perfused tissue the cytosolic ATP, ADP, and AMP concentrations are approximately 10 mM, 30 μM and 0.1 μM, respectively; and the energy charge is close to 1. Even when ADP and AMP concentrations increase (as in ischemia) to near millimolar levels, the energy charge does not change much. For the hypothetic case where ATP, ADP, and AMP concentrations are 8, 1, and 1 mM, respectively, the energy charge falls to only 0.85. (Note that the values given here for ADP and

AMP are estimates of cytosolic concentrations calculated from equilibrium expressions for creatine kinase and adenylate kinase and not amounts determined from acid extracts of freeze-clamped tissue. Amounts of ADP and AMP measured in acid extracts are at least an order of magnitude higher because acid extraction releases nucleotide bound to macromolecules. A good example of a source of releasable nucleotide is the ADP bound to each actin monomer in the thin filament.)

A variation of the energy charge more relevant to biologic conditions is the phosphorylation potential, defined as ATP/[ADP $\times$ Pi], where Pi represents inorganic phosphate. This term takes into account the ability of the end-products of ATP hydrolysis (i.e., Pi and ADP) to inhibit ATPase activity and, at least for ADP, to stimulate ATP synthesis pathways. Under most conditions the Pi concentration is low, less than 1 mM. However, under the extreme pathologic conditions where ATP is essentially fully hydrolyzed (e.g., severe ischemia and infarction), ADP can increase to values as high as 300 μM (most of the purine pool is in the form of AMP and nonphosphorylated purines), and the Pi concentration can be as high as 50 mM. The phosphorylation potential in well perfused myocardium is more than 300 mM^{-1}, and it decreases by four orders of magnitude to 0.01 mM^{-1} with severe ischemia (ATP, ADP, and Pi concentrations of 100 μM, 300 μM, and 50 mM, respectively). Thus the phosphorylation potential is a sensitive marker of the energy state of the cell. It is the critical component of the thermodynamic quantity representing the free energy of ATP hydrolysis.

The free energy of ATP hydrolysis defines the driving force for all ATP-utilizing reactions in the cell. It is calculated from the constant value for ATP hydrolysis under standard conditions, ΔG°, corrected for the actual concentrations of ATP, ADP, and Pi in the cytosol. The expression is

$$\Delta G = \Delta G^{\circ} - RT \ln [ATP]/[ADP][Pi]$$

where ΔG° is the standard free energy change of ATP hydrolysis (-30.5 kJ/mol under standard conditions of molarity, temperature, pH, and Mg^{2+}), R is the gas constant (8.3 J/mol·K), and T is the absolute temperature in Kelvin. The argument of the ln term is the phosphorylation potential. The value of ΔG for pyruvate-perfused rat heart with a typical rate–pressure product of 28,000 is -69.9 ± 2.0 kJ/mol; for a glucose-perfused heart, which has higher Pi concentration, ΔG becomes less negative, -57.7 ± 0.6 kJ/mol. The less negative value means that the glucose-only perfused heart has a lower driving force for ATP-utilizing reactions. Because it is often confusing to describe changes for a negative number, it is convenient to describe changes in ΔG in terms of its absolute value.

Given the critical need to maintain both a constant level and a high level of ATP and the ATP/[ADP $\times$ Pi] ratio, it is not surprising that the cell uses many reactions and pathways to synthesize ATP. The remarkable feature of intermediary metabolism is that constant ATP concentration is maintained by the integration of multiple pathways. Table 6-1, compiled from data reported elsewhere,[1-3] summarizes the rates of ATP synthesis from the major pathways for its synthesis.

HEART FAILURE

Although there have been conflicting results as to whether ATP concentration is the same or lower in the failing myocardium, results using the noninvasive tool of phosphorus 31 (^{31}P) nuclear magnetic resonance (NMR) spectroscopy to study rodent models of heart failure suggest that the ATP concentration is reduced in severely failing myocardium. In the rat heart model of moderate heart failure secondary to chronic myocardial infarction, the ATP concentration was indistinguishable from that in normal rat heart,[3] but in the severely failing hamster heart the ATP concentration was 28 percent lower than that in age-matched animals.[4] Whether the phosphorylation potential is lower depends on whether the enzymes responsible for maintaining low ADP and Pi contents function normally.

ATP SYNTHESIS DE NOVO AND FROM SALVAGE PATHWAYS

De novo synthesis of the purine ring of ATP from formate, carbon dioxide, and amino acids occurs slowly. Zimmer et al. estimated that this rate is in the order of nanomoles per second.[5] At this rate, it would take about 100 days to replace the entire ATP pool. Phosphorylation of preformed purine via sal-

Table 6-1. ATP Synthesis Rates in the Glucose-Perfused Intact Heart

Pathway	Synthesis rate (mM/s)[a]
De novo[5]	10^{-6}
Glycolysis[1]	0.04
Oxidative phosphorylation[2]	0.7
Creatine kinase[2]	10

The reference numbers indicate the study from which the data were obtained to calculate the figures here.

[a]Cystolic concentrations of ATP per second.

vage pathways is rapid, occurring with in seconds or minutes instead of days. Examples are salvage of ADP via the adenylate kinase reaction ($2ADP \leftrightarrow ATP + AMP$) and phosphorylation of purine nucleobases (e.g., hypoxanthine) or nucleosides (e.g., inosine or adenosine) by enzymes located in myocytes and endothelial cells.

There are no data relevant to these pathways for the *failing heart*. However, the loss in the total adenine pool suggests that myocytes in the failing heart are either unable to synthesize enough adenine or are unable to prevent ATP degradation (ATP → ADP → AMP → adenosine → inosine → hypoxanthine) and subsequent loss of diffusible purines (the nucleosides and bases).

ATP SYNTHESIS FROM CARBON-BASED FUELS

Adenosine triphosphate is generated by the metabolic breakdown of carbon-based fuels through two processes: (1) substrate-level phosphorylation and (2) the generation of reducing equivalents for oxidative phosphorylation. An example of substrate-level phosphorylation is the production of ATP from glucose in the cytosol. The generation of reducing equivalents from glycolysis and from the tricarboxylic acid (TCA) cycle contributes to the production of ATP via oxidative phosphorylation within the mitochondria. In the normal heart, oxidative production of ATP predominates over substrate-level phosphorylation. However, changes in work state or pathophysiology of the heart can result in a shift toward substrate-level phosphorylation.

The fuels of carbohydrates, fats, amino acids, or ketone bodies required for energy production are made available to the myocyte from either intracellular stores or circulating plasma levels. These fuels are referred to as *substrates* to indicate that they are converted to other reactants through a series of enzyme-catalyzed reactions. The normal heart preferentially utilizes fatty acids as the substrate for oxidative energy production, although nutritional, metabolic, and hormonal influences can induce a greater contribution from carbohydrates. Starches and sugars can enter glycolysis as the monomeric sugars glucose or fructose. Glycogen, a starch composed of polymerized glucose units, serves as an intracellular store of glucose. Amino acids and ketones can also serve as substrates but normally contribute little to total energy production. The regulation of intermediary pathways that determine the produc-

tion of energy from this menu of carbon-based fuels is summarized in Figure 6-1.

Glycolytic Pathway

Uptake of glucose by the heart is controlled by glucose transporters in the sarcolemmal membrane. No energy is required for glucose transport because the extracellular glucose concentration is much higher than the intracellular concentration. Glucose transport is regulated by: (1) demand for anaerobic glycolysis; (2) workload; (3) plasma glucose concentrations; and (4) the actions of the circulating hormone insulin. The glucose transporter responsive to insulin is GLUT 4; the transporter that is insulin-independent is GLUT 1.

Once glucose enters the myocyte, it is used for glycolysis, glycogen synthesis, or the pentose shunt. The pentose shunt is the least involved in the production of energy, although the five-carbon pentose phosphates from this pathway can reenter glycolysis. The pentose shunt supplies carbon chains for the formation of adenine nucleotides, such as AMP and GTP, and regenerates the cofactor $NADP^+$. Glycogen synthesis allows storage of glucose, a process regulated by a complex network of enzyme activation in response to metabolic and hormonal stimuli within the cell. It is the glycolytic pathway whereby glucose is converted to three-carbon units, yielding not only ATP but also products that can be used for further ATP production in the mitochondria.

For purposes of energy accounting, this pathway of glycolysis (Fig. 6-2) can be separated into two stages. The ATP-requiring stage consists of the formation of glucose-6-phosphate from glucose and the subsequent production of fructose-1, 6-biphosphate. If glucose-6-phosphate is produced from glucose via the hexokinase reaction, two ATP molecules are consumed. If glucose 6-phosphate is produced from glycogen breakdown, only one ATP is consumed. The ATP-yielding stage consists of the formation of two triose units per six-carbon sugar chain and ultimate formation of pyruvate, yielding four molecules of ATP. Thus the net energy yield of this pathway is two molecules of ATP from glucose and three molecules of ATP from glycogen. The net reaction of the glycolytic breakdown of glucose of pyruvate is:

$$Glucose + 2\ NAD^+ + 2\ Pi + 2\ ADP \rightarrow 2\ pyruvate$$
$$+ 2\ NADH + 2\ H^+ + 2\ ATP + 2\ H_2O$$

The two most important regulatory enzymes in the glycolytic pathway are glyceraldehyde-3-phosphate dehydrogenase and phosphofructokinase. The glyc-

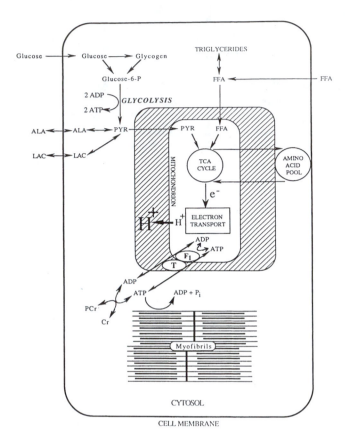

Fig. 6-1. Energy production from carbon-based fuels in the myocyte. Glucose uptake across the sarcolemmal membrane supplies both glycogen storage and substrate-level energy production via glycolysis. Cytosolic metabolism of pyruvate (PYR) produces lactate (LAC), which either leaves the cell or is reconverted to pyruvate for oxidation within the mitochondria. Free fatty acids (FFA) enter the cell by passive, facilitated diffusion across the sarcolemmal membrane and are either stored through triglyceride formation or transported into the mitochondria for oxidative metabolism. Both PYR and FFA are metabolized to form two-carbon acetyl groups, which enter oxidative metabolism within the tricarboxylic acid (TCA) cycle. The oxidative production of reducing equivalents from the TCA cycle supplies electrons (e⁻) to the electron transport chain, which generates a proton (H⁺) gradient across the inner mitochondrial membrane. This proton gradient drives F_1 ATPase (F_1), converting ADP to ATP, which is coupled to the nucleotide translocase (T). The high-energy phosphoryl group of ATP supports the energy requirements of excitation-contraction coupling. Energy is also supplied by phosphate transfer from phosphocreatine (PCr) to ADP to form ATP and creatine (Cr). (From Lewandowski and Ingwall,[6] with permission.)

eraldehyde-3-phosphate dehydrogenase reaction generates one NADH and a proton (H⁺) from NAD⁺ and the two molecules of glyceraldehyde-3-phosphate that are converted to 1,3-diphosphoglycerate (remember that one six-carbon glucose molecule produces two three-carbon units). This step is the only oxidative reaction within the glycolytic pathway, and the cytosolic supply of NAD⁺ must be replenished for the chain of reactions to continue beyond the formation of glyceraldehyde-3-phosphate. NAD⁺ is made available by either oxidation of NADH in the mitochondria or conversion of pyruvate to lactate as described below. Because of the requirement for NAD⁺, the glyceraldehyde-3-phosphate dehydrogenase reaction is one of the rate-limiting steps of glycolysis under anaerobic conditions. This enzyme is inhibited by 1,3-diphosphoglycerate and by the end-products of anaerobic glycolysis: NADH, protons, and lactate.

Phosphofructokinase, which is at the head of the pathway, converts fructose-6-phosphate to fructose-1, 6-biphosphate. Unlike glyceraldehyde-3-phosphate dehydrogenase, which is dependent on the redox state and the ability of the heart to undergo oxidative metabolism, this enzyme is more responsive to the energetic state of the cytosol. The phosphofructokinase reaction is irreversible and determines the intracellular content of glucose-6-phosphate. When phosphofructokinase is activated by a fall in ATP or by elevated levels of ADP, AMP, and Pi, the resultant drop in glucose-6-phosphate stimulates the activity of the hexokinase enzyme. The rate-limiting step in glycolysis then becomes the glyceraldehyde-3-phosphate dehydrogenase reaction. Phosphofructokinase can also become rate-limiting by an inhibitory response to high levels of ATP or changes in the TCA cycle intermediate citrate, which are metabolically translated to the cytosol.

Therefore although many enzymes are involved in the glycolytic pathway, the ability of the heart to regulate glycolytic flux in response to the energetic state of the heart and the rate of oxidative metabolism is primarily provided by the balance between the activity of two regulatory enzymes: phosphofructokinase and glyceraldehyde-3-phosphate dehydrogenase.

Anaerobic Versus Aerobic Glycolysis

The difference between aerobic and anaerobic glycolysis is the fate of pyruvate, the end-product of glycolysis. With *anaerobic glycolysis* pyruvate does not enter the TCA cycle but is converted to lactate via the lactate dehydrogenase (LDH) reaction. The reaction is rapid and reversible, and its equilibrium position is far to the right:

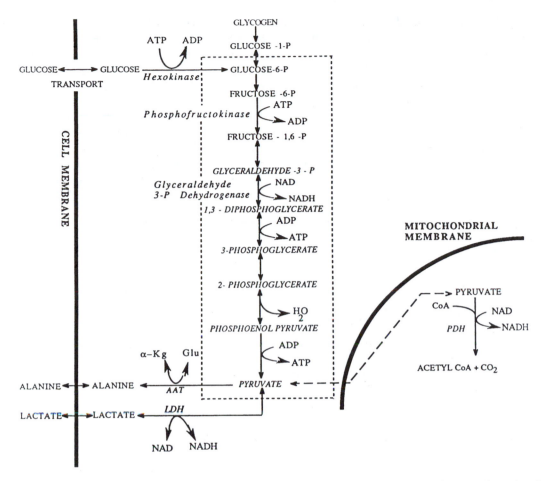

Fig. 6-2. Metabolism of glucose and pyruvate. Two triose units are produced from each molecule of glucose. Key enzymes of glucose metabolism are shown in italics. Pyruvate is the pivotal intermediate between nonoxidative metabolism in the cytosol via alanine aminotransferase (AAT) and lactate dehydrogenase (LDH) and the oxidative metabolism in the mitochondrial via the action of the pyruvate dehydrogenase enzyme complex (PDH). α-Kg, α-ketoglutarate; Glu, glutamate; CoA, coenzyme A. (From Lewandowski and Ingwall,[6] with permission.)

Pyruvate + NADH + H$^+$ $\leftrightarrow$ lactate + NAD$^+$

This reaction restores the cofactor NAD$^+$ necessary to maintain the rate-limiting glyceraldehyde-3-phosphate dehydrogenase reaction, thereby allowing glycolysis to continue even in the absence of oxygen. ATP that is produced independently of oxygen via the glycolytic breakdown of glucose in this way is what is meant by the term substrate-level phosphorylation.

With *aerobic glycolysis* pyruvate enters the TCA cycle as acetyl-coenzyme A (CoA) and is oxidized. Some lactate is also produced as the result of differential rates of glycolysis and pyruvate oxidation, which can result from altered metabolic demands (e.g., when glycolytic activity increases in response to increased work) or from competition with other substrates for entry into the TCA cycle. Under aerobic conditions, LDH allows lactate to be rapidly oxi-

dized following reconversion to pyruvate. Thus glycolysis does not refer solely to the anaerobic breakdown of glucose. Indeed, aerobic glycolysis is the normal condition in the heart. Under aerobic conditions the products of glycolysis (i.e., pyruvate and NADH) are used to support oxidative ATP production in the mitochondria.

HEART FAILURE

Although LDH was the first protein for which isozyme switches were identified in the compensated hypertrophied heart, little is known about the changes in tissue content and activity of the glycolytic proteins in failing heart. Some indirect information is available. Using the BIO 14.6 strain of hamsters, a model of hypertrophic cardiomyophathy, Wikman-Coffelt and colleagues[7,8] have shown that the phosphorylation potential, which is lower in failing than in nonfailing hearts, could be improved by supplying either pyruvate or β-adrenergic agonists to isolated glucose-perfused hearts. This finding was interpreted as a failure of glycolysis to provide sufficient pyruvate to support normal oxidative phosphorylation. Neither glucose uptake rates nor glycolytic rates have been directly measured in the failing myocardium, however. Because it is now possible to measure glucose uptake rates using Positron emission tomography (PET) and ^{31}P NMR (using 2-deoxyglucose) and glycolysis rates using radiolabeled glucose and carbon 13 (^{13}C) NMR in the intact heart, the contribution of glycolysis to overall ATP production can be directly measured.

Oxidative Metabolism

The heart derives more than 90 percent of its energy production from the oxidation of carbon-based fuels. Unlike glycolysis, which takes place in the cytosol, oxidative metabolism occurs in the mitochondria. The concentration of protein in mitochondria is much higher than in the cytosol, allowing rapid, efficient transfer of substrates between enzyme systems. The currency for oxidative energy production is the reducing equivalent derived from the carbon substrates and carried by the cofactors NAD$^+$ and FAD. In addition to the two ATPs produced by substrate-level phosphorylation during glycolysis, oxidation of the two NADHs produced during glycolysis generates six more molecules of ATP if these reducing equivalents move from the cytosol to the mitochondrial matrix. This change corresponds to a 300 percent increase in the energetic efficiency of the breakdown of glucose to two pyruvate molecules. The malate–aspartate shuttle exchanges cytosolic and mitochondrial NADH pools. The oxidation of the two pyruvate molecules produced from the glycolytic breakdown of glucose yields 30 molecules of ATP for a combined total of 38 molecules of ATP produced from the complete oxidative breakdown of one molecule of glucose by the heart.

Other substrates such as fatty acids can yield much greater amounts of ATP per molecule than is oxidized. For example, palmitate, a long-chain fatty acid comprised of 16 carbons, yields a total of 129 molecules of ATP per molecule oxidized, compared to 15 ATP molecules from the oxidation of one pyruvate molecule. The amount of oxygen utilized per ATP produced by fatty acid oxidation is more than that used with the oxidation of glucose or pyruvate. Thus not only is substrate oxidation an efficient source of energy for the heart but the availability of substrate to the heart and substrate preference by the heart

can influence the respiratory efficiency at a given level of cardiac performance.

FORMATION OF ACETYL-CoA BY PYRUVATE DEHYDROGENASE

The relative contributions of pyruvate and fatty acids to oxidative metabolism are regulated by the activity of the pyruvate dehydrogenase (PDH) complex. PDH, located in the inner mitochondrial membrane, decarboxylates the three-carbon pyruvate to the two-carbon fragment, acetyl-CoA, for incorporation into the TCA cycle:

$$\text{Pyruvate} + \text{CoA-SH} + \text{NAD}^+ \rightarrow \text{acetyl-CoA} + \text{CO}_2 + \text{NADH} + \text{H}^+$$

Inhibition of carbohydrate oxidation by fatty acid metabolism is mediated through PDH. PDH activity is regulated by (de)phosphorylation cycles, intramitochondrial ratios of NADH/NAD and acetyl-CoA/CoA, and mitochondrial calcium levels.

HEART FAILURE

Because of its central role in supplying substrate for the TCA cycle, PDH has been studied in the failing heart. Hansford and colleagues, using both the BIO 14.6 and TO-2 strains of cardiomyopathic hamsters, have elegantly shown that, although pyruvate concentration is normal, the control of PDH activity is altered in failing hearts of both strains.[9] They found that a smaller proportion of PDH is in the active form in failing myocardium, and they presented evidence that the underlying mechanism is a smaller rise in mitochondrial Ca^{2+} content during excitation.

FORMATION OF ACETYL-CoA FROM FATS BY β-OXIDATION

Free fatty acids are the predominant oxidative fuel for the heart. Circulating free fatty acids are bound to plasma proteins, primarily albumin. The uptake of fatty acid by the myocyte occurs by passive diffusion across the sarcolemmal membrane, facilitated by fatty acid carrier proteins. The rate of transport depends on the size of the gradient between plasma and myocyte fatty acid content. Triglycerides, which are composed of fatty acids bound to glycerol, are another source of fatty acids.

Once in the cytosol, the fatty acid must be activated to acyl-CoA prior to transport into the mitochondria for subsequent oxidation. The activated acyl-CoA in the cytosol is then converted to acyl-carnitine, which is transported into the mitochondria via the action of the acyl-carnitine transferases. This transfer is driven by the concentration differences in acyl-carnitine (high cytosolic levels) and acyl-CoA (high mitochondrial levels) across the outer mitochondrial membrane. The transferase reaction is mediated by the acyl-carnitine transferase system.

Once in the mitochondria, activated fatty acids are broken down by β-oxidation into two-carbon acetyl-CoA units by repeated cleavage of the chain at the β-carbon position—hence the name of this pathway. Each acetyl-CoA unit enters the TCA cycle at the citrate synthase step. During each round of β-oxidation, reducing equivalents are also produced that are available for oxidation via the respiratory chain. The action of β-oxidation on odd-numbered fatty acids results in the formation of the activated three-carbon fatty acid propionyl-CoA (from propionate). Propionyl-CoA enters oxidative metabolism by conversion to the TCA cycle intermediate succinyl-CoA.

TRICARBOXYLIC ACID CYCLE

The energy yield from one "turn" of the TCA cycle (also known as the Krebs cycle or the citric acid cycle), starting from the entry of acetyl-CoA at the citrate synthase step, is 12 ATP molecules. One of these ATP molecules is produced by substrate-level phosphorylation during the conversion of succinyl-CoA to succinate and the other 11 ATPs come from the oxidation of three NADHs and one FADH$_2$. During the process, the carbon pool, which is distributed among all of the TCA cycle intermediate pools, is conserved within the cycle. The net conversion of acetyl-CoA to carbon dioxide is:

$$Acetyl\text{-}CoA + 3\,NAD^+ + FAD + GDP + Pi + 2H_2O \rightarrow 2CO_2 \\ + 3\,NADH + FADH_2 + GTP + 2H^+ + CoA$$

The rate of NADH production by the TCA cycle subsequently used for the oxidative synthesis of ATP is closely matched to the energy requirement of cardiac work. This pathway is often represented as a spinning loop that speeds up in response to metabolic indicators of increased energy demands, largely mediated by TCA intermediate levels and the NADH/NAD ratio in the mitochondria (which decreases during increased work). However, this pathway is not a closed loop, and other points of entry into the cycle are available for precursors of TCA cycle intermediates in addition to the entry step for acetyl-CoA at the citrate synthase step (Fig. 6-3). Supply of TCA cycle intermediates to these alternative entry points also affects the TCA cycle rate and the rate of oxygen consumption, indicating a reciprocal relation between the physiologic demands of the heart and the metabolically induced redox (reduction/ oxidation) state of heart. It is important to emphasize that although the tissue concentrations of the TCA cycle intermediates affect activity within the cycle, the rate of energy utilization by the heart correlates with the flux of carbon passing through each intermediate pool. Flux rates closely correspond to the rate of oxygen consumed by the heart in response to workload.

HEART FAILURE

Metabolic disorders can lead to contractile failure of the heart if the span between citrate synthase and α-ketoglutarate dehydrogenase is metabolically dissociated from the span between succinyl-CoA synthase and citrate synthase (Fig. 6-3). As CoA is sequestered by the activation of ketones from the plasma, succinyl-CoA is formed. The carbon pool within this first span of the TCA cycle then accumulates, starving the second span of its carbon pool. Unless anaplerotic sources of carbon are available, in the form of pyruvate from carbohydrates or propionate from odd-numbered fatty acids, to replenish the TCA intermediate pool within the second span, citrate synthase becomes substrate-starved and the cycle grinds to a halt. Alternatively, redistribution of the TCA intermediate carbon pool could ensue, adjusting the TCA cycle rate via feedback inhibition. Such redistribution of the total carbon pool between the intermediates of either span of the TCA cycle provides internal regulation of cycle flux and the capability of adjusting the rate of oxidative substrate metabolism to the carbon flux through the multiple entry/exit points of the cycle. Thus the TCA cycle is in communication with other pathways within the mitochondria and between the cytosol and the mitochondria to maintain a balance between the metabolic state of the heart and the physiologic demand for oxidative energy production. It is not known if the TCA cycle flux is altered during heart failure.

Oxidative Phosphorylation

Oxidative phosphorylation is the process whereby ATP is formed as electrons are transferred from NADH or FADH$_2$ (which were made either by glycolysis in the cytosol or by fatty acid oxidation and the citric acid cycle in the nearby mitochondrial matrix) to molecular O$_2$ by a series of electron carriers (Fig. 6-1). The driving force of oxidative phosphorylation is derived from the oxidation of NADH and FADH$_2$ by O$_2$. Electrons are transferred from NADH to O$_2$ through a chain of three large protein complexes—NADH-Q reductase, cytochrome reductase,

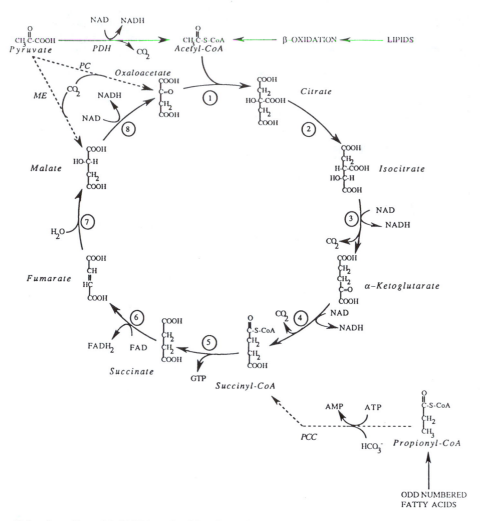

Fig. 6-3. Tricarboxylic acid (TCA) cycle. Numbered reactions within the TCA cycle are catalyzed by the following enzymes: 1, citrate synthase; 2, aconitase; 3, isocitrate dehydrogenase; 4, α-ketoglutarate dehydrogenase; 5, succinyl CoA synthase; 6, succinate dehydrogenase; 7, fumarase; 8, malate dehydrogenase. (From Lewandowski and Ingwall,[6] with permission.)

and cytochrome oxidase—interspersed with electron carriers coenzyme Q and cytochrome c. $FADH_2$ enters at the level of coenzyme Q. The specific electron-carrying groups are the flavins, iron-sulfur clusters, hemes, and copper ions. The net reaction is:

$$NADH + 0.5\ O_2 + H^+ \rightarrow H_2O + NAD^+$$

The flow of electrons through these three complexes leads to the pumping of protons from the matrix to the cytosolic side of the inner mitochondrial membranes, creating the proton-motive force.

Because O_2 has a high affinity for electrons, it provides a large thermodynamic driving force for oxidative phosphorylation. The oxidation of NADH and $FADH_2$ is coupled to the phosphorylation of ADP to form ATP via the ATPase complex, also known as H^+-ATPase, F_0, F_1-ATPase, or ATP synthase. This

ATPase is driven by the flow of protons back to the matrix. The net reaction is:

$$ADP^{3-} + Pi^{2-} + H^+ \rightarrow ATP^{4-} + H_2O$$

Oxidation of each NADH yields three ATPs, and each $FADH_2$ yields two ATPs.

The substances ATP and ADP are not permeable to the inner mitochondrial membrane. The coupled exchange of cytosolic ADP for mitochondrial ATP occurs via the ATP-ADP translocase. The result is a net transfer of one negative charge out of the matrix, decreasing the membrane potential. About 25 percent of the energy obtained from respiration is used to restore this membrane potential. The net reaction for the complete oxidation of glucose in heart is:

$$\text{Glucose} + 38\ ADP + 38\ Pi + 38\ H^+$$
$$+ 6\ O_2 \rightarrow 6\ CO_2 + 38\ ATP + 42\ H_2O$$

In this way, electron transport is tightly coupled to phosphorylation—hence the high efficiency of ATP synthesis via oxidative phosphorylation.

Respiration is controlled by availability of NADH, O_2, ADP, and Pi. Based on experiments using isolated mitochondria, the notion that ADP is the most important regulator became widely accepted. Using ^{31}P NMR spectroscopy to measure ATP, phosphocreatine, and pH in vivo, cytosolic ADP concentrations can now be calculated with reasonable confidence. Coordinate changes in ADP and respiration rates can be shown in some[2] but not all[10] experimental conditions. Thus regulators other than ADP must also function to regulate respiration in vivo. The choice is governed by the physiology and pathophysiology of the moment. The existence of multiple regulators minimizes fluctuations in ATP production and maintenance of a high phosphorylation potential, [ATP]/[ADP]/[Pi].

HEART FAILURE

It is critically important to understand how the pathways for ATP production combine to maintain ATP levels in the failing heart. It is highly likely that the relative contributions of the metabolic pathways described above integrate differently in the failing heart. How this process occurs during the development of compensated hypertrophy and then from compensated to decompensated hypertrophy requires application of the tools of biochemistry, biophysics, physiology, and cellular and molecular biology. A multidisciplinary approach was suggested by Sylven and colleagues,[11] who showed that mRNA for the adenine nucleotide translocator is up-regulated in ventricular biopsy specimens obtained from patients with dilated cardiomyopathy.

ATP Synthesis from Creatine Kinase

The major nonpurine high-energy phosphate-containing compound in the heart is phosphocreatine (PCr) (free energy − 10.3 kcal/mol). In heart the PCr concentration is twice the ATP concentration. Transfer of the phosphoryl group between PCr and ATP is not oxygen-consuming and is catalyzed by creatine kinase:

$$PCr + MgADP + H^+ \leftrightarrow creatine + MgATP$$

The overall equilibrium position is far to the right, kEq is approximately 144 at pH 7. Creatine kinase is abundant in excitable tissues. It exists as a family of five isozymes: BB, MB, MM, and the ubiquitous

and sarcomeric mitochondrial isoforms. The discovery that the mitochondrial creatine kinase isoenzyme is located on the inner mitochondrial membrane[12] and some of the MM isoenzyme in the M-band of the myofibril[13] has led to the hypothesis the creatine-PCr "shuttles" chemical energy between sites of ATP production (mitochondria) and sites of ATP utilization (myofibrils and ion transport across membranes).

Using the NMR technique of magnetization transfer, the unidirectional velocity of the creatine kinase reaction can be measured in vivo. The opportunity to measure the reaction velocity of a single protein in the intact beating heart is unique. This approach allows us to understand how this enzyme works. By comparing the measured reaction velocity to the reaction velocity predicted from the rate equation developed by solution biochemists, to the maximal capacity of the reaction (Vmax) measured in tissue homogenates under saturating substrate conditions, and to the rate of ATP synthesis from other pathways, several conclusions can be drawn: (1) ATP synthesis via creatine kinase is 10 times faster than the net ATP synthesis rate estimated from the physiologic index of oxygen consumption. Because its reaction velocity is high, creatine kinase effectively functions to (a) resupply ATP during high demand conditions, (b) keep [ADP] and [Pi] low thereby maintaining a high driving force for all ATPase reactions, and (c) buffer the intracellular hydrogen ion concentration. (2) The ratio of measured creatine kinase reaction velocity in the beating heart to Vmax is approximately 0.1, which means that most of the enzyme activity is not used. It is not known if enzyme activity can be recruited for use under times of high energy demand. (3) Comparison of measured and predicted reaction velocities are usually in good agreement. However, lack of agreement in the presence of hypoxia and ischemia, when the reaction velocity measured in vivo is *lower* than predicted from the rate equation,[14] and lack of agreement when failing, aged hearts are treated with angiotensin converting enzyme (ACE) inhibitors,[4] when the velocity is *higher* than predicted from the rate equation, show that the enzyme is regulated in vivo by mechanisms in addition to substrate control. A likely candidate is a (de)phosphorylation cycle.

ENERGY RESERVE AND CONTRACTILE PERFORMANCE

The creatine kinase system acts as an energy reserve mechanism, especially during high workload conditions. The link between energy reserve and contractile reserve is clearly shown for the ATP supply–demand mismatch that occurs with hypoxia and ischemia when phosphoryl transfer's from PCr to ADP slows the rate of tissue ATP depletion. The link has also been shown in three experiments designed to selectively perturb the creatine kinase reaction in intact striated muscle. First, acute and selective chemical inhibition of creatine kinase activity in intact rat hearts with the sulfydryl group modifier iodoacetamide resulted in decreased contractile reserve when the heart was inotropically stressed with either high extracellular $[Ca^{2+}]$ or norepinephrine.[15] Second, in rat hearts in which the myocardial PCr pool was replaced with a poorly hydrolyzable guanidino analog, β-guanidinopropionic, the PCr content, creatine kinase reaction velocity, and heart function all decreased under high workload conditions.[16] Third, depleting M creatine kinase by transgenic technology reduced the ability of skeletal muscle to sustain burst work.[17] Each of these experiments shows that decreasing energy reserve limits the ability of striated muscle to increase contractile performance. Moreover, the perturbations that result in *chronic* impairment of creatine kinase activity, such as the M creatine kinase knockout, elicit compensatory changes in other pathways for ATP synthesis. Most notably, glycolytic capacity and the fractional cell volume of mitochondria increased in striated muscle of the M creatine kinase knockout mouse.

These results illustrate the important principle that ATP synthesis occurs by the integration of all ATP-synthesizing pathways. When one pathway is diminished or eliminated (in this case the creatine kinase reaction), compensatory increases occur in the others. The biochemical remodeling of the myocyte also emphasizes the importance of the creatine kinase system for phosphoryl transfer. Taken together, and of great importance for understanding the bioenergetics of heart failure, these results also show that reducing the energy reserve of the heart by selectively inhibiting creatine kinase activity leads to decreased contractile reserve.

CREATINE KINASE SYSTEM IN FAILING MYOCARDIUM

Evidence obtained using myocardium obtained from patients with dilated cardiomyopathy suggests that the capacity for ATP resynthesis via the creatine kinase system is compromised in failing myocardium. This conclusion is based on measured decreases in both the tissue activity of creatine kinase (30 to 50 percent decrease in Vmax)[18,19] and in tissue content of the guanidino substrate for the reaction, that is, the sum of free creatine and PCr (60 percent decrease).[18] Consistent with the decrease in total cre-

atine content, ^{31}P NMR studies of the failing human myocardium by several groups[20-22] have shown that PCr is decreased in failing myocardium compared to that in nonfailing myocardium. These reports describe lower PCr/ATP resonance area ratios in the ^{31}P NMR spectrum. If (as occurs in at least some animal models of severe failure) ATP content is also lower in failing human myocardium, the decrease in PCr content would be even greater than indicated by the PCr/ATP ratio.

The changes in Vmax and guanidino pool observed with human heart failure are faithfully reproduced in animal models of heart failure. These results have been reviewed elsewhere.[23] One of the major advantages of studying small animal models of heart failure is that we can use ^{31}P NMR spectroscopy to measure the turnover rate of the phosphoryl group in the intact beating heart while simultaneously measuring contractile performance. We and our colleagues have observed decreased cardiac function or contractile reserve (or both) in several animal models of heart failure, each with a different etiology: the 18-month-old failing spontaneously hypertensive rat heart,[24] the 10-month-old failing hamster heart,[4] the rat heart 8 weeks after myocardial infarction,[3] and the furazolidone-treated turkey poult.[25] Consistent with depressed cardiac performance during congestive heart failure in humans and in other animal models of failure, isovolumic contractile performance measured as the rate–pressure product in hearts isolated from failing animals was much lower (typically 50 to 70 percent lower) than for hearts isolated from age-matched nonfailing animals perfused under the same conditions of load and coronary flow. In concert with the decrease in contractile performance, the tissue content of PCr, the capacity for ATP synthesis via the creatine kinase reaction measured as tissue enzyme activity (Vmax), and the rate of phosphoryl transfer measured as creatine kinase reaction velocity in vivo are all lower in the severely failing mammalian myocardium.

We conclude that the creatine kinase phenotype in failing myocardium can be described as large decreases in both total creatine kinase activity (Vmax) and the guanidino pool. These decreases are independent of species and etiology, strongly suggesting that it is a property of failing myocardium. Decreased Vmax and PCr content combine to limit the velocity of the creatine kinase reaction. We now know that this decrease in energy reserve limits the contractile reserve of the heart. In the normal heart, decreased energy reserve via creatine kinase reaction leads to compensatory increases in glycolysis and the machinery for oxidative phosphorylation, maintaining normal baseline contractile performance. The relevant question becomes: Does the heart fail because it cannot adapt?

ACKNOWLEDGMENTS

We acknowledge the help of our colleagues who have contributed to our work on heart failure: Paul D. Allen, John A. Bittl, Jan Friedrich, Julie K. Fetters, Judith K. Gwathmey, Baron Hamman, William E. Jacobus, Martha F. Kramer, Ronglih Liao, Luigino Nascimben, Stefan Neubauer, Janice Pfeffer, Ilana Reis, and Rong Tian.

REFERENCES

1. Christe M, Tian R, Hopkins JA, Ingwall JS: Elevated [ADP] increases end diastolic pressure in hearts with normal glycolytic rates. J Mol Cell Cardiol 1995;27:A50
2. Bittl JA, Ingwall JS: Reaction rates of creatine kinase and ATP synthesis in the isolated rat heart. A P-31 magnetization transfer study. J Biol Chem 1985;260:3512–3517
3. Neubauer S, Horn M, Naumann A et al: Impairment of energy metabolism in intact myocardium of rat hearts with chronic myocardial infarction. J Clin Invest 1995;95:1092–1100
4. Nascimben L, Friedrich J, Liao R et al: Enalapril treatment increases cardia performance and energy reserve via the creatine kinase reaction in myocardium of Syrian myopathic hamsters with advanced heart failure. Circulation 1995;91:1824–1833
5. Zimmer HG, Trendelenburg C, Kammermeier H, Gerlach E: De novo synthesis of myocardial adenine nucleotides in the rat. Circ Res 1973;32:635–642
6. Lewandowski ED, Ingwall JS: The physiological chemistry of energy production in the heart. p. 153. In Schlant RC, Alexander RW (eds): The Heart. 8th Ed. McGraw-Hill, New York, 1994
7. Camacho SA, Wikman-Coffelt J, Wu ST et al: Improvement in myocardial performance without a decrease in high energy phosphate metabolites after isoproterenol in Syrian cardiomyopathic hamsters. Circulation 1988;77:712–719
8. Wikman-Coffelt J, Sievers R, Parmley WW, Jasmin G: Cardiomyopathic and healthy acidotic hamster hearts. Mitochondrial activity may regulate cardiac performance. Cardiovasc Res 1986;20:471–481
9. Di Lisa F, Fan C-Z, Gambassi G et al: Altered pyruvate dehydrogenase control and mitochondrial free Ca^{+2} in hearts of cardiomyopathic hamsters. Am J Physiol 1993;264(Heart Circ Physiol 33):H2188–H2197
10. Katz LA, Swain JA, Portman MA, Balaban RS: The relation between phosphate metabolites and oxygen consumption in the heart in vivo. Am J Physiol 1989;256:H265–H274
11. Sylven C, Lin L, Jansson E et al: Ventricular adenine nucleotide translocator mRNA is upregulated in dilated cardiomyopathy. Cardiovasc Res 1993;27:1295–1299
12. Bessman SP, Fonyo A: The possible role of the mitochondrial bound creatine kinase in regulation of mitochondrial respiration. Biochem Biophys Res Commun 1966;22:597–602
13. Turner DC, Walliman T, Eppenberger HM: A protein that binds specifically to the M-line of skeletal muscle is identified as the muscle form of creatine kinase. Proc Natl Acad Sci USA 1973;70:702–705
14. Bittl JA, Balschi JA, Ingwall JS: Contractile failure and high-energy phosphate turnover during hypoxia.[31] P-NMR surface coil studies in living rat. Circ Res 1987;60:871–878
15. Hamman BL, Bittl JA, Jacobus WE, Ingwall JS: Inhibition of creatine kinase decreases the contractile reserve of the isolate rat heart. In: Proceedings of the 5th Annual Meeting of the Society for Magnetic Resonance Medicine 1986;WP:133
16. Zweier JL, Jacobus WE, Korecky B, Brandeis-Barry Y: Bioenergetic consequences of cardiac phosphocreatine depletion induced by creatine analogue feeding. J Biol Chem 1991;266:20296–20304
17. Van Deursen J, Heerschap, Oerlemans F et al: Skeletal muscles of mice deficient in muscle creatine kinase lack burst activity. Cell 1993;74:621–631
18. Nascimben L, Ingwall JS: Decreased energy reserve may cause pump failure in human dilated cardiomyopathy. Circulation 1991;84:II-563
19. Van der Laarse A, Hollaar L, Kok SW et al: Myocardial creatine kinase-MB concentration in normal and explanted human hearts and released from hearts of patients with acute myocardial infarction. Clin Physiol Biochem 1992;9:11–17
20. Conway MA, Allis J, Ouwerkerk R et al: Detection of low phosphocreatine to ATP ratio in failing hypertrophied human myocardium by ^{31}P magnetic resonance spectroscopy. Lancet 1991;338:973–976
21. Hardy CJ, Weiss RG, Bottomley PA, Gerstenblith G: Altered myocardial high-energy phosphate metabolites in patients with dilated cardiomyopathy. Am Heart J 1991;122:795–801
22. Neubauer S, Horn M, Schindler R et al: Clinical and hemodynamic correlates of impaired cardiac high-energy phosphate metabolism in patients with aortic valve disease [abstract]. p. 355. In: Proceedings of the 12th Annual Meeting of the Society for Magnetic Resonance Medicine, 1993
23. Ingwall JS: Is the failing myocardium energy starved? Heart Failure 1994;3:128–136
24. Ingwall JS: The hypertrophied myocardium accumulates the MB-creatine kinase isozyme. Eur Heart J, suppl. F 1984;5:129–139
25. Liao R, Nascimben L, Friedrich J et al: Decreased energy reserve in an animal model of dilated cardiomyopathy [abstract]. Circulation, suppl. I 1992;86:1121

7 Myocardial Mechanics

David A. Kass

The mechanical properties of the myopathic ventricle play a central role in the complex array of symptoms and abnormalities of clinical heart failure. Although attention has traditionally focused on contractile dysfunction, the failing heart also displays important alterations of diastolic properties, interactions with the systemic vasculature, myocardial and chamber energetics, and reserve mechanisms. Advances in the ability to study these changes in isolated tissues and intact humans have substantially improved our understanding of each of these factors. Furthermore, novel therapies for heart failure and their impact on cardiac mechanics can now be evaluated more specifically and in greater detail.

This chapter reviews myocardial mechanics, starting from the physiology of isolated muscle or myocytes and extending to intact chamber function of patients with cardiac disease. It focuses on recent developments in muscle mechanics, particularly those related to force–length and pressure–volume relations assessed in myocytes, isolated muscle, and the intact human heart. Cross-bridge structure and function and details of excitation–contraction coupling are covered elsewhere in this volume.

MUSCLE MECHANICS: BASIC ELEMENTS

Investigators of basic muscle mechanics have, like many biologists, begun to ask questions at the molecular level. Studies have reported the force of a single cross-bridge,[1,2] quantified the movement of myosin heads along a plate of actin monomers, and measured the force of this interaction with optical "tweezers."[3–5] Much of this work on "molecular motors" is in its infancy, and insights related to heart failure are only just evolving. For the purpose of this chapter, I have chosen to start at a more intact level: that of the muscle fiber. As it stands, much of our understanding of muscle function stems from studies performed at this level.

Four principal physiologic properties dominate the mechanical function of the cardiac muscle fiber. They can be expressed by the dependence of muscle force on (1) sarcomere length (both passive and active relations); (2) sarcomere shortening velocity (force–velocity relations); (3) the tension or load developed during the contraction (i.e., interactions between force and afterload); and (4) the rate of muscle stimulation (force–frequency dependence).

Force–Length Relation

The dependence of force generation on muscle length is generally depicted by a stress–strain or force–length relation. In the nonstimulated state, the force–length relation reflects passive properties of the constitutive proteins and elastic elements that comprise the muscle. Unlike skeletal muscle, cardiac muscle has a high internal resistance to stretch, rendering the passive force–length relation steep at sarcomere lengths of more than about 2.4 μm.[6,7] Figure 7-1A demonstrates an example of this behavior in a rat trabecula.[8] At a sarcomere length of more than 2.25 μm, the curve becomes nearly vertical. Studies of muscle fibers in which the external membrane is removed (skinned) have shown that although a sub-

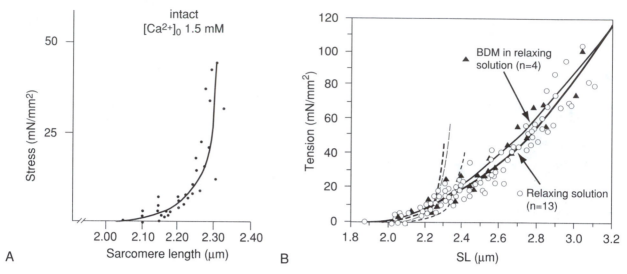

Fig. 7-1. **(A)** Passive force–sarcomere length relation of an intact rat cardiac trabecula. The relation is shallow at sarcomere lengths of 2.00–2.25 μm and then suddenly rises. The steep rise reflects the stiffness of structural proteins both within and exernal to myocytes. **(B)** Passive force–sarcomere length relation for a single myofibril. The open and closed symbols reflect, respectively, data with and without the addition of 2,3-butanedione monoxime (BDM), which inhibits cross-bridge interaction. In the normal operating sarcomere length range (1.8–2.3 μm), the data are similar to those for intact muscle, whereas at longer lengths the intact muscle is stiffer (*dashed lines*) demonstrating the contribution of structural factors. (Fig. A from Kentish et al.[8] and Fig. B from Linke et al.,[9] with permission.)

stantial component of the resistance to stretch resides in the cytoskeletal membrane proteins and extracellular matrix[8] a considerable fraction is due to internal cellular proteins. This is particularly relevant over the normal operating range of sarcomere lengths. When a single myofibril is studied[9] (Fig. 7-1B), the passive force–length relation is similar to that of more intact muscle (with or without skinning) at a sarcomere length of less than 2.3 μm, displaying much less stiffness only at longer lengths. One important and direct consequence of the inhibition to stretch at sarcomere lenghts above 2.3 μm[10] is that the classic "descending limb" of the force–length relation measured in skeletal muscle,[11] which typically occurs at sarcomere lengths of 2.4–3.7 μm, is rarely observed in the heart. Only at extraordinarily high diastolic pressures, likely incompatible with life, might one find a descending limb in cardiac muscle.

The active force-length relation reflects the influence of thick and thin myofilament interaction. The classic ultrastructural sliding filament theory of Gordon and colleagues,[11] developed from skeletal muscle data, related force development to the degree of actin and myosin overlap. The force was small at long sarcomere lengths owing to minimal overlap between thick and thin myofilaments, and it increased as the filaments became optimally overlapped (sarcomere length about 2.0 μm). At this range of lengths this mechanism best explained the *descending* limb of the force–length curve; yet as noted above, this portion

of the force–length curve is rarely reached in cardiac muscle. The *ascending* limb was ascribed to a disadvantageous double overlap of the thin filaments and deformation of the thick filaments at the Z lines at shorter sarcomere lengths.[11] More recent studies, however, have demonstrated that this behavior is primarily due to changes in the calcium sensitivity of the myofilament–regulatory protein complex as a function of sarcomere length.[8,12–14]

Figure 7-2A displays the phenomenon of length-dependent calcium sensitivity in a rat trabecula. The steady-state sigmoidal dependence of active force on [Ca^{2+}] is itself shown to be highly sensitive to the resting sarcomere length. For example, at a constant [Ca^{2+}] of 4 mmol the developed force changes profoundly as the sarcomere length is altered within the physiologic operating range (~1.65–2.10 μm). For these studies, sarcomere length was measured by laser diffraction. This methodology has proved valuable in muscle studies, as it controls for internal shortening resulting from series elasticity.[8] Length-dependent myofilament Ca^{2+} sensitivity produces a steep dependence of force on sarcomere length (systolic force–length relation). It also gives rise to a nonlinear shape of this relation, which becomes a function of Ca^{2+} concentration (or contractile state). Figure 7-2B displays systolic force data from an isolated cat trabecula at high and low Ca^{2+} concentration.[15] The passive force–length relation for this

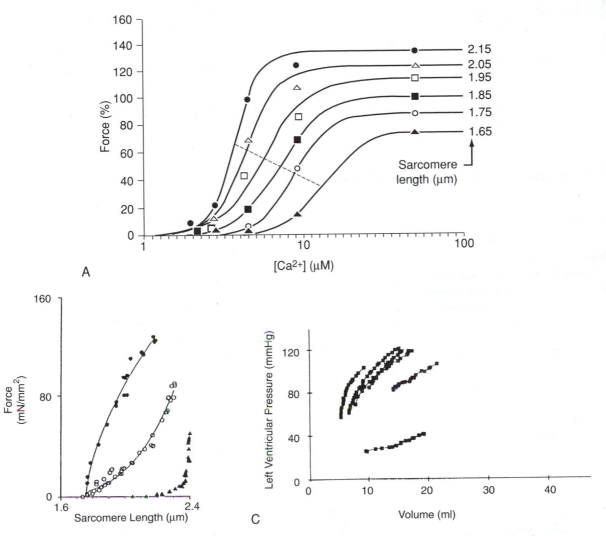

Fig. 7-2. **(A)** Length dependence of calcium activation in a skinned rat trabecula. The relation between developed force and calcium concentration in the bathing solution are plotted at six constant sarcomere lengths. The curves shift upward and to the left as the sarcomere length is increased, indicating enhanced calcium sensitivity. At a $[Ca^{2+}]$ of 4 μM, for example, force development is near zero at a sarcomere length of 1.65 μm and rises to near-maximal levels at a length of 2.15 μm. **(B)** Steady-state force–sarcomere length relations in a cat trabecula shown as a function of $[Ca^{2+}]$. ▲, passive relation; ○ and ●, data measured at 1.5 and 6.0 mM $[Ca^{2+}]$, respectively. The force–length relation shifts upward to the left with increased Ca^{2+}, and the nonlinear shape changes from concave (to the SL axis) to convex. This behavior can be explained by length-dependent Ca^{2+} activation. **(C)** Contractile dependence of the nonlinearity of end-systolic pressure–volume data of in vivo canine heart. As with isolated muscle, these relations take on concave or convex shapes depending on the level of inotropic stimulation. (Fig. A from Kentish et al.,[8] Fig. B from de Tombe et al.[15] and Fig. C from Kass et al.,[17] with permission.)

muscle is shown by the solid triangles in Figure 7-2B. At low $[Ca^{2+}]$, the force–length relation is nonlinear convex to the sarcomere length axis, analogous to the passive relation. At higher $[Ca^{2+}]$, the curve becomes concave. The dependence of the force–length relation nonlinearity on inotropic state has also been observed in the end–systolic pressure–volume relations of isolated or intact whole hearts[16–18] (Fig. 7-2C). In intact hearts with normal or enhanced inotropic stimulation, these relations are often concave,[19] whereas fail-

ing hearts take on a convex appearance. The latter has been reported, for example, in the tachycardia pacing model of dilated failure in the dog.[20]

Force–length data are analogous to stress–strain relations, except that the former are directly measurable, whereas the latter are generally not. Stress is force normalized per area of tissue, and strain is a dimensionless deformation. Stress–strain analysis is particularly valuable for assessing the properties of myocardium independent of its fiber or chamber geometry. In vivo three-dimensional strains have been measured by a variety of methods and can now be noninvasively obtained by magnetic resonance tissue tagging.[21] Stress, on the other hand, cannot yet be directly measured in the intact heart. For a cylindrical or planar sheet of muscle, relatively simple geometry can be assumed in order to estimate stress. More complex models are needed to make calculations for an intact ventricle.[22–24] To date, virtually all stress estimates at the chamber level rely on simplified models based on an axisymmetric ventricle with uniform wall properties. Sophisticated approaches in isolated canine septa have been employed by Yin and colleagues[25–27] involving a high frequency perpendicular indentor to estimate in-plane stresses. Practical extensions of this approach to the whole heart, however, remain to be developed.

Force–Velocity Relation

The hyperbolic force–velocity curve, usually generated by quick load-release experiments of isolated muscle, is thought to define the dependence of the cycling rate of the actin-myosin cross-bridge on load. Maximal unloaded shortening velocity (Vmax) was used for some time as a contractility index,[28–30] as the parameter varied with calcium concentration. Vmax was subsequently shown to be also influenced by sarcomere length, likely reflecting length-dependent Ca^{2+} activation,[9,31,32] and by internal viscous forces.[9,31,32] The latter was studied by de Tombe and ter Keurs,[31] who reported that viscous loads could largely explain the decline in Vmax at reduced levels of force generation (whether due to length or Ca^{2+} changes). Candidate proteins or structures suggested to be responsible for this viscous load include titin and microtubules. Cooper and colleagues reported that myocyte microtubular content profoundly alters unloaded cell shortening (the cellular correlate of Vmax) and can explain reduced shortening in hypertrophied failing myocytes.[33]

Although Vmax itself has found limited utility as a contractile index, the force–velocity relation has been usefully transformed into the fiber shortening (Vcf)–systolic wall stress relation[34] for contractile assessment of whole hearts (Fig. 7-3A). This function relation is analogous to the midportion of the force–velocity curve and has been employed to assess cardiac contractile performance in many clinical studies.[35–38] Vcf varies little with preload volume, whereas systolic stress changes considerably.[35] Thus the relation is preload-dependent,[34] and changes in chamber volumes must be accounted for in order to obtain meaningful interpretations. Nevertheless, it

has been useful in heart failure studies, as the data can be measured noninvasively.

Another parameter that is perhaps even easier to determine noninvasively is preload-adjusted maximal ventricular power.[39,40] Chamber power is the product of pressure and flow, as muscle power would be the product of force and shortening velocity. Maximal power is the instantaneous peak product of pressure and flow and is highly dependent on chamber preload. Dividing maximal power by the square of the end-diastolic volume. (PWRmax/EDV^2) yields a parameter that is minimally influenced by vascular loads[39,40] (Fig. 7-3B). We demonstrated that this parameter provides excellent discrimination in heart failure patients between inotropic and vasodilating drug influences (Fig. 7-3C),[40] and it has proved useful for testing novel cardiac inotropic agents.[41] Power-based assessments of cardiac function were introduced during the early 1970s, stemming from force–velocity mechanics theories.[42,43] Their renewed value derives from several studies that have established how to minimize load dependence and obtain the measurements noninvasively.[44]

Force–Afterload Dependence

In isolated muscle sudden perturbations in the active force during a twitch can have profound influences on the subsequent developed tension and relaxation.[45,46] Rapid shortening of myofibrils is thought to increase cross-bridge detachment and magnify internal viscous effects, thereby diminishing net force.[45–47] The level of isotonic developed tension also has a profound influence on the time course of the twitch, with a shorter onset and more rapid relaxation observed at reduced tensions.[45]

In the intact chamber there is no constant force (pressure or stress) experienced during ejection; however, there are parallels for both abrupt[48] and sustained afterload influences on the pressure–volume relation[49,50] and ventricular relaxation.[51] Studies have shown that the end-systolic pressure–volume relation (ESPVR) of the intact heart is altered by changes in vascular resistance; increasing resistance shifts the relation leftward,[49,50] and decreasing it shifts it to the right.[49] This behavior has been ascribed to negative effects of rapid shortening from internal viscous loads and cross-bridge detachment. Burkhoff et al. found that the ESPVR could also be favorably influenced by ejection.[52] This positive influence of shortening (compared to an isovolumic or isometric contraction) has now been shown at the sarcomere level as well and is ascribed to the influence of a higher end-diastolic length (or chamber vol-

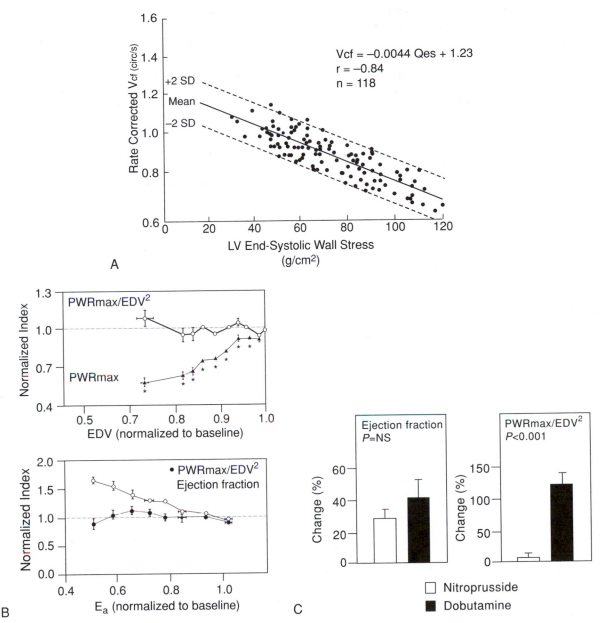

Fig. 7-3. Clinical relations that apply myocardial force–velocity behavior to the assessment of contractile function in patients. **(A)** Relation of heart rate-corrected velocity of circumferential fractional shortening (Vcf) and end-systolic wall stress from human subjects. As wall stress increases, the Vcf declines (much like the force–velocity relation of isolated muscle). The position and slope of this relation has been frequently used to index ventricular contractile function. **(B)** Preload and afterload independence of preload-adjusted maximal ventricular power (PWR_{max}/EDV^2) in patients with dilated cardiomyopathy. Data are normalized to initial baseline values of end-diastolic volume (EDV) or arterial load (E_a). (*Top*) Whereas PWR_{max} itself is highly preload-dependent, the PWR_{max}/EDV^2 ratio is minimally so. (*Bottom*) This ratio is afterload-insensitive over a physiologic range in max contrast to ejection fraction (EF).[40] **(C)** PWR_{max}/EDV^2 provides much greater specificity to inotropic change than the EF. Data are from 10 heart failure patients who received nitroprusside or dobutamine (random order). Whereas both drugs increased the EF by a similar amount, only dobutamine enhanced PWR_{max}/EDV^2, and by a much larger percent.[40] (Fig. A from Colan et al.,[34] with permission.)

ume) for the ejecting beats.[53] This phenomenon is countered by negative effects of shortening, with the net balance depending on the relative magnitude of these factors.[54] The extent and mechanisms by which this behavior may be altered in the failing heart are currently being explored.

Effects of afterload on relaxation have also been studied. As previously noted, isolated muscle demonstrates a marked prolongation of the time to the peak twitch and delay in the relaxation of tension at high afterloads. Similarly, intact hearts demonstrate that relaxation time depends on the afterload impedance: the higher the impedance, the longer the relaxation time.[51] One can also find parallels of acute load change experiments in the intact circulation. For example, vascular aging enhances late systolic reflected waves, which impose a sudden load increase on the heart during midejection. Such changes also prolong relaxation time.[55]

Force–Frequency Relation

In addition to varying its force with length, shortening velocity, and afterload tension, cardiac muscle also displays changes in systolic force due to varying stimulation frequency.[56–58] As a consequence of the E-C coupling processes by which Ca^{2+} enters and

exits the cell and is internally sequestered and released by the sarcoplasmic reticulum, myofilament Ca^{2+} availability changes with the cycle length.[58] Studies of isolated muscle have shown marked effects of heart rate on contractile function, yet in conscious animals and humans the role of the force–frequency dependence has been more controversial.[59,60] Experimental[61] and clinical[62] data based on less load-dependent pressure–volume analyses have demonstrated a nearly 100 percent increase in contractile function as the heart rate is increased from 70 bpm to 150 bpm. Furthermore, data measured in hearts with dilated[20,63] or hypertrophic cardiomyopathy[62] have shown marked blunting of this force–frequency relation.

Figure 7-4A displays data obtained from isolated muscle strips from hearts of patients with normal versus failing myopathic hearts,[64] and Figure 7-4B expresses data from intact humans with hypertrophic cardiomyopathy. In both instances there is marked depression of the contractile response to increased pacing rate in failing, compared to normal, ventricles. This depression is more fully characterized in the isolated-muscle data, which also reveals a leftward shift of the peak inotropic response to a lower frequency.[64] This abnormality may play an important role in limiting contractile reserve during heart failure. The blunted force–frequency relation

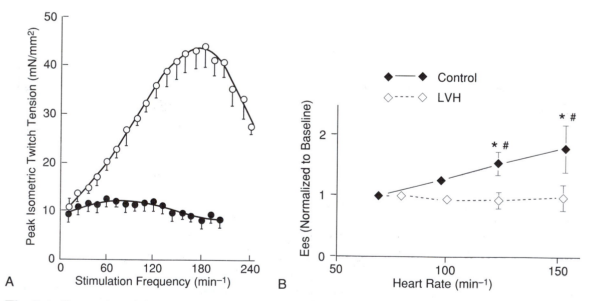

Fig. 7-4. Depression of the cardiac force–frequency relation in patients with dilated and hypertrophic cardiomyopathy. **(A)** Results from isolated muscle strips obtained from human ventricles and paced in a tissue bath. Normal hearts display a marked rise in developed isometric force peaking near 180/min. In contrast, failing hearts have a severely blunted response to a varying stimulation rate and a leftward shift of this peak. **(B)** Similar results from intact patients with congestive failure due to chronic hypertrophy. Contractile function assessed by the end-systolic elastance (E_{es}) increases with heart rate in normal subjects (●) but is markedly depressed in patients with left ventricular hypertrophy (◇). (Fig. A from Mulieri et al.,[64] and Fig. B from Liu et al.,[62] with permission.)

has been correlated with reductions in mRNA message and protein levels of the sarcoplasmic reticular ATPase.[65]

CHAMBER MECHANICS: PRESSURE–VOLUME RELATIONS

Ventricular pressure–volume data are the chamber level correlates of force–length relations of isolated muscle. Active and passive force–length relations correspond to the diastolic and end-systolic pressure–volume relations of an intact heart. The intact chamber data also embody properties of the extracellular matrix and vascular elements,[6,66,67] electrical activation sequence,[68] and three-dimensional fiber and chamber geometry,[69] so it is not as specific for myocyte function. Importantly, however, pressure–volume analysis provides a useful approach for examining each of the above described basic mechanical behaviors of cardiac muscle in intact patients.[70–72]

Figure 7-5A displays human pressure–volume data recorded at rest and during transient reduction of ventricular preload volume. It was accomplished by means of an intraventricular conductance catheter to measure volume[73,74] and vena caval inflow obstruction via a balloon catheter. This method results in a gradual decline in left ventricular volumes and stroke volumes. The rapidity of this unloading maneuver generally results in data with minimal reflex increase in heart rate despite the often substantial decline in systolic pressure. Systolic and diastolic pressure–volume relations are easily determined from this set of loops (Fig. 7-5B). These relations are analogous to the passive and active force–length relations, as shown in Figure 7-2B. To a large extent, changes in the slope or position of each boundary defines primary mechanical abnormalities in systolic pump function, diastolic chamber stiffness, and geometric remodeling.

Systolic Function and the ESPVR

Like the active force–length relation of muscle, the chamber ESPVR provides a measure of systolic pump performance. As discussed in the section Force–Length Relation, myofilament [Ca^{2+}] sensitivity varies with length[8,12–14] (or volume).[75] There is thus an implicit ambiguity in defining "contractility" from this relation (or for that matter from a systolic force–length relation, as shown in Figure 7-2B). When accepting this relation as a measure of contractile function for the whole chamber[76,77] it should be recognized that the preload dependency of [Ca^{2+}] activation is, by definition, *not* viewed as an alteration in inotropic state.

Emphasis has historically been placed on the ESPVR slope (Ees or Emax) as a measure of "contractility." As shown by the studies of Sagawa et al.[70] and Kass[71] in isolated hearts and by others in intact animals[78,79] and human hearts,[9,71,72,80] the ESPVR slope does indeed acutely vary with inotropic state, and it can be utilized as a fairly load-insensitive measurement of this change. An example in a patient with hypertrophic cardiomyopathy before and after receiving a 10 mg IV bolus of verapamil is shown in Figure 7-5C. This relation can also shift rightward or leftward with changes in contractile function, particularly when dysfunction is regional, as with dyssynchronous activation or ischemia.[81–84] Figure 7-5D displays this behavior in a patient during acute left anterior descending coronary artery occlusion. Thus a slope change is not required to indicate a decline (or improvement) in contractile performance; acute right and left parallel shifts of the ESPVR also convey this information.

Even more complex issues are raised when the ESPVR is examined in patients with chronic disease, as changes in chamber geometry and nonmyocyte composition of the wall contribute to the relation. Figure 7-6 displays data from a normal human subject as well as showing examples of chronic heart diseases: dilated cardiomyopathy, hypertrophic disease, and restrictive heart disease (amyloidosis). In each case, the slope or position of the ESPVR is altered. Hypertrophic and restrictive diseases result in steep ESPVRs, whereas dilated cardiomyopathy (DCM) hearts have shallow relations. Both DCM and restrictive hearts show a rightward shift of the relation. In the case of amyloidosis, this shift may reflect the influence of the infiltrative process that prevents the myocardium from contracting to lower systolic volumes. In the case of DCM, the rightward shift likely effects chronic chamber remodeling, which enables the heart to dilate to two to four times its resting size without reaching extraordinarily high diastolic pressures. It is virtually impossible to know the true contractile performance of the underlying myocytes based on such chamber data. Some investigators have applied stress–strain models to better account for chamber geometry[22–24]; however, this method has limitations, as the unstressed reference state cannot be measured, and many simplifying assumptions are required to estimate stress. Still, it often improves extrapolations from chamber to muscle level physiology.

In addition to the end-systolic pressure–volume relation, the same set of pressure–volume loops recorded at varying preloads can be used to derive other useful pump function relations. One such relation is a linear dependence of stroke work (SW) and

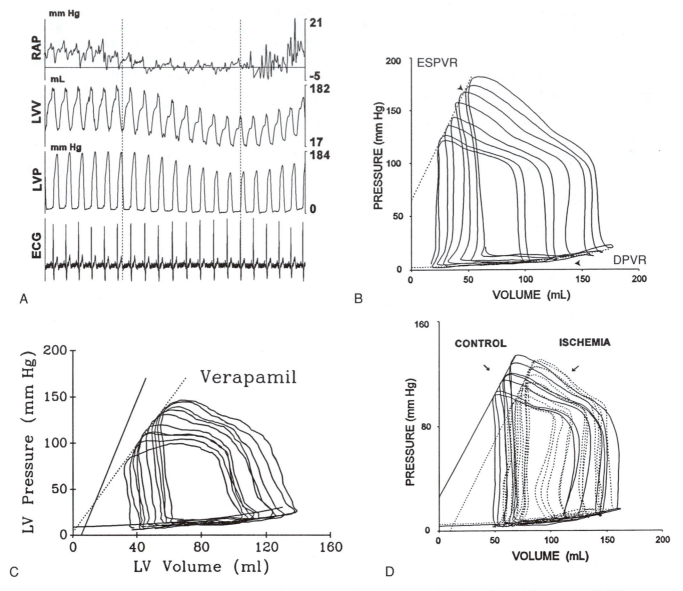

Fig. 7-5. **(A)** Time series plot of ventricular pressure (LVP), volume (LVV), right atrial pressure (RAP), and the electrocardiogram (ECG) before and during transient obstruction of inferior vena cava inflow (between *vertical dotted lines*) by a balloon catheter. There is a rapid decline in chamber preload and corresponding reductions in systolic pressures and stroke volumes due to this maneuver. Heart rate is minimally influenced owing to its rapidity. Pressure–volume relations are constructed from these data. **(B)** Pressure–volume loops generated during the transient decline in left ventricular preload. As with the force–sarcomere length relations of isolated muscle, these relations define passive (DPVR) and active (ESPVR) relations for the whole heart. **(C)** Acute global contractile changes such as produced by verapamil 10 mg IV manifest as a decline in the slope of the ESPVR relation. **(D)** Acute regional contractile changes, such as are produced by abrupt occlusion of the proximal left anterior descending artery, often manifest as rightward shifts of the relation with less change in slope. This change also is interpreted as a decline in systolic pump function. (From Kass,[71] with permission.)

end-diastolic volume (EDV).[85] This relation, often termed preload recruitable stroke work, is a modification of the Sarnoff curve,[86] itself a variant of the Starling relation. Stroke work integrates the data between diastolic and systolic pressure–volume boundaries and can therefore be altered by abnor-

malities in both.[87] Practically, it is far more influenced by systolic function changes. The SW–EDV relation has some advantages in clinical studies, as the slope of this relation (units of millimeters of mercury) is minimally changed by chamber size compared to the ESPVR. This slope has proved to be remarkably

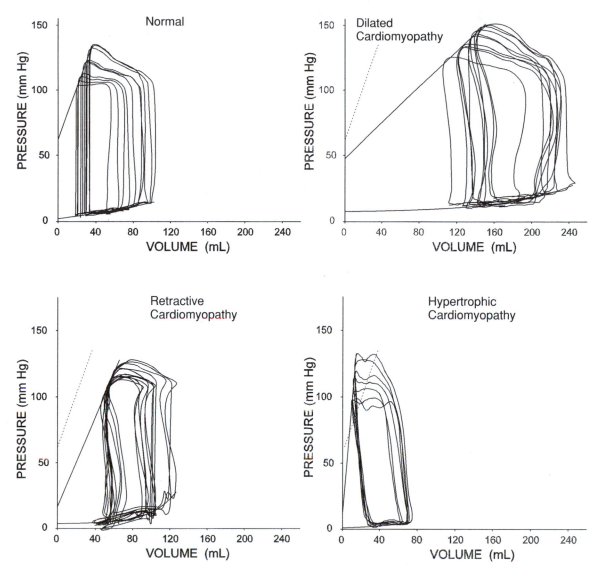

Fig. 7-6. Pressure–volume relations in a normal subject and patients with dilated, restrictive, and hypertrophic cardiomyopathy. Dilated cardiomyopathy typically reduces the ESPVR slope and shifts the relation rightward. Restrictive disease (amyloid in this instance) also shifts the ESPVR rightward, but the slope remains steep, reflecting stiffening of the myocardium. The diastolic relation is shifted upward and is steeper. Hypertrophic disease usually presents with small end-systolic volumes, a steep ESPVR slope, and variable changes in the diastolic function curve. (From Kass,[71] with permission.)

similar (75–80 mmHg) in normal hearts of humans and of small or large animals (Fig. 7-7).

Diastolic Function: End-Diastolic Pressure–Volume Relation

Diastolic chamber function can be conveniently separated into events that occur upon the initiation of relaxation and elastic recoil and those associated with chamber filling. Both properties have been studied extensively in isolated muscle and intact hearts. The relaxation time constant measured in adult humans is normally 35–50 ms. During various forms of heart failure this time constant can be prolonged to as much as 100 ms.[88–90] Although the role of relaxation abnormalities in clinical failure syndromes has been an area of intense study, it remains unclear just how important such changes are to net diastolic dysfunction. Clinical dilated and hypertrophic cardiomyopathy data suggest that relaxation times shorten normally[63,91] or even supranormally[62] in response to chronotropic or inotropic stimulation, making it less of a detrimental factor. Several therapies, particularly those acting via β-adrenergic activation or phosphodiesterase inhibition[91,92] or

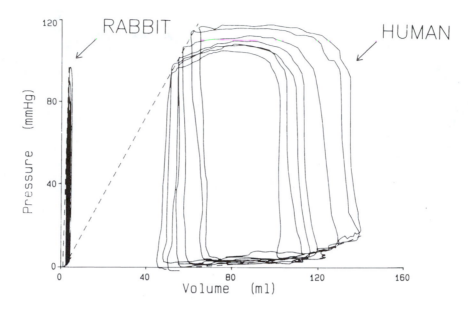

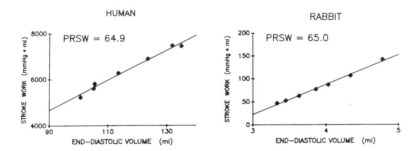

Fig. 7-7. Comparison of ESPVR (*Top*) and stroke work–end-diastolic volume (EDV) (*Bottom*) relations as a function of cardiac size. Data are shown from a normal rabbit heart and human ventricle. The marked disparity in chamber size yields a much steeper ESPVR slope (in millimeters of mercury per milliliter) for the rabbit heart. The slope of the relation between stroke work and EDV (PRSW), in millimeters of mercury, is independent of chamber size. Thus for normal myocardium in both instances one obtains similar results for this index. The index has proved useful when human hearts of variable chamber size are studied.

calcium channel blockade,[88,93] produce modest shortening of relaxation times. Yet baseline relaxation is often sufficiently brief that the dominant effect of any additional shortening manifests only during early filling. Relaxation delay may have a greater influence at faster heart rates or when filling times are abbreviated in heart failure patients with restrictive filling patterns.[94]

Another component of early diastolic function is elastic recoil. When the heart contracts to low end-systolic volumes, a portion of the contraction energy is stored in compressed elastic elements within the wall. As the myocytes relax, this stored energy is released in the form of an elastic recoil. In studies in which the heart is suddenly prevented from filling

after isovolumic relaxation, this restoring force manifests as negative chamber pressures.[95] Such energy is thought to play an important role in assisting early filling by "sucking" blood from the left atrium into the ventricle. The magnitude of negative "suction" relates to how small the chamber becomes during systole. Thus far, suction effects have been studied primarily in normal hearts; however, elastic recoil may well be abnormal in the presence of cardiomyopathy.

In addition to assisting the decline in ventricular pressure, elastic recoil also is likely responsible for a rapid reversal of systolic torsion[96–99] during early diastole. During systolic ejection the heart twists in a counterclockwise direction (relative to the base).

With early diastole there is an abrupt untwisting of the heart, reversing nearly half of the torsion within the first 15 percent of diastolic filling. Clinical studies have shown that early reverse *untwist* is reduced in disorders such as myocarditis associated with transplant rejection.[98] The development of magnetic resonance imaging methods to study torsion[99] may enable this intriguing component of early diastole to be further studied in various disease states and to explore how therapies may enhance this aspect of normal diastolic function.

The third major component of diastolic chamber mechanics, and perhaps the most important, is the passive force–length or diastolic pressure–volume relation (DPVR). The instantaneous dependence of chamber pressure on volume throughout cardiac filling provides measures of chamber elastic stiffness and compliance. Like the ESPVR, the DPVR intersects the volume axis at a positive volume. In experimental studies in which cardiac filling can be precisely controlled, this intercept, termed *equilibrium volume*, can be measured.[95] The utility of this parameter is that it can index chronic chamber remodeling[20] and provide the zero-stress reference strain for the heart. Unfortunately, in intact chambers the DPVR is influenced by the filling process, which, plus noise in the measured data, generally precludes accurate measurement of the equilibrium volume.

The slope and curvature of the DPVR can be measured using various model fits, including monoexponentials, polynomials, logarithmic equations, or even linear regression. More complex equations suffer from overparameterization in that the often limited data obtainable in an intact heart does not uniquely determine a set of fit parameters. Small perturbations at a single data point within the raw data may thereby lead to a completely different regression result. As with the ESPVR, chamber DPVR data do not reflect properties of the myocytes any more than they do the extracellular matrix, chamber geometry, and potentially the coronary vasculature.[67,100]

Whereas the relation between passive force and length (or stress–strain) is essentially unique for isolated muscle fibers or myofibrils, it is not for the intact chamber. The dependence of pressure on volume is also critically influenced by external constraining forces generated by the pericardium and by shared fibers between the right and left hearts.[101–103] In numerous animal studies, these influences have been rather small, but some studies in patients have shown that they can play a considerable role in the diastolic mechanical behavior of the heart.[104] Figure 7-8 shows diastolic pressure–volume data from resting steady state cardiac cycles (SS) as well as the data measured after the right heart was suddenly

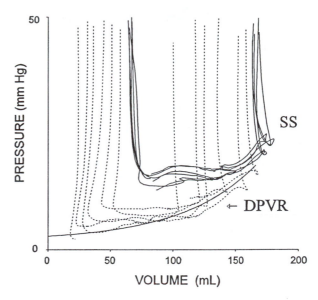

Fig. 7-8. Disparity between the steady-state resting diastolic pressure–volume relation, as is most often measured in human studies, and the diastolic pressure–volume relation obtained from many cardiac cycles during the preload reduction maneuver (i.e., Fig. 7-5B). The latter is typically at a lower pressure throughout, and the slope is somewhat steeper than that of the steady-state beat. The DVPR comes as close as is currently available to measuring the intrinsic chamber properties, with less influence of pericardial and right heart interactions.[71]

unloaded by inferior vena cava inflow obstruction (DPVR). The data are clearly different in that the latter is shifted downward. This shift primarily reflects the acute release of external forces that contributed to the resting elevated diastolic pressures. We have demonstrated that once resting diastolic left ventricular pressure exceeds 6 mmHg nearly one-third of the remaining diastolic pressure can be attributed to external forces. In other words, only about 65 percent of the resting diastolic pressure appears to reflect passive stiffness properties of the left heart.[104]

Analysis of DPVRs, as shown in Figure 7-8, has revealed several insights into human pathophysiology. For example, during acute coronary occlusion the steady-state (or resting) DPVR often shifts upward. This shift has been ascribed to ischemia-induced lowered chamber distensibility.[105,106] DPVR analysis revealed that the shift could be abruptly eliminated by right heart unloading (inferior vena cava inflow obstruction), and that the resulting DPVRs were in fact unchanged by coronary occlusion.[84,107] Furthermore, the initial resting upward shift was eliminated if the pericardium was first removed.[107] Other studies have revealed that Ca^{2+} channel or β-receptor blockers have minimal influence on the diastolic compliance of hypertrophied human hearts.[80] We reported that intravenous adenosine, which augments coronary flow and has been thought to increase pulmonary capillary wedge pressure by vascular engorgement within the myocardium,[67] also does not change the DPVR in normal human hearts.[108] Together, these and other studies indicate that most of the measured DPVR is dependent on structural components of the muscle wall. Future therapeutic efforts aimed at improving chamber compliance must be directed toward these factors.

LOADING: TRANSLATIONS FROM MUSCLE TO CHAMBER

As with isolated muscle, the two dominant components of cardiac load are the end-diastolic length (or preload) and the systolic tension (or afterload). Early muscle studies measured preload by the resting tension prior to a twitch. However, current paradigms focus on sarcomere length measured by laser diffraction because it is the length of the sarcomere rather than the tension required to obtain this length that primarily affects developed force. Similarly, at the chamber level preload has been primarily assessed by diastolic pressure, often using pulmonary capillary wedge pressure. As discussed above, there are several reasons these measures may be misleading. External forces that provide an offset to the resting diastolic pressure can alter its value independent of chamber filling. However, it is chamber stretch or volume that primarily determines cardiac performance. Second, the diastolic pressure–volume relation is often shallow in intact subjects (and animals) (Fig. 7-5B). The impact of this phenomenon is that substantial changes in preload (volume) often translate into fairly small (1–2 mmHg) changes in filling pressure. Given the inaccuracies of pressure measurement, particularly by right heart catheterization methods, it is not surprising to find that small but significant preload alterations have been frequently missed. Thus, end-diastolic volume and not pressure is the better measure of preload.

Chamber afterload is more difficult to relate to definitions pertaining to isolated muscle, as there is no fixed force against which the heart contracts. If one extends the model of a muscle contracting until a prefixed force is achieved and defines afterload as this force, the seemingly natural parallel for the intact chamber is arterial pressure or systolic stress. However, unlike isolated muscle, pressure or stress is not constant but varies considerably throughout the cardiac cycle. Furthermore, both arterial pressure and systolic stress are dependent on cardiac preload volume, as changes in preload alter ejected volumes and thus the developed pressures (Fig. 7-5B) and stresses. Figure 7-9A replots the data in Figure 7-5B employing a stress–strain formula. Note how peak stress occurs at the onset of ejection and then declines considerably during ejection. Furthermore, peak and end-systolic stress are highly influenced by preload strain alteration.

By defining afterload as arterial pressure or systolic stress, one automatically couples afterload with preload. Drugs that simultaneously influence arterial and venous vascular tones can thereby influence arterial pressures (or stress) in a complex way, making its interpretation ambiguous. To circumvent this problem, many physiology texts have imagined the pressure–volume equivalent of a "pure preload change" by a set of loops, each starting at a different preload volume but generating the identical systolic pressure (Fig. 7-9B). Although this may be the pressure–volume loop analog of an isolated muscle experiment, it is highly nonphysiologic. Indeed, it would be extraordinarily difficult to match changes in arterial impedance precisely to each preload change in order to generate such beats. Unfortunately, many investigators have embraced this notion, and there are numerous studies in which afterload is equated with arterial pressure,[109,110] yet still considered "independent" of preload.

Aortic input impedance is an alternative definition of cardiac afterload, which is far less dependent on cardiac preload than are systolic pressure and stress. Impedance characterizes both resistive (mean) and reactive (pulsatile) components of the vascular load. The dominant factor in impedance is systemic vascular resistance, although arterial compliance, the distributed geometry of the vasculature that gives rise to reflected waves, and proximal aortic properties, contribute.[111–114] The combination of these loads is typically depicted in the frequency domain based on Fourier analysis. Studies have shown that these spectra vary somewhat with mean arterial pressure, but the change is fairly small.[115]

The frequency-domain plot of impedance modulus and phase provides an accurate description of the arterial load, but it is difficult to link this description to time-based plots of cardiac function. Vascular impedance can also be represented in the pressure–volume diagram. Sunagawa et al.[116] first proposed that the end-systolic pressure/stroke volume (Pes/SV) ratio, termed effective arterial elastance (Ea), provides a measure of aortic input impedance. Kelly et al.[117] subsequently validated this measurement in patients. In their study simultaneous central aortic pressure–flow data were used to derive vascular impedance spectra, and an elastance index of total vascular load was derived from these spectra. This impedance-based parameter was compared to

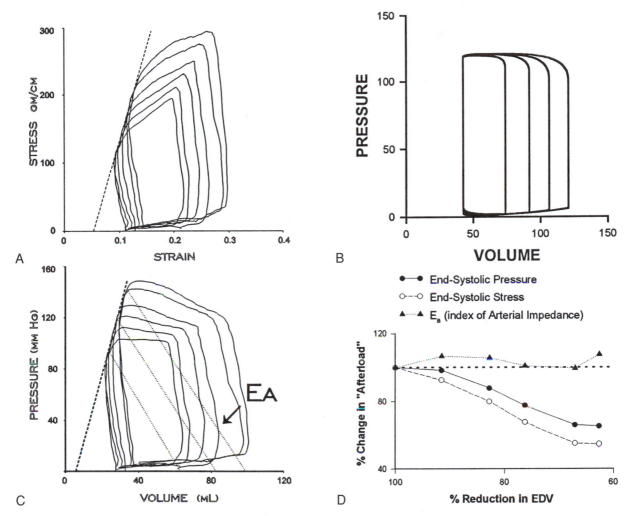

Fig. 7-9. Approaches to estimating ventricular "afterload" in the intact heart. **(A)** Systolic stress is frequently estimated. This panel shows stress–strain relations derived from the human pressure–volume loops data in **C**. Systolic stress is highest at the onset of ejection and declines thereafter; both end-systolic and peak systolic stresses are highly dependent on the preload (or end-diastolic strain) of the contraction. This situation is different from that of isolated muscle, in which afterload stress can be maintained constant during a twitch and is independent of preload strain. **(B)** This representation often appears in physiology texts to depict the effects of altered cardiac preload at a fixed "afterload." In this instance afterload is equated with systolic pressure, and thus all the loops generate identical systolic pressures and meet at the same end-systolic pressure–volume point regardless of the stroke volume ejected. This scheme is patterned after isolated muscle paradigms but is nonphysiologic. In the intact circulation there is no way in which only preload volume can be altered without arterial pressures also changing. **(C)** In addition to stress and arterial pressure, arterial impedance can be used to index the afterload. In the pressure–volume loop plane, it can be measured as the effective arterial elastance (Ea), drawn as the diagonal line connecting the end-systolic pressure–volume point to the (0,EDV) point. As shown, this slope is minimally influenced by changes in preload volume. **(D)** Percent change in various measures of chamber "afterload" as a function of preload. Unlike systolic stress or pressure, the arterial impedance, indexed in this case by E_a, is minimally affected by changes in preload volume. This method has advantages for analysis of ventricular–arterial interactions and specific characterizations of heart failure interventions.

the pressure–volume loop-derived Pes/SV ratio. The two estimates were nearly identical, confirming that Ea = Pes/SV embodies the major features of the vascular afterload system.

Arterial elastance is graphically depicted in Figure 7-9C. The long dashed diagonal line connects the end-systolic pressure–volume point with a point at (0, EDV). The absolute value of the slope of this line is (Pes − 0)/(EDV − ESV), or Pes/SV, which is the arterial elastance. In contrast to arterial pressure or systolic stress, arterial elastance is minimally altered by a pure preload change. Figure 7-9D displays the change in systolic pressure, end-systolic stress, and arterial elastance for the set of pressure–volume loops shown in Figure 7-5B. Whereas systolic pressure and stress are highly preload-sensitive, arterial elastance varies little.

Arterial elastance conveys two important aspects of ventricular loading: One is the vascular impedance, and the other is the effect of the number of beats per minute ejecting stroke volume into a given impedance load.[116] For a given mean peripheral vascular resistance, Ea ≈ R × HR, where HR is the heart rate. The influence of the heart rate stems from the fact that, for a given vascular impedance, the faster the heart rate the more stroke volumes are ejected per minute, the less time for arterial pressure decay between beats, and the higher the Pes. Because Ea = Pes/SV, this ratio rises. The heart rate dependence of arterial elastance has led some to criticize it as being equally determined by a cardiac property (i.e., heart rate) and a vasculature property. It does mean that interpretation of the arterial elastance changes as solely reflecting altered systemic vascular load is true only if heart rate is constant. However, from the cardiac load perspective, combining a rate–load interaction into a single variable is often helpful. For example, during exercise the heart rate change is a major determinant of the net effect of altered vascular resistance on a cardiac performance variable such as the ejection fraction.[118] Assessment of the vascular load by resistance (or impedance) does not adequately explain how the load ultimately influences integrated performance variables such as cardiac output and ejection fraction. This value of arterial elastance as a ventricular–vascular coupling parameter is being pursued by more and more heart failure investigators and is discussed in the next section.

VENTRICULAR–VASCULAR COUPLING

With each ejection the heart matches systolic force generation with the vascular loading system. The interaction of the two components ultimately deter-mines systemic variables, such as cardiac output, ejection fraction, external work, mechanical efficiency, and systolic pressure. Depending on the matching of cardiac and vascular properties, several of these variables can be maximized or become suboptimal. There are several ways to assess ventricular–vascular coupling, but the pressure–volume framework employing ESPVR and arterial elastance parameters has been particularly powerful. For this description, coupling is generally expressed by the arterial elastance/ESPVR slope ratio (Ea/Ees).

In a model heart, optimal transfer of energy or work (power or stroke work) is predicted to occur when the Ea/Ees ratio is 1.0.[116,119] Nonlinearity[16,17] and afterload dependencies of the ESPVR[49,52] can alter this ratio somewhat, and in isolated hearts the ratio was found to be 0.8 ± 0.16.[120] Similar data have been reported for conscious dogs[121] and in patients.[122] Figure 7-10A displays the nonlinear dependence of stroke work and metabolic efficiency on changes in the Ea/Ees ratio measured in isolated dog hearts.[120] The abscissa is shown using a log scale to clarify the relation over a wide range of ratios. The plateau of the relation is fairly broad, encompassing ratios from 0.4 to 1.2 (ejection fractions from about 40 to 80 percent). Chiu et al. reported analogous data in human subjects for ventricular power.[123] Again, many of these curves were shallow, but an optimal point was generally observed (Fig. 7-10B). Interestingly, in healthy individuals the coupling ratio is such that near-maximal power, efficiency, and stroke work are obtained. Furthermore, this condition of optimal matching is maintained during exercise.[124] The normal matching of the heart and vessels to achieve near-optimal power and efficiency has been suggested to relate to an evolutionary process designed to maintain a minimum relative heart/body size ratio.[125]

Work or power output is far from optimal, however, in hearts with depressed contractility and increased vascular loading, which is typical of congestive heart failure syndromes. Asanoi et al.[126] first reported coupling ratios in patients with normal and moderately or severely depressed left ventricular function. In the patients with ejection fractions of about 20 percent, the coupling ratio was more than 2.5. As shown by the isolated heart data (Fig. 7-10A), at such a ratio external work is nearly 50 percent below optimal (vertical dashed line). An example of how this can be important is shown in Figure 7-11. Panel A displays pressure–volume loops of a patient before and during an acute bolus injection of nitroglycerin 400 μg IV. There is a marked beat-to-beat decline in arterial load (arte-

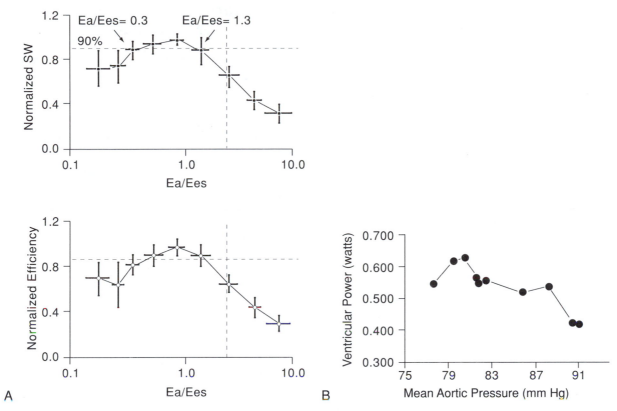

Fig. 7-10. **(A)** Influence of varying ventricular vascular coupling on cardiac stroke work (SW) and myocardial efficiency (EFFIC = SW/MVO$_2$). Both parameters have optimums that occur near an Ea/Ees coupling ratio of 1.0. The horizontal line represents 90 percent of optimum point, and ventricular-vascular coupling can vary considerably while maintaining 90 percent or more of this optimum. In heart failure patients the Ea/Ees ratio often exceeds 2.5. The vertical line demonstrates that with this interaction (i.e., high vascular resistance and reduced ventricular contractile function) both work and efficiency are compromised by nearly 40 percent of their potential maximum. These data were obtained in isolated canine ventricles. **(B)** Similar analysis in an intact dilated cardiomyopathy human heart, with a ventricular power (rate of work) plot versus mean arterial pressure (as a reflection of varied resistance). (Fig. A from de Tombe et al.,[120] and Fig. B from Chiu et al.,[123] with permission.)

rial elastance, solid lines, show a gradual decline in slope). Because the resting Ea/Ees ratio was high (near 4.5) this afterload reduction is predicted to enhance cardiac work, which was indeed the case, as shown in Figure 7-11B, where stroke work was plotted versus the natural log of the Ee/Ees ratio. The solid line shows the theoretic dependence of these variables based on reported coupling equations.[77] Thus one way to view vasodilator treatment in such a patient is that it can improve the matching of a depressed heart with the vascular load.[127,128] Whether optimizing cardiac work efficiency, or power output in heart failure patients improves long-term outcome and should thus be an important goal of therapy remains to be tested.

Energetic factors are also frequently considered in studies of ventricular–arterial interaction. Mechanical efficiency, defined by the cardiac work/total myocardial oxygen consumption ratio (SW/MVO$_2$), is also influenced by the Ea/Ees ratio[129] (Fig. 7-10A, *lower panel*). Thus another effect of adverse cardiovascular interaction is an increase in the amount of fuel needed to perform the same external work. The SW/MVO$_2$ ratio is more difficult to measure in humans, although several studies have reported such data.[129,130] As with external work, the SW/MVO$_2$ ratio is fairly constant over a broad range of coupling ratios, but it declines substantially as the ratio exceeds 2.0–3.0 (Fig. 7-10A).[120] Using a theoretic model, Burkhoff and Sagawa first suggested that the coupling ratios for maximal efficiency and work were sufficiently different that optimization of both was impossible.[119] In reality, there appears to be sufficient overlap and the dependence of both parameters on the Ea/Ees ratio are broad enough that this distinction is not meaningful.

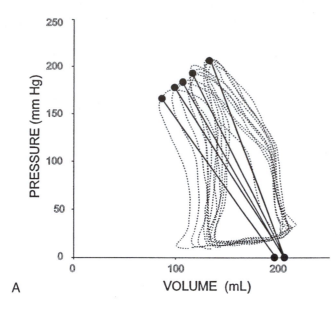

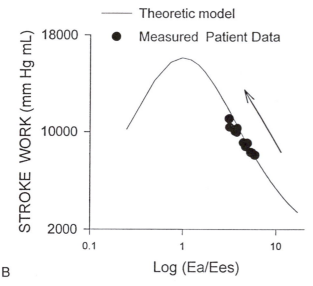

Fig. 7-11. Effect of afterload reduction on improving cardiac work in a patient with dilated cardiomyopathy. **(A)** An acute intravenous bolus of nitroglycerin was administered, resulting in a beat-to-beat decline in the vascular load (Ea). It was indexed by the gradual fall in the slope of the *dark diagonal lines* that depict Ea. This effect reduced the coupling ratio Ea/Ees. **(B)** Plot of stroke work (SW) versus Ea/Ees from the same data. Because the patient started with a high Ea/Ees ratio, the data fell along the steep portion of the relation, and improving coupling (reducing the ratio) increased the stroke work substantially. The *solid line* is a theoretic prediction based on an analytic coupling framework. In this patient, even more afterload reduction is predicted to yield further enhancements in cardiac work.

MYOCARDIAL MECHANOENERGETICS

The energy utilized to generate a given cardiac contraction is comprised of the oxygen costs for basal metabolism, excitation–contraction coupling, and external work. As with every aspect of myocardial mechanics, many methods are used to assess myocardial energetics and relate it to mechanical performance. Those most frequently employed are (1) the relation between myocardial oxygen consumption (MVO_2) and the force–time integral (the area under the force transient),[131,132] and (2) MVO_2 and the pressure–volume area (PVA).[133–136] The latter has the particular advantage of being defined by the same pressure–volume terms used to assess systolic and diastolic chamber properties as well as ventricular–vascular coupling.

Pressure–volume area is a mechanical term that combines the external work (or stroke work) with a potential energy area outlined by the ESPVR and DPVR between the end-systolic volume and the zero volume intercept of the ESPVR (Fig. 7-12A). If the heart were simply a spring with a time-varying stiffness (the notion embodied by a "time-varying elastance" model),[70,133–135] the pressure–volume area would represent both external work performed on the system (SW) and potential energy (PE) still within the spring at the end of ejection. If the heart contracts isovolumetrically, only the potential energy exists; thus all MVO_2 is potential energy and could be measured as heat. Even though this model is certainly oversimplified, the pressure–volume area has been repeatedly shown to embody the mechanical elements of total cardiac work. Studies have demonstrated that regardless of how the pressure–volume area is generated, including heartbeats that cycle backward[137] under a volume pump control, or beats in which the potential energy is turned into external work by rapidly reducing the chamber volume during the relaxation period,[138] the dependence of the pressure–volume area on MVO_2 remains fairly constant. Studies in isolated muscle have further confirmed that the potential energy is proportional to the recovery heat, adenosine triphosphate (ATP) utilization, or both during a muscle twitch.[139,140] The MVO_2–PVA relation yields a slope and intercept (Fig. 7-12B). The inverse of the slope is a measure of cardiac efficiency (work/O_2 consumption). Unlike the SW/MVO_2 ratio discussed earlier, this slope is minimally altered by ventricular–vascular coupling ratios or preload volumes. The intercept of the relation reflects non-work-related O_2 consumption, primarily that used for E-C coupling and basal metabolism.[133–135] In animal studies these components have

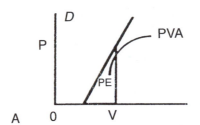
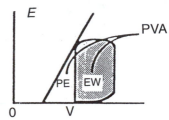

Fig. 7-12. (A) Myocardial energetics based on the pressure–volume area (PVA) concept. **(A)** PVA is calculated as the sum of external work (EW) and a potential energy term (PE). PE reflects the internal work performed if the contraction had been isovolumic at the end-systolic volume (*left panel*). **(B)** The total PVA is linearly correlated with myocardial oxygen consumption (MVO_2). Here data are shown from isolated canine hearts, in which this relation is obtained from both ejecting and isovolumic contractions. The data fall along a similar relation. **(C)** When the contractile state is increased by Ca^{2+} or epinephrine, for example, the MVO_2–PVA relation shifts upward in parallel, reflecting an increased O_2 cost for the enhanced contractile function. This analysis has proved useful for studying novel heart failure agents, particularly those that may sensitize the myofilaments to calcium and thus increase contractility without requiring an analogous upward shift of this relation. (From Suga et al.,[134] with permission.)

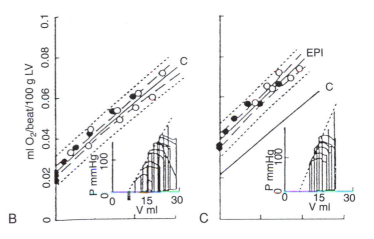

been separated by use of potassium cardioplegia[133–135] or 2,3-butanedione monoxime[141] to inhibit E-C coupling.

Whereas changes in the contraction pattern generally have a small influence on the MVO_2–PVA relation, changes in inotropic state,[136] pH,[142] and temperature[143] acutely alter the relation. Inotropic change, in particular, shifts the relation upward or downward in proportion to the contractile state (Fig. 7-12C). This relation defines the normal oxygen cost of Emax (i.e., Ees). Increasing Ca^{2+} availability to the myofilaments either directly or via the adrenergic cascade increases Ees as well as the O_2 cost of E-C coupling. The mechanometabolic conversion efficiency (MVO_2–PVA slope) is unaltered. If an intervention or disease state altered Ees without the anticipated change in MVO_2 at PVA = 0 (i.e., MVO_2–PVA relation intercept), this O_2 cost of Ees would be changed.

Conceivably, a pharmacologic agent that increased Ees without changing this intercept would be beneficial, as it could provide added contractile performance with less energy cost. Such agents are actively being sought, and it is thought that myofilament calcium sensitizers may prove to be one class of such agents. Thus far studies of pimobendan[144] and EMD[145] have not demonstrated such an effect, but this may reflect a greater than anticipated influence of phosphodiesterase inhibition from these agents. A more recent agent, MCI 154, appears more promising in this regard.[146] Acidosis has been shown to produce the opposite effect, with a decline in the Ees and minimal change in unloaded MVO_2.[142] Thus the O_2 cost of Ees is increased by acidosis.

So far few interventions have been found to alter the *slope* of the MVO_2–PVA relation (i.e., chemomechanical efficiency). One intriguing example in which the slope was altered is experimental canine dilated cardiomyopathy induced by tachycardia pacing.[20] In this instance the chemomechanical conversion efficiency was 32 percent in failing hearts compared to 23 percent in controls. However, as with acidosis, the O_2 cost of Ees was markedly increased by heart failure, offsetting this change in efficiency. Somewhat analogous improvement in myothermal economy has been reported from isolated muscle strips of failing human hearts.[131] The mechanism responsible for a change in efficiency with human or canine heart failure remains unknown. Some of the change may relate to associated alterations in the creatine kinase isoforms, with a shift toward an increase in the CKB isoform.[147,148] Changes in the thin regulatory filaments have also been suggested.

CONCLUSION

As new insights into molecular and biochemical mechanisms of heart failure come to light, understanding the relation they have to myocardial mechanical properties at both the tissue and intact organ level continue to be of prime importance. Novel methods for studying muscle function at the single actin–myosin molecular level are enabling studies of the force of a single cross-bridge, which is proving ideal for examining the effects of single gene mutations in contractile proteins on muscle function. At the opposite extreme, pressure–volume analysis is now being applied in patients with heart failure to determine the mechanisms of novel drugs and surgical therapies for heart failure, such as cardiomyoplasty.[149] Noninvasive advances may finally enable much of this theory to be applied to large-scale clinical trials, opening yet another important realm of understanding into heart failure.

REFERENCES

1. Finer JT, Simmons RM, Spudich JA: Single myosin molecule mechanics. Piconewton forces and nanometre steps. Nature 1994;368:113–119
2. Oiwa K, Kawakami T, Sugi H: Unitary distance of actin-myosin sliding studied using an in vitro force-movement assay system combined with ATP iontophoresis. J Biochem 1993;114:28–32
3. Kuo SC, Sheetz MP: Force of single kinesin molecules measured with optical tweezers. Science 1993;260:232–234
4. Svoboda K, Block SM: Force and velocity measured for single kinesin molecules. Cell 1994;77:773–784
5. Svoboda K, Schmidt CF, Schnapp BJ et al: Direct observation of kinesin stepping by optical trapping interferometry. Nature 1993;365:721–727
6. Borg TK, Ranson FA, Moslehy FA et al: Structural basis of ventricular stiffness. Lab Invest 1981;44:49–54
7. Julian FJ, Sollins MR, Moss RL: Absence of a plateau in length-tension relationship of rabbit papillary muscle when internal shortening is prevented. Nature 1976;260:340–342
8. Kentish JC, ter Keurs HEDJ, Ricciardi L et al: Comparison between sarcomere length-force relations of intact and skinned trabeculae from rat right ventricle. Circ Res 1986;58:755–768
9. Linke WA, Popov VI, Pollack GH: Passive and active tension in single cardiac myofibrils. Biophysic J 1994;67:782–792
10. Pollack GH, Krueger JW: Sarcomere dynamics in intact cardiac muscle. Eur J Cardiol 1976;4:53–65
11. Gordon AM, Huxley AF, Julian FJ: The variation in isometric tension with sarcomere length in vertebrate muscle fibers. J Physiol (Lond) 1966;184:170
12. Allen DG, Kentish JC: The cellular basis of the length-tension relation in cardiac muscle. J Mol Cell Cardiol 1985;17:821–840
13. Ter Keurs HEDJ, Rijnsburger WH, van Heuningen R et al: Tension development and sarcomere length in rat cardiac trabeculae. Circ Res 1980;46:703–714
14. Babu A, Scoiditis SP, Sonnenblick EH et al: The control of myocardial contraction with fast muscle troponin C. J Biol Chem 1987;262:5815–5822
15. De Tombe PP, ter Keurs HEDJ: Sarcomere dynamics in cat cardiac trabeculae. Circ Res 1991;68:588–596
16. Burkhoff D, Sugiura S, Yue DT et al: Contractility-dependent curvilinearity of end-systolic pressure-volume relations. Am J Physiol 1987;252:H1218–H1227
17. Kass DA, Beyar R, Lankford E et al: Influence of contractile state on curvilinearity of the in situ end-systolic pressure-volume relations. Circulation 1989;79:167–178
18. Noda T, Cheng CP, de Tombe PP et al: Curvilinearity of LV end-systolic pressure-volume and dP/dt$_{max}$-end-diastolic volume relations. Am J Physiol 1993;265:H910–H917
19. Kass DA, Maughan WL: From "Emax" to pressure-volume relations. A broader view. Circulation 1988;77:1203–1212
20. Wolff MR, de Tombe PP, Harasawa Y et al: Alterations in left ventricular mechanics, energetics, and contractile reserve in experimental heart failure. Circ Res 1992;70:516–529
21. Azhari H, Weiss JL, Rogers WJ et al: Non-invasive quantification of principal strains in normal canine hearts using tagged MRI images in 3-D. Am J Physiol 1993;264:H205–H216
22. Regen DM: Calculation of left ventricular wall stress. Circ Res 1990;67:245–252
23. Nakano K, Sugawara M, Ishihara K et al: Myocardial stiffness derived from end-systolic wall stress and logarithm of reciprocal of wall thickness. Circulation 1990;82:1352–1361
24. Arts T, Bovendeerd PHM, Prinzen FW et al: Relation between left ventricular cavity pressure and volume and systolic fiber stress and strain in the wall. Biophys J 1991;59:93–102
25. Strumpf RK, Humphrey JD, Yin FCP: Biaxial mechanical properties of passive and tetanized canine diaphragm. Am J Physiol 1993;265:H469–H475
26. Humphrey JD, Yin FCP: Biomechanical experiments on excised myocardium. Theoretical considerations. J Biomech 1989;22:377–383
27. Halperin HR, Chew PH, Weisfeldt ML et al: Transverse stiffness. A method for estimation of myocardial wall stress. Circ Res 1987;61:695–703
28. Henderson AH, Van Ocker E, Brutsaert DL: A reappraisal of force-velocity measurements in isolated heart muscle preparation. Eur J Cardiol 1973;1:105
29. Sonnenblick EH: Force-velocity relations in mammalian heart muscle. Am J Physiol 1962;202:931–939
30. Daniels M, Noble MIM, ter Keurs HEDJ: Velocity of sarcomere shortening in rat cardiac muscle. Relationship to force, sarcomere length, calcium and time. J Physiol (Lond) 1984;355:367–381
31. De Tombe PP, ter Keurs HE: An internal viscous element limits unloaded velocity of sarcomere shortening in rat myocardium. J Physiol (Lond) 1992;454:619–642
32. Wang K, McCarter R, Wright J et al: Regulation of skeletal muscle stiffness and elasticity by titin isoforms. A test of the segmental extension model of

resting tension. Proc Natl Acad Sci USA 1991;88: 7101–7105

33. Tsutsui H, Ishihara K, Cooper G IV: Cytoskeletal role in the contractile dysfunction of hypertrophied myocardium. Science 1993;260:682–687

34. Colan SD, Borow KM, Neumann A: Left ventricular end-systolic wall stress-velocity of fiber shortening relation. A load-independent index of myocardial contractility. J Am Coll Cardiol 1984;4:715–724

35. Mirsky I, Aoyagi T, Crocker VM et al: Preload dependence of fiber shortening rate in conscious dogs with left ventricular hypertrophy. J Am Coll Cardiol 1990; 15:899

36. Borow KM, Green LH, Grossman W et al: Left ventricular end-systolic stress-shortening and stress-length relations in humans. Am J Cardiol 1982;50: 1301–1308

37. Borow KM, Lang RM, Neumann A et al: Physiologic mechanisms governing hemodynamic responses to positive inotropic therapy in patients with dilated cardiomyopathy. Circulation 1988;77:625–637

38. Borow KM, Neumann A, Marcus RH et al: Effects of simultaneous alterations in preload and afterload on measurements of left ventricular contractility in patients with dilated cardiomyopathy. Comparisons of ejection phase, isovolumetric and end-systolic force-velocity indexes. J Am Coll Cardiol 1992;20:787–795

39. Kass DA, Beyar R: Evaluation of contractile state by maximal ventricular power divided by the square of end-diastolic volume. Circulation 1991;84: 1698–1708

40. Sharir T, Feldman MD, Haber H et al: Ventricular systolic assessment in patients with dilated cardiomyopathy by preload-adjusted maximal power. Validation and noninvasive application. Circulation 1994;89:2045–2053

41. Kass DA, van Anden E, Kiernan-Pownall K et al: Positive inotropic activity of vesnarinone in patients with dilated cardiomyopathy [abstract]. Circulation, suppl. II 1994;90:111

42. Russel RO, Porter CM, Frimer M et al: Left ventricular power in man. Am Heart J 1971;81:799–808

43. Unterberg RH, Korfer R, Politz B et al: Assessment of left ventricular function by a power index. An intraoperative study. Basic Res Cardiol 1989;79:423–431

44. Sharir T, Marmor A, Ting CT et al: Validation of a method for noninvasive measurement of central arterial pressure. Hypertension 1993;21:74–82

45. Gillebert TC, Sys SU, Brutsaert DL: Influence of loading patterns on peak length-tension relation and on relaxation in cardiac muscle. J Am Coll Cardiol 1989;13:483–490

46. Brutsaert DL, Sys SU: Relaxation and diastole of the heart. Physiol Rev 1989;69:1228–1315

47. Brutsaert DL, Claes VA, Sonnenblick EH: Velocity of shortening of unloaded heart muscle and the length-tension relation. Circ Res 1971;29:63–75

48. Campbell KB, Rahimi AR, Bell DL et al: Pressure response to quick volume changes in tetanized isolated ferret hearts. Am J Physiol 1989;257:H38–H46

49. Freeman GL, Little WC, O'Rourke RA: The effect of vasoactive agents on the left ventricular end-systolic pressure-volume relation in closed-chest dogs. Circulation 1986;74:1107–1113

50. Freeman GL: Effects of increased afterload on left ventricular function in closed-chest dogs. Am J Physiol 1990;259:H619–H625

51. Zile MR, Gaasch WH: Mechanical loads and the isovolumic and filling indices of left ventricular relaxation. Prog Cardiovasc Dis 1990;32:333–346

52. Burkhoff D, de Tombe PP, Hunter WC et al: Contractile strength and mechanical efficiency of left ventricle are enhanced by physiological afterload. Am J Physiol 1991;260:H569–H578

53. De Tombe PP, Little WC: Inotropic effects of ejection are myocardial properties. Am J Physiol 1994;266: H1202–H1213

54. Hunter WC: End-systolic pressure as a balance between opposing effects of ejection. Circ Res 1989;64: 265–275

55. Zatko FJ, Martin P, Bahler RC: Time course of systolic loading is an important determinant of ventricular relaxation. Am J Physiol 1987;252:H461–H466

56. Buckley NM, Penefsky ZJ, Litwak RS: Comparative force-frequency relationships in human and other mammalian ventricular myocardium. Pflugers Arch 1972;332:259–270

57. Burkhoff D, Yue DT, Franz MR et al: Mechanical restitution of isolated perfused canine left ventricles. Am J Physiol 1984;246:H8–H16

58. Wier WG, Yue DT: Intracellular calcium transients underlying the short-term force-interval relationship in ferret ventricular myocardium. J Physiol (Lond) 1986;376:507–530

59. Higgins CB, Vatner SF, Franklin D et al: Extent of regulation of the heart's contractile state in the conscious dog by alteration in the frequency of contraction. J Clin Invest 1973;52:1187–1194

60. Vatner SF, Braunwald E: Cardiac frequency. Control and adjustments to alterations [review]. Prog Cardiovasc Dis 1972;14:431–445

61. Freeman GL, Little WC, O'Rourke RA: Influence of heart rate on left ventricular performance in conscious dogs. Circ Res 1987;61:455–464

62. Liu CP, Ting CT, Lawrence W, et al: Diminished contractile response to increased heart rate in intact human left ventricular hypertrophy. Systolic versus diastolic determinants. Circulation 1993;88:1893–1906

63. Feldman MD, Alderman JD, Aroesty JM et al: Depression of systolic and diastolic myocardial reserve during atrial pacing tachycardia in patients with dilated cardiomyopathy. J Clin Invest 1988;82: 1661–1669

64. Mulieri LA, Hasenfuss G, Leavitt B et al: Altered myocardial force-frequency relation in human heart failure. Circulation 1992;85:1743–1750

65. Hasenfuss G, Reinecke H, Studer R et al: Relation between myocardial function and expression of sarcoplasmic reticulum Ca^{2+}-ATPase in failing and nonfailing human myocardium. Circ Res 1994;75: 434–442

66. Weber KT, Janicki JS, Pick R et al: Myocardial fibrosis and pathologic hypertrophy in the rat with renovascular hypertension. Am J Cardiol 1990;65:1G–7G

67. Vogel P, Mark W, Apstein CS et al: Acute alterations in left ventricular diastolic chamber stiffness. Role of the "erectile" effect of coronary arterial pressure and flow in normal and damaged hearts. Circ Res 1982; 51:465–478

68. Park RC, Little WC, O'Rourke RA: Effect of alteration

of the left ventricular activation sequence on the left ventricular end-systolic pressure-volume relation in closed-chest dogs. Circ Res 1985;57:706–717

69. Suga H, Hisano R, Goto Y et al: Normalization of end-systolic pressure-volume relation and Emax of different sized hearts. Jpn Circ J 1984;48:136–143

70. Sagawa K, Maughan WL, Suga H et al: Cardiac Contraction and the Pressure–Volume Relationship. Oxford University Press, New York, 1988

71. Kass DA: Clinical ventricular pathophysiology. A pressure-volume view. pp. 131–152. In Warltier DC (ed): Ventricular Function. Williams & Wilkins, Baltimore, 1995

72. Kass DA: Clinical evaluation of left heart function by conductance catheter technique. Eur Heart J, suppl E 1992;13:57–64

73. Baan J, Van der Velde ET, de Brun HG et al: Continuous measurement of left ventricular volume in animals and humans by conductance catheter. Circulation 1984;70:812–823

74. Kass DA, Midei M, Graves W et al: Use of a conductance (volume) catheter and transient inferior vena caval occlusion for rapid determination of pressure-volume relationships in man. Cathet Cardiovasc Diag 1988;15:192–202

75. Lew WY: Mechanisms of volume-induced increase in left ventricular contractility. Am J Physiol 1993;265: H1778–H1786

76. Sagawa K, Suga H, Shoukas AA et al: End-systolic pressure-volume ratio. A new index of ventricular contractility. Am J Cardiol 1979;40:748

77. Kass DA, Maughan WL, Guo ZM et al: Comparative influence of load versus inotropic states on indexes of ventricular contractility. Experimental and theoretical analysis based on pressure-volume relationships. Circulation 1987;76:1422–1436

78. Kass DA, Yamazaki T, Burkhoff D et al: Determination of left ventricular end-systolic pressure-volume relationships by the conductance (volume) catheter technique. Circulation 1986;73:586–595

79. Sodums MT, Badke FR, Starling MR et al: Evaluation of left ventricular contractile performance utilizing end-systolic pressure-volume relationships in conscious dogs. Circ Res 1984;54:731–739

80. Kass DA, Wolff MR, Ting CT et al: Diastolic compliance of hypertrophied ventricle is not acutely altered by pharmacologic agents influencing active processes. Ann Intern Med 1993;119:466–473

81. Sunagawa K, Maughan WL, Sagawa K: Effect of regional ischemia on the left ventricular end-systolic pressure-volume relationship of isolated canine hearts. Circ Res 1983;52:170–178

82. Little WC, O'Roarke RA: Effect of regional ischemia on the left ventricular end-systolic pressure-volume relation in chronically instrumented dogs. J Am Coll Cardiol 1985;5:297–302

83. Kass DA, Marino P, Maugman WL et al: Determinants of end-systolic pressure-volume relations during acute regional ischemia in situ. Circulation 1989; 80:1783–1794

84. Kass DA, Midei M, Brinker J et al: Influence of coronary occlusion during PTCA on end-systolic and end-diastolic pressure-volume relations in humans. Circulation 1990;81:447–460

85. Glower DD, Spratt JA, Snow ND et al: Linearity of the Frank-Starling relationship in the intact heart. The concept of preload recruitable stroke work. Circulation 1985;71:994–1009

86. Sarnoff SJ, Berglund E: Starling's law of the heart studied by means of simultaneous right and left ventricular function curves in the dog. Circulation 1954; 9:706

87. Liu CP, Ting CT, Yang TM et al: Reduced left ventricular compliance in human mitral stenosis. Role of reversible internal constraint. Circulation 1992;85: 1447–1456

88. Bonow RO: Effects of calcium-channel blocking agents on left ventricular diastolic function in hypertrophic cardiomyopathy and in coronary artery disease. Am J Cardiol 1985;55:172B–178B

89. Bonow RO: Left ventricular diastolic dysfunction as a cause of congestive heart failure. Mechanisms and management. Ann Intern Med 1992;117:502–510

90. Betocchi S, Bonow RO, Bacharach SL et al: Isovolumic relaxation period in hypertrophic cardiomyopathy. Assessment by radionuclide angiography. J Am Coll Cardiol 1986;7:74–81

91. Parker JD, Landzberg JS, Bittl JA et al: Effects of β-adrenergic stimulation with dobutamine on isovolumic relaxation in the normal and failing human left ventricle. Circulation 1991;84:1040–1048

92. Jaski BE, Fifer MA, Wright RF et al: Positive inotropic and vasodilator actions of milrinone in patients with severe congestive heart failure. Dose-response relationships and comparison to nitroprusside. J Clin Invest 1985;75:643–649

93. Lorell BH, Paulus WJ, Grossman W et al: Improved diastolic function and systolic performance in hypertrophic cardiomyopathy after nifedipine. N Engl J Med 1980;303:801–803

94. Pinamonti B, Di Lenarda A, Sinagra G et al: Restrictive left ventricular filling pattern in dilated cardiomyopathy assessed by Doppler echocardiography. Clinical echocardiographic and hemodynamic correlations and prognostic implications. J Am Coll Cardiol 1993;22:808–815

95. Nikolic S, Yellin EL, Tamura K et al: Passive properties of canine left ventricle. Diastolic stiffness and restoring forces. Circ Res 1988;62:1210–1222

96. Arts T, Meerbaum S, Reneman RS: Shear of the left ventricle during the ejection phase in the intact dog. Cardiovasc Res 1984;18:183–193

97. Beyar R, Yin FC, Hausknecht M et al: Dependence of left ventricular twist-radial shortening relations on cardiac cycle phase. Am J Physiol 1989;257: H1119–H1126

98. Yun KL, Niczyporuk MA, Daughters GT, et al: Alterations in left ventricular diastolic twist mechanics during acute human cardiac allograft rejection. Circulation 1991;83:962–973

99. Buchalter MB, Weiss JL, Rogers WJ et al: Noninvasive quantification of left ventricular rotational deformation in normal humans using magnetic resonance imaging myocardial tagging. Circulation 1990; 81:1236–1244

100. Gilbert JC, Glantz SA: Determinants of left ventricular filling and of the diastolic pressure-volume relation. Circ Res 1989;64:827–852

101. Tyberg JV, Misbach GA, Glantz SA et al: A mechanism for shifts in the diastolic, left ventricular, pressure-volume curve. The role of the pericardium. Eur J Cardiol, suppl. 1978;7:163–175

102. Smiseth O, Frais MA, Kingma I et al: Assessment of pericardial constraint. The relations between right ventricular filling pressure and pericardial pressure measured after pericardiocentesis. J Am Coll Cardiol 1986;7:307–314

103. Slinker BK, Goto Y, LeWinter MM: Systolic direct ventricular interaction affects left ventricular contraction and relaxation in the intact dog circulation. Circ Res 1989;65:307–315

104. Dauterman K, Pak PH, Nussbacher A et al: Contribution of external forces to left ventricle diastolic pressure. Implications for the clinical use of the Frank-Starling law. Ann Intern Med 1995;122:737–742

105. Serruys PW, Wijns W, van den Brand M et al: Left ventricular performance, regional blood flow, wall motion, and lactate metabolism during transluminal angioplasty. Circulation 1984;70:25–36

106. Bertrand ME, LeBlanche JM, Fourrier JL et al: Left ventricular systolic and diastolic function during acute coronary artery balloon occlusion in humans. J Am Coll Cardiol 1988;12:341–347

107. Applegate RJ: Load dependence of left ventricular diastolic pressure-volume relations during short-term coronary artery occlusion. Circulation 1991;83: 661–673

108. Nussbacher A, Arie S, Kalil R et al: Mechanism of adenosine induced elevation of pulmonary capillary wedge pressure in humans. Circulation 1995;92: 371–379

109. Varma SK, Owen RM, Smucker ML et al: Is tau a preload-independent measure of isovolumetric relaxation? Circulation 1989;80:1757–1765

110. Eichorn EJ, Willard JE, Alvarez L et al: Are contraction and relaxation coupled in patients with and without congestive heart failure? Circulation 1992; 85:2326–2328

111. O'Rourke MF: Vascular impedance in studies of arterial and cardiac function. Physiol Rev 1982;62: 570–623

112. Murgo JP, Westerhof N, Giolma JP et al: Aortic input impedance in normal man. Relationship to pressure waveforms. Circulation 1980;62:105–116

113. Pollack GH, Reddy RV, Noordergraff A: Input impedance, wave travel, and reflections in the human pulmonary arterial tree. Studies using an electrical analog. IEE Trans Biomed Eng 1968;15:151–164

114. Merillon JP, Fontenier GJ, Lerallut JF et al: Aortic input impedance in normal man and arterial hypertension. Its modification during changes in aortic pressure. Cardiovasc Res 1982;16:646–656

115. Alexander J Jr, Burkhoff D, Schipke J et al: Influence of mean pressure on aortic impedance and reflections in the systemic arterial system. Am J Physiol 1989; 257:H969–H978

116. Sunagawa K, Maughan WL, Burkhoff D et al: Left ventricular interaction with arterial load studied in isolated canine ventricle. Am J Physiol 1983;245: H773–H780

117. Kelly RP, Ting CT, Yang TM et al: Effective arterial elastance as index of arterial vascular load in humans. Circulation 1992;86:513–521

118. Sharir T, Fleg J, Kass DA: Mechanism of abnormal ejection fraction response to exercise in patients with moderate hypertension [abstract]. Circulation, suppl. II 1994;90:15

119. Burkhoff D, Sagawa K: Ventricular efficiency predicted by an analytical model. Am J Physiol 1986; 250:R1021–R1027

120. De Tombe PP, Jones S, Burkhoff D et al: Ventricular stroke work and efficiency both remain nearly optimal despite altered vascular loading. Am J Physiol 1993;264:H1817–H1824

121. Little WC, Cheng C: Left ventricular-arterial coupling in conscious dogs. Am J Physiol 1991;261: H70–H76

122. Starling MR: Left ventricular-arterial coupling relations in the normal human heart. Am Heart J 1993; 125:1659–1666

123. Chiu YC, Arand PW, Carroll JD: Power-afterload relation in the failing human ventricle. Circ Res 1992; 70:530–535

124. Little WC, Cheng CP: Effect of exercise on left ventricular-vascular coupling assessed in the pressure-volume plane. Am J Physiol 1993;264:H1629–H1633

125. Elzinga G, Westerhof N: Matching between ventricle and arterial load. An evolutionary process. Circ Res 1991;68:1495–1500

126. Asanoi H, Sasayama S, Kameyama T: Ventriculoarterial coupling in normal and failing heart in humans. Circ Res 1989;65:483–493

127. Kameyama T, Asanoi H, Ishizaka S et al: Ventricular load optimization by unloading therapy in patients with heart failure. J Am Coll Cardiol 1991;17: 199–207

128. Takaoka H, Takeuchi M, Odake M et al: Comparison of hemodynamic determinants for myocardial oxygen consumption under different contractile states in human ventricle. Circulation 1993;87:59–69

129. Ishihara H, Yokota M, Sobue T et al: Relation between ventriculoarterial coupling and myocardial energetics in patients with idiopathic dilated cardiomyopathy. J Am Coll Cardiol 1994;23:406–416

130. Nozawa T, Yasumura Y, Futaki S et al: Efficiency of energy transfer from pressure-volume area to external mechanical work increases with contractile state and decreases with afterload in the left ventricle of the anesthetized closed-chest dog. Circulation 1988; 77:1116–1124

131. Hasenfuss G, Mulieri LA, Blanchard EM et al: Energetics of isometric force development in control and volume-overload human myocardium. Circ Res 1991; 68:836–846

132. Hasenfuss G, Mulieri LA, Leavitt BJ et al: Alteration of contractile function and excitation-contraction coupling in dilated cardiomyopathy. Circ Res 1992; 70:1225–1232

133. Suga H: Ventricular energetics. Physiol Rev 1990;70: 247–277

134. Suga H, Hisano R, Goto Y et al: Effect of positive inotropic agents on the relation between oxygen consumption and systolic pressure volume area in canine left ventricle. Circ Res 1983;53:306–318

135. Goto Y, Futaki S, Kawaguchi O et al: Left ventricular contractility and energetic cost in disease models—an approach from the pressure-volume diagram. Jpn Circ J 1992;56:716–721

136. Suga H: Total mechanical energy of a ventricle model and cardiac oxygen consumption. Am J Physiol 1979; 236:H498–H505

137. Suga H, Goto Y, Yasumura Y et al: Oxygen saving effects of negative work in dog left ventricle. Am J Physiol 1988;254:H34–H44

138. Hata K, Goto Y, Suga H: External mechanical work during relaxation period does not affect myocardial oxygen consumption. Am J Physiol 1991;261: H1778–H1784

139. Hisano R, Cooper GIV: Correlation of force-length area with oxygen consumption in ferret papillary muscle. Circ Res 1987;61:318–328

140. Mast F, Elzinga G: Heat released during relaxation equals force-length area in isometric contractions of rabbit papillary muscle. Circ Res 1990;67:893–901

141. Yaku H, Slinker BK, Mochizuki T et al: Use of 2,3-butanedione monoxime to estimate nonmechanical VO_2 in rabbit. Am J Physiol 1993;265:H834–H842

142. Hata K, Goto Y, Kawaguchi O et al: Hypercapnic acidosis increases oxygen cost of contractility in the dog left ventricle. Am J Physiol 1994;266:H730–H740

143. Suga H, Goto Y, Igarashi Y et al: Cardiac cooling increases Emax without affecting relation between O_2 consumption and systolic pressure-volume area in dog left ventricle. Circ Res 1988;63:61–71

144. Hata K, Goto Y, Futaki S et al: Mechanoenergetic effects of pimobendan in canine left ventricles. Circulation 1992;82:1291–1301

145. De Tombe PP, Burkhoff D, Hunter WC: Effects of calcium and EMD–53998 on oxygen consumption in isolated canine hearts. Circulation 1992;86: 1945–1954

146. Mori M, Takeuchi M, Takaoka H et al: New Ca^{2+} sensitizer, MCI-154, reduces myocardial oxygen consumption for non-mechanical work in diseased human hearts [abstract]. Circulation, suppl. II 1994; 90:217

147. Williams RE, Kass DA, Kawagoe Y et al: Endomyocardial gene expression during development of pacing tachycardia-induced heart failure in the dog. Circ Res 1994;75:615–623

148. Ingwall JS: Is cardiac failure a consequence of decreased energy reserve? Circulation, suppl. VII 1993; 87:58–62

149. Kass DA, Baughman KL, Pak PH et al: Reverse remodeling from cardiomyoplasty in human heart failure. External constraint versus active assist. Circulation 1995;91:2314–2318

8 Remodeling, Hibernation, and Stunning

Robert A. Kloner
Jonathan Leor
Yochai Birnbaum

Coronary artery disease can contribute to left ventricular (LV) dysfunction in a number of ways. Acute ischemia, by inducing a regional wall motion abnormality of the left ventricle, can cause acute heart failure and pulmonary edema (often referred to as an "anginal equivalent"). A myocardial infarction (MI) results in the loss of viable myocytes and therefore limits the amount of ventricle (left, right, or both) capable of ejecting blood into the systemic circulation. When 40 percent or more of the left ventricle is lost, severe heart failure and shock ensue. If a ventricular aneurysm develops, heart failure may develop or worsen as a portion of blood is ejected into the aneurysmal sac rather than out the aorta. Other mechanical complications of acute MI that can contribute directly to heart failure include papillary muscle dysfunction or rupture with subsequent mitral regurgitation, ventricular septal defect, and myocardial rupture.

In addition to acute ischemia and infarction (and the direct consequences of necrotic cells) causing heart failure, there are a number of syndromes in which coronary artery disease contributes to heart failure. These syndromes involve viable myocytes that are neither acutely ischemic nor infarcted and include stunned and hibernating myocardium.[1] Another syndrome that involves changes in both necrotic and nonnecrotic, nonischemic myocardium is ventricular remodeling.[2] The purpose of this chapter

is to review the basic pathophysiology and the clinical relevance of these three phenomena.

POSTMYOCARDIAL INFARCTION VENTRICULAR REMODELING

The term ventricular remodeling has been variously defined. Postinfarction remodeling was described by Mitchell and Pfeffer as "left ventricular enlargement and distortion of regional and global ventricular geometry occurring after myocardial infarction."[3] Whittaker and Kloner defined it as "any architectural or structural change that occurs after myocardial infarction in either the infarcted or noninfarcted regions of the heart."[4] Such changes include infarct expansion (regional thinning and dilatation of the infarct zone) and both eccentric and concentric hypertrophy of noninfarcted muscle, with progressive LV dilation.[2–4] LV remodeling may involve not only the myocardial cells but the collagen network and vasculature as well.[4] Of course ventricular remodeling can occur with forms of heart disease other than coronary artery disease. Structural changes such as LV hypertrophy develop with long-standing hypertension or aortic stenosis. Mitral regurgitation induces structural changes in the left atrium and ventricle leading to enlargement of these chambers. For the purposes of this chapter we use the term ventricular remodeling as it relates to changes that occur in the left ventricle after an MI.

Pathophysiology

There are a series of physiologic and pathologic changes that occur during an acute MI that set the stage for ventricular remodeling (Fig. 8-1). Within seconds of an acute coronary artery occlusion of a proximal vessel, a regional wall motion abnormality develops in the muscle supplied by the occluded vessel. It is usually associated with paradoxical systolic bulging of the ischemic zone and physiologic or functional dilatation of the ventricle even before pathologic changes occur.[5] Dilatation of the ventricle contributes to increased wall stress. A wavefront of necrosis progresses from subendocardium to subepicardium in areas of severe ischemia. By 6 hours of permanent coronary artery occlusion, infarcts are nearly transmural. Damage occurs to not only the ventricular myocytes but also to the vasculature and native collagen. Whittaker et al., using polarized light microscopy, observed that there was a decrease in normally birefringent collagen fibers by 1 day after an experimental infarction; at 4 days there was a loss of intermyocyte collagen struts, which run perpendicular to myofibers.[6] This loss of collagen struts may then allow infarcting myocytes to slip past each other in a longitudinal direction.[7] The early phase of ventricular remodeling in which there is thinning and dilatation of the infarct was termed infarct expansion by Hutchins and Bulkley.[8] These investigators made the important distinction between the concept of infarct expansion (in which there is no additional myocardial cell death) versus infarct extension (in which there is additional myocyte death associated with recurrent chest pain, new Q waves, and an additional rise in creatine kinase).

The concept of infarct expansion has been confirmed in experimental and clinical studies. Experimentally, the phenomenon is typically observed within the first week of infarction in models of low coronary collateral flow, such as the rat.[9] In models of higher coronary collateral flow, a functional form of expansion with acute LV dilation can be observed early after coronary occlusion; but pathologic expansion with the slippage of myocytes and thinning of the ventricular wall is less common. Certain maneuvers, such as tying off visible epicardial collateral blood vessels, early exercise, or pharmacologic manipulation, such as administration of steroids or nonsteroidal antiinflammatory agents, may induce expansion in these models of high collateral flow.[10]

In clinical studies, infarct expansion has also been

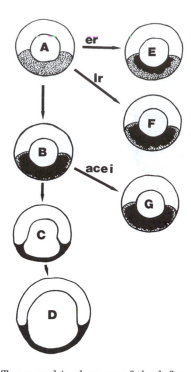

Fig. 8-1. Topographic changes of the left ventricle (LV) after myocardial infarction (MI) and potential therapies, represented in cross sections of the LV cavity. The capital letters are within the ventricular cavity. **(A)** Ischemic risk zone (*dotted area*) of the LV shortly after coronary artery occlusion. **(B–D)** Natural history of the nonreperfused moderately large infarction. **(B)** No reperfusion—no thrombolysis, failed thrombolysis, or failed angioplasty—results in a large percentage of the risk zone developing infarction (*confluent black area*). **(C)** Within 4–7 days early infarct expansion develops. The infarct thins and stretches, with regional LV dilation within the area of infarction. **(D)** Over a course of weeks to months, continued LV dilation occurs. The noninfarct and infarct zone lengthens. Eccentric hypertrophy (with dilation disproportionate to hypertrophy) develops similar to that which occurs with volume overload. **(E–G)** Potential therapy. **(E)** Early reperfusion (er) (thrombolysis, angioplasty, or both) after coronary occlusion reduces the MI size. The infarct (*confluent black area*) is subendocardial with salvage of tissue in the subepicardium of the risk zone (*dotted area*). Infarct expansion does not occur. **(F)** Late reperfusion (lr) (thrombolysis, angioplasty, or both) may result in a large infarct, but experimental studies suggest that less LV dilation and expansion occur with this therapy. If reocclusion occurs in this situation shown in ventricle E or F (and the previously patent infarct artery is no longer patent), LV dilation again may occur (as in ventricles B–D). **(G)** Finally, the situation indicates that angiotensin-converting enzyme inhibitors (acei) can prevent or reduce the degree of LV dilation after coronary artery occlusion. Nitrates can also prevent this LV dilation. These agents may be especially useful in cases of moderate to large infarction in which initial attempts at reperfusion were unsuccessful or reocclusion occurred after initially successful reperfusion. (From Kloner RA,[94] with permission.)

reported to occur within the first week of myocardial infarction and was observed in 59 percent of nonsurvivors of MI by pathologic diagnosis.[8] Typically it occurred with transmural and first MI and was associated with heart failure, cardiac rupture, and increased mortality. Easton et al. observed the progression of infarct expansion in 8 of 28 acute infarct patients utilizing two-dimensional echocardiography.[11] Infarct expansion was observed in acute anterior infarcts; during the first week there was a 25 percent increase in LV circumference due to expansion of the infarct segment; by 2 weeks lengthening of this segment accounted for a 50 percent increase in ventricular circumference. Several studies have suggested that the apical segment of the left ventricle is especially prone to infarct expansion.

Lamas and coworkers developed a "sphericity index" to study early shape changes of the left ventricle following acute MI. They described this index as "a ratio of observed biplane ventricular volume divided by the volume of a theoretical ventricle with the same biplane circumference but perfectly spherical geometry.[12]" Normal hearts had a diastolic sphericity index of 0.66 and a systolic index of 0.55, whereas patients with a large first anterior wall Q wave MI typically had an increase in this index, reflecting volume enlargement during the first 3 weeks of infarction. Patients with higher sphericity indices (more global shape) had lower ejection fractions, higher filling pressures, more heart failure, and poorer exercise capacity.[12] During the first few weeks of infarction most remodeling seems to occur within the infarct zone, although some lengthening and thinning of noninfarcted myocardium may occur owing to distension of the ventricle.

Beyond 3 to 6 weeks of infarction changes in the nonischemic myocardium become even more important. With large infarcts eccentric hypertrophy of surviving myocardium is common. This hypertrophy is a "lengthwise" type with series replication of sarcomeres that increase ventricular volume and compliance.[2,3] Concentric hypertrophy (parallel replication of sarcomeres) may also occur in areas of high systolic wall stress (e.g., at the border zone of the infarct). An increase in wall stress may contribute to alterations in myocyte organization.[13,14] Whittaker et al. observed disarray of viable myocytes and collagen fibers at the border of scars after 6 weeks of coronary artery occlusion in the dog.[14]

Ventricular remodeling may initially serve as an adaptive process. By Starling's law, an increase in ventricular volume would initially improve forward output. Eccentric hypertrophy would improve ventricular compliance, stabilizing filling pressures despite increases in volumes. Concentric hypertrophy, by increasing LV wall thickness, would tend to re-duce wall stress. However, such adaptation can only partially compensate for muscle loss; eventually, if the infarct is large enough, these topographic changes become severe and decompensation occurs. Not all patients decompensate. Some have small degrees of ventricular enlargement and do well. In some patients, shrinkage of the scar may contribute to compensation.

In other patients progressive ventricular enlargement due to eccentric hypertrophy of noninfarcted tissue may continue for months to years after an MI.[15] Patients showing early and severe LV dilation during the first month after infarction are the patients most likely to develop progressive LV dilation.[3] Several studies have now shown that LV dilation during the first month of infarction, as determined by measurements of LV end-diastolic and end-systolic volumes, was associated with increased cardiovascular death at 1 year.[16,17] Progressive LV dilation is associated with the development of clinical heart failure over weeks to months after infarction, which may not have been present during the early days of infarction.

Therapy

Early coronary artery reperfusion interrupts the wavefront of necrosis and converts what would have become a transmural infarction (with permanent occlusion) into a subendocardial infarction (Fig. 8-1). This maneuver alone should reduce infarct expansion, which, as noted above, is usually associated with transmural MI. In addition, reperfusion, by inducing contraction bands, may tend to shrink the infarct zone, and it may allow exposure of dead myocytes to blood elements and macrophages, which are crucial for the removal of necrotic debris. Thus early reperfusion not only reduces infarct size but may speed the healing and shrinkage of the scar.

An intriguing concept is that reperfusion too late to reduce the MI size may nevertheless reduce ventricular remodeling and speed the healing phase.[9,18] Several studies in the rat model have observed that reperfusion after either 2 hours or 90 minutes of proximal coronary occlusion did not reduce infarct size but did reduce the degree of infarct expansion compared with permanent coronary artery occlusions.[17,19] Studies in rats and dogs have suggested that reperfusion too late to reduce necrosis nevertheless hastens the resorption of necrotic myocytes.

Several studies in humans have supported the concept that opening an infarcted artery (even if opening occurs relatively late) may improve postinfarct survival and LV function. White et al. observed that infarct vessel patency at 1 month after a first MI predicted the 3-year survival.[17] Leung and Lau[20] determined vessel patency in patients at 7 to 10 days after MI. At 1 week after MI, the LV function was similar in patients with patent and occluded vessels. At 1 year, patients who had occluded vessels were most likely to demonstrate ventricular dilatation and decreased ejection fractions. Pfeffer et al.[21] observed that a major risk factor for late ventricular dilatation after MI was persistent occlusion of the infarct-related artery. Other clinical studies have suggested that infarct vessel patency (even if measured 3 to 5 weeks after MI) was an important predictor of less late LV dilatation and better ejection fraction. Nidorf et al.[22] suggested that late reperfusion, at a mean 5 days after infarct, was associated with a reduction in regional wall motion abnormalities and less LV dilatation at 3 months. Several studies, such as the ISIS II and LATE trials, have suggested that reperfusion, presumably too late to salvage substantial myocardium, nevertheless reduced mortality.

Angiotensin-converting enzyme (ACE) inhibition has clearly been shown to reduce ventricular remodeling. Pfeffer et al. showed that rats with moderate to large transmural infarction had improved survival and less ventricular dilatation when they were treated chronically with the ACE inhibitor captopril.[23] They then showed, in a clinical study of 52 patients with large, first anterior MIs, that captopril administered from 3 weeks to 1 year after an MI prevented late ventricular volume enlargement and resulted in improved exercise tolerance.[21] In the Survival and Ventricular Enlargement (SAVE) trial, captopril given 3 to 16 days after MI for 2 to 5 years reduced total mortality by 19 percent and decreased the incidence of congestive heart failure and recurrent MI.[24] Patients with adverse cardiac events tended to have more progressive enlargement of the left ventricle.[25]

The CONSENSUS II investigators,[26] in contrast, observed that enalapril, administered within 24 hours of MI, did not improve survival at 6 months. It has been suggested that if ACE inhibitors are given too early post-infarction, hypotension may adversely affect coronary artery perfusion pressure. Another potential explanation for the negative results in the CONSENSUS study is that 6 months is too short a time during which to see beneficial effects. Our own experimental studies with captopril showed that when this agent was administered early after infarction it reduced infarct size, improved coronary collateral blood flow, and reduced the functional form of infarct expansion that occurs during the early hours of coronary artery occlusion.[5,27] Studies with captopril—(ISIS-4), lisinopril (GISS-3), and Zofenopril (SMILE)[28]—have suggested that early administration of ACE inhibitors after infarction is not only safe but effective and may improve survival and limit heart failure.

The exact mechanism whereby ACE inhibitors exert their protective effect on remodeling is not clear. The beneficial effect may simply reflect improved hemodynamics: Lower preload and afterload may prevent progressive ventricular remodeling. Less ventricular dilation and a smaller ventricular radius would tend to decrease wall stress and hence reduce oxygen demand, which could lead to the lower frequency of ischemic events observed in the SAVE trial. Other theories include the concept that ACE inhibitors are favorably altering postinfarct neurohumoral mechanisms, are acting on the local renin-angiotensin system within the myocardium or vasculature, or are reducing preload, afterload, and augmenting coronary flow by a bradykinin-dependent mechanism.

In summary, LV remodeling occurs early after infarction in the form of infarct expansion followed by later eccentric and concentric hypertrophy of noninfarcted myocardium with progressive LV dilatation in some patients. LV dilatation is associated with more heart failure and mortality. The two best therapies to prevent ventricular remodeling appear to be early coronary artery reperfusion and chronic administration of ACE inhibitors. Clearly, the ACE inhibitors need not be given until a few days after infarction. Whether early administration of ACE inhibitors confers added benefit compared to late administration remains to be determined.

HIBERNATING MYOCARDIUM

Hibernating myocardium is identified as persistent myocardial dysfunction at rest that is due to reduced coronary perfusion. Although myocardial contraction is depressed, myocytes remain viable; and myocardial dysfunction can be restored with myocardial revascularization. Whether hibernating myocardium represents a form of ischemia remains controversial.[29]

Unlike other ischemia-related phenomena, such as myocardial stunning, ischemic preconditioning, or no reflow, which were first described in animal models, this unique phenomenon was first recognized from clinical observations. In 1973, Chatterjee et al.[30] were among the first to report a significant incidence of improved segmental myocardial wall motion after coronary bypass graft surgery. In 1985 Rahimtoola,[31] in a commentary on the results of coronary bypass surgery trials, suggested the concept of hibernating myocardium as a protective mechanism. He hypothesized that the myocardium down-regulates its function and metabolism in order to survive in the setting of reduced oxygen supply.[32] The hypothesis of hibernating myocardium was not accepted immediately, and the mechanism behind this phenomenon is still questioned and debated.[33] However, the recovery of regional and global LV function at rest after revascularization in a large subset of patients with chronic LV dysfunction suggests that many myocardial regions that are asynergic before revascularization represent viable myocardium.[34–41]

This section reviews the concept of hibernating myocardium, the basic data derived from animal models and human patients, the controversy regarding the concept of hibernating myocardium, the novel methods for assessment of myocardial viability, and the therapy for hibernating myocardium.

Animal Studies

There is no perfect animal model that can mimic prolonged hibernation as occurs in the clinical setting. However, several animal models of short-term hibernation (several hours up to 1 week) have provided considerable insight into the processes that follow mild to moderate ischemia and have given support to the concept that hibernation is a process of myocardial adjustment or adaptation.

Myocardial ischemia is defined as inadequate blood perfusion leading to anaerobic metabolism.

Following acute coronary artery occlusion there is a rapid fall in myocardial high-energy phosphates, an increase in anaerobic glycolysis, a rise in lactate content, a fall in cytosolic pH, and the accumulation of inorganic phosphate (Pi).[42] Ventricular function in the ischemic area is impaired within a few seconds after coronary artery occlusion.[42] This initial sudden dysfunction occurs before depletion of the high-energy phosphates. Although the precise mechanism is unknown, it may be related to alterations in calcium flux,[43] acidosis,[42] reduced levels of ATP,[42] or increased intracellular Pi, which is due to phosphocreatine breakdown.[44] It is now believed that the increasing concentrations of Pi and hydrogen ion are the major causes of contractility depression following ischemia.[42–44]

The metabolic and hemodynamic changes during mild and moderate ischemia produced by experimental coronary stenosis are different from those produced by complete coronary occlusion. Short-term hibernation models are characterized by a decrease in contractile function in proportion to the reduced myocardial blood flow.[45–48] Myocardial creatine phosphate content, which is initially decreased during the first minutes of ischemia, returns to a near-normal value by 60 to 85 minutes.[46,47] The ischemia-induced net lactate production is attenuated[45,49] (Figs. 8-2 and 8-3), and the myocardium remains via-

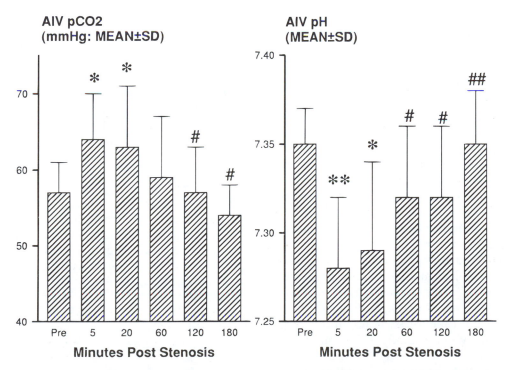

Fig. 8-2. Bar graphs of **(A)** PCO_2 and **(B)** pH of anterior interventricular vein (AIV) blood. Both variables exhibit substantial worsening 5 minutes after stenosis placement with gradual return to prestenosis levels over 3 hours. *$P < 0.05$ vs. prestenosis, **$P < 0.01$ vs. prestenosis. #$P < 0.05$ vs. 5 minutes poststenosis. ## $P < 0.01$ vs. 5 minutes poststenosis. STNS, stenosis. (From Fedele et al.,[49] with permission.)

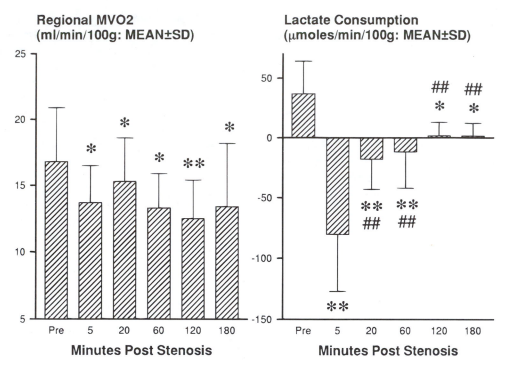

Fig. 8-3. Bar graphs of **(A)** regional myocardial oxygen (MVO$_2$) and **(B)** lactate consumption. Oxygen consumption declined 5 minutes after stenosis placement and then remained unchanged for the duration of the study. Lactate production was maximal immediately after stenosis insertion and then reversed toward consumption during the next 3 hours. *$P < 0.05$ vs. prestenosis. ** $P < 0.01$ vs. prestenosis. ##$P < 0.01$ vs. 5 minutes poststenosis. STNS, stenosis. (From Fedele et al.,[49] with permission.)

ble despite ongoing hypoperfusion and contractile dysfunction.

Based on the metabolic and hemodynamic changes in animal models, several investigators have proposed that hibernating myocardium is a protective process that down-regulates energy requirements, thereby reducing the supply–demand imbalance and allowing reaccumulation of high-energy phosphates during ongoing low coronary blood flow.[50,51] This response prevents irreversible myocardial cell damage.

Schulz et al.[47] showed that short-term hibernating myocardium retains contractile reserve and transiently responds to short-term intracoronary dobutamine infusion with increased work. This inotropic response, however, interfered with the metabolic equilibrium achieved during hibernation and was associated with increased metabolic products of myocardial ischemia.[47,48] Furthermore, in a model of severe ischemia (with an 80 to 90 percent reduction in regional myocardial function), the enhanced oxygen demand induced by dobutamine infusion impaired the supply–demand balance and precipitated MI.[48] The results of this experimental study may have therapeutic implications for management of patients with LV dysfunction due to hibernating myocardium: An increase in oxygen demand in the setting of ongoing ischemia may worsen the ischemic insult.

Human Studies

Hibernating myocardium is a significant component of LV dysfunction in patients with coronary artery disease. The prevalence rate is as high as 42 percent of patients with coronary artery disease.[52,53] Clinical evidence supporting the concept of hibernating myocardium comes largely from clinical observations that showed resolution of chronic wall motion abnormalities after coronary artery bypass surgery or angioplasty. Some of these studies suggested that the improvement in wall motion occurred immediately,[38,39,54] but other studies[36,37,55,56] demonstrated gradual recovery, suggesting that the revascularized hibernating myocardium underwent a phase of stunning. An alternative explanation is that myocyte atrophy occurred during the phase of hibernation and required time to resolve.[57,58] It is of interest that a significant proportion of patients referred for cardiac transplantation because of ischemic cardiomyopathy and severe LV dysfunction met the criteria of hibernating myocardium and benefited from coronary artery bypass surgery.[41]

The morphologic changes of the hibernating regions have been investigated in patients undergoing coronary bypass surgery. The data were collected from regions corresponding to the dysfunctional but viable zone and showed loss of sarcomeres, abundant glycogen granules, rough endoplasmic reticulum, and mitochondria, a tortuous nucleus, and an increase in connective tissue strands. The number of affected cells was greater in endocardial portions than in epicardial ones.[57–59]

Identification of Viable Myocardium

Ventricular function is a major factor influencing survival in patients with coronary artery disease. The available data suggest that an improvement in ventricular function translates into improved prognosis. Thus it is essential to identify patients with viable myocardium who may benefit from coronary revascularization. The ultimate gold standard for diagnosis of hibernating myocardium is recovery of function following coronary revascularization and restoration of normal perfusion, which can be determined, however, only retrospectively, after the patient has undergone revascularization.

Advances in imaging medicine have allowed assessment of myocardial viability prospectively. The current modalities to assess viability are listed in Table 8-1.

Table 8-1. Current Methods for Identifying Myocardial Viability

Electrocardiography
    Absence of Q waves in the dysfunctional regions
Venticulography
    Postextrasystolic potentiation
    Enhancement of wall motion after nitroglycerin
    Enhancement of wall motion after catecholamines
Thallium 201 Scintigraphy
    Delayed thallium 201 uptake during an exercise-redistribution test
    Thallium uptake on 24-hour imaging
    Defect reversibility after thallium 201 reinjection
    Thallium uptake during rest-redistribution imaging
Technetium 99m Sestamibi
    Sestamibi uptake in zones of myocardial dysfunction
Positron emission tomography
    Metabolic activity
Echocardiography
    Enhanced systolic thickening and function after low dose dobutamine test
    Enhanced systolic thickening and function after dipyridamole test
    Evidence of microcirculatory flow reserve by contrast echocardiography
Magnetic resonance imaging
    Preserved diastolic thickness or evidence of systolic thickening

---

ELECTROCARDIOGRAPHY

Absence of the Q wave on the electrocardiogram (ECG) in the territory of dysfunctional myocardium was suggested as a marker of viability.[60] This method is not specific, however, and many of the myocardial segments showing Q waves are still viable.[60]

THALLIUM MYOCARDIAL IMAGING

Thallium myocardial imaging is used clinically to assess myocardial perfusion and cell membrane function. Two clinical approaches can be applied to the detection of viability: stress-redistribution-reinjection imaging or rest-redistribution imaging.[61,62] The latter method may be more suitable for patients with ischemic cardiomyopathy with severe LV dysfunction who cannot exercise or who have contraindications to stress testing[62] (Fig. 8-4). Dilsizian and Bonow[61] and Ragosta et al.[62] found that addition of quantitative analysis can enhance the sensitivity for predicting viability in patients with fixed thallium defects. Viability is likely to be present if the delayed images show only a mild or moderate defect in thallium 201 activity relative to activity in the normal zone.[62]

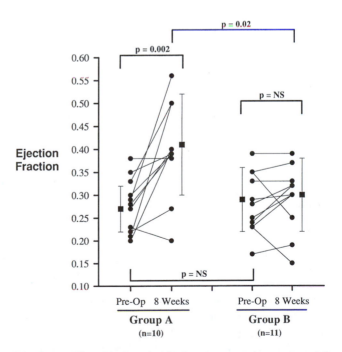

Fig. 8-4. Ejection fraction before surgery (pre-op) and 8 weeks after coronary artery bypass surgery in group A and group B patients. Group A patients had more than seven viable but asynergistic segments, whereas group B patients had seven or fewer such segments. (From Ragosta et al.,[62] with permission.)

TECHNETIUM 99M SESTAMIBI

One of the most widely used new perfusion agents is technetium 99m sestamibi. It has been suggested to be an excellent agent for investigating stunned myocardium, but sestamibi may have limitations in the setting of hibernating myocardium: The uptake of sestamibi is flow-dependent. Moreover, as sestamibi does not redistribute, in theory it underestimates the magnitude of viable myocardium, compared with thallium assessment, under conditions of hypoperfusion.

POSITRON EMISSION TOMOGRAPHY

Positron emission tomography (PET) has evolved as the noninvasive standard for determining viability. The PET criterion for viability is the demonstration of glucose metabolism in hypofunctioning myocardium using the radiolabeled glucose analogue fluorine 18 (^{18}F)-fluorodeoxyglucose. The positive predictive value is up to 85 percent and the negative predictive value up to 92 percent.[41,63,64] PET provides enhanced image resolution and routine correction for body attenuation, thereby overcoming the two major limitations of thallium imaging.

Although PET technology may be superior to thallium imaging, it is expensive and not readily available. On the other hand, thallium is widely available for clinical use and provides a less expensive alternative to PET assessment of regional metabolic activity. Based on studies published to date, the predictive accuracy of thallium reinjection studies approaches that of PET.[61]

ECHOCARDIOGRAPHY TO ASSESS CONTRACTILE RESERVE

The presence of contractile reserve as assessed during nitroglycerin administration,[65] during postextrasystolic potentiation,[66] during low-dose catecholamine infusion,[67] by the dipyridamole test,[68] or immediately after exercise[69] has been proposed to identify viable myocardium in patients with chronic regional dysfunction.

Echocardiography is emerging as a useful modality for evaluating contractile reserve and myocardial viability. The wall motion response during dobutamine echocardiography can identify viable myocardium, a useful test for predicting recovery of ventricular function after revascularization in patients with stable coronary artery disease and LV dysfunction.[70] The biphasic response (e.g., improvement at low doses and deterioration at high doses of dobutamine) has been suggested to have the best predictive value

for the presence of hibernating myocardium.[71] In addition, echocardiography can provide real-time assessment of segmental wall motion, systolic wall thickening, and various myocardial functions, such as valve competence and diastolic function.

MYOCARDIAL CONTRAST ECHOCARDIOGRAPHY

Myocardial contrast echocardiography has been suggested as a promising method for evaluating flow reserve and myocardial viability and for predicting restoration of myocardial function after revascularization.[72] More clinical data are needed before conclusions can be drawn about the clinical utility of this test.

Hibernating Myocardium or Repetitive Stunning?

Hibernating myocardium is similar to stunned myocardium in that both terms refer to contractile dysfunction of viable tissue. The crucial difference between the two phenomena is the status of blood flow to the tissue: "Stunned myocardium" refers to contractile dysfunction following reperfusion, whereas "hibernating myocardium" refers to contractile dysfunction during low perfusion. Furthermore, stunned myocardium is transient (i.e., wall motion gradually improves over hours to days following reperfusion), whereas hibernating myocardium persists throughout chronic low blood flow. Experimental and clinical studies have indicated that hibernating myocardium, once reperfused, may go through a phase of postischemic dysfunction or stunning prior to eventual improvement in contractile performance.[36,37,55,56]

There is controversy regarding whether hibernating myocardium represents an active process of down-regulation of metabolic demand due to severe chronic, silent, low blood flow or represents repetitive stunning after discrete episodes of ischemia.[29,33,53] Vanoverschelde et al.[73] investigated the mechanism of regional dysfunction in patients with coronary artery disease. They selected patients who had total occlusion of the coronary artery with corresponding myocardial dysfunction and in whom myocardial perfusion to the area of dysfunction depended entirely on collateral blood flow supply. They found significant morphologic abnormalities in myocardial tissue samples obtained at the time of bypass surgery in dysfunctioning collateral-dependent segments. These abnormalities included cellular swelling, loss of myofibrillar content, and accumulation of glycogen. On PET study, however, these collateral-dependent but dysfunctional myocardial segments were found to have nearly normal resting flow and oxygen consumption. The authors concluded that repetitive stunning, rather than chronic hibernation, was responsible for the myocardial dysfunction. Based on the PET studies, the dysfunctional segments did not fulfill the conventional criteria for hibernation.

Therapy

The ultimate therapy for hibernating myocardium is revascularization by percutaneous transluminal angioplasty or coronary bypass surgery. One study[40] suggested that hibernating myocardium acts as an "unstable substrate" for later ischemic events. This and other studies[30,35,41] suggested that revascularization and improvement in ventricular function can translate into improved prognosis. Many patients referred for heart transplantation because of severe LV dysfunction have a significant component of hibernating myocardium and can benefit from revascularization.[35,41] Medical alternatives (until revascularization can be performed) include administration of nitroglycerin and cautious use of β-adrenergic blocking agents to reduce oxygen demand and to prevent ischemia and infarction. The results of animal experiments[48] raise concern that inotropic stimulation in the presence of severe hibernation may interfere with the metabolic equilibrium and may precipitate ischemia and infarction, which may partly explain the deleterious effects of several inotropic agents on survival of patients with heart failure and coronary artery disease.

Comment

The major importance of the hibernating myocardium concept is that chronic dysfunction of the myocardium is not necessarily indicative of irreversible injury. Patients with coronary artery disease and significant LV dysfunction who previously had a poor prognosis can improve their outcome by undergoing revascularization. For an appropriate decision in regard to the selection of patients for revascularization, it is essential to be aware of the pathophysiology of the LV dysfunction in the individual patient. Scarring, ischemia, stunning, and hibernation may coexist in the same patient and contribute to LV dysfunction and to the clinical picture of heart failure. The decision-making process is often complex when the LV function is low, and diagnostic procedures reliably differentiating viable from nonviable myocardium are required for a potential approach to treatment. Once hibernating myocardium has been identified, revascularization should be considered, as it can improve myocardial function and the prognosis.

More basic research is needed to determine whether hibernating myocardium is a down-regulation of cardiac function in the setting of reduced flow and represents true ischemia or is the consequence of repetitive stunning, as some investigators have suggested. Data derived from histologic studies and new imaging techniques may help to elucidate the mechanism behind this phenomenon.

The advances in modalities for assessing myocardial viability allow more appropriate selection of patients for myocardial revascularization. With the advance in myocardial revascularization techniques and myocardial protection, it is likely that the prognosis of patients with LV dysfunction due to hibernating myocardium will be consistently improved.

STUNNED MYOCARDIUM

Myocardial stunning, or postischemic dysfunction, is defined as delayed recovery of myocardial function despite restoration of coronary flow to previously ischemic myocardium in the absence of irreversible damage.[74-76] The hallmarks of stunned myocardium encompass both systolic and diastolic dysfunction.[77-80] The phenomenon of myocardial stunning, first described in 1975 by Heyndrickx et al. in a conscious dog model of acute ischemia,[77] was followed by numerous reports of transient myocardial dysfunction following various types of myocardial ischemia/reperfusion in several animal models.[76] However, only after introduction of reperfusion modalities for the treatment of acute MI did the clinical importance of distinguishing reversible from irreversible regional impairment of contractility become apparent. Moreover, the introduction of invasive and noninvasive imaging tools for assessing function, perfusion, and metabolism has revealed that reversible dysfunction of viable myocardial regions is more common than previously thought.

Dysfunction of viable myocardium may be caused by any one of several distinct mechanisms: subendocardial ischemia, repetitive episodes of silent ischemia (resulting in severe limitation of coronary flow reserve), hibernation, stunning, or superimposition of two or more of these causes.[81] The major difference between stunning and the former is that blood flow is normal or near-normal with stunning, whereas it is reduced with ischemia or hibernation.[81]

Metabolic Aspects

In addition to the transient mechanical impairment that follows a nonlethal ischemic/reperfusion insult, several metabolic derangements occur: changes in myocardial oxygen consumption, oxidative phosphorylation, and glucose and lipid metabolism.[82] After reperfusion there is a paradoxical transient increase in myocardial oxygen consumption, despite continuous impairment of mechanical function that may last 4 hours or more. There is an association between the degree of mechanical dysfunction and the magnitude of the increase of oxygen consumption. Myocardial oxygen consumption may be elevated even in reperfused myocardium with areas of ultrastructural evidence of irreversible damage.[82] Although oxygen consumption is elevated, maximal oxygen consumption is reduced. Administration of inotropic agents causes an exaggerated increase in myocardial oxygen consumption out of proportion to the augmentation in mechanical function. The mechanisms of the elevated oxygen consumption are not clear. Inefficient utilization of adenosine triphosphate (ATP) by the contracting elements, probably due to altered Ca^{2+} sensitivity of the contractile regulatory proteins or myosin ATPase, is the most plausible explanation. Most of the experimental data do not support mitochondrial uncoupling of oxygen consumption from ATP synthesis as the mechanism. There is no evidence for increased ATP utilization by noncontracting processes.[82] The nonesterified fatty acid metabolites, accumulated during ischemia, are preferentially utilized upon reperfusion, despite the presence of high concentrations of lactate. Accumulation of fatty acid intermediates reduces mechanical function during ischemia, but it is not clear if these metabolites influence stunning during reperfusion.[82] After reperfusion there is increased glucose uptake in the postischemic zone that may persist for days after a severe insult. Immediately after reperfusion, glycolysis may be an important source of ATP production. However, after the initial few minutes, fatty acid oxidation continues to be the primary source for energy production, and utilization of lactate and pyruvate is decreased.[82]

Mechanisms of Myocardial Stunning

Myocardial stunning is probably a multifactorial process. Several mechanisms may be involved in the generation of this phenomenon. Two major hypotheses have been proposed to explain the etiology of postischemic myocardial dysfunction: oxygen free radical generation or abnormal calcium homeostasis (or some combination of the two) (Fig. 8-5).

OXYGEN FREE RADICAL GENERATION

Oxygen free radicals are produced at the time of reperfusion after a short ischemic period that does not result in myocardial necrosis. The burst of free radicals appears in the venous blood draining the ischemic-reperfused area, peaks within 2 to 4 minutes of reperfusion, and persists up to 3 hours.[83] Administration of various free radical scavengers, such as combination of superoxide dismutase and catalase, dimethylthiourea, desferrioxamine, and N-2-mercaptopropionyl glycine inhibits the production of these radicals and attenuates myocardial stunning.[76,84] The injury mediated by the free radicals probably occurs immediately upon reperfusion. When various antioxidant agents were infused later than 1 minute after reflow, the stunning was not attenuated.[84] The source of these free radicals is still unresolved. Data concerning the role of free radicals in myocardial stunning after a prolonged ischemic period, such as that associated with subendocardial infarction, are conflicting.[76,84] It may be that the pathophysiologic mechanisms of delayed recovery of function after long ischemic periods differ from those associated with short episodes.

The mechanisms whereby oxygen free radicals mediate stunning are not clear. Some studies suggest that free radical-induced damage to cell membranes such as the sarcoplasmic reticulum or the sarcolemma may be the cause. Free radicals may disrupt membrane Ca^{2+}/Mg^{2+}-ATPase and Na^{+}/K^{+}-ATPase function.[76,84]

ALTERED CALCIUM HOMEOSTASIS

During ischemia and the early reperfusion period there is a rise in cytosolic Ca^{2+} concentrations. The mechanism for this transient calcium rise is still unresolved. Oxygen free radicals, generated upon reperfusion, are able to damage the sarcoplasmic reticulum or the sarcolemma and may contribute to an increase in membrane permeability and calcium overload. Transient increase in intracytosolic Ca^{2+} concentrations can cause myocardial dysfunction similar to stunning. The mechanism is probably damage to the contractile elements by activating various protein kinases, phospholipases, and other degradative enzymes, or by triggering production of free radicals via xanthine oxidase activation.[76,84] An alternative hypothesis is that transiently elevated Ca^{2+} concentrations, by activating protein kinases, change the Ca^{2+} sensitivity and maximal Ca^{2+} acti-

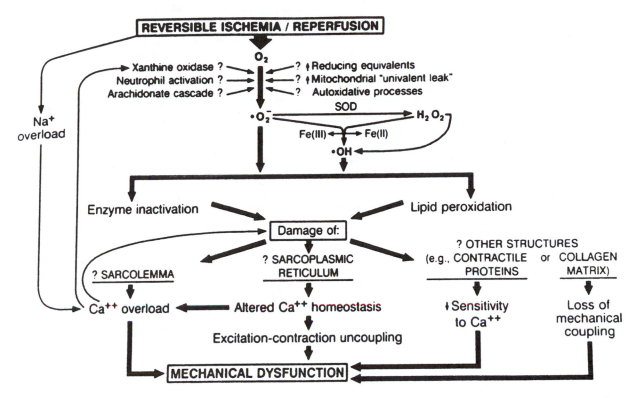

Fig. 8-5. Proposed pathogenesis of postischemic myocardial dysfunction. This proposal integrates and reconciles various mechanisms into a unifying pathogenetic hypothesis. Transient reversible ischemia followed by reperfusion could result in increased production of superoxide radicals ($\bullet O_2$-) through several mechanisms, including (1) increased activity of xanthine oxidase, (2) activation of neutrophils, (3) activation of arachidonate cascade, (4) accumulation of reducing equivalents during oxygen deprivation, (5) derangements of intramitochondrial electron transport system resulting in increased univalent reduction of oxygen, and (6) autoxidation of catecholamines and other substances. Superoxide dismutase (SOD) dismutates $\bullet O_2$- to hydrogen peroxide (H_2O_2); in the presence of catalytic iron, $\bullet O_2$- and H_2O_2 interreact in a Haber-Weiss reaction to generate the hydroxyl radical ($\bullet OH$). H_2O_2 can also generate $\bullet OH$ in the absence of $\bullet O_2$- through a Fenton reaction that other substances (e.g., ascorbate) reduce Fe(III) to Fe(II). $\bullet O_2$- and $\bullet OH$ attack proteins and polyunsaturated fatty acids, causing enzyme inactivation and lipid peroxidation, respectively. With reversible ischemia, the intensity of this damage is not sufficient to cause cell death but is sufficient to produce dysfunction of key cellular organelles. Postulated targets of free radical damage include (1) the sarcolemma, with consequent loss of selective permeability, impairment of calcium-stimulated ATPase activity and calcium transport out of the cell, and impairment of Na+, K+-ATPase activity (the net result of these perturbations would be increased transarcolemmal calcium influx and cellular calcium overload); (2) the sarcoplasmic reticulum, with consequent impairment of calcium-stimulated ATPase activity and calcium transport (which would result in impaired calcium homeostasis—specifically decreased calcium sequestration, contributing to increased free cytosolic calcium and decreased calcium release during systole, in turn causing excitation-contraction uncoupling); and (3) possibly other structures, such as the extracellular collagen matrix (with consequent loss of mechanical coupling) or the contractile proteins (with consequent decreased sensitivity to calcium). At the same time, reversible ischemia/reperfusion could cause cellular Na+ overload due to (1) inhibition of sarcolemmal Na+, K+-ATPase and (2) acidosis and Na+-H+ exchange. This situation could further exaggerate calcium overload by the increased Na+-Ca2 exchange. An increase in free cytosolic calcium would activate phospholipases and other degradative enzymes and further exacerbate the injury to the aforementioned key subcellular structures (sarcolemma, sarcoplasmic reticulum, and contractile proteins). Thus calcium overload could serve to amplify the damage initiated by oxygen radicals. In addition, calcium overload could itself impair contractile performance and contribute to mechanical dysfunction. It is also possible that the increase in free cytosolic calcium could increase oxyradical production by promoting conversion of xanthine dehydrogenase to xanthine oxidase. The ultimate consequence of this complex series of perturbations is a reversible depression of contractility. (From Bolli,[76] with permission.)

vated force through phosphorylation of various contractile proteins, making the myofilaments less sensitive to subsequent calcium.

Factors Determining Severity and Duration

The severity and duration of postischemic dysfunction are closely related to the duration and severity of the preceding ischemia. The presence of residual flow to the ischemic zone via collaterals attenuates stunning. Short ischemic episodes, lasting less than a few minutes, are not sufficient to cause stunning and may even result in a transient hypercontractility state after reperfusion.[85] After longer episodes of ischemia, a short period of increased contractility was demonstrated upon reperfusion, lasting 1 to 3 minutes, followed by a gradual decline of function. The longer the ischemic insult, the greater and more prolonged is the ensuing dysfunction. Thus brief ischemic episodes, as seen during variant angina or balloon occlusion during angioplasty, are not expected to be associated with prolonged dysfunction, whereas recovery of myocardial function after reperfusion therapy for acute MI or after cardiac surgery may be delayed for several days to weeks.

Myocardial Stunning in the Clinical Setting

AFTER REPERFUSION FOR MI

Early coronary reperfusion, spontaneous or after intervention (thrombolytic therapy or mechanical recanalization), salvages variable amounts of midmyocardial and subepicardial myocardium otherwise destined to die. Numerous studies, using various imaging techniques, have demonstrated delayed recovery of regional systolic and diastolic myocardial function despite successful reperfusion (Fig. 8-6). Function is recovered gradually over 10 days to even several weeks in most of the studies. Greater and faster improvement in function was obtained in patients reperfused within 4 hours than in those reperfused more than 4 hours from the onset of cardiac pain.[81,85] Studies have shown that infusion of inotropic agents results in augmentation of regional and global systolic function, and it was more pronounced in patients who were successfully reperfused than in those in whom reperfusion failed. This reversible regional dysfunction could be demonstrated as early as 3 days after reperfusion of an acute anterior wall MI.[85] However, because spontaneous delayed recovery of function can be related to improved perfusion by either delayed recanalization or recruitment of collaterals, hibernation and stunning cannot always be distinguished by these studies.[85]

UNSTABLE ANGINA

Unstable angina is a heterogeneous syndrome, from new-onset effort angina to severe angina at rest. Luminal stenosis produced by intracoronary thrombus fluctuates over time. Thus repeated simultaneous demonstration of reduced regional function in a normally perfused segment is mandatory for the diagnosis of stunning and for ruling out chronic ischemia as the cause of dysfunction in this setting. Most of the previous studies, which demonstrated an improved

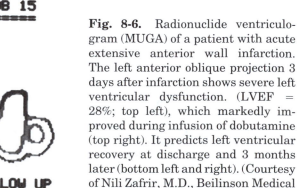

GLOBAL LVEF

REST ✴ 28%

DOB15 ✴ 55%

PD ✴ 49%

FU ✴ 58%

PRE DOB

DOB 15

PRE DISCHARGE

FOLLOW UP

Fig. 8-6. Radionuclide ventriculogram (MUGA) of a patient with acute extensive anterior wall infarction. The left anterior oblique projection 3 days after infarction shows severe left ventricular dysfunction. (LVEF = 28%; top left), which markedly improved during infusion of dobutamine (top right). It predicts left ventricular recovery at discharge and 3 months later (bottom left and right). (Courtesy of Nili Zafrir, M.D., Beilinson Medical Center, Petach Tikva, Israel.)

regional wall motion score between admission and a later time point after conservative therapy, angioplasty, or coronary artery bypass grafting, failed to fulfill these criteria.[81–84] Jeroudi et al. demonstrated delayed recovery of regional wall motion abnormalities after resolution of chest pain in six patients with unstable angina pectoris. They noted that during short ischemic episodes (about 10 minutes) the recovery was almost complete 2 hours after the chest pain, whereas longer episodes of pain resulted in delayed recovery, over more than 24 hours.[85] As mentioned above, because no direct evidence of restoration of flow after resolution of pain is presented, persistent (silent) subendocardial ischemia or hibernation as the cause of the dysfunction cannot be ruled out.

VARIANT ANGINA

Evidence for myocardial stunning after episodes of vasospastic (Prinzmetal's) angina is sparse. This lack is probably because most of the ischemic episodes are too short to produce stunning.[81]

AFTER EXERCISE

Immediately following exercise-induced ischemia there may be improvement in regional wall motion abnormalities in some patients. During the next 10 to 20 minutes, however, function in previously ischemic zones gradually deteriorates in some patients, especially in those in whom effort-induced ischemia is severe and prolonged (i.e., individuals with multivessel disease and severe luminal narrowing). These wall motion impairments may last at least 30 to 45 minutes.[86] Ambrosio et al. studied seven patients with coronary artery disease. Two-dimensional echocardiography was performed at baseline, immediately after exercise, and following recovery. ^{99m}Tc-sestamibi was injected 30 minutes into recovery for assessment of late perfusion. Regional wall thickening remained depressed for at least 30 minutes, at a time when no perfusion defects were demonstrated. Thus there was evidence of persistent systolic impairment despite restoration of flow (flow–function mismatch).[87]

AFTER CORONARY ANGIOPLASTY

Occlusion periods by balloon inflation, as commonly practiced, are probably too short to induce prolonged systolic stunning. Indeed, prompt return of systolic function has been observed after angioplasty, although diastolic dysfunction may persist.[88] Prolongation of the balloon inflation to 4 to 7 minutes resulted in delayed recovery of regional wall motion and thickening that lasted 3 days in some patients.[89]

AFTER CARDIAC SURGERY

Numerous studies have reported transient deterioration of regional and global myocardial function after cardiac surgery that may last 24 to 48 hours.[81]

During the course of cardiac transplantation the heart is exposed to periods of global ischemia followed by reperfusion, so a component of myocardial stunning should be expected. Indeed, transient hemodynamic instability is commonly observed during the immediate posttransplantation period.

NEUROGENIC MYOCARDIAL STUNNING

Transient ECG changes, consisting of ST segment deviation resembling acute MI, occur in 0.8 to 10.2 percent of patients with subarachnoid hemorrhage. Transient wall motion abnormalities during the acute phase have been reported in the absence of angiographic evidence of either fixed or vasospastic coronary occlusion. The mechanism of neurogenic myocardial stunning has not been elucidated, but vasoconstriction induced by increased levels of catecholamines may be the cause.

Diagnosis

Stunned myocardium retains its ability to augment contraction after infusion of β-mimetic agents. Indeed, low-dose dobutamine infusion (10 $\mu g \cdot kg^{-1} \cdot min^{-1}$ or less) coupled with echocardiography or radionuclide ventriculography is a reliable method for detecting viable myocardium with reversible dysfunction following an ischemic insult[61,90] (Fig. 8-6). However, because hibernating myocardium may improve its contractility the same way, the diagnosis of stunning should rely on demonstrating normal or near-normal perfusion in the dysfunctional region after the ischemic insult. Perfusion can be assessed invasively by coronary angiography or contrast echocardiography after intracoronary infusion of contrast agents, or it can be evaluated noninvasively by radionuclide techniques.[61] Imaging with thallium 201 (^{201}Tl) and the technetium-based agents ^{99m}Tc-sestamibi and ^{99m}Tc-teboroxime is reliable for estimating regional myocardial perfusion. However, immediately upon reperfusion there may be a transient hyperemic state resulting in excessively high thallium uptake, even in necrotic zones.[61] Hence thallium injection during the first few hours after reperfusion may overestimate the amount of viable myocardium.[61] However, because necrotic myocardium cannot retain thallium, there is early washout from the necrotic zones that can be appreciated with late redistribution imaging.[61]

Metabolic imaging with PET using ^{18}F-fluorodeoxyglucose can accurately distinguish viable from necrotic zones. However, this technique overestimates the extent of viable myocardium after acute MI.[61]

Treatment

PREVENTION

According to experimental models, myocardial stunning can be prevented by administering antioxidative agents just prior to reperfusion. In the clinical setting the goal is to prevent the severe, prolonged stunning episodes that follow prolonged ischemic episodes, as seen with acute MI or after cardiac surgery. The role of free radicals in preventing myocardial stunning induced by prolonged ischemic periods is less clear. Several authors have reported that allopurinol, a blocker of free radical production, improved the cardiac performance and reduced cardiac complications in patients who underwent coronary artery bypass surgery,[91] but these studies included only a small number of patients. Up to the present, no other controlled clinical trial has documented the efficacy of antioxidants in the clinical setting of myocardial ischemia-reperfusion.

Calcium antagonists have a potential role in preventing stunning by blocking the hypercalcemic phase and by their free radical-scavenging effect.[92] Various experimental models of global, brief regional myocardial ischemia and reperfusion have demonstrated that calcium antagonists, given especially before occlusion but also during reperfusion, enhance the recovery of contractile function. However, the results after long ischemic episodes are conflicting.[92] The effect of calcium antagonists on myocardial stunning has been evaluated only in small clinical trials. Adding nifedipine or diltiazem to cardioplegic solutions resulted in improved myocardial metabolism and hemodynamic status.[92] Calcium antagonists improved myocardial stunning induced by prolonged balloon inflation during angioplasty.[89]

Evidence that β-blockers enhance recovery after postischemic dysfunction is equivocal. Several studies have shown that stable analogues of prostacyclin enhanced the recovery of myocardial function upon reperfusion, and ACE inhibitors have been demonstrated to enhance recovery of function after ischemic/reperfusion insult, but the mechanism is not clear. The SH-containing agents captopril and zofenopril have been shown consistently to ameliorate stunning, possibly by their antioxidant properties. However, even other ACE inhibitors that do not contain the SH group are effective in some experimental models of stunning.

AUGMENTATION OF MYOCARDIAL FUNCTION

Stunned myocardium retains its contractile reserves. After infusion of various positive inotropic agents, transient augmentation of global and regional function is observed. Various β-mimetic agents have been reported to enhance contractility and improve diastolic relaxation in the ischemia/reperfusion zone, without further depletion of ATP stores.[93] However, due to down-regulation by β-receptors, the effect is lost after 24 hours of infusion.

REFERENCES

1. Kloner RA, Przyklenk K, Patel B: Altered myocardial states. Am J Med, suppl. 1A 1989;86:14
2. McKay RG, Pfeffer MA, Pasternak RC et al: Left ventricular remodeling following myocardial infarction. A corollary to infarct expansion. Circulation 1986;74:693
3. Mitchell GF, Pfeffer MA: Left ventricular remodeling after myocardial infarction. p. 317. In Kloner RA (ed): The Guide to Cardiology. 3rd Ed. LeJacq Communication, New York 1995
4. Whittaker P, Kloner RA: Ventricular remodeling of the heart. Curr Opin Cardiol 1991;6:346
5. Mehta PM, Alker KJ, Kloner RA: Functional infarct expansion, left ventricular dilation and isovolumic relaxation time following coronary occlusion. A two-dimensional echocardiographic study. J Am Coll Cardiol 1988;11:630
6. Whittaker P, Boughner DR, Kloner RA: Role of collagen in acute myocardial infarct expansion. Circulation 1991;84:2123
7. Weisman HF, Bush DE, Mannisi JA, Weisfeldt ML, Healy B: Cellular mechanisms of myocardial infarct expansion. Circulation 1988;78:186
8. Hutchins GM, Bulkley BH: Infarct expansion versus extension. Two different complications of acute myocardial infarction. Am J Cardiol 1978;41:1127
9. Hochman JS, Choo H: Limitation of myocardial infarct expansion by reperfusion independent of myocardial salvage. Circulation 1987;75:299
10. Hammerman H, Schoen FJ, Braunwald E, Kloner RA: Drug induced expansion of infarct. Morphologic and functional correlations. Circulation 1984;69:611
11. Easton LW, Weiss JL, Bulkley BH et al: Regional cardiac dilatation after acute myocardial infarction. Recognition by two-dimensional echocardiography. N Engl J Med 1979;300:57
12. Lamas GA, Vaughan DE, Parisi AF et al: Effects of left ventricular shape and captopril therapy on exercise capacity after anterior wall acute myocardial infarction. Am J Cardiol 1989;63:1167
13. Olivetti G, Ricci R, Begeri C et al: Response of the border zone to myocardial infarction in rats. Am J Pathol 1986;125:476
14. Whittaker P, Boughner DR, Kloner RA: Analysis of healing after myocardial infarction using polarized light microscopy. Am J Pathol 1989;134:879
15. Erlebacher JA, Weiss JL, Eaton LW et al: Late effects of acute infarct dilation on heart size. A two dimen-

sional echocardiographic study. Am J Cardiol 1982;49:1120

16. Hammermeister KE, DeRouen TA, Dodge HT: Variables predictive of survival in patients with coronary artery disease. Selection by univariate and multivariate analyses from clinical, electrocardiographic, exercise, arteriographic and quantitative angiographic evaluations. Circulation 1979;59:421

17. White HD, Norris RM, Brown MA et al: Left ventricular end-systolic volume as the major determinant of survival after recovery from myocardial infarction. Circulation 1987;76:44

18. Braunwald E: Myocardial reperfusion, limitation of infarct size, reduction of left ventricular dysfunction, and improved survival. Should the paradigm be expanded? Circulation 1989;79:441

19. Hale SL, Kloner RA: Left ventricular topographic alterations in the completely healed rat infarct caused by early and late coronary artery reperfusion. Am Heart J 1988;116:1508

20. Leung WH, Lau CP: Effects of severity of the residual stenosis of the infarct-related coronary artery on left ventricular dilation and function after acute myocardial infarction. J Am Coll Cardiol 1992;20:307

21. Pfeffer MA, Lamas GA, Vaughan DE et al: Effect of captopril on progressive ventricular dilatation after anterior myocardial infarction. N Engl J Med 1988;319:80

22. Nidorf SM, Siu SC, Galambos G, Weyman AE, Picard MH: Benefit of late coronary reperfusion on ventricular morphology and function after myocardial infarction. J Am Coll Cardiol 1993;21:683

23. Pfeffer MA, Pfeffer JM, Steinberg C et al: Survival following an experimental myocardial infarction. Beneficial effects of chronic captopril therapy. Circulation 1985;72:406

24. Pfeffer MA, Braunwald E, Moye LA et al: Effect of captopril on mortality and morbidity in patients with left ventricular dysfunction after myocardial infarction. Results of the survival and ventricular enlargement trial. N Engl J Med 1992;327:669

25. St. John Sutton M, Pfeffer MA, Plappert T et al: Quantitative two dimensional echocardiographic measurements are major predictors of adverse cardiovascular events following acute myocardial infarction. The protective effects of captopril. Circulation 1994;89:68

26. Swedberg K, Held P, Kjekshus J et al: Effects of the early administration of enalapril on mortality in patients with acute myocardial infarction. Results of the Cooperative New Scandinavian Enalapril Survival Study II (CONSENSUS II). N Engl J Med 1992;327:678

27. Ertl G, Kloner RA, Alexander RW, Braunwald E: Limitation of experimental infarct size by angiotensin converting enzyme inhibitor. Circulation 1982;65:40

28. Ambrosioni E, Borghi C, Magnani B et al: The effect of the angiotensin-converting-enzyme inhibitor zofenopril on mortality and morbidity after anterior myocardial infarction. N Engl J Med 1995;332:80

29. Hearse DJ: Myocardial ischemia. Can we agree on a definition for the 21st century? Cardiovasc Res 1994;28:1737

30. Chatterjee K, Swan HJC, Parmley WW et al: Influence of direct cardiac revascularization on left ventricular asynergy and function in patients with coronary heart disease. Circulation 1973;47:276

31. Rahimtoola SH: A perspective on three large multicenter randomized clinical trials of coronary bypass surgery for chronic stable angina. Circulation, suppl. V 1985;72:123

32. Rahimtoola SH: The hibernating myocardium. Am Heart J 1989;117:211

33. Buxton DB: Dysfunction in collateral-dependent myocardium. Hibernation or repetitive stunning? Circulation 1993;87:1756

34. Rankin JS, Newman GE, Mulhbaier LH et al: The effect of coronary revascularization on ventricular function in ischemic heart disease. J Thorac Cardiovasc Surg 1985;90:818

35. Califf RM, Harrel FE, Lee KL et al: Changing efficacy of coronary revascularization. Implications for patients selections. Circulation 1988;78:S185

36. Takeishi Y, Tono-oka I, Kubota I et al: Functional recovery of hibernating myocardium after coronary bypass surgery. Does it coincide with improvement in perfusion? Am Heart J 1991;122:665

37. Nienaber CA, Brunken RC, Sherman CT et al: Metabolic and functional recovery of ischemic human myocardium after coronary angioplasty. J Am Coll Cardiol 1991;18:996

38. Carlson EB, Cowely WJ, Wolfgang TC, Vetrovec GW: Acute changes in global and regional rest left ventricular function after successful coronary angioplasty. Comparative results in stable and unstable angina. J Am Coll Cardiol 1989;13:1262

39. Cohen M, Charney R, Hershman R et al: Reversal of chronic ischemic myocardial dysfunction after transluminal coronary angioplasty. J Am Coll Cardiol 1988;12:1193

40. Lee KS, Marwick TH, Cook SA et al: Prognosis of patients with left ventricular dysfunction, with and without viable myocardium after myocardial infarction. Relative efficacy of medical therapy and revascularization. Circulation 1994;90:2687

41. Loui HW, Laks H, Milgalter E et al: Ischemic cardiomyopathy. Criteria for coronary revascularization and cardiac transplantation. Circulation, suppl. III 1991;84:290

42. Jennings RB, Murry CE, Steenbergen C, Reimer KA: Development of cell injury in sustained acute ischemia. Circulation, suppl. II 1990;82:2

43. Lee JA, Allen DG: Mechanism of acute ischemic contractile failure of the heart. Role of intracellular calcium. J Clin Invest 1991;88:361

44. Kentish JC: The effects of inorganic phosphate and creatine phosphate on force production in skinned muscles from rat ventricle. J Physiol (Lond) 1986;370:585

45. Arai AE, Pantely GA, Anselone CG, Bristow J, Bristow JD: Active downregulation of myocardial energy requirements during prolonged moderate ischemia in swine. Circ Res 1991;69:1458

46. Pantely GA, Maloney SA, Rhen WS et al: Regeneration of myocardial phosphocreatine in pigs despite continued moderate ischemia. Circ Res 1990;67:1481

47. Shulz R, Guth BD, Pieper K, Martin C, Heuch G: Requirement of an inotropic reserve in moderately ischemic myocardium. A model of short-term hibernation. Circ Res 1992;70:1282

48. Shulz R, Rose J, Martin C, Brodde OE, Heuch G: Development of short-term myocardial hibernation. Its

limitation by the severity of ischemia and inotropic stimulation. Circulation 1993;88:684

49. Fedele FA, Gewirtz H, Capone RJ, Sharaf B, Most AS: Metabolic response to prolonged reduction of myocardial blood flow distal to a severe coronary artery stenosis. Circulation 1988;78:729

50. Ross J Jr: Myocardial perfusion-contraction matching. Circulation 1991;83:1076

51. Bristow JD, Arai AE, Anselone CG, Pantely GA: Response to myocardial ischemia as a regulated process. Circulation 1991;84:2580

52. Lewis SJ, Sawada SG, Ryan T et al: Segmental wall motion abnormalities in the absence of clinically documented myocardial infarction. Clinical significance and evidence of hibernating myocardium. Am Heart J 1991;121:1088

53. Schelbert H, Buxton D: Insight into coronary artery disease gained from metabolic imaging. Circulation 1988;78:496

54. Topol EJ, Weiss JL, Guzman PA et al: Immediate improvement of dysfunctional myocardial segments after coronary revascularization. Detection by intraoperative transesophageal echocardiography. J Am Coll Cardiol 1984;4:1123

55. Kloner RA, Przyklenk K: Hibernation and stunning of the myocardium. N Engl J Med 1991;325:1877

56. Przyklenk K, Bauer B, Kloner RA: Reperfusion of hibernating myocardium. Contractile function, high-energy phosphate content and myocyte injury after 3 hours of sublethal ischemia and 3 hours of reperfusion in the canine model. Am Heart J 1992;123:575

57. Flameng W, Suy R, Schwarz F et al: Ultrastructural correlates of left ventricular contraction abnormalities in patients with chronic ischemic heart disease. Determinants of segmental asynergy post revascularization surgery. Am Heart J 1981;102:846

58. Borgers M, Thone F, Wouters L et al: Structural correlates of regional myocardial dysfunction in patients with critical coronary artery stenosis. Chronic hibernation? Cardiovasc Pathol 1993;2:237

59. Maes A, Flameng W, Nuyts J et al: Histological alterations in chronically hypoperfused myocardium. Correlation with PET findings. Circulation 1994;90:735

60. Hashimoto T, Kambara H, Fudo T et al: Non Q wave versus Q wave myocardial infarction. Regional myocardial metabolism and blood flow assessed by positron emission tomography. J Am Coll Cardiol 1988;12:88

61. Dilsizian V, Bonow RO: Current diagnostic techniques of assessing myocardial viability in patients with hibernating and stunned myocardium. Circulation 1993;87:1

62. Ragosta M, Beller GA, Watson DD et al: Quantitative planar rest-redistribution 201-thallium imaging in detection of myocardial viability and prediction of improvement in left ventricular function after coronary bypass surgery in patients with severely depressed left ventricular function. Circulation 1993;87:1630

63. Tillisch J, Brunken R, Marshall R et al: Reversibility of cardiac motion abnormalities predicted by positron tomography. N Engl J Med 1986;314:884

64. Tamaki N, Yonekura Y, Yamashita K et al: PET using F-18 deoxyglucose in evaluation of coronary artery bypass grafting. Am J Cardiol 1989;64:860

65. Helfant RH, Pine R, Meister SG et al: Nitroglycerin to unmask reversible asynergy. Correlation with post

coronary bypass ventriculography. Circulation 1974; 50:108

66. Popio KA, Gorlin R, Bechtel D, Levine JA: Postextrasystolic potentiation as a predictor of potential myocardial viability. Preoperative analysis compared with studies after coronary bypass surgery. Am J Cardiol 1977;39:944

67. Horn HR, Teichholz LE, Cohn PF, Herman MV, Gorlin R: Augmentation of left ventricular contraction pattern in coronary artery disease by an inotropic catecholamine. The epinephrine ventriculogram. Circulation 1974;49:1063

68. Picano E, Marzullo P, Gigli G et al: Identification of viable myocardium by dipyridamole-induced improvement in regional left ventricular function assessed by echocardiography in myocardial infarction and comparison with thallium scintigraphy at rest. Am J Cardiol 1992;70:703

69. Rozanski A, Berman D, Gray R et al: Preoperative prediction of reversible myocardial asynergy by postexercise radionuclide ventriculography. N Engl J Med 1982;307:212

70. Cigarroa CG, deFilippi CR, Brickner ME et al: Dobutamine stress echocardiography identifies hibernating myocardium and predicts recovery of left ventricular function after coronary revascularization. Circulation 1993;88:430

71. Afridi I, Kleiman NS, Raizner AE, Zoghbi WA: Dobutamine echocardiography in myocardial hibernation. Optimal dose and accuracy in predicting recovery of left ventricular function after coronary angioplasty. Circulation 1995;91:663

72. Camarano G, Ragosta M, Gimple LW et al: Identification of viable myocardium with contrast echocardiography in patients with poor left ventricular systolic function caused by recent or remote myocardial infarction. Am J Cardiol 1995;75:215

73. Vanoverschelde J-LJ, Wijns W, Depre C et al: Mechanisms of chronic regional postischemic dysfunction in humans. New insight from the study of noninfarcted collateral-dependent myocardium. Circulation 1993; 87:1513

74. Patel B, Kloner RA, Przyklenk K, Braunwald E: Postischemic myocardial "stunning". A clinically relevant phenomenon. Ann Intern Med 1988;108:627

75. Braunwald E, Kloner RA: The stunned myocardium. Prolonged postischemic ventricular dysfunction. Circulation 1982;66:1146

76. Bolli R: Mechanism of myocardial "stunning." Circulation 1990;82:723

77. Heyndrickx GR, Millard RW, McRitchie RJ et al: Regional myocardial function and electrophysiological alterations after brief coronary artery occlusion in conscious dogs. J Clin Invest 1975;56:978

78. Kloner RA, Przyklenk K: First evidence. Postischemic dysfunction of viable myocardium. p. 17. In Kloner RA, Przyklenk K (eds): Stunned Myocardium. Properties, Mechanisms and Clinical Manifestations. Marcel Dekker, New York, 1993

79. Charlat ML, O'Neill PG, Hartley CJ et al: Prolonged abnormalities of left ventricular diastolic wall thinning in the "stunned" myocardium in conscious dogs. Time course and relation to systolic function. J Am Coll Cardiol 1989;13:185

80. Przyklenk K, Kloner RA: Diastolic abnormalities of

postischemic stunned myocardium. Am J Cardiol 1987;60:1211

81. Bolli R: Myocardial "stunning" in man. Circulation 1992;86:1671

82. Zimmer SD, Bache RJ: Metabolic correlates of reversibly injured myocardium. p. 41. In Kloner RA, Przyklenk K (eds): Stunned Myocardium. Properties, Mechanisms and Clinical Manifestations. Marcel Dekker, New York, 1993

83. Zughayb M, Sekili A, Li XY et al: Detection of free radical generation in the "stunned" myocardium in the conscious dog using spin trapping techniques. FASEB J 1991;5:A704

84. Bolli R: Role of oxygen radicals in myocardial stunning. p. 155. In Kloner RA, Przyklenk K (eds): Stunned Myocardium. Properties, Mechanisms and Clinical Manifestations. Marcel Dekker, New York, 1993

85. Jeroudi M, Cheirif J, Habib G, Bolli R: Prolonged wall motion abnormalities after chest pain at rest in patients with unstable angina. A possible manifestation of myocardial stunning. Am Heart J 1994;127:1241

86. Kloner RA, Allen J, Cox TA, Zheng Y, Ruiz CE: Stunned left ventricular myocardium following exercise treadmill testing in coronary artery disease. Am J Cardiol 1991;68:329

87. Ambrosio G, Losi MA, Perrone-Filardi P et al: Persistence of contractile impairment in the absence of flow abnormalities after exercise. Evidence for myocardial stunning in patients with stable angina. Circulation, suppl. I 1993;88:646

88. Wijns W, Serruys PW, Slager CJ et al: Effect of coronary occlusion during percutaneous transluminal angioplasty in humans on left ventricular chamber stiffness and regional diastolic pressure-radius relations. J Am Coll Cardiol 1986;7:455

89. Sheiban I, Tonni S, Marini A, Trevi GP: Left ventricular dysfunction following transient ischaemia induced by transluminal coronary angioplasty. Beneficial effects of calcium antagonists against post-ischaemic myocardial stunning. Eur Heart J, suppl. A 1993;14:14

90. Watada H, Ito H, Oh H et al: Dobutamine stress echocardiography predicts reversible dysfunction and quantitates the extent of irreversibly damaged myocardium after reperfusion of anterior myocardial infarction. J Am Coll Cardiol 1994;24:624

91. Coghlan JG, Flitter WD, Clutton SM et al: Allopurinol pretreatment improves postoperative recovery and reduced lipid peroxidation in patients undergoing coronary artery bypass grafting. J Thorac Cardiovasc Surg 1994;107:248

92. Przyklenk K, Kloner RA: Calcium antagonists as treatment for the stunned myocardium. p. 281. In Kloner RA, Przyklenk K (eds): Stunned Myocardium. Properties, Mechanisms and Clinical Manifestations. Marcel Dekker, New York, 1993

93. Becker LC: Inotropic agents and stimulation of stunned myocardium. p. 267. In Kloner RA, Przyklenk K (eds): Stunned Myocardium. Properties, Mechanisms and Clinical Manifestations. Marcel Dekker, New York, 1993

94. Kloner RA: Coronary angioplasty. A treatment option for left ventricular remodeling after myocardial infarction? J Am Coll Cardiol 1992;20:314–316

9 Neurohormonal Receptors in the Failing Heart

William T. Abraham

J. David Port

Michael R. Bristow

A number of neurotransmitter and hormone receptors have been identified in the mammalian heart (Table 9-1). Stimulation of these neurohormonal receptors by their cognate agonists influences myocardial contractility, heart rate and conduction, cardiac metabolism, cellular growth, and ventricular remodeling. Thus these cardiac neurohormonal receptors undoubtedly play important roles in cardiac physiology and myocyte growth in health and disease. For example, cardiac hypertrophy is produced by a combination of increased myocyte stretch, neurotransmitter release, and several types of autocrine, paracrine, and hormonal stimulation that mediate myocyte growth. In this context, the α_1-adrenergic receptor pathway, the angiotensin II AT_1 receptor pathway, the endothelin 1 receptor pathway, and the β-adrenergic receptor pathways have all been implicated in the pathogenesis of myocyte hypertrophy.

In the setting of left ventricular systolic dysfunction, alterations in the function of myocardial receptor-effector mechanisms may be particularly important, as various neurohormonal systems are markedly activated in response to low-output cardiac failure and have been shown to play a role in the onset and progression of the clinical syndrome of chronic heart failure. Activation of the adrenergic nervous system and the renin-angiotensin system appears to be of primary importance in producing some of the major adaptive cardiac receptor-signal transduction changes observed in the failing heart.

As reviewed below, during heart failure it appears that changes in the expression of these receptors as well as alterations in the function of their signal transduction pathways occur so as to withdraw the heart from the potentially deleterious effects of adrenergic stimulation and increased angiotensin II. It is the purpose of this chapter to review the alterations in myocardial receptors, particularly adrenergic and angiotensin II receptors, that occur in the failing human heart.

CONTRACTILE FUNCTION OF THE HEART

Mechanisms governing the contractile function of the human heart may be divided into two general categories. *Intrinsic contractile function* accounts for the ability of the cardiac myocyte to respond to stretch and is utilized in the normal heart to maintain pump performance under resting conditions. Among other subcellular mechanisms, intrinsic function depends on contractile proteins and the various processes responsible for excitation-contraction coupling. *Modulated cardiac function* permits the heart to markedly increase or decrease its performance nearly instantaneously in response to various stimuli. For example, in the nonfailing heart cardiac output can be increased by 2- to 10-fold within a matter of seconds to meet the circulatory demands of in-

Table 9-1. Some Neurohormonal Receptors Found in the Human Heart

Adrenergic
   α_1
   β_1
   β_2
   β_3
Muscarinic
   M_1
   M_2
Histaminic
   H_1
   H_2
Angiotensin II
   AT_1
   AT_2
Endothelin
   ET_1
Serotonergic
   5-Hydroxytryptamine
Adenosine
   A_1
Mineralocorticoid
   Mineralocorticoid receptor
Miscellaneous
   Vasoactive intestinal polypeptide
   Glucagon
   Somatostatin
   Dihydropyridine
   Oubain

creased activity.[1] Modulated cardiac function depends on the adrenergic nervous system, adrenergic receptor–effector mechanisms, and a prominent force–frequency response.

When the heart begins to fail, modulated function mechanisms that increase cardiac performance are activated to stabilize cardiac output by increasing the heart rate and cardiac contractility (Fig. 9-1). The most important modulated function mechanisms responsible for the acute stimulation of cardiac function are the adrenergic signal transduction pathways. These pathways and their alteration as a consequence of heart failure are discussed in detail below. Immediate stimulation of cardiac performance by adrenergic mechanisms is subsequently aided by two additional means of stabilizing or increasing pump function: an increase in plasma volume, resulting in an increased ventricular preload, and an increase in cardiac myocyte hypertrophy, which results in more contractile elements, increased wall thickness, and decreased wall tension. The former mechanism is accomplished by neuroendocrine signaling and intrarenal mechanisms, where

activation of renal nerves and increased circulating angiotensin II and aldosterone enhance sodium and water reabsorption in both the proximal and distal renal tubule.[2] Myocyte hypertrophy is produced by the aforementioned mechanisms of myocyte stretch, neurotransmitter release, and autocrine, paracrine, and hormonal stimulation. Here again, stimulation of the adrenergic nervous system and increased angiotensin II production play a predominant role in the cardiac response.

ACTIVATION OF THE ADRENERGIC AND RENIN-ANGIOTENSIN SYSTEMS DURING HEART FAILURE

The adrenergic nervous system is activated early during the course of heart failure. Numerous studies have documented elevated peripheral venous plasma norepinephrine concentrations in heart failure patients as well as a positive correlation between the severity of the heart failure and the plasma norepinephrine concentration.[3–7] With advanced heart failure, using tritiated norepinephrine to determine norepinephrine kinetics, Hasking et al.[5] and Davis and coworkers[6] demonstrated that both increased norepinephrine spillover and decreased norepinephrine clearance contribute to the elevated venous plasma norepinephrine levels seen in patients with heart failure, suggesting that increased adrenergic nerve activity is at least partially responsible for the high circulating norepinephrine. A subsequent report[7] indicates that during the earlier stages of heart failure the rise in peripheral venous plasma norepinephrine in patients with heart failure is due solely to increased norepinephrine secretion, supporting the notion that adrenergic nervous system activity is increased early in the course of heart failure. Significantly, in these heart failure patients with mild to moderate symptoms, plasma epinephrine, a marker of adrenal activation, was not substantially elevated, confirming the neuronal source of the increased norepinephrine.[7] The observation of adrenergic activation during mild to moderate heart failure has been extended to patients with asymptomatic left ventricular dysfunction studied by the SOLVD investigators.[8] This substudy of the SOLVD trials demonstrated a 35 percent increase in plasma norepinephrine concentration in subjects with asymptomatic left ventricular dysfunction compared to healthy controls. Finally, studies employing peroneal nerve microneurography to directly assess sympathetic nerve activity to skeletal muscle have

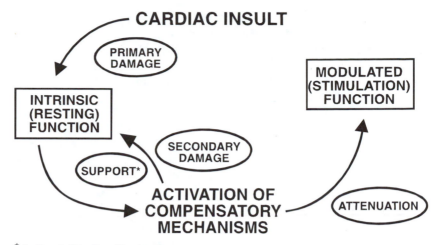

CARDIAC INSULT

PRIMARY DAMAGE

INTRINSIC (RESTING) FUNCTION

MODULATED (STIMULATION) FUNCTION

SECONDARY DAMAGE

SUPPORT*

ACTIVATION OF COMPENSATORY MECHANISMS

ATTENUATION

Fig. 9-1. Hypothetic model of the development of myocardial failure, demonstrating the roles of intrinsic versus modulated cardiac function.

* 1. **Frank-Starling Mechanism**
2. **Adrenergic Stimulation**
3. **Hypertrophy**

also confirmed increased adrenergic nerve traffic in patients with heart failure.[9]

The aforementioned study by Hasking et al.[5] also demonstrated the presence of selective cardiorenal adrenergic activation in patients with heart failure. This study of whole-body and organ-specific norepinephrine kinetics demonstrated that cardiac and renal norepinephrine spillovers were increased 504 and 206 percent, respectively, and norepinephrine spillover from the lungs was normal in patients with advanced cardiac failure. Furthermore, there appears to be chamber-specific adrenergic activation in failing right ventricles versus nonfailing left ventricles from patients with right heart failure due to primary pulmonary hypertension.[10] These observations of organ-specific[5] and cardiac chamber-specific[10] increases in adrenergic activity in heart failure support an important role for local presynaptic control of cardiac adrenergic activity. Thus in the failing human heart, increased cardiac adrenergic activity may occur as a consequence of increased central sympathetic outflow, presynaptic facilitation of norepinephrine release, or decreased neuronal norepinephrine reuptake (uptake$_1$). The observation of a substantial decrease in uptake$_1$ in the failing human heart suggests a role for decreased neuronal norepinephrine reuptake in the pathogenesis of increased cardiac adrenergic activity.[11]

Presynaptic facilitation of norepinephrine release by angiotensin II may also play an important role in cardiac adrenergic activation,[12] thus demonstrating a positive feedback of angiotensin II on cardiac adrenergic activity. Conversely, the adrenergic nervous system provides a major stimulus for activation of the renin-angiotensin system, as activation of renal nerves results in renal renin release[13,14] and in-

creased norepinephrine may increase angiotensin-converting enzyme (ACE) and angiotensinogen gene expression in human coronary smooth muscle cells.[15] Indeed, in heart failure patients, assessment of plasma renin activity and plasma aldosterone indicates that activation of the renin-angiotensin system also occurs early during the course of cardiac failure.[4,8] Thus activation of the adrenergic and renin-angiotensin systems appears to be co-regulated during heart failure, such that activation of one system stimulates the other and maneuvers that decrease the activity of one system may inhibit the other (Fig. 9-2).[16] For example, administration of an ACE inhibitor to patients with heart failure results not only in a fall in plasma angiotensin II concentrations but

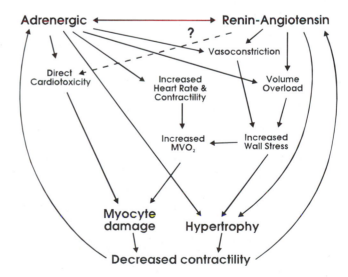

Fig. 9-2. Role of the co-activated/co-regulated adrenergic and renin-angiotensin systems in the setting of cardiac failure.

also in a decrease in circulating and transmyocardial norepinephrine.[17,18] It is the activation of these two neurohormonal vasoconstrictor systems at both the systemic and cardiac levels that seems to produce the changes in cardiac receptor-signal transduction function observed in the failing human heart (discussed below).

ADRENERGIC RECEPTORS

Two major classes of adrenergic receptors, the α-adrenergic and the β-adrenergic receptor (AR) families, are present in the human heart.[19] The two AR families can be further divided into multiple subclassifications: α_1-AR family and the α_2-AR family, each with at least three receptor subtypes. Currently, there are also three subtypes of β-ARs described. Each receptor pathway elicits a spectrum of biochemical and physiologic activities that may be either additive or antagonistic to one another. As previously mentioned, the β-AR pathways are perhaps the most powerful stimuli of modulated cardiac function. The relevance of these adrenergic receptor pathways and the consequences of heart failure on each pathway are discussed below. Here we emphasize the role and modulation of the β-AR pathway(s).

α-Adrenergic Receptors

The two major categories of α-ARs, the α_1 and α_2-ARs, have distinctly different signal transduction pathways. There appears to be no significant density of α_2-AR in the heart,[20] and so this class of adrenergic receptor is not discussed further. Currently, the three subtypes of the α_1-AR that have been described are the $\alpha_{1a/d}$, α_{1b}, and α_{1c} subtypes.[21] Unfortunately, the subtype classification scheme now used is being revised, causing some confusion because of differences between traditional pharmacologic characterization of the receptors versus the properties of cloned receptors. The prevalent subtype of α_1-AR expressed in the heart as determined pharmacologically appears to be the α_{1b}-AR. In contrast, analysis of subtype expression at the level of messenger RNA (mRNA) indicates that the α_{1c}-subtype may be the most abundant isoform. The α_{1c}-subtype appears to be more prevalent in human myocardium and many other human tissues than in tissues from other species.[21]

Receptors of the α_1-AR subclass have been demonstrated to be coupled to the G_q/G_{11} family of guanine-nucleotide regulatory proteins (G proteins). Stimulation of the α_1-AR pathway causes activation of phospholipase C (PLC), which catalyzes the breakdown of phosphoinositol-bis-phosphate (PIP_2) into inositol-tris-phosphate (IP_3) and diacylglycerol (DAG). IP_3 causes the release of Ca^{2+} from intracellular stores within the sarcoplasmic reticulum (SR). Changes in the intracellular cytoplasmic Ca^{2+} concentration modulate a variety of Ca^{2+}-sensitive regulatory proteins including a variety of enzymes and protein kinases. In contrast, DAG stimulates protein kinase C (PKC). Both PLC and PKC exist as multiple isoforms. Expression of PLC and PKC is dependent on tissue, species, and developmental stage.[22] Activated PKC phosphorylates a number of intracellular substrates. These targets include nuclear transcription factors, enzymes, activated transporters, and cell surface receptors including both the β_1- and β_2-ARs.[23] Stimulation of the α_1-AR has also been associated with activation of the phospholipases PLD and PLA_2[24] as well as the activation of Ca^{2+} channels and the inhibition of certain K^+ channels. Finally, α_1-AR stimulation appears to affect the rates of the Na^+/H^+ and Na^+/Ca^{2+} exchangers.[24] It is therefore apparent that stimulation of the α_1-AR pathways may be an important modulator of heart rate, contractility, systolic and diastolic wall tension, and vascular compliance and tone. In this regard, it should be noted that the magnitude of the positive inotropic effect of myocardial α_1-AR stimulation may be attenuated during heart failure.[25]

Like angiotensin II receptors, α_1-adrenergic receptors are central to the induction of cardiac hypertrophy,[26–28] an effect that may be direct or indirect. The "cause and effect" relation between α_1-AR stimulation and activation of the signal transduction pathways ultimately responsible for producing myocyte hypertrophy have been worked out in animals and in cell culture, they appear to be obligate components of the model systems. Data indicate that G_q, p21[ras], and Raf signal transduction pathways are necessary for the indication of hypertrophy.[26] α_1-AR also stimulates the mitogen-activated protein (MAP) kinase cascade, a pathway that seems to be ubiquitously involved in the regulation and expression of numerous transcription factors, cell-cycle proteins, and proto-oncogenes, which ultimately result in remodeling and hypertrophy of the ventricle. More recent evidence calls into question the requirement of the MAP kinase pathway in myocardial hypertrophy and remodeling. In other words, although MAP kinase pathways are activated, it is not apparent that in all circumstances MAP kinase activation is necessary for producing cardiac hypertrophy.[29] In cardiac myocytes from neonatal rat heart, Takahashi et al.[28] demonstrated that α_1-AR-stimulated myocyte hypertrophy is dependent on Ca^{2+} influx and is associated with Ca^{2+} influx-dependent modulation of the expression of mRNAs for sarcoplasmic reticulum Ca^{2+}-ATPase, Ca^{2+} release channel, and associated growth factors. In this regard, it is worth noting that overexpression of a constitutively activated α_1-AR in transgenic mice has been shown to produce gross myocardial hypertrophy.[30]

Stimulation of the α_1-AR pathways by norepinephrine also causes cardiomyocytes to contract. Moreover, deformation and mechanical stress have been shown to cause the release of angiotensin II, which in turn can cause hypertrophy through stimulation of AT_1 receptors.[31,32] The role of cardiac angiotensin II receptors is discussed below.

The relative abundance of α_1-AR subtypes is usually less in human myocardium than in other species. For example, myocardial α_1-AR density is considerably lower in humans than in rodents, a fact that is relevant, as rodents are a frequently used model for studying myocardial hypertrophy.[20] Thus, as might be anticipated, the inositol phosphate pathway appears to be less well stimulated in the human myocardium than in the rodent model.[33,34] Interestingly, the abundance of α_1-AR increases modestly during heart failure,[35] and it is possible that an increase in α_1-AR density leads to a greater hypertrophic stimulus. However, the correlation between α_1-AR density and the rate of progression or severity of the hypertrophy phenotype remains untested. On the other hand, there may be an important clinical association of α_1-AR stimulation and an increased frequency of cardiac arrythmias.[36] In this context and in the context of heart failure, it is important to note that the presence of ischemia or hypoxia has been shown to acutely up-regulate α_1-AR density.[20]

Selective α_1-AR antagonists have been used as a therapeutic intervention for management of heart failure. A frequently cited investigation is the VHeFT-1 (First Vasodilator Heart Failure Trial),[37] which compared the effects of placebo versus the α_1-blocker prazosin versus the combination of hydralazine and isosorbide dinitrate on the survival of patients with symptomatic heart failure. Whereas the combination of hydralazine and isosorbide dinitrate improved survival in this trial, prazosin was no better than placebo. Of note, Colucci and colleagues[38] showed that the chronic administration of prazosin to patients with symptomatic heart failure results in a marked, highly significant increase in plasma norepinephrine, thereby exacerbating the degree of adrenergic activation. On a more positive note and as discussed below, combined α-/β-blockers used in the treatment of heart failure seem to exert an anti-adrenergic effect[39] and to be of clinical benefit for treatment of heart failure.[40,41]

β-Adrenergic Receptors

Three subtypes of β-AR have been described: β_1, β_2, and β_3-ARs. Although present in human myocardium,[42] the role of the β_3-AR seems confined to body metabolism and diabetes[43,44] and therefore is not discussed further in this chapter.

In the human heart as well as in other tissues, β-ARs produce their effects by interacting with the stimulatory G protein G_s (Fig. 9-3). The presence of β-AR agonist causes dissociation of the heterotrimeric G protein into its α- and $\beta\gamma$-subunits.[45] Stimulation of adenylyl cyclase by $G_{s\alpha}$ catalyzes the conversion of adenosine triphosphate (ATP) to cyclic adenosine monophosphate (cAMP), which in turn binds to the regulatory subunit of PKA, stimulating the dissociation of the active catalytic subunits. As with PKC, there are numerous intracellular substrates for PKA-mediated phosphorylation within the myocardium. Targets of particular importance include L-type Ca^{2+} channels, cell-surface receptors including α- and β-ARs and muscarinic receptors, nuclear transcription factors, and regulatory proteins associated with the myocardial contractile apparatus. In this context, it should again be acknowledged that stimulation of the β-AR pathways is perhaps the single most important regulatory mechanism for determining the rate and force of myocardial contraction.

Although it has long been recognized that β-AR stimulates adenylyl cyclase activity via $G_{s\alpha}$, it has been discovered that the β-AR pathways can also stimulate the MAP kinase cascade, an effect that appears to be mediated by the $\beta\gamma$-subunit of G_s.[46] This finding suggests a mechanism by which the β-AR pathway may be mitogenic.

As described above, the β_1- and β_2-AR pathways are both coupled to stimulation of G_s and to stimulation of adenylyl cyclase. However, the coupling efficiency of the two receptor subtypes appears to be significantly different. In preparations of human ventricular myocardium, the β_2-AR is approximately 5 to 15 times more efficiently coupled to the production of cAMP than is the β_1-AR.[47] In contrast, the relation between β-AR density and contractility appears to be more direct; that is, subtype selectivity of myocardial contractility does not appear to be stoichiometrically different between the β_1-AR and the β_2-AR.[47,48] The lack of correlation between cAMP mass and contractility for each receptor subtype argues in favor of intracellular compartmentalization of cAMP.

The normal human heart expresses a mixed population of β-ARs, with approximately 70 to 80 percent β_1-subtype and 20 to 30 percent β_2-subtype.[49–51] As

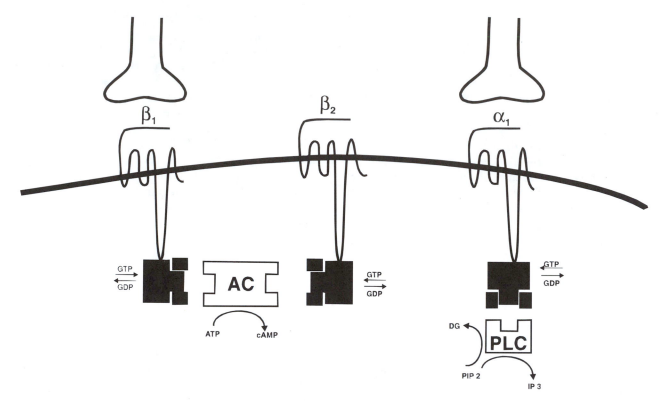

Fig. 9-3. Three adrenergic receptors coupled to two positive inotropic effector enzymes in the cell surface membrane of human ventricular myocytes. AC, adenylyl cyclase; ATP, adenosine triphosphate; cAMP, cyclic adenosine monophosphate; DG, diacylglycerol; GDP, guanine diphosphate; GTP, guanosine triphosphate; IP3, inositol triphosphate; PIP2, phosphotidylinositol biphosphate; PLC, phospholipase C.

shown in Table 9-2, several alterations in the β-adrenergic/G protein signal transduction pathways occur in the chronically failing human heart. One of the most well described changes and, in fact, a hallmark of clinical heart failure is the selective down-regulation of the β_1-AR subtype[50,51] a finding that has obvious therapeutic implications (discussed below). Although there may be some differences in β_1-AR density based on the etiology of the heart failure (Table 9-2), the extent of β_1-AR down-regulation correlates well with the severity of the heart failure regardless of cause.[49] The absolute density of myocardial β_1-AR also correlates well with systemic or coronary sinus plasma norepinephrine concentrations.

In contrast to the β_1-AR, the β_2-AR is not down-regulated in the failing human heart. There are at least two potential explanations for this finding. First, the endogenous catecholamine norepinephrine is somewhere between 10- and 60-fold more selective for the β_1-AR than for the β_2-AR. Second, the β_1-AR appears to be most commonly localized with the vicinity of the synaptic cleft, which suggests that the β_1-AR is exposed to higher sustained concentrations of norepinephrine. Because of the subtype-selective

down-regulation of the β_1-AR in the failing human heart, the proportion of β-ARs of the β_2-AR subtype variety increases to roughly 40 percent of the total β-AR density.[52] Thus although selective β_1-AR antagonists, such as metoprolol or bisoprolol, may be of benefit for treatment of chronic heart failure[53,54] nonselective agents that are also better tolerated during heart failure due to desirable ancillary cardiovascular effects (e.g., carvedilol, bucindolol) may be qualitatively and quantitatively better.[39–41] This issue is discussed below (see also Ch. 47).

As indicated in Table 9-2, with heart failure due to ischemic cardiomyopathy, the β_1-AR is not only significantly down-regulated it is uncoupled from its signal transduction pathway. The β_2-AR is uncoupled from its signal-transduction pathway in the presence of all kinds of cardiomyopathy studied to date. For both of the β-AR subtypes, uncoupling has been associated with phosphorylation of the receptor.[23,55,56] Both β_1-AR and β_2-AR subtypes are phosphorylated by PKA, PKC, and several members of the G protein-coupled receptor kinase (GRK) family. These kinase are also referred to as β-adrenergic receptor kinases (βARKs). Each of these kinases phosphorylate the β-ARs at serine or threonine residues

Table 9-2. Abnormalities in the Adrenergic Receptor/G Protein Signal Transduction Pathways Associated with Myocardial Failure

Abnormality	Extent of effect (0 to 3 +)	Type of heart disease
β_1-AR down-regulation	+ +	IDC
	+	ISC
	+ + +	PPH (RV only)
β_1-AR uncoupling	NSC	IDC
	+	ISC
β_2-AR uncoupling	+	IDC
	+ +	ISC
Decrease in $G_{\alpha s}$ activity	−	−
Increase in $G_{\alpha i}$ activity	+	IDC, ISC
Increased βARK activity	+	−
Decrease in AC activity	+	IDC (RV only)
	NSC	ISC
	+ +	PPH (RV only)

Abbreviations: AR, adrenergic receptor; NSC, not significantly different; IDC, idiopathic dilated cardiomyopathy; ISC, ischemic cardiomyopathy; AC, adenylyl cyclase; RV, right ventricle; PPH primary pulmonary hypertension; βARK, β-adrenergic receptor kinase.
(Modified from Bristow et al.,[49] with permission.)

within the third intracytoplasmic loop or on the intracellular carboxy-terminus of the receptor protein. It has been determined that βARK protein and activity are up-regulated in the failing human heart.[57,58] Finally, activity of the inhibitory G protein G_i is increased[49,58] and adenylyl cyclase activity decreased[10,49] in the failing human heart.

One factor accounting for altered β-adrenergic receptor and G_i changes in the failing human heart is chronically elevated adrenergic drive,[59] based on data from both model systems and the intact human heart. Chronic exposure to β-agonists consistently produces β-receptor desensitization phenomena, which include receptor uncoupling[60] down-regulation,[61] and increased activity of G_i.[62] In the failing human heart the degree of adrenergic drive, as assessed by coronary sinus norepinephrine levels[63] or tissue norepinephrine depletion,[64] correlates with β-receptor down-regulation. Finally, removal of adrenergic drive by β-blockade[65-67] or partial attenuation of it by ACE inhibition[18] partially reverses β-AR down-regulation,[65,66] and β-blockade may reverse β-receptor uncoupling.[67]

The mechanism by which the β_1-AR is down-regulated in the failing human heart has been explored.[57] It has been demonstrated that down-regulation of the receptor correlates well with a decline in the steady-state abundance of human β_1-AR mRNA.[57,68] β-AR mRNA abundance can be measured using the reverse-transcription/quantitative polymerase chain reaction (RT-qPCR). This technique represents a sig-

nificant advantage over other more conventional quantitative methodologies such as Northern blotting and even ribonuclease protection assays in that it is sufficiently sensitive and requires such minimal tissue as to allow gene expression to be accurately measured from endomyocardial biopsy specimens.[69] This methodologic advantage permits serial measurements of gene expression in patients before and after therapeutic intervention. The results of these experiments may eventually lead to a significantly better understanding of the time course of gene regulation of receptor density and function during heart failure. Moreover, it may allow assignment of more specific markers of heart failure, and it may also elucidate new therapeutic targets for the treatment of heart failure.

At a mechanistic level, the steady-state abundance of an mRNA, such as that of the human β_1-AR, can be altered in several ways. It is has been assumed that steady-state mRNA abundance is regulated at the level of mRNA transcription (i.e., the rate of mRNA synthesis). mRNA turnover or "stability" may also be regulated. In fact, it is well established that the half-life of many mRNAs encoding proto-oncogenes and cytokines are regulated by mRNA stability,[70] a regulatory paradigm that has now been observed for a number of G protein-coupled receptors including the human β_1-AR. As demonstrated previously for the hamster β_2-AR, it has been shown that β-agonist exposure decreases the half-life of the β_1-AR mRNA approximately 50 percent, a value that correlates well with the observed decrease in receptor density at the protein level.[71] For mRNAs regulated at the level of stability, work is now continuing in the direction of defining specific nucleotide sequences within the mRNA that may interact with specific mRNA binding proteins. The ultimate goal is to understand more completely how these nucleotide sequences and mRNA binding proteins that bind to the sequences may regulate β-agonist-mediated destabilization of specific mRNAs, such as the mRNA encoding β_1-AR.

The role of the β-AR in producing heart failure has begun to be investigated using transgenic mouse technology. Using an α-myosin heavy chain promoter to direct cardiac selective expression, Milano et al.[72] developed transgenic mice overexpressing the wild-type β_2-AR as well as a constitutively activated β_2-AR. In each case the mice are significantly hyperdynamic,[72] and diastolic relaxation appears to be altered as well.[73] Of considerable interest is the specific pathophysiologic effects of long-term overstimulation of the β_2-AR pathway on these hearts. Kobilka and colleagues (B. Kobilka, personal communication) have produced by homologous recombination transgenic mice deficient in the expression of either β_1-AR or β_2-AR genes. The morphologic and functional phenotype of these mice are of considerable interest to the heart failure research community.

Clinical Significance of Altered β-Receptor/G Protein/Adenylyl Cyclase Pathway in the Human Heart

As previously mentioned, the β-receptor/G protein/adenylyl cyclase pathway is the means by which myocardial performance is changed rapidly, and this pathway exerts powerful positive inotropic and chronotropic effects in the human heart. In the innervated heart, contractility can be increased literally within a matter of seconds by occupancy of β-adrenergic receptors. However, there is a negative component to this powerful stimulating pathway; that is, chronic activation of the adrenergic drive is potentially cardiotoxic, possibly by overloading the cell with Ca^{2+} and subsequent adverse effects on macromolecular synthesis.[74] It is therefore fortuitous that this pathway is highly regulated, with desensitization being an important and probably adaptive process.

As shown in Figure 9-4, the desensitization changes involving the β-receptor/G protein/adenylyl cyclase pathway lead to attenuation of the systolic tension response to β-agonists including isoproterenol and dobutamine and the phosphodiesterase inhibitor enoximone, but not to the sodium channel agonist BDF-9148.[75] β-Agonist responses are decreased because of the aforementioned β_1-receptor down-regulation, receptor uncoupling, and increased tonic inhibition by G_i, whereas phosphodiesterase inhibitor responses are decreased because there is less substrate (i.e., cAMP) available owing to the collective desensitization process.

Clinically, specific abnormalities in stimulated cardiac function involving the β-receptor/G protein signal transduction system can be demonstrated in the intact human heart.[76] Figure 9-5 presents data on contractility estimated by change in pressure/change in time (dP/dt) measurements with a left ventricular Millar catheter during infusion of the β-agonist dobutamine. As shown in Figure 9-4, dobutamine is a nonselective partial agonist in human ventricular myocardium, with an intrinsic activity of about 0.5.[77] There are two groups of subjects in Figure 9-5: those with no or mild heart failure and ejection fractions of more than 0.40, and those with severe heart failure and ejection fractions of less than 0.25. As can be seen, there is a marked reduction in the dobutamine contractility response in subjects with advanced heart failure. After dobutamine is washed out and Ca^{2+} is infused, there is no difference in contractility response between control and failing hearts. Another point to be made here is that even though dobutamine is a partial agonist the degree of increase in systolic performance conferred by it is still substantial and comparable to the increase seen with Ca^{2+} in failing hearts. In other words, the β-adrenergic pathways are powerful enhancers of contractility even when β-adrenergic activity is partially lost during heart failure.

The above-mentioned adrenergic receptor changes that occur in the failing human heart may represent an adaptive response that attempts to limit the adverse effects of cardiac adrenergic stimulation. That is, changes at the level of these receptors and G proteins may serve to restrict the amount of inotropic stimulation and biologic effect that can be produced through these pathways. Quantitatively, approximately one-half of the combined adrenergic pathways appear to be subject to such regulation; and despite these desensitization changes the adrenergic pathways, particularly the β-receptor/G protein/adenylyl cyclase pathway, are still capable of producing formidable effects. In this regard, it should be acknowledged that a number of counterregulatory hormones may also attempt to limit the activity of

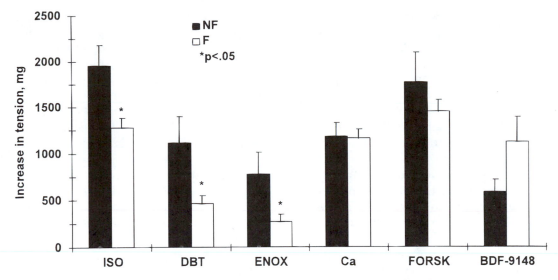

Fig. 9-4. Systolic tension response to the β-agonists isoproterenol (ISO) and dobutamine (DBT), the phosphodiesterase inhibitor enoximone (ENOX), calcium (Ca), forskolin (FORSK), and the Na⁺ channel agonist BDF-9148 in isolated right ventricular trabeculae taken from nonfailing (NF) and failing (F) human heart.

the β-receptor/G protein signal transduction pathway during heart failure by producing either a decrease in β-AR responsiveness (nitric oxide[78,79]) or a decrease in neuronal norepinephrine release (natriuretic peptides[80,81]).

The deleterious clinical manifestations of this increase in cardiac adrenergic activity comprise three major components of the natural history of heart failure: loss of exercise tolerance, progression of left ventricular dysfunction, and an increased prevalence of arrhythmias including a high incidence of sudden death as the cause of demise in 20 to 50 percent of subjects. Although the desensitization changes that occur in adrenergic receptor pathways limit the functional capacity of the failing heart by compromising its modulated function capability, chronically increased adrenergic stimulation provides an explanation for the progressive pump dysfunction by virtue of a generally cardiotoxic mechanism. Support for this hypothesis comes from the observations that β-blockade consistently improves left ventricular function in heart failure patients,[65,66,82] and some β-blockers may also improve clinical outcome (i.e., survival).[39–41]

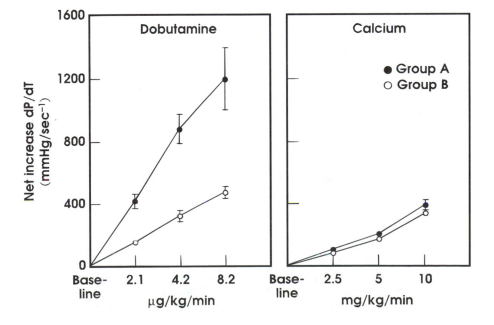

Fig. 9-5. Comparison of the positive inotropic response of the partial β-agonist dobutamine or calcium in subjects with advanced heart failure (group B) or controls with no heart failure (group A). (From Fowler et al.,[76] with permission.)

In this regard, it should be noted that the survival benefits of β-blockers appear variable. For example, the second-generation selective β_1-adrenergic receptor blockers metoprolol and bisoprolol seem to reduce mortality only slightly[54] or not at all[53] in patients with nonischemic dilated cardiomyopathy and have little effect on the outcome of those with ischemic cardiomyopathy.[54] In contrast, the third-generation nonselective β-blocking agent carvedilol appears to have a substantial effect on reducing the mortality associated with both ischemic and nonischemic cardiomyopathies and, unlike the two second-generation compounds, reduces the incidence of sudden death.[40,41] These observations are compatible with the adaptive nature of cardiac adrenergic desensitization phenomena in that carvedilol, compared to metoprolol, appears to more completely antagonize cardiac adrenergic mechanisms.[39] Using the third-generation nonselective β-blocking agent bucindolol, the ongoing Beta-Blocker Evaluation of Survival Trial (BEST) should provide further insight into the importance of antagonizing cardiac adrenergic activity in patients with chronic symptomatic heart failure.

ANGIOTENSIN II RECEPTORS

Angiotensin II receptors are subdivided into two major classes: AT_1 and AT_2 receptor subtypes. In rodents, AT_1 receptors are further subdivided into the AT_{1a} and AT_{1b} subtypes.[24] It is not yet clear that more than one subtype of the AT_1 receptor exists in humans. Although not yet explored in great depth, differences have not been detected in the signaling of the AT_{1a} and AT_{1b} subtypes. The angiotensin II AT_{1a} receptor is expressed in a variety of tissues, and its presence has been confirmed in human ventricular myocardium.[83] In this organ, angiotensin II AT_1 and AT_2 receptors are expressed at low density, approximately 2 to 10 fmol/mg of protein, a volume considerably lower than that of β-ARs.

Like the α_1-AR, the angiotensin II AT_1 appears to be coupled to the G_q family of G proteins. Agonist binding leads to phosphatidylinositol hydrolysis and to the activation of a number of protein kinases, including PKC, MAP kinase, JNK (jun N-terminal kinase), and uniquely tyrosine kinase activity. The AT_{1a} receptor appears to be unique among the G protein-coupled receptors in that tyrosine kinase activation is normally associated with growth factor receptors such as those for epidermal growth factor, fibroblast growth factor, platelet-derived growth factor, and insulin. Furthermore, the AT_{1a} receptor appears to activate protein tyrosine kinase activity by a pathway similar to that utilized by growth factor receptors. More specifically, angiotensin II appears to activate the translocation of p21^{ras} as well as affecting the SH2/SH3 or Src-homology adapter proteins Shc, Grb2, and Sos.[32,84,85] The mitogenic and hypertrophic effects of angiotensin II on the heart and vasculature are most likely due to the tyrosine kinase activity of the AT_{1a} receptor. In contrast to the AT_{1a} receptor, the signaling pathways of the AT_2 receptor are relatively poorly defined. Some evidence suggests that the AT_2 receptor is coupled to phospholipases such as PLD and PLA$_2$.[32,86] However, most recently, the AT_2 receptor has been shown to antagonize hypertrophic and mitogenic effects mediated by the AT_1 receptor.[87]

In humans, the effects of chronic heart failure and renin-angiotensin system activation on the AT_1 receptor have begun to be investigated. It is now appreciated that the AT_1 receptor undergoes subtype-specific down-regulation in the failing human heart (Fig. 9-6).[83] Interestingly, angiotensin II AT_1 receptor down-regulation appears to be related to the etiology of the heart failure. That is, AT_1 receptor down-regulation seems to occur only in patients with idiopathic dilated cardiomyopathy rather than ischemic cardiomyopathy. Similar to the β_2-AR, the angiotensin II AT_2 receptor does not appear to down-regulate during any type of heart failure. Like the β-AR, there appears to be regional specificity of angiotensin II receptor distribution in the heart. The AT_2 receptor appears to be highly expressed in fibroblasts, whereas the AT_1 receptor appears to be more ubiquitously distributed.[88] Functional changes associated with down-regulation of the AT_1 receptor in the human heart have not yet been investigated.

Like the β-AR, transgenic mouse technology is now being exploited to more completely understand the influence and role of the AT_1 receptor. A transgenic mouse overexpressing the AT_1 receptor in the heart has been reported. Its phenotype is one of gross atrial hypertrophy and death within the first week or two of life.[89] The phenotype may be due to the developmental expression pattern of the α-myosin heavy chain (α-MHC) promoter that was used to express the AT_1 receptor in the mouse model.

The use of inhibitors and antagonists of the renin-angiotensin system are of proved benefit for treatment of chronic heart failure.[90,91] Moreover, the prophylactic administration of ACE inhibitors to subjects with asymptomatic left ventricular dysfunction or after a myocardial infarction has been shown to exert favorable effects on ventricular remodeling and dilation, progression to overt heart failure, and clinical outcome.[92,93] Thus down-regulation of the angiotensin II AT_1 receptor seen with some forms of heart

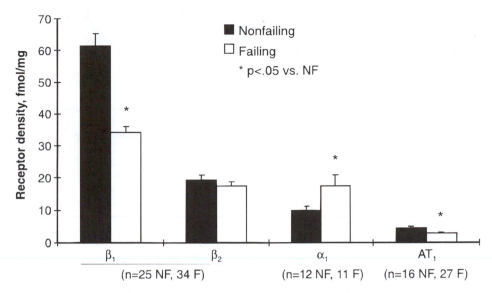

Fig. 9-6. Receptor densities for four major G protein-coupled adrenergic or angiotensin receptors in crude membrane preparations from nonfailing and failing human left ventricles. Failing left ventricles were obtained from class III–IV heart failure patients with idiopathic dilated cardiomyopathy who were not being supported by intravenous inotropes or mechanical assist devices. The mean age of nonfailing subjects was similar to that of the heart failure patients (36.5 ± 3.2 vs. 37.1 ± 2.5 years; $p =$ NS).

failure may also be viewed as a part of the adaptive cardiac response to myocardial failure. The use of ACE inhibitors for treating left ventricular dysfunction and heart failure is discussed in Chapter 45.

OTHER CARDIAC RECEPTORS DURING HEART FAILURE

To date, many of the other cardiac receptors listed in Table 9-1 have been incompletely studied during heart failure. The H_2 histamine receptor does not appear to change during heart failure.[94,95] The vasoactive intestinal peptide receptor down-regulates substantially, by 70 percent.[96] Many other receptors in the failing heart do not appear to be significantly regulated, including the dihydropyridine,[97] oubain,[98] and histamine[94,90] receptors. Therefore most cell surface receptors coupled to a positive inotropic response are unchanged during heart failure. The clinical significance of this observation remains unclear.

SUMMARY

Changes occur in cardiac adrenergic receptor pathways in the failing human heart. In ventricular myocardium, receptor pathway changes are observed only in failing chambers. The implication is that the myocardial changes are under local or regional con-

trol; that is, the regulatory factors are not related to systemic factors. Of the changes in myocardial adrenergic receptors, β-receptor phenomena are the most striking; and of the changes in β-adrenergic receptors, β_1-receptor down-regulation is the most prominent. Most of the changes in adrenergic receptors appear to be related to increased adrenergic drive. In heart failure patients with idiopathic dilated cardiomyopathy, the angiotensin II AT_1 receptor is also down-regulated. In both cases, this receptor down-regulation and other desensitization phenomena may represent an adaptive cardioprotective response in the setting of increased cardiac adrenergic drive and elevated angiotensin II. The fact that inhibitors and antagonists of the adrenergic and renin-angiotensin systems improve left ventricular function and outcome in patients with heart failure supports the notion that activation of these neurohormonal systems exerts a net long-term detrimental effect on the natural history of chronic cardiac failure.

ACKNOWLEDGMENTS

Studies reported in this chapter were supported, in part, by U.S. Public Health Service grants HL51239 (JDP) and HL48013 (MRB); grants CBG-015-93 and CHA COGB-22-95 from the Colorado Heart Association (JDP); and grant M01-RR00051 from the Division of Research Resources, National Institutes of

Health, General Clinical Research Centers Program (WTA and MRB). Dr. Abraham is supported by the Clinical Associate Physician Award from the General Clinical Research Centers Program, National Institutes of Health (3 M01-RR00051-33S1).

REFERENCES

1. Guyton AC: Cardiac output, venous return, and their regulation. pp. 273–286. In: Textbook of Medical Physiology. WB Saunders, Philadelphia, 1986
2. Abraham WT, Schrier RW: Renal salt and water handling in congestive heart failure. pp. 161–173. In Hosenpud JD, Greenberg JH (eds): Congestive Heart Failure. Pathophysiology, Diagnosis, and Comprehensive Approach to Management. Springer-Verlag, New York, 1994
3. Thomas JA, Marks BH: Plasma norepinephrine in congestive heart failure. Am J Cardiol 1978;41:233–243
4. Levine TB, Francis GS, Goldsmith SR., Simon AB, Cohn JN: Activity of the sympathetic nervous system and renin-angiotensin system assessed by plasma hormone levels and their relation to hemodynamic abnormalities in congestive heart failure. Am J Cardiol 1982;49:1659–1666
5. Hasking GJ, Esler MD, Jennings GL et al: Norepinephrine spillover to plasma in patients with congestive heart failure. Evidence of increased overall and cardiorenal sympathetic nervous activity. Circulation 1986;73:615–621
6. Davis D, Baily R, Zelis R: Abnormalities in systemic norepinephrine kinetics in human congestive heart failure. Am J Physiol 1988;254:E760–E766
7. Abraham WT, Hensen J, Schrier RW: Elevated plasma noradrenaline concentrations in patients with low-output cardiac failure. Dependence on increased noradrenaline secretion rates. Clin Sci 1990;79:429–435
8. Francis GS, Benedict C, Johnstone EE et al: Comparison of neuroendocrine activation in patients with left ventricular dysfunction with and without congestive heart failure. A substudy of the studies of left ventricular dysfunction (SOLVD). Circulation 1990;82:1724–1729
9. Leimbach WN, Wallin BG, Victor RG et al: Direct evidence from intraneural recordings for increased central sympathetic outflow in patients with heart failure. Circulation 1986;73:913–919
10. Bristow MR, Minobe W, Rasmussen R et al: β-Adrenergic neuroeffector abnormalities in the failing human heart are produced by local, rather than systemic mechanisms. J Clin Invest 1992;89:803–815
11. Abraham WT, Lowes BD, Roden RL et al: Evidence for decreased neuronal norepinephrine reuptake in the intact failing human heart. Submitted
12. Abraham WT, Lowes BD, Rose CP, Larrabee P, Bristow MR: Angiotensin II selectively increases cardiac adrenergic activity in patients with heart failure. J Am Coll Cardiol 1994;23:215A
13. Berl T, Henrich WL, Erickson AL, Schrier RW: Prostaglandins in the beta adrenergic and baroreceptor-mediated secretion of renin. Am J Physiol 1979;235:F472–F477
14. Weber F, Brodde OE, Anlauf M, Bock KD: Subclassification of human beta-adrenergic receptors mediating renin release. Clin Exp Hypertens 1983;5:225–238
15. Hattler B, Raynolds MV: Differential regulation of angiotensin-converting enzyme and angiotensinogen gene expression in human coronary smooth muscle cells. p. 472. In: Proceedings of the 76th Annual Meeting of the Endocrine Society, 1994
16. Bristow MR, Abraham WT: Anti-adrenergic effects of angiotensin converting enzyme inhibitors. Eur Heart J, suppl. K 1995;16:37–41
17. Cody RJ, Franklin KW, Kluger J, Laragh JH: Sympathetic responsiveness and plasma norepinephrine during therapy of chronic congestive heart failure with captopril. Am J Med 1982;72:791–797
18. Gilbert EM, Sandoval A, Larrabee P et al: Lisinopril lowers cardiac adrenergic drive and increases β-receptor density in the failing human heart. Circulation 1993;88:472–480
19. Ahlquist R: A study of the adrenotropic receptors. Am J Physiol 1948;153:586–600
20. Fedida D, Braun AP, Giles WR: α_1-Adrenoceptors in myocardium. Functional aspects and transmembrane signaling mechanisms. Physiol Rev 1993;73:469–487
21. Price DT, Lefkowitz RJ, Caron MG, Berkowitz D, Schwinn DA: Localization of mRNA for three distinct alpha-1 adrenergic receptor subtypes in human tissues. Implications for human alpha-adrenergic physiology. Mol Pharmacol 1994;45:171–175
22. Steinberg SF, Goldberg M, Rybin VO: Protein kinase C isoform diversity in the heart. J Mol Cell Cardiol 1995;27:141–153
23. Hausdorff WP, Caron MG, Lefkowitz RJ: Turning off the signal. Desensitization of β-adrenergic receptor function. FASEB J 1990;4:2881–2889
24. Ruffolo RR, Hollinger MA (eds): G-Protein Coupled Transmembrane Signaling Mechanisms. pp. 1–34. CRC Press, Boca Raton, FL, 1995
25. Landzberg JS, Parker JD, Gauthier DF, Colucci WS: Effects of myocardial α_1-adrenergic receptor stimulation and blockade on contractility in humans. Circulation 1991;84:1608–1614
26. LaMorte VJ, Thorburn J, Absher D et al: Gq- and ras-dependent pathways mediate hypertrophy of neonatal rat ventricular myocytes following α_1-adrenergic stimulation. J Biol Chem 1994;269:13490–13496
27. Simpson P: Norepinephrine-stimulated hypertrophy of cultured rat myocardial cells is an alpha-1 adrenergic response. J Clin Invest 1993;83:732–738
28. Takahashi N, Thaik CM, Calderone A, Colucci WS: α_1-Adrenergic receptor-mediated hypertrophy and gene expression in cardiac myocytes are mediated by calcium influx [abstract]. Circulation, suppl. I 1995;92:384
29. Thorburn J, Frost JA, Thorburn A: Mitogen-activated protein kinases mediate changes in gene expression, but not cytoskeletal organization associated with cardiac muscle cell hypertrophy. J Cell Biol 1994;126:1565–1572
30. Milano CA, Dolber PC, Rockman HA et al: Myocardial expression of a constitutively active α_{1b}-adrenergic receptor in transgenic mice induces cardiac hypertrophy. Proc Natl Acad Sci USA 1994;91:10109–10113
31. Sadoshima J-I, Izumo S: Mechanical stretch rapidly activates multiple signal transduction pathways in cardiac myocytes. Potential involvement of an

autocrine/paracrine mechanism. EMBO J 1993;12: 1681–1692

32. Sadoshima J-I, Izumo S: The heterotrimeric Gq protein-coupled angiotensin II receptor activates p21ras via the Src-family tyrosine kinase-Shc-Grb2-Sos pathway in cardiac myocytes. Circulation, suppl. I 1995; 92:7

33. Bohm M, Diet F, Feiler G, Kemkes B, Erdmann E: α-Adrenoceptors and α-adrenoceptor-mediated positive inotropic effects in failing human myocardium. J Cardiovasc Pharmacol 1988;12:357–364

34. Bristow MR, Minobe W, Rassmussen R, Hershberger RE, Hoffman BB: Alpha-1 adrenergic receptors in the nonfailing and failing human heart. J Pharmacol Exp Ther 1988;247:1039–1045

35. Bristow MR, Gilbert EM: Improvement on cardiac myocyte function by biological effects of medical therapy. A new concept in the treatment of heart failure. Eur Heart J, suppl. F 1995;16:20–31

36. Jahnel U, Jakob H, Nawrath H: Electrophysiologic and inotropic effects of alpha-adrenoceptor stimulation in human isolated atrial heart muscle. Naunyn Schmiedebergs Arch Pharmacol 1992;346:82–87

37. Cohn JN, Archibald DG, Ziesche S et al: Effect of vasodilator therapy on mortality in chronic congestive heart failure. Results of a Veterans Administration cooperative study. N Engl J Med 1986;314:1547–1552

38. Colucci WS, Williams GH, Braunwald E: Increased plasma norepinephrine levels during prazosin therapy for severe congestive heart failure. Ann Intern Med 1980;93:452–453

39. Gilbert EM, Abraham WT, Olsen S et al: Comparative hemodynamic, LV functional, and anti-adrenergic effects of chronic treatment with metoprolol vs. carvedilol in the failing heart. Submitted

40. Packer M, Bristow MR, Cohn JN et al: The effect of carvedilol on morbidity and mortality in patients with chronic heart failure. N Engl J Med 1996; 334: 1349–1355

41. Bristow MR, Gilbert EM, Abraham WT et al: Multicenter oral carvedilol heart failure assessment (MOCHA). A six-month dose-response evaluation in class II–IV patients. Circulation, suppl. I 1995;92:142

42. Gauthier C, Charpentier F, Laurent K, Trochu J-N, Le Marec H: Pharmacologic evidence for the presence of β_3-adrenoceptors in human ventricular cells. Circulation, suppl. I 1995;92:639

43. Widén E, Lehto M, Kanninen T et al: Association of a polymorphism in the β_3-adrenergic-receptor gene with features of the insulin resistance syndrome in Finns. N Engl J Med 1995;333:348–351

44. Clément K, Vaisse C, Manning B et al: Genetic variation in the β_3-adrenergic receptor and an increased capacity to gain weight in patients with morbid obesity. N Engl J Med 1995;333:352–354

45. Gilman AG: G proteins. Transducers of receptor-generated signals. Annu Rev Biochem 1987;56:615–649

46. Crespo P, Cachero TG, Xu N, Gutkind JS: Dual effect of β-adrenergic receptors on mitogen-activated protein kinase. Evidence for a $\beta\gamma$-dependent activation and a Gαs-cAMP-mediated inhibition. J Biol Chem 1995; 270:25259–25265

47. Bristow MR, Hershberger RE, Port JD, Minobe W, Rasmussen R: β_1 & β_2 Adrenergic receptor mediated adenylate cyclase stimulation in nonfailing and failing human ventricular myocardium. Mol Pharmacol 1989; 35:295–303

48. Kaumann AJ, Lemoine H: β_2-Adrenoceptor-mediated positive inotropic effect of adrenaline in human ventricular myocardium. Quantitative discrepancies with binding and adenylate cyclase stimulation. Naunyn-Schmiedebergs Arch Pharmacol 1987;335:403–411

49. Bristow MR, Anderson FL, Port JD et al: Differences in β-adrenergic neuroeffector mechanisms in ischemic versus idiopathic dilated cardiomyopathy. Circulation 1991;84:1024–1039

50. Bristow MR, Ginsberg R, Fowler M et al: β_1- and β_2-Adrenergic receptor subtype populations in normal and failing human ventricular myocardium. Circ Res 1986;59:297–309

51. Brodde O-E, Zerkowski HR, Doetsch N et al: Myocardial beta-adrenoceptor changes in heart failure. Concomitant reduction in beta$_1$-and beta$_2$-adrenoceptor function related to the degree of heart failure in patients with mitral valve disease. J Am Coll Cardiol 1989;14:323–331

52. Brodde OE, Schuler S, Kretsch R et al: Regional distribution of β-adrenoceptors in the human heart. Coexistence of function β_1- and β_2-adrenoceptors in both atria and ventricles in severe congestive cardiomyopathy. J Cardiovasc Pharmacol 1986;8:1235–1242

53. Waagstein F, Bristow MR, Swedberg K et al: Beneficial effects of metoprolol in idiopathic dilated cardiomyopathy. Lancet 1993;342:1441–1446

54. CIBIS Investigators: A randomized trial of beta-blockade in heart failure. The cardiac insufficiency bisoprolol study (CIBIS). CIBIS Investigators and Committees. Circulation 1994;90:1765–1773

55. Bouvier M, Collins S, O'Dowd BF et al: Two distinct pathways for cAMP-mediated down-regulation of the β_2-adrenergic receptor. Phosphorylation of the receptor and regulation of its mRNA level. J Biol Chem 1989;264:16786–16792

56. Freedman NJ, Ligget SB, Drachman DE et al: Phosphorylation and desensitization of the human β_1-adrenergic receptor. J Biol Chem 1995;270:17953–17961

57. Ungerer M, Bohm M, Elce S, Erdmann E, Lohse MJ: Altered expression of β-adrenergic receptor kinase and β_1-adrenergic receptors in the failing human heart. Circulation 1993;87:454–463

58. Feldman AM, Gates AE, Veazey WB et al: Increase of the M_r 40,000 pertussis toxin substrate (G protein) in the failing human heart. J Clin Invest 1988;82: 189–197

59. Bristow MR, Hershberger RE, Port JD et al: β-Adrenergic pathways in nonfailing and failing human ventricular myocardium. Circulation, suppl. I 1990;82: 12–25

60. Bobik A, Campbell JH, Carson V, Campbell GR: Mechanism of isoprenaline-induced refractoriness of the β-adrenoceptor-adenylate cyclase system in chick embryo cardiac cells. J Cardiovasc Pharmacol 1981;3: 541–553

61. Linden J, Patel A, Spanier AM, Weglicki WB: Rapid agonist-induced decrease of ^{125}I-pindolol binding to β-adrenergic receptors. Relationship to desensitization of cyclic AMP accumulation in intact heart cells. J Biol Chem 1984;259:15115–15122

62. Reithmann C, Werdan K: Homologous vs. heterologous desensitization of the adenylate cyclase system in heart cells. Eur J Pharmacol 1988;154:99–104

63. Bristow MR, Sandoval AB, Gilbert EM et al: Myocar-

dial alpha- and beta-adrenergic receptors in heart failure. Is cardiac-derived norepinephrine the regulatory signal? Eur Heart J 1988;9:35–40

64. Sandoval A, Gilbert EM, Ginsburg R et al: β_1 Receptor down-regulation in the failing human heart. The result of exposure to cardiac derived norepinephrine? J Am Coll Cardiol 1988;11:117A

65. Heilbrunn SM, Shaw P, Bristow MR et al: Increased β-receptor density and improved hemodynamic response to catecholamine stimulation during long-term metoprolol therapy in heart failure from dilated cardiomyopathy. Circulation 1989;79:483–490

66. Waagstein F, Caidahl K, Wallentin I, Bergh CH, Hjalmarson AÅ: Long-term beta-blockade in dilated cardiomyopathy. Effects of short- and long-term metoprolol treatment followed by withdrawal and readministration of metoprolol. Circulation 1989;80:551–563

67. Hall JA, Petch MC, Brown MJ: In vivo demonstration of cardiac β_2-adrenoreceptor sensitization by β_1-antagonist treatment. Circ Res 1991;69:959–964

68. Bristow MR, Minobe W, Raynolds MV et al: Reduced β_1 receptor messenger RNA abundance in the failing human heart. J Clin Invest 1993;92:2737–2745

69. Minobe W, Lowes BD, Abraham WT, Feldman AM, Bristow MR: In vivo measurement of myocardial gene expression in the human heart. J Am Coll Cardiol 1995;25:277A

70. Brawerman G: mRNA degradation in eukaryotic cells. In Belasco J, Brawerman G (eds): Control of mRNA Stability. Academic Press, San Diego, 1993

71. Tremmel KD, Pende A, Bristow MR, Port JD: Regulation of human β_1-adrenergic receptor mRNA stability by agonist exposure. J Cell Biochem (in press)

72. Milano CA, Allen LF, Rockman HA et al: Enhanced myocardial function in transgenic mice overexpressing the β_2-adrenergic receptor. Science 1994;264:582–586

73. Rockman HA, Hamilton RA, Milano CA et al: Enhanced myocardial relaxation in vivo in transgenic mice overexpressing the β_2-adrenergic receptor. J Am Coll Cardiol 1995;25:26A

74. Mann DL, Kent RL, Parsons B, Cooper G IV: Adrenergic effects on the biology of the adult mammalian cardiocyte. Circulation 1992;85:790–804

75. Schwinger RH, Bohm M, Mittmann C, LaRosee K, Erdmann E: Evidence for a sustained effectiveness of sodium-channel activators in failing human myocardium. J Mol Cell Cardiol 1991;23:461–471

76. Fowler MB, Laser JA, Hopkins GL, Minobe WA, Bristow MR: Assessment of the β-adrenergic pathway in the intact human heart. Progressive receptor down-regulation and subsensitivity to agonist response. Circulation 1986;74:1290–1302

77. Wollmering MM, Wiechmann RJ, Port JD et al: Dobutamine is a partial agonist with an intrinsic activity of 0.5 in human myocardium. J Am Coll Cardiol 1991; 17:283A

78. Hare JM, Keaney JF Jr, Balligand J-L et al: Role of nitric oxide in parasympathetic modulation of β-adrenergic myocardial contractility in normal dogs. J Clin Invest 1995;95:360–366

79. Hare JM, Givertz MM, Creager MA, Colucci WS: Nitric oxide attenuates myocardial β-adrenergic responsiveness in humans with heart failure. Circulation, suppl. I 1995;92:567

80. Holtz J, Sommer O, Bassenge E: Inhibition of sympa-thoadrenal activity by atrial natriuretic factor in dogs. Hypertension 1987;9:350–354

81. Münzel T, Kurz S, Holtz J, et al: Neurohormonal inhibition and hemodynamic unloading during prolonged inhibition of ANF degradation in patients with severe chronic heart failure. Circulation 1992;86:1089–1098

82. Gilbert EM, Anderson JL, Deitchman D et al: Long-term β-blocker vasodilator therapy improves cardiac function in idiopathic dilated cardiomyopathy. A double-blind, randomized study of bucindolol versus placebo. Am J Med 1990;88:223–229

83. Asano K, Dutcher DL, Port JD et al: Selective down-regulation of the angiotensin II AT_1 receptor subtype in failing human left ventricles with idiopathic dilated but not ischemic cardiomyopathy. Submitted

84. Bhat GJ, Thekkumkara TJ, Thomas WG, Conrad KM, Baker KM: Activation of the STAT pathway by angiotensin II in T3CHO/ATA1A cells. Cross-talk between angiotensin II and interleukin-6 nuclear signaling. J Biol Chem 1995;270:19059–19065

85. Schorb W, Peeler TC, Madigan NN, Conrad KM, Baker KM: Angiotensin II-induced protein tyrosine phosphorylation in neonatal rat cardiac fibroblasts. J Biol Chem 1994;269:19626–19632

86. Booz GW, Taher MM, Baker KM, Singer HA: Angiotensin II induces phosphatidic acid formation in neonatal rat cardiac fibroblasts. Evaluation of the roles of phospholipases C and D. Mol Cell Biochem 1994; 141:135–143

87. Nakajima M, Hutchinson HG, Fujinaga M et al: The angiotensin II type 2 (AT_2) receptor antagonizes the growth effects of the AT_1 receptor. Gain-of-function study using gene transfer. Proc Natl Acad Sci USA 1995;92:10663–10667

88. Brink M, de Gasparo M, Rogg H, Schmid A, Bullock G: Localization of the angiotensin II AT_2 receptor subtype in the human heart. Circulation, suppl. I 1995; 92:63

89. Hein L, Stevens ME, Barsh GS et al: Cardiac remodeling in transgenic mice expressing angiotensin AT_{1a} receptors under the control of the α-myosin heavy chain promoter. Circulation, suppl. I 1995;93:63

90. CONSENSUS Trial Study Group: Effects of enalapril on mortality in severe congestive heart failure. Results of the North Scandinavian Enalapril Survival Study (CONSENSUS). N Engl J Med 1987;316:1429–1435

91. SOLVD Investigators: Effect of enalapril on survival in patients with reduced left ventricular ejection fractions and congestive heart failure. N Engl J Med 1991; 325:293–302

92. SOLVD Investigators: Effect of enalapril on mortality and the development of heart failure in asymptomatic patients with reduced left ventricular ejection fractions. N Engl J Med 1992;327:685–691

93. Pfeffer MA, Braunwald E, Moyé LA et al: Effect of captopril on mortality and morbidity in patients with left ventricular dysfunction after myocardial infarction. Results of the Survival and Ventricular Enlargement Trial. N Engl J Med 1992;327:669–677

94. Bristow MR, Cubicciotti R, Ginsburg R, Stinson EB, Johnson C: Histamine-mediated adenylate cyclase stimulation in human myocardium. Mol Pharmacol 1982;21:671–679

95. Baumann G, Mercader D, Busch U et al: Effects of the H_2-receptor agonist impromidine in human myocardium from patients with heart failure due to mitral

and aortic valve disease. J Cardiovasc Pharmacol 1983;5:618–625

96. Hershberger RE, Anderson FL, Bristow MR: Vasoactive intestinal peptide receptor in failing human ventricular myocardium exhibits increased affinity and decreased density. Circ Res 1989;65:283–294

97. Rasmussen RP, Minobe W, Bristow MR: Calcium antagonist binding sites in failing and non-failing human ventricular myocardium. Biochem Pharmacol 1990; 39:691–696

98. Schwinger RH, Böhm M, Erdmann E: Effectiveness of cardiac glycosides in human myocardium with and without "downregulated" β-adrenoceptors. J Cardiovasc Pharmacol 1990;15:692–697.

Humoral Control of the Kidney During Congestive Heart Failure: Role of Cardiac Natriuretic Peptides and Angiotensin II

Roland R. Brandt
John C. Burnett, Jr.

10

A hallmark of overt congestive heart failure (CHF) is renal retention of sodium, which results in signs and symptoms of congestion. Renal retention of sodium also may contribute to the progression of ventricular dysfunction through increases in cardiac preload. Reinforcing cardiac overload is the release of renin by the kidney in patients with overt CHF, which culminates in the generation of angiotensin II (ANG II). ANG II is a key humoral mediator of renal and cardiovascular maladaptations in overt CHF. ANG II has direct vascular and tubular actions in the kidney in CHF that promote sodium retention. Such actions are reinforced by ANG II-mediated adrenal release of the sodium-retaining hormone aldosterone. It is now apparent that ANG II may also contribute to progressive ventricular dysfunction not only via its sodium-retaining properties but also by direct vascular actions to increase preload and direct myocardial actions that may contribute to ventricular hypertrophy and cardiac fibrosis.

The renin-angiotensin system (RAS) plays a fundamental role in the control of renal hemodynamics and tubular sodium reabsorption in CHF; and it is now well established that the heart as an endocrine gland synthesizes and releases two peptide hormones that are activated with the onset of left ventricular dysfunction (LVD). These cardiac natriuretic peptides play a homeostatic role, maintaining sodium excretion and inhibiting activation of the RAS during the progression of CHF from the initial period of asymptomatic LVD to overt CHF. These two peptides, atrial (ANP) and brain (BNP) natriuretic peptides, share structural similarities but are genetically distinct. They are complemented by a third structurally similar peptide, CNP, of endothelial cell origin; this peptide functions in control of vascular tone and vascular smooth muscle cell growth; it is not reviewed here as it has no known renal action.

This chapter explores the interactions of two cardiovascular humoral systems—natriuretic peptides and the RAS—in the adaptations of the kidney during the progression of CHF. We begin with a review of ANP and BNP, which are activated early in CHF, and then address interactions with ANG II.

CARDIAC NATRIURETIC PEPTIDES IN CHF

Physiologic Role of ANP and BNP in Cardiorenal Homeostasis

Kisch[1] first suggested an endocrine role for the heart with the observation of membrane-bound storage granules, referred to as specific granules in atrial cardiocytes. The density of these granules was reported to be affected by various experimental procedures, such as changes in fluid and electrolyte balance. The physiologic significance of these atrial granules was established when de Bold et al.[2] observed in their seminal study a natriuretic and hypotensive effect in response to intravenous injection of atrial extracts into rats. These hallmark investigations led to the characterization of ANP as a 28-residue C-terminal peptide that is derived from the 126-

amino-acid precursor pro-ANP, which is the principal storage form.[3] Repeated studies have demonstrated that ANP has unique biologic actions, including natriuretic, vasodilator, renin- and aldosterone-inhibiting, and antimitogenic actions.[4] BNP is now the second member of the natriuretic peptide family, complementing ANP.[5] Like ANP, BNP is synthesized in cardiac myocytes and released in response to atrial and ventricular stretch.[6] BNP has biologic actions similar to those of ANP. Therefore the two peptides function as a dual cardiac natriuretic peptide system.[7]

The cellular mechanism for ANP and BNP synthesis and processing continues to emerge, Edwards et al.,[8] in an elegant study creating cardiac tamponade in animals, showed that atrial stretch is the principal stimulus for ANP secretion. Cardiac tamponade produced a balanced increase in intraatrial and pericardial pressures with no change in atrial transmural pressure or atrial stretch. No change in circulating ANP was observed. In contrast, great artery constriction resulted in increased transmural pressure and atrial stretch in association with elevated plasma ANP concentrations. This mechanism explains ANP release evoked by a variety of maneuvers and conditions associated with central volume overload.[9] The cellular mechanism underlying stretch-mediated ANP release is dependent on increases in cytosolic calcium with activation of the phosphoinositide pathway.[10] Release of BNP involves similar mechanisms. However, increases in circulating BNP occur hours or days after increases in cardiac filling pressures, suggesting that BNP may serve as a complementary natriuretic peptide that is recruited only if increases in cardiac filling are sustained.

Two receptors have been identified that interact with ANP and BNP[11] (Figure 10-1). A biologically active receptor termed the NPR-A receptor is linked to the activation of particulate guanylyl cyclase. Binding of ANP and BNP to this receptor results in increases in guanosine 3′,5′-cyclic monophosphate (cGMP), which leads to the biologic actions of the natriuretic peptides. The most abundant receptor for ANP and BNP, however, is a biologically silent clearance receptor termed the NPR-C receptor, which functions to bind and clear ANP and BNP from the circulation.[12] After binding, receptor-mediated endocytosis occurs with intracellular degradation. Additionally, the natriuretic peptides are degraded by a membrane ectoenzyme neutral endopeptidase. This enzyme is also co-localized and widely distributed with angiotensin-converting enzyme (ACE). Although natriuretic peptides function via the second messenger cGMP, evidence supports an additional mechanism of action, which is activation of potas-

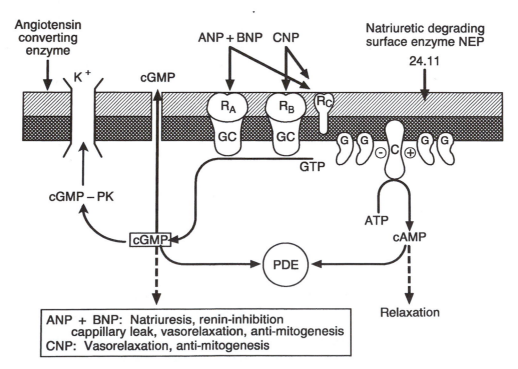

Fig. 10-1. Natriuretic peptide receptor organization and signal transduction mechanisms for atrial (ANP), brain (BNP), and endothelial cell (CNP) natriuretic peptides with localization of neutral endopeptidase (NEP) and angiotensin-converting enzyme (ACE) at the cell surface.

Table 10-1. Mechanisms of ANP and BNP Natriuresis: Renal Sites and Actions

Site	Action
Glomerulus	Increases glomerular filtration rate via increases in glomerular hydrostatic pressure and in Kf
Proximal tubule and inner medullary collecting duct	Decreases tubular reabsorption of sodium
Vasa recta	Increases vasa recta blood flow
Juxtaglomerular cell	Decreases renin release

Abbreviation: Kf, glomerular capillary ultrafiltration coefficient.

sium channels.[13] Lastly, CNP, which lacks renal action, functions via a separate receptor, NPR-B.

The renal actions and sites of action for ANP and BNP are noted in Table 10-1 and Figure 10-2. ANP and BNP have been demonstrated to enhance the glomerular filtration rate (GFR), decrease proximal

and distal reabsorption, increase medullary blood flow, and inhibit renin release by the kidney. These actions are mediated via the NPR-A receptor and are secondary to cGMP accumulation within the target cell.

Cardiac Endocrine Response to Ventricular Dysfunction: Increased Cardiac Synthesis and Release of ANP and BNP

A hallmark of chronic CHF is elevation of circulating ANP and BNP.[14,15] This elevation is secondary to enhanced cardiac synthesis and release, which are activated by increased cardiac volume and pressure overload. Investigations also support the role of humoral stimulation of natriuretic peptide synthesis and release by other local and circulating humoral factors.[16] During early CHF the increase of circulating ANP is secondary to release of stored ANP and BNP, with enhanced cardiac synthesis maintaining elevated levels with more sustained ventricular failure.[17] In the cardiomyopathic strain of the Syrian hamster, the content of ANP granules within the cardiac atria varies inversely with the circulating

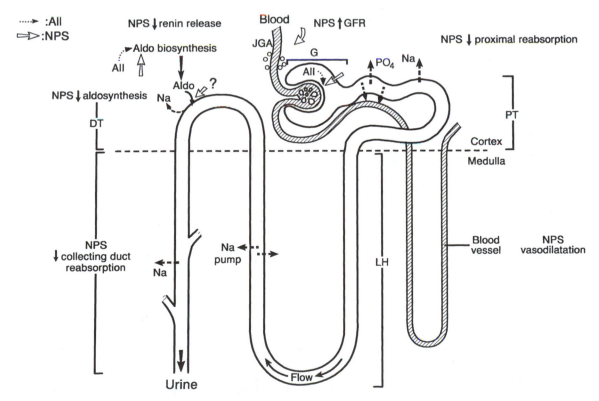

Fig. 10-2. Vascular and tubular sites of actions of the atrial and brain natriuretic peptides (ANP and BNP) and angiotensin II (ANG II). The antagonism of angiotensin II on the natriuretic actions of ANP and BNP are facilitated by similar sites of actions of these hormones.

plasma level of ANP, consistent with increased atrial synthesis and release.[18] It is possible that the synthetic capacity of the atria is overwhelmed relative to the demands of the system, leading to a state of relative deficiency with chronic and severe ventricular dysfunction. Indeed, Redfield et al.[19] demonstrated in dogs with chronic CHF an impaired capacity to release ANP in response to acute volume expansion with increases in atrial pressures. Volpe et al.[20] have also demonstrated impaired release of ANP in humans with dilated cardiomyopathy and mild CHF. Thus a relative deficiency may occur in patients with chronic CHF and produce biologic consequences.

In humans and animals CHF is characterized by the presence of ventricular ANP and BNP.[15,21] Because ventricular ANP and BNP are present in primitive organisms, the occurrence in higher species may represent the reactivation of fetal genes. Proto-oncogenes that regulate the hypertrophic process during cardiomyopathy may also control the recruitment of ventricular ANP and BNP synthesis.[22] It has been shown in cardiomyopathic hamsters that ventricular myocardium becomes the principal source of the natriuretic peptides.[23]

A portion of total immunoreactive ANP in the severe failing human heart is composed of β-ANP, an antiparallel dimer with reduced biologic activity. Wei et al.[24] have reported that this altered biologic form of ANP is also elevated in the circulation of patients with severe CHF. Thus β-ANP exists with overt heart failure and may have biologic significance for this sodium-retaining and vasoconstrictive state. Such a concept is supported by evidence that β-ANP may not effectively bind to the NPR-A receptor, resulting in reduced ability to activate cGMP production.[25]

Based on its elevation in chronic CHF, circulating ANP has emerged as an important diagnostic and prognostic serum marker for CHF. Repeated studies have demonstrated that elevated ANP correlates with the functional class of symptomatic CHF. Gottlieb et al.[26] reported that ANP provides prognostic data on survival, ventricular ectopy, and hemodynamic abnormalities. Davis et al.[27] extended these findings and identified ANP as a specific and sensitive test for predicting CHF in elderly subjects. These investigators reported that ANP could identify patients at risk for CHF, suggesting that its use in the elderly could be utilized for prevention, early detection, and treatment in this population.

We and others have focused on the N-terminus of pro-ANP (N-ANP) which is the nonbiologically active fragment of the pro-hormone and co-released with the biologically active 28-amino-acid C-terminal ANP (C-ANP). N-ANP is cleared more slowly and thus circulates at higher concentrations than the biologically active C-ANP. Moreover, it is more stable in vitro than is C-ANP. We examined its specificity and sensitivity as a diagnostic test for identifying subjects with asymptomatic left ventricular dysfunction (ALVD) as documented prospectively with radionuclide angiography and clinical characterization.[28] These studies demonstrated that N-ANP was elevated consistently in New York Heart Association (NYHA) class I patients with ALVD and was more sensitive and specific than C-terminal ANP, thus emerging as a important noninvasive serum marker for the identification of patients with ALVD. The diagnostic importance of N-ANP was underscored by Hall and coworkers,[29] who reported that N-ANP is the most powerful independent prognostic indicator in patients with ALVD following acute myocardial infarction.

Functional Role of ANP and BNP in the Regulation of Sodium Homeostasis and Inhibition of the Renin-Angiotensin System in CHF

Several well designed therapeutic trials have demonstrated drug efficacy in terms of improving functional capacity and survival in humans with CHF.[30-33] The fact that patients classified as NYHA functional class I or II experienced significant benefit and that drug intervention was not completely effective in halting the progressive worsening process leading to death has shifted interest to the early stages of heart failure. The National Institutes of Health (NIH) sponsored Studies of Left Ventricular Dysfunction (SOLVD) in patients with chronic left ventricular dysfunction but without signs of overt CHF (i.e., ALVD) demonstrated humoral activation, characterized by increases in circulating ANP without activation of the circulating RAS in the absence of diuretic treatment.[34] Based on the known biology of ANP and BNP, this cardiac peptide system may play a key role in preserving the compensated state of ALVD.

Evidence supports an important role for the natriuretic peptide system in ALVD to preserve cardiorenal homeostasis and contribute to the maintenance of sodium balance and inhibit activation of the RAS despite ventricular dysfunction. In a low-ANP model of acute CHF produced by thoracic inferior vena caval constriction characterized by decreased cardiac output without increases in atrial pressures or ANP, marked sodium retention, vasoconstriction, and activation of the RAS resulted. These findings were not observed in a high-ANP model produced by rapid ventricular pacing despite similar reductions in cardiac output and mean arterial pressure.[35] Exogenous administration of ANP in the caval-constricted dogs to mimic circulating concentrations encountered in the high-ANP heart failure model prevented sodium retention, vasoconstriction, and activation of the RAS. Margulies et al.[36] observed with the onset of ventricular dysfunction a significant natriuresis and renal cGMP generation with elevation of plasma ANP. Awazu et al.[37] tested the effect of anti-ANP antibodies in a model of chronic CHF in rats. Bolus injection of ANP neutralizing antibodies resulted in further sodium retention without affecting the systemic blood pressure or GFR. Redfield et al.[38] have reported cardiorenal function in a conscious canine model of ALVD. This model mimics the humoral profile of patients with ALVD reported in SOLVD and was characterized by significant ventricular dysfunction but without sodium retention in association with elevated ANP and no activation of the RAS. In response to acute intravascular volume expansion, normal release of ANP and an intact renal natriuretic response were observed. Stevens et al. established that the transition from experimental ALVD to overt CHF could be accelerated utilizing a natriuretic peptide receptor antagonist, which in ALVD led to premature sodium retention, impaired renal natriuretic response to volume expansion, and activation of the RAS.[39] These investigators concluded that increased ANP and probably BNP are activated with cardiac volume overload during early CHF and contribute to the maintenance of sodium balance and inhibition of the RAS in ALVD. They speculated that therapeutic strategies that potentiate the biologic actions of ANP and BNP may prolong the asymptomatic phase of ventricular dysfunction and delay to progression to overt CHF.

Renal Hyporesponsiveness to ANP and BNP in CHF

Overt CHF is a syndrome characterized by sodium retention and activation of the RAS with elevation of both circulating ANP and BNP. Humans and animal models of chronic CHF are characterized by an attenuated natriuretic response to endogenous and exogenous ANP.[39–41] It has been suggested that the diminished renal response to the hormone plays an important role in the pathophysiology of sodium retention and systemic and renal vasoconstriction observed with overt heart failure. The mechanism(s) responsible for the renal hyporesponsiveness to the cardiac natriuretic peptides in CHF are most likely multifactorial and include decreases in renal perfu-

sion pressure,[42] increases in renal sympathetic nerve activity,[43] receptor down-regulation,[44] and possibly enhanced enzymatic degradation of ANP and BNP.[45] A key role for the RAS in mediating the renal hyporesponsiveness to the natriuretic peptide system appears to be fundamental to CHF.

ANGIOTENSIN II AND CONTROL OF RENAL HEMODYNAMICS AND TUBULAR SODIUM REABSORPTION IN CHF

Angiotensin II and the Kidney in CHF

Many reviews have extensively summarized the biology of the RAS and generation of ANG II with a focus on the kidney.[46] Briefly, in response to a number of stimuli (e.g., decreased renal perfusion pressure, increased renal sympathetic nerve activity, and decreased delivery of sodium to the macula densa) the juxtaglomerular cells of the kidney release renin. Renin is an enzyme that then, within the kidney or at extrarenal sites, cleaves angiotensinogen to ANG I. Angiotensin-converting enzyme (ACE), which is widely expressed, converts ANG I to ANG II. Repeated investigations have established multiple actions of ANG II (Table 10-2, Fig. 10-2) that are mediated after binding of ANG II to specific receptor subtypes.

The importance of the RAS in the evolution of CHF and the effects of blocking the formation of ANG II were highlighted by the classic experiment of Watkins and coworkers.[47] After heart failure induced by thoracic inferior vena cava constriction, the plasma renin activity and aldosterone concentrations were markedly elevated during the initial stages of impaired cardiac output. During this period, the initial sudden decrease in arterial blood pressure was restored to baseline, whereas sodium excretion decreased to less than 5 mEq per day and plasma volume increased by 50 percent. The response of this intense sodium and water retention to maintain arterial blood pressure was marked ascites and peripheral edema. Preventing the formation of ANG II with an ACE inhibitor from the onset of caval constriction resulted in a greater degree of hypotension but less sodium retention and no ascites or edema. This study provided some of the first evidence for the role of ANG II in maintaining blood pressure and decreasing sodium excretion during the initial stages of heart failure. It also demonstrated that preventing the formation of this peptide may have significant beneficial effects, particularly in terms of edema formation. A similar pattern of activation of the RAS also has been found in humans with CHF, with the plasma renin activity, ANG II, and aldosterone levels increasing during acute or decompensated chronic heart failure and decreasing to normal with stabilization of cardiac function.

Angiotensin II and Glomerular Hemodynamics in CHF

The renal adaptations that accompany heart failure can occur with relatively minor impairment in cardiac function and include alterations in glomerular hemodynamics mediated by the action of ANG II (Fig. 10-3, Table 10-2). In an animal model of experimental heart failure induced by myocardial infarction, Hostetter et al. found that rats with small to moderate-sized infarcts (24 percent) and baseline arterial and ventricular pressures no different from controls had an impaired ability to excrete a sodium load despite only mild reductions in renal hemodynamics.[48] This impairment in sodium excretion was even greater with large infarctions (50 percent), where the GFR and renal plasma flow (RPF) were

Table 10-2. Renal Vascular Actions of Angiotensin II

Effect	Result
Afferent arteriolar vasoconstriction	Decreases glomerular hydrostatic pressure
Efferent arteriolar vasoconstriction	Increases glomerular hydrostatic pressure
Mesangial cell contraction	Decreases Kf and glomerular filtration rate
Vasa recta vasoconstriction	Decreases papillary plasma flow

Abbreviation: Kf, glomerular capillary ultrafiltration coefficient.

decreased to a much greater extent and renal vascular resistance was significantly increased. Similar results have been reported in humans with mild heart failure in response to both an acute intravenous saline load and increased oral sodium intake. Thus the propensity for sodium retention can begin early during heart failure even when there is only mild impairment in cardiac function.

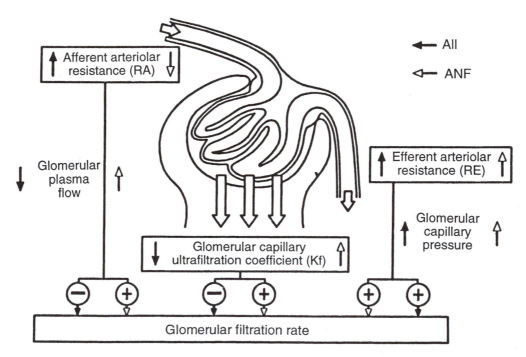

Fig. 10-3. Effector sites of angiotensin II and atrial natriuretic factor (ANF) within the glomerular microcirculation. The constriction of angiotensin II raises afferent (RA) and efferent (RE) arteriolar resistance and reduces the glomerular capillary ultrafiltration coefficient Kf. An increase in RA and a reduction in Kf tend to reduce the glomerular filtration rate (GFR), whereas an increase in RE, in some circumstances, serves to increase the GFR. ANF has opposite effects, which serve to enhance the GFR and are largely opposed by angiotensin II.

Intrarenal hemodynamics and the role of ANG II in this model of heart failure was more extensively evaluated by Ichikawa and Harris.[49] Despite only a small reduction in total kidney GFR, single nephron GFR (SNGFR) was significantly decreased along with a much greater reduction in glomerular capillary plasma flow rate. This greater decrease in glomerular capillary plasma flow rate than SNGFR led to a significant increase in single nephron filtration fraction (SNFF), glomerular capillary hydraulic pressure, and mean transcapillary hydraulic pressure difference. These changes were the consequence of profound constriction of the efferent arterioles. In addition to plasma flow and transcapillary hydraulic pressure another determinant of SNGFR is the ultrafiltration coefficient (Kf), a product of the permeability of the glomerular basement membrane and the glomerular capillary endothelial surface area. Again in an animal model of heart failure, Kf was uniformly lower in the experimental than the control group and thus contributed to the decrease in SNGFR. ACE inhibition resulted in a return to or toward control levels in all of these renal microvascular indices and an increase in SNGFR, suggesting ANG II as the predominant mediator of these changes. Although ANG II can also cause vasoconstriction of the afferent arteriole and thus decrease glomerular capillary plasma flow, hydraulic pressure, and GFR, there was only a mild, nonsignificant increase in this parameter in this model of heart failure. Thus ANG II modulates GFR by contracting vascular smooth muscle cells of both the afferent and efferent arteriole, modifying the filtration fraction, and contracting mesangial cells of the glomerulus modifying Kf. The overall effect of ANG II on GFR depends on the balance of these three factors, which certainly changes as mild heart failure evolves into severe failure. Even with severe congestive heart failure, chronic ACE inhibition, at doses that avoid excessive reductions in renal perfusion pressure, may improve renal hemodynamics to enhance sodium excretion.

Angiotensin II and Tubular Sodium Reabsorption in CHF

In addition to its actions on renal hemodynamics, ANG II may cause sodium and water retention by direct actions on tubular sodium reabsorption (Table 10-3). In the proximal tubule, the phenomenon of glomerulotubular balance dictates that changes in GFR are accompanied by proportional changes in the rate of fluid reabsorption by the proximal tubule. Thus the rate of fluid delivery to the proximal tubule is thought to affect the rate of fluid absorbed across the proximal tubule epithelial cells. The ability to increase fluid reabsorption occurs primarily by two mechanisms. One is through an increase in the Na^+/H^+ antiporter on the luminal aspect of proximal tubule epithelial cells, which appears to be regulated by the amount of filtered bicarbonate present in tubular fluid. The presence of large amounts of bicarbonate due to an increase in GFR enhances H^+ secretion in exchange for Na^+ reabsorption. The other mechanism is through changes in peritubular capillary Starling forces. Changes in GFR and RPF result in changes in the filtration fraction. An increase in the filtration fraction increases the glomerular ultrafiltrate and decreases the amount of plasma that eventually enters the peritubular capillaries. Because little protein is filtered at the glomerulus, this action increases the peritubular capillary oncotic pressure and favors reabsorption of fluid from the proximal tubule.

Angiotensin II has effects on both of these mechanisms independent of the GFR and RPF and thus has the unique ability to disrupt glomerulotubular balance. Fractional proximal sodium reabsorption is enhanced by ANG II through activation of the Na^+/H^+ antiporter, probably by inhibiting intracellular cyclic

Table 10-3. Renal Tubular Actions of Angiotensin II

Site	Effect	Result
Proximal tubule	Activation of Na^+/H^+ antiporter on luminal aspect of cell Increased peritubular oncotic pressure by increasing filtration fraction	Enhanced sodium and water reabsorption
Loop of Henle	Vasoconstriction of vasa recta	Increased medullary hypertonicity and increased sodium reabsorption
Collecting ducts	Increased production of aldosterone by adrenal gland	Increased sodium reabsorption

adenylate cyclase activity and by raising peritubular capillary oncotic pressure via increasing the filtration fraction through efferent arteriole vasoconstriction. The role of ANG II in tubular function in the presence of heart failure was reported by Ichikawa et al.[50] Despite decreases in SNGFR and glomerular plasma flow, fractional proximal sodium reabsorption was increased in an animal model of heart failure, suggesting disruption of the normal glomerulotubular balance. It occurred through an increase in filtration fraction and subsequently a rise in peritubular capillary oncotic pressure. Treatment with an ACE inhibitor resulted in a significant decrease in filtration fraction and peritubular oncotic pressure as well as a decrease in fractional proximal sodium reabsorption, again implicating ANG II as the mediator of these important changes.

A direct effect of ANG II on other nephron segments has been studied less extensively. Receptors for ANG II have been found in every nephron segment, but the highest concentrations are found in the proximal tubule, consistent with this nephron segment being the major tubular site of action.[51] ANG II, however, can regulate sodium reabsorption in other nephron segments (Table 10-3). One mechanism is through changes in the medullary circulation via alterations in papillary plasma flow (PPF).[52] By decreasing the PPF, ANG II may increase sodium reabsorption in the long loops of Henle via changes in Starling forces and medullary tonicity. In the thoracic inferior vena cava constriction model of congestive failure (which is characterized by marked activation of the RAS) the GFR, renal blood flow, and intracortical blood flow distribution are similar to that in normal controls. However, PPF is markedly reduced and papillary tissue solute content is increased both during hydropenia and after acute saline loading, resulting in an inability to excrete a sodium load due to increased sodium and water reabsorption in the loops of Henle.

The actions of ANG II to maintain the GFR, increase the filtration fraction, and thus increase the filtered sodium load seem paradoxical in relation to its other action of increasing sodium and water reabsorption. This paradox may reflect the unique ability of this hormone to maintain renal excretion of nitrogenous wastes, on one hand, while contributing to the maintenance of systemic hemodynamics through sodium and water retention on the other.

Angiotensin II and Interactions with Cardiac Natriuretic Peptides in CHF

Another way RAS may modulate renal function during heart failure is through antagonizing the action other hormones, specifically ANP and BNP. As can be seen in Figures 10-2 and 10-3, the cardiac natriuretic peptides and ANG II have renal actions at the same vascular and tubular sites within the kidney. The attenuated natriuretic effect of ANP that characterized CHF in both humans and experimental animal models has been implicated as an important factor in the pathogenesis of the sodium retention and edema formation seen with CHF.[40,41] Studies in both normal animals and experimental models of heart failure have provided convincing evidence that the attenuated response to ANP is mediated in part by an activated RAS. These studies support the concept that ANG II modulates the renal effects of ANP at the level of both the glomerulus and the level of the renal tubule, preventing the full natriuretic activity of this peptide. This concept provides yet another mechanism for the sodium retention and edema formation of CHF.

Several studies further support the concept that increased ANG II plays a key role in mediating the blunted renal response to the natriuretic peptides during overt CHF. The natriuretic response to exogenous ANP in salt-retaining rats with a chronic arteriovenous fistula could be restored with chronic treatment using the ACE inhibitor enalapril.[53] This response occurred despite a decrease in mean arterial blood pressure and was unrelated to changes in endogenous levels of ANP. The mechanism of this enhancement secondary to decreased generation of ANG II probably includes reductions in renal vascular resistance and decrements in cGMP phosphodiesterase. Indeed, the opposing action of ANG II on ANP is importantly supported by the work of Showalter et al.,[54] who observed a blunting of the natriuretic effect to systematically administered ANP when ANG II was infused via the renal artery at a dose without systemic effects, indicating that at normal renal perfusion pressure intrarenal ANG II can antagonize the natriuretic response to ANP.

Results from our laboratory indicate that sodium retention during the evolution of CHF occurs in association with a loss of the previously enhanced renal generation of cGMP and occurs with activation of the RAS.[36] Smith and Lincoln[55] observed in cultured vascular smooth muscle cells that angiotensin II decreased ANP-stimulated intracellular cGMP accumulation by stimulating cGMP hydrolysis. This augmented hydrolysis of cGMP appeared to be mediated via a Ca^{2+}-activated cGMP phosphodiesterase. Studies have demonstrated that cGMP phosphodiesterase inhibition markedly potentiates the effect of acute volume expansion and low dose ANP infusion on urinary sodium and cGMP excretion, an effect that was attenuated by administration of a monoclonal antibody directed against ANP.[56,57] These studies support an important role of renal cGMP phosphodiesterase modulation in the biologic response to endogenous and exogenous ANP and a key role for ANG II in this alteration.

As previously mentioned, moderate heart failure in the thoracic inferior vena cava constriction model is characterized initially by elevated renin (and hence ANG II), which return to normal in the compensated state. Similar observations have been seen in other models of heart failure, including myocardial infarction-induced heart failure.[58] In this model there is an inability to excrete sodium and water after a volume load, despite normal circulating renin. Furthermore, low dose intrarenal infusions of an ACE inhibitor or an ANG II receptor antagonist can improve the GFR and sodium excretion.[53]

To help explain this phenomenon, the concept of a local intrarenal RAS, independent from the circulating system, has emerged. All components of the RAS have been identified in the kidney.[59] In addition, proximal tubular fluid contains ANG II concentrations 1000-fold higher than plasma concentrations, suggesting local synthesis of ANG II. In animals with stable, compensated heart failure and normal levels of circulating angiotensinogen, ANG II, and plasma renin concentrations, renal angiotensinogen mRNA levels are increased 47 percent and renal ANG II levels twofold compared to sham control rats, suggesting local activation of this system. Chronic treatment with enalapril results in marked attenuation of renal angiotensinogen mRNA. These and other studies certainly suggest that the intrarenal RAS may play an important role in the regulation of renal function during heart failure.

Therapeutic Potentiation of ANP and BNP for Treatment of CHF

Since the discovery of ANP and subsequently BNP, strategies have emerged to utilize these peptides for treatment of disorders of cardiorenal function such as CHF. Therapeutic strategies have included infusion of the peptide and potentiation of its actions by inhibitors of cGMP phosphodiesterases. Therapeutic approaches have focused on inhibition of the enzyme that degrades the natriuretic peptide neutral endopeptidase 24.11, which is co-localized with ACE (Fig. 10-2).

Two pathways exist for ANP and BNP metabolism: enzymatic clearance via the ectoenzyme neutral endopeptidase 24.11 (NEP) and receptor clearance via the clearance receptor. NEP is a well characterized ectoenzyme that is present in numerous tissues including kidney, lung, brain, and endothelial cells.[60]

Repeated studies have demonstrated that ANP and BNP are substrates for NEP. Kenny and Stephenson,[61] in part based on the high concentration of NEP in renal brush border membranes, suggested that renal tubular NEP serves a physiologic function: It rapidly and efficiently degrades filtered ANP to prevent biologically intact peptide from reaching the terminal nephron, which is a major site of action. Evidence also suggests that NEP activity may be regulated. Such a phenomenon may be relevant to disease states in which ANP and BNP may be elevated, such as CHF, and increased NEP could attenuate the full biologic actions of elevated endogenous natriuretic peptides.

With acute experimental CHF, we found a parallel increase of urinary cGMP excretion and urinary sodium excretion after NEP inhibition together with an increase in urinary ANP, suggesting that delivery of ANP to the terminal nephron indeed may activate cGMP and contribute to a natriuretic response.[57,62] This finding supports the conclusion that NEP may limit the full natriuretic action of elevated endogenous ANP in CHF. Such observations are also supported by studies demonstrating a luminal action of ANP in the inner medullary collecting duct to inhibit sodium transport.[63]

With chronic experimental CHF, NEP inhibition produces a decrease in atrial pressures and an initial maintenance of cardiac output. NEP inhibition potentiated the natriuretic action of endogenous ANP by a mechanism independent of systemic or renal hemodynamics.[45] More striking, this natriuretic action occurred in a model of severe CHF that was resistant to the natriuretic action of exogenous ANP, underscoring the potential efficacy of this form of therapy. The observed biologic responses in these studies of acute and chronic experimental CHF were also greater than that predicted from any increase in circulating ANP, indicating local tissue potentiation of ANP. The unique natriuretic action of NEP inhibition may also be associated with cardiovascular and humoral effects. Elsner and coworkers[64] reported that chronic NEP inhibition in humans with chronic CHF resulted in favorable hemodynamic responses together with suppression of vasoconstrictor humoral systems.

We already discussed the antagonism of ANP and BNP by ANG II. Such an antagonism is observed in severe CHF to limit the full natriuretic action of NEP inhibition. Chronic angiotensin antagonism with ACE inhibition potentiated renal hemodynamic and excretory responses to NEP inhibition, an effect that was abolished by intrarenal infusion of low dose ANG II.[65] These results support the concept that co-inhibition of NEP and ACE may emerge as a unique form of therapy for CHF. Indeed, based on knowledge of the delay in onset of symptoms with ACE inhibition in ALVD, one could speculate that co-inhibition of these ectoenzyme systems may indeed emerge as the optimal therapy for delaying the onset of overt CHF.

CONCLUSION

The syndrome of CHF is characterized by activation of many neurohumoral systems. Of major importance is the RAS, which modulates renal function by decreasing SNGFR and glomerular plasma flow; increasing efferent arteriole resistance, filtration fraction, and tubular sodium reabsorption; and attenuating the effects of other hormones, such as ANP and BNP.[66] Acutely, the RAS is necessary to help maintain blood pressure and systemic hemodynamics, but chronically the continued antinatriuretic action eventually leads to profound edema formation. Even with compensated heart failure, when the circulating RAS is not activated a local renal RAS may continue to regulate renal function. ACE inhibition and ANG II receptor antagonists may effectively prevent the renal actions of ANG II, which may be an important reason this therapy improves survival in patients with heart failure.

The natriuretic peptides ANP and BNP emerge as a humoral mechanism that delays the progression of CHF in part by its renal actions to enhance GFR, decrease tubular sodium reabsorption, and inhibit renin release.[5] Pharmacologic potentiation of this system via inhibition of its degradation by NEP inhibition may complement ACE inhibition in the treatment of CHF. Clearly, the kidney plays a key role in CHF, a role modulated by these counterregulatory hormones.

REFERENCES

1. Kisch B: Electron microscopy of the atrium of the heart. I. Guinea pig. Exp Med Surg 1956;14:99–112
2. De Bold AJ: Heart atria granularity effects of changes in water-electrolyte balance. Proc Soc Exp Biol Med 1979;161:508–511
3. Bloch KD, Zisfein JB, Margolies MN et al: A serum protease cleaves proANF into 14-kilodalton peptide and ANF. Am J Physiol 1987;252:E147–E151
4. De Bold AJ, Borenstein HB, Veress AT, Sonnenberg H: A rapid and potent natriuretic response to intravenous injection of atrial myocardial extract in rats. Life Sci 1981;28:89–94
5. Burnett JC Jr, Granger JP, Opgenorth TJ: Effects of synthetic atrial natriuretic factor on renal function and renin release. Am J Physiol 1984;247:F863–F866
6. Matsuo H, Nakazato H: Molecular biology of atrial na-
triuretic peptides. Endocrinol Metab Clin North Am 1987;16:43–61
7. Itoh H, Pratt RE, Dzau VJ: Interaction of atrial natriuretic polypeptide and angiotensin II on protooncogene expression and vascular cell growth. Biochem Biophys Res Commun 1991;176:1601–1609
8. Edwards BS, Zimmerman RS, Schwab TR, Heublein DM, Burnett JC Jr: Atrial stretch, not pressure, is the principal determinant controlling the acute release of atrial natriuretic factor. Circ Res 1988;62:191–195
9. Schwab TR, Edwards BS, Heublein DM, Burnett JC Jr: Role of atrial natriuretic peptide in volume-expansion natriuresis. Am J Physiol 1986;251:R310–R313
10. Sonnenberg H. Mechanisms of release and renal tubular action of atrial natriuretic factor. Fed Proc 1986; 45:2106–2110
11. Koller KJ, Lowe DG, Bennett GL et al: Selective activation of the B natriuretic peptide receptor by C-type natriuretic peptide (CNP). Science 1991;252:120–123
12. Almeida FA, Suszuki M, Scarborough RM, Lewicki JA, Maack T: Clearance function of type C receptors of atrial natriuretic factor in rats. Am J Physiol 1989; 256:R469–R475
13. Wei C, Hu S, Miller V, Burnett JC Jr: Vascular actions of C-type natriuretic peptide in isolated porcine arteries and coronary vascular smooth muscle cells. Biochem Biophys Res Commun 1994;205:765–771
14. Burnett JC Jr, Kao PC, Hu DC et al: Atrial natriuretic peptide elevation in congestive heart failure in the human. Science 1986;231:1145–1147
15. Mukoyama M, Nakao K, Hosoda K et al: Brain natriuretic peptide as a novel cardiac hormone in humans. Evidence for an exquisite dual natriuretic peptide system, atrial natriuretic peptide and brain natriuretic peptide. J Clin Invest 1991;87:1402–1412
16. Schiebinger RJ, Greening KM: Interaction between stretch and hormonally stimulated atrial natriuretic peptide secretion. Am J Physiol 1992;262:H78–H83
17. Perrella MA, Schwab TR, O'Murchau B et al: Cardiac atrial natriuretic factor during evolution of congestive heart failure. Am J Physiol 1992;262:H1248–H1255
18. Edwards BS, Ackermann DM, Schwab TR et al: The relationship between atrial granularity and circulating atrial natriuretic peptide in hamsters with congestive heart failure. Mayo Clin Proc 1986;61:517–521
19. Redfield MM, Edwards BS, McGoon MD et al: Failure of atrial natriuretic factor to increase with volume expansion in acute and chronic congestive heart failure in the dog. Circulation 1989;80:651–657
20. Volpe M, Tritto C, De Luca N et al: Failure of atrial natriuretic factor to increase with saline load in patients with dilated cardiomyopathy and mild heart failure. J Clin Invest 1991;88:1481–1489
21. Edwards BS, Ackermann DM, Lee MU et al: Identification of atrial natriuretic factor within ventricular tissue in hamsters and humans with congestive heart failure. J Clin Invest 1988;81:82–86
22. Izumo S, Nakal-Ginard B, Mahdavi V: Protooncogene induction and reprogramming of cardiac gene expression produced by pressure overload. Proc Natl Acad Sci USA 1988;85:339–343
23. Thibault G, Nemer M, Drouin J et al: Ventricles as a major site of atrial natriuretic factor synthesis and release in cardiomyopathic hamsters with heart failure. Circ Res 1989;65:71–82
24. Wei CM, Kao PC, Lin JT et al: Circulating β-atrial

natriuretic factor in congestive heart failure in humans. Circulation 1993;88:1016–1020

25. Kambayashi Y, Nakajimia S, Ueda M, Inouye K: A dicarba analog of beta-atrial peptide inhibits cGMP induced by ANP in cultured rat vascular smooth muscle cells. FEBS Lett 1989;248:23–38

26. Gottlieb SS, Kukin ML, Ahern D, Packer M: Prognostic importance of atrial natriuretic peptide in patients with chronic heart failure. J Am Coll Cardiol 1989;13:1534–1539

27. Davis KM, Fish LC, Elahi D, Clark BA, Minaker KL: Atrial natriuretic peptide levels in the prediction of congestive heart failure risk in frail elderly. JAMA 1992;267:2625–2629

28. Lerman A, Gibbons RJ, Rodeheffer RJ et al: Circulating N-terminal atrial natriuretic peptide as a marker for symptomless left-ventricular dysfunction. Lancet 1993;341:1105–1109

29. Hall C, Rouleau JL, Klein M et al: N-terminal proatrial natriuretic factor (PRO-ANF)—a uniquely powerful predictor of long term outcome after myocardial infarction [abstract]. J Am Coll Cardiol 1993;21:270A

30. Cohn JN, Archibald DG, Ziesche S et al: Effect of vasodilator therapy on mortality in chronic congestive heart failure. Results of a Veterans Administration Cooperative Study. N Engl J Med 1986;314:1547–1552

31. Cohn JN, Johnson G, Ziesche S et al: A comparison of enalapril with hydralazine-isosorbide dinitrate in the treatment of chronic congestive heart failure. N Engl J Med 1991;325:303–310

32. CONSENSUS Trial Study Group: Effects of enalapril on mortality in severe congestive heart failure. Results of the Cooperative North Scandinavian Enalapril Survival Study (CONSENSUS). N Engl J Med 1987;316:1429–1435

33. SOLVD Investigators: Effect of enalapril on survival in patients with reduced left ventricular ejection fractions and congestive heart failure. N Engl J Med 1991;325:293–302

34. Francis GS, Benedict C, Johnstone DE et al: Comparison of neuroendocrine activation in patients with left ventricular dysfunction with and without congestive heart failure. A substudy of the Studies of Left Ventricular Dysfunction (SOLVD). Circulation 1990;82:1724–1729

35. Lee ME, Miller WL, Edwards BS, Burnett JC Jr: Role of endogenous atrial natriuretic factor in acute congestive heart failure. J Clin Invest 1989;84:1962–1966

36. Margulies KB, Heublein DM, Perrella MA, Burnett JC Jr: ANF-mediated renal cGMP generation in congestive heart failure. Am J Physiol 1991;260:F562–F568

37. Awazu M, Imada T, Kon V, Inagami T, Ichikawa I: Role of endogenous atrial natriuretic peptide in congestive heart failure. Am J Physiol 1989;257:R641–R646

38. Redfield MM, Aarhus LL, Wright RS, Burnett JC Jr: Cardiorenal and neurohumoral function in a canine model of early left ventricular dysfunction. Circulation 1993;87:2016–2022

39. Stevens TL, Burnett JC Jr, Kinoshita M, Matsuda Y, Redfield MM: A functional role of endogenous atrial natriuretic peptide in a canine model of early left ventricular dysfunction. J Clin Invest 1995;95:1101–1108

40. Scriven TA, Burnett JC Jr: Effects of synthetic atrial natriuretic peptide on renal function and renin release in acute experimental heart failure. Circulation 1985;72:892–897

41. Cody RJ, Atlas SA, Laragh JH et al: Atrial natriuretic factor in normal subjects and heart failure patients. Plasma levels and renal, hormonal, and hemodynamic responses to peptide infusion. J Clin Invest 1986;78:1362–1374

42. Redfield MM, Edwards BS, Heublein DM, Burnett JC Jr: Restoration of renal response to atrial natriuretic factor in experimental low-output heart failure. Am J Physiol 1989;257:R917–R923

43. Morgan DA, Pueler JD, Koepke JP, Mark AL, DiBona GF: Renal sympathetic nerves attenuate the natriuretic effects of atrial peptide. J Lab Clin Med 1989;114:538–544

44. Schiffrin EL: Decreased density of binding sites for atrial natriuretic peptide on platelets of patients with severe congestive heart failure. Clin Sci 1988;74:213–218

45. Cavero PG, Margulies KB, Winaver J et al: Cardiorenal actions of neutral endopeptidase inhibition in experimental congestive heart failure. Circulation 1990;82:196–201

46. Hall JE: Control of sodium excretion by angiotensin II. Intrarenal mechanisms and blood pressure regulation. Am J Physiol 1986;250:R960–R972

47. Watkins L, Burton JA, Haber E et al: The renin-angiotensin-aldosterone system in congestive failure in conscious dogs. J Clin Invest 1976;57:1606–1617

48. Hostetter TH, Pfeffer JM, Pfeffer MA et al: Cardiorenal hemodynamics and sodium excretion in rats with myocardial infarction. Am J Physiol 1983;245:H98–H103

49. Ichikawa I, Harris RC: Angiotensin actions in the kidney. Renewed insight into the old hormone. Kidney Int 1991;40:583–596

50. Ichikawa I, Pfeffer JM, Pfeffer MA, Hostetter TH, Brenner BM: Role of angiotensin II in the altered renal function of congestive heart failure. Circ Res 1984;55:669–675

51. Ichikawa I, Harris RC: Renal actions of angiotensin revisited. Kidney Int 1991;40:583–596

52. Chou S, Faubert PF, Porush JG: Contribution of angiotensin to the control of medullary hemodynamics. Fed Proc 1986;45:1338–1443

53. Abassi Z, Haramati A, Hoffman A, Burnett JC Jr, Winaver J: Effect of converting-enzyme inhibition on renal response to ANF in rats with experimental heart failure. Am J Physiol 1990;259:R84–R89

54. Showalter CJ, Zimmerman RS, Schwab TR et al: Renal response to atrial natriuretic factor is modulated by intrarenal angiotensin II. Am J Physiol 1988;254:R453–R456

55. Smith JB, Lincoln TM: Angiotensin decreases cyclic GMP accumulation produced by atrial natriuretic factor. Am J Physiol 1987;253:C147–C150

56. Wilkins MR, Settle SL, Needleman P: Augmentation of the natriuretic activity of exogenous and endogenous atriopeptin in rats by inhibition of guanosine 3′,5′-cyclic monophosphate degradation. J Clin Invest 1990;85:1274–1279

57. Margulies KB, Burnett JC Jr: Inhibition of cyclic GMP phosphodiesterases augments renal responses to atrial natriuretic factor in congestive heart failure. J Card Failure 1994;1:71–80

58. Wilkins MR, Settle SL, Stockmann PT, Needleman P:

Maximizing the natriuretic effect of endogenous atriopeptin in a rat model of heart failure. Proc Natl Acad Sci USA 1990;87:6465–6469

59. Schunkert H, Ingelfinger JR, Hirsch AT et al: Evidence for tissue specific activation of renal angiotensinogen mRNA expression in chronic experimental heart failure. J Clin Invest 1992;90:1523–1529

60. Margulies KB, Burnett JC Jr: Neutral endopeptidase 24.11. A modulator of natriuretic peptides. Semin Nephrol 1993;13:71–77

61. Kenny AJ, Stephenson SL: Role of endopeptidase-24.11 in the inactivation of atrial natriuretic peptide. FEBS Lett 1988;232:1–8

62. Perrella MA, Schwab TR, O'Murchu B et al: Cardiac atrial natriuretic factor during the evolution of congestive heart failure. Am J Physiol 1992;262:H1248–H1255

63. Sonnenberg H, Honrath U, Wilson DR: In vivo microperfusion of inner medullary collecting ducts in rats. Effect of amiloride and ANF. Am J Physiol 1990;259:F222–F226

64. Elsner D, Muntze A, Kromer EP, Riegger GAJ: Effectiveness of endopeptidase inhibition (candoxatril) in congestive heart failure. Am J Cardiol 1992;70:494–498

65. Margulies KB, Perrella MA, McKinley LJ, Burnett JC Jr: Angiotensin inhibition potentiates the renal responses to neutral endopeptidase inhibition in dogs with congestive heart failure. J Clin Invest 1991;88:1636–1642

66. Mattingly MT, Burnett JC Jr: Angiotensin II as a modulator of renal function in cardiovascular disease. Choices Cardiol 1995;9:10–13

11 Pathogenesis of Salt and Water Retention in the Congestive Heart Failure Syndrome

Inder S. Anand

During the natural history of chronic heart disease, many patients accumulate fluid, develop edema, and occasionally develop anasarca, a syndrome referred to as congestive heart failure (CHF). The study of mechanisms of fluid retention in this syndrome has a checkered history dating back to the early nineteenth century. A succession of complicated theories attempted to explain why patients with heart disease develop edema. Historical concepts such as backward failure[1] and a number of theories of forward failure[2,3] have been summarized by Harris is an excellent review[4] and are not discussed here. The fundamental features of edema formation have, however, been known for many years and were discovered by simple observations. At the turn of the century, Starling[2] was probably aware that blood volume was increased in patients with edema, and measurements made by Wollheim[5] in 1931 confirmed that he was correct. Then, more than a half-century ago, Starr et al.[6,7] showed that edema could not occur unless the venous pressure was elevated, and Warren and Stead[8] made the simple observation that during the early stages of CHF an increase in weight precedes a rise in venous pressure. A few years later Merrill[9,10] found that weight gain in these patients was a result of salt and water retention by the kidney due to decreased renal blood flow. Thus for more than 50 years we have known that edema in the syndrome of CHF depends on retention of salt and water by the kidney. What causes the kidney to start to retain fluid has, however, remained less clear.

In normal subjects, extracellular volume (ECV) and its intravascular (plasma volume) and extravas-cular (interstitial space) compartments remain remarkably constant despite alterations in dietary sodium and water intake.[11,12] Sodium is largely confined to the extracellular space and comprises more than 90 percent of the total solute of the extracellular fluid. It therefore largely determines the oncotic pressure of the extracellular fluid. Control of the ECV is thus dependent on the regulation of sodium balance. Because sodium is primarily excreted by the kidneys, regulation of sodium balance is determined by sodium intake and its excretion by the kidney. If the ECV is increased in normal subjects, kidneys excrete extra salt and water, returning the ECV to normal. In CHF with edema, avid retention of sodium and water by the kidney persists despite expansion of the ECV and increases in total body water and total body sodium.

The mechanisms responsible for this continued retention of salt and water by the kidney have been the subject of intense study. In patients with CHF the kidneys are intrinsically normal, and when transplanted to a normal environment they function normally. Therefore the renal efferent mechanisms that operate to conserve sodium and water must remain abnormally active in CHF patients despite overt expansion of the ECV. The afferents that signal the kidney to retain salt and water have been vigorously debated. A decrease in blood volume and cardiac output were initially considered to trigger fluid retention. However, blood volume, as discussed above, is increased, not decreased, with CHF. Although cardiac output is low in most patients with CHF, there is a distinct group with edema whose cardiac output is either normal or increased. Causes of "high output failure" include severe anemia, chronic cor pulmonale, thyrotoxicosis, chronic arteriovenous (AV) fistula, Paget's disease, and beri-beri. Any explanation of the mechanisms of salt and water retention by the kidneys in the presence of CHF must take these conditions into account.

During the late 1940s and early 1950s Peters[13,14] developed the concept that in patients with CHF there is "under-filling of the arterial tree," and that this condition modulated renal retention of sodium and water. Because blood volume is increased with CHF, Peters proposed a hypothetical effective blood volume as a measure of fullness of the arterial compartment. He believed that the effective blood volume was reduced even though total blood volume and the volume of the venous compartment were increased. More recently, Schrier[15] popularized this idea as a unifying hypothesis to explain salt and water retention in CHF, cirrhosis, certain forms of nephrotic syndrome, and pregnancy. Unfortunately, effective blood volume is a poorly defined entity because there are no known mechanisms by which the body can directly monitor its adequacy, and it cannot be measured. Until we can measure effective blood volume, this concept must remain hypothetic.

In this chapter, some data on the determinants of salt and water retention in a number of syndromes of low and high cardiac output states are reviewed,[16–20] and our current understanding of the sensor and effector mechanisms involved in the CHF syndrome are discussed. It becomes apparent that salt and water retention in the CHF syndrome is a long-term consequence of the body's attempt to maintain normal arterial blood pressure.

LOW OUTPUT HEART FAILURE

Dilated Cardiomyopathy

Analysis of data on the determinants of salt and water retention in patients with the CHF syndrome provide considerable insight into the altered physiology of edema. However, such data are useful only when obtained from patients who have not been treated because treatment has profound effects on the mechanisms being studied. Unfortunately, few such data are available. Changes in hemodynamics, body fluid compartments, and plasma hormones in a group of patients with severe untreated left ventricular (LV) dysfunction due to ischemic cardiomyopathy[16] are shown in Table 11-1 and Figures 11-1 to 11-3. As might be expected, these patients had resting tachycardia and increased right- and left-sided filling pressures. Despite a severe reduction in cardiac output (50 percent of normal), arterial blood pressure was normal due in part to an increase in systemic vascular resistance. Total body water (TBW) was 16 percent above normal, and the excess

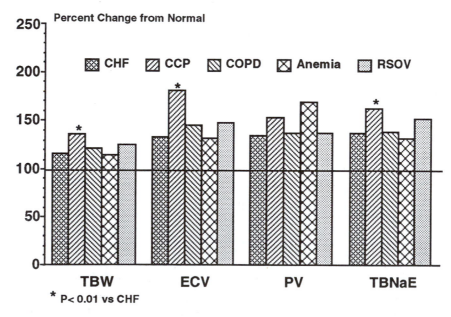

Fig. 11-1. Increase in body fluid compartments in various untreated low and high output states with edema. Data are expressed as a percent of normal. CHF, congestive heart failure due to dilated cardiomyopathy; CCP, chronic constrictive pericarditis; COPD, chronic obstructive pulmonary disease; RSOV, ruptured aneurysm of a sinus of Valsalva; TBW, total body water; ECV, extracellular volume; PV, plasma volume; TBNa$_E$, total body exchangeable sodium. * Significant difference from the valve for dilated cardiomyopathy.

Table 11-1. Average Hemodynamics in Various Syndromes of Low and High Output Congestive Heart Failure

Output state	Heart rate (beats/min)	Mean RAP (mmHg)	Mean PAP (mmHg)	Mean PAW (mmHg)	Mean ABP (mmHg)	Cardiac index (L/min/m^2)	SVR (dynes·s·cm^{-5})
Low output							
Cardiomyopathy[16]	115	15	44	30	99	1.75	2495
Pericarditis[17]	104	23	30	24	91	1.98	1844
High output							
COPD[18]	113	11	41	11	83	3.8	1046
Chronic anemia[19]	89	8	21	13	81	6.1	603
RSOV[20]	110	16	30	24	72	12	220

Abbreviations: RAP, right atrial pressure; PAP, pulmonary arterial pressure; PAW, pulmonary arterial wedge pressure; ABP, arterial blood pressure; SVR, systemic vascular resistance; COPD, chronic obstructive pulmonary disease; RSOV, ruptured aneurysm of a sinus of Valsalva.

fluid was accommodated almost entirely in the extracellular space, which increased by 33 percent (Fig. 11-1). The increase in ECV was accommodated in the extravascular and intravascular compartments in proportion to their normal volumes, so the plasma volume increased by an equal amount (34 percent). Total body exchangeable sodium (TBNa$_E$) was also increased by a similar amount (37 percent). Effective renal plasma flow (ERPF) was severely decreased, amounting to only 30 percent of normal (Fig. 11-2). The reduction in ERPF was substantially greater than the decrease in cardiac output, implying particularly severe renal vasoconstriction. On the other hand, the glomerular filtration rate (GFR) was re-

duced to a lesser extent than renal blood flow, so the filtration fraction (GFR/ERPF ratio) increased. This situation suggests greater efferent than afferent arteriolar vasoconstriction. Plasma norepinephrine was consistently increased and on average was more than six times normal (Fig. 11-3). Plasma renin activity (PRA) and aldosterone levels varied a great deal but, on average, were nine and six times normal, respectively. The plasma atrial natriuretic peptide (ANP) level was elevated in every patient with the average value more than 15 times normal. Although plasma arginine vasopressin (AVP) was normal, the levels were inappropriately high with respect to the hyponatremia (serum Na 133 mmol/L).

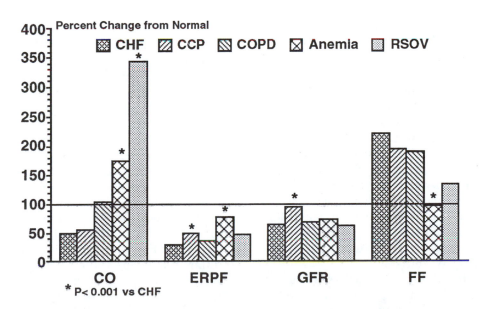

Fig. 11-2. Changes in cardiac output (CO), effective renal plasma flow (ERPF), glomerular filtration rate (GFR), and filtration fraction (FF) in various untreated low and high output states with edema. Data are expressed as a percent of normal. Abbreviations are as in Figure 11-1. *Significant difference from the valve for CHF.

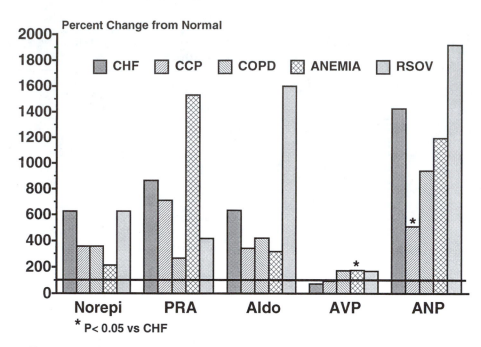

Fig. 11-3. Changes in plasma norepinephrine (Norepi), renin activity (PRA), aldosterone (Aldo), arginine vasopressin (AVP), and atrial natriuretic peptide (ANP) in various untreated low and high output states with edema. Data are expressed as a percent of normal. Abbreviations are as in Figure 11-1. *Significant difference from the valve for CHF.

Chronic Constrictive Pericarditis

Similar compensatory responses are seen with all low output cardiac failure irrespective of whether systolic or diastolic dysfunction is responsible. The classic example of pure diastolic dysfunction with low cardiac output is chronic constrictive pericarditis, where the rigid, often calcified pericardium restricts ventricular filling. The underlying myocardium is usually normal. The compensatory changes of constrictive pericarditis are similar to those seen with dilated cardiomyopathy with some subtle differences.[17] Hemodynamic changes are classic and reflect restricted ventricular filling with equalization of end-diastolic pressures in all cardiac chambers (Table 11-1). Right-sided filling pressures are usually higher and left-sided filling pressures lower than those seen with cardiomyopathy. Here too, despite low cardiac output, arterial pressure is maintained although the systemic vascular resistance does not increase to the same extent as it does with cardiomyopathy. These patients, however, retain more salt and water than do those with cardiomyopathy, resulting in higher TBW and $TBNa_E$ and greater expansion of the extracellular and blood volumes (Fig. 11-1). Therefore blood pressure in patients with constrictive pericarditis is maintained more by expansion of blood volume than by an increase in systemic vascular resistance. Apart from ANP, the neurohormonal response of constrictive pericarditis is similar

to that seen with cardiomyopathy (Fig. 11-3). Plasma ANP is significantly lower than that seen with cardiomyopathy because the constrictive process limits distension of the atria and thus release of ANP. The markedly lower concentrations of ANP of constrictive pericarditis may explain why, despite a higher renal plasma flow and glomerular filtration rates and a similar decrease in cardiac output (Fig. 11-2), significantly more salt and water accumulate than in patients with cardiomyopathy.

These data permit us to reconstruct the sequence of events that lead to salt and water retention in severe low output CHF. The purely mechanical effects of a weakened myocardium in LV systolic dysfunction or a restriction to cardiac filling with diastolic dysfunction causes a decrease in cardiac output (Fig. 11-4). The reduced cardiac output "threatens" arterial blood pressure and evokes a series of neurohormonal responses, the predominant effects of which are vasoconstriction, antidiuresis, and antinatriuresis. Renal blood flow and to a lesser extent the GFR decrease, and the kidneys start to retain salt and water. The TBW and $TBNa_E$ increase, and the extracellular and plasma volumes expand, contributing to elevated intracardiac filling pressures, which may in turn help increase cardiac output through the Frank-Starling mechanism. All these effects help support arterial blood pressure, which is maintained partly by an increase in systemic vascular resistance and partly by expansion of the plasma volume. The ex-

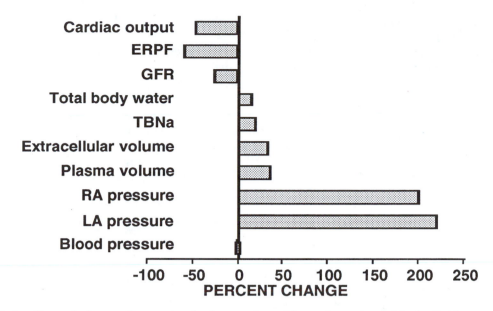

Fig. 11-4. Percent change from normal of a number of hemodynamic and body fluid compartment parameters in patients with untreated dilated cardiomyopathy. With severe untreated heart failure, compensatory changes in hemodynamics and body fluids help to maintain a normal arterial blood pressure. ERPF, effective renal plasma flow; GFR, glomerular filtration rate; TBNa, total body sodium.

panded plasma volume and increased venous pressures eventually lead to edema. These data confirm that the primary role of cardiovascular homeostasis is to maintain arterial blood pressure in order to optimize tissue perfusion. The chronic "threat" to arterial pressure therefore appears to be the stimulus for salt and water retention in patients with reduced cardiac output. If a threat to arterial blood pressure is the cause of neurohormonal activation and if activation of the neurohormones over a prolonged period of time is the stimulus to salt and water retention in the low output states, what is the stimulus for fluid retention in "high output failure"?

HIGH OUTPUT FAILURE

Cor Pulmonale

The hemodynamics of a group of patients with untreated cor pulmonale due to chronic obstructive pulmonary disease (COPD)[18] are shown in Table 11-1. The heart rate and right atrial and pulmonary arterial pressures are increased to the same extent as seen in patients with untreated cardiomyopathy. On the other hand, the left ventricle is usually normal in COPD, as shown by a normal pulmonary wedge pressure and cardiac output.[21] Despite normal cardiac output, blood pressure may be threatened by vasodilatation when there is carbon dioxide retention. It is interesting that patients with COPD retain

fluid and develop edema only when a chest infection worsens the ventilation-perfusion mismatch and leads to hypercarbia.[22-24] The neurohormonal response evoked in these patients is similar to that seen with low output heart failure (Fig. 11-3); and despite normal cardiac output, there is a similar reduction in renal blood flow and GFR (Fig. 11-2) and an identical pattern of salt and water retention (Fig. 11-1).

Chronic Severe Anemia

In patients with chronic severe anemia with edema, the arterial blood pressure is low despite a considerable increase in cardiac output.[19] The heart is often hyperdynamic. The threat to blood pressure comes from low systemic vascular resistance (Table 11-1), which is reduced partly because of low blood viscosity and partly because of enhanced basal activity of endothelium-derived relaxing factor.[25,26] The same neurohormonal response is found in these patients as well (Fig. 11-3). Renal blood flow and GFR decrease and salt and water retention is similar to that seen in low output states (Figs. 11-1 and 11-2).

Chronic Arteriovenous Fistula

Patients with chronic arteriovenous (AV) fistula often develop severe fluid retention. In these patients, even temporary manual compression of the

AV fistula elevates the blood pressure and increases renal excretion of sodium.[27] A unique example of an AV fistula is a ruptured aneurysm of a sinus of Valsalva (RSOV).[20] The hemodynamics of a patient with untreated RSOV and severe fluid retention are shown in Table 11-1. LV function was normal; and despite an increase in cardiac output to 12 $L \cdot min^{-1} \cdot sq\, m^{-1}$ the arterial blood pressure remained low. Again, neurohormonal response and changes in ERPF, GFR, and fluid retention were similar to that seen in low output states.

Comment

An identical neurohormonal response and similar retention of salt and water occur with low and high output states, which have different hemodynamics. The common factor appears to be a tendency toward low arterial blood pressure. Blood pressure is "threatened" in low output states because of low cardiac output and in high output states because of a decrease in systemic vascular resistance.

The neurohormonal response described above, however, is not unique to CHF syndrome. The same response is seen whenever blood pressure is threatened or reduced for whatever reason, for example during acute reduction of arterial pressure with nitroprusside.[28] A similar response is seen during physical exercise,[29] where blood pressure is threatened by marked vasodilatation in exercising muscles. These findings therefore support the theory proposed by Harris[4,30] that the neurohormonal response evoked during CHF is the same that evolved to support survival of the species under two main circumstances that threatened life (i.e., hemorrhage and physical exercise). With these conditions, a short-term threat to blood pressure evokes a baroreceptor-mediated increase in sympathetic activity, which causes venoconstriction, tachycardia, stimulation of the myocardium, and regional vasoconstriction. When blood pressure is threatened by reduced cardiac output due to LV dysfunction, the body has no way to distinguish whether the threat is from hemorrhage, exercise, or heart disease and therefore uses the same stereotyped response for which it is programmed. With heart disease (and other sustained vasodilated high output states), however, blood pressure is threatened over a prolonged period. Therefore the effector mechanisms continue to operate so long as the threat persists. An examination of various afferent and efferent mechanisms involved in these responses is necessary to better understand the pathophysiology of this syndrome.

AFFERENT MECHANISMS

In the foregoing discussion it was argued that of the three possible hemodynamic parameters—cardiac output, blood flow, blood pressure—a decrease in arterial blood pressure was the most likely primary event that initiates sodium and water retention by the kidney. How is this condition sensed? Table 11-2 outlines various afferent mechanisms available to the body. Receptors that monitor stretch are located at a number of sites in the arterial tree, great veins, and cardiac chambers. In low pressure chambers stretch of these receptors reflects primarily volume information, whereas in the high pressure arterial tree it reflects blood pressure.

Low Pressure or Volume Cardiopulmonary Receptors

Low pressure receptors are located in the atria and great veins. Because these structures are compliant, changes in stretch of the atria can effectively monitor changes in intracardiac volume. Atrial distension by rapid fluid infusion in animals[31–34] and by head-out water immersion in humans[35,36] induces prompt diuresis, natriuresis, and a decrease in systemic vascular resistance, suggesting that these receptors serve as sensing mechanisms for control of central volume. Two types of mechanoreceptor that sense atrial volume and heart rate have been identified in the atria.[37,38] Signals from these receptors are transmitted via the glossopharyngeal and vagal nerves to the hypothalamus and medullary centers, where there is integrated control of renal sympathetic discharge,[39,40] systemic vascular resistance,[41] and release of arginine vasopressin (AVP).[42,43] An increase in atrial size causes a decrease in renal nerve discharge, AVP release, and peripheral resistance.

In addition to neural mechanisms, the existence of

Table 11-2. Afferent Mechanisms

Low pressure or volume receptors:
    Atrial receptors
    Neural pathways
    Hormonal factors
High pressure baroreceptors
    Carotid sinus and aortic arch baroreceptors
    Renal sensors
        Juxtaglomerular cells
        Macula densa
        Renal parenchymal mechanoreceptors
Other receptors
    Central nervous system and liver

a hormonal factor in the atria became clear when De Bold et al.[44,45] published a landmark report showing that infusion of atrial extracts produce diuresis and natriuresis, leading to the discovery of ANP. ANP is stored in atrial tissue[44] and is released following atrial stretch.[46,47] A number of agents, including norepinephrine, angiotensin II, and AVP, have been shown to facilitate its release.[48–50] Thus the diuretic, natriuretic, and vasodilator effects of atrial distension are mediated by both activation of low pressure volume receptors and ANP.

High Pressure Baroreceptors

High pressure baroreceptors are stretch receptors located at several sites in the arterial tree. The carotid sinus and aortic arch baroreceptors respond to changes in arterial pressure by modulating their discharge transmitted in the glossopharyngeal and vagal nerves to the vasomotor center. A decrease in arterial pressure inhibits baroreceptor discharge, which activates the sympathetic nervous system, particularly the renal sympathetics nerves[51,52] which ultimately promote renal retention of sodium and water.[53–55] An increase in arterial pressure and stimulation of the carotid sinus baroreceptors have the opposite effect.[55,56] These baroreceptor responses can be modified by the volume status of the animal due to central integration with afferent stimuli from other cardiopulmonary stimuli.[57,58]

Renal Sensors

At least two types of sensor exist in the kidney.[59] The first are stretch receptors located in the juxtaglomerular cells, which are specialized myoepithelial cells cuffing the afferent arterioles. They act as baroreceptors and sense renal perfusion pressure. A decrease in perfusion pressure causes a corresponding decrease in arteriolar stretch leading to release of renin. The second type are the macula densa cells, a group of specialized distal convoluted tubular epithelial cells lying in apposition to the juxtaglomerular cells.[59] The macula densa and juxtaglomerular cells together form the juxtaglomerular apparatus. Macula densa cells function as chemoreceptors for the juxtaglomerular cells, monitoring the sodium load presented to the distal tubules. A decrease in tubular sodium load at the macula densa results in prompt release of renin by the juxtaglomerular cells. Renin release from the juxtaglomerular cells is also modulated by renal sympathetic nerves[60] and a variety of paracrine (angiotensin II,[61] prostaglandin,[62,63] aden-

osine[64]) and systemic (catecholamines,[61] AVP,[65] ANP[65,66]) humoral agents. Release of renin from the kidney and the ensuing production of angiotensin II and aldosterone are important effector mechanisms for sodium homeostasis. A third type of renal sensor is the mechanoreceptor within the renal parenchyma, which may also influence sodium excretion.[67]

Other Sensors

A number of other sensory afferents, of doubtful significance, have been localized in the central nervous system and liver. Selective infusion of hypertonic saline into the carotid artery or cerebral aqueduct induces natriuresis and diuresis.[58,68] Likewise, infusion of saline into the portal vein induces sodium and water excretion.[69]

Abnormalities of Afferent Mechanisms in CHF

Normally, atrial distension after intravascular volume expansion causes natriuresis, diuresis, and thereby a decrease in circulatory congestion. In patients with CHF, there is impaired diuresis and natriuresis despite a chronic increase in atrial pressures. In dogs with chronic heart failure a resetting of the low pressure atrial receptors with a consequent decrease in the firing of these receptors has been reported.[70,71] It is believed that it is due to structural alterations and the decreased atrial compliance that accompanies prolonged left atrial enlargement. This situation may contribute to the decrease in diuresis and natriuresis during chronic heart failure. Patients with CHF experience a similar resetting of arterial baroreceptor function that is reversed by cardiac transplantation.[72] Abnormal baroreceptor function may contribute to the chronic increase in sympathetic nervous activity seen with CHF.[73–75] The mechanisms responsible for resetting the baroreceptors are not clear but may be related to alterations in the nerve endings themselves or to the mechanical properties of the vessel wall,[76] possibly induced by catecholamines.[77,78] The decrease in atrial compliance seen with CHF may also explain why during exercise the increase in ANP is not proportional to the increase in right atrial pressure.[79]

EFFERENT MECHANISMS

Some of the efferent mechanisms active in CHF and that help to retain sodium and water are listed in Table 11-3. The main effect, as discussed previously,

Table 11-3. Efferent Mechanisms
Sympathetic nervous system
Renal sympathetic nerves
Neurohormones
Renin-angiotensin-aldosterone system
Vasopressin
Atrial natriuretic peptides
Intrarenal hormones
Prostaglandins
Kallikrein-kinin system
Renal responses
Glomerular filtration
Peritubular capillary Starling forces

is to help maintain arterial blood pressure by inducing peripheral vasoconstriction and by increasing plasma volume. Some of these mechanisms are discussed in greater detail in other chapters of this book and have been reviewed extensively elsewhere.[80] Here the role of these effector mechanisms in sodium and water retention is briefly summarized.

Sympathetic Nervous System and Renal Nerves

The sympathetic nervous system is activated early in response to heart failure[81] via the low and high pressure baroreceptors.[73] Direct intraneural recordings in patients with CHF confirm increased neural discharge, which correlates with the increased levels of plasma norepinephrine.[82,83] The result is tachycardia, increased myocardial contractility, and arteriolar vasoconstriction, particularly in the cutaneous, splanchnic, and renal beds. In the kidney, sympathetic stimulation and catecholamines increase sodium reabsorption by renal hemodynamic and tubular effects similar to those produced by angiotensin II.[84-86] Catecholamines also stimulate secretion of renin and antagonize the counterregulatory effects of vasodilator neurohormones.[87] In dogs with low output CHF, ganglion blockers markedly increase sodium excretion.[88] In rats with experimental CHF, efferent renal sympathetic nerve activity is increased and fails to suppress normally during an acute intravenous saline load.[89] Bilateral renal denervation attenuates progressive renal sodium retention[90] and increases single-nephron renal plasma flow and GFR.[91] These data confirm an important role of the sympathetic nervous system and renal nerves in the retention of sodium during clinical and experimental heart failure.

Neurohormones

RENIN-ANGIOTENSIN-ALDOSTERONE SYSTEM

The mechanisms for the release of renin were discussed in the section on afferent mechanisms. Renin is released from the kidney and possibly from other vascular sites.[55] It acts on renin substrate (angiotensinogen) to form the decapeptide angiotensin I, which is converted to the octapeptide angiotensin II by angiotensin-converting enzyme (ACE) present in the lungs, kidneys, vascular endothelium, and other sites. Angiotensin II has important renal and extrarenal effects. The two main direct renal effects of angiotensin II occur at low concentrations: 10- to 100-fold lower than what produces extrarenal effects.[92,93] The first effect is vasoconstriction of efferent arterioles of the glomerulus,[92] which increases the filtration fraction and helps to preserve the GFR.[84,94] The hemodynamic consequences of this effect are also responsible for enhanced proximal tubular reabsorption of sodium (discussed later). During heart failure with a severe reduction in perfusion pressure, introduction of ACE inhibitors may cause severe deterioration of renal function by reversing efferent arteriolar vasoconstriction, thereby decreasing the GFR.[95] The second renal effect of angiotensin II is on the proximal tubular epithelial cells, causing a direct increase in sodium reabsorption.[93]

The extrarenal actions of angiotensin II include systemic vasoconstriction,[96] release of norepinephrine from sympathetic nerve terminals, central stimulation of thirst, and stimulation of aldosterone production by the adrenal cortex,[96,97] all of which help to maintain arterial blood pressure. Aldosterone acts principally on the cortical collecting tubules to conserve sodium,[98] but its antinatriuretic and kaliuretic effects depend largely on the volume of filtrate reaching the collecting tubules. This delivery of filtrate (discussed later) depends on other effector mechanisms acting on the proximal tubules. Factors that may be implicated in the "escape" from the continued sodium-retaining effects of aldosterone include increases in GFR, blood pressure, local levels of bradykinin, prostaglandins, and ANP.[94,99,100] Although the renin-angiotensin-aldosterone system plays an important role in the pathogenesis of salt and water retention, most experimental and clinical studies have shown no consistent relation between the renin-angiotensin-aldosterone axis and any of the indices of fluid retention.[101-105] The elegant experiments of Watkins et al.[104] on dogs with inferior vena caval and pulmonary arterial constriction may provide an explanation for the variability and lack of consistency of the renin-angiotensin-aldosterone system in

CHF. They showed that plasma renin activity increased immediately after constriction but returned to normal as the plasma volume and arterial blood pressure were restored to normal. The negative feedback control of the renin-angiotensin-aldosterone system through blood volume and arterial blood pressure may explain the great variability in the renin-angiotensin-aldosterone axis in CHF. These hormone levels would therefore depend on the phase of fluid retention in a particular patient. Those who avidly retain sodium and water would be expected to have higher levels of the hormones than those who have reached a new steady state.

ARGININE VASOPRESSIN

Arginine vasopressin is released in response to a decrease in intracellular fluid volume (osmotic stimulus) or to a threat to ECV or blood pressure (nonosmotic stimulus). The afferent signals for nonosmotic release of AVP originate in the low and high pressure cardiopulmonary receptors. AVP enhances reabsorption of water at the level of the distal tubule and the cortical and medullary collecting ducts. AVP also constricts vascular smooth muscle. It is elevated after hemorrhage,[106] in animals with low cardiac output due to inferior vena caval constriction,[107,108] and with CHF.[109–111] The exact role of AVP in the pathogenesis of CHF is not clear. With severe CHF, administration of AVP antagonists may result in reduced peripheral vascular resistance and increased cardiac output.[112,113] AVP may also contribute to dilutional hyponatremia, a finding indicating a poor prognosis for the CHF patient.[87] Additional studies with specific AVP antagonists are required before the exact role of AVP in CHF can be defined.

ATRIAL NATRIURETIC PEPTIDES

Atrial natriuretic peptides have a variety of extrarenal and renal actions. A number of these peptides have been discovered and are described in detail elsewhere in this book. These peptides cause vasodilatation, which is most evident in vessels preconstricted with angiotensin II, AVP, and norepinephrine.[114,115] They decrease cardiac filling pressures and enhance fluid transduction into interstitial compartments.[116] ANP inhibits renin and AVP release and inhibits angiotensin II-stimulated aldosterone secretion.[117–119] In the kidney the most prominent effect of ANP is promotion of natriuresis and diuresis.[45] ANP dilates afferent arterioles and constricts efferent arterioles so the GFR increases without a change in renal blood flow.[120,121] ANP also inhibits sodium reabsorption in

the medullary collecting tubules[122] and angiotensin II-stimulated reabsorption in the proximal tubules.[123] ANP is one of the earliest neurohormones to increase with the development of LV dysfunction,[81,124] and circulating levels of ANP during heart failure correlate with atrial pressures.[79] Despite greatly increased circulating ANP, patients with CHF retain salt and water, suggesting an attenuation of its effect in patients with this condition. Infusion of synthetic ANP in experimental animals[125,126] and humans[127,128] has consistently confirmed attenuation of the renal response in CHF. The mechanisms of this attenuated response are unclear but may be related to the inability of ANP to antagonize the renal effects of angiotensin II and the sympathetic nervous system[87,126] when renal blood flow is decreased. Data suggest that the defect leading to ANP resistance may lie in an intracellular site distal to the production of cyclic guanosine monophosphate (cGMP) because ANP infusion in dogs with CHF increases cGMP without having any renal or hemodynamic effects.[129]

Intrarenal Hormones

A number of intrarenal hormonal systems may be activated during CHF. The important hormones belong to the arachidonic acid cascade and the kallikrein-kinin system.

PROSTAGLANDINS

The renal arterioles, glomeruli, and some parts of the renal tubules and collecting ducts synthesize the vasodilator prostaglandins (PG) I_2, E_2, and $F_{2\alpha}$.[130–132] Renal glomeruli also synthesize thromboxane A_2, which causes platelet aggregation and vasoconstriction.[130,133] The prominent effect of prostaglandins is to protect the glomerular microcirculation during states of renal vasoconstriction by causing vasodilation,[134] predominantly in the afferent arterioles,[135] thereby promoting sodium excretion. In addition to their hemodynamic effects, prostaglandins can also directly inhibit sodium transport in the cortical tubules[130,133] and medullary collecting ducts[136–138] and can blunt the AVP-induced reabsorption of water in cortical collecting ducts.[139] Prostaglandin synthesis is increased during activation of the renin-angiotensin system and renal sympathetic nerves[140,141] and during clinical and experimental heart failure.[141,142] Prostaglandins probably do not modulate renal hemodynamics or sodium excretion in normal subjects but may play a major role in situations with heightened renin-angiotensin and sympathetic activity, as is seen with CHF. In such settings inhibition of prostaglandins with cyclooxygenase inhibitors may induce a marked reduction of cardiac output and renal blood flow and an increase in peripheral vascular resistance and sodium retention.[142–144]

KALLIKREIN-KININ SYSTEM

The distal tubules in the kidney synthesize kallikrein, a protease that acts on its substrate kininogen to form the peptides bradykinin and kalliden. These peptides are destroyed by the enzyme kininase II, which is the same as angiotensin-converting enzyme. Both peptides produce vasodilation and natriuresis, and bradykinin also stimulates the production of prostaglandins.[145] Although the exact role of this system in CHF is unknown, urinary secretion of kallikrein and kinins change during alterations in sodium balance.[145,146]

Renal Responses

The changes in renal function during heart failure include adjustments in glomerular hemodynamics and tubular transport. They are brought about by alterations in the sympathetic nervous system and other effector hormones described above.

GLOMERULAR FILTRATION AND PERITUBULAR STARLING FORCES

The glomerular filtration rate is determined by the balance of pressures acting across the capillary wall (glomerular capillary hydrostatic and Bowman space oncotic pressures favor filtration, whereas glomerular capillary oncotic and Bowman space hydrostatic pressures oppose filtration), surface area, and permeability of the capillary membrane. Urinary excretion of sodium is determined by the difference between the amount of sodium filtered by the glomerulus and reabsorbed by the tubules. The amount of sodium filtered by the glomerulus is in turn determined by the GFR. In normal subjects, fluctuations in GFR throughout the day (e.g., due to changes in posture) result in considerable variations in the load of sodium filtered. Urinary excretion of sodium remains relatively constant, however, because the sodium reabsorbed by the tubules tends to parallel the filtered load, and the fraction of the filtrate reabsorbed remains relatively constant because of a process termed glomerular-tubular balance. It tends to reduce wide fluctuations in sodium excretion when renal hemodynamics are altered.

The mechanisms responsible for this coupling between GFR and sodium reabsorption are due to alterations in the Starling forces along the peritubular capillaries, which are the important determinants of proximal tubular reabsorption.[147] In this regard, the anatomic relation between glomerular and peritubular capillaries is important. The glomerular capillary bed is connected in series with the peritubular capillary network through the efferent arterioles, such that changes in the physical determinants of GFR critically influence the hydrostatic and oncotic pressures in peritubular capillaries. Therefore the hydrostatic pressure in the peritubular capillary network is lower than in the glomerular capillaries. Vasoconstriction of the efferent arteriole by the sympathetic nerves or angiotensin II[148,149] can further decrease the hydrostatic pressure in the peritubular capillaries. Also because peritubular capillaries receive blood from the glomerulus, the plasma oncotic pressure is high. An increase in efferent arteriolar tone, and therefore the filtration fraction (GFR/renal blood flow), increases not only the amount of sodium filtered by the glomerulus but also the peritubular oncotic pressure. The absolute rate of reabsorption of the proximal tubule absorbate by the peritubular capillaries is again given by the Starling forces.

With CHF syndromes, as discussed above, afferent signals are activated, leading to sympathetic stimulation, renin-angiotensin activation, and an increase in AVP and ANP. At the level of the kidneys, alterations in renal hemodynamics and tubular reabsorption ensue. Renal blood flow declines, in part due to a decrease in cardiac output and also because of an increase in renal vascular resistance; it returns toward normal when cardiac performance improves.[8,9,16–20,150] The increase in renal vascular resistance can be partly reversed by intrarenal infusion of α-adrenergic blocking agents, angiotensin II receptor antagonists, and ACE inhibitors, suggesting a role for renal sympathetic nerves and the renin-angiotensin system in increasing renal vascular resistance.[104,151–155] The GFR is usually not decreased with mild or early heart failure; and even during late stages of heart failure the decrease in GFR is proportionately smaller than the decrease in renal blood flow.[8,10,16–20] The filtration fraction is increased, implying greater efferent than afferent arteriolar vasoconstriction. Similar changes have also been observed at the level of the single nephron in the rat model of coronary artery ligation.[156] Compared with normal rats, the single-nephron GFR in rats with CHF is lower, but the single-nephron plasma flow is reduced disproportionately, so the single-nephron filtration fraction is markedly elevated because of a greater increase in efferent than afferent arteriolar

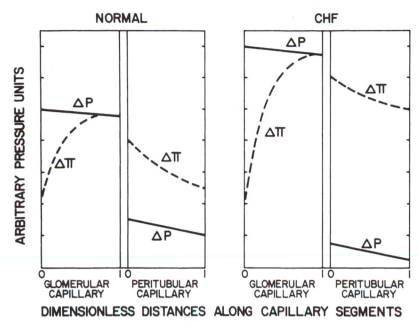

Fig. 11-5. Glomerular and peritubular microcirculations in the normal state **(left)** and in congestive heart failure (CHF) **(right)**. The afferent arteriolar end of the glomerular capillary bed is depicted as 0 and the efferent arteriolar end as 1. For the peritubular capillary, 0 represents the efferent arteriolar and 1 the renal venous end. ΔP and $\Delta \Pi$ are, respectively, the transcapillary hydraulic and oncotic pressures operating across the glomerular and peritubular capillaries. ΔP is relatively constant across the glomerular capillaries, whereas the net driving force for ultrafiltration ($\Delta P - \Delta \Pi$) diminishes as the opposing colloid osmotic pressure difference ($\Delta \Pi$) increases owing to the formation of an essentially protein-free ultrafiltrate. In the peritubular capillaries, as a result of the drop in hydraulic pressure (ΔP) along the efferent arterioles and an increase in the colloid osmotic pressure ($\Delta \Pi$), the net driving pressure ($\Delta P - \Delta \Pi$) becomes negative, favoring resorption. With CHF decreased renal blood flow is associated with a compensatory increase in ΔP due to greater efferent than afferent arteriolar vasoconstriction. This situation leads to a greater ultrafiltrate and hence a greater rise in the plasma protein and $\Delta \Pi$ at the distal end of the glomerular capillary and ultimately in the peritubular capillaries. This increase in $\Delta \Pi$ results in an increase in the net driving pressure responsible for enhanced proximal tubular salt and water reabsorption in CHF. (From Humes HD, Gottlieb M, Brenner BM,[163] with permission.)

resistance. Figure 11-5 compares the glomerular capillary hemodynamics profiles of normal and CHF states. The transmural hydrostatic pressure gradient (ΔP) declines along the distance of the glomerular capillary in both normal and CHF states, but the ΔP in CHF is much higher because of increased efferent arteriolar vasoconstriction. The transmural plasma oncotic pressure gradient ($\Delta \Pi$) increases over the length of the glomerular capillary in both states, as fluid is filtered in Bowman's space; but it increases to a greater extent in the presence of CHF because of the increased filtration fraction. Therefore the major component of glomerular hemodynamic alteration is due to the disproportionate increase in efferent, compared to afferent, arteriolar vasoconstriction; and this situation helps to maintain the GFR. At the tubular level, the $\Delta \Pi$ along the peritubular capillary is increased with CHF, compared to that in normals, whereas ΔP is decreased. The bal-

ance of hemodynamic forces in the peritubular capillaries thus favors increased reabsorption of sodium and fluid by the proximal tubules in CHF.

Thus although sodium retention during heart failure occurs mainly at the level of the proximal tubules in response to changes in intrarenal hemodynamics induced by an increase in sympathetic stimulation and angiotensin II, there is evidence that enhanced sodium reabsorption also occurs at other tubular sites. Indirect evidence during experimental low and high output failure suggests that sodium reabsorption is increased in the ascending limb of the loop of Henle.[157–159] The increased levels of aldosterone found during heart failure could act to promote sodium retention in cortical and medullary collecting ducts, although its exact role in CHF remains less clear. Experimental studies suggest that alterations in collecting duct sodium transport may also contribute to sodium excretion during heart failure.[160,161]

Finally, studies of clinical and experimental heart failure using inert gases have shown that renal blood flow is diverted away from the outer regions of the cortex to the juxtamedullary regions.[162] Whether this process has an effect on sodium retention remains uncertain.

SUMMARY

A review of hemodynamic and neurohormonal data from patients with untreated low and high output CHF leads to the conclusion that the primary afferent signal that initiates salt and water retention is most likely a threat to arterial blood pressure. The body responds to this threat in a consistent way, identical to its response to hemorrhage, for which it has been primed far back in evolution (Fig. 11-6). A threat to arterial blood pressure, as encountered with low cardiac output or in persistently vasodilated states, leads to a baroreceptor-mediated increase in sympathetic activity and activation of the renin-an-

giotensin-aldosterone system by the juxtaglomerular apparatus. A chronic increase in sympathetic activity follows the resetting of baroreceptors. The greatly enhanced sympathetic activity increases peripheral vascular resistance, reduces renal blood flow, and may contribute to the nonosmotic release of vasopressin. The intrinsic intrarenal mechanisms for salt and water retention are also set in motion. Superimposed on these mechanisms are the influences of the renin-angiotensin-aldosterone system and vasopressin, further favoring retention of sodium and water.

The net effect is expansion of the ECV and blood volume, which help maintain arterial pressure; and its negative feedback explains the great variability in the renin-angiotensin-aldosterone response in those with CHF. The expanded blood volume also increases intracardiac pressures, causing atrial distension, which in turn leads to release of atrial natriuretic peptides, which have natriuretic and vasodilator properties. Atrial distension also activates the low pressure volume receptors, which tend to attenuate sympathetic activity and AVP release. With heart

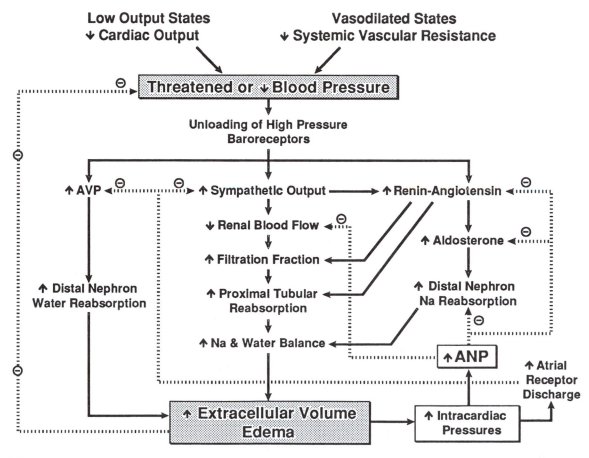

Fig. 11-6. Sequence of events by which conditions with a decrease in cardiac output (low output states) or reduced systemic vascular resistance (in persistently vasodilated states) initiate salt and water retention by the kidney.

disease, however, a decrease in arterial pressure is accompanied by an increase in venous pressure. Therefore in contrast to hemorrhage, low pressure volume receptor and high pressure baroreceptor systems oppose one another in the presence of heart disease. However, the natriuretic and vasodilator effects of ANP and the attenuating effects of volume receptors on sympathetic nerves and AVP are clearly overwhelmed by opposing influences, and the overall effect is one of salt and water retention. It is therefore clear that the high pressure baroreceptor and the renin-angiotensin-aldosterone control system predominate and play a dominant role in the pathophysiology of salt and water retention in CHF syndromes

REFERENCES

1. Hope JA: Treatise on the Disease of the Heart and Great Vessels. John Churchill, London, 1832
2. Starling EH: On the absorption of fluids from the connective tissue spaces. J Physiol (Lond) 1896;19:312–326
3. Mackenzie J: Diseases of the Heart. 3rd Ed. Oxford Medical Publications, Oxford, 1913
4. Harris P: Congestive cardiac failure. Central role of the arterial blood pressure. Br Heart J 1987;58:190–203
5. Wollheim E: Die Zirkulierende Blutmenge und ihre Bedeutung fur Kompensation und Dekompensation des Kreislaufs. Z Klin Med 1931;116:269–397
6. Starr I, Rawson AJ: Role of the "static blood pressure" in abnormal increments of venous pressure, especially in heart failure. I. Theoretical studies on an improved circulation schema whose pump obeys Starling's law of the heart. Am J Med Sci 1940;199:27–39
7. Starr I: Role of the "static blood pressure" in abnormal increments of venous pressure, especially in heart failure. II. Clinical and experimental studies. Am J Med Sci 1940;199:40–55
8. Warren JV, Stead EA Jr: Fluid dynamics in chronic congestive failure. Arch Intern Med 1944;73:138–147
9. Merrill AJ: Edema and decreased renal blood flow in patients with chronic congestive heart failure. Evidence of "forward failure" as the primary cause of edema. J Clin Invest 1946;25:389–400
10. Merrill AJ: Mechanisms of salt and water retention in heart failure. Am J Med 1949;6:357–367
11. McCance RA: Experimental sodium chloride deficiency in man. Proc R Soc Lond B 1936;119:245
12. Luft FC, Rankin LI, Block R et al: Cardiovascular and humoral responses to extremes of sodium intake in normal black and white men. Circulation 1979;60:697–706
13. Peters JP: The role of sodium in the production of edema. N Engl J Med 1948;239:353–362
14. Peters JP: The problem of cardiac edema. Am J Med 1952;12:66–76
15. Schrier RW: Pathogenesis of sodium and water retention in high-output and low-output cardiac failure, nephrotic syndrome, cirrhosis, and pregnancy. N Engl J Med 1988;319:1065–1072 (part I), 1127–1134 (part II)
16. Anand IS, Ferrari R, Kalra GS et al: Edema of cardiac origin. Studies of body water and sodium, renal function, hemodynamic indexes, and plasma hormones in untreated congestive cardiac failure. Circulation 1989;80:299–305
17. Anand IS, Ferrari R, Kalra GS, et al: Pathogenesis of edema in constrictive pericarditis. Circulation 1991;83:1880–1887
18. Anand IS, Chandrashekhar Y, Ferrari R et al: Pathogenesis of congestive state in chronic obstructive pulmonary disease. Circulation 1992;86:12–21
19. Anand IS, Chandrashekhar Y, Ferrari R, Poole-Wilson PA, Harris P: Pathogenesis of edema in chronic anaemia. Studies of body water and sodium, renal function, haemodynamics and plasma hormones. Br Heart J 1993;70:357–362
20. Anand IS, Chandrashekhar Y, Ferrari R, Poole-Wilson PA, Harris P: Edema in high output state of AV fistula. Study of a case with ruptured aneurysm of sinus of Valsalva. Am J Cardiol (in press)
21. Wade OL, Bishop JM: Cardiac Output and Regional Blood Flow. Blackwell Scientific Publications, Oxford, 1962
22. Cambell EJM, Short DS: The cause of oedema in cor pulmonale. Lancet 1960;1:1184–1186
23. Richens JM, Howard P: Oedema in cor pulmonale. Clin Sci 1982;62:255–259
24. Harris P: Are pulmonary haemodynamics of importance to survival in chronic obstructive lung disease? Eur Respir J 1989;7:674–677
25. Anand IS, Chandrashekhar Y: Reduced inhibition of endothelial-derived relaxing factor causes the hyperdynamic circulation of chronic severe anemia. Med Hypotheses 1993;41:225–228
26. Anand IS, Chandrashekhar Y, Wander G, Chawla LS: Endothelium-derived relaxing factor is important in mediating the high output state in chronic severe anemia. J Am Coll Cardiol 1995;25:1402–1407
27. Epstein FH, Post RS, McDowell M: Effects of an arteriovenous fistula on renal hemodynamics and electrolyte excretion. J Clin Invest 1953;32:233–241
28. Ferarri R, Ceconi C, De Guili F, Panzail A, Harris P: Temporal relations of the endocrine response to hypotension with sodium nitroprusside. Cardioscience 1992;3:51–60
29. Ferrari R, Ceconi C, Rodella A et al: Temporal relations of the endocrine response to exercise. Cardioscience 1991;2:131–139
30. Harris P: Role of arterial pressure in the oedema of heart disease. Lancet 1988;1:1036–1038
31. Gauer OH, Henry JP, Behn C: The regulation of extracellular fluid volume. Annu Rev Physiol 1970;32:547–595
32. Henry JP, Gauer OH, Reeves JL: Evidence of the atrial location of receptors influencing urine flow. Circ Res 1956;4:85
33. Linden RJ: Atrial reflexes and renal function. Am J Cardiol 1979;44:879–883
34. Kaczmarczyk G, Drake A, Eisele R et al: The role of the cardiac nerves in the regulation of sodium excretion in conscious dogs. Pflugers Arch 1981;390:125–130
35. Epstein M: Cardiovascular and renal effects of head-

out water immersion in man. Circ Res 1976;39: 619–628

36. Arborelius M, Balldin UI, Lilja B, Lundgren CEG: Hemodynamic changes in man during immersion with the head above water. Aerospace Med 1972;43: 592–598

37. Coleridge HM, Coleridge JCG, Kidd C: Cardiac receptors in the dog, with particular reference to two types of apparent endings in the ventricular wall. J Physiol (Lond) 1964;174:323

38. Paintal AS: Vagal sensory receptors and their reflex effects. Physiol Rev 1973;53:159–227

39. Shepherd JT: Intrathoracic baroreflexes. Mayo Clin Proc 1973;48:426–437

40. Myers BD, Peterson C, Molina C et al: Role of cardiac atria in the human renal response to changing plasma volume. Am J Physiol 1988;254:F562–F573

41. Linden RJ, Kappagoda CT: Atrial Receptors. Monographs of the Physiological Society No 39. Cambridge University Press, Cambridge, 1982

42. De Torrente A, Robertson G, McDonald KM, Schrier RW: Mechanism of diuretic response to increased left atrial pressure in the anesthetized dog. Kidney Int 1975;8:355–361

43. Quail AW, Woods RL, Korner PI: Cardiac and arterial baroreceptor influences in release of vasopressin and renin during hemorrhage. Am J Physiol 1987;252: H1120–H1126

44. De Bold AJ: Heart atrial granularity. Effects of changes in water-electrolyte balance. Proc Soc Exp Biol Med 1979;161:508–511

45. De Bold AJ, Borenstein HB, Veress AT, Sonnenberg H: A rapid and potent natriuretic response to intravenous injection of atrial myocardial extract in rats. Life Sci 1981;28:89–94

46. Schiebinger RJ, Linden J: The influence of resting tension on immunoreactive atrial natriuretic peptide secretion by rat atria superfused in vitro. Circ Res 1986;59:105–109

47. Agnoletti G, Rodella A, Ferrari R, Harris P: Release of atrial natriuretic peptide-like immunoreactive material during stretching of the rat atrium. J Mol Cell Cardiol 1987;19:217–222

48. Inoue M, Kimura T, Ota K et al: Effect of vasopressin on atrial natriuretic peptide release and renal function in dogs. Am J Physiol 1988;255:E449–E455

49. Rankin AJ, Wilson N, Ledsome JR: Effects of autonomic stimulation on plasma immunoreactive atrial natriuretic peptide in the anesthesized rabbit. Can J Physiol Pharmacol 1987;65:532–537

50. Manning PT, Schwartz D, Katsube NC, Holmberg SW, Needleman P: Vasopressin-stimulated release of atriopeptin. Endocrine antagonists in fluid homeostasis. Science 1985;229:395–397

51. Kezdi P, Geller E: Baroreceptor control of post-ganglionic sympathetic nerve discharge. Am J Physiol 1968;214:427–435

52. Kirchheim HR: Systemic arterial baroreceptor reflexes. Physiol Rev 1976;56:100–177

53. DiBona GF: Neurogenic regulation of renal tubular sodium reabsorption. Am J Physiol 1977;233: F73–F81

54. Davis JO: The control of renin release. Am J Med 1973;55:333–350

55. Guyton A, Scanlon CJ, Armstrong GG: Effects of

56. Keeler R: Natruiresis after unilateral stimulation of carotid receptors in unanesthetized rats. Am J Physiol 1974;226:507–511

57. Tramposch A, Brosnihan KB, Ferrario CM: Reduced role of cardiopulmonary receptors in modulation of carotid sinus reflexes in sodium-loaded dogs [abstract]. Physiologist 1984;27:283

58. Ferrario CM, Tramposch A, Kawano Y, Brosnihan KB: Sodium balance and the reflex regulation of baroreceptor function. Circulation, suppl. I 1987;75: 141–148

59. Davis JO, Freeman RH: Mechanisms regulating renin release. Physiol Rev 1976;56:1–56

60. Vander AJ, Miller R: Control of renin secretion in the dog. Am J Physiol 1964;207:537–546

61. Keeton TK, Pettinger WA, Campbell WB: The effects of altered sodium balance and adrenergic blockade on renin release induced in rats by angiotensin antagonism. Circ Res 1976;38:531–539

62. Oates JA, Whorton AR, Gerkins JF et al: The participation of prostaglandins in the control of renin release. Fed Proc 1979;38:72–74

63. Henrich WL: Role of prostaglandins in renin secretion. Kidney Int 1981;19:822–830

64. Itoh S, Carretero OA, Murray RD: Possible role of adenosine in the macula densa mechanism of renin release in rabbits. J Clin Invest 1985;76:1412–1417

65. Johnson MD, Kinter LB, Beeuwkes R III: Effects of AVP and DDAVP on plasma renin activity and electrolyte excretion in conscious dogs. Am J Physiol 1979;236:F66–F76

66. Maack T, Marion DN, Camargo MJF et al: Effects of auriculin (atrial natriuretic factor) on blood pressure, renal function, and the renin-aldosterone system in dogs. Am J Med 1984;77:1069–1075

67. Burnett JC, Granger JP, Opgenorth TJ: Effects of synthetic atrial natriuretic factor on renal function and renin release. Am J Physiol 1984;247:F863–F866

68. Andersson B, Olsson K: On central control of body fluid homeostasis. Conditional Reflex 1973;8: 147–159

69. Passo SS, Thornborough JR, Rothballer AB: Hepatic receptors in control of sodium excretion in anesthetized cats. Am J Physiol 1972;224:373–375

70. Greenberg TT, Richmond WH, Stocking RA et al: Impaired atrial receptor responses in dogs with heart failure due to tricuspid insufficiency and pulmonary artery stenosis. Circ Res 1973;32:424–433

71. Zucker IH, Earle AM, Gilmore JP: The mechanism of adaptation of left atrial stretch receptors in dogs with chronic congestive heart failure. J Clin Invest 1977;60:323–331

72. Ellenbogen KA, Mohanty PK, Szentpetery S, Thames MD: Arterial baroreflex abnormalities in heart failure. Reversal after orthotropic cardiac transplantation. Circulation 1989;79:51–58

73. Ferguson DW, Abboud FM, Mark AL: Selective impairment of baroreflex-mediated vasoconstrictor responses in patients with ventricular dysfunction. Circulation 1984;75:451–460

74. Hirsch AT, Dzau VJ, Creager MA: Baroreceptor function in congestive heart failure. Effect on neurohumoral activation and regional vascular resistance. Circulation, suppl. IV 1987;75:36–48

75. Ferguson DW, Berg WJ, Roach PJ, Oven RM, Mark AL: Effect of heart failure on baroreflex control of sympathetic activity. Am J Cardiol 1992;69:523–531

76. Zucker IH, Wang W, Brandle M: Baroreceptor abnormalities in congestive heart failure. News Physiol Sci 1993;8:87–90

77. Anand IS, Bergel DH: Mechanical factors affecting baroreceptor function. Proc Int Union Physiol Sci 1971;9:17–18

78. Bergel DH, Anand IS, Brooks DE et al: Carotid sinus wall mechanics and baroreceptor function in the dog. pp. 1–5. In Sleight P (ed): Baroreceptors and Hypertension. Oxford University Press, Oxford, 1980

79. Raine AEG, Erne P, Burgisser E et al: Atrial natriuretic peptide and atrial pressure in patients with congestive heart failure. N Engl J Med 1986;315:553

80. Moe GW, Legault L, Skorecki KL: Control of extracellular fluid volume and pathophysiology of edema formation. pp. 623–676. In Brenner BM, Rector FC (eds): The Kidney. WB Saunders, Philadelphia, 1991

81. Francis GS, Benedict C, Johnstone D et al: Comparison of neuroendocrine activation in patients with and without congestive heart failure. Circulation 1990; 82:1724–1729

82. Leimbach WN, Wallin G, Victor RG et al: Direct evidence from intraneural recordings for increased central sympathetic outflow in patients with heart failure. Circulation 1986;73:913–919

83. Hasking GJ, Esler MD, Jennings GL, Burton D, Korner PI: Norepinephrine spillover to plasma in patients with congestive heart failure. Evidence of increased overall cardiorenal sympathetic nervous activity. Circulation 1986;73:615–621

84. Myers ED, Dean WM, Brenner DM: Effects of norepinephrine and angiotensin II on the determinants of glomerular ultrafiltration and proximal tubule fluid reabsorption in the rat. Circ Res 1975;37:101–110

85. DiBona GF: The functions of the renal nerves. Rev Physiol Biochem Pharmacol 1982;94:75–94

86. Bello-Reuss E: Effect of catecholamines on fluid reabsorption by the isolated proximal convoluted tubule. Am J Physiol 1980;238:F347–F352

87. Packer M: Neurohormonal interactions and adaptations in congestive heart failure. Circulation 1988; 77:721–730

88. Gill JR, Carr AA, Fleischmann LE, Casper AG, Bartter FC: Effects of pentolium on sodium excretion in dogs with constriction of the vena cava. Am J Physiol 1967;212:191–196

89. DiBona GF, Herman PJ, Swan LL: Neural control of renal function in edema forming states. Am J Physiol 1988;254:R1017–R1024

90. DiBona GF, Swan LL: Role of renal nerves in sodium retention of cirrhosis and congestive heart failure. Am J Physiol 1991;260:R298–R305

91. Kon V, Yared A, Ichikawa I: Role of sympathetic nerves in mediating acute extracellular fluid volume depletion of renal cortical microcirculation in experimental congestive heart failure and in systemic circulatory impairment. J Clin Invest 1985;76:1913–1920

92. Edwards RM: Segmental effects of norepinephrine and angiotensin II on isolated renal microvessels. Am J Physiol 1983;244:F526–F534

93. Schuster VL, Kokko GP, Jacobson HR: Angiotensin II directly stimulates transport in rabbit proximal convoluted tubules. J Clin Invest 1984;73:507–515

94. Hall JE, Guyton AC, Jackson TE et al: Control of glomerular filtration rate by renin-angiotensin system. Am J Physiol 1977;233:F366–F372

95. Murphy BF, Whitworth JA, Kincaid-Smith P: Renal insufficiency with combinations of angiotensin-converting enzyme inhibitors and diuretics. BMJ 1984; 288:844–845

96. Laragh JH, Sealey JE: The renin-angiotensin-aldosterone hormonal system and regulation of sodium, potassium and blood pressure homeostasis. pp. 831–908. In Orloff J, Berliner RW (eds): Handbook of Physiology. Renal Physiology. American Physiological Society, Washington, DC, 1973

97. Hall JE, Granger JP: Role of peripheral sympathetic nervous system in mediating chronic blood pressure and renal hemodynamic effects of angiotensin II [abstract]. Fed Proc 1983;42:589

98. Gross JB, Kokko JP: Effects of aldosterone and potassium sparing diuretics on electrical potential difference across the distal nephron. J Clin Invest 1977; 59:82–89

99. Harris PJ, Young JA: Dose dependence stimulation and inhibition of proximal tubular reabsorption by angiotensin II in the rat kidney. Pflugers Arch 1977; 367:295–297

100. Durr J, Favre L, Gaillard R, Riondel AM, Vallotton MB: Mineralocorticoid escape in man. Role of renal prostaglandins. Acta Endocrinol (Copenh) 1982;99: 474–480

101. Chonko AM, Bay WH, Stein JH, Ferris TF: The role of renin and aldosterone in the salt retention of edema. Am J Med 1977;63:881–890

102. Sanders LL, Melby JC: Aldosterone and the edema of congestive heart failure. Arch Intern Med 1964; 113:331–338

103. Dzau VJ, Colucci WS, Hollenberg NK, William GH: Relation of the renin-angiotensin-aldosterone system to clinical state in congestive heart failure. Circulation 1981;63:645–651

104. Watkins L Jr, Burton JA, Haber E et al: The renin-angiotensin-aldosterone system in congestive heart failure in conscious dogs. J Clin Invest 1976;57: 1606–1617

105. Anand IS, Chandrashekhar Y, Ferrari R, Poole-Wilson PA, Harris P: Aldosterone in untreated heart failure. In Ferrari R (ed): Aldosterone and Heart Failure. Canal Press, Venice, 1995

106. Johnston JA, Moore WW, Segar WE: Small changes in left atrial pressure and plasma antidiuretic hormone titers in dogs. Am J Physiol 1969;217:210–214

107. Anderson RJ, Cadnapahornchai P, Harbottle JA, McDonald K, Schrier R: Mechanism of effect of thoracic inferior vena cava constriction on renal water excretion. J Clin Invest 1974;54:1473–1479

108. Ishikawa S, Saito T, Okada K, Tsutaui K, Kuzuya T: Effect of vasopressin antagonist on water excretion in inferior vena cava constriction. Kidney Int 1986; 30:49–55

109. Cowley AW, Quillen EW, Skelton MM: Role of vasopressin in cardiovascular regulation. Fed Proc 1983; 42:3170–3176

110. Goldsmith SR, Francis GS, AW Cowley, Levine T, Cohn J: Increased plasma arginine vasopressin levels in patients with congestive heart failure. J Am Coll Cardiol 1983;1:1385–1390

111. Riegger GAJ, Liebau G, Kochsiek K: Antidiuretic

hormone in congestive heart failure. Am J Med 1982; 72:49–52

112. Nicod P, Biollaz J, Waeber B et al: Hormonal, global, and regional hemodynamic responses to a vascular antagonist of vasopressin in patients with congestive heart failure with or without hyponatremia. Br Heart J 1986;56:433–439

113. Creager MA, Faxon DP, Cutler S et al: Contribution of vasopressin to vasoconstriction in patients with congestive heart failure. Comparison with the renin-angiotensin system and sympathetic nervous system. J Am Coll Cardiol 1986;7:758–765

114. Kleinert HD, Maack T, Atlas SA et al: Atrial natriuretic factor inhibits angiotensin-, norepinephrine-, and potassium-induced vascular contractility. Hypertension, suppl. 1 1984;6:143–147

115. Bolli P, Muller FB, Linder L et al: The vasodilator potency of atrial natriuretic peptide in man. Circulation 1987;75:221–228

116. Roy LF, Ogilvie RI, Larochelle P, Hamet P, Leenen FH: Cardiac and vascular effects of atrial natriuretic factor and sodium nitroprusside in healthy men. Circulation 1989;79:383–392

117. Shenker Y: Atrial natriuretic hormone effect on renal function and aldosterone secretion in sodium depletion. Am J Physiol 1988;255:R867–R873

118. Isales CM, Bollag WB, Kiernan LC, Barrett PQ: Effect of ANP on sustained aldosterone secretion stimulated by angiotensin II. Am J Physiol 1989;256:C89–C95

119. Allen MJ, Ang VT, Bennett ED, Jenkins JS: Atrial natriuretic peptide inhibits osmolality-induced arginine vasopressin release in man. Clin Sci 1987;75:35–39

120. Borenstein HB, Cupples WA, Sonnenberg H, Veress A: The effect of natriuretic atrial extract on renal hemodynamics and urinary excretion in anaesthetized rats. J Physiol (Lond) 1983;334:133–140

121. Dunn BR, Ichikawa I, Pfeffer JM, Troy JL, Brenner BM: Renal and systemic hemodynamic effects of synthetic atrial natriuretic peptide in the anesthetized rat. Circ Res 1986;59:237–246

122. Sonnenberg H, Honrath U, Chong CK, Wilson DR: Atrial natriuretic factor inhibits sodium transport in medullary collecting duct. Am J Physiol 1986;250:F963–F966

123. Harris PJ, Thomas D, Morgan TO: Atrial natriuretic peptide inhibits angiotensin-stimulated proximal tubular sodium and water reabsorption. Nature 1987;326:697–698

124. Redfield MM, Aarhus LL, Wright RS, Burnett JC Jr: Cardiorenal and neurohumoral function in a canine model of early left ventricular dysfunction. Circulation 1993;87:2016–2022

125. Scriven TA, Burnett JC: Effects of synthetic atrial natriuretic peptide on renal function and renin release in acute experimental heart failure. Circulation 1985;72:892–897

126. Kohzuki M, Hodsman P, Johnston C: Attenuated response to atrial natriuretic peptide in rats with myocardial infarction. Am J Physiol 1989;25:H533–H538

127. Anand IS, Kalra GS, Ferrari R et al: Hemodynamic, hormonal, and renal effects of atrial natriuretic peptide in untreated congestive heart failure. Am Heart J 1989;118:500–505

128. Cody JR, Atlas SA, Laragh JH et al: Atrial natriuretic factor in normal subjects and heart failure patients. J Clin Invest 1986;78:1362–1374

129. Riegger GAJ, Elsner D, Kromer EP et al: Atrial natriuretic peptide in congestive heart failure in the dog. Plasma levels, cyclic guanosine monophosphate, ultrastructure of atrial myoendocrine cells, and hemodynamic, hormonal, and renal effects. Circulation 1988;77:398–406

130. Hassid A, Konieczkowski M, Dunn MJ: Prostaglandin synthesis in isolated rat kidney glomeruli. Proc Natl Acad Sci USA 1979;76:1155–1159

131. Schlondorff D, Satriano JA, Schwartz GJ: Synthesis of prostaglandin PGE_2 in different segments of isolated collecting tubules from adult and neonatal rabbits. Am J Physiol 1985;248:F134–F144

132. Schlondorff D, Ardailloui R: Prostaglandins and other arachidonic acid metabolites in the kidney. Kidney Int 1986;29:108–119

133. Stahl RA, Paravicini M, Schollmeyer P: Angiotensin II stimulation of PGE_2 and 6-keto-PGF_1 formation by isolated human glomeruli. Kidney Int 1984;26:30–34

134. Scharschmidt L, Simonson M, Dunn MJ: Glomerular prostaglandins. AII, and non-steroidal anti-inflammatory drugs. Am J Med, suppl. 20 1986;81:30–42

135. Edwards RM: Effects of prostaglandins and vasoconstrictor action in isolated renal arterioles. Am J Physiol 1985;248:F779–F784

136. Fine LG, Trizna W: Influence of prostaglandins on sodium transport of isolated medullary nephron segments. Am J Physiol 1977;232:F383–F390

137. Lino J, Imai M: Effects of prostaglandins on Na transport in isolated collecting tubules. Pflugers Arch 1978;373:125–132

138. Stokes JB, Kokko JP: Inhibition of sodium transport by prostaglandin E_2 across the isolated, perfused rabbit collecting tubule. J Clin Invest 1977;59:1099–1104

139. Holt WF, Lechene C: ADH-PGE_2 interactions in cortical collecting tubule. I. Depression of sodium transport. Am J Physiol 1981;241:F452–F460

140. Oliver JA, Pinto J, Sciacca RR, Cannon P: Increased renal secretion of norepinephrine and prostaglandin E_2 during sodium depletion in the dog. J Clin Invest 1980;68:748–756

141. Oliver JA, Sciacca RR, Pinto J, Cannon P: Participation of the prostaglandins in the control of renal blood flow during acute reduction of cardiac output in the dog. J Clin Invest 1981;67:229–237

142. Dzau VJ, Packer M, Lilly LS et al: Prostaglandins in severe congestive heart failure. N Engl J Med 1984;310:347–352

143. Ichikawa I, Pfeffer J, Pferffer MA et al: Glomerular response to severe congestive heart failure [abstract]. Kidney Int 1983;23:245A

144. Walshe JJ, Venuto RC: Acute oliguric renal failure induced by indomethacin. Possible mechanisms. Ann Intern Med 1979;91:47–49

145. Stein JH, Congbaly RC, Karsh DL, Osgood RW, Ferris TF: The effect of bradykinin on proximal tubular sodium reabsorption in the dog. Evidence for functional nephron heterogeneity. J Clin Invest 1972;51:1709–1721

146. Margolies HG, Horwitz D, Pisano JJ et al: Urinary kallikrein excretion in hypertensive man. Relationship to sodium intake and sodium-retaining steroids. Circ Res 1974;35:820–825

147. Brenner BM, Troy JL, Daugharty TM: Quantitative importance of changes in post-glomerular colloid osmotic pressure in mediating tubular balance in the rat. J Clin Invest 1973;52:190–197

148. Ichikawa I, Brenner BM: Importance of efferent arteriolar vascular tone in regulation of proximal tubule fluid reabsorption and glomerulotubular balance in the rat. J Clin Invest 1980;65:1192–1201

149. Meyers BD, Deen WM, Brenner BM: Effects of norepinephrine and angiotensin II on the determinants of glomerular ultrafiltration and proximal tubule fluid reabsorption in the rat. Circ Res 1975;37:101–110

150. Barger AC: Renal hemodynamics in congestive heart failure. Ann NY Acad Sci 1966;139:276–284

151. Brod J, Fejfar Z, Fejfarova MH: The role of neurohumoral factors in the genesis of renal hemodynamic changes in heart failure. Acta Med Scand 1954;148:273–290

152. Creager MA, Halperin JL, Bernard DB et al: Acute regional circulatory and renal hemodynamic effects of converting enzyme inhibition in patients with congestive heart failure. Circulation 1981;64:483–489

153. Dzau VJ, Colucci WS, Williams GH et al: Sustained effectiveness of converting enzyme inhibition in patients with severe congestive heart failure. N Engl J Med 1980;302:1373–1379

154. Mokotoff RG, Ross G: The effect of spinal anesthesia on the renal ischemia in congestive heart failure. J Clin Invest 1948;27:335–339

155. Freeman RH, Davis JO, Williams GM et al: Effects of the oral converting enzyme inhibitor SQ14225 in a model of low cardiac output in dogs. Circ Res 1979;45:540–545

156. Ichikawa I, Pfeffer JM, Pfeffer MA, Hostetter TH, Brenner BM: Role of angiotensin II in the altered renal function of congestive heart failure. Circ Res 1984;55:669–675

157. Levy M: Effects of acute volume expansion and altered hemodynamics on renal tubular function in chronic caval dogs. J Clin Invest 1972;5:922–938

158. Mandin H: Cardiac edema in dogs. I. Proximal tubular and renal function. Kidney Int 1976;10:591–598

159. Stumpe KO, Solle H, Klein H, et al: Mechanism of sodium and water retention in rats with experimental heart failure. Kidney Int 1973;4:309–317

160. Osgood RW, Reineck HJ, Stein JH: Further studies in segmental sodium transport in rat kidney during expansion of extracellular volume. J Clin Invest 1978;62:311–320

161. Stein JH, Reineck HJ: The role of collecting duct in the regulation of excretion of sodium and other electrolytes. Kidney Int 1974;6:1–9

162. Kilcoyne MM, Schmidt DH, Cannon PJ: Intrarenal blood flow in congestive heart failure. Circulation 1973;47:787–797

163. Humes HD, Gottlieb M, Brenner BM: The kidney in congestive heart failure. pp. 51–72. In Brenner BM, Stein JH (eds): Sodium and Water Homeostasis. Churchill Livingstone, New York, 1978

12 Endothelial Factors

Helmut Drexler

The endothelium plays an important role in the regulation of vascular tone by releasing relaxing and contracting factors under basal conditions and, when activated, by neurotransmitters, hormones, autacoids, or physical stimuli (Fig. 12-1). Located between the lumen and the underlying media of the vascular wall, the endothelium represents both a target and a modulator of blood pressure or hormonal influences (or both). Alterations in endothelial function, such as impaired release of endothelium-derived relaxing factors or increased release of endothelium-derived contracting factors emerge in numerous pathophysiologic conditions, including all known risk factors for atherosclerosis.

ENDOTHELIUM-DEPENDENT CONTROL OF VASCULAR TONE

Endothelium-Derived Relaxing Factors

Numerous factors such as neurotransmitters, hormones, platelet-derived factors, and substances involved in homeostasis of thrombosis and fibrinolysis can elicit endothelium-dependent relaxations[1] by stimulating the release of endothelium-derived factors, in particular EDRF,[2] a yet to be identified endothelium-hyperpolarizing factor (EDHF),[3] and prostaglandin (PGI$_2$). Importantly, shear stress exerted by the circulating blood represents an important stimulus for endothelium-dependent vasodilation.[4–7] To a large extent, endothelium-dependent relaxations are mediated by EDRF, whose biologic activity is pro-

vided by nitric oxide[8] or a closely related substance that incorporates nitric oxide (i.e., a nitrosylated compound).[9]

ENDOTHELIUM-DERIVED NITRIC OXIDE

Nitric oxide is formed from L-arginine by oxidation of the guanidine-nitrogen terminal of L-arginine[10] by an endothelial nitric oxide synthase.[11,12] This calcium-dependent enzyme generates picomoles of nitric oxide. Early observations suggested that this endothelial nitric oxide synthase is constitutively expressed, but more recent studies have shown that several stimuli, such as estrogens or shear stress, affect expression of the endothelial (constitutive) nitric oxide synthase (cNOS).[13,14] Other isoforms of the enzyme have been identified and cloned, one occurring in the brain, peripheral nerves, and skeletal muscle (bNOS).[15] A calcium-independent, highly inducible nitric oxide synthase (iNOS)[16,17] has also been found that produces large amounts of nitric oxide (i.e., nanomoles) and is expressed only upon stimulation by cytokines. iNOS has been identified in numerous tissues, including endothelial cells, smooth muscle cells, cardiac myocytes, macrophages, and hepatocytes. The synthesis of nitric oxide from L-arginine can be inhibited in vivo by analogs of L-arginine, such as L-N^G-monomethyl arginine (L-NMMA) and are restored by L-arginine but not D-arginine.[18] When infused in humans, L-NMMA causes long-lasting increases in vascular resistance that are reversed by L-arginine,[19] indicating that the vasculature is in a constant state of vasodilation as a result of the continuous release of nitric oxide from

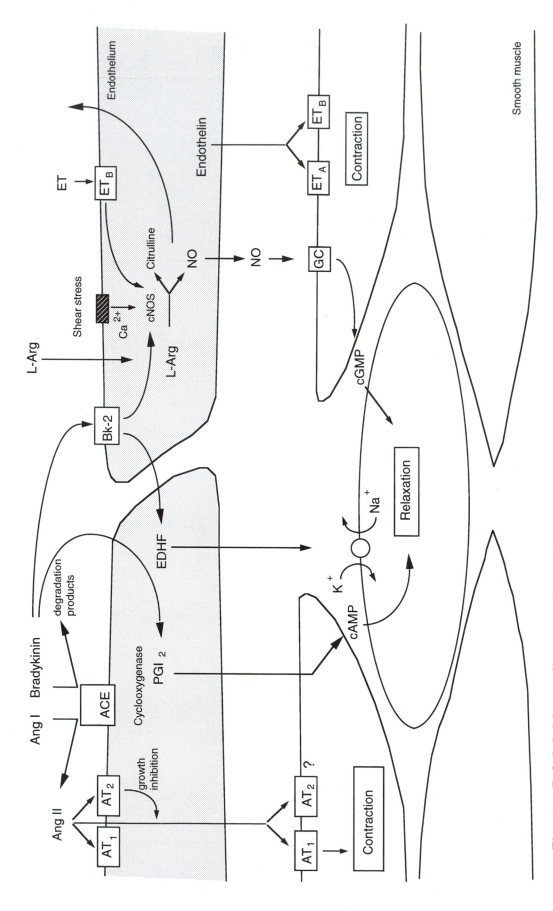

Fig. 12-1. Endothelial factors affecting vascular tone by relaxing or constricting the underlying smooth muscle cells. Ang II and I, angiotensin I and II; AT$_1$ and AT$_2$, angiotensin II receptors; ACE, angiotensin-converting enzyme; PG$_2$, prostacyclin; EDHF, endothelium-derived hyperpolarization factor; BK-2, brady-kinin 2 receptor L-Arg, L-arginine; cNOS, endothelial nitric oxide synthase; NO, nitric oxide; ET, endothelin; ET$_A$ and ET$_B$ endothelin receptors. For further explanation see text.

the endothelium. The systemic administration of L-NMMA in humans has confirmed animal studies showing that the basal release of nitric oxide is involved in maintaining normal blood pressure and vascular resistance in humans.[20,21] The trigger for the basal release of nitric oxide is provided by basal blood flow eliciting a baseline stress at the endothelial surface.[22] Nitric oxide acts by activating guanylate cyclase at the vascular smooth muscle, causing an increase in cyclic 3'5'-guanosine monophosphate (cGMP) and subsequently relaxation of vascular smooth muscle. Platelets express nitric oxide synthase,[23] and soluble guanylate cyclase is also present in platelets and can be activated by nitric oxide. Increased levels of cGMP in platelets are associated with reduced adhesion and aggregation. Thus nitric oxide causes vasodilatation and prevents platelet activation, providing an important antithrombotic feature of the endothelium.

VASCULAR SMOOTH MUSCLE-DERIVED NITRIC OXIDE

Although the blood vessel wall normally does not produce nitric oxide, vascular smooth muscle cells can express iNOS upon stimulation by cytokines with subsequent production of nitric oxide in smooth muscle.[24] Activation of the L-arginine pathway in smooth muscle cells by endotoxin, tumor necrosis factor, and interleukins may play a role in septic shock and may explain why the cardiovascular system becomes resistant to catecholamines under these conditions.

PROSTACYCLIN

Prostacyclin is the major product of vascular cyclooxygenase.[25] It is formed primarily in the intima but also in the media and adventitia in response to shear stress, hypoxia, and several mediators that also lead to the formation of nitric oxide. However, the contribution of prostacyclin to endothelium-dependent relaxation appears to be modest or even negligible in different circulatory beds. Prostacyclin increases cyclic 3'5'-adenosine monophosphate (cAMP) in smooth muscle and platelets, where it inhibits platelet aggregation. In human platelets, nitric oxide and prostacyclin synergistically inhibit platelet aggregation.[26]

ENDOTHELIUM-DERIVED HYPERPOLARIZATION FACTORS

Several observations strongly suggest the existence of an additional endothelium-derived relaxing factor(s). It has been shown that bradykinin or acetylcholine elicits endothelium-dependent relaxation following pretreatment with L-NMMA and indomethacin. These pretreatments block the potential contribution of nitric oxide and prostaglandin. Several candidates for these responses have been proposed, including an endothelium-dependent hyperpolarizing factor,[3,4] which may be derived from the cytochrome P-450 pathway. Acetylcholine and bradykinin cause an endothelium-dependent relaxation not only by releasing nitric oxide but also by endothelium-dependent hyperpolarization of vascular smooth muscle; however, the nature of the putative endothelium-derived relaxing factors has not been identified. The endothelium-derived hyperpolarizing factor appears to activate adenosine triphosphate (ATP)-sensitive K^+ channels and Na^+,K^+-ATPase in smooth muscle.[27] The hyperpolarization may contribute to endothelium-dependent relaxations or reduce the sensitivity of vascular smooth muscle to vasoconstrictor stimuli.

Endothelium-Derived Contracting Factors

CYCLOOXYGENASE-DEPENDENT ENDOTHEKIUM-DERIVED CONTRACTING FACTOR

Exogenous arachidonic acid can elicit endothelium-dependent contractions, which can be prevented by indomethacin, an inhibitor of cyclooxygenase.[28] In the human saphenous vein, acetylcholine and histamine evoke endothelium-dependent contractions; in the presence of indomethacin, however, endothelium-dependent relaxations are unmasked.[29] Acetylcholine-induced contractions are mediated by cyclooxygenase-dependent substances, such as thromboxane A_2, or endoperoxides (prostaglandin H_2) in the case of histamine-induced constriction.[29] Thromboxane A_2 and endoperoxide activate both vascular smooth muscle and platelets. Furthermore, the cyclooxygenase pathway is a source of superoxide anions that can mediate endothelium-dependent contractions by either the breakdown of nitric oxide or direct effects on vascular smooth muscle.[30,31] Thus the cyclooxygenase pathway produces a variety of endothelium-derived contracting factors (EDCFs).

ENDOTHELIN

Endothelial cells produce the 21-amino-acid peptide endothelin 1 (ET-1).[32] Two other forms, endothelin 2 and endothelin 3, have been characterized and differ in two and five residues from ET-1.[33] Translation

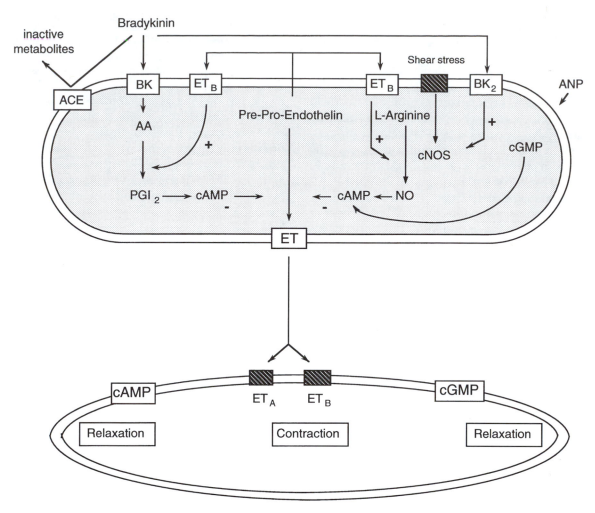

Fig. 12-2. Endothelin, its receptors, and its interactions with other endothelium-derived factors. cNOS, endothelial nitric acid synthase; NO, nitric oxide; cGMP, cyclic guanosine monophosphate ACE, angiotensin-converting enzyme.

of messenger RNA generates preproendothelin, which is converted to big endothelin. The conversion of big endothelin to ET-1 by the endothelin-converting enzyme is necessary for the development of full vascular activity. The expression of messenger RNA and the release of the peptide is stimulated by several factors including thrombin, transforming growth factor β (TGFβ), interleukin 1, epinephrine, and angiotensin II.

Endothelin 1 is a potent vasoconstrictor in vitro and in vivo, acting on endothelin A and B receptors (Fig. 12-2). Infusion of endothelin in humans causes marked vasoconstriction; but at lower concentrations endothelin causes vasodilation by releasing nitric oxide and prostacyclin, which may represent a negative feedback mechanism.[34,35] The circulating levels of ET-1 are low. This finding suggests either that little of the peptide is synthesized under physiologic conditions (i.e., in the absence of stimuli or the presence of potent inhibitory mechanisms) or that endothelin is released predominantly toward smooth muscle cells.[36] Endothelin synthesis can be inhibited by several mechanisms, including cGMP-dependent inhibition and cAMP-dependent inhibition.[37] The cGMP-dependent mechanism can be activated by nitric oxide and atrial natriuretic peptide, which activates particularly guanylate cyclase. It has been shown that after inhibition of the endothelial L-arginine pathway the thrombin-induced production of endothelin is augmented.[37] Moreover, inhibition of nitric oxide synthesis unmasks a tonic pressor influence of endothelin in vivo,[38] suggesting that this peptide is likely to play a major role in pathophysiologic conditions such as chronic heart failure associated with impaired formation of nitric oxide (see below). Based on these and other (experimental) observations one must consider that regional vasoconstriction may develop secondary to removal of vasodilating actions by nitric oxide (or prostaglandins),[39] which then gives rise to the actions of increasing levels of vasoconstricting factors such as endothelin (whose synthesis is enhanced in the absence of nitric oxide).[40] It should be emphasized that vascular tone is the net effect of interactions between vasodilating and vasoconstricting factors. In this respect, the application of endothelin antagonists have provided convincing evidence that ET-1 exerts a continuous influence on the human vascular system. Inhibition of the conversion of proendothelin to ET-1 and the administration of a selective ET-1 antagonist resulted in a substantial increase in forearm blood flow in normal volunteers.[41] These observations clearly indicate that ET-1 is released under physiologic conditions and is involved in the regulation of peripheral vascular tone in humans.

ENDOTHELIUM DURING HEART FAILURE

During chronic heart failure, systemic compensatory mechanisms are activated to maintain arterial blood pressure in the face of reduced cardiac output. In particular, the sympathetic system and the renin-angiotensin system are activated, contributing to increased systemic vasoconstriction.[42] Yet short-term α-adrenergic blockade or angiotensin-converting enzyme (ACE) inhibition is not accompanied by increased blood flow to skeletal muscle during exercise, indicating that factors other than norepinephrine or angiotensin II are involved in the impaired blood flow response during exercise.[43,44] Whereas neurohumoral factors have been studied extensively in the past, the impact of local factors regulating peripheral vasomotor tone and tissue perfusion during heart failure remain poorly defined.

Endothelium-Dependent Relaxation During Chronic Heart Failure

Based on observations in animal models of heart failure, depression of endothelium-dependent vasodilation was proposed to represent one local mechanism involved in the impaired metabolic vasodilation in patients with chronic heart failure. Kaiser et al. first noted that endothelium-dependent relaxations of the femoral artery in response to acetylcholine are impaired in the pacing dog model of heart failure.[45] These observations were confirmed in other models of heart failure; reduced endothelial dependent dilations were demonstrated in the aorta of rats with myocardial infarction and failure.[46] There is some

evidence that endothelial dysfunction emerges slowly over time after infarction.[47] Moreover, impaired endothelium-dependent relaxations have been shown to occur in peripheral resistance vessels in this model,[48] which raised the possibility that endothelial dysfunction may be involved in the impaired tissue perfusion during heart failure. Several clinical studies have now studied endothelial function in patients with heart failure. By assessing the blood flow response to acetylcholine in the forearm or hindlimb, these studies have demonstrated an impaired acetylcholine-induced increase in blood flow in patients with severe heart failure.[49–51] There is evidence that the release of EDRF in humans is stimulated by acetylcholine.[19] Although an interaction of acetylcholine and α-adrenergic receptors cannot be totally excluded during heart failure, the effect of acetylcholine in normal individuals was not inhibited by pretreatment with phentolamine,[52] which indicates that EDRF is involved in the endothelium-dependent relaxation by acetylcholine. Indeed, the vascular responses to acetylcholine can be blocked in part by L-NMMA, a selective inhibitor of nitric oxide from L-arginine.[19]

In addition, impaired endothelium-dependent dilation was documented in peripheral conduit vessels in patients with severe heart failure. Although the response to acetylcholine in human conduit vessels is modest in normal volunteers and patients with heart failure, flow-dependent dilation appears to be a sensitive measure of endothelium-dependent dilation in human conduit vessels. Experimental studies have shown that flow-dependent dilation is mediated by the endothelium, that is, by the release of EDRF.[5,6] There is preliminary evidence that flow-dependent dilation in humans is mediated, to a large extent, by the release of nitric oxide, as flow-dependent dilation can be blunted to 60 to 70 percent by N-monomethyl-L-arginine, an inhibitor of nitric oxide synthesis.[53] Using this approach, our studies have shown that flow-dependent dilation during reactive hyperemia is reduced in patients with chronic heart failure.[54] Because both the dilator response to the endothelium-independent agent nitroglycerin and to the endothelium-dependent intervention (increased flow) are impaired, abnormalities of both the cGMP signal pathway (or structural alterations associated with a decreased vasodilatory capacity) and endothelial dysfunction appear to be present in human conduit vessels in CHF. Consistent with this interpretation, Arnold et al. demonstrated impaired vascular compliance of large conduit arteries in patients with chronic heart failure.[55] Endothelial dysfunction of conduit vessels may have functional consequences, as it impairs the elastic properties of large conduit vessels and has a negative feedback on the pumping performance of the left ventricle.[56] There is preliminary evidence that EDRF dynamically controls large artery distensibility, suggesting a physiologic role for EDRF in reducing cardiac work relative to tissue perfusion by affecting arterial impedence.[57] However, it remains to be shown that the impaired large artery compliance in patients with chronic heart failure[55] is related to endothelial dysfunction or which factors are involved in this vascular abnormality.

Notably, coronary artery disease is the primary underlying cause of chronic heart failure, followed by hypertension. Risk factors for coronary artery disease, such as hypercholesterolemia, are associated with endothelial dysfunction. To establish heart failure as a causal factor for the presence of endothelial dysfunction, these other conditions associated with endothelial dysfunction must be ruled out. However, endothelial dysfunction of peripheral resistance and conduit vessels do occur in patients with dilated cardiomyopathy without a history of hypertension, diabetes, or other risk factors,[50,51] indicating that heart failure per se is associated with endothelial dysfunction.

Basal Release of Nitric Oxide During Chronic Heart Failure

As discussed above, endothelium-dependent dilation of forearm resistance vessels in response to acetylcholine is impaired with chronic heart failure, suggesting a reduced *stimulated release* of nitric oxide in response to acetylcholine. In contrast to the responses elicited by acetylcholine, it appears that the basal release of nitric oxide from peripheral resistance vessels is enhanced during advanced stages of heart failure rather than impaired. This tentative conclusion is derived from three approaches. In patients with chronic heart failure, the decrease in forearm blood flow by L-NMMA was enhanced in patients with chronic heart failure compared to that of age-matched normal volunteers[51]; that is, blockade of the basal release resulted in an exaggerated vasoconstrictor response in heart failure patients (Fig. 12-3). Similarly, after systemic administration of L-NMMA, Habib et al. observed that the increase in systemic vascular resistance was greatest in those patients with heart failure who already had the highest basal systemic vascular resistance.[58] Moreover, Winlaw et al. measured plasma nitrate, the stable end-product of nitric oxide production, and reported increased levels in patients with heart failure.[59] Taken together, these observations suggest that the *basal release*

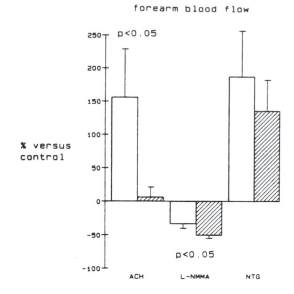

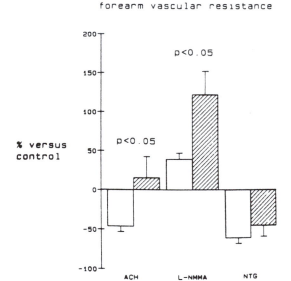

Fig. 12-3. Maximal percent change in forearm blood flow and vascular resistance versus control induced by acetylcholine (ACH) (endothelium-dependent), *N*-monomethyl-L-arginine (L-NMMA) (inhibitor of nitric oxide synthesis), and nitroglycerin (NTG) (endothelium-independent) in control subjects ($n = 6$) and patients with congestive heart failure (CHF) ($n = 6$). Data are mean ± SEM. The *p* values donote statistical significance between percent changes in control subjects and patients with heart failure. □, normal, ▨, CHF. (From Drexler et al.,[51] with permission.)

of nitric oxide, in an compensatory manner, is enhanced. It should be noted, however, that heightened vasoconstrictor tone is present during heart failure, and therefore the effect of any additional vasoconstrictor agent may be enhanced in this setting; however, the demonstration of increased plasma levels of nitrates in patients with heart failure (not treated with nitrates!) and the relation between nitrate levels and NYHA class of these patients[60] support the principal concept.

It should be noted that some investigators have found no differences between patients with and without heart failure,[61] and one group reported that the effect of L-NMMA was attenuated.[62] More studies are needed to clarify whether the conflicting results with L-NMMA are related to different patient populations (i.e., severity of heart failure, treatment regimens, or cytokine activation). Nevertheless, taken together, these observations raise the possibility that basal nitric oxide may play a counteracting role in patients with chronic heart failure; that is, the increased basal release of nitric oxide from resistance vessels may contribute, in a compensatory manner, to the maintenance of adequate tissue perfusion at rest, providing an important local "endogenous" vasodilator system to antagonize neurohumoral vasoconstrictor forces. The source of nitric oxide in response to cytokinine activation remains to be determined. The induction of iNOS in vascular smooth muscle represents one possibility, but induction of iNOS may occur in leukocytes, particularly monocytes.

Potential Mechanisms for Development of Endothelial Dysfunction During Heart Failure

Notably, endothelial dysfunction appears to be a time-dependent alteration, occurring slowly over time, particularly with more advanced stages of heart failure. Although endothelium-dependent relaxations stimulated by acetylcholine (presumably by the release of nitric oxide) are impaired during heart failure, the basal release of nitric oxide may be enhanced, particularly with more advanced stages of chronic heart failure. Circulating cytokines, particularly, tumor necrosis factor (TNF), are increased in severe chronic heart failure.[63] Experimental evidence suggests that TNF-α is able to impair the stimulated release of EDRF[64] and the stability of the endothelial nitric oxide synthase mRNA[65] (the enzyme that cleaves nitric oxide from L-arginine). Katz et al. showed that plasma levels of TNF in patients with heart failure are related to the degree of endothelial dysfunction as tested by acetylcholine.[66] Thus the impaired endothelium-dependent relaxations stimulated by agents such as acetylcholine may be attributed to increased plasma levels of cytokines. In contrast, TNF-α has been shown to induce iNOS in vascular smooth muscle,

endothelium, or both. Although speculative at present, the induction of iNOS could provide a molecular mechanism for the increased basal release of nitric oxide in patients with chronic heart failure and elevated plasma levels of cytokines (Fig. 12-4).

Other potential mechanisms involved in the pathogenesis of endothelial dysfunction during heart failure include chronically decreased blood flow,[67] increased tissue ACE activity, or inactivation of nitric oxide by increased radical formation during chronic heart failure. Increased oxygen free radicals have been indirectly implicated in chronic heart failure and its severity by demonstrating increased levels of plasma lipid peroxides and thiols.[68] Increased radical activity in chronic heart failure may be related to autoxidation of increased levels of catecholamines[69] due to increased radical formation in response to angiotensin II[70] or may be provided by polymorphonuclear leukocytes.[71] The oxygen-derived free radical superoxide has been shown to inactivate nitric oxide[30] and inhibit endothelial-dependent relaxations.[72] In addition, a decreased capacity of free radical scavenging may emerge during chronic heart failure.

There is some experimental evidence that hemodynamics play a determinant role in the altered vasodilator response in heart failure,[73,74] possibly related to reduced expression of endothelial nitric oxide synthase, which is regulated by shear stress. Flow-dependent dilation is thought to be endothelium-dependent due to the release of EDRF.[7,75] Indeed, flow-dependent dilation can be inhibited by L-NMMA in humans, indicating that the dilation in response to increased flow in humans is mediated by nitric oxide.[53] Conceivably, chronically reduced blood flow would result in impaired flow-dependent dilation. Changes in flow affect both the expression of nitric oxide synthase and endothelin, which is down-regulated with increased shear stress. Chronic increases in blood flow enhance the release of EDRF from the endothelium, and a 10-day exercise program increased the expression of the endothelial cNOS in normal dogs. Vice versa, chronic inactivation of patients with chronic heart failure may be associated with decreased expression of cNOS and consequently impaired release of nitric oxide. Indeed, flow-dependent dilation during reactive hyperemia is reduced in patients with chronic heart failure,[54] and preliminary data from our laboratory suggest that intermittent physical exercise over 4 weeks improves flow-dependent dilation in patients with chronic heart failure.

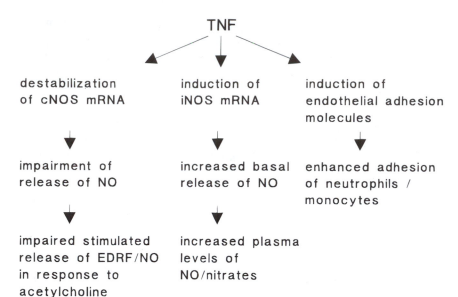

Fig. 12-4. Potential role of cytokines, including tumor necrosis factor (TNF), for endothelial dysfunction in chronic heart failure. cNOS, endothelial nitric oxide synthase; NO, nitric oxide; iNOS, inducible nitric oxide synthase; EDRF, endothelium-derived relaxing factor.

Endothelium-Derived Contracting Factors

CYCLOOXYGENASE-DEPENDENT ENDOTHELIUM-DERIVED CONTRACTING FACTOR

It should be noted that the vasomotor response to acetylcholine in patients with heart failure cannot be merely attributed to the release of EDRF. Acetylcholine-stimulated release of a cyclooxygenase-dependent vasoconstrictor substance has been reported previously in a femoral artery preparation from a canine model of heart failure.[45] More recently, evidence was presented that the reduced vasodilator response to acetylcholine in patients with chronic heart failure includes abnormal production and release of a cyclooxygenase-dependent vasoconstrictor.[76] Moreover, the vasodilatory response to nitroglycerin may be reduced in these patients with severe heart failure, suggesting decreased vascular smooth muscle responsiveness to cGMP-mediated vasodilation. Although there are conflicting data concerning the regional vascular dilator response to nitrates in patients with heart failure, the controversy may be reconciled by acknowledging the different patient populations studied. During the compensated stage of heart failure, the response of peripheral resistance vessels to nitroglycerin is usually preserved, whereas in severe cases, particularly at an edematous stage, the vasodilator response to nitroglycerin or nitroprusside is impaired. A potential mechanism involved in the impaired nitrate-induced dilation of peripheral resistance vessels during chronic heart failure includes a vascular stiffness component owing to the increased vascular sodium content, which can be in part reduced with diuretic therapy during decompensated heart failure.[77] However, a generalized defect within the guanylate cyclase system appears unlikely to account for the abnormal vascular responses seen in patients with chronic heart failure, as a blunted response to acetylcholine has been observed in patients with normal blood flow responses to nitroglycerin or sodium nitroprusside.[49,50]

ENDOTHELIN

Plasma endothelin levels are increased in animal models of heart failure and in patients with chronic heart failure. The degree of plasma elevation of plasma endothelin correlates with the magnitude of alterations in cardiac hemodynamics and functional class. Cardiac tissue endothelin is not increased in patients with heart failure, suggesting that the heart is not the source but, rather, a target of increased circulating endothelin concentrations.[78] By calculating the endothelin spillover in the lungs, data suggest that the main source of circulating plasma ET-1 is the pulmonary bed in patients with heart failure.[79] A close correlation between ET-1 levels and pulmonary vascular resistance was observed, and therefore this peptide may act mainly as a local factor. In contrast, endothelium-dependent dilation in response to acetylcholine appears to be attenuated in patients with chronic heart failure and pulmonary hypertension (or the vasoconstricting effects of acetylcholine are enhanced owing to the diminished release of nitric oxide).[80]

Numerous studies have evaluated plasma levels of endothelin during heart failure and the vasomotor responses to exogenous endothelin; the more recent approaches utilized endothelin receptor antagonists and inhibitors of endothelin-converting enzyme. In preliminary studies antiendothelin interventions were associated with increases in forearm blood flow in patients on medical therapy including ACE inhibitors.[81] When administered systemically, a significant fall in left ventricular filling pressures and a modest increase in cardiac output was observed in patients with chronic heart failure.[82] These observations suggest that the increased circulating plasma levels of endothelin during heart failure exert vascular effects. An experimental study demonstrated that endothelin is involved in the maintenance of blood pressure in rats with chronic heart failure[83]; in this study, long-term administration of an orally active endothelin antagonist reduced blood pressure even in rats treated with an ACE inhibitor, indicating a vasoactive role of endothelin independent of ACE inhibition. As noted above, it remains to be determined whether the increase in endothelin plasma levels is an event secondary to the impaired availability of nitric oxide or an independent event (i.e., in response to tissue hypoxia).

Functional Consequences of Endothelial Dysfunction During Heart Failure

Significant relations between peripheral endothelial function and peak oxygen consumption and ventilatory threshold have been documented raising the possibility that endothelial function may contribute to exercise capacity in patients with chronic heart failure.[84] A key issue is to what extent abnormalities of local endothelial function are involved in the impaired vasodilator response of the peripheral vasculature in patients with chronic heart failure. It is possible that the increased basal release of nitric oxide from resistance vessels may contribute, in a compensatory manner, to maintain adequate tissue perfusion at rest, thereby providing an important local "endogenous" vasodilator system to antagonize neurohumoral vasoconstrictor forces. However, the stimulated release of nitric oxide (i.e., during exercise) may be limited and therefore could affect tissue perfusion during exercise.

Previous observations suggest that impaired calf blood flow during exercise is associated with reduced exercise capacity, although intrinsic abnormalities of skeletal muscle contribute to reduced exercise capacity in this patient population. Hirooka et al. provided some evidence that defective endothelial function contributes to impaired ischemic vasodilator

capacity during heart failure.[85] In this study, reactive hyperemic blood flow was attenuated in patients with heart failure compared to that of normal individuals. After intraarterial infusion of L-arginine, minimal forearm vascular resistance during reactive hyperemia was significantly decreased in patients with heart failure but not in normal individuals. Similarly, L-arginine significantly augmented maximal vasodilation evoked by acetylcholine. These observations suggest that decreased maximal vasodilation in response to ischemic stimuli in patients with heart failure may be partly due to a defect in the release (or synthesis) of nitric oxide from the endothelium. These findings are consistent with experimental data indicating that nitric oxide partly regulates vascular resistance during exercise in conscious dogs.[86] Conflicting observations have been reported in humans: One study failed to document a contribution of EDRF to exercise-induced vasodilation in humans,[87] whereas others claim a role of nitric oxide, albeit modest, in exercise-induced hyperemia.[88] Notably, the beneficial effect of L-arginine was observed only in patients with heart failure, not in normal individuals,[85] but the benefit was modest at best.

Interventions To Improve Endothelial Dysfunction During Heart Failure

Other potential mechanisms, listed in Table 12-1, include increased tissue ACE activity. The latter may increase the local degradation of bradykinin, as ACE acts also as kinase II and degrades circulating kinins (kinins act as a stimulus for the release of EDRF).

Long-term but not short-term ACE inhibition im-

Table 12-1. Putative Mechanisms for Endothelial Dysfunction in Heart Failure

Increased levels of cytokines (i.e., tumor necrosis factor—impairs the synthesis of endothelial NO synthase)

Increased angiotensin-converting enzyme activity (increased breakdown of bradykinin)

Increased levels of oxygen radicals ($\rightarrow$ inactivation of EDRF/NO)

Chronically reduced blood flow (decreased expression of endothelial NO synthase)

Increased endothelial-dependent vasoconstrictor agents (i.e., cyclooxygenase-dependent)

Impaired endothelial receptor-signal transduction pathways (i.e., dysfunctional muscarinic receptor)

Abbreviations: NO, nitric oxide; EDRF, endothelium-derived relaxing factors.

proves skeletal muscle blood flow and oxygen extraction during exercise.[43,89] Given experimental observations that long-term treatment with ACE inhibitors improves aortic endothelial dysfunction in experimental heart failure,[90] one might expect that long-term ACE inhibition improves skeletal muscle flow by correcting endothelial dysfunction. Preliminary data suggest that the increase in forearm blood flow elicited by acute administration of enalapril is mediated by prostaglandins, as the effect of enalapril was attenuated after pretreatment with indomethacin or aspirin.[91,92] The contribution of bradykinin and nitric oxide remains uncertain. One clinical study reported that captopril given acutely improves impaired endothelium-dependent vasodilation in hypertensive patients.[93] This finding is surprising, as the beneficial effect on the acetylcholine-induced increase in flow is independent of bradykinin. Based on experimental findings, the beneficial effect of ACE inhibitors can be best explained by the interference with the breakdown of bradykinin. Inhibition of the ACE may increase local tissue levels of bradykinin, which in turn stimulates the release of nitric oxide (which accounts for the biologic activity of the endothelium-derived relaxing factor EDRF) and vasodilating prostaglandins.[94,95] Thus the beneficial effect of ACE inhibitors on endothelial function might be due to inhibition of the breakdown of bradykinin, which is degraded by the ACE. The significance of an acute effect of captopril on endothelial function for the long-term treatment of hypertension awaits clinical trials with chronic ACE inhibitor therapy. Preliminary data from our laboratory suggest that long-term ACE inhibition improves (but does not completely restore) endothelial function (as tested by acetylcholine) in patients with chronic heart failure (unpublished observations). Similarly, physical training has the potential to improve peripheral endothelial dysfunction in patients with chronic heart failure. Several studies are under way to address this important issue. Endothelium-dependent dilation has been demonstrated to improve after cardiac transplantation, again indicating that endothelial dysfunction is reversible.[96] Because that beneficial effect of cardiac transplantation occurred in the setting of overall improved responsiveness of the peripheral vasculature, the independent effect of improved cardiocirculatory status on endothelial function remains to be established.

ENDOTHELIAL DYSFUNCTION IN THE CORONARY CIRCULATION

Coronary artery disease and hypertension, two major causes of heart failure, are associated with endothelial dysfunction of the coronary circulation. Impaired relaxation of the microvasculature has been demonstrated in patients with dilated cardiomyopathy in response to the endothelium-dependent vasodilator acetylcholine.[97,98] This impairment was out of proportion to the modestly impaired response to adenosine, an endothelium-independent dilator of vascular smooth muscle. The impaired relaxation in response to acetylcholine with an almost normal relaxation response to adenosine suggests that extravascular factors do not completely explain the different responses of normal and cardiomyopathic patients to acetylcholine. These observations suggest that endothelial dysfunction emerges in the microvasculature of hearts with dilated cardiomyopathy, although extravascular influences may also contribute to the impaired coronary blood flow responses.[98] This view is supported by preliminary observations suggesting that myocardial endothelial nitric oxide activity is reduced in patients with dilated cardiomyopathy,[99] although the genetic expression of endothelial nitric oxide synthase is not decreased in these patients.[100]

The underlying mechanism for endothelial dysfunction in the coronary microvessels of patients with dilated cardiomyopathy remains to be defined. It is possible that the coronary endothelium is dysfunctional because of severe heart failure[101] or severe left ventricular (LV) hypertrophy. The patients studied by Treasure et al. were in a well compensated state[97]; therefore heart failure appears unlikely to account for these alterations. Previous studies have documented endothelial dysfunction in patients with systemic hypertension and LV hypertrophy, but it is impossible to differentiate whether hypertension, LV hypertrophy, or both were responsible for endothelial dysfunction in the coronary circulation in these patients. Notably, experimental data suggest that LV hypertrophy in the absence of hypertension can be associated with endothelial dysfunction of the coronary circulation.[102] Alternatively, endothelial dysfunction may represent an intrinsic abnormality in patients with dilated cardiomyopathy, and the resulting impaired endothelium-mediated vascular regulation could be involved in the progression of the disease.

In this respect, there is experimental evidence for cell–cell signaling between cardiac myocytes and microvascular endothelial cells[103]; for example, co-culture of endothelial cells and myocytes is associated with increased expression of preproendothelin RNA levels in endothelial cells, which in turn may affect cardiac function.[104] In addition, experimental evidence has indicated that endothelial cells are required for the cAMP-dependent regulation of cardiac proteins.[105] Nitric oxide has been shown to abbreviate myocardial contraction and modulate relaxation, possibly via cGMP-mediated pathways, resulting in a reduced, relative myofilament response to Ca^{2+}.[106] Indeed, Paulus et al. have provided data indicating that nitric oxide affects LV relaxation and diastolic distensibility in humans.[107] Thus it appears that the endothelium has some influence on myocardial performance by releasing relaxing factors such as nitric oxide and constricting factors such as endothelin (which has been shown to be released under hypoxic conditions). Future studies will undoubtedly identify the impact of endothelium-derived factors on cardiac performance (for review see Paulus[108]). Moreover, it has been shown that cardiac myocytes can express both the endothelial[109] and inducible nitric oxide synthases (upon stimulation with cytokines),[110,111] thereby representing an autocrine system to modulate cardiac performance. cNOS and iNOS mRNA activities have been shown to be present in patients with ischemic and dilated cardiomyopathy,[99,100,112] in particular in patients with myocarditis.[113] Future studies are needed to elucidate the functional significance of these observations.

REFERENCES

1. Lüscher TF, Vanhoutte PM: The Endothelium Modulator of Cardiovascular Function. pp. 1–215. CRC Press, Boca Raton, Fl, 1990
2. Furchgott RF, Zawadzki JV: The obligatory role of endothelial cells in the relaxation of arterial smooth muscle by acetylcholine. Nature 1980;299:373
3. Feletou M, Vanhoutte PM: Endothelium-dependent hyperpolarization of canine coronary smooth muscle. Br J Pharmacol 1988;93:515
4. Taylor SG, Weston AH: Endothelium-derived hyperpolarizing factor. A new endogenous inhibitor from the vascular endothelium. TIPS 1988;9:272
5. Pohl U, Holtz J, Busse R, Basenge E: Crucial role of endothelium in the vasodilator response to increased flow in vivo. Hypertension 1986;8:37
6. Rubanyi GM, Romero JC, Vanhoutte PM: Flow-induced release of endothelium-derived relaxing factor. Am J Physiol 1986;231:H405
7. Holtz J, Förstermann U, Pohl U, Giesler M, Bassenge E: Flow-dependent, endothelium-mediated dilation of epicardial coronary arteries in conscious dogs. Effects of cyclooxygenase inhibition. J Cardiovasc Pharmacol 1984;6:1161
8. Palmer RMJ, Ferrige AG, Moncada S: Nitric oxide release accounts for the biological activity of endothelium-derived relaxing factor. Nature 1987;327:524
9. Myers PR, Minor RL Jr, Guerra R Jr et al: Vasorelaxant properties of the endothelium-derived relaxing factor more closely resemble S-nitrocysteine than nitric oxide. Nature 1990;345:161
10. Palmer RMJ, Ashton DS, Moncada S: Vascular endothelial cells synthesize nitric oxide from L-arginine. Nature 1988;333:664

11. Sessa WC, Harrison JK, Durieux ME et al: Molecular cloning and expression of a cDNA encoding endothelial cell nitric oxide synthase. J Biol Chem 1992;267:15274
12. Lamas S, Marsden PA, Li GK, Tempst P, Michel T: Endothelial nitric oxide synthase. Molecular cloning and characterization of a distinct constitutive enzyme isoform. Proc Natl Acad Sci USA 1992;89:6348
13. Weiner CP, Lizasoain I, Baylis SA et al: Induction of calcium-dependent nitric oxide synthases by sex hormones. Proc Natl Acad Sci USA 1994;91:5212
14. Nishida K, Harrison DG, Navas JP et al: Molecular cloning and characterization of the constitutive bovine aortic endothelial cell nitric oxide synthase. J Clin Invest 1992;90:2092
15. Bredt DS, Hwang PM, Glatt CE et al: Cloned and expressed nitric oxide synthase structurally resembles cytochrome P-450 reductase. Nature 1991;351:714
16. Xie Q, Cho HJ, Calaycay J et al: Cloning and characterization of inducible nitric oxide synthase from mouse macrophages. Science 1992;256:225
17. Geller DA, Lowenstein CJ, Shapiro RA et al: Molecular cloning and expression of inducible nitric oxide synthase from human hepatocytes. Proc Natl Acad Sci USA 1993;90:3491
18. Moncada S, Palmer RMJ, Higgs EA: Biosynthesis of nitric oxide from L-arginine. A pathway for the regulation of cell function and communication. Biochem Pharmacol 1989;38:1709
19. Vallance P, Collier J, Moncada S: Effects of endothelium-derived nitric oxide on peripheral arteriolar tone in man. Lancet 1989;ii:997
20. Stamler JS, Loh E, Roddy MA, Currie KE, Creager MA: Nitric oxide regulates basal systemic and pulmonary vascular resistance in healthy humans. Circulation 1994;89:2035
21. Haynes WG, Noon JP, Walker BR, Webb DJ: Inhibition of nitric oxide synthesis increases blood pressure in healthy humans. J Hypertens 1993;11:1375
22. Buga GM, Gold ME, Fukuto JM, Ignarro LJ: Shear stress-induced release of nitric oxide from endothelial cells grown on beads. Hypertension 1991;17:187
23. Radomski MW, Palmer RMJ, Moncada S: An L-arginine/nitric oxide pathway present in human platelets regulates aggregation. Proc Natl Acad Sci USA 1990;87:5193
24. Nunokawa Y, Ishida N, Tanaka S: Cloning of inducible nitric oxide synthase in rat vascular smooth muscle cells. Biochem Biophys Res Commun 1993;191:89
25. Moncada S, Vane JR: Pharmacology and endogenous roles of prostaglandin endoperoxides, thromboxane A_2 and prostacyclin. Pharmacol Rev 1979;30:292
26. Macdonald PS, Read MA, Dusting GJ: Synergistic inhibition of platelet aggregation by endothelium-derived relaxing factor and prostacyclin. Thromb Res 1988;49:437
27. Standen NB, Quayle JM, Davies NW et al: Hyperpolarising vasodilators activate ATP-sensitive K^+ channels in arterial smooth muscle. Science 1989;245:177
28. Miller VM, Vanhoutte PM: Endothelium-dependent contractions to arachidonic acid are mediated by products of cyclooxygenase in canine veins. Am J Physiol 1985;248:H432
29. Yang Z, von Segesser L, Bauer E et al: Different acti-

vation of the endothelial L-arginine and cyclooxygenase pathway in the human internal mammary artery and saphenous vein. Circ Res 1991;68:52

30. Gryglewski RJ, Palmer RMS, Moncada S: Superoxide anion is involved in the breakdown of endothelium-derived relaxing factor. Nature 1986;320:454

31. Katusic ZS, Vanhoutte PM: Superoxide anion is an endothelium-derived contracting factor. Am J Physiol 1989;357:H33

32. Yanagisawa M, Kurihara H, Kimura S et al: A novel potent vasoconstrictor peptide produced by vascular endothelial cells. Nature 1988;332:411

33. Inoue A, Yanagisawa M, Kimura S et al: The human endothelin family. Three structurally and pharmacologically distinct isopeptides predicted by three separate genes. Proc Natl Acad Sci USA 1989;86:2863

34. Kiowski W, Lüscher TF, Linder L, Bühler FR: Endothelin-1 induced vasoconstriction in man. Reversal by calcium channel blockade but not by nitrovasodilators or endothelium-derived relaxing factor. Circulation 1991;83:469

35. Kasuya Y, Ishikawa T, Yanagisawa M et al: Mechanism of contraction to endothelin in isolated porcine coronary artery. Am J Physiol 1989;257:H1828

36. MacCumber MW, Ross CA, Glaser BM, Sny SH: Endothelin. Visualization of mRNAs by in situ hybridization provides evidence for local action. Proc Natl Acad Sci USA 1989;86:7285

37. Boulanger C, Lüscher TF: Release of endothelin from the porcine aorta. Inhibition by endothelium-derived nitric oxide. J Clin Invest 1990;85:587

38. Richard V, Hogie M, Clozel M, Löffler B-M, Thuillez C: In vivo evidence of an endothelin-induced vasopressor tone after inhibition of nitric oxide synthesis in rats. Circulation 1995;91:771

39. Moncada S, Palmer RMJ, Higgs EA: Nitric oxide. Physiology, pathophysiology, and pharmacology. Pharmacol Rev 1991;43:109

40. Vanhoutte PM: A matter of life and breath. Nature 1994;368:693

41. Haynes WG, Webb DJ: Contribution of endogenous generation of endothelin-1 to basal vascular tone. Lancet 1994;344:852

42. Zelis R, Flaim SF: Alterations in vasomotor tone in congestive heart failure. Prog Cardiovasc Dis 1982; 24:437

43. Drexler H, Banhardt U, Meinertz T et al: Contrasting peripheral short-term and long-term effects of converting enzyme inhibition in patients with congestive heart failure. A double-blind, placebo-controlled trial. Circulation 1989;79:491

44. LeJemtel TH, Maskin CS, Lucido D, Chadwick BJ: Failure to augment maximal limb blood flow in response to one-leg versus two-leg exercise in patients with severe heart failure. Circulation 1986;74:245

45. Kaiser L, Spickard RC, Olivier NB: Heart failure depresses endothelium-dependent responses in canine femoral artery. Am J Physiol 1989;256:H962

46. Ontkean M, Gay R, Greenberg B: Diminished endothelium-derived relaxing factor activity in an experimental model of chronic heart failure. Circ Res 1991; 69:1088

47. Teerlink JR, Clozel M, Fischli W, Clozel J-P: Temporal evolution of endothelial dysfunction in a rat model of chronic heart failure. J Am Coll Cardiol 1993;22:615

48. Drexler H, Lu W: Endothelial dysfunction of hindquarter resistance vessels in experimental heart failure. Am J Physiol 1992;262:H1640

49. Katz SD, Biasucci L, Sabba C et al: Impaired endothelium-mediated vasodilation in the peripheral vasculature of patients with congestive heart failure. J Am Coll Cardiol 1992;19:918

50. Kubo SH, Rector TS, Bank AJ, Williams RE, Heifetz SM: Endothelium-dependent vasodilation is attenuated in patients with heart failure. Circulation 1991; 84:1589

51. Drexler H, Hayoz D, Münzel T et al: Endothelial function in chronic heart failure. Am J Cardiol 1991;69: 1596

52. Linder L, Kiowski W, Bühler FR, Lüscher TF: Indirect evidence for release of endothelium-derived relaxing factors in human forearm circulation in vivo. Blunted response in essential hypertension. Circulation 1990;81:1762–1767

53. Joannides R, Haefeli WE, Linder L et al: Nitric oxide is responsible for flow-dependent dilatation of human peripheral conduit arteries in vivo. Circulation 1995; 91:1314

54. Hayoz D, Drexler H, Münzel T et al: Flow-mediated arterial dilation is abnormal in congestive heart failure. Circulation, suppl. VII 1993;87:92

55. Arnold JMO, Marchiori GE, Imrie JR et al: Large artery function in patients with chronic heart failure. Circulation 1991;84:2418

56. Ramsey MJ, Jones CJH: Large arteries are more than passive conduits. Br Heart J 1994;72:3

57. Ramsey MW, Jones CJH, Steward W, Lewis MJ, Henderson AH: Endothelium-derived relaxing factor dynamically controls large artery distensibility in normal subjects [abstract]. Eur Heart J 1993;14:274

58. Habib F, Dutka D, Crossman D, Oakley CM, Cleland JGF: Enhanced basal nitric oxide production in heart failure. Another failed counter-regulatory vasodilator mechanism? Lancet 1994;344:371

59. Winlaw DS, Smythe GA, Keogh AM et al: Increased nitric oxide production in heart failure. Lancet 1994; 344:373

60. Winlaw DS, Smythe GA, Keogh AM et al: Nitric oxide production and heart failure. Lancet 1995;345:390

61. Kubo SH, Rector TSA, Bank AJ et al: Lack of contribution of nitric oxide to basal vasomotor tone in heart failure. Am Cardiol 1994;74:1144

62. Katz SD, Krum H, Packer M: Resting and exercise-induced release of endothelium-derived nitric oxide is impaired in patients with heart failure [abstract]. J Am Coll Cardiol 1994;23:272A

63. Levine B, Kalman J, Mayer L, Fillit HM, Packer M: Elevated circulating levels of tumor necrosis factor in severe chronic heart failure. N Engl J Med 1990; 323:236

64. Aoki N, Siegfried M, Lefer AM: Anti-EDRF effect of tumor necrosis factor in isolated, perfused cat carotid arteries. Am J Physiol 1989;256:H1509

65. Yoshizumi M, Perrella MA, Burnett JC, Lee M-E: Tumor necrosis factor downregulates an endothelial nitric oxide synthase mRNA by shortening its half-life. Circ Res 1993;73:205

66. Katz SD, Ramanath Rao, Berman JW et al: Pathophysiological correlates of increased serum tumor necrosis factor in patients with congestive heart failure.

Relation to nitric oxide-dependent vasodilation in the forearm circulation. Circulation 1994;90:12

67. Miller VM, Vanhoutte PM: Enhanced release of endothelium-derived factor(s) by chronic increases in blood flow. Am J Physiol 1988;255:H446

68. Belch JJF, Bridges AB, Scott N, Chopra M: Oxygen free radicals and congestive heart failure. Br Heart J 1991;65:245

69. Graham DG, Tiffany SM, Bell WR, Gutkencht WF: Autoxidation versus covalent binding of quinones as the mechanism of toxicity of dopamine, 6-hydroxydopamine and related compounds toward C1300 neuroblastoma cells in vitro. Mol Pharmacol 1978;14:644

70. Griendling KK, Minieri CA, Ollerenshaw JD, Alexander RW: Angiotensin II stimulates NADH and NADPH oxidase activity in cultured vascular smooth muscle cells. Circ Res 1994;74:1141

71. Prasad K, Kalra J, Bharadwaj B: Phagocytic activity in blood of dogs with chronic heart failure. Clin Invest Med 1987;10:1354

72. Steward DJ, Pohl U, Bassenge W: Superoxide anions and hypoxia inactivate endothelium-dependent dilation in the coronary resistance bed. Am J Physiol 1988;255:H765

73. Arnal JF, Schott C, Stoclet JC, Michel JB: Vascular relaxation and cyclic guanosine monophosphate in a rat model of high output heart failure. Cardiovasc Res 1993;27:1651

74. Miller VM, Burnett JC: Modulation of NO and endothelin by chronic increase in blood flow in canine femoral arteries. Am J Physiol 1992;263:H103

75. Cooke JP, Stamler J, Andon N et al: Flow stimulates endothelial cells to release a nitrovasodilator that is potentiated by reduced thiol. Am J Physiol 1990;259:H804

76. Katz SD, Schwarz M, Yuen J, LeJemtel TH: Impaired acetycholine-mediated vasodilation in patients with congestive heart failure. Role of endothelium-derived vasodilating and vasoconstricting factors. Circulation 1993;88:55

77. Sinoway LI, Minotti J, Musch T et al: Enhanced metabolic vasodilation secondary to diuretic therapy in decompensated congestive heart failure secondary to coronary artery disease. Am J Cardiol 1987;60:107

78. Wei CM, Lerman A, Rodeheffer RJ et al: Endothelin in human congestive heart failure. Circulation 1994;89:1580

79. Tsutamoto T, Wada A, Maeda Y, Adachi T, Kinoshita M: Relation between endothelin-1 spill over in the lungs and pulmonary vascular resistance in patients with chronic heart failure. J Am Coll Cardiol 1994;23:1427

80. Porter TR, Taylor DO, Cycan A et al: Endothelium-dependent pulmonary artery responses in chronic heart failure. Influence of pulmonary hypertension. J Am Coll Cardiol 1993;22:1418

81. Love MP, Haynes WG, Webb DJ, McMurray JJV: Anti-endothelin therapy is of potential benefit in heart failure [abstract]. Circulation, suppl. I 1994;90:47

82. Kiowski W, Sütch G, Hunzikes P, et al: Evidence for endothelial mediated vasoconstriction in severe chronic heart failure. Lancet 1995;346:732

83. Teerlink JR, Löffler B-M, Hess P et al: Role of endothelin in the maintenance of blood pressure in conscious rats with chronic heart failure. Acute effects of the endothelin receptor antagonist Ro 47-0203 (Bosentan). Circulation 1994;90:2510

84. Nakamura M, Ishikawa M, Funakoshi T et al: Attenuated endothelium-dependent peripheral vasodilation and clinical characteristics in patients with chronic heart failure. Am Heart J 1994;128:1164

85. Hirooka Y, Imaizumi T, Tagawa T et al: Effects of L-arginine on impaired acetylcholine-induced and ischemic vasodilation of the forearm in patients with heart failure. Circulation 1994;90:658

86. Shen W, Lundborg M, Wang J et al: Role of EDRF in the regulation of regional blood flow and vascular resistance at rest and during exercise in conscious dogs. J Appl Physiol 1994;77:165

87. Wilson JR, Kapoor S: Contribution of endothelium-derived relaxing factor to exercise-induced vasodilation in humans. J Appl Physiol 1993;75:2740

88. Meredith IT, Jain RK, Anderson TJ, Ganz P, Creager MA: Endothelium-derived nitric oxide contributes to exercise-induced hyperemia in the human forearm [abstract]. Circulation, suppl. I 1994;90:295

89. Mancini DM, Davis L, Wexler JP, Chadwick B, LeJemtel TH: Dependence of enhanced maximal exercise performance on increased peak skeletal muscle perfusion during long-term captopril therapy in heart failure. J Am Coll Cardiol 1987;10:845

90. Ontkean MT, Gay R, Greenberg B: Effects of chronic captopril therapy on endothelium-derived relaxing factor activity in heart failure [abstract]. J Am Coll Cardiol 1992;19:207A

91. Hirsch H, Bijou R, Yuen J et al: Enalapril-mediated vasodilation is attenuated by indomethacin in congestive heart failure and completely abolished in normal subjects. Circulation, suppl. I 1993;88:293

92. Nakamura M, Funakoshi T, Chiba M et al: Effect of ACE-inhibitors on endothelium-dependent peripheral vasodilation in patients with chronic heart failure. J Am Coll Cardiol 1994;24:1321

93. Hirooka Y, Imaizumi T, Masaki H et al: Captopril improves impaired endothelium-dependent vasodilation in hypertensive patients. Hypertension 1992;20:175

94. Mombouli J-V, Naphtali M, Vanhoutte PM: Effects of the converting enzyme inhibitor cilazaprilat on endothelium-dependent responses. Hypertension, suppl. II 1991;18:22

95. Wiemer G, Schölkens, BA, Becker RHA, Busse R: Ramiprilat enhances endothelial autacoid formation by inhibiting breakdown of endothelium-derived bradykinin. Hypertension 1991;18:558

96. Kubo SH, Rector TS, Bank AJ et al: Effects of cardiac transplantation on endothelium-dependent dilation of the peripheral vasculature in congestive heart failure. Am J Cardiol 1993;71:88

97. Treasure CB, Vita JA, Cox DA et al: Endothelium-dependent dilation of the coronary microvasculature is impaired in dilated cardiomyopathy. Circulation 1990;81:772

98. Inoue T, Sakai Y, Morooka S et al: Vasodilatory capacity of coronary resistance vessels in dilated cardiomyopathy. Am Heart J 1994;127:376

99. DeBelder AJ, Radomski MW, Why HJF et al: Nitric oxide synthase activities in human myocardium. Lancet 1993;341:84

100. Studer R, Kästner S, Just H, Drexler H: Myocardial

gene expression of endothelial nitric oxide synthase in ischemic and dilated cardiomyopathy [abstract]. Circulation, suppl. I 1994;90:547

101. Wang J, Seyedi N, Xu X-B, Wolin MS, Hintze TH: Defective endothelium-mediated control of coronary circulation in conscious dogs after heart failure. Am J Physiol 1994;266:H670

102. Drexler H, Hablawetz E, Lu W, Riede U, Christes C: Effect of inhibition of nitric oxide formation on regional blood flow in experimental myocardial infarction. Circulation 1992;86:255

103. Nishida M, Springhorn JP, Kelly RA, Smith TW: Cell-cell signaling between adult rat ventricular myocytes and cardiac microvascular endothelial cells in heterotypic primary culture. J Clin Invest 1993;91: 1934

104. Mebazza A, Mayoux E, Maeda K et al: Paracrine effects of endocardial endothelial cells on myocyte contraction mediated via endothelin. Am J Physiol 1993; 265:H1841

105. McClellan G, Weisberg A, Lin L-E et al: Endothelial cells are required for the cAMP regulation of cardiac contractile proteins. Proc Natl Acad Sci USA 1993; 90:2885

106. Shah AM, Spurgeon HA, Sollott SJ, Talo A, Lakatta EG: 8-Bromo-cGMP reduces the myofilament re-sponse to Ca^{2+} in intact cardiac myocytes. Circ Res 1994;74:970

107. Paulus WJ, Vantrimpont PJ, Shah AM: Acute effects of nitric oxide on left ventricular relaxation and diastolic distensibility in humans. Assessment by bicoronary sodium nitroprusside infusion. Circulation 1994;89:2070

108. Paulus WJ: Endothelial control of vascular and myocardial function in heart failure. Cardiovasc Drug Ther 1994;8:437

109. Balligand J-L, Kelly RA, Marsden PA, Smith TW, Michel T: Control of cardiac muscle cell function by an endogenous nitric oxide signaling system. Proc Natl Acad Sci USA 1993;90:347

110. Tsujino M, Hirata Y, Imai T et al: Induction of nitric oxide synthase gene by interleukin 1β in cultured rat cardiocytes. Circulation 1994;90:375

111. Balligand J-L, Ungureanu-Longrois D, Simmons WW et al: Cytokine-inducible nitric oxide synthase (iNOS) expression in cardiac myocytes. J Biol Chem 1994;269:27580

112. Haywood GA, Tsao PS, von der Leyen HE et al: Expression of inducible nitric oxide synthase in human failing heart. Circulation 1996; 93:1087

113. Hiroe M, Ishiyama S, Nishikawa T et al: Expression of inducible nitric oxide synthase in the myocardium of acute myocarditis—a serial cardiac biopsy study [abstract]. J Am Coll Cardiol 1995;25:131

13 Regional Vascular Control

Thierry H. LeJemtel
Irving H. Zucker

During the progression of the syndrome of congestive heart failure (CHF), the peripheral circulation undergoes substantial changes, which have been extensively reviewed by Zelis et al.[1-5] The well recognized pattern of cardiac output redistribution during the syndrome of CHF results from vasoconstriction in the regional circulation, which is most affected by α-adrenoreceptor stimulation (i.e., cutaneous, renal, and splanchnic), and relative preservation of blood flow in circulations, which is mostly governed by metabolic demands (i.e., cerebral and coronary). The changes in the skeletal muscle circulation are not as easily characterized as the mechanisms that regulate skeletal muscle blood flow changes from rest to exercise.[6]

Overall, although the peripheral circulation has been a highly successful therapeutic target for the pharmacologic management of CHF with the introduction of angiotensin-converting enzyme (ACE) inhibitors, little progress has been made in developing a better understanding of the mechanisms that mediate alterations in regional vascular control and the resulting abnormalities of the peripheral circulation in CHF. For example, it is well known that, in contrast to left ventricular performance, the impaired vasodilatory response of the skeletal muscle beds is not immediately improved by ACE inhibition.[7,8] Several weeks of ACE inhibition are required to observe an increase in skeletal muscle blood flow during exercise in patients with CHF. The cellular and molecular mechanisms that mediate this delayed response of the skeletal muscle vasculature to ACE inhibition

are largely unknown. With regard to the sympathetic adrenergic system, the stimuli for and control of increased α-adrenergic stimulation, which characterizes the syndrome of CHF, are still unknown. Moreover, the resulting cellular and molecular changes that may occur in the vascular smooth muscle cells have not been studied in patients with CHF.[9,10]

Since the early 1980s, our understanding of regional vascular control in patients with CHF has progressed in three areas. The first area is the role played by the vasodilatory substances released by the vascular endothelium in response to changes in wall shear stress. The second area of concern is a better understanding of the time course of the abnormalities of regional vascular control in patients with CHF. The syndrome of left ventricular (LV) systolic dysfunction/CHF is a dynamic process. Patients with asymptomatic LV systolic dysfunction are free of major peripheral circulatory abnormalities. When the syndrome of CHF progresses and patients become symptomatic, regional vascular control is reprogrammed; and the resulting abnormalities of the peripheral circulation play a major role in the pathophysiology of the syndrome of severe CHF. Of note many controversies regarding the state of the peripheral circulation in patients with CHF can be explained by the nonhomogeneity of patients studied in regard to the stage of CHF (i.e., early versus late stage).

The third area of progress has been the coronary circulation. Substantial abnormalities of the coronary circulation, including the coronary microvascu-

187

lature, have been increasingly reported in patients with idiopathic dilated cardiomyopathy, as well as in those with ischemic cardiomyopathy. The present chapter essentially focuses on the developments that have occurred since the mid-1980s.

As previously mentioned, the overall alterations in regional vascular control have already been extensively reviewed, with updates, by Zelis and collaborators.[1-5] The contribution of endothelial dilating substances to the overall vasodilatory response of the skeletal muscle beds to exercise is reviewed in the first part of this chapter. In the second part the importance of staging the syndrome of CHF when evaluating regional vascular control is emphasized. It is essential when reviewing data concerning the peripheral circulation in patients with CHF to have a precise knowledge of what stage of the syndrome patients have reached. Failure to do so has led to the selection of improper endpoints in pharmacologic trials and therapeutic failures. Lastly, the abnormalities of the coronary circulation are reviewed, with special emphasis on recent measurements of myocardial blood flow in patients undergoing cardiac transplantation.

DILATING ENDOTHELIAL SUBSTANCES AND SKELETAL MUSCLE VASCULATURE

Experimental and Human Studies

Soon after the crucial role of the vascular endothelium in mediating flow-dependent vasodilation was recognized, the functional status of the vascular endothelium was assessed in experimental models and patients with CHF.[11-13] The rationale for such studies was that chronic increases in blood had been shown to enhance the release of endothelium-derived factors (EDRF).[14] Conversely, clinical conditions associated with reduced peripheral blood flow (e.g., CHF) were thought to lead to endothelial dysfunction, apart from other associated conditions known to depress vascular endothelial function (e.g., diffuse atherosclerosis, diabetes mellitus, hypercholesterolemia, hypertension, and smoking).

Kaiser et al. demonstrated that endothelium-dependent vascular responses are depressed in the rapid pacing canine model of heart failure.[15] These investigators observed a significant depression of relaxation induced by local administration of acetylcholine in the femoral artery, whereas the responses to regional administration of norepinephrine and nitroglycerin were intact.

Kubo et al. demonstrated that in patients with CHF administration of acetylcholine in the brachial artery does not increase forearm blood flow to the same extent it does in normal subjects of similar age.[16] In contrast, forearm blood flow responses to local administration of nitroprusside were similar in patients and normal subjects.[16] The data of Kubo et al. are in agreement with the experimental findings of Kaiser et al. and suggest that attenuation of endothelium-mediated vasodilation may in part mediate the abnormalities that are characteristically present in the peripheral circulation of patients with chronic heart failure. In contrast to the findings of Kubo et al.,[16] Katz et al. reported that abnormalities of the peripheral circulation were not limited to the vascular endothelium in patients with CHF.[17] In agreement with Kaiser et al.[15] and Kubo et al.,[16] Katz et al. observed that the vasodilatory responses to acetylcholine were decreased in the lower limb circulation of patients with severe CHF when compared to that noted in normal subjects of similar age. However, Katz et al. also found that the vasodilatory response to nitroglycerin, an endothelium-independent dilator, was markedly depressed in patients with CHF when compared to that in normal subjects.[17] Consequently, intrinsic abnormalities of vascular smooth muscle relaxation must be taken into account when evaluating the vasodilatory responses to endothelium-dependent stimuli.

Limitations and Implications of Current Studies

Notwithstanding the technical difficulties of noninvasively measuring vascular reactivity and regional blood flow, the study of vascular endothelial function is complex. Several pathways that are interacting are responsible for flow-mediated vasodilation. The changes in shear stress on the endothelial cell that accompany alterations in blood flow are responsible for the release of nitric oxide (the first EDRF identified) and prostaglandins.[18,19] The modifications in intracellular calcium associated with nitric oxide release are in turn responsible for the release of endothelium-derived hyperpolarizing factor (EDHF).[20] The latter factor has not yet been characterized.

In most clinical studies the vascular responses to stimulation or blockage of one pathway, often the nitric oxide pathway, are determined without evaluating the effect these changes have on the other pathways. For example, patients are rarely pretreated with indomethacin when the vasodilatory responses to local administration of acetylcholine are studied. When blood flow (i.e., shear stress) is increased, rat gracilis muscle arterioles have been shown to release nitric oxide and prostaglandins. These two substances act additively to dilate skeletal muscle arterioles. The relative contribution of nitric oxide and prostaglandins in promoting dilation appears to vary in different vascular beds. Of interest, in canine models of heart failure the vascular response to low doses of acetylcholine are amplified by pretreatment with indomethacin.[15] The interaction between nitric oxide and prostaglandin pathways may be relevant to understanding the behavior of the vascular endothelium at rest and during stress.[21]

Basal Versus Stimulated Release of Endothelial Factors

Current knowledge of the vascular endothelial function in patients with CHF is mostly derived from the vascular responses to nonphysiologic situations involving local administration of acetylcholine or substance P. Investigators have attempted to study the behavior of vascular endothelium in more physiologic circumstances by specifically inhibiting nitric oxide synthesis with N-monomethyl-L-arginine (L-NMMA) at rest and during exercise.[22,23] The data are controversial. Whereas Katz et al. reported that resting forearm blood flow does not change after administration of L-NMMA,[24] a finding compatible with depressed vascular endothelial function, Drexler et al. observed an exaggerated response at rest,[22] a finding compatible with enhancement of vascular endothelial function. Similarly, Kubo et al. reported that the vasoconstrictor response to inhibition of nitric oxide production with L-NMMA is unchanged or even increased in the forearm circulation of patients with CHF when compared to that in normal subjects.[23] Although the data concerning inhibition of nitric oxide production in the basal state are conflicting, all investigators agree that the vasodilatory response to acetylcholine is decreased in patients with CHF.[16,17,22] As previously mentioned, the interpretation of data regarding specific inhibition of the nitric oxide pathway by L-NMMA is complicated in the absence of concomitant blockade of prostaglandin synthesis and characterization of the EDHF.[20] Koller and Kaley suggested that the primary role of the vascular endothelium is to maintain shear stress close to control by a negative feedback mechanism.[25] In that perspective, specifically inhibiting one pathway may stimulate an alternate pathway, as the vascular endothelium compensates in order to maintain a relatively constant shear stress.

In addition, the severity of the syndrome of CHF may contribute to the disparate findings regarding basal versus stimulated vascular endothelial function during heart failure. At an early stage in a rat model of heart failure, Teerlink et al. demonstrated normal vascular endothelial function in aortic rings.[26] At a later stage in the model when heart failure is more severe, the same investigators documented vascular endothelial dysfunction in aortic rings. When evaluated under stimulated conditions, vascular endothelial function appears to deteriorate as the syndrome of CHF progresses. However, as occurs with cardiac output, basal and stimulated vascular endothelial function may be differently altered in response to the severity of CHF. The cardiac output response to exercise is reduced well before cardiac output is clearly reduced at rest. Similarly, the ability of the vascular endothelium to maximally release nitric oxide and prostaglandins may be reduced before basal release is affected.

Differences in vascular endothelial responsiveness in the basal state and during stimulation may also be partly explained by the interaction between α-adrenergic vasoconstriction and vascular endothelial function.[27,28] The interaction between the vascular endothelium and the sympathetic adrenergic system may be particularly relevant during physical exercise, which is associated with early stimulation of the sympathetic system in CHF. The increased vascular responsiveness to norepinephrine of intact vessels from rats with heart failure results from decreased basal release of nitric oxide.[29] Interestingly, the vascular responsiveness to norepinephrine is already reduced when the basal vascular endothelial function appears to be normal early in the syndrome of heart failure, as mentioned earlier. Thus the dissociation of basal and stimulated nitric oxide release is an important characteristic of vascular endothelial dysfunction during the syndrome of CHF.

Amplification of Nitric Oxide Pathway

To assess vascular endothelial function under as physiologic conditions as possible the flow-mediated component of the increase in blood flow induced by a specific vasodilator such as phentolamine was compared in patients with heart failure and normal subjects of similar age.[30] Rather than inhibiting production of nitric oxide with L-NMMA, we elected to enhance the vascular effects of the nitric oxide pathway by simultaneously infusing nitroglycerin at a dose that had been shown to have no direct vasodilatory effect.[31] The net effect of combining such low dose nitroglycerin to phentolamine was to heighten the endothelial nitric oxide pathway and therefore amplify, flow-mediated vasodilation. The concomitant administration of phentolamine and low dose nitroglycerin increased blood flow over that noted with phentolamine alone in normal subjects, but it did not in patients with CHF.[30] The findings indicate that the flow-mediated component of the increase in blood flow induced by a specific vasodilator is reduced in patients with CHF. Combining low dose nitroglycerin with a specific vasodilator or other intervention that increases blood flow is a simple method for amplifying the spontaneously occurring flow-mediated dilation, which is part of the vasodilatory response to any vascular smooth muscle relaxant to exercise or arterial occlusion (i.e., peak reactive hyperemia). This method has the advantage of assessing vascular endothelial function in response to an increase in shear stress, which is the most relevant stimulus in humans. The amplification method is not flawed by the previously mentioned limitations of exogenous stimuli such as acetylcholine or substance P or of inhibition of the nitric oxide pathway with L-NMMA. By clearly demonstrating reduced vascular endothelial function under physiologic conditions, the amplification method resolves the controversy generated by the contrasting findings with administration of acetylcholine and substance P in patients with CHF.[32]

The normal vascular endothelial response appears to be impaired in patients with CHF under physiologic conditions involving a mild increase in blood flow. To what extent such impairment in vascular endothelial function contributes to the heightened vascular resistance that characterizes late stages of the syndrome of CHF is unclear. However, preliminary data regarding the benefits of physical training on vascular endothelial function indicate that reversal of the vascular endothelial dysfunction is associated with a significant but mild increase in maximal oxygen uptake.[33] Such a mild increase suggests that the role of the vascular endothelium in the overall vasodilatory response to exercise is modest.

Mechanisms of Vascular Endothelial Dysfunction

The determinants of progressive vascular endothelial dysfunction during the syndrome of CHF are not well understood. As initially alluded to, chronically reduced peripheral blood flow may reduce the synthesis and release of EDRF by the endothelial cell. Enhancement of vascular endothelial function, which specifically develops in the trained circulation during progressive exercise training, strongly supports the view that local hemodynamic conditions are responsible for vascular endothelial function.[34]

A short program of daily exercise has been shown to augment flow-dependent dilation in the gracilis muscle arterioles of rats.[35] Such augmentation appears to be due to increased sensitivity of the arteriolar endothelium to wall shear stress, which in turn is elicited by augmented release of both nitric oxide and prostaglandins.[36] The increased sensitivity of the vascular endothelium is likely to result from periodic exposures to high skeletal muscle blood flows during repeated bouts of daily exercise rather than to circulating metabolites.[36]

In agreement with the findings in the skeletal muscle vasculature, the vasoreactivity of rat abdominal aorta to acetylcholine has been found to increase after a treadmill training program of 10–12 weeks duration.[37] The increased vascular responsiveness to acetylcholine induced by physical training was completely blocked by the arginine analog L-NAME. Thus enhancement of acetylcholine-induced vasodilation is likely to be related to adaptation in the nitric oxide synthase pathway.

Katz et al. demonstrated in normal subjects that an intense physical training program, resulting in an average increase of 26 percent in maximal oxygen uptake, was associated with an enhanced vasodilatory response to acetylcholine but not to nitroglycerin.[38] The vascular benefits of physical training are limited to the vascular endothelium, as the response to nitroglycerin was unchanged. The mechanisms responsible for the training-induced enhancement in vascular endothelial function are poorly understood. Periodic increases in blood flow may be sufficient to steadily increase production and release of nitric oxide when the endothelial cell is stimulated by acetylcholine. Production of vasoactive substances by vascular endothelial cells are clearly related to the wall shear stress conditions experienced by these cells.[13,36] Gene expression of nitric oxide synthase has been shown to be reduced in patients with clinical conditions associated with reduced blood flow, such as CHF.[39] Endothelial cell nitric oxide synthase gene expression was reduced by approximately 50 percent in thoracic aorta endothelial cells obtained from failing dogs who underwent 4 weeks of LV pacing.[39] As discussed later, chronic exercise has been shown to increase endothelial cell nitric oxide synthase gene expression in endothelial aortic cells.[40] Thus part of the benefits of physical training may be to up-regulate endothelial vasodilator gene products.

The benefits of physical training on vascular endothelial function have also been demonstrated in patients with severe CHF. Eight weeks of hand grip exercise were shown to increase forearm blood flow response to local administration of acetylcholine but not of nitroglycerin.[41] Of interest, the vascular response to acetylcholine was enhanced as early as after 4 weeks of hand grip training, when forearm strength and peak reactive hyperemia had not changed. Thus enhancement of endothelial function appears to be an early and specific vascular effect of vascular physical training. Conversely, chronic reduction in regional blood flow, as witnessed during progression of the syndrome of CHF, is likely to progressively and negatively affect vascular endothelial function.

VASCULAR CONTROL, CIRCULATORY ABNORMALITIES, AND SEVERITY OF CHF

Forearm Vasculature

The abnormal responses of the forearm and calf circulation to vasodilator stimuli were first reported by Zelis et al.[42] After 5 minutes of brachial or femoral artery occlusion, peak hyperemic blood flow was substantially reduced in the forearm and calf of patients with decompensated CHF when compared to that recorded in normal subjects. Intraarterial administration of phentolamine, an α-adrenergic blocker did not restore the abnormal hyperemic blood flows to normal; therefore increased sympathetic vasoconstrictor activity is not likely to be responsible for the abnormal hyperemic response. Interestingly, once patients had been treated and were in a compensated state of heart failure, the hyperemic blood flow returned toward normal values. Zelis et al., in their initial report, pointed out that the derangements of the peripheral circulation were clearly related to the severity of the process. Subsequently, the same investigators demonstrated that forearm blood flows were markedly reduced during dynamic exercise in patients with CHF compared to those measured in normal subjects during similar exercise.[43] The augmented oxygen extraction by the forearm skeletal muscles of patients with CHF was not sufficient to prevent them from shifting early to anaerobic metabolism.[43] Zelis et al., who also studied cutaneous blood flow at rest and during exercise, demonstrated that cutaneous blood vessels do not dilate normally during exercise in patients with CHF.[44]

The abnormal response of the forearm vasculature during dynamic exercise was extended to static exercise by Longhurst et al.[45] The observations by Zelis et al. and Longhurst et al. are of seminal importance, as these investigators were the first to point out that an abnormal vasodilating response of the skeletal muscle vasculature to exercise may be the primary mechanism limiting exercise capacity in patients

with severe CHF. Interpretation of these observations is somewhat limited, however, as the abnormalities of the skeletal muscle vasculature were demonstrated during exercise, which involved a relatively small muscle mass and did not test cardiopulmonary reserve.

Lower Limb Vasculature

The abnormal behavior of the skeletal muscle vasculature during exercise involving a large muscle mass (i.e., treadmill) was demonstrated by Cowley et al.[46] These investigators concluded that reduced calf blood flow was a major reason for decreased exercise capacity in patients with CHF. A similar conclusion was reached during bicycle exercise in patients with severe CHF.[47] Using the model of one-leg versus two-leg bicycle exercise, patients with severe CHF were unable to augment maximal limb blood flow during one-leg bicycle exercise over that reached during two-leg bicycle exercise. In contrast, normal subjects are able to reach a greater maximal limb blood flow during one-leg bicycle exercise than during two-leg bicycle exercise.[47] The fixed capacity of the skeletal muscle vasculature to dilate in response to maximal exercise appears to be independent of cardiac performance in patients with severe CHF and thus may be the primary determinant of exercise intolerance. The comparison of one-leg versus two-leg bicycle exercise provides a physiologic intervention by which the peripheral versus the central components of the exercise response can be evaluated.[47]

Vascular Control of Oxygen Extraction by Skeletal Muscles

Reduced capacity of skeletal muscles to maximally extract oxygen during exercise—which in turn can result from abnormal skeletal muscle metabolism—could also contribute to decreased exercise capacity in patients with CHF. However, the oxygen content of the deep femoral vein (which almost exclusively drains blood from the skeletal muscles) is extremely low, corresponding to a PO_2 of 20 mmHg in patients with severe CHF.[48] The near-complete extraction of oxygen by the skeletal muscles during maximal symptoms-limited exercise rules out that abnormalities of the skeletal muscle metabolism impairs oxygen utilization in patients with severe CHF. Whether mechanical efficiency is reduced in patients with CHF has not been thoroughly investigated. From the data available regarding oxygen uptake at low workloads in normal subjects and in patients with CHF, mechanical efficiency appears to be normal in patients with CHF. Oxygen delivery to the skeletal muscles is essentially flow-dependent, as oxygen extraction is almost maximal.

Near-maximal oxygen extraction by the skeletal muscles of patients with severe CHF also indicates that at peak exercise arteriovenous shunting does not occur across the skeletal muscle bed vasculature and only arterioles perfusing metabolically active muscle fibers are dilated. Severe local hypoxia may mediate the arteriolar dilatation in patients with CHF. Severe local hypoxia is associated with release of vasodilating substances such as potassium and adenosine.[49] Adenosine activates K+-ATP channels on the skeletal muscle fibers via adenosine receptors that may be coupled to the channels via a G protein. The release of potassium relaxes vascular smooth muscle and thereby dilates the arterioles. At modest levels of hypoxia, the vasoconstrictor influence predominates. As previously mentioned, increased sympathetic nerve activity and norepinephrine release, as well as levels of vasopressin and angiotensin II, are responsible for the vasoconstriction.[49] In summary, in patients with CHF severe local hypoxia resulting from severely impaired skeletal muscle perfusion during exercise may explain the dilatation of the arterioles perfusing metabolically active fibers, whereas intense arteriolar vasoconstriction predominates in metabolically inactive fibers. Such local control of the microvasculature during exercise prevents oxygen waste in a manner similar to that seen in highly trained athletes.

Forearm and Lower Limb Vasculature

The interaction between active skeletal muscle mass and cardiopulmonary reserve can be assessed by measuring peak oxygen consumption (VO$_2$) attained during maximal exercise involving the lower limbs alone (i.e., upright bicycling) and the lower and upper limbs (i.e., upright bicycling and arm cranking).[50] Normal subjects do not further increase their peak VO$_2$ during lower and upper limb exercise over that reached with lower limb exercise alone.[50] In contrast, patients with severe CHF, as evidenced by exertional symptoms compatible with New York Heart Association (NYHA) functional class III–IV reach a substantially greater peak VO$_2$ during exercise combining lower and upper limbs than during exercise with the lower limbs alone.[50] Patients with less severe CHF, as evidenced by exertional symptoms compatible with NYHA functional class I–II, behave like normal subjects. They do not reach a higher peak

VO$_2$ during exercise involving the lower and upper limbs compared to that with the lower limbs alone.[50] Thus patients with severe CHF do not have enough skeletal muscle mass in their lower limbs to reach their true maximal cardiac output due to circulatory abnormalities, or they are unable to perfuse a sufficient amount of skeletal muscles to exhaust the limit of the cardiac output response to exercise. The increase in calf diameter that has been demonstrated after prolonged therapy with ACE inhibition suggests that derangements of the peripheral circulation may be the primary determinant of the peripheral abnormalities.[51] Regression of the peripheral vascular abnormalities during long-term administration of ACE inhibitors leads to regression of disuse-induced skeletal muscle atrophy.[51] The contrasting behavior of patients with severe and moderate CHF during exercise involving the lower limbs and the upper and lower limbs clearly points out that the derangements of the periphery in patients with CHF are predominantly related to the severity of the process.

Experimental Studies

Skeletal muscle blood flow has been measured at rest and during exercise in rats with chronic myocardial infarction (MI).[52] Skeletal muscle blood flow was measured by radioactive microspheres in rats with small and large infarctions and in sham-operated rats. Blood flow to the hind limb musculature was significantly less during a given level of treadmill exercise in rats with MI than that of their sham counterparts. The blood flow deficits were more pronounced in rats with large MIs than in rats with small MIs. In rats with large MIs the blood flow deficits positively correlated with the percentage of fast-twitch oxidative glycolytic fibers and negatively with the percentage of fast-twitch glycolytic fibers found in the individual muscles. In rats with MI, the degree of skeletal muscle blood flow abnormalities also appears to depend on the severity of LV dysfunction. These more recent data confirm that the rat model of chronic heart failure is characterized by reduced skeletal muscle perfusion at rest and during exercise.[53,54]

Conflicting Human Studies

The vasodilatory behavior of the skeletal muscle arterioles was evaluated during forearm exercise and after transient ischemia in nonedematous patients with chronic heart failure by Wilson et al.[55] In contrast to the previous findings of Zelis et al. and Cowley et al., the responses of the forearm vasculature to exercise and ischemia were found to be similar to those of age-matched controls. Even patients with the most severe CHF, as evidenced by a peak VO_2 of less than $14 \; ml \cdot kg^{-1} \cdot min^{-1}$, were found to have normal forearm vasculature responses.

The clinical characteristics of the patients studied by Wilson et al. are briefly mentioned and therefore cannot be reviewed in great detail.[55] Abnormalities of the peripheral circulation are predominantly observed during the syndrome of CHF in patients whose CHF is due to LV systolic, not diastolic, dysfunction and in patients whose forward output is reduced by poor contractile performance, not by severe mitral valve regurgitation.[56] When studying a group of patients whose symptoms of CHF were clearly secondary to severe LV systolic dysfunction, Wilson et al. reported that lower limb blood flow was markedly reduced during maximal symptoms-limited exercise.[57] In each patient these investigators reported a significant correlation between leg blood flow attained during exercise and peak oxygen uptake.[58]

Arnold et al. reported forearm blood flow to be decreased at rest in patients with severe CHF when compared to that of normal subjects.[59] During exercise, however, forearm blood flows were not statistically different in patients with severe CHF from those in normal subjects, although the values were consistently lower in patients; moreover, statistical significance might have been reached with a larger patient population.[59] Notwithstanding the difficulties involved when comparing different workloads in patients and normal subjects, the data of Arnold et al. pointed out the limitations of extrapolating from the results of exercise studies that involve small skeletal muscle mass.[59] In contrast to the findings of Arnold et al., prolonged ACE inhibition has been well documented to increase peak aerobic capacity by enhancing the vasodilatory response of the lower limb skeletal muscle beds to exercise.[7,8] Whether such changes can be demonstrated when exercise involves only a small skeletal muscle mass, as is the case with upper limb exercise, is unclear.

Mechanisms of Abnormal Vascular Control and Circulating Abnormalities

SYSTEMIC MECHANISMS

The mechanisms that alter regional vascular control and mediate the derangements of the peripheral circulation in patients with CHF are still poorly understood. The stimulus for increased sympathetic vaso-motor tone in patients with CHF has not yet been elucidated. Enhanced "central command" vasoconstrictor reflex is presently the most likely mechanism.[60,61] At the start of exercise, a central reflex increases the heart rate and sympathetic vasoconstrictor activity. In view of the limited rise in cardiac output, the enhanced central command reflex prevents systemic hypotension by increasing vascular resistance in exercising and nonexercising skeletal muscles. Skeletal muscle meta-boreceptor activity is markedly attenuated during exercise in patients with CHF.[62] Because sympathetic outflow is not decreased but, to the contrary, is increased in these patients, an alternative pathway to sympathoexcitation may be recruited, or the activity of the existing pathway must be enhanced. Central volitional neural influences (i.e., central command) may compensate the attenuation of meta-baroreceptors as the syndrome of CHF evolves. Depressed baroreflex sensitivity is no longer held responsible for the augmented sympathetic tone during heart failure.[63] The role of the arterial baroreceptors in mediating the sympathoexcitation that accompanies the syndrome of CHF was evaluated in the canine pacing model of heart failure.[63] Plasma norepinephrine levels were compared in failing dogs who previously underwent sinoaortic denervation and in failing dogs who did not. Surprisingly, plasma norepinephrine levels were increased to similar levels in failing dogs regardless of whether they had undergone sinoaortic denervation. Whether mechanosensitive and chemosensitive cardiopulmonary reflexes are involved in the sympathoexcitation that develops and progresses during the syndrome of CHF is still being investigated.[64]

The role of the renin-angiotensin system in mediating the derangements of the peripheral circulation has been indirectly investigated. During prolonged ACE inhibition the vasodilating response of the skeletal muscle beds substantially improves, although it remains well below that of normal subjects of similar age. Whether this improvement is directly mediated by lower tissue levels of angiotensin II or by a pharmacologic training-induced phenomenon secondary to the relief of symptoms is currently unknown.[65] Because of its interaction with the sympathetic adrenergic system, the renin-angiotensin system may stimulate sympathoexcitation during the syndrome of CHF. Angiotensin II increases sympathetic outflow and augments norepinephrine release from sympathetic nerve terminals.[66–68]

LOCAL MECHANISMS

In addition to systemic neurohumoral activation, local factors may play a preponderant role in mediating the derangements of the peripheral circulation.

Jondeaú et al.[69] compared peak reactive hyperemic blood flows in the forearm and calf of patients with CHF due to LV systolic dysfunction with that in age- and gender-matched normal subjects. Calf peak reactive hyperemic blood flows were significantly lower in patients with CHF than in normal subjects, whereas forearm peak reactive hyperemic blood flows were similar in patients and normal subjects. Calf peak reactive hyperemic flow and peak VO_2 were linearly related, but forearm peak reactive hyperemic flow was not related to peak VO_2. Lastly, forearm and calf peak hyperemic flows were not related.

The mechanisms responsible for the regional specificity of the limb peak reactive hyperemic response are still unclear, but physical deconditioning is likely to be involved. Differences in forearm peak hyperemic blood flow responses have been documented in tennis players by Sinoway et al.,[70] who also reviewed the effects of conditioning and deconditioning stimuli in metabolically determined blood flows in humans.[71] Activity-related vascular changes may be mediated in part by changes in vascular endothelial function, which in turn may structurally affect blood vessels.[72] In that regard, local factors may explain why inhibition of heightened sympathetic and renin-angiotensin systems do not rapidly reverse the abnormalities of the peripheral circulation in patients with CHF. These abnormalities are reversed only by steadily increasing physical activity, thereby restoring a normal blood flow response to exercise.

ABNORMALITIES OF THE CORONARY CIRCULATION WITH CHF

Human Studies

One would expect that abnormalities of the coronary circulation, and thereby myocardial perfusion, are primarily dependent on the nature of the disease that leads to the syndrome of heart failure. Parodi et al., however, demonstrated that myocardial blood flow is similarly depressed in failing hearts with both ischemic and idiopathic dilated cardiomyopathy despite the significantly lesser amount of fibrosis and the lack of coronary stenosis in patients with idiopathic dilated cardiomyopathy.[73] In addition, these authors failed to find a correlation between the degree of myocardial blood flow impairment and the extent of myocardial fibrosis. The presence of substantial myocardial underperfusion with both idiopathic dilated cardiomyopathy and myocardial areas

not dependent on underlying coronary lesions and the tissue fibrosis in ischemic cardiomyopathy is poorly understood. Parodi et al.[73] suggested that functional and structural damage of myocytes may down-regulate myocardial blood flow at lower levels to meet the reduced metabolic needs. However, the well documented lack of coronary blood flow reserve in patients with ischemic and idiopathic dilated cardiomyopathy suggest that in addition to adjusting to lower metabolic needs, abnormalities of the coronary microcirculation are responsible for decreased myocardial perfusion.

Pathophysiologic Implications

In addition to its important implications for thallium imaging in patients with idiopathic dilated cardiomyopathy, the reduction in resting myocardial blood flow in patients with CHF suggest that functional abnormalities of the microcirculation may be major mechanisms responsible for the steady progression of the syndrome of CHF.[74] An alternative explanation to the lack of correlation between the amount of fibrosis and myocardial blood flow impairment is that myocyte death may not always be associated with fibrosis. The reduction in myocardial blood flow could be more related to myocyte loss than to the amount of fibrosis. In that regard, for a given amount of remaining myocardial tissue, myocyte loss due to necrosis, which is associated with myocardial fibrosis, may result in less reduction in myocardial blood flow than myocyte loss due to apoptosis, which is not associated with fibrosis. With both necrosis and apoptosis, the remaining viable myocytes are expected to hypertrophy substantially. Combining measurement of myocardial blood flow (as done by Parodi et al.[73] in patients undergoing cardiac transplantation) with morphometric sampling, including counting the total number of myocyte nuclear profiles (as done by Beltrami et al.),[75,76] should lead to a better understanding of the mechanisms responsible for myocardial underperfusion.

Beltrami et al. reported that in patients with ischemic cardiomyopathy replacement fibrosis affected the noninfarcted myocardium of both ventricles. Moreover, myocyte loss was similar in the two ventricles despite marked differences in the fractional volumes of the collagen compartment. These findings confirm the results of Parodi et al.,[73] who as previously mentioned could not find a relation between the myocardial perfusion impairment and the degree of myocardial fibrosis. Whether this lack of correlation between perfusion and fibrosis is consistent with primary abnormalities in the coronary microcirculation or is related to the various processes responsible for cell death is currently under investigation.

Coronary Vasculature and Myocardial Hypertrophy

Dilated cardiomyopathy involves extensive myocardial damage, with accumulation of collagen in the ventricular wall and myocyte hypertrophy. Myocardial hypertrophy is associated with abnormalities of the coronary circulation characterized by a decreased coronary reserve.[77,78] However, as the syndrome of CHF worsens, the abnormalities of the coronary circulation associated with myocardial hypertrophy could progress on their own and lead to the marked underperfusion at rest that characterizes the late stages of CHF. Cardiac hypertrophy is accompanied by abnormalities of myocardial perfusion, including decreased coronary reserve, increased minimal coronary vascular resistance, and underperfusion of the subendocardium.[79] Reduction in the luminal diameter of resistance vessels, coupled with inadequate proliferation of arterioles and capillaries, may limit myocardial perfusion. The myocyte hypertrophy that develops after myocardial damage must be accompanied by sufficient angiogenesis. In the absence of angiogenesis and capillary growth, hypertrophied myocytes are likely to be underperfused, which may reduce contractile function and promote further cell death.

The primary determinant of pathologic hypertrophy (in contrast to physiologic hypertrophy) may be the vascular component, as insufficient arteriolar and capillary growth may initiate the chain of events leading to the reduced contractile function, increased collagen production, and abnormal relaxation that characterize pathologic hypertrophy.

Coronary Endothelial Function in CHF

Severely impaired relaxation of the coronary microvasculature in response to acetylcholine has been demonstrated in patients with dilated cardiomyopathy, whereas the response to adenosine is only mildly impaired.[80] This finding suggests that the vascular endothelium is dysfunctional in the microvasculature of dilated hearts. The mechanisms responsible for vascular endothelial dysfunction in the coronary microvasculature of patients with dilated cardiomyopathy is unclear. An early primary genetic defect that affects the vascular endothelium cannot be ruled out. However, experimental evidence points out that a reduction in regional blood flow similar to that observed in the skeletal muscle vasculature may be the primary determinant of endothelial dysfunction.

Experimental studies using the canine pacing model of heart failure have shown that vascular endothelial dysfunction is observed in the coronary vessels only when the failure is overt.[81] During the early weeks of chronic pacing (i.e., weeks 1–3) endothelial function is enhanced and not reduced in the coronary vasculature.[82] This time dependence of coronary endothelial function in the pacing model of heart failure may explain the disparate findings initially reported.[82]

An overt state of CHF should be documented by precise measurement of cardiac function before assessing the vascular responses to endothelium dependent and independent stimuli. In addition, the time dependence of the coronary endothelial findings in the pacing model of cardiac failure argues that reduced blood flow may be responsible for the reduced endothelial function. During the first weeks of pacing, when coronary blood flow is increased, vascular endothelial function is enhanced. After 4 weeks of pacing, when CHF is overt, as demonstrated by abnormal cardiac output at rest, coronary blood flow is reduced and the vascular endothelium dysfunctional.

The enhanced endothelium-mediated dilatation of epicardial coronary arteries that occurs after 7 days of physical training in normal conscious dogs supports the view that blood flow is the important modulator of endothelial function and nitric oxide release.[83] The training-induced enhancement of endothelium-mediated dilatation in the coronary artery was demonstrated by an increased vasodilatory response to local administration of acetylcholine.[83] Chronic exercise appears to provide a stimulus for the enhanced production of endothelial dilating substances including nitric oxide. Endothelial cell nitric oxide synthase gene expression was shown to increase by two- to threefold in the aortic endothelial cells of failing dogs after 10 days of daily running on a treadmill.[84] Daily exercise increased endothelial cell nitric oxide synthase gene expression by presumably increasing endothelial shear stress.

CLINICAL IMPLICATIONS

During the late 1970s and early 1980s excessive systemic vasoconstriction was the major rationale behind the impetus for reducing cardiac afterload in patients with CHF. Nonspecific vasodilator agents such as hydralazine or minoxidil were used to improve LV cardiac performance by reducing cardiac afterload, thereby relieving the exertional symptoms of patients with CHF. Advances in the understanding of regional vascular control and circulatory abnormalities in patients with CHF have led to questioning the therapeutic validity of the excessive vasoconstriction pathophysiologic construct.

Among the pharmacologic agents that lower cardiac afterload, ACE inhibitors are the most beneficial. Interestingly, their clinical benefits appear to be mediated through specific cellular and molecular pathways. ACE inhibitors relieve symptoms and enhance peak exercise capacity by improving the vasodilatory response to exercise, which in turn results from regression of circulatory abnormalities and not by enhancing LV performance, which when present is modest. The therapeutic importance of the effects of ACE inhibitors in the vasculature is further illustrated by a significant reduction of reinfarction rates in patients with ischemic cardiomyopathy and by their absence of benefits on peak exercise capacity in patients with modest CHF who do not have substantial circulatory abnormalities. In these mildly symptomatic patients, ACE inhibitors beneficially affect LV remodeling but not symptoms.

The regional nature of vascular control is being increasingly recognized in patients with CHF. The regional nature of vascular control is particularly relevant to the skeletal muscle vasculature. The periodic increases in skeletal muscle blood flow that accompany physical training are sufficient to steadily improve the peripheral circulation, as evidenced by augmentation of maximal dilatory capacity (i.e., peak reactive hyperemia). Of note, the vascular benefits of physical training are observed even in patients who are treated with ACE inhibitors at recommended doses. Maintenance of near-normal vascular capacity allows patients with LV systolic dysfunction to remain free of exertional symptoms, although their peak oxygen uptake is reduced compared to that of age-matched normal subjects.[85] Thus the clinical paradox of severely depressed LV systolic function and unimpaired physical activity can, to a large extent, be explained by the absence of circulatory derangements. Patients who were physically trained before they developed LV dysfunction and who remained active despite the fall in ejection fraction are likely to be less symptomatic than patients who were sedentary before they developed LV dysfunction and further reduced their activities. Additional research regarding vascular control and circulatory derangements in patients with CHF may not solve the primary problem of heart failure, but it may allow patients to remain asymptomatic for longer periods of time.

REFERENCES

1. Zelis R, Longhurst J: The circulation in congestive heart failure. pp. 283–314. In Zelis R (ed): The Peripheral Circulations. Grune & Stratton, Orlands, 1975
2. Zelis R, Flaim SF, Liedtke J, Nellis SH: Cardiocirculatory dynamics in the normal and failing heart. Annu Rev Physiol 1981;43:455–476
3. Zelis R, Flaim SF: Alterations in vasomotor tone in congestive heart failure. Prog Cardiovasc Dis 1982;24:437–459
4. Zelis R, Sinoway L, Musch T, Davis D: Vasoconstrictor mechanisms in congestive heart failure. Part 1. Mod Concepts Cardiovasc Dis 1989;58(2):7–12
5. Zelis R, Sinoway L, Musch T et al: Metabolic and neurogenic determinants of blood flow in congestive heart failure. pp. 385–395. In Lewis BS, Kimchi A (eds): Heart Failure Mechanisms and Management. Springer, Berlin, 1991
6. Costin JC, Skinner NS Jr: Competition between vasoconstrictor and vasodilator mechanisms in skeletal muscle. Am J Physiol 1971;220:462–468
7. Mancini DM, Davis L, Wexler JP, Chadwick B, LeJemtel TH: Dependence of enhanced maximal exercise performance on increased peak skeletal muscle perfusion during long-term captopril therapy in heart failure. J Am Coll Cardiol 1987;10:845–850
8. Drexler H, Banhardt U, Meinertz T et al: Contrasting peripheral short-term and long-term effects of converting enzyme inhibition in patients with congestive heart failure. A double-blind, placebo-controlled trial. Circulation 1989;79:491–502
9. Cohn JN: Abnormalities of peripheral sympathetic nervous system control in congestive heart failure. Circulation, suppl. I 1990;82:59–67
10. Leier CV, Binkley PF, Cody RJ: α-Adrenergic component of the sympathetic nervous system in congestive heart failure. Circulation, suppl. I 1990;82:68–76
11. Pohl U, Holtz J, Busse R, Bassenge E: Crucial role of endothelium in the vasodilator response to increased flow in vivo. Hypertension 1986;8:37–44
12. Vane JR, Anggard EE, Botting RM: Regulatory functions of the vascular endothelium. N Engl J Med 1990;323:27–36
13. Davies PF, Tripathi SC: Mechanical stress mechanisms and the cell. An endothelial paradigm. Circ Res 1993;72:239–245
14. Miller VM, Vanhoutte PM: Enhanced release of endothelium-derived factor(s) by chronic increases in blood flow. Am J Physiol 1988;255:H446–H451
15. Kaiser L, Spickard RC, Olivier NB: Heart failure depresses endothelium-dependent responses in canine femoral artery. Am J Physiol 1989;256:H962–H967
16. Kubo SH, Rector TS, Bank AJ, Williams RE, Heifetz SM: Endothelium-dependent vasodilation is attenuated in patients with heart failure. Circulation 1991;84:1589–1596
17. Katz SD, Biasucci L, Sabba C et al: Impaired endothelium-mediated vasodilation in the peripheral vasculature of patients with congestive heart failure. J Am Coll Cardiol 1992;19:918–925
18. Moncada S, Radomski MW, Palmer RMJ: Endothelium-derived relaxing factor. Identification as nitric oxide and role in the control of vascular tone and platelet function. Biochem Pharmacol 1988;37:2495–2501
19. Koller A, Sun D, Huang A, Kaley G: Corelease of nitric oxide and prostaglandins mediates flow-dependent di-

lation of rat gracilis muscle arterioles. Am J Physiol 1994;267:H326–332

20. Cohen RA, Vanhoutte PM: Endothelium-dependent hyperpolarization. Beyond nitric oxide and cyclic GMP. Circulation 1995;92:3337–3349

21. Katz SD, Schwarz M, Yuen J, LeJemtel TH: Impaired acetylcholine-mediated vasodilation in patients with congestive heart failure. Role of endothelium-derived vasodilating and vasoconstricting factors. Circulation 1993;88:55–61

22. Drexler H, Hayoz D, Munzel T et al: Endothelial function in chronic congestive heart failure. Am J Cardiol 1992;69:1596–1601

23. Kubo SH, Rector TS, Bank AJ et al: Lack of contribution of nitric oxide to basal vasomotor tone in heart failure. Am J Cardiol 1994;74:1133–1136

24. Katz SD, Krum H, Khan T: Exercise-induced vasodilation in the forearm circulation of normal subjects and patients with congestive heart failure. Role of endothelium-derived nitric oxide. J Am Coll Cardiol (1996, in press)

25. Koller A, Kaley G: Endothelial regulation of wall shear stress and blood flow in skeletal muscle microcirculation. Am J Physiol 1991;260:H862–868

26. Teerlink JR, Clozel M, Fischli W, Clozel J-P: Temporal evolution of endothelial dysfunction in a rat model of chronic heart failure. J Am Coll Cardiol 1993;22:615–620

27. Teerlink JR, Gray GA, Clozel M, Clozel J-P: Increased vascular responsiveness to norepinephrine in rats with heart failure is endothelium dependent. Dissociation of basal and stimulated nitric oxide release. Circulation 1994;89:393–401

28. Main JS, Forster C, Armstrong PW: Inhibitory role of the coronary arterial endothelium to α-adrenergic stimulation in experimental heart failure. Circ Res 1991;68:940–946

29. Forster C, Campbell PM, Armstrong PW: Temporal alterations in peripheral vascular responsiveness during both the development and recovery from pacing-induced heart failure. J Cardiovasc Pharmacol 1992;20:206–215

30. Hirsch H, Demopoulos LA, Woo D, Jones M, LeJemtel T: Flow-mediated vasodilatation is impaired in congestive heart failure [abstract]. J Am Coll Cardiol 1994;1A–484A:271A

31. Schwarz M, Katz SD, Demopoulos L et al: Enhancement of endothelium-dependent vasodilation by low-dose nitroglycerin in patients with congestive heart failure. Circulation 1994;89:1609–1614

32. Hirooka Y, Imaizumi T, Harada S et al: Endothelium-dependent forearm vasodilation with acetylcholine but not that with substance P is impaired in patients with heart failure. J Cardiovasc Pharmacol, suppl. 12 1992;20:221–225

33. Katz SD: The role of endothelium-derived vasoactive substances in the pathophysiology of exercise intolerance in patients with congestive heart failure. Prog Cardiovasc Dis 1995;38:23–50

34. Noris M, Morigi M, Donadelli R et al: Nitric oxide synthesis by cultured endothelial cells is modulated by flow conditions. Circ Res 1995;76:536–543

35. Sun D, Huang A, Koller A, Kaley G: Short-term daily exercise activity enhances endothelial NO synthesis in skeletal muscle arterioles of rats. J Appl Physiol 1994;76:2241–2247

36. Koller A, Huang A, Sun D, Kaley G: Exercise training augments flow-dependent dilation in rat skeletal muscle arterioles. Role of endothelial nitric oxide and prostaglandins. Circ Res 1995;76:544–550

37. Delp MD, McAllister RM, Laughlin MH: Exercise training alters endothelium-dependent vasoreactivity of rat abdominal aorta. J Appl Physiol 1993;75:1354–1363

38. Katz SD, Klapholz M, Jondeau G et al: Endothelium-dependent vasodilation is improved by physical training in normal subjects. pp. 229–237. In Brouset JB (ed): Proceedings of the Vth World Congress on Cardiac Rehabilitation. Intercept, Andover, Hampshire, 1993

39. Smith CJ, Sun D, Hoegler C et al: Reduced gene expression of vascular endothelial NO synthase and cyclooxygenase-1 in heart failure. Circ Res 1996;78:58–64

40. Sessa WC, Pritchard K, Seyedi N, Wang J, Hintze TH: Chronic exercise in dogs increases coronary vascular nitric oxide production and endothelial cell nitric oxide synthase gene expression. Circ Res 1994;74:349–353

41. Katz SD, Yuen J, Bijou R, LeJemtel TH: Physical training specifically improves endothelium-dependent control of vascular reactivity in resistance vessels of patients with congestive heart failure. Circulation (in press)

42. Zelis R, Mason DT, Braunwald E, Winterhalter M, King C: A comparison of the effects of vasodilator stimuli on peripheral resistance vessels in normal subjects and in patients with congestive heart failure. J Clin Invest 1968;47:960–970

43. Zelis R, Longhurst J, Capone RJ, Mason DT: A comparison of regional blood flow and oxygen utilization during dynamic forearm exercise in normal subjects and patients with congestive heart failure. Circulation 1974;50:137–143

44. Zelis R, Maston DT, Braunwald E: Partition of blood flow to the cutaneous and muscular beds of the forearm at rest and during leg exercise in normal subjects and in patients with heart failure. Circ Res 1969;24:799–806

45. Longhurst J, Gifford W, Zelis R: Impaired forearm oxygen consumption during static exercise in patients with congestive heart failure. Circulation 1976;54:477–480

46. Cowley AJ, Stainer K, Rowley JM, Hampton JR: Abnormalities of the peripheral circulation and respiratory function in patients with severe heart failure. Br Heart J 1986;55:75–80

47. LeJemtel TH, Maskin CS, Lucido D, Chadwick BJ: Failure to augment maximal limb blood flow in response to one-leg versus two-leg exercise in patients with severe heart failure. Circulation 1986;74:245–251

48. LeJemtel TH, Maskin CS, Chadwick B, Sinoway L: Near maximal oxygen extraction by exercising muscles in patients with severe heart failure. A limitation to benefits of training [abstract]. J Am Coll Cardiol 1983;1:662

49. Marshall JM: Skeletal muscle vasculature and systemic hypoxia. NIPS 1995;10:274–280

50. Jondeau G, Katz SD, Zohman L et al: Active skeletal muscle mass and cardiopulmonary reserve. Failure to attain peak aerobic capacity during maximal bicycle exercise in patients with severe congestive heart failure. Circulation 1992;86:1351–1356

51. Jondeau G, Dib J-C, Dubourg O, Bourdarias J-P: Func-

tional improvement in heart failure after ACE inhibition. Relation with peripheral limitation. Am J Cardiol (in press)

52. Musch TI, Terrell JA: Skeletal muscle blood flow abnormalities in rats with a chronic myocardial infarction. Rest and exercise. Am J Physiol 1992;262: H411–419

53. Drexler H, Flaim SF, Toggart EJ, Glick MR, Zelis R: Cardiocirculatory adjustments to exercise following myocardial infarction in rats. Basic Res Cardiol 1986; 81:350–360

54. Drexler H, Toggart EJ, Glick MR et al: Regional vascular adjustments during recovery from myocardial infarction in rats. J Am Coll Cardiol 1986;8:134–142

55. Wilson JR, Wiener DH, Fink LI, Ferraro N: Vasodilatory behavior of skeletal muscle arterioles in patients with nonedematous chronic heart failure. Circulation 1986;74:775–779

56. Mancini DM, LeJemtel TH, Factor S et al: Central and peripheral components of heart failure. Am J Med, suppl. 28 1986;80:2–13

57. Wilson JR, Martin JL, Ferraro N: Impaired skeletal muscle nutritive flow during exercise in patients with congestive heart failure. Role of cardiac pump dysfunction as determined by the effect of dobutamine. Am J Cardiol 1984;53:1308–1315

58. Wilson JR, Martin JL, Ferraro N, Weber KT: Effect of hydralazine on perfusion and metabolism in the leg during upright bicycle exercise in patients with heart failure. Circulation 1983;68:425–432

59. Arnold JMO, Ribeiro J, Colucci WS: Muscle blood flow during forearm exercise in patients with severe heart failure. Circulation 1990;82:465–472

60. Zucker IH, Brandle M, Schultz HD, Patel KP: Neural regulation of sympathetic nerve activity in heart failure. Prog Cardiovasc Dis 1995;37:397–414

61. Mark AL: Sympathetic dysregulation in heart failure. Mechanisms and therapy. Clin Cardiol, suppl. I 1995; 18:3–8

62. Sterns DA, Ettinger SM, Gray KS et al: Skeletal muscle meta-baroreceptor exercise responses are attenuated in heart failure. Circulation 1991;84:2034–2039

63. Brandle M, Patel K, Wang W, Zucker IH: Hemodynamic and norepinephrine responses to pace-induced heart failure in conscious sino-aortic denervated dogs. J Appl Physiol 1996 (in press)

64. Brandle M, Wang W, Zucker IH: Ventricular mechanoreflex and chemoreflex alterations in chronic heart failure. Circ Res 1994;74:262–270

65. Lonn EM, Yusuf S, Jha P et al: Emerging role of angiotensin-converting enzyme inhibitors in cardiac and vascular protection. Circulation 1994;909:2056–2069

66. Zimmerman BG, Gomer SK, Liao JC: Action of angiotensin on vascular adrenergic nerve endings. Facilitation of norepinephrine release. Fed Proc 1972;31: 1344–1350

67. Dibona GF, Jones SY, Brooks VL: Ang II receptor blockade and arterial baroreflex regulation of renal nerve activity in cardiac failure. Am J Physiol 1995; 269:R1189–R1196

68. Murakami H, Liu J-L, Zucker IH: Blockade of AT_1 receptors enhances baroreflex control of heart rate in conscious rabbits with heart failure. Am J Physiol 1996;271:R303–R309.

69. Jondeau G, Katz SD, Toussaint J-F et al: Regional specificity of peak hyperemic response in patients with congestive heart failure. Correlation with peak aerobic capacity. J Am Coll Cardiol 1993;22:1399–1402

70. Sinoway LI, Musch TI, Minotti JR, Zelis R: Enhanced maximal metabolic vasodilation in the dominant forearms of tennis players. J Appl Physiol 1986;61: 673–678

71. Sinoway LI: Effect of conditioning and deconditioning stimuli on metabolically determined blood flow in humans and implications for congestive heart failure. Am J Cardiol 1988;62:45E–48E

72. Langille BL, O'Connell F: Reductions in arterial diameter produced by chronic decreases in blood flow are endothelium-dependent. Science 1986;231:405–407

73. Parodi O, DeMaria R, Oltrona L et al: Myocardial blood flow distribution in patients with ischemic heart disease or dilated cardiomyopathy undergoing heart transplantation. Circulation 1993;88:509–522

74. Bulkley BH, Hutchins GM, Bailey I, Strauss HW, Pitt B: Thallium 201 imaging and gated cardiac blood pool scans in patients with ischemic and idiopathic congestive cardiomyopathy. A clinical and pathologic study. Circulation 1977;55:753–760

75. Beltrami CA, Finato N, Rocco M et al: Structural basis of end-stage failure in ischemic cardiomyopathy in humans. Circulation 1994;89:151–163

76. Beltrami CA, Finato N, Rocco M et al: The cellular basis of dilated cardiomyopathy in humans. J Mol Cell Cardiol 1995;27:291–305

77. Tomanek RJ: Response of the coronary vasculature to myocardial hypertrophy. J Am Coll Cardiol 1990;15: 528–533

78. Wangler RD, Peters KG, Marcus ML, Tomanek RJ: Effects of duration and severity of arterial hypertension and cardiac hypertrophy on coronary vasodilator reserve. Circ Res 1982;51:10–18

79. Cannon RO III, Cunnion RE, Parrillo JE et al: Dynamic limitation of coronary vasodilator reserve in patients with dilated cardiomyopathy and chest pain. J Am Coll Cardiol 1987;10:1190–1200

80. Treasure CB, Vita JA, Cox DA et al: Endothelium-dependent dilation of the coronary microvasculature is impaired in dilated cardiomyopathy. Circulation 1990; 81:772–779

81. Wang J, Seyedi N, Xu X-B, Wolin MS, Hintze TH: Defective endothelium-mediated control of coronary circulation in conscious dogs after heart failure. Am J Physiol 1994;266:H670–680

82. Hintze TH, Wang J, Seyedi N, Wolin MS: Role of EDRF/NO in chronic high coronary blood flow states during myocardial dysfunction and failure. In Bevan J, Kaley G, Rubanyi G (eds): Flow Velocity Control of the Circulation. Oxford University Press, New York, 1995

83. Wang J, Wolin MS, Hintze TH: Chronic exercise enhances endothelium-mediated dilation of epicardial coronary artery in conscious dogs. Circ Res 1993;73: 829–838

84. Sessa WC, Pritchard K, Seyedi N, Wang J, Hintze TH: Chronic exercise in dogs increases coronary vascular nitric oxide production and endothelial cell nitric oxide synthase gene expression. Circ Res 1994;74:349–353

85. LeJemtel TH, Liang C-s, Stewart DK et al: Reduced peak aerobic capacity in asymptomatic left ventricular systolic dysfunction. A substudy of the Studies of Left Ventricular Dysfunction (SOLVD). Circulation 1994; 90:2757–2760

14 Sympathetic Nervous System

Guido Grassi
Bianca Maria Cattaneo
Giuseppe Mancia

In the past congestive heart failure (CHF) was usually regarded as a clinical syndrome primarily due to and characterized by an impairment of systolic and diastolic function of cardiac muscle tissue. That is, CHF has been associated primarily with impairment of the heart as a pump (and therefore with an imbalance between oxygen supply and oxygen needs). Hence the attention of investigators and clinicians has been directed mainly to the causes and mechanisms of myocardial damage.

Evidence that CHF is accompanied by major alterations of the peripheral circulation has been growing rapidly along with the observation that these alterations include a major mechanism of cardiovascular control (i.e., the autonomic nervous system[1,2]). In their pioneering work performed during the 1950s, Bridgen and Sharpey-Schafer[3] demonstrated that patients with CHF display a reduction of the sympathetically mediated vascular responses on assumption of the upright posture. It was then shown in several studies that in the "failing-heart syndrome" sympathetic tone is markedly increased[2,4,5] and that abnormalities in reflex cardiovascular control often occur.[2,6] Finally, research performed in animal models of CHF and in humans have defined the extent and time course of the changes in autonomic cardiovascular control that take place during heart failure, shedding light on their mechanisms, clinical significance, and reversal with treatment.[7–10]

The aim of this chapter is to review the sympathetic abnormalities and the alterations in autonomic cardiovascular control that characterize the CHF state, followed by an analysis of the pathophysiologic implications and clinical relevance of these phenomena. Finally, the effects of nonpharmacologic and pharmacologic interventions on the sympathetic disturbances that characterize CHF are discussed.

SYMPATHETIC ACTIVATION

Urinary and Plasma Norepinephrine

The first direct evidence that sympathetic activity is increased during CHF goes back to the demonstration that urinary catecholamines and their metabolites are increased in this condition compared to that in healthy subjects.[2,5] When technical refinement allowed the sensitivity of catecholamine assessments to be markedly increased so they can be measured in plasma, this finding was confirmed by plasma catecholamine values as well. That is, it was shown in a large number of studies that the plasma norepinephrine concentration is greater in resting patients with CHF than in controls.[4,5,7,8] This finding pertains when measurements are obtained from venous or arterial blood.[5,7,8] It is also the case when plasma norepinephrine is measured during dynamic exercise; indeed, the greater increase in plasma norepinephrine during exercise in patients with CHF

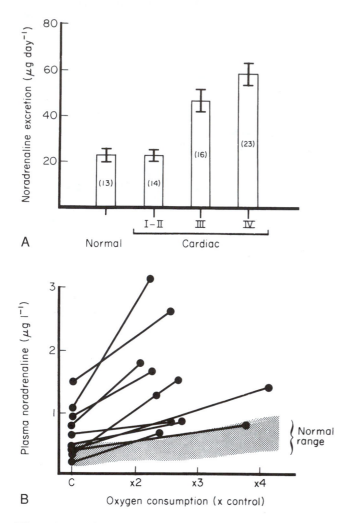

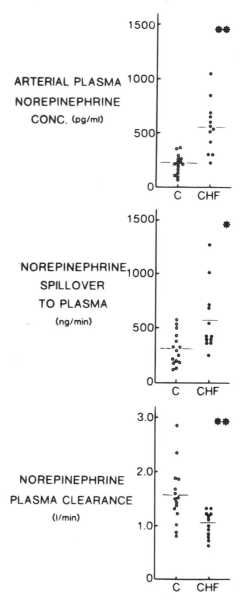

overcome by a technique developed by Esler and co-workers.[13] These investigators made use of intravenous infusions of small amounts of radiolabeled norepinephrine to measure directly the tissue clearance of this neurotransmitter and thus calculate (by subtracting the clearance from the plasma norepinephrine value) the net "spillover" of norepinephrine from the neuroeffector junctions. This test allowed an elegant demonstration that with CHF norepinephrine clearance is indeed reduced but that its "spillover" is definitively increased and that this increase accounts for more than half of the overall increase in

Fig. 14-1. **(A)** Urinary and **(B)** plasma norepinephrine values in normal subjects and in patients with congestive heart failure (CHF). **(B)** Plasma norepinephrine values in patients with CHF are compared to the normal range at rest and during an increase in oxygen consumption induced by exercise. Cardiac, congestive heart failure. Roman numbers refer to NYHA functional class. (From Mancia,[8] with permission.)

makes the difference from control subjects even more apparent[11,12] (Fig. 14-1).

Norepinephrine Spillover Technique

With CHF an increased plasma norepinephrine level does not per se prove the occurrence of a sympathetic activation because the plasma level of this adrenergic neurotransmitter depends not only on the amount secreted from sympathetic nerve terminals but also on its "clearance" from the peripheral circulation. The latter is a function of blood flow and cardiac output and is thus reduced in the presence of a failing heart. This limitation, however, has been

Fig. 14-2. Arterial plasma norepinephrine, norepinephrine spillover rate, and norepinephrine clearance in control subjects (C) and patients with congestive heart failure (CHF). *$P < 0.02$ and **$P < 0.002$ for mean values of the two groups. (From Hasking et al.,[14] with permission.)

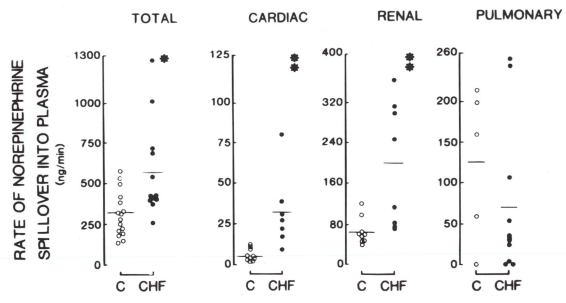

Fig. 14-3. Norepinephrine spillover rate into plasma from the systemic circulation, heart, kidney, and lungs in control subjects (C) and congestive heart failure (CHF) patients. (From Hasking et al.,[14] with permission.)

plasma norepinephrine[14] (Fig. 14-2). These findings have been confirmed in other studies,[15,16] and calculation of the norepinephrine spillover rate independently in several vascular districts (by collecting blood samples from various arteries and regional veins) has demonstrated that it occurs to a marked extent in vital organs, such as the heart and the kidney (Fig. 14-3). The norepinephrine spillover rate is increased also in the brain and skeletal muscle,[17] which suggests that this phenomenon involves most of the cardiovascular system.

Microneurographic Recording

Efferent postganglionic nerve activity can be measured in conscious humans by a microneurographic technique that employs a tungsten microelectrode inserted in the fascicles of the peroneal or brachial nerve innervating skeletal muscle.[18] This method has three advantages over the technique based on plasma norepinephrine assay: (1) Microneurographic assessment displays a greater sensitivity for detecting changes in sympathetic activity than plasma norepinephrine measurement.[19] (2) Reproducibility of the measurements in the same session or at an interval of several weeks is greater for the microneurographic approach.[20] (3) Microneurography provides a direct assessment of sympathetic nerve traffic rather than the indirect estimate provided by the plasma norepinephrine assay, thereby avoiding the confounding effect of peripheral factors[19] (e.g., reuptake and clearance of norepineph-

rine, variable secretion rate of neurotransmitter, variable responsiveness of adrenergic receptors and effector mechanisms) when interpreting the data.

Several microneurographic studies have found that heart failure patients are characterized by a resting muscle sympathetic nerve activity that is markedly greater than that displayed by age-matched healthy subjects.[21-24] This is true not only when data are expressed as burst frequency over time, but also when they are corrected for the accompanying heart rate values to account for a possible increase in nerve traffic due to a heart failure-related tachycardia. It has also been found that the magnitude of the muscle nerve sympathetic activation correlates (1) directly with the severity of symptoms of congestive heart failure, that is, with the New York Heart Association (NYHA) functional class of the patient[25], and (2) inversely with measures of left ventricular function such as left ventricular stroke work, stroke volume, and ejection fraction.[22,25] This leaves no doubt that sympathetic activity is increased with CHF. It does not dispose of all questions related to this increase, however, because one limitation of microneurography is that it allows measurement only of muscle sympathetic nerve traffic, which leaves open the question whether muscle sympathetic activation reflects sympathetic activation in other vascular districts. There is a linear correlation between the sympathetic nerve traffic occurring with CHF and the concomitant plasma norepinephrine levels.[21] The value of this observation, however, is limited by the fact that plasma norepinephrine probably originates mainly from skeletal muscle tissues[26,27] and thus may also be a selective, rather than an overall, marker of sympathetic activity.[19] Indeed, microneurographic assessment of skin efferent sympathetic activity has provided values that are superimposable on those found in age-matched healthy controls.[28] As discussed below, it may be explained by the fact that skin sympathetic nerve traffic is controlled by mechanisms (e.g., thermoregulation, emotion) that are probably preserved during CHF and not by reflex influences that are impaired in this condition.[29,30] At any rate, it clearly indicates a certain amount of between-vascular beds heterogeneity in the sympathetic activation that occurs during CHF, a subject that needs to be explored more deeply and precisely characterized.

Heart Rate and Blood Pressure Variability

Sympathetic activity decreases and vagal activity increases at night, leading to marked hypotension and bradycardia.[31] Both of these changes have been shown to be blunted with CHF,[32] again pointing to an abnormal autonomic modulation of the heart and the peripheral circulation.

Further evidence of this abnormality has been provided by spectral analysis of heart variations[19] in bands that are reported as specific for vagal (high frequency band, 0.2 to 0.4 Hz) and sympathetic (low frequency band, 0.02 to 0.07 Hz) modulation of the sinus node. In patients with CHF (NYHA functional class II or III) due to coronary heart disease, the spectral power of the low frequency and high frequency heart rate variations was found to be increased and reduced, respectively.[33] Similar findings were observed in other studies on patients with CHF of various etiologies and severities,[34–37] suggesting an overall enhanced sympathetic and impaired parasympathetic control of the heart under all these conditions. In one study[38] 8 weeks of physical training reduced the low frequency power of the R-R interval on the electrocardiogram (ECG) while concomitantly increasing the high frequency R-R interval power, indicating the possibility of reversing these changes by treating the CHF nonpharmacologically.

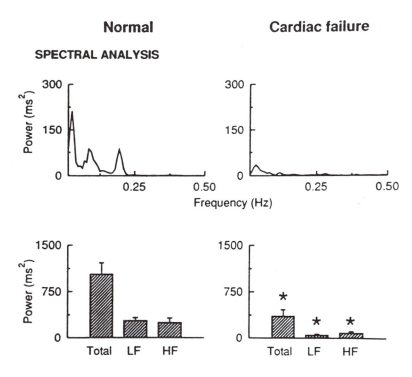

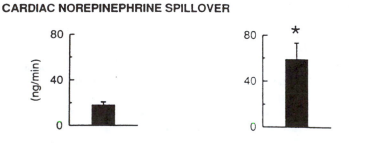

Fig. 14-4. Mean total power, low frequency (LF, 0.1 Hz) power, and high frequency (HF, 0.2–0.4 Hz) heart rate power in normal subjects and patients with congestive heart failure of NYHA class III or IV. Data (means ± SEM) are compared with cardiac norepinephrine spillover rate for the same two groups. (From Kingwell et al.,[40] with permission.)

No information is available on the critical issue of low and high frequency blood pressure powers in CHF. Furthermore, the effects of drug treatment on low and high frequency heart rate powers have never been systematically investigated. Finally, and most importantly, no definite conclusion is available on the overall value of the power spectral approach to quantity precisely the autonomic influences on the heart and blood vessels. There is no question that by considering heart rate and blood pressure responses this approach addresses actual autonomic cardiovascular influences rather than intermediate steps in the chain of events expressing autonomic activa-

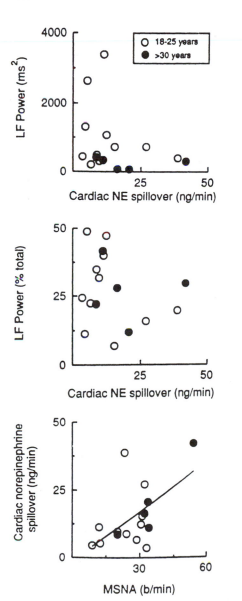

Fig. 14-5. Relation between LF heart rate power, cardiac norepinephrine spillover, and muscle sympathetic nerve activity (MSNA) in normal subjects. (From Kingwell et al.,[40] with permission.)

tion.[19] There is evidence, however, that the sensitivity, specificity, and reproducibility of high and low power values as autonomic markers may be limited.[19,39] For CHF this point has been emphasized by the report of a reduction in the low frequency heart rate power concomitant with a marked increase in the norepinephrine "spillover" rate from the coronary sinus[40] (Fig. 14-4). It has been additionally emphasized by the observation that cardiac norepinephrine "spillover" correlates with muscle sympathetic nerve traffic but that neither correlates with low frequency power for heart rate[40] (Fig. 14-5).

ADRENERGIC RECEPTORS

Bristow and coworkers reported that the inotropic responses to the in vitro administration of isoproterenol were blunted in ventricular myocytes from failing human hearts compared to those from healthy donors.[41] Their finding was confirmed by in vivo studies[42,43] on the contractile and tachycardic effects of adrenergic stimuli, which also showed that the impaired responses involved the β_1-adrenergic receptors (i.e., the receptors innervated by sympathetic fibers). It established the concept that the responsiveness of cardiac β-adrenoreceptors is impaired in CHF due to a reduced receptor density in the myocyte surface or to a reduced receptor sensitivity (or both).

The mechanisms of these β-adrenoreceptor abnormalities are not clear, but because a failing heart shows a normal inotropic response to calcium[44] it is believed that the mechanisms are specific for adrenergic stimuli and that they mainly consist of down-regulation of β_1-adrenergic receptors accompanying their long-lasting exposure to enhanced sympathetic activation.[42,44] Whether a similar down-regulation involves other adrenergic receptors is less clear; and indeed the responsiveness of β_2-adrenergic receptors to agonist stimulation has been shown to be better preserved in the presence of CHF,[45] possibly because these receptors lack sympathetic innervation and therefore are not exposed to the marked local increase in catecholamine concentrations due to an increased sympathetic drive. It is also not clear if down-regulation involves α-adrenergic receptors.[45] For the purpose of the present chapter the reduced responsiveness of β_1-adrenergic receptors to sympathetic stimuli implies that with CHF there are local factors that limit the effect of a continuing sympathetic activation, at least on the heart. The overall sympathetic activation is thus less than predicted on the basis of the increase in sympathetic nerve traffic and the secretion of plasma norepinephrine. This state may become more evident as the CHF worsens, not only because of a progressive increase in the adrenoreceptor down-regulation but also because of exhaustion of the norepinephrine stores in the sympathetic nerve terminals, which leads to a marked reduction of cardiac catecholamine content.

CLINICAL AND PROGNOSTIC IMPLICATIONS OF SYMPATHETIC ACTIVATION

With CHF, sympathetic activation represents a homeostatic mechanism that preserves tissue perfusion. As shown in Table 14-1, it can be achieved through a variety of effects: (1) An increase in sympathetic drive enhances heart rate and myocardial contractility, thereby acting to maintain the output of the failing heart. (2) Sympathetic activation causes arteriolar vasoconstriction, which maintains arterial blood pressure despite cardiac output reduction. (3) This activation leads to systemic venoconstriction and sodium and water retention (through increased secretion of renin, reduced renal blood flow, and increased sodium and water reabsorption), which enhances venous return to the heart and augments cardiac filling pressure, further helping cardiac performance through the Starling mechanism. However, the sympathetic activation that occurs with CHF may also exert a wide range of adverse effects. For example, an increase in heart rate and myocardial contractility enhances cardiac work while reduc-

Table 14-1. Compensatory and Adverse Effects of Sympathetic Activation During CHF

Compensatory effects
    Increased heart rate and myocardial contractility
    Arteriolar vasoconstriction
    Systemic venoconstriction and sodium and water retention
Adverse effects
    Increased cardiac work
    Reduced coronary perfusion
    Increased cardiac afterload and preload
    Fluid retention and circulatory congestion
    Myocardial necrosis
    Potassium loss and cardiac arrhythmias

ing coronary perfusion. Furthermore, arteriolar constriction and venoconstriction increases cardiac afterload and preload, increasing cardiac work and myocardial oxygen consumption while reducing, via a direct increase in coronary vascular resistance, myocardial oxygen supply. In addition, renal sympathetic effects cause sodium and water retention, contributing, with the venoconstriction, to circulatory congestion. Finally, when plasma catecholamine levels are extremely high, myocardial necrosis is produced.[46] These conditions explain the clinical observation that in CHF patients plasma norepinephrine values are inversely related to the patient's survival[47,48] (Fig. 14-6). It also provides a pathophysiologic background for the evidence that cardiac ar-

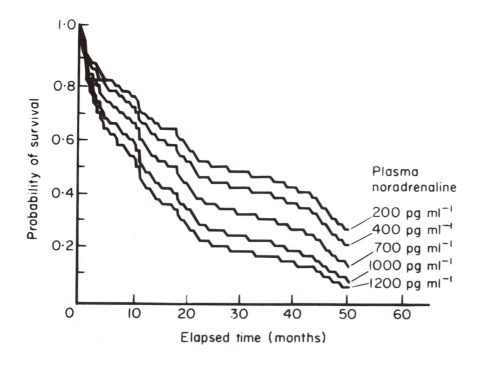

Plasma noradrenaline

200 pg ml^{-1}
400 pg ml^{-1}
700 pg ml^{-1}
1000 pg ml^{-1}
1200 pg ml^{-1}

Fig. 14-6. Relation between plasma norepinephrine values and probability of survival in patients with congestive heart failure. (From Cohn et al.,[47] with permission.)

rhythmias, even of a life-threatening type, are common events with CHF, possibly accounting for the high rate of sudden death typical of this condition.[49]

SYMPATHETIC ACTIVATION IN CHF: EARLY OR LATE PHENOMENON?

The important implications of sympathetic activation during CHF pose three questions: At what stage in the evolution of CHF does sympathetic activation appear? Why does this activation lead to adverse consequences? When do these consequences prevail over the compensatory effects of an increased sympathetic tone? No information is available on the last two questions, although it is possible to speculate that the continuing (and perhaps excessive) activation of a system whose homeostatic involvement is normally episodic is a major factor. In contrast, several studies agree that although the sympathetic activation is related to the severity of the CHF an increased sympathetic tone can be seen in CHF patients with mild or no symptoms at all. A large database on this issue comes from the SOLVD trial, in which plasma norepinephrine was slightly but significantly increased, even when patients belonging to the prevention group (NYHA functional class I) were considered[50] (Fig. 14-7). Similar results were

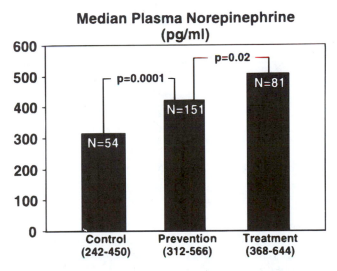

Fig. 14-7. Mean plasma norepinephrine values in control subjects, patients with NYHA class II–II congestive heart failure (SOLVD Prevention Study), and patients with NYHA class II–III congestive heart failure (SOLVD Treatment Study). Numbers with histograms refer to subjects studied. Numbers within parentheses refer to the range of plasma norepinephrine values. (From Francis et al.,[50] with permission.)

obtained in the SAVE study, which recruited patients with a left ventricular dysfunction due to myocardial infarction but who were largely asymptomatic.[51]

Straightforward evidence of early sympathetic activation during CHF has been obtained by our group[25] in patients belonging to NYHA functional class I or II who had much less impairment of left ventricular function than the patients recruited in the SOLVD and the SAVE studies. That is, our patients had a left ventricular ejection fraction amounting to 44.9 ± 3.3 percent (mean ± SEM) rather than less than 35 percent and 40 percent as in previous studies.[50,51] Other notable features were that, in addition to being age-matched with a control group, the recruited patients had no history of hypertension and no treatment with angiotensin-converting enzyme (ACE) inhibitors, vasodilators, or digitalis, which removed several confounding influences when interpreting the results. As shown in Figure 14-8, sympathetic activity as measured by microneurography was significantly greater with mild CHF failure than in control individuals, a further significant increase being observed in a third group of age-matched patients with more severe CHF and altered cardiac function. Plasma atrial natriuretic peptide also showed a progressive increase from the controls to those with mild and severe CHF, and plasma norepinephrine, plasma renin activity, and plasma vasopressin increased significantly only in those with severe CHF.

Taken together these studies leave no doubt that sympathetic activation is an early phenomenon of CHF, and that if a sensitive marker such as microneurography is used sympathetic activation can be recognized in an asymptomatic stage when left ventricular function is only moderately depressed. The results also suggest that it is the case for atrial natriuretic peptide, whereas stimulation of the renin-angiotensin system and vasopressin secretion is a later event (see Ch. 15).

MECHANISMS OF SYMPATHETIC ACTIVATION

The mechanisms responsible for the sympathetic activation that occurs during CHF are not completely understood. One possibility is that the activation is secondary to activation of the renin-angiotensin system, given the marked stimulatory influence exerted by angiotensin II on central sympathetic modulation, norepinephrine secretion from sympathetic nerve terminals, and adrenergic receptor responsiveness.[52,53] This possibility is made unlikely, however,

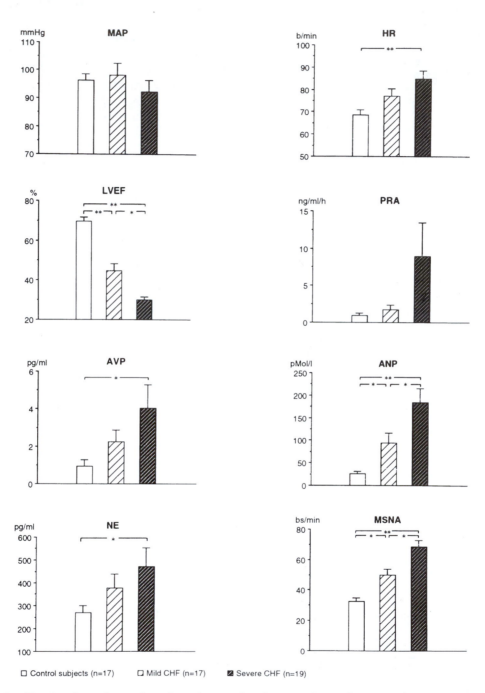

Fig. 14-8. Resting hemodynamic values, humoral values, and muscle sympathetic nerve activity in control subjects (open histograms), patients with mild congestive heart failure (dashed histograms), and patients with severe congestive heart failure (dark histograms). Data are shown as means ± SE. *$P <$ 0.05, **$P <$ 0.01. MAP, mean arterial pressure; HR, heart rate; LVEF, left ventricular ejection fraction; PRA, plasma renin activity; AVP, plasma arginine vasopressin; ANP, plasma atrial natriuretic peptide; NE, plasma norepinephrine; MSNA, muscle sympathetic nerve activity. (Data from Grassi et al.[25])

by the observation that with mild CHF sympathetic activation precedes rather than follows activation of the renin-angiotensin system.[25,50,51]

An alternative possibility is that the sympathetic activation characterizing CHF has a reflex origin.[7,8,21] This possibility has received experimental support in both animals and humans and thus is discussed in greater detail.

Arterial Baroreflex

Arterial baroreceptor signals may be reduced with CHF owing to a reduction in pulse pressure, pulse dP/dt, and mean arterial pressure.[7,8] With early CHF, however, these changes are often barely visible, which means that a "physiologic" baroreceptor deactivation cannot easily explain the concomitantly marked sympathetic overactivity. It is more likely to be accounted for by a striking reduction of baroreflex sensitivity, which makes the reflex unable to exert its inhibitory and excitatory influences on sympathetic and vagal tone, respectively.[7,8,54] Eckberg and coworkers[6] first documented this reduction by showing that in heart failure patients the reflex vagal bradycardia induced by stimulating arterial baroreceptors via an intravenous bolus of phenylephrine was reduced by more than 75 percent compared to the response seen in healthy controls. A similar reduction was then observed for the tachycardia induced by deactivating arterial baroreceptors via an intravenous bolus or an infusion of a nitrate.[55] Finally, the changes in sympathetic nerve activity (microneurography) induced by prolonged baroreceptor stimulation and deactivation brought about by increasing and reducing blood pressure via phenylephrine and nitroprusside infusions were also found to be impaired in those with CHF.[24]

Evidence regarding the relation between baroreflex impairment and the stage of the heart failure has been provided by our group.[25] Resting sympathetic nerve traffic was measured in control subjects, CHF patients of NYHA classes I–II and only moderate ventricular dysfunction, and CHF patients of NYHA classes III–IV. As shown in Figure 14-9, when baroreceptors were progressively stimulated by stepwise increases in blood pressure (phenylephrine infusion), the reflex bradycardia and sympathoinhibition were virtually abolished in patients with severe CHF but were almost as strikingly attenuated in those with mild CHF. The same results were seen regarding the tachycardia and sympathoexcitation induced by progressive baroreceptor deactivation that accompanies a stepwise reduction in blood pressure (nitroprusside infusion), although in this in-

stance the alteration observed with mild CHF was less pronounced.

There is therefore no question that the ability of arterial baroreceptors to enhance vagal tone and restrain sympathetic tone is compromised in the presence of CHF, and that the impairment involves the entire reflex stimulus–response curve. This phenomenon is already marked at an early phase of CHF.

Cardiopulmonary Reflex

Sympathetic tone is under tonic restraint from stretch receptors located in the heart and lungs[56] (in humans mainly in the heart[57,58]) that respond predominantly to changes in central blood volume. At variance with arterial baroreceptors, these receptors exert a major restraint also on renal secretion of renin and central secretion of vasopressin.[58–60] Similar to arterial baroreceptors, however, their reflex sympathetic modulation is virtually abolished in the presence of severe CHF[61,62] and is strikingly reduced with mild CHF.[23,63] This point is illustrated in Figure 14-10, which shows that the reflex increase in forearm vascular resistance induced by deactivating cardiac volume receptors through a reduction of central venous pressure and blood volume brought about by lower body negative pressure was markedly less in patients with NYHA class II CHF than in controls.[23] A similar impairment was observed when forearm vascular resistance was reflexly reduced by stimulating cardiac receptors through an increase in central venous pressure induced by passive leg raising.

Thus both reflexogenic areas involved in restraint of sympathetic tone are compromised at an early stage of CHF. This finding implies a condition of "functional afferent denervation,"[62,64] which may be responsible, at least in part, for the early appearance and subsequent progression of sympathetic activation. As far as the cardiopulmonary reflex is concerned, it may also lead to a derangement of humoral mechanisms involved not only in blood pressure modulation but also in blood volume control, accounting for other alterations of CHF.

Arterial Compliance

The reflex impairment characterizing CHF is not due to a nonspecific reduction of effector responsiveness to autonomic stimuli because the cardiac and vascular effects of the cold pressor test are preserved in this condition.[25,61,65] Other possibilities are impairment of the central integration of afferent barorecep-

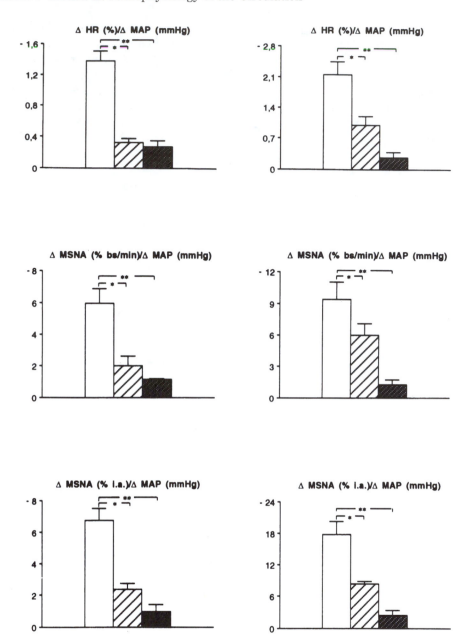

Fig. 14-9. Sensitivity of the baroreceptor–heart rate and sympathetic reflex in the three groups of subjects of Figure 14-8. Baroreflex sensitivity was calculated separately for baroreceptor stimulation (phenylephrine infusion, *left*) and deactivation (nitroprusside infusion, *right*). In either instances, ratios between the HR or MSNA changes and the corresponding MAP changes were calculated. Data are shown as means ± SE. Symbols are as in preceding figures. i.a., integrated MSNA activity. (From Grassi et al.,[25] with permission.)

tor or cardiopulmonary receptor signals, receptor structural or functional damage, and reduced compliance of the vascular structure in which the receptors are located.[23] The last possibility has received support by studies that have shown that the radial artery diameter was similar in patients with CHF and control subjects throughout the systodiastolic blood pressure range.[66–68] In contrast, radial artery compliance (which showed a curvilinear reduction

from diastolic to systolic pressure) was markedly diminished in the former compared to the latter condition[68] (Fig. 14-11). Radial artery compliance showed some impairment also in mild CHF in which the normally occurring increase in arterial compliance brought about by release of prolonged forearm ischemia was blunted.[67,68]

If it is assumed that reduced radial artery compliance reflects a similar reduction of compliance of

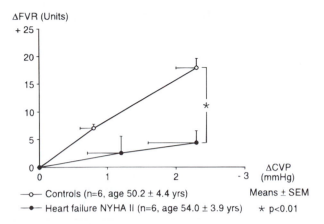

Fig. 14-10. Changes in forearm vascular resistance (FVR: ratio between mean arterial pressure and forearm blood flow) induced by reducing central venous pressure (CVP, right atrial catheter) by lower body suction in congestive heart failure patients (closed circles) and age-matched controls (open circles). The stimuli did not cause significant mean arterial pressure changes. (From Mancia et al.,[23] with permission.)

large elastic arteries (i.e., the arteries where baroreceptors are anatomically located), the hypothesis can be advanced that in CHF patients arterial stiffness prevents baroreceptor signals from being properly altered in response to blood pressure changes, thereby being responsible for the baroreflex impairment. This point agrees with the observation that in CHF patients radial artery compliance values were directly related to the ability of baroreceptors to modulate sympathetic nerve traffic.[69] Hence the lower the radial artery compliance, the greater is the reflex impairment (Fig. 14-12).

Which mechanisms are responsible for the reduction of arterial compliance with CHF, and does a reduction of cardiac compliance account for the impairment of the cardiopulmonary reflex? Concerning the first question, the mechanisms responsible for reduced arterial compliance (e.g., arterial wall edema, increased vessel wall tone by catecholamines, angiotensin II, and other vasoconstrictor substances, reduced secretion of endothelial relaxing factors) are at present only hypothetical.[66–68] This statement is true also for the second question, although the responsiveness of cardiac receptors not only to changes in stretch due to changes in cardiac volume and dis-

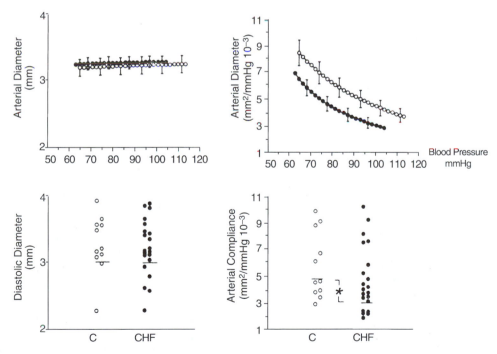

Fig. 14-11. Mean (± SEM) and individual radial artery diameter and compliance values in 21 patients with congestive heart failure (closed circles) and 11 control subjects (open circles). Data are shown as the diameter or compliance values over the systodiastolic pressure range (*Top*) and as the diameter at diastolic pressure or compliance index (*Bottom*) (i.e., the area under the compliance-pressure curve normalized for pulse pressure). *$P < 0.05$. (From Giannattasio et al.,[68] with permission.)

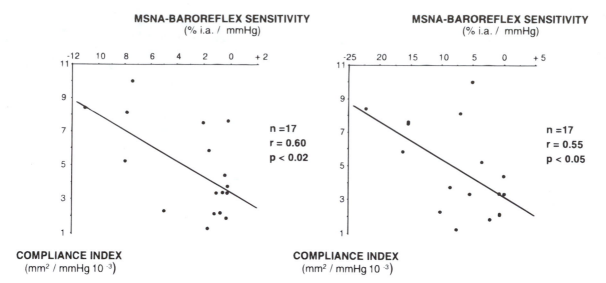

Fig. 14-12. Scatterplots showing the direct relation between radial artery compliance and the sensitivity of the baroreceptor control of MSNA (Phenylephrine: *left panel*; Nitroprusside: *right panel*) in patients with congestive heart failure. Compliance is expressed as the compliance index. For other symbols and explanations see Figures 14-9 and 14-11. (From Grassi et al.,[69] with permission.)

tension but also to changes in myocardial contractility[70] makes it likely that factors more complex than a simple reduction in the compliance of cardiac structures are involved.

Other Cardiovascular Reflexes

Several other reflexes participate in cardiovascular control, but the modification of these reflexes in the presence of CHF has not been studied extensively. An exception is the reflex originating from skeletal muscle metaboreceptors.[71] Although the precise mechanisms activating these receptors are unknown (lactid acid production? reduction in muscle pH?), there is evidence that their stimulation increases sympathetic outflow to skeletal muscle much less in CHF patients than in healthy subjects.[72] It is also the case for the concomitant increase in heart rate. It has been suggested that with CHF an impairment of this metaboreflex contributes to the altered cardiovascular adjustments that occur during exercise and to the reduced exercise tolerance.[72]

TREATMENT

It has been repeatedly shown that physical training favorably affects the hemodynamic profile (decreased blood pressure, bradycardia, systemic vasodilatation, increased arterial compliance). It also reduces sympathetic activity with an increase in

cardiac vagal influences and in the autonomic control exerted by arterial baroreceptors.[73–75] Some of these potentially beneficial effects can also be seen when physical training is implemented in CHF patients,[38] although the various indices of sympathetic and vagal tone show a poor correlation to each other.[76] Thus nonpharmacologic treatment may partially reverse the autonomic derangement seen with CHF.

This derangement can be even more clearly reversed with drug treatment of CHF by digitalis and ACE inhibitors. The evidence comes from studies showing that in CHF patients administration of a digitalis preparation or an ACE inhibitor is accompanied by a reduction in plasma norepinephrine.[77–81] It has also been shown that in these patients muscle sympathetic nerve traffic can be acutely reduced by intravenous digitalis[82] and chronically reduced by administration of an ACE inhibitor on top of conventional digitalis and diuretic therapy.[83] These data support the view that the reduction of plasma norepinephrine induced by digitalis and ACE inhibitors reflects not just increased clearance of this neurotransmitter brought about by increased cardiac output and tissue perfusion, but real sympathetic deactivation.

The effects of treatment of CHF on sympathetic activity are far from being satisfactorily characterized, however, and several important questions remain totally or partially unanswered. As shown in Table 14-2, although reduced by digitalis and ACE inhibitors, sympathetic activity can be increased by other drugs employed for CHF (i.e., diuretics, vasodi-

Table 14-2. Effects of Pharmacologic Treatment on Sympathetic Activity and Reflex Cardiovascular Control in Congestive Heart Failure

| Drug | Sympathetic activity | | | | Reflex control | |
| | Plasma NE | | MSNA | | | |
	Acute	Chronic	Acute	Chronic	Acute	Chronic
Diuretics	↑	↑	?	?	?	?
Vasodilators	↑	↑	?	?	→	?
Digitalis	↓	↓	↓	?	↑	?
Inotropes	↑	↑	?	?	→	?
ACE inhibitors	↓	↓	?	↓	↑	↑

Abbreviations: NE, norepinephrine; MSNA, muscle sympathetic nerve activity; ACE, angiotensin-converting enzyme; ↑, increase; ↓, reduction; ?, effect unknown.

lators, and adrenergic and nonadrenergic inotropes). It has been shown that not all vasodilators exert the same sympathoexcitatory effect[84–86]: (1) among the calcium antagonists, some (amlodipine) produce less excitation than others[86,87]; and (2) a vasodilator such as ibopamine has been associated with reduced plasma norepinephrine values.[88] Thus the spectrum of effects of various drugs employed to treat CHF on sympathetic activity is complex.

It is largely unknown why ACE inhibitors and digitalis reverse the sympathetic activation of CHF. In normal subjects digitalis preparations enhance the sensitivity of the baroreflex,[89] presumably by sensitizing baroreceptors via activation of the ouabain-dependent sodium-potassium pump.[90] They also enhance the sensitivity of the cardiopulmonary reflex, an effect that has been documented in humans with CHF.[61] It can thus be speculated that the sympathetic deactivation caused by digitalis originates from restoration of reflex cardiovascular control. There is some evidence that a restoration of reflex cardiovascular control can play a role also in the sympathetic deactivation induced by ACE inhibitor treatment of CHF.[91] The mechanisms of this restoration, however, may be different from those due to digitalis, because ACE inhibitors reverse the alteration of arterial compliance that occurs with CHF[92], thereby increasing the baroreceptor responsiveness to physiological stimuli and their ability to restrain sympathetic activity. Furthermore, in this instance the sympathetic deactivation may depend, to a considerable extent, on removal of the sympathoexcitatory effect of angiotensin II production.[52,53]

Finally, no definitive conclusion can be drawn about the prognostic value of the changes in plasma norepinephrine and sympathetic activity induced by treatment of CHF, except for the circumstantial evidence that drugs that reduce sympathetic activity tend to reduce cardiovascular morbidity and mortal-ity more than drugs that enhance or leave this activity unaltered.[80,93–96] Future studies on this important issue should await collection of less sketchy information on the short- and long-term effects on autonomic activity and reflex control during the treatment of CHF.

REFERENCES

1. Zelis R, Flain SE: Alterations in vasomotor tone in congestive heart failure. Prog Cardiovasc Dis 1982;24:437
2. Braunwald E: Pathophysiology of heart failure. p.393. In Braunwald E (ed): Heart Disease WB Saunders, Philadelphia, 1992
3. Bridgen W, Sharpey-Schafer EP: Postural changes in peripheral blood flow in cases with left heart failure. Clin Sci 1950;9:93
4. Thomas JA, Marks BH: Plasma norepinephrine in congestive heart failure. Am J Cardiol 1978;41:233
5. Francis GS, Goldsmith SR, Levine TB et al: The neurohumoral axis in congestive heart failure. Ann Intern Med 1984;101:370
6. Eckberg DL, Drabinsky M, Braunwald E: Defective cardiac parasympathetic control in patients with heart disease. N Engl J Med 1971;285:877
7. Mancia G: Neurohumoral activation in congestive heart failure. Am Heart J 1990;120:1532
8. Mancia G: Sympathetic activation in congestive heart failure. Eur Heart J, suppl. A 1990;11:3
9. Packer M: The neurohormonal hypothesis. A theory to explain the mechanism of disease progression in heart failure. J Am Coll Cardiol 1992;20:248
10. Packer M: Pathophysiology of chronic heart failure. Lancet 1992;340:88
11. Chidesy CA, Harison DC, Braunwald E: Augmentation of the plasma norepinephrine response to exercise in patients with congestive heart failure. N Engl J Med 1962;267:650
12. Francis GS, Goldsmith SR, Ziescke SM et al: Response to plasma norepinephrine and epinephrine to dynamic exercise in patients with congestive heart failure. Am J Cardiol 1982;49:1152

13. Esler H, Jackman G, Bobok A et al: Determination of norepinephrine apparent release rate and clearance in humans. Life Sci 1979;25:1461

14. Hasking GJ, Esler MD, Jennings JL et al: Norepinephrine spillover to plasma in patients with congestive heart failure. Evidence of increased overall and cardiorenal sympathetic nervous activity. Circulation 1986;73:615

15. Davis D, Baily R, Zelis R: Abnormalities in systemic norepinephrine kinetics in human congestive heart failure. Am J Physiol 1988;254:760E

16. Meredith IT, Eisenhofer G, Lambert GW et al: Cardiac sympathetic nervous system activity in congestive heart failure. Evidence for increased neuronal norepinephrine release and preserved neuronal uptake. Circulation 1993;88:136

17. Kaye DM, Lambert GW, Lefkovits J et al: Neurochemical evidence of cardiac sympathetic activation and increased central nervous system norepinephrine turnover in severe congestive heart failure. J Am Coll Cardiol 1994;23:570

18. Vallbo AB, Hagbarth KE, Torebjork HE et al: Somatosensory, proprioceptive and sympathetic activity in human peripheral nerves. Physiol Rev 1979;59:919

19. Mancia G, Grassi G, Parati G et al: Evaluating sympathetic activity in human hypertension. J Hypertens Suppl 5 1993;11:S13

20. Grassi G, Bolla GB, Seravalle G et al: Short-and long-term reproducibility of techniques employed to assess sympathetic tone in humans. A preliminary report. J Hypertens Suppl 5 1993;11:S166

21. Leimbach WN, Wallin BG, Victor RG et al: Direct evidence from intraneural recording of increased central sympathetic outflow in patients with heart failure. Circulation 1986;73:913

22. Ferguson DW, Berg WJ, Sanders JS et al: Clinical and hemodynamic correlates of sympathetic nerve activity in normal humans and patients with heart failure. Evidence from direct microneurographic recordings. J Am Coll Cardiol 1990;16:1125

23. Mancia G, Seravalle G, Giannattasio C et al: Reflex cardiovascular control in congestive heart failure. Am J Cardiol 1992;69:17G

24. Ferguson DW, Berg WJ, Roach PJ et al: Effects of heart failure on baroreflex control of sympathetic neural activity. Am J Cardiol 1992;69:523

25. Grassi G, Seravalle G, Cattaneo BM et al: Sympathetic activation and loss of reflex sympathetic control in mild congestive heart failure. Circulation 1995;92:3206

26. Folkow B, DiBona G, Hjemdahl P et al: Measurement of plasma norepinephrine concentrations in human primary hypertension. Hypertension 1983;5:399

27. Mancia G, Ferrari A, Gregorini L et al: Plasma catecholamines do not invariably reflect sympathetically induced changes in blood pressure in man. Clin Sci 1983;65:227

28. Middlekauff HR, Hamilton MA, Stevenson LW et al: Independent control of skin and muscle sympathetic nerve activity in patients with heart failure. Circulation 1994;90:1794

29. Delius W, Hagbarth KE, Hongel A et al: Manoeuvers affecting sympathetic outflow in human muscle nerves. Acta Physiol Scand 1972;84:82

30. Delius W, Hagbarth KE, Hongel A et al: Manoeuvers affecting sympathetic outflow in human skin nerves. Acta Physiol Scand 1972;84:177

31. Mancia G, Ferrari A, Gregorini L et al: Blood pressure and heart rate variability in normotensive and hypertensive human beings. Circ Res 1983;53:96

32. Caruana MP, Lahiri A, Cashman PM et al: Effects of chronic congestive heart failure secondary to coronary artery disease on the circadian rhythm of blood pressure and heart rate. Am J Cardiol 1988;62:755

33. Saul JP, Arai Y, Berger RD et al: Assessment of autonomic regulation in chronic congestive heart failure by heart rate spectral analysis. Am J Cardiol 1988;61:1292

34. Casolo G, Balli E, Fazi A et al: Twenty-four hour spectral analysis of heart rate variability in congestive heart failure secondary to coronary artery disease. Am J Cardiol 1991;67:1154

35. Woo MA, Stevenson WG, Moser DK et al: Patterns of beat-to-beat heart rate variability in advanced heart failure. Am Heart J 1992;123:704

36. Woo MA, Stevenson WG, Moser DK et al: Complex heart rate variability and serum norepinephrine levels in patients with advanced heart failure. J Am Coll Cardiol 1994;23:565

37. Panina G, Khot UN, Nunziata E et al: Assessment of autonomic tone over a 24-hour period in patients with congestive heart failure. Am Heart J 1995;129:748

38. Coats A, Adamopoulos S, Radaelli A et al: Controlled trial of physical training in chronic heart failure. Exercise performance, hemodynamics, ventilation and autonomic function. Circulation 1992;85:2119

39. Parati GF, Saul JP, DiRienzo M et al: Spectral analysis of blood pressure and heart rate variability in evaluating cardiovascular regulation. A critical appraisal. Hypertension 1995;25:1276

40. Kingwell BA, Thompson JM, Kaye DM et al: Heart rate spectral analysis, cardiac norepinephrine spillover, and muscle sympathetic nerve activity during human sympathetic nervous activation and failure. Circulation 1994;90:234

41. Bristow MR, Ginsburg R, Minobe W et al: Decreased catecholamine sensitivity and β-adrenergic receptor pathway in the intact failing human heart. Progressive receptor down regulation and subsensitivity to agonist response. Circulation 1986;74:1290

42. Fowler MB, Laser JA, Hopkins GL et al: Assessment of the β-adrenergic receptor pathway in the intact failing human heart. Progressive receptor down regulation and subsensitivity to agonist response. Circulation 1986;74:1290

43. Colucci WS, Denniss AR, Leatherman GF et al: Intracoronary infusion of dobutamine to patients with and without severe congestive heart failure. J Clin Invest 1988;81:1103

44. Bristow MR, Hershberger RE, Port JD et al: β-Adrenergic pathways in nonfailing and failing human ventricular myocardium. Circulation, suppl. I 1990;82:12

45. Bristow MR: Changes in myocardial and vascular receptors in heart failure. J Am Coll Cardiol, suppl. A 1993;22:61

46. Cruickshank JM, Degante JP, Kuurne T et al: Reduction of stress catecholamines induces cardiac necrosis by beta$_1$-selective blockade. Lancet 1987;2:585

47. Cohn JN, Levine TB, Olivari MT et al: Plasma norepinephrine as a guide to prognosis in patients with

chronic congestive heart failure. N Engl J Med 1984; 311:819

48. Rector TS, Olivari MT, Levine TB et al: Predicting survival for an individual with congestive heart failure using the plasma norepinephrine concentration. Am Heart J 1987;114:148

49. Bigger JT: Why patients with congestive heart failure die. Arrhythmias and sudden death. Circulation, suppl. IV 1987;75:28

50. Francis GS, Benedict C, Johnstone DE et al: Comparison of neuroendocrine activation in patients with left ventricular dysfunction with and without congestive heart failure. A substudy of the studies of left ventricular dysfunction (SOLVD). Circulation 1990;82:1724

51. Rouleau JL, De Champlaiin J, Klein M et al: Activation of neurohumoral system in postinfarction left ventricular dysfunction. J Am Coll Cardiol 1993;22:390

52. Zimmerman BG: Actions of angiotensin on adrenergic nerve endings. Fed Proc 1978;37:199

53. Mancia G, Giannattasio C, Grassi G et al: Reflex control of circulation and ACE inhibition in man. J Hypertens Suppl 3 1988;6:S45

54. Mancia G, Mark AL: Arterial baroreflex in humans. p. 755 In Shepherd JT, Abboud FM (eds): Handbook of Physiology. Sec. 2. The Cardiovascular System. Vol. 3 (part 2). American Physiological Society, Bethesda, 1983

55. Goldstein RE, Beiser GD, Stampfer M: Impairment of autonomically mediated heart rate control in patients with cardiac dysfunction. Circ Res 1975;36:571

56. Mark AL, Mancia G: Cardiopulmonary baroreflex in humans. p. 795. In Shepherd JT, Abboud FM (eds): Handbook of Physiology. Sect. 2. The Cardiovascular System. Vol. 3 (part 2). American Physiological Society, Bethesda, 1983

57. Mohanty PK, Thames MD, Arrowood JA et al: Impairment of cardiopulmonary baroreflex after cardiac transplantation in humans. Circulation 1987;75:914

58. Grassi G, Giannattasio C, Saino A et al: Cardiopulmonary receptor modulation of plasma renin activity in normotensive and hypertensive subjects. Hypertension 1988;11:92

59. Grassi G, Giannattasio C, Cuspidi C et al: Cardiopulmonary receptor regulation of renin release. Am J Med, suppl. 3A 1988;84:97

60. Giannattasio C, Del Bo A, Cattaneo BM et al: Reflex vasopressin and renin modulation by cardiac receptors in humans. Hypertension 1993;21:461

61. Ferguson DW, Abboud FM, Mark AL: Selective impairment of baroreflex-mediated vasoconstrictor responses in patients with ventricular dysfunction. Circulation 1984;69:451

62. Mohanty PK, Arrowood JA, Ellenbogen KA et al: Neurohumoral and hemodynamic effects of lower body negative pressure in patients with congestive heart failure. Am Heart J 1989;118:78

63. Osculati G, Giannattasio C, De Ceglie S et al: Asymmetry of the cardiopulmonary reflexes in patients with dilated cardiomyopathy [abstract]. Eur Heart J 1993; 14:18

64. Abboud FM, Thames MD, Mark AL: Role of cardiac afferent nerves in regulation of circulation during coronary occlusion and heart failure. p. 65. In Abboud FM, Fozzard HA, Gilmore JP et al. (eds): Disturbances in Neurogenic Control of the Circulation. American Physiological Society, Bethesda, 1981

65. Oren RM, Roach PJ, Schobel HP: Sympathetic responses of patients with congestive heart failure to the cold pressor stimulus. Am J Cardiol 1991;67:993

66. Drexler H, Hayoz D, Munzel T et al: Endothelial function in congestive heart failure. Am J Cardiol 1992; 69:1596

67. Hayoz D, Drexler H, Munzel T et al: Flow-mediated arterial dilation is abnormal in congestive heart failure. Circulation, suppl. VII 1993;87:92

68. Giannattasio C, Stella ML, Failla M et al: Alterations of radial artery compliance in patients with mild and severe congestive heart failure. Am J Cardiol 1995;76: 381

69. Grassi G, Giannattasio C, Failla M et al: Sympathetic modulation of radial artery compliance in congestive heart failure. Hypertension 1995;26:348

70. Zoller RP, Mark AL, Abboud FM et al: The role of low pressure baroreceptors in reflex vasoconstrictor responses in man. J Clin Invest 1972;51:2967

71. Mitchell JH, Schmidt RF: Cardiovascular reflex control by afferent fibers from skeletal muscle receptors. p. 623. In Shepherd JT, Abboud FM (eds): Handbook of Physiology. Sect. 2. The Cardiovascular System. Vol. 3 (part 2). American Physiological Society, Bethesda, 1983

72. Stems DA, Ettinger SM, Gray KS et al: Skeletal muscle metaboreceptor exercise responses are attenuated in heart failure. Circulation 1991;84:2034

73. Grassi G, Seravalle G, Calhoun DA et al: Physical exercise in essential hypertension. Chest 1992;101:312S

74. Giannattasio C, Cattaneo BM, Mangoni A et al: Changes in arterial compliance induced by physical training in hammer throwers. J Hypertens Suppl 5 1992;10:S53

75. Grassi G, Seravalle G, Calhoun DA et al: Physical training and baroreceptor control of sympathetic nerve activity in humans. Hypertension 1994;23:294

76. Adamopoulos S, Piepoli M, McCance A et al: Comparison of different methods for assessing sympathovagal balance in chronic congestive heart failure secondary to coronary artery disease. Am J Cardiol 1992;70:1576

77. Gillis RA, Quest JA: Neural action of digitalis. Annu Rev Med 1978;29:73

78. Gheorghiade M, Hall V, Lakier JB et al: Comparative hemodynamic and neurohormonal effects of intravenous captopril and digoxin and their combination in patients with severe heart failure. J Am Coll Cardiol 1989;12:134

79. Swedberg K, Eneroth P, Kjeksmus J et al: Hormones regulating cardiovascular function in patients with severe congestive heart failure and their relation to mortality. Circulation 1990;82:1730

80. Cohn JN, Johnson G, Ziesche S et al: A comparison of enalapril with hydralazine-isosorbide dinitrate in the treatment of chronic congestive heart failure. N Engl J Med 1991;325:303

81. Goldsmith SR, Simon AB, Miller E: Effect of digitalis on norepinephrine kinetics in congestive heart failure. J Am Coll Cardiol 1992;20:858

82. Ferguson DW, Berg WJ, Sanders JS et al: Sympathoinhibitory responses to digitalis glycosides in heart failure patients. Direct evidence from sympathetic neural recordings. Circulation 1989;80:65

83. Grassi G, Lanfranchi A, Seravalle G et al: Effects of chronic angiotensin converting enzyme inhibition on

sympathetic nerve traffic in congestive heart failure [abstract]. Eur Heart J 1994;15:447

84. Packer M: Treatment of chronic heart failure. Lancet 1992;340:92

85. Cohn JN: Efficacy of vasodilators in the treatment of heart failure. J Am Coll Cardiol, suppl. A 1993;22:135A

86. Elkayam V, Shotan A, Mehra A et al: Calcium channel blockers in heart failure. J Am Coll Cardiol, suppl. A 1993;22:139A

87. Packer M, Nicod P, Khandheria BR et al: Randomized, multicenter, double-blind, placebo-controlled evaluation of amlodipine in patients with mild-to-moderate heart failure [abstract]. J Am Coll Cardiol 1991;17:274A

88. Raifer SI, Rossen JD, Douglas FL et al: Effect of long-term therapy with oral ibopamine on resting and exercise capacity in patients with heart failure. Relationship to the generation of N-methyldopamine and to plasma norepinephrine levels. Circulation 1986;73:740

89. Ferrari A, Gregorini L, Ferrari MC et al: Digitalis and baroreceptor reflexes in man. Circulation 1981;63:279

90. Sarum WR, Brown AM, Tuley FH: An electrogenic sodium pump and baroreceptor function in normotensive and spontaneously hypertensive rats. Circ Res 1976;39:497

91. Lanfranchi A, Cattaneo BM, Bolla GB et al: Effects of angiotensin converting enzyme inhibition on baroreflex control of circulation in congestive heart failure [abstract]. Eur Heart J 1995;16:454

92. Giannattasio C, Failla M, Stella ML et al: ACE-inhibition and radial artery compliance in patients with congestive heart failure. Hypertension 1995;26:491

93. Cohn JN, Archibald DG, Ziesche S et al: Effect of vasodilator therapy on mortality in chronic congestive heart failure. Results of a Veterans Administration cooperative study. N Engl J Med 1986;314:1547

94. CONSENSUS Trial Study Group: Effects of enalapril on mortality in severe congestive heart failure. Results of the Cooperative North Scandinavian Enalapril Survival Study (CONSENSUS). N Engl J Med 1987;316:1429

95. SOLVD Investigators: Effect of enalapril on survival in patients with reduced left ventricular ejection fraction and congestive heart failure. N Engl J Med 1991;325:293

96. Pfeffer MA, Braunwald E, Moye LA et al: Effect of captopril on mortality and morbidity in patients with left ventricular dysfunction after myocardial infarction. Results of the survival and ventricular enlargement trial. N Engl J Med 1992;327:669

15 Vasoactive Hormone Systems

Gary S. Francis

The idea that neurohormones are important in control of the circulation is old. Starling and other physiologists recognized the concept during the halcyon days of physiology at the turn of the century. With further enlightenment regarding myocardial mechanics and pathogenesis behind them, a number of investigators during the 1960s began to study endocrine systems and hormones in patients and experimental animal models of heart failure.[1,2] As many laboratories acquired the ability to measure neurohormones with precise methodology using radioimmunoassays, radioenzymatic assays, and high pressure liquid chromatography, the role of neuroendocrine factors in the pathogenesis of heart failure became more obvious.[3] These early observations set the stage for development of therapy designed to block excessive neurohormone activation. Angiotensin-converting enzyme (ACE) inhibitors, which have proved highly successful for treatment of heart failure,[4–8] have emerged as the cornerstone of therapy.

The concept that neuroendocrine activation is important in the pathogenesis and prognosis of heart failure is now well established.[9–15] One could even argue that neuroendocrine activation is the centerpiece of heart failure,[16] but we should not forget that the syndrome of heart failure is primarily a problem of pump dysfunction. Nevertheless, as we move away from the "hemodynamic model" of heart failure popularized from 1960 to 1980 to the more current "neurohormone model," our current understanding suggests that neuroendocrine systems are associated with progression of heart failure from the point of early injury to the myocardium and its "adaptation" by remodeling,[17,18] through the development of abnormalities of the regional circulation,[19–23] and finally to end-stage pump failure[24] and sudden death.[25] Neurohormones influence the myocardium directly and indirectly. In the direct sense they may be toxic.[26–32] Neurohormones also affect the peripheral circulation,[19–23] where they are important to vascular remodeling[33–36] and regional blood flow distribution.[37] The role of neuroendocrine activation in heart failure is therefore difficult to overstate. Importantly, many of these neuroendocrine systems in heart failure are highly interactive and integrated with the brain, heart, kidneys, and periphery[16–23] (Fig. 15-1). Therefore to describe them in the sole context of the "circulation" is by definition incomplete. Nevertheless, an appreciation of each neurohormone "system" (Table 15-1) should provide some additional enlightenment regarding the pathophysiology of this complex syndrome.[38]

SYMPATHETIC NERVOUS SYSTEM

The sympathetic nervous system is an early evolutionary development, probably antedating the renin-angiotensin-aldosterone system.[39] Its evolutionary conservation undoubtedly relates to the importance of maintenance of cardiac output, blood pressure, and filling pressure. It is designed to make up for deficiency of blood volume and to contribute to the "defense reaction" that accompanies exercise and other conditions of "stress." Homeostasis is achieved through protection of blood pressure.[40] Why should there be such a wide variation in blood pressure

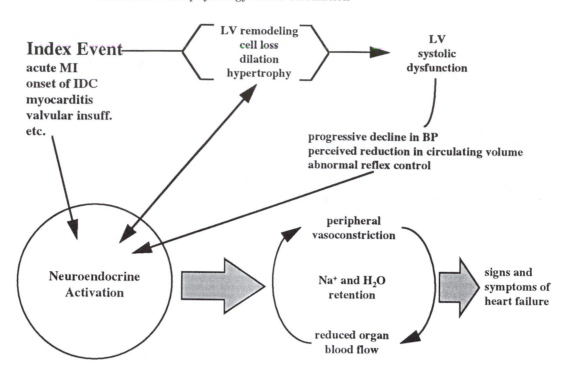

Fig. 15-1. Heart failure is a highly complex clinical syndrome characterized by neuroendocrine activation. The many neuroendocrine systems that are activated are highly interactive with each other and are in turn integrated with the heart, peripheral circulation, brain, and kidneys.

among living beings? Harris argued that the fourfold difference in arterial pressure between fishes and mammals corresponds approximately to a fourfold increase in cardiac output.[39] He believed that the need to conserve arterial resistance and to develop rather high blood pressure in mammals (e.g., in gi-

Table 15-1.
Neurohormones Reported
To Be Increased in
Congestive Heart Failure

Norepinephrine
Epinephrine
Renin activity
Angiotensin II
Aldosterone
Arginine vasopressin
Neuropeptide Y
Vasoactive intestinal peptide
Prostaglandins
Atrial natriuretic peptide
Endothelin
β-Endorphins
Calcitonin gene-related peptide
Growth hormone
Cortisol
Tumor necrosis factor α
Neurokinin A
Substance P

raffes the mean arterial pressure is 200–300 mmHg) was imposed indirectly because of the need for redistribution of blood flow during exercise.[39] Heart failure, however one cares to define it, is also characterized by a redistribution of blood flow at rest (Fig. 15-2). This redistribution maintains coronary and skeletal muscle blood flow at the expense of skin, renal, splanchnic, and cerebral blood flow (Fig. 15-3).[41] As with shock and hemorrhage, a reduced cardiac output is somehow sensed to be a hazardous circumstance, and nature has allowed for the evolution of special provisions that maintain perfusion to the heart and skeletal muscles. As heart failure begins to ensue from any cause, plasma concentrations[42] and urinary excretion of norepinephrine (NE) increase[43] presumably in an attempt to protect blood pressure and redistribute flow.

It had long been suspected that sympathetic activity was increased in heart failure, Starling having recognized it as early as 1895.[44] Introduction of the microneurographic recording technique by Hagbarth and Valbo during the 1960s was a methodologic tour de force in that it introduced the concept of sympathetic differentiation.[45] This concept challenged the earlier dogma of uniform "sympathetic tone." Rather, microneurography demonstrated clear differences between sympathetic traffic in cutaneous and visceral nerves. With these findings, the tradi-

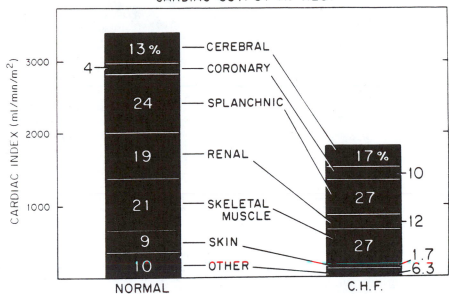

CARDIAC OUTPUT AT REST

Fig. 15-2. Distribution of cardiac output or blood flow to regional vascular beds in normal individuals and a patient with heart failure. (Adapted from Zelis et al.[19] and Wade and Bishop,[41] with permission.)

tional view of a global sympathetic outflow was no longer tenable and had to be discarded. The new concept was that data from one sympathetic effector could not be generalized to other conditions without experimental support. Nevertheless, NE is the main sympathetic neurotransmitter, and there is a significant positive correlation between venous plasma levels and total body spillover of norepinephrine.[46] This is because skeletal muscle is a large tissue accounting for about 20 percent of total NE, and NE from skeletal muscle is likely overrepresented in forearm venous blood. Microneurographic muscle sympathetic activity and NE spillover in the heart and kidney are also significantly correlated in normal subjects and patients with heart failure,[46] suggesting that even though sympathetic outflow is differen-

tiated, several sympathetic subdivisions can nevertheless be activated in parallel at rest.

A different methodologic concern regarding plasma NE was the spontaneous variation of values. Day-to-day variation in plasma NE in patients with heart failure, however, is relatively modest,[9] provided patients are clinically stable. Baseline measurement of plasma NE in patients with heart failure correlates with clinical[42] and hemodynamic[47] status, although the correlation coefficients are consistently modest. Sequential measurement of plasma NE correlates with change in clinical status[48,49] and mechanism of death.[50] Plasma NE has consistently been shown to associate with survival in patients with heart failure[10,51] (Fig. 15-4).

The traditional concept had been that patients with heart failure are dependent on the sympathetic nervous system to support the circulation.[52] From the early work of Chidsey and colleagues it was apparent that patients with heart failure have increased plasma NE in the basal state and greatly augmented plasma NE during exercise.[53] It was logically assumed that the failing circulation was dependent on the sympathetic nervous system to augment cardiac output and redistribute blood flow.[52] Although the assumption implied that this was an adaptive response to a major change in homeostasis, thinking eventually began gradually to embrace a somewhat different view that neuroendocrine activation in general could be detrimental over time, and that inhibition of these "vasoactive hormone systems" might be therapeutically beneficial for some patients.[3,16] A major dilemma arose in that it was unclear if sympathetic activation (and other neu-

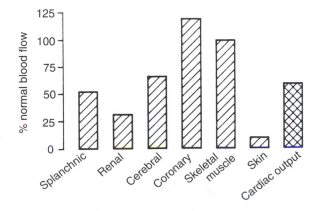

Fig. 15-3. Distribution of regional blood flow in a patient with heart failure at rest expressed as a percent of normal flow. (Adapted from Wade and Bishop,[41] with permission.)

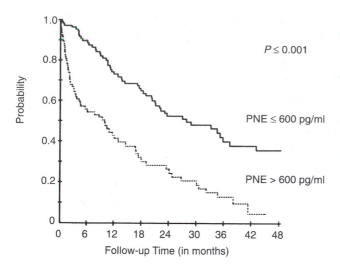

Fig. 15-4. Survival curves for two plasma norepinephrine strata with the most prognostic information. (From Rector et al.,[51] with permission.)

roendocrine activity) was simply an epiphenomenon without pathophysiologic importance, or this activation occurred early, before overt heart failure, and therefore was contributory to the pathogenesis of heart failure. It now seems evident from the SOLVD trials (Studies of Left Ventricular Dysfunction)[5,6] that augmentation of plasma NE occurs during the

early phase of left ventricular dysfunction prior to the onset of overt heart failure[14] (Fig. 15-5). These observations suggest that activation of the sympathetic nervous system occurs gradually during the syndrome of heart failure even before symptoms ensue. If progressively increasing circulating catechamines are indeed toxic to the myocardium,[30-32] inhibition of the sympathetic nervous system at an early stage of heart failure remains an intriguing therapeutic possibility.[54,55]

Although a number of potential mechanisms have been put forth to explain excessive sympathetic nervous system activation in heart failure, the fundamental mechanism has remained elusive.[38] When cardiac output is low, there is reduced clearance of plasma NE,[56,57] but the prevailing view is that the NE secretion rate is excessive in patients with heart failure.[58-62] A long-standing controversy has developed regarding neuronal reuptake of NE in the heart, with evidence favoring both preserved neuronal reuptake[63] and hypofunction of neuronal reuptake[64] in the heart. These differences are possibly due to methodologic differences and differences in how the data are expressed. The fact remains that the precise sequence of events that leads to enhanced sympathetic drive during heart failure is undetermined.

Baroreceptor reflex abnormalities during heart failure are well described,[65-72] but their quantitative

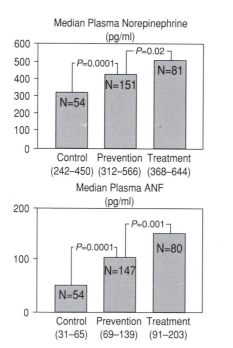

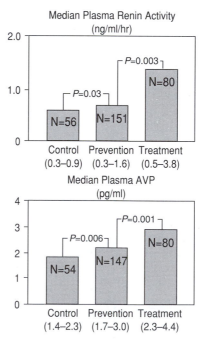

Fig. 15-5. Incremental and significant increases in plasma norepinephrine, plasma renin activity, plasma arginine vasopressin (AVP), and plasma atrial natriuretic factor (ANF) in control subjects, prevention patients, and treatment patients. Treatment values are higher than control values for each neurohormone. Median values and interquartile ranges, 25 percent to 75 percent, are shown. (From Francis et al.,[14] with permission.)

importance in causing abnormal sympathetic drive in heart failure has never been entirely clear. There may be an afferent and target organ abnormality in heart failure, but there does not appear to be a central abnormality of the baroreceptor control of sympathetic outflow.[72] A major abnormality of baroreflex function probably resides at the afferent baroreceptor endings. There is an apparent increase in Na^+/K^+-ATPase in baroreceptor neuronal structures in experimental heart failure, but the cause is unknown. Blunted baroreceptor responses to high cardiac filling pressures or depressed cardiac function reduce afferent signals that normally inhibit efferent sympathetic activity, vasopressin release, and indirectly renin secretion. The resulting increase in neuroendocrine activity presumably helps modulate the redistribution of blood flow, which is well known to occur in heart failure.[41] The regulation of regional blood flow to skeletal muscle and the liver in response to orthostasis is markedly blunted in patients with heart failure.[73] However, critical experiments linking baroreflexes to sympathetic outflow during heart failure have yet to be undertaken. Such studies would require removing arterial baroreceptors with direct recording from sympathetic nerves in an experimental model of heart failure. If sympathetic outflow remains enhanced despite sinoaortic denervation and cardiac denervation, other as yet undefined peripheral signals must be involved.

Abnormal baroreceptor control mechanisms during heart failure are seemingly functional and not due to structural changes in the reflex arc. This concept is supported by the observation that reflex impairment appears to reverse when the clinical condition is improved[74] and following heart transplantation.[75–77] However, impaired vasodilation may be delayed for several months after transplant.[77,78] This area of study remains active.

In summary, it is now clear that heart failure is characterized by heightened sympathetic nervous system activity. Plasma NE levels are increased early in the syndrome and progressively rise with worsening heart failure. The extent of sympathetic nervous system activation is related to the prognosis in a powerful and consistent fashion.[79] The progressive rise in plasma NE can be attenuated by ACE inhibitor therapy.[79] In addition to impairing peripheral vascular dilatation,[80] catecholamines may have a direct toxic effect on the heart. The importance of the sympathetic nervous system in the pathogenesis of heart failure now seems undoubted. However, the signals[5] whereby augmented catecholamines are released, how the signals are processed, and their independent contribution to the syndrome of heart failure remain unclear and need further study.

RENIN-ANGIOTENSIN-ALDOSTERONE SYSTEM

In 1946 Merrill and colleagues identified an increased concentration of renin in blood samples obtained from the renal veins of patients with chronic heart failure.[81] At the time it was believed that the release of renin was a compensatory response to diminished renal blood flow. The role of the renin-angiotensin-aldosterone system (RAAS) in the pathogenesis of heart failure was later suggested by Davis[82] and Laragh.[1] Renin is a large enzyme that appears to limit the production of angiotensin II (Fig. 15-6). Angiotensin II, although perhaps known primarily as a potent vasoconstrictor, has a vast array of biologic activities (Fig. 15-7). A variety of factors stimulate renin release (Table 15-2). Indeed, reduced renal blood flow is an important determinant of renin release. The sympathetic nervous system is also well known to stimulate renin release.[83,84] A hyponatremic perfusate to the macula densa is also a powerful stimulus for renin release.[85] Hyponatremia is a common complication of advanced heart failure,[86,87] and patients with severe heart failure are presumed to have decreased sodium delivery to the distal tubule.[83–85] The kidney senses the hyponatremia and perceives a reduction in total body sodium, resulting in stimulation of renin release. Diuretics are a potent stimulus for renin release[88] and are likely responsible for much of the hyperreninemia that occurs in early or mild heart failure.[14] Diuretic-induced renin release forms part of the pharmacologic rationale for using ACE inhibitors in the early stages of heart failure.

Angiotensinogen, an α_2-globulin, is the substrate for renin (Fig. 15-6). The liver is probably the primary source of the substrate in the circulation. Renin and angiotensinogen interact to cleave and release a small decapeptide, angiotensin I. This decapeptide is converted by "converting enzyme" (ACE or kininase II) primarily as it passes through the lungs to angiotensin II, an octapeptide. Angiotensin II is a major contributor to the pathophysiology of heart failure via its multiple mechanisms (Fig. 15-7). The octapeptide is relatively difficult to measure, as the antibody tends to cross react with other peptides. Therefore plasma renin activity has traditionally been measured as an index of RAAS activity. The normal supine plasma renin activity (PRA) is 1–3 $ng \cdot ml^{-1} \cdot h^{-1}$ and normally increases with upright posture. In the SOLVD study, PRA was only minimally "elevated" in patients with mild or "asymptomatic" heart failure compared with that in normal subjects[14] (Fig. 15-5), and the slight increment is probably related to concomitant diuretic use by a

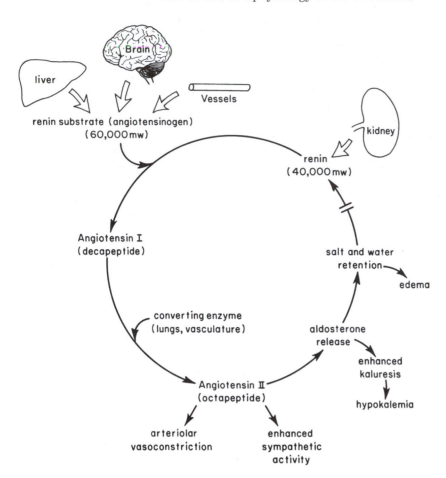

Fig. 15-6. Renin-angiotensin-aldosterone system. Circulating renin is primarily produced by the kidney. Plasma renin interacts with renin substrate (angiotensinogen) to produce angiotensin I, which is cleaved by angiotensin-converting enzyme to angiotensin II, a peptide of major importance in the syndrome of heart failure.

small number of hypertensive patients. However, in patients with untreated overt heart failure PRA is usually elevated,[89] and it progressively rises in states of decompensated heart failure.[90] In the study by Anand and colleagues of untreated patients with heart failure, PRA and aldosterone varied widely, but renin was increased on average 9.5-fold and aldosterone 6.4 times control.[89]

Angiotensin II causes direct peripheral vasoconstriction and further augmentation of the sympathetic nervous system, probably via a presynaptic angiotensin II receptor mechanism.[91,93] However, the importance of the sympathetic augmentation mechanism in humans has been questioned.[94,95] Nevertheless, it is possible that local concentrations of angiotensin II that occur during heart failure contribute to the intense sympathetic drive characteristic of the syndrome. Angiotensin II also acts on the adrenal cortex to stimulate release of aldosterone, which in turn acts on the kidney to promote salt and water retention and to stimulate potassium excretion. Patients with heart failure who are receiving potent diuretics thus are at great risk of developing hypokalemia, cardiac arrhythmias, and sudden death. Drugs such as ACE inhibitors are highly effective

in the treatment of heart failure in part because in principle they block production of angiotensin II and all of its multiple mechanisms, thus highlighting the central role of the RAAS in the pathogenesis of the syndrome.

The impressive effectiveness of ACE inhibitors in the treatment of heart failure suggests that the RAAS is somehow maladaptive. However, this system evolved over many millions of years as an evolutionary advantage in the preservation of circulatory homeostasis. Angiotensin II supports systemic blood pressure via direct vasoconstriction, enhancement of the sympathetic nervous system, sodium and water retention through aldosterone secretion, and increasing total body volume through stimulation of thirst and arginine vasopressin. In addition, angiotensin II has evolved an important role in the preservation of the glomerular filtration rate (GFR) when the kidney is underperfused.[96] Angiotensin II causes intense vasoconstriction of the efferent glomerular arterioles, thus maintaining intraglomerular hydraulic pressure and GFR in low-flow states. Therefore the RAAS in patients with heart failure is an important element in the preservation of circulatory homeostasis of the systemic and regional vascular

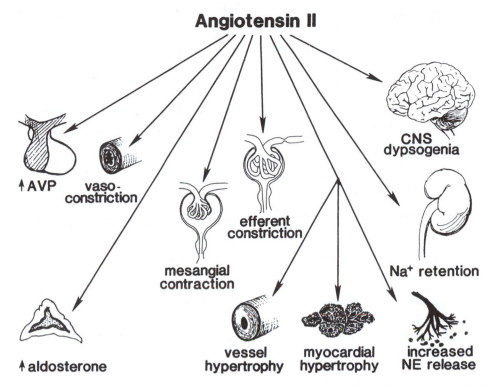

Fig. 15-7. Angiotensin II has a large number of important biologic effects that are basically helpful in maintaining circulatory homeostasis by restoring blood pressure and blood volume. At the tissue level angiotensin II is believed to have important growth activity, which is probably important for remodeling of the heart and peripheral vasculature. (From Francis,[289] with permission.)

beds. There may be a price to be paid in the form of hypotension, azotemia, and hyperkalemia when the RAAS is pharmacologically blocked in the setting of severe heart failure, and these problems are indeed occasional complications of ACE inhibitor therapy.

Although hyponatremia identifies those patients most likely to experience symptomatic hypotension during ACE inhibitor therapy,[86] substantial patient-to-patient variability limits the predictive value of these correlations, and they cannot be relied on to make major inferences regarding the severity of

heart failure.[97] Heart failure is a dynamic syndrome characterized by wide swings in the state of circulatory compensation and treatment. Though the RAAS is markedly activated during decompensated cardiac failure, it may return to near normal during periods of stabilization even when severe cardiac dysfunction persists.[90] This is why no single laboratory measurement (e.g., serum sodium, angiotensin II, or PRA) and no single measurement of cardiac function (e.g., cardiac output, pulmonary capillary wedge pressure, or systemic vascular resistance) can accurately portray the patient with heart failure. The picture can be constantly changing, and a neurohumoral or hemodynamic "snapshot" fails to provide a meaningful representation. Overall, it is difficult to overstate the importance of the RAAS in the clinical syndrome of heart failure.

Table 15-2. Stimuli for Renin Release in Heart Failure

Decreased renal perfusion pressure or renal blood flow
Enhanced sympathetic activity
Decreased macula densa Na^+ concentration
Diuretic therapy
Abnormal reflex control mechanisms
Vasopressin
Direct-acting vasodilators
Low Na^+ diet
Prostaglandins

ARGININE VASOPRESSIN

Plasma arginine vasopressin (AVP) levels are frequently increased in patients with heart failure,[14,98–102] although there is great variation and levels are not increased in all patients.[89] AVP is a powerful vasoconstrictor[103] and exerts its effects by interacting with a vascular (V-1) receptor that is functionally distinct from the renal tubular (V-2) receptor, where it subserves reduced clearance of free water.[104] It is also likely that AVP can produce peripheral vasodilation via a vascular V-2 receptor,[105] with possible contribution from a positive inotropic effect. For many years the vascular effects of vasopressin were thought not to be physiologically important, as only large pharmacologic increases in circulating AVP produced changes in blood pressure. However, as sensitive radioimmunoassays were developed that could measure AVP at low physiologic concentrations, it has become clear that AVP does exert important vascular effects within the normal circulating range.[106] Support for this concept also derives from the development of specific V-1 receptor antagonists, which are associated with improvement in hemodynamic status in some patients with heart failure.[101,102] This work has led to the development of orally effective nonpeptide vasopressin V-1 receptor antagonists.[107–109] Theoretically, increased levels of AVP could contribute to both fluid retention and vasoconstriction in patients with heart failure.

The control of AVP secretion is highly complex and involves both osmotic and nonosmotic stimuli.[110] Factors known to influence vasopressin release include plasma osmolality, intracardiac and intraarterial pressure, circulating angiotensin II levels, atrial natriuretic factor, central α_2-adrenoceptors, central opioid and dopaminergic receptors, and central prostaglandin-related stimuli.[111] Under most circumstances AVP is tightly coupled to increases and decreases in osmolality, making the osmoreceptor the dominant determinant of vasopressin levels. However, reflex control systems are important determinants of AVP release,[112] and both low pressure cardiopulmonary and high pressure sinoaortic baroreceptors participate in this regulation. When pressure within the heart or arterial system decreases, tonic inhibitory restraint of vasopressin is normally diminished, and plasma AVP levels rise. Conversely, increased circulatory pressure normally increases this restraint, leading to decreased plasma AVP, although this finding is not observed during heart failure.[113–115] Despite their hypoosmolar hyponatremia, a large percentage of patients with heart failure have inappropriately elevated plasma AVP levels.[98–100] In general, the nonosmotic stimuli may be more important in driving increased AVP release in the syndrome of heart failure.[116]

In our laboratory normal plasma AVP levels range from 2.5 to 4.0 pg/ml. Patients with heart failure have an average value of approximately 9.0 pg/ml, although severely ill patients with heart failure may have values up to 40 pg/ml. The physiologic increases in AVP observed during heart failure are associated with modest but statistically significant adverse effects on the systemic vascular resistance and cardiac output.[106] Patients with high levels of plasma AVP respond to V-1 antagonists with hemodynamic improvement,[101,102] and those with extremely high levels of AVP may have striking improvement in response to AVP receptor antagonists.[102] However, modest elevations in plasma AVP, which are most common, may not be associated with much reduction in systemic vascular resistance when an AVP receptor antagonist is given, suggesting that AVP contributes to heightened vascular tone in heart failure only in those cases where it is most elevated.

Hyponatremia is common in severe heart failure, and plasma AVP and renal water excretion are normally tightly coupled to maintain normal tonicity of blood.[110] Increases in plasma AVP diminish the ability of the kidney to excrete free water and could conceivably contribute to the hyponatremia of heart failure. However, other factors can lead to impaired water excretion during heart failure, such as reduced renal blood flow and polydypsia. We have found no correlation between plasma AVP and either serum sodium or osmolality in patients with heart failure,[100] suggesting that hyponatremia is not a simple product of enhanced AVP secretion in this syndrome. The osmoreceptor-mediated suppression of AVP is intact during heart failure but is probably shifted to a new set point.[117] That is, plasma AVP decreases when osmolality falls during heart failure, but residual levels remain above what they should be for the prevailing osmolality. Because patients with heart failure can apparently dilute their urine normally despite an elevated plasma AVP, the plasma AVP level cannot be the sole determinant of hyponatremia.

NEUROPEPTIDE Y

Neuropeptide Y (NPY) is a peptide with 36 amino acid residues that was originally isolated from porcine brain in 1982.[118,119] It is derived from a 97 amino acid precursor that is abundant in sympathetic perivascular nerves throughout the circulation and brain. NPY is co-localized with norepinephrine in sympathetic ganglia and sympathetic fibers that innervate arterioles, veins, and the heart.[120,121] In addition to being a potent vasoconstrictor, NPY may have vagolytic activity.[122] The storage of NPY in sympathetic neurons is primarily in the large vesicles, and it is normally co-released with NE only during intense sympathetic stimulation, such as might occur during dynamic exercise. Whereas high frequency stimulation releases both NPY and NE, low frequency stimulation of sympathetic nerves preferentially releases NE from the small granules.

Neuropeptide acts on presynaptic receptors (Y-2) to inhibit NE release from sympathetic neurons and on postsynaptic effector organs, such as vascular tissue and the heart (Y-1 receptors), to inhibit cGMP via a Gi (guanosine triphosphate) regulatory protein.[123] Both veins and arterioles constrict in response to NPY, whereas myocardial performance is depressed[124,125] and the heart rate slows.[126] Because coronary vasoconstriction can occur in response to NPY, some of the reduction in inotropy may be indirectly due to myocardial ischemia. NPY can also reduce plasma renin activity in the setting of experimental heart failure.[127]

Human conditions known to be associated with high plasma levels of NPY include birth (neonates upon vaginal delivery), cardiopulmonary bypass,[128] hypertension and pheochromocytoma,[129] and congestive heart failure.[130] Maisel and colleagues studied plasma NPY in 17 patients with heart failure and 14 healthy control subjects.[130] Both radioimmunoassay and high-pressure liquid chromatography were used, which indicated basal levels of NPY to be increased in patients with heart failure (551 ± 48 versus 311 ± 22 pg/ml). During dynamic exercise NPY failed to increase in patients with heart failure, whereas it rose significantly during exercise in normal subjects. Although it is still not clear if NPY has a pathophysiologic role in heart failure, it is possible that increased levels contribute to a negative inotropic state by facilitating myocardial Gi activity, which is known to be increased in the failing heart muscle.[131-133] Support for this hypothesis must await the availability of a specific NPY antagonist.[134]

VASOACTIVE INTESTINAL PEPTIDE

Whereas NPY is a potent vasoconstrictor, vasoactive intestinal peptide (VIP) is associated with parasympathetic nerves and acts as a vasodilator.[135] It is a 28 amino acid peptide isolated from porcine intestine that is structurally related to the gastrointestinal peptides secretin and glucagon. In addition to its vasodilator properties, it may have positive inotropic activity. VIP-immunoreactive neurons have been identified in mammalian heart tissue, including that of humans. The myocardial concentration of VIP is reduced with heart failure,[136] and plasma levels can be enhanced by ACE inhibitor therapy.[137] VIP, like substance P, co-localizes with calcitonin gene related

peptide (CGRP) and when released induces peripheral vasodilation. It is present in cardiac neurons[138] mainly in the right atrium.[139] When VIP is infused in humans there is associated dilation of peripheral[140] and coronary[141] arteries. Although plasma levels of VIP are increased with shock and heart failure,[142] the role this peptide plays in the pathogenesis of heart failure remains unclear.

PROSTAGLANDINS

Normal healthy people are not dependent on prostaglandin (PG) synthesis, as evidenced by the widespread use of aspirin and nonsteroidal antiinflammatory drugs (NSAIDs). However, patients with advanced heart failure are keenly dependent on prostaglandins to maintain normal renal function including adequate sodium excretion.[143] Prostaglandins are not true hormones but are autocoids (i.e., they are synthesized and biologically active locally). However, some metabolites such as PGI_2 and PGE_2 do circulate and are known to be increased in patients with heart failure.[143-145] When patients with advanced heart failure are treated with an NSAID such as indomethacin, the cardiac index may fall and the systemic vascular resistance and pulmonary capillary wedge pressure can increase.[143]

As with vasoconstrictor peptides, prostaglandin activity rises as heart failure worsens. There are important interactions between neurohormones and prostaglandins. Renin release is enhanced by prostaglandins, and PGE_2 and PGI_2 modulate the constrictor effects of angiotensin II. Prostaglandins are in turn released by angiotensin II, NE, and AVP.[146] Atrial natriuretic peptide is also released by prostaglandins. During heart failure renal homeostasis is highly dependent on prostaglandin synthesis.[147] The adverse effects of NSAIDs on kidney function in the setting of heart failure is now well established.[148,149] Aspirin, unlike NSAIDs, seems well tolerated by patients with heart failure, although some concerns have been raised regarding the dependence of ACE inhibitor efficacy on the integrity of prostaglandin metabolism.[150]

ATRIAL NATRIURETIC PEPTIDES

There have been thousands of reports on atrial natriuretic factor (ANF) since the seminal report of DeBold et al.[151] In fact, the existence of a natriuretic system regulating salt and water balance and opposing the action of the RAAS had been suspected for many years.[152,153] Although the primary functions of cardiac cells are excitation, conduction, and contraction, the concept that the heart might act as a volume controlling system with "atrial stress receptors" was considered by Henry and Pearse in 1956.[154] Intracellular granules were reported in atrial myocytes in 1956,[155] and the granules were later demonstrated to be associated with water and sodium intake.[156] In 1985 Lang and colleagues demonstrated circulating ANF.[157] In 1987 the International Society for Hypertension, the American Heart Association, and the World Health Organization agreed on the current terminology: atrial natriuretic factor, which refers to the circulating form of a 28 amino acid peptide derived from the C-terminus pro-ANF (i.e., 99–126). ANF has been the subject of several reviews.[158–162] We now know that ANF belongs to a family of peptides including brain natriuretic peptide (BNP)[163] and central nervous system natriuretic peptide (CNP),[164] both of which were isolated from porcine brain.

The biosynthesis of ANF is still not completely understood but includes transcription of a large molecule that undergoes multiple cleavage steps before achieving the 28 amino acid status of the biologically active moiety.[159] Granules of ANF are clustered as pro-ANF in the nuclear poles of atrial cardiocytes. However, granules can be found in ventricular myocytes of hearts that are dilated or hypertrophied[165] and correlate with the size of the myocytes.

The principal stimulus to ANF release is right atrial distension or stretch, not pressure.[166–168] ANF acts as a diuretic[169] and a vasodilator[170] in humans. The circulating half-life is about 2.5 minutes, and it is cleared in the kidney by neutral endopeptidase and specific clearance receptors.[171,172] ANF acts through its primary receptors to generate guanylate cyclase.[172] ANF receptors may down-regulate in the syndrome of heart failure,[173] analogous to β-adrenoceptors.

In 1986 Burnett and colleagues reported that plasma ANF was increased in patients with heart failure.[174] These observations set into motion a number of clinical studies that further characterized the role of ANF during normal homeostasis and in pathologic states.[175–179] Meanwhile, the more basic biology of the ANF system gradually became better understood. The predominant ANF receptor subpopulation appears on vascular tissue, renal glomeruli, and the adrenal cortex. These receptors are coupled to cyclic guanosine monophosphate (cGMP) (soluble) and subserve vasodilation, natriuresis, and reduced aldosterone production, respectively.[180,181] The clearance receptors[171,172] are primarily in the kidney[182] and are not coupled to soluble cGMP. The major circulating form of ANF in patients with heart failure may

be β-ANF (an antiparallel dimer of α-ANF), which has reduced biologic activity.[183]

The BNP is stored mainly as a 32 amino acid residue in the heart from where it is secreted. There is considerable interspecies variation in BNP structure.[184] In tandem with ANF, BNP forms a dual control system,[185] although their actions are rather similar.[186] Like ANF, BNP is increased during heart failure[186–188] and may correlate better with left ventricular performance than ANF.[189,190]

The CNP is primarily in the central nervous system rather than the heart[191] and like ANF is highly conserved among species.[192] In addition to being concentrated in cerebral fluid[193] CNP is a potent vasodilator, especially in the brain.[194,195] The natriuretic action of CNP is rather weak,[196] as it lacks a C-terminal tail structure. Plasma levels of CNP are low and are not apparently increased during heart failure.[197] With more structure–function information available, genetic engineering of "designer peptides" may open the door for more therapeutically effective ANF family members.[198,199]

The interaction of ANF with other neuroendocrine systems has been studied extensively.[200–204] ANF appears to reduce sympathetic activity through a central or ganglionic effect.[205] Of interest, few or modest neuroendocrine effects are seen when large doses of exogenous ANF are infused into patients with heart failure,[206,207] suggesting a lack of responsiveness at the cellular level.[208] The hemodynamic effects of ANF infusions are also somewhat variable. Pulmonary capillary wedge pressure usually falls, but cardiac output may increase[209] or remain unchanged.[210] Patients with heart failure demonstrate a blunted hemodynamic and renal response to ANF.[211,212] Related therapies may emerge in the future, such as orally effective endopeptidase inhibitors that enhance plasma levels of ANF[213–217] or "designer peptides" (e.g., ANF 95–126), which preserve renal excretory function during heart failure because they are not easily degraded by the kidney.[218] It is also possible that the antihypertrophy or antigrowth properties of ANF or its analogs will be of eventual therapeutic value,[219] though much research is still required in this arena.

ENDOTHELINS

A potent vasoconstrictor peptide produced by vascular endothelial cells was described in 1988 by Masaki's laboratory.[220] Termed "endothelin," we now know endothelins (ETs) are a family of 21 amino acid peptides found in at least four distinct isoforms (ET-1, ET-2, ET-3, and vasoactive intestinal contractor).[221–224] Although originally thought to be secreted only by the endothelium, it is now apparent that many diverse tissues synthesize and release ET. Like many hormones and neuropeptides, ET arises from posttranslational processing of longer prohormones and is secreted primarily by a constitutive pathway. A converting enzyme is involved[225] that is similar to angiotensin.

Once released, ET has a large variety of biologic actions involving the cardiovascular, renal, pulmonary, and neuroendocrine systems (Table 15-3). The mature, active endothelins act on two distinct, seven-membrane domain receptors,[226–228] ET_A and ET_B. The ET_A receptor is selective for endothelins, whereas the ET_B receptor is more promiscuous. Intracellular signaling by endothelins is complex. Both stimulate phosphatidylinositol hydrolysis and arachidonic acid release, but the effects on cyclic adenosine monophosphate (cAMP) production vary according to cell type.[229] The ET_A receptor subserves mitogenic activity, including hypertrophy and proliferation in vascular cells, fibroblasts, and glomerular mesangial cells,[230] as well as hypertrophy in cultured neonatal rat cardiomyocytes.[231] A number of ET_A receptor blockers have been developed,[232–235] opening up a number of interesting treatment possibilities.

Increasing evidence suggests that in addition to its known role as an autocoid, ET circulates in plasma.[236] It is increased about threefold during clinical heart failure[237–242] and twofold during experimental (rapid pacing) heart failure.[243] Plasma ET is also modestly increased in essential hypertension and transplantation-associated hypertension, and

more so in cardiogenic shock. Circulating concentrations in the range of 5–40 pg/ml are vasoactive,[241] with normal values being variably reported at 1.8 pg/ml. Plasma ET varies substantially in patients with severe heart failure[237] but is usually in the range of 20–25 pg/ml, where it is principally big-ET.[242] ET is present in both nonfailing and failing heart muscle and is unchanged in failing heart muscle. The degree of plasma ET elevation correlates with functional class[237,242] and with the degree of pulmonary hypertension.[244] As ET_A blockers and ET converting enzyme inhibitors are developed, the quantitative role of ET in the pathophysiology of heart failure should begin to unfold. These pharmacologic tools may take on growing importance in the face of mounting evidence supporting the existence of a dynamic interaction in vivo between cardiac myocytes and adjacent microvascular endothelial cells,[245] thus linking coronary blood flow and myocardial contractility.

ENDOTHELIUM-DERIVED RELAXATION FACTORS AND NITRIC OXIDE

Strictly speaking, endothelial derived relaxation factor (EDRF) and nitric oxide (NO) are not neurohormones or cytokines. Yet their biologic activity is fundamental to the pathophysiology of heart failure in both the myocardium[246] and the peripheral circulation.[247] They behave as "neurohormones" in this regard. The concept of a vasodilating substance being released from the endothelium in response to acetylcholine was reported by Furchgott and Zawadzki in 1980.[248] Since then it has become apparent that a host of biologic amines and peptides can release EDRF,[249] and the flow itself may activate endogenous vasodilator substance via potassium channels.[250,251] Moreover, EDRF can apparently be released from vascular smooth muscle.[252] Although the current view is that EDRF is largely NO,[253] there may be other vasorelaxant nitrosothiols that differ from NO and may be more potent.[254] EDRF or NO is released from endothelial cells following interaction with ligands such as bradykinin or acetylcholine. It diffuses to adjacent vascular smooth cells where it subserves vasodilation via cGMP.

Kaiser and associates demonstrated a lack of responsiveness to acetylcholine in the rapid pacing canine model of heart failure.[255] It subsequently became clear that EDRF release was attenuated in patients with a variety of cardiovascular conditions including hypertension,[256,257] atherosclerosis,[258] cor-

Table 15-3. Biologic Actions of Endothelin

Cardiovascular
    Potent and sustained pressor action
    Markedly positive inotropic action
    Reflex bradycardia
Renal
    Increased renal artery resistance
    ↓ GFR, ↓ RBF, ↓ UNaV
    Mesangial hypertrophy
Pulmonary
    Potent bronchoconstrictor
Neuroendocrine
    ↑ ANF, prostaglandins, renin, aldosterone
    ↑ Neurotransmitter release
    ↑ AVP

Abbreviations: GFR, glomerular filtration rate; RBF, renal blood flow; ANF, atrial natriuretic factor; AVP, arginine vasopressin.

onary artery disease,[259,260] and diabetes mellitus.[261] It is now also widely recognized that left ventricular hypertrophy, dilated cardiomyopathy, and post-transplantation hearts are associated with reduced coronary vascular reserve, possibly related to deficient EDRF or NO release. Clearly, regulation of the vascular[262,263] and myocardial[264] endothelial function plays an important role in circulatory homeostasis, and its impairment is probably critical to the development of many pathologic conditions.

Although basal release of NO may be normal in patients with heart failure,[247,265] endothelium-dependent vasodilation is impaired or attenuated,[266–269] which may be one of the factors contributing to exercise intolerance in patients with chronic heart failure.[270] Of interest, impaired peripheral vasodilation in patients with heart failure can be reversed to some extent with L-arginine,[271] a precursor of nitric oxide. Moreover, ACE inhibitors can potentiate endothelium-dependent vasodilation induced by cholinergic stimuli.[272] Experimentally, the type of heart failure does not seem to matter, as both the pacing model[255] and the rat myocardial infarction model[273–275] are associated with endothelial dysfunction. Abnormal endothelium-dependent responses during heart failure are reversible following heart transplantation.[276] As more is learned about how endothelium-dependent vasodilation is governed, it is expected that its pharmacologic manipulation may play a more prominent role in the treatment of heart failure, such as nitrates have had in the treatment of coronary disease for more than 100 years. The interest in NO synthase, which is both constitutive and inducible depending on the tissue, is great—as one might expect given the potential therapeutic possibilities. It is likely that NO participates in numerous biologic responses including inflammation, neutrotransmission, immune rejection, sepsis, and myocardial and vascular control mechanisms: hence the intense interest by a broad spectrum of the scientific community.

TUMOR NECROSIS FACTOR α

Clinical observations indicate that patients with advanced heart failure express elevated circulating levels of a proinflammatory cytokine called tumor necrosis factor α (TNFα).[277,278] The clinical significance of this observation is somewhat obscure, but there is growing awareness that proinflammatory cytokines may play some role in modulating the structure and function of the adult heart. Cytokines are not true "hormones" but a family of diverse, relatively small molecular weight proteins (generally 15–30 kDa) se-creted by "producer cells" that influence the biologic behavior of "target cells." They bind to specific receptors, usually in a complex fashion that involves oligodimerization of the receptor.[279] The TNFs, cloned in 1984, were among the first cytokines to be unambiguously defined. During heart failure TNFα elevation is associated with advanced disease, cachexia, and marked activation of the renin-angiotensin system.[277] One member of the TNF receptor family (Fas) transduces the apoptotic signal into cells.[280] Because cell dropout is an essential component of progressive heart failure[281] and apoptosis is known to occur in the human heart,[282] it is possible that TNFα is important in the syndrome of progressive left ventricular remodeling. There are now 12 identifiable TNF receptors that subserve a host of biologic activities. If is therefore likely that future developments will include therapies for heart failure that are designed to modulate excessive cytokine activity.

CALCITONIN GENE-RELATED PEPTIDE AND β-ENDORPHINS

A number of peptides reported to be increased in patients with heart failure have undergone far less study. Calcitonin gene-related peptide (CGRP) is a potent endogenous vasodilator substance that co-localizes with substance P and VIP in parasympathetic nerves. It is located in the central and peripheral nervous systems, as well as the heart and blood vessels. Plasma levels are increased in patients with untreated heart failure.[283] Short-term[284] and long-term[285] infusion of CGRP into patients with heart failure is associated with a beneficial hemodynamic effect.

β-Endorphin levels are also reported to be increased in patients with heart failure[286] and reflect to some extent the severity of the syndrome. As with many other peptides, their role in the pathophysiology of heart failure is unclear.

CONCLUSION

It is difficult to know when the idea of heart failure first arose, but it now seems clear that neurohumoral influences play an important role in this common clinical syndrome. Whether there is high output heart failure,[287] cor pulmonale,[288] or more conventional left heart failure,[14] neurohormones are released presumably in an attempt to preserve blood pressure and maintain circulatory homeostasis. Neuroendocrine hyperactivity is associated with a poor prognosis and, at the very least, is an important marker of disease severity. It is now clear that drugs designed to block excessive neurohormones have the potential to markedly improve clinical well-being and survival in patients with heart failure. As we come to understand neuroendocrine mechanisms and their role in the pathogenesis of heart failure, we can look forward to even better and more imaginative therapies.

REFERENCES

1. Laragh JH: Hormones and the pathogenesis of congestive heart failure: vasopressin, aldosterone, and angiotensin II. Circulation 1962;25:1015
2. Genest J, Granger P, De Champlain J: Endocrine factors in congestive heart failure. Am J Cardiol 1968; 22:35
3. Francis GS, Goldsmith SR, Levine TB et al: The neurohumoral axis in congestive heart failure. Ann Intern Med 1984;101:370
4. Cohn JN, Johnson G, Ziesche S et al: A comparison of enalapril with hydralazine-isosorbide dinitrate in the treatment of chronic congestive heart failure. N Engl J Med 1991;325:303
5. SOLVD Investigators: Effect of enalapril on survival in patients with reduced left ventricular ejection fractions and congestive heart failure. N Engl J Med 1991;325:293
6. SOLVD Investigators: Effect of enalapril on mortality and the development of heart failure in asymptomatic patients with reduced left ventricular ejection fraction. N Engl J Med 1992;327:685
7. CONSENSUS Trial Study Group: Effects of enalapril on mortality in severe congestive heart failure. Results of the Cooperative North Scandinavian Enalapril Survival Study (CONSENSUS). N Engl J Med 1987;316:1429
8. Pfeffer MA, Braunwald E, Moyé LA et al: Effect of captopril on mortality and morbidity in patients with left ventricular dysfunction after myocardial infarction. N Engl J Med 1992;327:669
9. Levine TB, Francis GS, Goldsmith SR et al: Activity of the sympathetic nervous system and renin-angiotensin system assessed by plasma hormone levels and their relation to hemodynamic abnormalities in congestive heart failure. Am J Cardiol 1982;49:1659
10. Cohn JN, Levine TB, Olivari MR et al: Plasma norepinephrine as a guide to prognosis in patients with chronic congestive heart failure. N Engl J Med 1984; 311:819
11. Packer M, Lee WH, Kessler PD et al: Role of neurohormonal mechanisms in determining survival in patients with severe chronic heart failure. Circulation, suppl. IV 1987;75:80
12. Packer M: Neurohormonal interactions and adaptations in congestive heart failure. Circulation 1988; 77:721
13. Swedberg K, Eneroth P, Kjekshus J et al: Hormones regulating cardiovascular function in patients with severe congestive heart failure and their relation to mortality. Circulation 1990;82:1730
14. Francis GS, Benedict C, Johnstone D et al: Comparison of neuroendocrine activation in patients with left ventricular dysfunction with and without congestive heart failure. Circulation 1990;82:1724
15. Kubo SH: The role of neurohormonal activation in the pathophysiology and prognosis of patients with congestive heart failure. Coronary Artery Dis 1993; 4:4
16. Packer M: The neurohormonal hypothesis. A theory to explain the mechanism of disease progression in heart failure. J Am Coll Cardiol 1992;20:248
17. Francis GS, McDonald KM: Left ventricular hypertrophy. An initial response to myocardial injury. Am J Cardiol 1992;69:3G–9G
18. Francis GS, McDonald KM, Cohn JN: Neurohumoral activation in preclinical heart failure. Remodeling and the potential for intervention. Circulation, suppl. IV 1993;87:90–96
19. Zelis R, Nellis SH, Longhurst J et al: Abnormalities in the regional circulations accompanying congestive heart failure. Prog Cardiovasc Dis 1975;18:181
20. Zelis R, Flaim SF, Liedtke AJ: Cardiocirculatory dynamics in the normal and failing heart. Annu Rev Physiol 1981;43:455
21. Zelis R, Flaim SF: The circulations in congestive heart failure. Mod Concepts Cardiovasc Dis 1982;51: 79
22. Zelis R, Flaim SF: Alterations in vasomotor tone in congestive heart failure. Prog Cardiovasc Dis 1982; 24:437
23. Leier CV: Regional blood flow in human congestive heart failure. Curr Cardiol 1992;124:726
24. Francis GS, Boosalis PJ: Mechanism of death in patients with congestive cardiac failure. The change in plasma norepinephrine and its relation to sudden death. Cardioscience 1990;1:29
25. Francis GS: Modulation of peripheral sympathetic nerve transmission. Am J Coll Cardiol 1988;12:250
26. Francis GS, Cohn JN: The autonomic nervous system in congestive heart failure. Annu Rev Med 1986;37: 235
27. Katz AM: Cardiomyopathy of overload. A major determinant of prognosis in congestive heart failure. N Engl J Med 1990;322:100
28. Tan L, Jalil JE, Pick R et al: Cardiac myocyte necrosis induced by angiotensin II. Circ Res 1991;69:1185
29. Ratajska A, Campbell SE, Sun Y et al: Angiotensin II associated cardiac myocyte necrosis. Role of adrenal catecholamines. Cardiovasc Res 1994;28:684
30. Mann DL, Kent RL, Parsons B et al: Adrenergic effects on the biology of the adult mammalian cardiocyte. Circulation 1992;85:790
31. Rona G: Catecholamine cardiotoxicity. J Mol Cell Cardiol 1985;17:291
32. Jiang JP, Downing SE: Catecholamine cardiomyopathy. Review and analysis of pathogenetic mechanisms. Yale J Biol Med 1990;63:581
33. Dzau VJ, Gibbons GH: Endothelium and growth factors in vascular remodeling of hypertension. Hypertension, suppl. III 1991;18:115
34. Mulvaney MJ: Vascular growth in hypertension. J Cardiovasc Pharmacol 1992;20:S7
35. Gibbons GH, Dzau VJ: The emerging concept of vascular remodeling. N Engl J Med 1994;330:1431
36. Ratajska A, Campbell SE, Cleutjens JPM et al: An-

giotensin II and structural remodeling of coronary vessels in rats. J Lab Clin Med 1994;124:408

37. Leithe JE, Margorien RD, Hermiller JB et al: Relationship between central hemodynamics and regional blood flow in normal subjects and in patients with congestive heart failure. Circulation 1984;69:57

38. Francis GS: Neurohormones in congestive heart failure. Cardiol Rev 1989;1:278

39. Harris P: Evolution and the cardiac patient. Cardiovasc Res 1989;17:3

40. Harris P: Congestive cardiac failure. Central role of the arterial blood pressure. Br Heart J 1987;58:190

41. Wade OL, Bishop JM: Cardiac Output and Regional Blood Flow. Blackwell Scientific, Oxford, 1962

42. Thomas JA, Marks BH: Plasma norepinephrine in congestive heart failure. Am J Cardiol 1978;41:233

43. Braunwald E: Congestive heart failure. Ann Intern Med 1966;64:904

44. Starling EH: Points on pathology of heart disease. Lancet 1897;1:569

45. Hagbarth K-E, Vallbo AB: Pulse and respiratory grouping of sympathetic impulses in human muscle nerves. Acta Physiol Scand 1968;74:96

46. Wallin BG, Elam M: Insights from intraneural recordings of sympathetic nerve traffic in humans. NIPS 1994;9:203

47. Francis GS, Goldsmith SR, Cohn JN: Relationship of exercise capacity to resting left ventricular performance and basal plasma norepinephrine levels in patients with congestive heart failure. Am Heart J 1982;104:725

48. Kao W, Gheroghiade M, Hall V et al: Relation between plasma norepinephrine and response to medical therapy in men with congestive heart failure secondary to coronary artery disease or idiopathic dilated cardiomyopathy. Am J Cardiol 1989;64:609

49. Francis GS, Rector TS, Cohn JN: Sequential neurohumoral measurements in patients with congestive heart failure. Am Heart J J 1988;116:1464

50. Francis GS, Boosalis PJ: Mechanism of death in patients with congestive cardiac failure. The change in plasma norepinephrine and its relation to sudden death. Cardioscience 1990;1:29

51. Rector TS, Olivari MT, Levine B, Francis GS, Cohn JN: Predicting survival for an individual with congestive heart failure using the plasma norepinephrine concentration. Am Heart J 1987;114:148

52. Gaffney TE, Braunwald E: Importance of the adrenergic nervous system in the support of circulatory function in patients with congestive heart failure. Am J Med 1962;34:320

53. Chidsey CA, Harrison DC, Braunwald E: Augmentation of the plasma norepinephrine response to exercise in patients wi congestive heart failure. N Engl J Med 1962;267:650

54. Waagstein F, Bristow MR, Swedberg K et al: Beneficial effects of metoprolol in idiopathic dilated cardiomyopathy. Lancet 1993;342:1441

55. CIBIS Investigators and Committees: A randomized trial of β-blockade in heart failure. Circulation 1994; 90:1754

56. Christensen NJ, Galbo H, Gjerris A et al: Whole body and regional clearances of noradrenaline and adrenaline in man. Acta Physiol Scand 1984;527:17

57. Nishioka A, Kubo S, Hirota Y et al: A clinical study on the role of the renin-angiotensin-aldosterone system

and catecholamines in chronic congestive heart failure. Jpn Heart J 1982;23:527

58. Hasking GJ, Esler MD, Jennings GL et al: Norepinephrine spillover to plasma in patients with congestive heart failure. Evidence of increased overall and cardiorenal sympathetic nerve activity. Circulation 1986;73:615

59. Leimbach WN, Wallin BG, Victor RG et al: Direct evidence from intraneural recordings for increased central sympathetic outflow in patients with heart failure. Circulation 1986;73:913

60. Kramer RS, Mason DT, Braunwald E: Augmented sympathetic neurotransmitter activity in the peripheral vascular bed of patients with congestive heart failure and cardiac norepinephrine depletion. Circulation 1968;37:629

61. Ferguson DW, Berg WJ, Sanders JS: Clinical and hemodynamic correlates of sympathetic nerve activity in normal humans and patients with heart failure. Evidence from direct microneurographic recordings. J Am Coll Cardiol 1990;16:1125

62. Abraham WT, Hensen J, Schrier RW: Elevated plasma noradrenaline concentrations in patients with low-output cardiac failure. Dependence on increased noradrenaline secretion rates. Clin Sci 1990; 79:429

63. Meredith IT, Eisenhofer G, Lambert GW: Cardiac sympathetic nervous activity in congestive heart failure. Circulation 1993;88:136

64. Rose CP, Burgess JH, Cousineau: Tracer norepinephrine kinetics in coronary circulation of patients with heart failure secondary to chronic pressure and volume overload. J Clin Invest 1985;76:1740

65. Goldstein RE, Beiser GD, Stampfer M et al: Impairment of autonomically mediated heart rate control in patients with cardiac dysfunction. Circ Res 1975;36: 571

66. Eckberg D, Drabinsky M, Braunwald E: Defective cardiac parasympathetic control in patients with heart disease. N Engl J Med 1971;265:877

67. Ferguson DW, Abboud FM, Mark AL: Selective impairment of baroreflex-mediated vasoconstrictor responses in patients with ventricular dysfunction. Circulation 1984;69:451

68. Francis GS, Cohn JN: The autonomic nervous system in congestive heart failure. Annu Rev Med 1986;37: 235

69. Hirsch AT, Dzau VJ, Creager MA: Baroreceptor function in congestive heart failure. Effect on neurohumoral activation and regional vascular resistance. Circulation, suppl. IV 1987;75:36

70. Ferguson DW, Berg WJ, Roach PJ: Effects of heart failure on baroreflex control of sympathetic neural activity. Am J Cardiol 1992;69:523

71. Dibner-Dunlap ME, Thames MD: Control of sympathetic nerve activity by vagal mechanoreflexes is blunted in heart failure. Circulation 1992;86:1929

72. Zucker IH, Wang W, Brandle M: Baroreflex abnormalities in congestive heart failure. NIPS 1993;8:87

73. Goldsmith SR, Francis GS, Levine TB et al: Regional blood flow response to orthostasis in patients with congestive heart failure. J Am Coll Cardiol 1983;1: 1391

74. Marin-Neto JA, Pintya AO, Gallo L et al: Abnormal baroreflex control of heart rate in decompensated

congestive heart failure and reversal after compensation. Am J Cardiol 1991;67:604

75. Levine TB, Olivari MT, Cohn JN: Effects of orthotopic heart transplantation on sympathetic control mechanisms in congestive heart failure. Am J Cardiol 1986; 58:1035

76. Mohanty PK, Thames MD, Arrowood JA: Impairment of cardiopulmonary baroreflex after cardiac transplantation in humans. Circulation 1987;75:914

77. Ellenbogen KA, Mohanty PR, Szentpetery S et al: Arterial baroreflex abnormalities in heart failure. Circulation 1989;79:51

78. Sinoway LI, Minotti JR, Davis D et al: Delayed reversal of impaired vasodilation in congestive heart failure after heart transplantation. Am J Cardiol 1988; 61:1076

79. Francis GS, Cohn JN, Johnson G et al: Plasma norepinephrine, plasma renin activity, and congestive heart failure. Circulation, suppl. VI 1993;87:40

80. Creager MA, Faxon DP, Cutler SS et al: Contribution of vasopressin to vasoconstriction in patients with congestive heart failure. Comparison with the renin-angiotensin system and the sympathetic nervous system. J Am Coll Cardiol 1986;7:758

81. Merrill AJ, Morrison JR, Brannon ES: Concentration of renin in renal venous blood in patients with congestive heart failure. Am J Med 1946;1:468

82. Davis JO: Mechanism of salt and water retention in congestive heart failure. The role of aldosterone. Am J Med 1960;19:486

83. Davis JO: What signals the kidney to release renin? Circ Res 1971;28:301

84. Davis JO: The control of renin release. Am J Med 1973;55:333

85. Vander AJ, Miller R: Control of renin secretion in the anesthetized dog. Am J Physiol 1964;207:537

86. Packer M, Medina N, Yushak M: Relation between serum sodium concentration and the hemodynamic and clinical responses to converting enzyme inhibition with captopril in severe heart failure. J Am Coll Cardiol 1984;3:1035

87. Lee WH, Packer M: Prognostic importance of serum sodium concentration and its modification by converting-enzyme inhibition in patients with severe chronic heart failure. Circulation 1986;73:257

88. Ikram H, Chan W, Espiner EA, Nicholls MG: Haemodynamic and hormone response to acute and chronic furosemide therapy in congestive heart failure. Clin Sci 1980;59:443

89. Anand IS, Ferrari R, Kalra GS et al: Edema of cardiac origin. Circulation 1989;80:299

90. Dzau VJ, Colucci WS, Hollenberg NK, Williams GH: Relation of the renin-angiotensin-aldosterone system to clinical state in congestive heart failure. Circulation 1981;63:645

91. Zimmerman BG, Sybertz EJ, Wong PC: Interaction between the sympathetic and renin-angiotensin system. Hypertension 1984;2:581

92. Fujii AM, Vatner SF: Direct versus indirect pressor and vasoconstrictor actions of angiotensin in conscious dogs. Hypertension 1985;7:253

93. Hilgers KF, Veelken R, Rupprecht G et al: Angiotensin II facilitates sympathetic transmission in rat hind limb circulation. Hypertension 1993;21:322

94. Goldsmith SR, Hasking GJ: Subpressor angiotensin II infusions do not stimulate sympathetic activity in humans. Am J Physiol 1990;258:H179

95. Goldsmith SR, Hasking GJ: Effect of a pressor infusion of angiotensin II on sympathetic activity and heart rate in normal humans. Circ Res 1991;68:263

96. Hall JE, Guyton AC, Jackson TE et al: Control of glomerular filtration rate by renin-angiotensin system. Am J Physiol 1977;233:F366

97. Schaer GL, Covit AB, Laragh JH, Cody RF: Association of hyponatremia with increased renin activity in chronic congestive heart failure. Impact of diuretic therapy. Am J Cardiol 1983;51:1635

98. Szatalowicz VL, Arnold PE, Chaimovitz C et al: Radioimmunoassay of plasma arginine vasopressin in hyponatremic patients with congestive heart failure. N Engl J Med 1981;305:263

99. Riegger GAJ, Liebau G, Kochsiek K: Antidiuretic hormone in congestive heart failure. Am J Med 1982; 72:49

100. Goldsmith SR, Francis GS, Cowley AW, Levine TB, Cohn JN: Increased plasma arginine vasopressin levels in patients with congestive heart failure. J Am Coll Cardiol 1983;1:1385

101. Creager MA, Faxon DP, Cutler SS et al: Contribution of vasopressin to vasoconstriction in patients with congestive heart failure. Comparison with the renin-angiotensin system and the sympathetic nervous system. J Am Coll Cardiol 1986;7:758

102. Nicod P, Waeber B, Bussien J-P et al: Acute hemodynamic effect of a vascular antagonist of vasopressin in patients with congestive heart failure. Am J Cardiol 1985;55:1043

103. Monos E, Cox RH, Peterson CH: Direct effect of physiologic doses of arginine vasopressin on the arterial wall in vivo. Am J Physiol 1978;243:H167

104. Pruszcynski W, Vahanian A, Ardaillou R, Acar J: Role of antidiuretic hormone in impaired water excretion of patients with congestive heart failure. J Clin Endocrinol Metab 1984;58:599

105. Liard J-F: Peripheral vasodilatation induced by a vasopressin analogue with selective V_2-agonism in dogs. J Physiol (Lond) 1989;256:H1621

106. Goldsmith SR, Francis GS, Cowley AW, Goldenberg IF, Cohn JN: Hemodynamic effects of infused arginine vasopressin in congestive heart failure. J Am Coll Cardiol 1986;8:779

107. Yamamura Y, Ogawa H, Chihara T et al: OPC-21268, an orally effective, nonpeptide vasopressin V_1 receptor antagonist. Science 1991;252:572

108. Imaizumi T, Harada S, Hirooka Y et al: Effects of OPC-21268, an orally effective vasopressin V_1 receptor antagonist in humans. Hypertension 1992;20:54

109. Ohnishi A, Ko Y, Fujihara H et al: Pharmacokinetics, safety, and pharmacologic effects of OPC-21268, a nonpeptide orally active vasopressin V_1 receptor antagonist, in humans. J Clin Pharmacol 1993;33:230

110. Schrier RW, Berl T, Anderson RJ: Osmotic and nonosmotic control of vasopressin release. Am J Physiol 1979;236:F321

111. Share L: Role of vasopressin in cardiovascular regulation. Physiol Rev 1988;68:1248

112. Aylward PE, Floras JS, Phil D, Leimbach WN, Abboud FM: Effects of vasopressin on the circulation and its baroreflex control in healthy men. Circulation 1986;73:1145

113. Goldsmith SR: Baroreflex loading maneuvers do not

suppress increased plasma arginine vasopressin in patients with congestive heart failure. J Am Coll Cardiol 1992;19:1180

114. Goldsmith SR, Francis GS, Cowley AW, Cohn JN: Response of vasopressin and norepinephrine to lower body negative pressure in humans. Am J Physiol 1982;243:H970

115. Goldsmith SR, Cowley AW, Francis GS, Cohn JN: Effects of increased intracardiac and arterial pressure on plasma vasopressin in humans. Am J Physiol 1984;246:H647

116. Goldsmith SR: Vasopressin as vasopressor. Am J Med 1987;82:1213

117. Goldsmith SR, Francis GS, Cowley AW: Arginine vasopressin and the renal response to water loading in congestive heart failure. Am J Cardiol 1986;58:295

118. Tatemoto K, Neuropeptide Y: Complete aminoacid sequence of the brain peptide. Proc Natl Acad Sci USA 1982;89:5485

119. Tatemoto K, Carlquist M, Mutt V: Neuropeptide Y. A novel brain peptide with the structural similarity to peptide YY and pancreatic polypeptide. Nature 1982;296:659

120. Potter EK: Neuropeptide Y as an autonomic neurotransmitter. Pharmacol Ther 1988;37:251

121. Lehmann J: Neuropeptide Y. An overview. Drug Dev Res 1990;19:329

122. Warner MR, Levy MN: Neuropeptide Y as a putative modulator of the vagal effects on heart rate. Circ Res 1989;64:882

123. Walker P, Grouzmann E, Burnier M, Waeber B: The role of neuropeptide Y in cardiovascular regulation. Trends Pharmacol Sci 1991;12:111

124. Zukowska-Grojec Z, Marks ES, Haass M: Neuropeptide Y is a potent vasoconstrictor and a cardiodepressant in rat. Am J Physiol 1987;253:H1234

125. Minson RB, McRitchie RJ, Chalmers JP: Effects of neuropeptide Y on left ventricular function in the conscious rabbit. Clin Exp Pharmacol Physiol 1987;14:263

126. Warner MR, Levy MN: Neuropeptide Y as a putative modulator of the vagal effects on heart rate. Circ Res 1989;64:882

127. Zelis R, Nussberger J, Clemson B et al: Neuropeptide Y infusion decreases plasma renin activity in postmyocardial infarction rats. J Cardiovasc Pharmacol 1994;24:896

128. Pernow J, Lundberg M, Kayser L: Plasma neuropeptide Y-like immunoreactivity and catecholamines during various degrees of activation in man. Clin Physiol (Oxford) 1986;6:561

129. Allen JM, Bloom SR: Neuropeptide Y. A putative neurotransmitter. Neurochem Int 1986;8:1

130. Maisel AS, Scott NA, Motulsky HJ et al: Elevation of plasma neuropeptide Y levels in congestive heart failure. Am J Med 1989;86:43

131. Feldman AM, Cates AE, Veazey WB et al: Increase of the 40,000-mol wt pertussis toxin substrate (G protein) in the failing human heart. J Clin Invest 1988;82:189

132. Heumann J, Scholz H, Doring V et al: Increase in myocardial Gi-proteins in heart failure. Lancet 1988;2:936

133. Bohm M, Gierschik P, Jakobs K-H et al: Increase of $G_{i\alpha}$ in human hearts with dilated but not ischemic cardiomyopathy. Circulation 1990;82:1249

134. Wahlestedt C, Reis DJ: Neuropeptide Y-related peptides and their receptors—are the receptors potential therapeutic drug targets? Annu Rev Pharmacol Toxicol 1993;32:309

135. Lundberg JM, Anggard A, Fahrenkrug J, Hokfelt T, Mutt V: Vasoactive intestinal polypeptide in cholinergic neurons of exoctine glands. Functional significance of coexisting transmitters for vasodilation and secretion. Proc Natl Acad Sci USA 1980;77:1651

136. Unverferth DV, O'Dorisio TM, Miller MM et al: Human and canine ventricular vasoactive intestinal polypeptide. Decrease with heart failure. J Lab Clin Med 1986;108:11

137. Woie L, Dickstein K, Kaada B: Increase in vasoactive intestinal polypeptides (VIP) by the angiotensin converting enzyme (ACE) inhibitor lisinopril in congestive heart failure. Relation to haemodynamic and hormonal changes. Gen Pharmacol 1987;18:577

138. All JM, Gjorstrup P, Bjorkman JA, Abrahamsson T, Bloom SR: Studies on cardiac distribution and function of neuropeptide Y. Acta Physiol Scand 1986;126:405

139. Karasawa Y, Furukawa Y, Ren L-M et al: Cardiac responses to VIP and VIP-ergic-cholinergic interaction in isolated dog heart preparations. Eur J Pharmacol 1990;187:9

140. Frase LL, Gaffney A, Lane LD et al: Cardiovascular effects of vasoactive intestinal peptide in healthy subjects. Am J Cardiol 1987;60:1356

141. Smitherman TC, Popma JJ, Said SI, Krejs GJ, Dehmer GJ: Coronary hemodynamic effects of intravenous vasoactive intestinal peptide in humans. Am J Physiol 1989;257:H1254

142. Clark AJL, Adrian TE, McMichael HB, Bloom SR: Vasoactive intestinal peptide in shock and heart failure [letter]. Lancet 1983;1:539

143. Dzau VJ, Packer M, Lilly LS et al: Prostaglandins in severe congestive heart failure. Relation to activation of the renin-angiotensin system and hyponatremia. N Engl J Med 1984;310:347

144. Stanek B, Punzengruber C, Silberbauer K: Increase in bicycloprostaglandin E_2 metabolite in congestive heart failure in response to captopril. Clin Cardiol 1989;12:97

145. Punzengruber C, Stanek B, Sinzinger H, Silberbauer K: Bicyclo-prostaglandin E_2 metabolite in congestive heart failure and relation to vasoconstrictor neurohumoral principles. Am J Cardiol 1986;57:619

146. Scharschmidt L, Simonson M, Dunn MJ: Glomerular prostaglandins, angiotensin II, and nonsteroidal anti-inflammatory drugs. Am J Med, suppl. 2B 1986;81:30

147. Schlondorff D: Renal prostaglandin synthesis. Sites of production and specific actions of prostaglandins. Am J Med, suppl. 2B 1986;81:1

148. Cannon PJ: Prostaglandins in congestive heart failure and the effects of nonsteroidal anti-inflammatory drugs. Am J Med, suppl. 2B 1986;81:123

149. Oates JA: Antagonism of antihypertensive drug therapy by nonsteroidal anti-inflammatory drugs. Hypertension, suppl. II 1988;11:4

150. Hall D, Zeitler H, Rudolph W: Counteraction of the vasodilator effects of enalapril by aspirin in severe heart failure. J Am Coll Cardiol 1992;20:1549

151. De Bold AJ, Borenstein HB, Veress AT, Sonnenberg H: A rapid and potent natriuretic response to intrave-

nous injection of atrial myocardial extracts in rats. Life Sci 1981;28:89

152. Henry JP, Gauer ON, Reeves JL: Evidence on the atrial location of receptors influencing urine flow. Circ Res 1956;5:85

153. De Wardener HE: Natriuretic hormone. Clin Sci Mol Med 1977;53:1

154. Henry JP, Pearse JW: The possible role of cardiac atrial stress receptors in the induction of changes in urine blood flow. Am J Physiol 1956;131:572

155. Kisch B: Electron microscopy of the atrium of the heart in guinea pig. Exp Med 1956;14:99

156. Marie JP, Guillement H, Hatt PY: Le degré de granulation des cardiocytes auricularies. Étude planimetrique aucours de differents apports d'au et de sodium chez le rat. Pathol Biol (Paris) 1976;24:549

157. Lang RE, Tholken H, Ganten D et al: Atrial natriuretic factor. A circulating hormone stimulated by volume loading. Nature 1985;314:264

158. Burnett JC: Atrial natriuretic factor in congestive heart failure. p. 141. In Brenner BM, Laragh JH (eds): Advances in Atrial Peptide Research. Vol. II. American Society of Hypertension Symposium Series, 1988

159. Ballermann BJ, Brenner BM: Biologically active atrial peptides. J Clin Invest 1985;76:2041

160. Maack T, Camargo MJF, Kleinert HD, Laragh JH, Atlas SA: Atrial natriuretic factor. Structure and function properties. Kidney Int 1985;27:607

161. Palluk R, Gaida W, Hoefke W: Atrial natriuretic factor. Life Sci 1985;36:1415

162. Athanassopoulos G, Cokkinos DV: Atrial natriuretic factor. Prog Cardiovasc Dis 1991;31:313

163. Sudoh T, Minamino N, Kangawa K, Matsuo H: BNP-32, N-terminally six amino acid extended form of BNP identified in porcine brain. Biochem Biophys Res Commun 1988;155:726

164. Sudoh T, Minamino N, Kangawa K, Matsuo H: CNP: a new member of the natriuretic peptide family identified in porcine brain. Biochem Biophys Res Commun 1990;168:863

165. Takemura G, Fujiwara H, Horike K et al: Ventricular expression of atrial natriuretic polypeptide and its relations with hemodynamics and histology in dilated human hearts. Immunohistochemical study of the endomyocardial biopsy specimens. Circulation 1989;80:1137

166. Edwards BS, Zimmerman RS, Schwab TR, Heublein DM, Burnett JC: Atrial stretch, not pressure, is the principal determinant controlling the release of atrial natriuretic factor. Circ Res 1988;62:191

167. Ong ACM, Handler CE, Slater JDH: ANP response to atrial stretch and not to atrial pressure. Observation during pericardiocentesis in a young woman. Eur Heart J 1990;11:368

168. Au J, Brown JE, Lee MR, Boon NA: Effect of cardiac tamponade on atrial natriuretic peptide concentrations. Influence of stretch and pressure. Clin Sci 1990;79:377

169. Brenner BM, Ballerman BJ, Gunning ME et al: Diverse biological actions of ANP. Physiol Rev 1990;20:665

170. Fujita T, Ito Y, Noda H et al: Vasodilatory actions of alpha-human atrial natriuretic peptide and high Ca^{2+} effects in normal man. J Clin Invest 1987;80:832

171. Yandel TG, Richards AM, Nicholls MG et al: Metabolic clearance rate and plasma half-life of alpha-human atrial natriuretic peptide in man. Life Sci 1986;38:1827

172. Anand-Srivastava MB, Trachte GJ: Atrial natriuretic factor receptors and signal transduction mechanisms. Pharmacol Rev 1993;45:455

173. Tsutamoto T, Kanamori T, Morigami N et al: Possibility of downregulation of atrial natriuretic peptide receptor coupled to guanylate cyclase in peripheral vascular beds of patients with chronic severe heart failure. Circulation 1993;87:70

174. Burnett JC, Kao PC, Hu C et al: Atrial natriuretic peptide elevation in congestive heart failure in the human. Science 1986;231:1145

175. Raine AEG, Erne P, Burgisser E et al: Atrial natriuretic peptide and atrial pressure in patients with congestive heart failure. N Engl J Med 1986;315:533

176. Rodeheffer RJ, Tanaka I, Imada T et al: Atrial pressure and secetion of atrial natriuretic factor into human central circulation. J Am Coll Cardiol 1986;8:18

177. Hodsman GP, Phillips PA, Ogawa K, Johnston CI: Atrial natriuretic factor in normal man. Effects of tilt, posture, exercise and haemorrhage. J Hypertens Suppl 6 1986;4:503

178. Bilder GE, Siegl PKS, Schofield TL, Friedman PA: Chronotropic stimulation. A primary effector for release of atrial natriuretic factor. Circ Res 1989;64:799

179. Gottlieb SS, Kukin ML, Ahern D, Packer M: Prognostic importance of atrial natriuretic peptide in patients with chronic heart failure. J Am Coll Cardiol 1989;13:1534

180. Schiffrin EL, Poissant L, Cantin M, Thibault G: Receptors for atrial natriuretic factor in cultured vascular smooth muscle cells. Life Sci 1986;38:817

181. Schiffrin EL, St-Louis J, Garcia R et al: Vascular and adrenal binding sites for atrial natriuretic factor. Effects of sodium and hypertension. Hypertension Suppl I 1986;8:141

182. Maack T, Suzuki M, Almeida FA et al: Physiological role of silent receptors of atrial natriuretic factor. Science 1987;238:675

183. Wei C-M, Kao PC, Lin J-T et al: Circulating β-atrial natriuretic factor in congestive heart failure in humans. Circulation 1993;88:1016

184. Lang CC, Choy A-MJ, Struthers AD: Atrial and brain natriuretic peptide. A dual natriuretic peptide system, potentially involved in circulatory homeostasis. Clin Sci 1992;83:519

185. Mukoyama M, Nakao K, Hosoda K et al: Brain natriuretic peptide as a novel cardiac hormone in humans. Evidence for an exquisite dual natriuretic peptide system, atrial natriuretic peptide and brain natriuretic peptide. J Clin Invest 1991;87:1402

186. Cheung BMY, Dickerson JEC, Ashby MJ, Brown JM, Brown J: Effects of physiological increments in human α-atrial natriuretic peptide and human brain natriuretic peptide in normal male subjects. Clin Sci 1994;86:723

187. Lang CC, Motwani JG, Coutie WJR, Struthers AD: Clearance of brain natriuretic peptide in patients with chronic heart failure. Indirect evidence for a neutral endopeptidase mechanism but against an

atrial natriuretic peptide clearance receptor mechanism. Clin Sci 1992;82:619

188. Mukoyama M, Nakao K, Saito Y et al: Increased human brain natriuretic peptide in congestive heart failure. N Engl J Med 1990;323:757

189. Davis M, Espiner E, Richards G et al: Plasma brain natriuretic peptide in assessment of acute dyspnoea. Lancet 1994;343:440

190. Struthers AD: Plasma concentration of brain natriuretic peptide. Will this new test reduce the need for cardiac investigations? Br Heart J 1993;70:397

191. Kamatsu Y, Nakao K, Suga S et al: C-type natriuretic peptide (CNP) in rats and humans. Endocrinology 1991;129:1104

192. Tawaragi Y, Fuchimura K, Tanaka S et al: Gene and precursor structure of human C-type natriuretic peptide. Biochem Biophys Res Commun 1991;175:645

193. Kaneko T, Shirakami G, Nakao K et al: C-type natriuretic peptide (CNP) is the major natriuretic peptide in human cerebrospinal fluid. Brain Res 1993;612:104

194. Clavell AL, Stingo AJ, Wei C-M, Heublein DM, Brunett JC: C-type natriuretic peptide. A selective cardiovascular profile. Am J Physiol 1993;264:R290

195. Vigne P, Frelin C: C-type natriuretic peptide is a potent activator of guanylate cyclase in endothelial cells from brain microvessels. Biochem Biophys Res Commun 1992;183:640

196. Wei C-M, Aarhus LL, Miller VM, Brunett JC: Action of C-type natriuretic peptide in isolated canine arteries and veins. Am J Physiol 1993;264:H71

197. Wei C-M, Heublein DM, Perrella MA et al: Natriuretic peptide system in human heart failure. Circulation 1993;88:1004

198. Wei C-M, Kim CH, Miller VM, Brunett JC: Vasonatrin peptide. A unique synthetic natriuretic and vasorelaxing peptide. J Clin Invest 1993;92:2048

199. Gardner DG: Designer natriuretic peptides: J Clin Invest 1993;92:1606

200. Maack T, Marion D, Camargo MJF et al: Effects of auriculin (atrial natriuretic factor) on blood pressure, renal function, and the renin-aldosterone system in dogs. Am J Med 1984;77:1069

201. Burnett JC, Granger JP, Opgenorth TJ: Effects of synthetic atrial natriuretic factor on renal function and renin release. Am J Physiol 1984;247:F863

202. Scriven TA, Burnett JC: Effects of synthetic atrial natriuretic peptide on renal function and renin release in acute experimental heart failure. Circulation 1985;72:892

203. Zimmerman RS, Schirger JA, Edwards BS et al: Cardio-renal endocrine dynamics during stepwise infusion of physiologic and pharmacologic concentrations of atrial natriuretic factor in the dog. Circ Res 1987;60:63

204. Deray G, Branch RA, Herzer WA, Ohnishi A, Jackson EK: Effects of atrial natriuretic factor on hormone-induced renin release. Hypertension 1987;9:513

205. Floras JS: Sympathoinhibitory effects of atrial natriuretic factor in normal humans. Circulation 1990;81:1860

206. Riegger GAJ, Kromer EP, Kochsiek K: Human atrial natriuretic peptide. Plasma levels, hemodynamic, hormonal, and renal effects in patients with severe congestive heart failure. J Cardiovasc Pharmacol 1986;8:1107

207. Anand IS, Kalra GS, Ferrari R, Harris P, Poole-Wilson PA: Hemodynamic, hormonal, and renal effects of atrial natriuretic peptide in untreated congestive cardiac failure. Am Heart J 1989;118:500

208. Riegger GAJ, Elsner D, Kromer EP et al: Atrial natriuretic peptide in congestive heart failure in the dog. Plasma levels, cyclic guanosine monophosphate cells, and hemodynamic, hormonal, and renal effects. Circulation 1988;77:398

209. Woods RL, Oliver JR, Korner PI: Direct and neurohumoral cardiovascular effects of atrial natriuretic peptide. J Cardiovasc Pharmacol 1989;13:177

210. Takeshita A: Effects of atrial natriuretic factor on baroreceptor reflexes. Hypertension 1990;15:168

211. Cody RJ, Atlas SA, Laragh JH et al: Atrial natriuretic factor in normal subjects and heart failure patients. Plasma levels and renal, hormonal, and hemodynamic responses to peptide infusion. J Clin Invest 1986;78:1362

212. Munzel T, Drexler H, Holtz J, Kurtz S, Just H: Mechanisms involved in the response to prolonged infusion of atrial natriuretic factor in patients with chronic heart failure. Circulation 1991;83:191

213. Northridge DB, Alabaster CT, Connell JMC et al: Effects of UK 69 578. A novel atriopeptidase inhibitor. Lancet 1989;2:591

214. Cavero PG, Margulies KB, Winaver J et al: Cardiorenal actions of neutral endopeptidase inhibition in experimental congestive heart failure. Circulation 1990;82:196

215. Seymour AA, Norman JA, Asaad MM et al: Possible regulation of atrial natriuretic factor by neutral endopeptidase 24.11 and clearance receptors. J Pharmacol Exp Ther 1991;256:1002

216. Wilkins MR, Settle SL, Stockmann PT, Needleman P: Maximizing the natriuretic effect of endogenous atriopeptin in a rat model of heart failure. Proc Natl Acad Sci USA 1990;87:6465

217. Richards M, Espiner E, Frampton C et al: Inhibition of endopeptidase EC 24.11 in humans. Renal and endocrine effects. Hypertension 1990;16:269

218. Riegger GAJ, Elsner D, Forssmann W-G, Kromer EP: Effects of ANP (95–126) in dogs before and after induction of heart failure. Am J Physiol 1990;259:H1643

219. Itoh H, Pratt RE, Dzau VJ: Atrial natriuretic polypeptide inhibits hypertrophy of vascular smooth muscle cells. J Clin Invest 1990;86:1690

220. Yanagisawa M, Kurihara H, Kimura S et al: A novel potent vasoconstrictor peptide produced by vascular endothelial cells. Nature 1988;332:411

221. Rubanyi GM, Botelho LHP: Endothelins. FASEB J 1991;5:2713

222. Simonson MS, Dunn MJ: Endothelins. A family of regulatory peptides. Hypertension 1991;17:856

223. Lerman A, Hildebrand FL, Maruilies KB et al: Endothelin. A new cardiovascular regulatory peptide. Mayo Clin Proc 1990;65:1441

224. Thomas CP, Simonson MS, Dunn MJ: Endothelin. Receptors and transmembrane signals. NIPS 1992;7:207

225. Opgenorth TJ, Wu-Wong JR, Shiosaki K: Endothelin-coverting enzymes. FASEB J 1992;6:2653

226. Sakurai T, Yanagisawa M, Takuwa Y et al: Cloning of a cDNA encoding a non-isopeptide-selective subtype of the endothelin receptor. Nature 1990;348:732

227. Arai H, Hori S, Aramori I, Ohkubo H, Nakanishi S: Cloning and expression of a cDNA encoding an endothelin receptor. Nature 1990;348:730

228. Sakurai T, Yanagisawa M, Masaki T: Molecular characterization of endothelin receptors. TIPS 1992;13:103

229. Vogelsang M, Broede-Sitz A, Schafer E, Zerkowski H, Brodde O: Endothelin ET$_A$-receptors couple to inositol phosphate formation and inhibition of adenylate cyclase in human right atrium. J Cardiovasc Pharmacol 1994;23:344

230. Shichiri M, Hirata Y, Nakajima T et al: Endothelin-1 is an autocrine/paracrine growth factor for human cancer cells lines. J Clin Invest 1991;87:1867

231. Ito H, Hirata Y, Hiroe M et al: Endothelin-1 induces hypertrophy with enhanced expression of muscle-specific genes in cultured neonatal rat cardiomyocytes. Circ Res 1991;69:209

232. Clozel M, Breu V, Gray GA, Loffler B: In vivo pharmacology of Ro 46-2005, the first synthetic nonpeptide endothelin receptor antagonist. Implications for endothelin physiology. J Cardiovasc Pharmacol 1993;22:5377

233. Sogabe K, Nirei H, Shoubo M et al: Pharmacological profile of FR139317, a novel, potent endothelin ET$_A$ receptor antagonist. J Pharmacol Exp Ther 1992;264:1040

234. Clozel M, Breu V, Burri K et al: Pathophysiological role of endothelin revealed by the first orally active endothelin receptor antagonist. Nature 1993;365:759

235. Hiroshi I, Hiroe M, Hirata Y et al: Endothelin ET$_A$ receptor antagonist blocks cardiac hypertrophy provoked by hemodynamic overload. Circulation 1994;89:2198

236. Lerman A, Hildebrand FL, Aarhus LL, Burnett JC: Endothelin has biological actions at pathophysiological concentrations. Circulation 1991;83:1808

237. Hiroe M, Hirata Y, Fujita N et al: Plasma endothelin-1 levels in idiopathic dilated cardiomyopathy. Am J Cardiol 1991;68:1114

238. Rodeheffer RJ, Lerman A, Heublein DM, Burnett JC: Increased plasma concentrations of endothelin in congestive heart failure in humans. Mayo Clin Proc 1992;67:719

239. Lerman A, Kubo SH, Tschumperlin LK, Burnett JC: Plasma endothelin concentrations in humans with end-stage heart failure and after heart transplantation. J Am Coll Cardiol 1992;20:849

240. Stewart DJ, Cernacek P, Costello KB, Rouleau JL: Elevated endothelin-1 in heart failure and loss of normal response to postural change. Circulation 1992;85:510

241. McMurray JJ, Ray SG, Abdullah I, Dargie HJ, Morton JJ: Plasma endothelin in chronic heart failure. Circulation 1992;85:1374

242. Wei C-M, Lerman A, Rodeheffer RJ et al: Endothelin in human congestive heart failure. Circulation 1994;89:1580

243. Margulies KB, Hildebrand FL, Lerman A, Perrella MA, Burnett JC: Increased endothelin in experimental heart failure. Circulation 1990;82:2226

244. Cody RJ, Haas GJ, Binkley PF, Capers Q, Kelley R: Plasma endothelin correlates with the extent of pulmonary hypertension in patients with chronic congestive heart failure. Circulation 1992;85:504

245. Kramer BK, Nishida M, Kelly RA, Smith TW: Endothelins. Circulation 1992;85:350

246. Brutsaert KL, Andries LJ: The endocardial endothelium. Am J Physiol 1992;263:H985

247. Drexler H, Hayoz D, Munzel T et al: Endothelial function in chronic congestive heart failure. Am J Cardiol 1992;69:1596

248. Furchgott RF, Zawadzki JV: The obligatory role of endothelial cells in the relaxation of arterial smooth muscle by acetylcholine. Nature 1980;288:373

249. Vanhoutte PM: Endothelium and control of vascular function. Hypertension 1989;13:658

250. Cooke JP, Rossitch E, Andon NA, Loscaizo J, Dzau VJ: Flow activates an endothelial potassium channel to release an endogenous nitrovasodilator. J Clin Invest 1991;88:1663

251. Ohno M, Gibbons GH, Dzau VJ, Cooke JP: Shear stress elevates endothelial cMGP. Circulation 1993;88:193

252. Ignarro LJ, Wood KS, Fukuto JM: Continuous basal formation of endothelium-derived relaxing factor and muscle-derived relaxing factor, both of which are nitric oxide. J Cardiovasc Pharmacol 1991;17:S229

253. Moncada S, Palmer RMJ, Higegs EA: The discovery of nitric oxide as the endogenous nitrovasodilator. Hypertension 1988;12:365

254. Myers PR, Minor RL, Guerra R, Bates JN, Harrison DG: Vasorelaxant properties of the endothelium-derived relaxing factor more closely resemble S-nitrosocysteine than nitric oxide. Nature 1990;345:161

255. Kaiser L, Spickard RC, Olivier NB: Heart failure depresses endothelium-dependent responses in canine femoral artery. Am J Physiol 1989;256:H962

256. Panza JA, Quyyumi AA, Brush JE, Epstein SE: Abnormal endothelium-dependent vascular relaxation in patients with essential hypertension. N Engl J Med 1990;323:22

257. Panza JA, Casino PR, Kilcoyne CM, Quyyumi AA: Role of endothelium-derived nitric oxide in the abnormal endothelium-dependent vascular relaxation of patients with essential hypertension. Circulation 1993;87:1468

258. Casino PR, Kilcoyne CM, Quyyumi AA, Hoeg JM, Panza JA: Investigation of decreased availability of nitric oxide precursor as the mechanism responsible for impaired endothelium-dependent vasodilation in hypercholesterolemic patients. J Am Coll Cardiol 1994;23:844

259. El-Tamimi H, Mansour M, Wargovich TJ et al: Constrictor and dilator responses to intracoronary acetylcholine in adjacent segments of the same coronary artery in patients with coronary artery disease. Circulation 1994;89:45

260. Zeihjer AM, Drexler H, Wollschlager, Just H: Modulation of coronary vasomotor tone in humans. Circulation 1991;83:391

261. Johnstone MT, Creager SJ, Sacles KM et al: Impaired endothelium-dependent vasodilation in patients with insulin-dependent diabetes mellitus. Circulation 1993;88:2510

262. Vane JR, Anggard EE, Botting RM: Regulatory functions of the vascular endothelium. N Engl J Med 1990;323:27

263. Rubanyi GM: The role of endothelium in cardiovascular homeostasis and diseases. J Cardiovasc Pharmacol 1993;22:S1

264. Shah AM, Lewis MJ: Modulation of myocardial contraction by endocardial and coronary vascular endothelium. Trends Cardiovasc Med 1993;3:98

265. Kubo SH, Rector TS, Bank AJ et al: Lack of contribution of nitric oxide to basal vasomotor tone in heart failure. Am J Cardiol 1994;74:1133

266. Kubo SH, Rector TS, Bank AJ, Williams RE, Heifetz SM: Endothelium-dependent vasodilation is attenuated in patients with heart failure. Circulation 1991; 84:1589

267. Katz SD, Schwarz M, Yuen J, LeJemtel TH: Impaired acetylcholine-mediated vasodilation in patients with congestive heart failure. Circulation 1993;88:55

268. Angus JA, Ferrier CP, Krishnankutty S, Kay DM, Jennings GL: Impaired contraction and relaxation in skin resistance arteries from patients with congestive heart failure. Cardiovasc Res 1993;27:204

269. Zelis R, Hayoz D, Drexler H et al: Arterial dilatory reserve in congestive heart failure. J Hypertens Suppl 6 1992;10:565

270. Nakamura M, Ishikawa M, Funakoshi T et al: Attenuated endothelium-dependent peripheral vasodilation and clinical characteristics in patients with chronic heart failure. Am Heart J 1994;128:1164

271. Hirooka Y, Imaizumi T, Tagawa T et al: Effects of L-arginine on impaired acetylcholine-induced and ischemic vasodilation of the forearm in patients with heart failure. Circulation 1994;90:658

272. Nakamura M, Funakoshi T, Arakawa N et al: Effect of angiotensin-converting enzyme inhibitors on endothelium-dependent peripheral vasodilation in patients with chronic heart failure. J Am Coll Cardiol 1994;24:1321

273. Lindsay DC, Jiang C, Brunotte F et al: Impairment of endothelial dependent responses in a rat model of chronic heart failure. Effects of an exercise training protocol. Cardiovasc Res 1992;26:694

274. Teerlink JR, Clozel M, Fischli W, Clozel J-P: Temporal evaluation of endothelial dysfunction in a rat model of chronic heart failure. J Am Coll Cardiol 1993;22:615

275. Drexler H, Lu W: Endothelial dysfunction of hindquarter resistance vessels in experimental heart failure. Am J Physiol 1992;262:H1640

276. Kubo SH, Rector TS, Bank AJ et al: Effects of cardiac transplantation on endothelium-dependent dilation of the peripheral vasculature in congestive heart failure. Am J Cardiol 1993;71:88

277. Levine B, Kalman J, Mayer L, Fillit HM, Packer M: Elevated circulating levels of tumor necrosis factor in severe chronic heart failure. N Engl J Med 1990; 323:236

278. McMurray J, Abdullah I, Dargie HJ, Shapiro D: Increased concentrations of tumor necrosis factor in "cachectic" patients with severe chronic heart failure. Br Heart J 1991;66:356

279. Smith CA, Farrah T, Goodwin RG: The TNF receptor superfamily of cellular and viral proteins. Activation, costimulation, and death. Cell 1994;76:959

280. Suda T, Takahashi T, Golstein P, Nagata S: Molecular cloning and expression of the fas ligand, a novel member of the tumor necrosis factor family. Cell 1993;75:1169

281. Anversa P, Zhang X, Li P, Capusso JM: Chronic coronary artery constriction leads to moderate myocyte loss and left ventricular dysfunction and failure in rats. J Clin Invest 1992;89:618

282. James TN: Normal and abnormal consequences of apoptosis in the human heart. From postnatal morphogenesis to paroxysmal arrhythmias. Circulation 1994;90:556

283. Ferrari R, Panzali AF, Poole-Wilson PA, Anand IS: Plasma CGRP-like immunoreactivity in treated and untreated congestive heart failure [letter]. Lancet 1991;338:1084

284. Ando K, Ito Y, Ogata E, Fujita T: Vasodilating actions of calcitonin gene-related peptide in normal man. Comparison with atrial natriuretic peptide. Am Heart J 1992;123:111

285. Chandrashekhar Y, Anand IS, Sarma R et al: Effects of prolonged infusion of human alpha calcitonin gene-related peptide on hemodynamics, renal blood flow and hormone levels in congestive heart failure. Am J Cardiol 1991;67:732

286. Kawashima S, Fukutake N, Nishian K, Asakuma S, Iwasaki T: Elevated plasma beta-endorphin levels in patients with congestive heart failure. J Am Coll Cardiol 1991;17:53

287. Anand IS, Chandrashekhar Y, Ferrari R, Poole-Wilson PA, Harris PC: Pathogenesis of oedema in chronic severe anaemia. Studies of body water and sodium, renal function, haemodynamic variables, and plasma hormones. Br Heart J 1993;70:357

288. Anand IS, Chandrashekhar Y, Ferrari R et al: Pathogenesis of congestive state in chronic obstructive pulmonary disease. Circulation 1992;86:12

289. Francis GS: The relationship of the sympathetic nervous system and the renin-angiotensin system in congestive heart failure. Am Heart J 1989;118:642

16 Skeletal Muscle Abnormalities

Derek Harrington
Andrew J. S. Coats

The syndrome of chronic heart failure (CHF) is characterized by exercise intolerance usually associated with breathlessness or fatigue. Historically it was believed that this exercise intolerance was simply a result of reduced cardiac output or increased ventricular filling pressures. However, many investigators have demonstrated a poor correlation between central hemodynamic disturbance and exercise capacity.[1–3] These findings, in addition to the observation that an acute increase in cardiac output did not immediately increase exercise capacity,[4–6] led to a more detailed examination of the periphery, including the skeletal musculature.

The observation that skeletal muscle is abnormal in CHF is not a new one. Around 400 BC an author from the school of Hippocrates described heart failure as a condition in which "the shoulders, clavicles, chest and thighs melt away,"[7] and in 1795 William Withering described his patient as one whose "body was greatly emaciated."[8] Only during recent years, however, have these changes been documented in any detail. Widespread abnormalities of skeletal muscle function, metabolism, and structure have been demonstrated. Moreover, the possibility that these changes are not simply a consequence of the disturbed hemodynamics of CHF, but that they may contribute to the generation of symptoms in this disabling condition has been considered.[9–12] This chapter reviews these abnormalities and the evidence for their role in the generation of symptoms suffered by patients with CHF.

SKELETAL MUSCLE ATROPHY

Despite the marked muscle atrophy observed with cardiac cachexia (see Ch. 18), only recently has muscle bulk in CHF patients without documented weight loss been assessed. Mancini et al.,[13] using a creatinine/height index and midarm muscle circumference, estimated muscle bulk in 76 patients. They demonstrated the presence of severe muscle atrophy in 68 percent, though they were unable to show significant abnormalities of protein synthesis (measuring serum albumin, prealbumin, or transferrin) or of body fat stores (using triceps skinfold thickness or percent ideal body weight). Using magnetic resonance imaging (MRI) they also estimated calf muscle volume and confirmed that it is significantly reduced compared with that of normal controls, even when this volume is normalized for body surface area. Other groups have confirmed these findings. Minotti et al.[14] calculated the maximal cross-sectional area of the thigh muscles, also using MRI, and demonstrated a reduction compared with normal controls. Dual energy x-ray absorptiometry (DEXA) has also demonstrated reduced leg muscle mass,[15] an observation confirmed by unpublished data from our institution. Biopsy studies (described in detail later) have in some instances reported atrophy of individual fibers.[16–18]

There have been attempts to correlate muscle atrophy with the extent of exercise intolerance. Some have shown modest correlations between peak oxygen consumption ($\dot{V}O_2$max) and indices of muscle bulk[13,14]; and Volterrani et al.[19] reported a strong correlation between midfemur quadriceps cross-sectional area, total muscle cross-sectional area, and peak oxygen consumption.

SKELETAL MUSCLE STRENGTH

With the observed reduction in muscle bulk, abnormalities of muscle performance may be expected. Quadriceps muscle strength has been assessed by several groups of investigators. Early small studies, using a twitch interpolation technique in an attempt to ensure maximal effort, suggested that maximal isometric strength was reduced,[16,20] and that this maximal strength correlated with $\dot{V}O_2$max. Subsequent studies, however, found no significant difference in maximal isometric or isokinetic quadriceps strength when compared to controls, though in most studies there has been a trend toward weakness.[14,21] Several groups of investigators have, however, reported that quadriceps strength per unit area is normal. The observed differences may be explained if the weaker patients had more muscle atrophy, as a strong correlation between quadriceps muscle size and maximal strength has been demonstrated.[14]

As noted, muscle atrophy has been widely described in CHF, and one would thus expect a reduction in strength in many patients if strength per unit area remains constant. The lack of weakness reported may simply reflect the small size of these studies with a trend toward weakness but not reaching statistical significance. Whether any observed weakness is simply a consequence of muscle atrophy or reflects a qualitative abnormality of muscle performance is unclear.

Although strength per unit area is reported to be normal, the normal range cited by Buller et al.[20] was derived from a study of 20 patients only 11 of whom were male.[22] Minotti et al.[14] studied 12 normal controls. Unpublished data gathered at our institution from more than 100 patients suggest that quadriceps weakness is a feature of these patients with a modest correlation between strength and $\dot{V}O_2$max. Other muscle groups have been assessed but in much smaller studies. No significant weakness has been demonstrated in the adductor pollicis, foot dorsiflexors, or wrist flexors.[16,23,24]

SKELETAL MUSCLE FATIGUE

In daily life the ability to perform repeated submaximal exercise is more important than tests of maximal strength. Fatigue has been assessed using various protocols by different groups. All have reported an increase in skeletal muscle fatigue in patients with CHF. Buller et al.[20] assessed quadriceps fatigue in 10 patients by asking them to perform repeated submaximal contractions and reassessing maximal strength after each 5 minutes of this 20-minute protocol. They demonstrated increasing fatigue with increasing severity of CHF and a good correlation between percentage fatigue and $\dot{V}O_2$max. Minotti et al.[14] evaluated isokinetic endurance in 21 patients by comparing the mean of the force generated in three 2-second maximal contractions with the mean of another three contractions after an intervening nine maximal contractions. They calculated fatigue as the reduction observed in these maximal contractions. CHF patients became fatigued to a greater extent than controls, and in patients there was excellent correlation with $\dot{V}O_2$max. This group also assessed isometric endurance by asking subjects to maintain a maximal contraction and noting the time required for the force generated to decay to 60 percent. They reported an increase in this fatigue in CHF patients but no correlation with $\dot{V}O_2$max. Similar results have been noted in the foot dorsiflexors.[24] Adductor pollicis fatigue has been assessed using supramaximal ulnar stimulation and observing the decay in force generated by multiple stimulations. No difference was noted between controls and patients during either normal conditions or ischemia (achieved by inflating a cuff at suprasystolic pressure around the upper arm). The relative increase in fatigue during ischemia was greatest in patients with severe heart failure.[20]

Wilson et al.[25] demonstrated fatigue using surface electomyograms. They calculated the root-mean-square (RMS) of the voltage recorded per contraction (increases in it being due to either additional fiber recruitment or increased frequency of motor unit firing) and recorded changes in the average firing frequency of motor units. In normal individuals they observed no increase in the average frequency of firing throughout exercise, although the RMS voltage per contraction initially increased only at the beginning of each workload. At the maximal and preceding stage there was an increase in the RMS voltage throughout the stage, suggesting continuous recruitment of new fibers to assist fatiguing fibers. In CHF patients similar changes in the RMS voltage were observed, though at significantly lower workloads than in normals, suggesting an earlier onset of muscular fatigue. Additionally, in CHF patients the average firing frequency was lower.

The reduced endurance does not appear to be a result of impaired neuromuscular transmission. A superimposed tetanic stimulus, applied either during maximal foot dorsiflexion or after a maximal contraction has decayed to 60 percent, results in similar increases in force generation both in normal individuals and CHF patients.[24] Minotti et al.[21] examined the role of reduced blood flow by assessing isokinetic endurance during ischemic conditions (by inflating a thigh cuff to a suprasystolic pressure). They demonstrated the persistence of differences between patients and controls during ischemia. The increased fatigue seen with CHF cannot be explained solely by differences in blood flow, suggesting the involvement of intrinsic abnormalities of skeletal muscle.

HISTOLOGY

With the observed abnormalities of skeletal muscle function, various groups have attempted to define a characteristic underlying histologic pattern; their findings are summarized in Table 16-1. Most reports have been of leg muscle histology (generally quadriceps), obtained using the needle biopsy technique first described by Bergstrom.[26] The distribution of the fiber types has been described. Generally there is an increase in the percentage of type II fibers.[16,18,27,28] Similar changes in fiber distribution were reported in animal models of CHF.[29] When type II fibers have been subtyped, the alteration in distribution appears to be due to an increase in type IIb fibers with no alteration in type IIa frequency. One group reported an increase in type IIc fibers[17]; others have not subtyped these fibers or, in one case, reported no change.[18] Type I fibers are mostly reported to be reduced or with a strong trend toward reduction.

Fiber size has been documented. Lipkin et al.[16] reported atrophy of both type I and II fibers, whereas other investigators have described a reduction only in type II fiber size. The subtype affected varies: Some report that only type IIb fibers[18] are reduced in size, whereas others describe a reduction in the size of both subtypes.[17,30] Despite these alterations in muscle composition and fiber size, Mancini et al.[17] noted in their study that the percentage of the total muscle area occupied by each fiber type was normal.

The vascularity of skeletal muscle has also been assessed, though reports are inconsistent. Some have described capillary numbers as normal.[16] Others describe a reduction in capillaries per fiber but a normal number per unit area[18] or a reduction in capillaries per unit volume of muscle.[28] Mancini et al.[17] described the opposite (i.e., no change in capillary number per fiber but an increase in capillaries per unit area), whereas Yancy et al.[27] described a reduction in all measures of capillary density. The net effect, when taken in concert with reduced muscle bulk, is a reduction in skeletal muscle vascular conductance.

Mitochondrial morphology and density have been considered in detail. Drexler et al.[28] calculated the volume density of mitochondria (mitochondrial volume fraction per unit volume of muscle tissue) and the surface density of mitochondrial cristae (surface fraction of mitochondrial cristae per unit volume of muscle). They observed that both of these indices were reduced in CHF patients when compared to normal controls. Some workers have also described other abnormalities of histology, such as increased intracellular lipid[16] and reduced glycogen content.[18] These abnormalities were not described by Drexler et al.,[28] who reported normal myofibrils and sarcoplasmic reticulum but an increased volume density of sarcoplasmic triads in all severe CHF patients and in patients with idiopathic dilated cardiomyopathy.

Table 16-1. Skeletal Muscle Biopsies in CHF

	Lipkin[16]	Mancini[17]	Yancy[27]	Sullivan[18]	Drexler[28]
Fiber type					
I	⇓	⇔	⇓	⇓	⇓
IIa		⇓		⇔	
IIb	⇑*	⇑	⇑*	⇑	⇑*
IIc		⇑		⇔	
Glycolytic pathway		⇔	⇔	⇔	
Krebs cycle		⇔	⇓	⇓	
Lipid oxidation		⇓		⇓	
Mitochondria					⇓ Volume ⇓ Cristae
Cap dens fiber/mm²		⇔	⇓	⇓	
		⇑	⇓	⇔	⇓

* In these studies Type II fibers were not subtyped, data is given for all type II fibers.

A characteristic histologic pattern has thus not been defined. At best, similar abnormalities have been described by the various investigators, with a trend toward decreased aerobic capacity being suggested. The marked differences in histology reported may be partially explained by the small number of patients studied, the variation in the severity of heart failure, and the underlying diagnosis in the patient groups. In their study of mitochondria Drexler et al.[28] noted that a subgroup of idiopathic dilated cardiomyopathy patients with near-normal exercise tolerance ($\dot{V}O_2$max > 25) had no apparent mitochondrial abnormalities. Mancini et al.[17] noted that 4 of their 22 patients had completely normal biopsies, and that these patients were all young and either New York Heart Association (NYHA) class I or II. This group also attempted to correlate the histologic changes with the extent of exercise intolerance. They observed a positive correlation between $\dot{V}O_2$max and percent type I fibers and a good negative correlation between percent type IIb fibers and $\dot{V}O_2$max. There was no correlation with fiber size. A correlation between mitochondrial indices and $\dot{V}O_2$max has been noted.

Only one group has reported histology of the diaphragm.[31] They reported no alteration in fiber type distribution, though there was a mild increase in fiber size variability in six patients with ischemic heart disease. There were histologic abnormalities in 10 of 14 patients with pathologic cores, tubular aggregates, and bizarre myosin types.

SKELETAL MUSCLE METABOLISM IN CHF

Muscle metabolism has been studied at rest and during exercise by analyzing biopsy specimens, measuring metabolites in femoral venous blood, and using magnetic resonance spectroscopy.

Biopsy Studies

Metabolism has been investigated in biopsy material by assessing enzyme and metabolite levels in muscle homogenates and staining biopsy specimens for enzymes of the metabolic pathways. Muscle composition assessments have suggested normal protein and myoglobin content, with normal or reduced high-energy phosphate levels.[18,32] Reduced glycogen levels associated with normal levels of glycolytic intermediates and lactate but increased pyruvate levels have been reported, suggesting an increased level of glycolysis.[17,18] Most studies have reported a decrease in the oxidative enzymes of Krebs cycle (succinate dehydrogenase, citrate synthetase),[18,27,28] though Mancini et al.[17] reported normal citrate synthetase activity. The ability to oxidize fat appears to be impaired, as β-hydroxyacyl coenzyme A (CoA) dehydrogenase levels are reduced.[17,18] The activity of the glycolytic pathway, however, has been consistently reported as normal.[17,18,27] Drexler et al.[28] examined mitochondrial cytochrome oxidase activity, noting a reduction in positively staining mitochondria. They observed the most marked changes in patients with severe CHF ($\dot{V}O_2$max < 16 ml·min^{-1}·kg^{-1}), who had a reduced mitochondrial volume density and positive staining (from 62.0 percent to 17.5 percent). Patients with moderate CHF ($\dot{V}O_2$max $16–25$ ml·min^{-1}·kg^{-1}), though having a normal mitochondrial density, also had reduced cytochrome oxidase staining. Generally reports have been consistent, with reduced oxidative capacity but preserved glycolytic capacity.

In a provisional report some data have been provided about diaphragmatic metabolism.[33] Citrate synthetase activity was higher than that in normal individuals, but lactate dehydrogenase levels were lower. The authors attempted to explain this finding by suggesting that as a result of the hyperventilation seen with CHF the diaphragm is effectively being trained; further evidence for this comes from the finding that myosin heavy-chain isoform I is increased but isoform IIb is decreased.

Magnetic Resonance Spectroscopy

Using phosphorus 31 (^{31}P) magnetic resonance spectroscopy, skeletal muscle metabolism can be monitored noninvasively at rest and during exercise. Analysis of the spectra allows evaluation of the relative concentrations of inorganic phosphate (Pi), phosphocreatine (PCr), and adenosine triphosphate (ATP) in intact tissues. Additionally, the technique can be used to assess intracellular pH, and the rate of PCr utilization can be followed with changes in the [PCr]/([PCr] + [Pi]) ratio (this normalized ratio is used to minimize the effect of any limb movement). With the breakdown of ATP and PCr, adenosine diphosphate (ADP) and Pi are released, which stimulate mitochondrial respiration and glycolysis. Mitochondrial respiration is closely related to the ADP level, which in turn is directly related to the Pi/PCr ratio. This ratio correlates linearly with the velocity of mitochondrial oxidation. Thus the relation between Pi/PCr and power output (or workload) is also linear (at least at low workloads) and is an index of metabolic efficiency. Finally, the rate of recovery of PCr following exercise can be assessed. It is an important measure of oxidative metabolism, as it is independent of both workload and muscle mass.

Initial studies in CHF analyzed the forearm muscles during protocols of gradually increasing workload. Wilson et al.[23] observed similar spectra at rest in normal controls and nine CHF patients. With low level exercise the PCr decreased and Pi increased, though the changes (reflected in the Pi/PCr ratio) were much greater in patients despite equivalent workloads. It resulted in a significantly higher slope in the relation between the Pi/PCr ratio and power output. In normal individuals there was no change in pH until the peak workload was reached; whereas in CHF patients there was a progressive decrease in pH at all workloads; the pH at peak exercise (and identical workloads) was similar. PCr recovery was normal. There was no correlation between the Pi/PCr to power output slope and $\dot{V}O_2$max, though a modest correlation between the subjectively assessed degree of fatigue experienced and the pH and Pi/PCr ratio was noted.

This study was repeated and extended by Massie et al.[34] They observed a similar early reduction in pH and PCr levels in patients. At peak exercise patients were significantly more acidotic even though probably exercising at a lower workload. PCr recovery was normal in 7 of 11 patients but markedly abnormal in the remaining 4; additionally, loss of ATP was noted in 4 patients. The reduced PCr implies reduced ATP and PCr synthesis, which in conjunction with a loss of ATP suggests impaired oxidative metabolism. The early fall in pH suggests excessive dependence on glycolysis for ATP synthesis. If PCr recovery is delayed, it would also imply impaired oxidative phosphorylation.

Clearly, these observations must be extended to the legs, as fatigue of these weight-bearing muscles is commonly responsible for exercise limitation in CHF patients. Mancini et al.[35] first studied the calf muscle. Patients were exercised either with stair climbing or repeated plantar flexion. After completing a workload the metabolic state of the muscle was "frozen" by inflating a thigh cuff to a suprasystolic pressure. The subject was then transferred to a magnet with the cuff still inflated, and spectra were obtained. Recovery could also be followed once the cuff was deflated. Again there was no abnormality of the resting spectra. With stair climbing the pH did not alter in either group, whereas the Pi/PCr increased in all subjects. When this finding was correlated with the $\dot{V}O_2$, a linear relation was observed; the slope of this relation was significantly steeper in CHF patients. Plantar flexion resulted in similar changes, though the difference between slopes was greater; additionally, although the pH remained constant in

controls, there was a fall in patients. Recovery of PCr took longer in patients, although generally they achieved a higher ratio at peak exercise. To correct for this result, recovery from all exercise that led to a peak Pi/PCr ratio of 0.8 was compared; a prolonged recovery time was still apparent in patients.

Subsequently calf muscle metabolism has been assessed with a magnet that permits analysis while leg work is being performed.[13,36] Similar results have been obtained with an early and greater fall in the Pi/PCr ratio and a more marked drop in pH in CHF patients. Mancini et al.[13] reported prolonged recovery of PCr, whereas Arnolda et al.[36] described only a trend to longer recovery.

Correlations between spectroscopic abnormalities and clinical characteristics have been reported. No association existed between the Pi/PCr and $\dot{V}O_2$ slope and age, $\dot{V}O_2$max, NYHA class, or left ventricular ejection fraction (LVEF).[13,37] Having established that muscle metabolism during exercise is abnormal, several groups have investigated the underlying cause. Reduced blood flow could account for the observations, as patients with peripheral vascular disease also have abnormalities of PCr metabolism.[38] To investigate the potential role of reduced blood flow, two groups[37,39] estimated forearm blood flow using plethysmography during an exercise protocol identical to that used for acquiring the phosphorus spectra. At equivalent workloads patients and controls exhibited no difference in blood flow. Massie et al.[39] also noted no difference in blood flow at a specific workload, postischemic blood flow, or rate of increase of flow when comparing patients with normal and abnormal PCr metabolism. They observed that patients with an abnormally low pH at 50 percent workload had higher blood flows than patients whose pH was normal. These studies suggested that reduced blood flow did not underlie the metabolic abnormalities. As plethysmography measures blood flow per unit of tissue, it is possible that while this flow remains normal, total muscle blood flow is actually reduced. Further evidence suggesting an abnormality independent of blood flow comes from spectroscopy studies performed under ischemic conditions.[40] Subjects performed work at 33 percent of their previously determined maximum. Basal aerobic exercise was compared with the same exercise performed during ischemic conditions induced by inflating an upper arm cuff to a suprasystolic pressure. During ischemic exercise the pH fell farther and faster in patients. PCr also fell farther in patients, though this decrease was principally due to a greater fall during the first minute of exercise when fully anaerobic conditions may not have been achieved. After 1 minute of exercise patients had a consistently lower pH. The spectra from the ischemic exercise were also analyzed with a number of assumptions that allowed calculation of PCr usage, lactate production, and ATP consumption. Patients and controls had similar rates of PCr usage, but lactate production was markedly higher with an associated greater level of ATP consumption. They demonstrated no difference in the rate of PCr recovery following ischemic exercise and no difference in the rate of pH recovery.

In summary, spectroscopy studies suggest that exercising muscle of patients with CHF exhibits increased glycolytic metabolism and appears to be metabolically less efficient in relation to external work performed. Because these abnormalities are present when limb blood flow appears normal and they persist under ischemic conditions, they cannot be explained on the basis of acutely abnormal blood flow alone, although chronic flow impairment could play a role in the genesis of the responsible muscle changes. One study, repeating quadriceps biopsies at submaximal and peak exercise, has confirmed the increase in glycolysis, though lactate accumulation and PCr depletion at peak exercise were less in patients.[41] The reason for this disparity is unclear.

LACTATE PRODUCTION DURING EXERCISE

The onset of anaerobic metabolism has been assessed by many groups noting changes in femoral venous, mixed venous, and arterial lactate concentration. An early onset of lactic acid release has been recognized for many years[42-44] and has been a consistent finding among more recent investigations.[45-47] It has thus been suggested that the nutritive blood flow to skeletal muscle (as assessed by lactate production) is reduced.[45] It could occur as a result of decreased oxygen delivery (potentially the result of reduced cardiac output response to exercise or abnormal local vasodilatation) or an impaired ability of exercising muscle to utilize oxygen. Wilson et al.[45] considered 23 patients and graded them according to their peak oxygen consumption. They measured leg blood flow using femoral venous catheters and observed that with increasing exercise intolerance there was a progressively earlier increase in femoral venous lactate associated with a lower cardiac output response to exercise, lower leg blood flow, and higher leg vascular resistance. Their results suggested that the reduced nutritive flow could be explained by both a pump failure and impaired vasodilatation in the exercising muscle group. Further work by this group and others has suggested that the early onset of lactate produc-

tion is not solely a result of reduced muscle perfusion. Wilson et al.[48] identified a subgroup of previously studied patients who had normal leg blood flow during exercise. Compared with their other CHF patients, this group had a better cardiac output response to exercise, and their leg arteriovenous oxygen differences were normal. The group still had an abnormal lactate response to exercise, suggesting that in some patients at least the abnormal lactate release is a result of intrinsic muscle abnormalities, not simply a consequence of impaired muscle perfusion. Further evidence for these intrinsic metabolic abnormalities comes from experiments in which leg blood flow has been acutely improved.

Hydralazine increases cardiac output and leg blood flow at rest and during exercise in CHF patients when given intravenously.[5] This increase was not associated with any change in lactate production. Furthermore hydralazine decreased leg oxygen extraction, suggesting that the increased oxygen supplied as a consequence of increased flow is not utilized by the ischemic muscle.

Similar experiments have been conducted using dobutamine. Maskin et al.[4] observed no change in exercise capacity or lactate levels but a small increase in $\dot{V}O_2$max following an infusion of dobutamine. They suggested that it was a result of dobutamine failing to increase leg blood flow. Wilson et al.[6] subsequently disproved this assumption by measuring leg blood flow with a thermodilution technique during exercise before and after dobutamine. They demonstrated increased leg blood flow associated with a reduced leg vascular resistance. There was no increase in exercise duration or $\dot{V}O_2$max, lactate production was unchanged, and leg oxygen extraction decreased. Thus either there is shunting of blood within the leg or abnormality of muscle such that oxygen utilization is impaired.

Of relevance to these studies are the observations of Katz et al.[49] Using an infusion of isotopically labeled lactate they were able to calculate lactate turnover and the rate of lactate clearance. They demonstrated that at submaximal (below the anaerobic threshold) exercise in CHF patients, despite the lack of change in femoral venous or arterial lactate, there was a marked increase in systemic lactate metabolism. They also observed that, unlike what occurs in normal individuals, there was no correlation between arterial lactate concentrations and systemic lactate metabolism. The previously described studies that measure blood lactate may thus be measuring an index, which is a poor measure of the metabolic state of exercising muscle.

RESPIRATORY MUSCLE ABNORMALITIES

Respiratory muscle weakness can result in dyspnea.[50] Given the documented abnormalities of skeletal muscle in CHF and the often severe dyspnea that patients may suffer, it is surprising that only recently have abnormalities of the respiratory musculature been sought. Hammond et al.[51] observed reduced maximal inspiratory and expiratory mouth pressures (MIP, MEP) in CHF patients compared with controls. This weakness has been confirmed by some groups,[52–55] whereas others have demonstrated only a trend toward MIP and MEP weakness[56,57] or the presence of weakness only in more symptomatic patients.[58] These investigators have attempted to assess the significance of this finding by correlating the weakness with exercise tolerance. McParland et al.[52] observed a correlation between the Mahler dyspnea index and MIP though no correlation with MEP. Similarly, Mancini et al.[56] demonstrated a correlation between Borg score at 25 Watts workload and MIP. Others have reported a correlation between $\dot{V}O_2$max and MIP with no correlation with MEP[55,58] or a correlation with the resting cardiac index and MIP.[58] Associations have been inconsistent, with some groups reporting no correlation between exercise capacity, symptoms, or hemodynamic disturbance and respiratory muscle strength.[53,54] Additionally a poor association between respiratory muscle weakness and other skeletal muscle weakness has been noted.[51,55]

Diaphragm strength has been assessed[56] using the twitch interpolation technique of Bellemare and Bigland-Richie.[59] Briefly, as diaphragm activation becomes maximal, the twitch elicited by bilateral maximal phrenic nerve stimulation (and hence the change in transdiaphragmatic pressure) tends to become zero as all motor units are recruited. If twitch height is plotted against transdiaphragmatic pressure, the theoretic point at which twitch height is zero and hence transdiaphragmatic pressure is maximal can be extrapolated even in patients who are unable to achieve maximal diaphragm activation. Mancini et al. used this technique in 10 patients and 6 controls.[56] They demonstrated no difference in transdiaphragmatic peak pressure and no difference in maximal rates of contraction or relaxation. They also calculated the time–tension index for the diaphragm of each patient (defined as the fraction of a breathing cycle spent during inspiration multiplied by the mean transdiaphragmatic pressure divided by the maximal voluntary transdiaphragmatic pressure), an index of diaphragmatic work. The time–tension index was significantly greater in patients at rest and throughout exercise, as was the transdiaphragmatic pressure. Fatigue of the diaphragm and respiratory muscles has been considered. Following exercise, Davies et al.[60] reported a fall in MIP and MEP only in patients, not controls, but others have described falls in mouth pressures in both patients and controls.[56] Maximal voluntary ventilation and maximal sustainable ventilation (ventilation using a 3-minute incremental work rate program while maintaining isocapnia) have been documented as indices of diaphragm endurance. Both are significantly reduced in CHF patients.[57]

The perfusion of the respiratory muscles at rest and during exercise has been assessed using near-infrared spectroscopy.[61] Normal individuals experience a small drop in serratus anterior saturation at near-peak exercise, whereas CHF patients had more marked desaturation at all levels of exercise. There was, however, no correlation between the extent of desaturation and either $\dot{V}O_2$max or MIP, though a correlation with the time–tension index (as defined earlier) was noted.

In addition to the modest correlations between exercise tolerance and indices of respiratory muscle function, the significance of the abnormalities has been suggested by two other studies. In a novel approach based on experience in patients with chronic obstructive pulmonary disease (COPD), respiratory muscle training has been employed in CHF patients.[62] A total of 14 patients, of whom only 8 completed the trial, had thrice-weekly 90-minute supervised training sessions for 3 months. Compared with an untrained group they had significant increases in MIP, MEP, and maximum voluntary and maximum sustainable ventilation. These increases were associated with an increase in $\dot{V}O_2$max, exercise time, and the $\dot{V}E/\dot{V}CO_2$ ratio at 1 liter and a reduction in the sensation of dyspnea. In another, provisional report this group reduced the work of breathing by exercising patients and controls while breathing room air or a mixture of 21 percent oxygen (the balance being helium). This mixture is 70 percent less dense than room air, and it reduces the work of breathing. Although it had no effect on normal subjects, exercise duration was significantly prolonged in the patients, and they subjectively assessed exercise as being easier.[63]

Abnormalities of skeletal muscle have thus been well documented in CHF. The abnormalities are present in patients with heart failure due to ischemic heart disease and dilated cardiomyopathy. It is thus unlikely that, as previously suggested, they are simply a reflection of a generalized myopathy. Though most studies are small, it appears that these changes are common. Further issues must thus be considered. What is the origin of the abnormalities, what is the evidence that they contribute to the symptoms experienced by patients with CHF, and how may these symptoms be generated? Prior to considering these issues data obtained from various studies describing the effects of physical training on muscle in CHF patients are worth reviewing, as the findings are pertinent to these questions.

SKELETAL MUSCLE AND PHYSICAL TRAINING OF CHF PATIENTS

The management of CHF has traditionally involved rest. Some groups, however, have observed that patients with impaired left ventricular function could benefit from rehabilitation programs.[64–66] These observations, coupled with the observed peripheral abnormalities seen in CHF, have led other groups to formally assess exercise training. Sullivan et al.[67] first demonstrated an improvement in exercise tolerance in patients with severe left ventricular dysfunction; subsequently, Coats et al.,[68,69] in a controlled crossover trial, confirmed these findings. Many other groups using differing training regimens and intensities of exercise have reproduced these results.[30,70] The mechanisms underlying the improvement have been considered. At rest there appears to be little change in hemodynamics, whereas at peak exercise there is an increase in cardiac output and leg blood flow (both at a greater absolute workload). There are also, however, significant improvements in the skeletal muscle abnormalities. Muscle metabolism improves at submaximal workloads. Despite no alteration in cardiac output or leg blood flow there is a reduction in both arterial and venous lactate levels.[66] Further evidence for this independence from central hemodynamic changes comes from Minotti et al.[71] In a study of five patients they examined the effect of a training regimen for the nondominant arm (using the untrained dominant arm as a control) on phosphorus spectra. Using a training regimen that did not lead to any change in cardiac output or norepinephrine or lactate levels, they demonstrated an improvement in the trained arm in the spectra abnormalities with a decrease in the Pi/PCr–work slope, though no alteration in the pH changes. There was no change in limb blood flow, but a 260 percent increase in forearm flexor endurance. Adamapoulos et al.[72] reported similar results in calf muscle exercise spectra in patients who were undergoing home-based cycle training. They additionally observed an increase in the PCr recovery rate, suggesting an improvement in the maximal mitochondrial ATP synthesis rate.

The histologic changes underlying these metabolic improvements have received limited attention. Hambrecht et al.[70] performed quadriceps biopsies in 18 patients, half of whom underwent a training program. Training resulted in an increase in the total volume density of mitochondria and an increase in the volume density of cytochrome oxidase-positive mitochondria (an objective measure of cytochrome oxidase activity). They were also able to demonstrate an excellent correlation between the improvement in $\dot{V}O_2$max and anaerobic threshold and the changes in cytochrome oxidase-positive mitochondria.

Belardinelli et al.[30] studied the effect of training on histology. Patients were enrolled in a low-level exercise program such that their training was at a level below the anaerobic threshold. There was no change in resting or exercise hemodynamics, whereas $\dot{V}O_2$max increased and lactate levels at submaximal exercise were lower. This study suggests that improvements were a result of peripheral alterations. Histology revealed an increase in type I and II fiber size after training, though there was no change in fiber distribution (which was abnormal) or capillary density. This group also observed an increase in mitochondrial volume density and a high correlation between change in mitochondrial volume density and change in $\dot{V}O_2$max and anaerobic threshold.

Exercise training thus results in improved exercise tolerance in CHF. This benefit, which appears largely independent of central hemodynamic changes, is associated with improvements in many of the observed skeletal muscle abnormalities.

ORIGINS OF SKELETAL MUSCLE CHANGES

Inactivity results in alterations in skeletal muscle similar to those observed in CHF. It is possible to envisage a cycle during which muscle change leads to inactivity, which in turn leads to greater change in skeletal muscle. The training studies outlined suggest that inactivity has a role, as training is at least in part able to reverse the abnormalities. The explanation is unlikely to be this simple. Changes have been documented in the hand flexors, a muscle group in which normal use may be expected. Moreover, abnormalities of the respiratory musculature have been documented, and these muscles are more likely to experience increased rather than decreased usage. Further evidence refuting inactivity as the sole cause of muscle changes comes from biopsy studies. Vescovo et al.[73] described an electrophoretic technique for subtyping myosin heavy chains. They compared inactive patients (following a stroke) and CHF patients and noted lower levels of myosin heavy-chain 1 and higher levels of myosin heavy-chain 2b in the CHF patients. In a rat model of heart failure, changes in muscle phenotype were unrelated to the degree of locomotor inactivity.[74]

Some authors have suggested malnutrition as a potential cause[13,32] and have documented a reduced calorific intake or a negative net energy balance in some patients. Broquist et al.[32] documented abnormalities of muscle composition and repeated biopsies after 8 weeks of high energy dietary supplementation. They observed no change in their patients' weight, skeletal muscle composition, or exercise capacity; this study, though, involved only a small number of patients, only two of whom were malnourished by their criteria.

Abnormalities of muscle blood flow outlined previously may play an important role despite many of the observed metabolic and functional abnormalities that appear to be independent of blood flow and persist in a situation in which blood flow is temporarily halted. Additionally, some of the training studies have resulted in an improvement in muscle abnormalities with no change in total limb blood flow. The possibility that shunting of blood within skeletal muscle is improved has not been excluded.

Another explanation is that CHF constitutes a catabolic state and the observed muscle changes are a result of this state. There is sympathetic activation; and in addition to documented insulin resistance,[75] some catabolic factors (e.g., tumor necrosis factor and human growth hormone) are known to be elevated in severe CHF.[76–78] CHF clearly can become a highly catabolic state with the development of the severe muscle wasting that is seen with cardiac cachexia (see Ch. 18).

SKELETAL MUSCLE ABNORMALITIES AND SYMPTOM GENERATION IN CHF

Indices of skeletal muscle structure and function in some instances correlate well with exercise intolerance as measured by peak oxygen consumption. Additionally, improvements in exercise tolerance can occur with changes in muscle abnormalities but no improvement in the hemodynamic disturbance. There are several other lines of evidence suggesting that muscle may contribute to the exercise intolerance experienced by some patients. The addition of arm exercise to near-peak leg exercise results in an

increase in $\dot{V}O_2$max in CHF patients but not in controls.[79] Patients who have muscular atrophy as a result of other conditions suffer breathlessness and fatigue similar to CHF patients. Individuals who suffer from mitochondrial myopathies have deletions or mutations in their maternally inherited mitochondrial DNA, resulting in abnormalities of their respiratory chain activity, in some cases similar to those observed in CHF. Limited studies have suggested that they have a hyperdynamic circulatory response to exercise. Despite this situation, they have reduced exercise capacity, low peak oxygen consumption, and an increased slope of the relation between $\dot{V}E$ and $\dot{V}CO_2$, similar to that seen in CHF.[80] Interestingly, these ventilatory abnormalities persisted in two patients who had undergone cardiac transplantation for a dilated cardiomyopathy.[81] Finally, patients undergoing mitral valvoplasty have been studied as a model for correctable CHF. Despite immediate improvements in hemodynamics, the improvement in exercise tolerance appears delayed, the late improvement being associated with changes in skeletal muscle bulk, strength, and histology.[82]

POSSIBLE MECHANISMS OF SYMPTOM GENERATION

Patients with CHF are usually limited by either breathlessness or muscular fatigue. These two symptoms have been considered discrete entities. The mode of exercise (cycle versus treadmill), however, appears to affect the symptoms that limit exercise. A comparison of patients limited by breathlessness or fatigue shows them to have nearly identical clinical characteristics and ventilatory responses to exercise.[83] The same process may thus be generating the two symptoms.

Intuitively, one would expect the sensation of fatigue to relate to the metabolic state of the exercising muscle. Lactate does not appear to generate the sensation. A reduction in lactate production in CHF achieved by infusing dichloroacetate does not result in an increase in exercise capacity.[84] Local levels of potassium may be important,[85] and abnormalities of potassium handling have been observed in CHF.[86] The method by which such a metabolic disturbance is sensed is unknown. Small myelinated and unmyelinated nerve fibers originating from skeletal muscle have been identified. It is possible that these fibers receive input from work-sensitive (ergosensitive) receptors, and that the impulses from these fibers help generate the sensation of fatigue and perhaps the sensation of dyspnea.

Some evidence for this hypothesis exists. Minotti

et al.[71] observed an improvement in single arm exercise tolerance after localized training. This work has been extended by Piepoli et al.[87] They observed the blood pressure, pulse, and ventilatory responses during circulatory occlusion after a period of hand grip exercise, comparing these responses with those following exercise without circulatory occlusion. Any difference between the two responses is due to a non-humoral signal, the "ergoreflex." They observed that the ergoreflex-dependent components of ventilation—diastolic blood pressure and nonexercising limb vascular resistance—were greater in CHF patients, implying that this reflex was more active in these patients. Additionally, a 6-week period of local forearm training was able to reduce the activity of this reflex in CHF patients.[88]

CONCLUSIONS

Hemodynamic disturbance correlates poorly with exercise tolerance in CHF. This observation, in conjunction with the failure of acute increases in cardiac output to improve exercise tolerance, has led to examination of the periphery. Extensive abnormalities of lower limb musculature have been described, with a reduction in muscle bulk and endurance. Metabolic and histologic studies have demonstrated a shift toward anaerobic metabolism that cannot be explained solely by reduced limb blood flow. Intrinsic abnormalities of skeletal muscle appear to exist.

There is some evidence to suggest that these muscle changes contribute to the exercise intolerance characteristic of CHF. It is possible that symptoms are generated by these muscle abnormalities via an exaggerated ergoreflex. The prime importance of such a hypothesis is its relevance to potentially novel therapies aimed at treating the mechanism of symptom generation rather than attempting to correct the hemodynamic abnormalities.

REFERENCES

1. Franciosa JA, Park M, Levine TB: Lack of correlation between exercise capacity and indices of resting left ventricular performance in heart failure. Am J Cardiol 1981;47:33–39
2. Higginbotham MB, Morris KG, Conn EH, Coleman RE, Cobb FR: Determinants of exercise performance among patients with congestive heart failure. Am J Cardiol 1983;51:52–60
3. Szlachcic J, Massie BM, Kramer BL, Topic N, Tubau J: Correlates and prognostic implication of exercise capacity in chronic congestive heart failure. Am J Cardiol 1985;55:1037–1363
4. Maskin CS, Forman R, Sonnenblick EH, Frishman WH, LeJemtel TH: Failure of dobutamine to increase exercise capacity despite haemodynamic improvement in severe chronic heart failure. Am J Cardiol 1983;51: 177–182
5. Wilson JR, Martin JL, Ferraro N, Weber KT: Effect of hydralazine on perfusion and metabolism in the leg during upright bicycle exercise in patients with heart failure. Circulation 1983;68:425–432
6. Wilson JR, Martin JL, Ferraro N: Impaired skeletal muscle nutritive flow during exercise in patients with congestive heart failure. Role of cardiac pump dysfunction as determined by the effect of dobutamine. Am J Cardiol 1984;53:1308–1315
7. Katz AM, Katz PB: Diseases of the heart in works of Hippocrates. Br Heart J 1962;24:257–264
8. Aronson JK: An Account of the Foxglove and Its Medical Uses. pp. 11–100. Oxford University Press, London, 1985
9. Drexler H: Skeletal muscle failure in heart failure. Circulation 1992;85:1621–1623
10. Minotti JR, Christoph I, Massie BM: Skeletal muscle function, morphology and metabolism in patients with congestive heart failure. Chest, suppl. 1992;101: 333S–338S
11. Coats AJS, Clark AL, Piepoli M, Volterrani M, Poole-Wilson P: Symptoms and quality of life in heart failure. The muscle hypothesis. Br Heart J, suppl. 1994;72: S36–S39
12. Wilson JR: Exercise intolerance in heart failure. Importance of skeletal muscle. Circulation 1995;91: 559–561
13. Mancini DM, Walter G, Reichnek N et al: Contribution of skeletal muscle atrophy to exercise intolerance and altered muscle metabolism in heart failure. Circulation 1992;85:1364–1373
14. Minotti JR, Pillay P, Oka R et al: Skeletal muscle size. Relationship to muscle function in heart failure. J Appl Physiol 1993;75:373–381
15. Miyagi K, Asanoi H, Ishizak S, Kameyama T, Sasayama S: Loss of skeletal muscle mass is a major determinant of exercise tolerance in chronic heart failure. Circulation, suppl. II 1991;84:74
16. Lipkin D, Jones D, Round J, Poole-Wilson P: Abnormalities of skeletal muscle in patients with chronic heart failure. Int J Cardiol 1988;18:187–195
17. Mancini DM, Coyle E, Coggan A et al: Contribution of intrinsic skeletal muscle changes to ^{31}P NMR skeletal muscle abnormalities in patients with chronic heart failure. Circulation 1989;80:1338–1346
18. Sullivan MJ, Green HJ, Cobb FR: Skeletal muscle biochemistry and histology in ambulatory patients with long-term heart failure. Circulation 1990;81:518–527
19. Volterrani M, Clark AL, Ludman PF et al: Determinants of exercise capacity in chronic heart failure. Eur Heart J 1994;15:801–809
20. Buller NP, Jones D, Poole-Wilson PA: Direct measurements of skeletal muscle fatigue in patients with chronic heart failure. Br Heart J 1991;65:20–24
21. Minotti JR, Christoph I, Oka R et al: Impaired skeletal muscle function in patients with congestive heart failure. Relationship to systemic exercise performance. J Clin Invest 1991;88:2077–2082
22. Chapman SJ, Grindrod SR, Jones DA: Cross-sectional area and force production of the quadriceps muscle. J Physiol (Lond) 1984;53:53P
23. Wilson JR, Fink L, Maris J et al: Evaluation of energy

metabolism in skeletal muscle of patients with heart failure with gated phosphorus-31 nuclear magnetic resonance. Circulation 1985;71:57–62

24. Minotti JR, Pillay P, Chang L, Wells L, Massie BM: Neurophysiological assessment of skeletal muscle fatigue in patients with congestive heart failure. Circulation 1992;86:903–908

25. Wilson JR, Mancini DM, Simson M: Detection of skeletal muscle fatigue in patients with heart failure using electromyography. Am J Cardiol 1992;70:488–493

26. Bergstrom J: Muscle electrolytes in man. Scand J Clin Lab Invest Suppl 1962;68:7–100

27. Yancy CW Jr, Parsons D, Lane L et al: Capillary density, fiber type and enzyme composition of skeletal muscle in congestive heart failure. J Am Coll Cardiol, suppl. 1989;13:38A

28. Drexler H, Riede U, Munzel T et al: Alterations of skeletal muscle in chronic heart failure. Circulation 1992; 85:1751–1759

29. Sabbah HN, Hansen-Smith F, Sharov VG et al: Decreased proportion of type I myofibers in skeletal muscle of dogs with chronic heart failure. Circulation 1993; 87:1729–1737

30. Belardinelli R, Georgiou D, Scocco V, Barstow TJ, Puracaro A: Low intensity exercise training in patients with chronic heart failure. J Am Coll Cardiol 1995;26: 975–982

31. Lindsay DC, Lovegrove CA, Dunn MJ et al: Histological abnormalities of diaphragmatic muscle may contribute to dyspnea in heart failure. Circulation, suppl. I 1992;86:514

32. Broquist M, Arnquist H, Dahlstrom U et al: Nutritional assessment and muscle energy metabolism in severe chronic heart failure. Effects of long term dietary supplementation. Eur Heart J 1994;15: 1641–1650

33. Tikunov B, Levine S, Mancini D: Chronic congestive heart failure elicits adaptations of endurance exercise in diaphragmatic muscle. Circulation, suppl. I 1995; 92:541

34. Massie BM, Conway M, Yonge R et al: ^{31}P nuclear magnetic resonance evidence of abnormal skeletal muscle metabolism in patients with congestive heart failure. Am J Cardiol 1987;60:309–315

35. Mancini DM, Ferraro N, Tuchler M, Chance B, Wilson JR: Detection of abnormal calf muscle metabolism in patients with heart failure using phosphorus-31 nuclear magnetic resonance. Am J Cardiol 1988;62: 1234–1240

36. Arnolda L, Conway M, Dolecki M et al: Skeletal muscle metabolism in heart failure: a ^{31}P nuclear magnetic resonance spectroscopy study of leg muscle. Clin Sci 1990;79:583–589

37. Wiener DH, Fink LI, Maris J et al: Abnormal skeletal muscle bioenergetics during exercise in patients with heart failure. Role of reduced muscle blood flow. Circulation 1986;73:1127–1136

38. Hands LJ, Bore PJ, Galloway G, Morris PJ, Radda GK: Muscle metabolism in patients with peripheral vascular disease, investigated by ^{31}P nuclear magnetic resonance spectroscopy. Clin Sci 1986;71:283–290

39. Massie BM, Conway M, Yonge R et al: Skeletal muscle metabolism in patients with congestive heart failure. Relation to clinical severity and blood flow. Circulation 1987;76:1009–1019

40. Massie BM, Conway M, Rajagopalan BM et al: Skele-

tal muscle metabolism during exercise under ischaemic conditions in congestive heart failure. Evidence for abnormalities unrelated to blood flow. Circulation 1988;78:320–326

41. Sullivan MJ, Green HJ, Cobb FR: Altered skeletal muscle metabolic response to exercise in chronic heart failure. Relation to skeletal muscle aerobic enzymes activity. Circulation 1991;84:1597–1607

42. Meakins J, Lang CNH: Oxygen consumption, oxygen debt and lactic acid in circulatory failure. J Clin Invest 1927;4:273–293

43. Huckabee WK, Judson WE: The role of anaerobic metabolism in the performance of mild muscular work. I. Relationship to oxygen consumption and cardiac output and the effect of congestive heart failure. J Clin Invest 1958;37:1577–1592

44. Donald KW, Gloster J, Harris EA, Reeves J, Harris P: The production of lactic acid during exercise in normal subjects and patients with rheumatic heart disease. Am Heart J 1961;62:494–510

45. Wilson JR, Martin JL, Schwartz D, Ferraro N: Exercise intolerance in patients with chronic heart failure. Role of impaired nutritive flow to skeletal muscle. Circulation 1984;69:1079–1087

46. Weber KT, Janicki JS: Lactate production during maximal and submaximal exercise in patients with chronic heart failure. J Am Coll Cardiol 1985;6:717–724

47. Sullivan MJ, Higginbotham MB, Cobb FR: Increased exercise ventilation in patients with chronic heart failure. Intact ventilatory control despite hemodynamic and pulmonary abnormalities. Circulation 1988;77: 552–559

48. Wilson JR, Mancini DM, Dunkman WB: Exertional fatigue due to skeletal muscle dysfunction in patients with heart failure. Circulation 1993;87:470–475

49. Katz SD, Bleiberg B, Wexler J et al: Lactate turnover at rest and during submaximal exercise in patients with heart failure. J Appl Physiol 1993;75:1974–1979

50. Manning HL, Schwartzstein RM: Pathophysiology of dyspnea. N Engl J Med 1995;333:1547–1553

51. Hammond MD, Bauer KA, Sharp JT, Rocha RD: Respiratory muscle strength in congestive heart failure. Chest;98:1091–1094

52. McParland C, Krishnan B, Wang Y, Gallagher CG: Inspiratory muscle weakness and dyspnea in chronic heart failure. Am Rev Respir Dis 1992;146:467–472

53. Evans SA, Watson L, Hawkins M et al: Respiratory muscle strength in chronic heart failure. Thorax 1995; 50:625–628

54. Ambrosino N, Opasich C, Crotti P et al: Breathing pattern, ventilatory drive and respiratory muscle strength in patients with chronic heart failure. Eur Respir J 1994;7:17–22

55. Chua TP, Anker SD, Harrington D, Coats AJS: Inspiratory muscle strength is a determinant of maximum oxygen consumption in chronic heart failure. Br Heart J 1995;74:381–385

56. Mancini DM, Henson D, LaManca J, Levine S: Respiratory muscle function and dyspnea in patients with chronic congestive heart failure. Circulation 1992;86: 909–918

57. Mancini DM, Henson D, LaManca J, Levine S: Evidence of reduced respiratory muscle endurance in patients with heart failure. J Am Coll Cardiol 1994;24: 972–981

58. Nishimura Y, Maeda H, Tanaka K et al: Respiratory

muscle strength and hemodynamics in chronic heart failure. Chest 1994;105:355–359

59. Bellemare F, Bigland-Richie B: Assessment of human diaphragm strength and activation using phrenic nerve stimulation. Respir Physiol 1984;58:263–277

60. Davies SW, Jordan SSL, Pride NB, Lipkin DP: Respiratory muscle failure in chronic heart failure. Circulation, suppl. III 1990;82:24

61. Mancini DM, Ferraro N, Nazzaro D, Chance B, Wilson JR: Respiratory muscle deoxygenation during exercise in patients with heart failure demonstrated with near-infrared spectroscopy. J Am Coll Cardiol 1991;18: 492–498

62. Mancini DM, Henson D, LaManca J, Donchez L, Levine S: Benefit of selective respiratory muscle training on exercise capacity in patients with chronic congestive heart failure. Circulation 1995;91:320–329

63. Mancini D, Donchez L, Foray A, Aaronson K, Levine S: Acute unloading of the work of breathing extends exercise duration in patients with heart failure. Circulation, suppl. I 1995;92:402

64. Letac B, Cribier A, Desplanches JF: A study of left ventricular function in coronary patients before and after physical training. Circulation 1977;56:375–378

65. Lee AP, Ice R, Blessey R, Sanmarco ME: Long-term effects of physical training in coronary patients with impaired left ventricular function. Circulation 1979; 60:1519–1526

66. Conn EH, Williams RS, Wallace AG: Exercise responses before and after physical conditioning in patients with severely depressed left ventricular function. Am J Cardiol 1982;49:296–300

67. Sullivan MJ, Higginbotham MB, Cobb FR: Exercise training in patients with severe left ventricular dysfunction. Hemodynamic and metabolic effects. Circulation 1988;78:506–516

68. Coats AJS, Adamopoulos S, Meyer T, Conway J, Sleight P: Physical training in chronic heart failure. Lancet 1990;335:63–66

69. Coats AJS, Adamopoulos S, Radaelli A et al: Controlled trial of physical training in chronic heart failure. Exercise performance, hemodynamics, ventilation, and autonomic function. Circulation 1992;85: 2119–2131

70. Hambrecht R, Niebauer J, Fiehn E et al: Physical training in patients with stable chronic heart failure. Effects on cardiopulmonary fitness and ultrastructural abnormalities of leg muscles. J Am Coll Cardiol 1995;25:1239–1249

71. Minotti JR, Johnson EC, Hudson TL et al: Skeletal muscle response to exercise training in congestive heart failure. J Clin Invest 1990;86:751–758

72. Adamopoulos S, Coats AJS, Brunotte F et al: Physical training improves skeletal muscle metabolic abnormalities in patients with chronic heart failure. J Am Coll Cardiol 1993;23:1101–1106

73. Vescovo G, Facchin L, Tenderini P et al: A new micromethod for assessing myosin heavy chain composition in skeletal muscle needle biopsies. Differences between chronic heart failure and disuse muscle atrophy. Eur Heart J, suppl. 1995;16:357

74. Simioni A, Long CS, Yue P et al: Heart failure in rats causes changes in skeletal muscle phenotype and gene expression unrelated to locomotor activity. Circulation, suppl. 1 1995;92:259

75. Swan JW, Walton C, Godsland IF, Clark AL, Coats AJS: Insulin resistance in chronic heart failure. Eur Heart J 1994;15:1528–1532

76. Levine B, Kalman J, Mayer L, Fillit H, Packer M: Elevated circulating levels of tumour necrosis factor in severe chronic heart failure. N Engl J Med 1990;323: 236–241

77. McMurray J, Abdullah I, Dargie HJ, Shapiro D: Increased concentrations of tumour necrosis factor in "cachectic" patients with severe chronic heart failure. Br Heart J 1991;66:356–368

78. Anker SD, Volterrani M, Swan JW et al: Hormonal changes in cardiac cachexia. Eur Heart J, suppl. 1995; 16:359

79. Jondeau G, Katz SD, Zohman L et al: Active skeletal muscle mass and cardiopulmonary reserve. Failure to attain peak aerobic capacity during maximal bicycle exercise in patients with severe congestive heart failure. Circulation 1992;86:1351–1356

80. Haller RG, Lewis SF, Estabrook RW et al: Exercise intolerance, lactic acidosis and abnormal cardiopulmonary regulation in exercise associated with adult skeletal muscle cytochrome oxidase deficiency. J Clin Invest 1989;84:155–161

81. Bussieres LM, Plugfelder PW, Guiraudon C et al: Exercise responses after cardiac transplantation in mitochondrial myopathy. Am J Cardiol 1993;71:1003–1006

82. Barlow CW, Long JEH, Brown G et al: Exercise capacity and skeletal muscle changes after balloon mitral valvuloplasty. Circulation, suppl. 1 1995;92:210

83. Clark AL, Sparrow JL, Coats AJS: Muscle fatigue and dyspnea in chronic heart failure. Two sides of the same coin? Eur Heart J 1995;16:49–52

84. Wilson JR, Mancini DM, Ferraro N, Egler J: Effect of dichloroacetate on the exercise performance of patients with heart failure. J Am Coll Cardiol 1988;12: 1464–1469

85. Sjogaard G: Role of exercise-induced potassium fluxes underlying muscle fatigue. A brief review. Can J Physiol Pharmacol 1991;69:238–245

86. Barlow CW, Qayyum MS, Davey PP et al: Effect of physical training on exercise-induced hyperkalemia in chronic heart failure. Relation with ventilation and catecholamines. Circulation 1994;89:1144–1152

87. Piepoli M, Clark AL, Coats AJS: Muscle metaboreceptors in hemodynamic, autonomic and ventilatory responses to exercise in men. Am J Physiol 1995; 269(Heart Circ Physiol 38):H1428–H1436

88. Piepoli M, Clark AL, Volterrani M et al: Contribution of muscle afferents to the hemodynamic, autonomic, and ventilatory responses to exercise in patients with chronic heart failure. Effects of physical training. Circulation 1996;93 (in press)

17 Involvement of the Lungs

Peter D. Wagner

This chapter considers pulmonary involvement during heart failure, and at the outset two major subdivisions of this topic should be recognized. The first addresses how primary cardiac diseases may affect the structure and function of the lungs. The second, complementary area relates to the effects of primary pulmonary diseases on cardiac function. With the heart and lungs not only interconnected by the circulation but also competing for space within the thorax, cardiopulmonary interactions can become complex. Both organs are subject to similar environmental (i.e., intrathoracic) pressures; and although the lungs functionally separate the right and left ventricles, the anatomic ventricular connections and pericardial containment can lead to functional effects of one chamber on the other.

LUNGS DURING FAILURE OF THE LEFT VENTRICLE

Normal Respiratory Physiology Relevant to Cardiac Function

Ventilation occurs as a result of voluntary contraction of the diaphragm and intercostal muscles. Working together, these muscles elongate the craniocaudal and enlarge the lateral and anteroposterior dimensions of the thoracic cavity. Volume enlargement reduces intrapleural pressure around the lungs, which causes lung volume to passively increase, drawing air into the alveoli for exchange of O_2 and CO_2. The necessary reduction in intrapleural pressure in resting normal humans is trivial, at no

more than 5 cm of water, due to the low resistance of the airways and tissues and to the highly compliant nature of lung tissue. Consequently, this small negative pressure swing has negligible effects on myocardial function. With lung diseases, when lung resistance rises or compliance falls, larger pressure swings are required to provide lung expansion. This situation may oppose ventricular contractile function by effectively increasing ventricular afterload.

Despite the enormously complex structure of the lung as a collection of some 300 million alveoli, all of which receive some ventilation to ensure gas exchange,[1] the distribution of ventilation in health is remarkably well matched to the distribution of blood flow. This situation is evidenced by the nearly perfect gas exchange behavior of normal lungs,[2] which could not occur if ventilation and blood flow were not similarly distributed throughout the lungs.

Whereas ventilation is necessarily bidirectional, or "tidal," owing to airway structure, *perfusion* of the lungs with pulmonary arterial blood is unidirectional, from the right atrium and ventricle via the pulmonary circulation to the left atrium and ventricle. In contrast to the high pressure systemic circulation, the pulmonary circulation operates at sixfold (or more) lower pressures.[3] Both circulations must accommodate the entire cardiac output; but whereas the mean systemic arterial pressure may average 100 mmHg in health, the mean pulmonary arterial pressure is only about 15 mmHg. Right and left atrial pressures are similar, the left usually being slightly greater than the right, averaging 5–10 mmHg. Vascular resistance, calculated as arterial minus atrial mean pressures divided by cardiac output, reveals values some 10-fold lower in the pulmonary than the systemic circulation. This ratio is critical to lung health because the microvascular walls of the pulmonary capillary network are necessarily thin to ensure adequate exchange of O_2 and CO_2 between gas and blood. Were the microvascular pressures not so low, physical damage to the capillary network would occur, and blood would leak into the alveolar spaces of the lungs.[4]

A key feature of the normal pulmonary circulation is its capacity to maintain a low pressure in the face of either increased blood flow or vascular obstruction. At rest, not all capillaries are perfused, and those that are, are not fully distended. Thus both recruitment of unperfused and distension of perfused capillaries are substantial when there is increased flow or vascular obstruction, which is how a low pressure is maintained even when blood flow is normal. By implication, pulmonary vascular resistance normally falls when in health blood flow rises, and the capacity for recruitment and distension even in disease limits the utility of measures of pulmonary vascular resistance per se as an index of pulmonary vascular disease: The value depends on overall blood flow.

Figure 17-1A shows that in patients with pulmonary embolism even major vascular occlusion raises pulmonary artery pressure only modestly. Figure 17-1B, from the same patients, serves to point out that failure of the pulmonary artery pressure to rise substantially is not attributable by and large to reduced total pulmonary blood flow. The ability to preserve low pressures in the face of vascular restriction is probably important for maintaining the integrity of the remaining perfused pulmonary vasculature.

The normally slightly subatmospheric intratho-

racic pressures associated with the elastic nature (i.e., collapsibility) of the lungs means that perivascular pressures are also generally subatmospheric. Yet the intravascular pressures, although low, remain above the atmospheric level, as mentioned. There is thus a transmural pressure gradient that constantly produces net outward *fluid movement* from the microvasculature into the pulmonary interstitium.[6] Although it is somewhat counteracted by the higher osmotic pressure of plasma compared to pulmonary interstitial fluid, albumin moves relatively freely across the capillary wall in the lungs such that pulmonary lymph/plasma protein ratios typically average 0.7–0.9.[6] The well known Starling equation expresses the balance between the hydrostatic and osmotic forces responsible for net fluid movement:

$$J = K \left[(P_{MV} - P_{INT}) - \rho (\Pi_{MV} - \Pi_{INT}) \right]$$

Here J is the rate of fluid movement across the capillary wall into the interstitial (INT) space, and K is a filtration coefficient proportional to surface area of the microvasculature (MV). P_{MV} and P_{INT} are the corresponding hydrostatic pressures and Π_{MV} and Π_{INT} the associated protein oncotic pressures. ρ is an overall reflection coefficient describing the ease of protein escape from the capillaries ($\rho = 0$ if the capillary is freely permeable, 1 if impermeable). The balance of forces results in net fluid escape from the capillaries. Figure 17-2 shows how edema develops when intravascular pressures are raised above about 25 mmHg, unbalancing the Starling equation. So long as pressures are lower than this level, edema

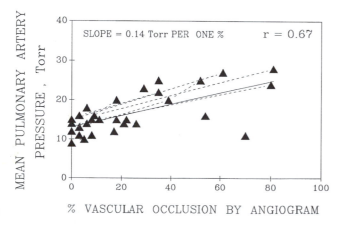
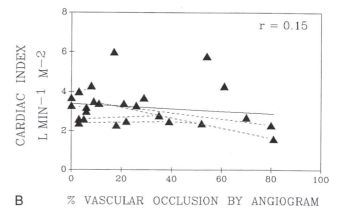

A   % VASCULAR OCCLUSION BY ANGIOGRAM

B   % VASCULAR OCCLUSION BY ANGIOGRAM

Fig. 17-1. Relation between mean pulmonary artery pressure and percentage occlusion of the pulmonary vasculature detected by angiography in pulmonary embolism. Dashed lines connect sequential measurements in individual patients. **(A)** The rise in pulmonary artery pressure is modest even when occlusion is extensive. **(B)** This is in general not due to a systematic reduction in cardiac output in the same patients. (Adapted from Wilson et al.,[5] with permission.)

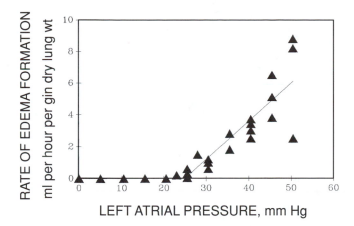

Fig. 17-2. Development of pulmonary edema when left atrial pressure exceeds about 25 mmHg. Below this critical value, pulmonary edema does not occur. (Adapted from Guyton and Lindsey,[7] with permission.)

can be avoided, even when transcapillary fluid flux is increased, because of the lymphatic system in the lungs that conducts lymph back to the systemic venous system. Without an efficient lymphatic drainage system in the lungs, fluid would rapidly accumulate to the point of edema. With lymph flow rates of about 0.25–1.00 ml/min (estimated from Meyer[8]) and a lung weight of about 600 g, it would take only 10–40 hours to double the weight of the lungs were there no lymph drainage. The pulmonary lymphatic system is well developed in humans and contains valves[9] that allow advantage to be taken of pressure and volume changes in the lungs during tidal breathing to assist lymphatic drainage back to the systemic venous system. Thus tidal breathing effectively pumps lymph out of alveoli and back to the superior vena cava. The lymphatic pathway from the alveoli closely tracks the major arteries (and neighboring airways) from distal to proximal branches and out of the lungs at the hilum. When fluid movement out of the capillaries occurs too rapidly for the lymphatic drainage system to keep pace, this arrangement makes these blood vessels and airways subject to compression by excess perivascular fluid and thus increases blood and gas flow resistance (Fig. 17-3). Under these conditions, fluid may also accumulate in the pulmonary parenchymal interstitial space (Fig. 17-4). When such accumulation occurs, compliance of the lungs falls: The alveoli become stiffer and require greater negative pressure to provide a given degree of lung inflation. Consequently, pulmonary fluid accumulation negatively affects the two primary mechanical determinants of ventilation: resistance and compliance.

Normally, however, the low pulmonary vascular pressures and efficient lymphatic drainage keep the lungs from accumulating fluid. Because the alveolar epithelial cells (Fig. 17-4) are joined much more tightly than the capillary endothelial cells, transcapillary fluid does not generally move all the way from endothelium through interstitial space and alveolar epithelium to the alveolar gas spaces (Fig. 17-4). Thus in disease states alveoli may remain gas-filled even while interstitial fluid accumulates. Only when vascular transmural pressures reach high levels or when alveolar cell integrity has been compromised by disease does the epithelial lining give way and produce alveolar flooding.[10] This resilience of the pulmonary epithelium to fluid movement is an important defense mechanism for keeping the lungs dry; although interstitial fluid can be rapidly cleared by lymphatic drainage as mentioned, clearance of alveolar fluid is slow, requiring movement up the airways (and eventually expectoration or swallowing) or reabsorption into the capillaries, which can occur only when the high pressure or cell damage (causing edema in the first place) has been reversed.

The tight alveolar epithelium helps keep the alveoli free from edema, but a supplementary mechanism exists as well: the alveolar surfactant system. Surfactant is a mixture of lipoprotein complexes, synthesized by alveolar type II epithelial cells, that greatly reduces the air–liquid interfacial surface tension in the alveoli from 70 dynes/cm (of water) to 5–10 dynes/cm. This reduction helps prevent alveolar collapse from such surface tension forces and reduces the amount by which the perivascular pressure would otherwise fall if surface tension were high (Fig. 17-5). A vicious cycle of events usually occurs with alveolar damage because transcapillary leak of protein into the alveolar space inactivates surfactants, which by the above mechanism worsens the problem of fluid movement and pulmonary edema.

Because blood has significant density (about equal to that of water) intravascular pressures become greater the lower down in the lungs one looks. The roughly 30 cm height of normal lungs makes the capillary pressure some 30 cm (or 20 mmHg) greater at the lung base than at the apex of normal upright humans. Generally, this factor explains the relatively greater transcapillary fluid movement at the lung bases in both health and disease. However, factors other than gravity may play a role in the distribution of fluid movement, such as regional differences in cellular damage in disease states.

Gas exchange (i.e., the uptake of O_2 by, and removal of CO_2 from, the blood) depends critically on ventilation and blood flow.[2] Thus the better matched are the local levels of ventilation and blood flow the

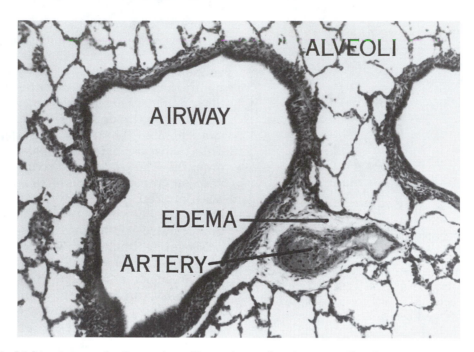

Fig. 17-3. Light micrograph of a section of lung tissue showing a small pulmonary artery surrounded by perivascular edema. Note that there is no peribronchial edema. Thus the pulmonary artery lumen may be compressed by edema, but it does not occur in the bronchus.

more efficient is gas exchange. When ventilation ($\dot{V}A$) is less than blood flow ($\dot{Q}$) in a small area of the lungs, the ratio of the two ($\dot{V}A/\dot{Q}$) is reduced. Local alveolar and capillary PO_2 are reduced, and corresponding values of PCO_2 are elevated.[2] The converse occurs when the $\dot{V}A/\dot{Q}$ ratio is increased. Because cardiac function can affect those lung properties that determine distribution of ventilation (i.e., lung compliance and resistance) and of blood flow (pulmonary arterial and venous pressures, local fluid accumulation in the lungs), and thus the number of areas of low or high $\dot{V}A/\dot{Q}$ ratio, it is easy to see that gas exchange can be greatly affected by cardiac function.

The matching of ventilation to blood flow throughout the lungs is normally surprisingly well preserved despite the many potential factors that could disrupt their even distribution. The supporting evidence is the nearly perfect gas exchange performance with the difference in alveolar gas and arterial blood PO_2 ($AaPO_2$) being only 5–10 mmHg in healthy young subjects. It is a trivial departure from perfection (an $AaPO_2$ of zero) because it takes place at an arterial PO_2 of 90–100 mmHg. At such PO_2 values, the O_2-hemoglobin dissociation curve is virtually flat, such that the difference in O_2 concentration of arterial blood is almost immeasurably small. Thus at $PO_2 =$ 100 mmHg, the arterial $[O_2]$ would normally be 20.6 $ml \cdot dl^{-1}$. At a PO_2 of 90 mmHg under the same conditions, it would be 20.5 $ml \cdot dl^{-1}$, only 0.5 percent less. This is of absolutely no importance to O_2 transport.

Altered distribution of ventilation or blood flow (such as may occur with heart failure) significantly impairs gas exchange and results therefore in hypoxemia.

The remaining important functional component of respiration is the *control of breathing*. How ventilation is controlled is a complex matter, and several neural pathways connecting specialized sensory cells to the brain combine to produce the final result: (1) Peripheral chemoreceptors in the carotid bodies sense arterial PO_2. Hypoxemia, especially below a PO_2 of about 50–60 mmHg, stimulates breathing by this mechanism. (2) Central nervous system sensors oppose it acutely (i.e., over several minutes) but not over longer periods. (3) The carotid body chemoreceptors also respond to arterial PCO_2 and pH, stimulating respiration as PCO_2 rises or pH falls and diminishing ventilation as PCO_2 falls or pH rises. (4) The ventral medulla houses neurons sensitive to pH that stimulate ventilation during acidosis and inhibit ventilation during alkalosis. This reaction is mediated via PCO_2 in arterial blood and thus cerebrospinal fluid, as CO_2 molecules but not H^+ ions can cross from the blood to the chemosensitive regions. (5) Higher brain center activity permits voluntary control of breathing within limits and may be responsible for anxiety-related hyperventilation. (6) For example, nonmyelinated pulmonary C fibers may transmit J receptor (juxtacapillary receptor) signals from the alveolar interstitial region via the vagus nerve when distortion or edema is present, which

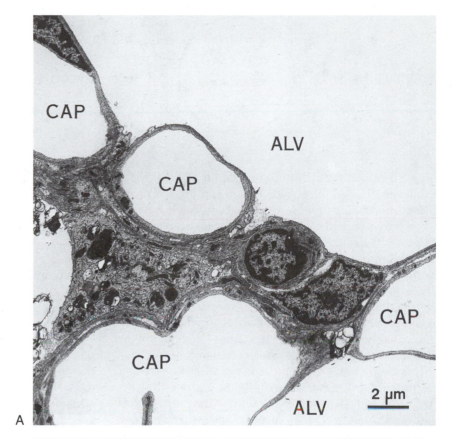

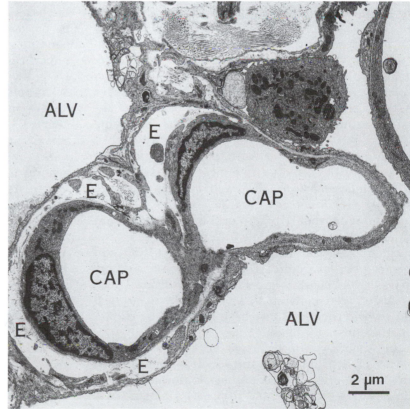

Fig. 17-4. Transmission electron micrographs of normal lung tissue (**A**) and edematous lung tissue (**B**) showing alveolar gas spaces (ALV), alveolar wall capillaries (CAP), and interstitial edema (E). Edema can be seen to separate the capillary endothelium from the alveolar epithelium. Capillaries are devoid of cells because of the perfusion fixation technique.

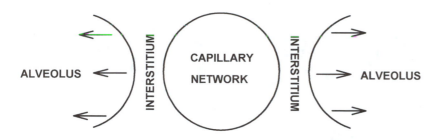

Fig. 17-5. Concept of how surface tension forces reduce interstitial pressure around the alveolar capillary network. Thus surfactants, which lower surface tension, protect against undue reduction in interstitial hydrostatic pressure. Arrows indicate the direction of the surface forces acting to reduce interstitial pressure.

may stimulate ventilation independently of PO_2, PCO_2, or pH.[11] (7) Both slowly and rapidly adapting receptors feeding myelinated nerves in the large airways may respond to venous congestion or extravascular fluid around the large airways and transmit their signals via the vagus nerve to the respiratory centers in the brain.[12,13] (8) A variety of inputs from other sources, such as muscles and joints, may affect ventilation, particularly during exercise. (9) Various activators of ion channels, indeed K^+ itself, may play a role, as the basic receptor transduction mechanism reflects ion channel responses of sensing cells.[14]

It is clear that several pulmonary afferent systems could transmit signals during heart failure that affect ventilation by controlling tidal volume and respiratory frequency.[15] How deeply and how often we breathe determines alveolar ventilation, which in turn has immediate consequences for local PO_2 and PCO_2 in the alveoli and hence for arterial PO_2 and PCO_2. Hyperventilation increases PO_2 and decreases PCO_2 in all alveoli and thus in arterial blood. Just how beneficial it is to O_2 transport depends on where one is operating in the O_2 dissociation curve and therefore how much ventilation–blood flow distribution mismatching is present. Thus improving the arterial PO_2 from 90 to 100 mmHg by hyperventilation insignificantly affects arterial oxygenation (see above), but a similar 10 mmHg increase from 40 to 50 mmHg in arterial PO_2, would increase arterial the $[O_2]$ by 15 percent from 15.5 to 17.9 ml $\cdot$ dl^{-1} (assuming normal [Hb] and acid-base status). That calculation assumes no leftward shift in the O_2-hemoglobin dissociation curve from the lower PCO_2 and higher pH that would accompany hyperventilation. When those changes are factored in, arterial $[O_2]$ would be even higher at 18.7 ml $\cdot$ dl^{-1}. In all, arterial $[O_2]$ would therefore have been improved by 20 percent, a substantial gain.

In summary, the principal physiologic determinants or attributes of lung function—mechanical properties and ventilation, blood flow, fluid exchange, gas exchange, and respiratory control—are all to a greater or lesser extent vulnerable to abnormalities in left heart function. More details on these relations in heart failure follow.

Effects of Left Ventricular Failure on Lung Function

LUNG MECHANICAL PROPERTIES AND VENTILATION

As left atrial pressure increases as a consequence of left-sided ventricular failure, pulmonary venous pressure must passively follow, as also must pulmonary arterial pressure, in order to maintain forward circulation of blood through the lungs. Because both pulmonary arterial and venous pressures increase, the pulmonary microvascular pressure has to rise as well. From normal mean pulmonary arterial and venous pressures of, for example, 15 and 5 mmHg, respectively, 20 mmHg increases in both are not infrequently seen with left heart failure. Prior to such increases, the pulmonary vasculature is not fully perfused at rest, with considerable opportunity to expand its volume by a combination of recruitment of unperfused microvessels and distension of others. Despite years of research, it is uncertain how much of the volume increase is due to recruitment versus distension, but this question may be largely academic. By whatever means, an increase in microvascular blood volume reduces alveolar compliance (because the microvessels are in the alveolar walls). In general, because of the weight of the blood, the effects are greatest in dependent lung regions (i.e., at the bases in an upright posture). However, additional nongravitational influences may cause a more patchy distribution of effects. These regions of reduced compliance expand less for a given inspiratory effort, producing lower regional ventilation, which causes local alveolar hypoxia and thus systemic arterial hypoxemia. Reduced compliance also tends to cause a reduction in lung volume. Because an important mechanism preserving airway diameters is elastic radial traction from attached alveoli,[16,17] which is greater at high than low lung volumes, airway lumen reduction may occur, increasing airflow resistance and reducing local ventilation.

Increased transcapillary fluid movement with fluid accumulation in the interstitial spaces (Fig. 17-4) also contributes to reduced compliance and ventilation. Perivascular or peribronchial fluid accumulation may develop (Fig. 17-3), which leads to further loss of airway cross-sectional area, increasing airways resistance.

All of these changes reflect only interstitial edema, the alveoli in the preceding discussion remaining free of fluid. Even so, the changes described increase the work of breathing and may contribute to a sense of dyspnea felt by the patient. Via vagally transmitted signals not yet fully understood (see below), ventilation may be stimulated and be clinically detectable as hyperpnea and arterial hypocapnia.

When frank alveolar edema has developed, generally requiring substantial microvascular pressures of 25 mmHg or more (Fig. 17-2), the flooded alveoli receive no fresh gas, the alveolar fluid not being displaceable by air during ventilation. Compliance of the lung is therefore further reduced compared to values during interstitial edema. Simple spirometric and other indices of lung function—residual volume (RV), vital capacity (VC), forced expiratory volume at 1 second (FEV_1), maximal flow rates during the middle half of expiration (FEF_{25-75}), for example—show a combination of usually mild obstructive and restrictive features. Thus FEV_1/VC and FEF_{25-75} fall below predicted norms, reflecting obstruction, whereas a fall in lung volumes [RV, VC, and total lung capacity (TLC = RV + VC)] reflects the restrictive components. Of course any preexisting lung disease (many heart failure patients have a substantial smoking history, and many have chronic obstructive lung disease) yield typical changes in addition to the above lung function values.

In extreme cases, pleural fluid accumulation can occur, presumably owing to the high systemic venous pressures when right failure accompanies left heart failure. Such fluid in the intrapleural space, transudative in nature, further compromises lung expansion and may also cause alveolar collapse. Additional fluid accumulation in the abdomen (ascites) is even less common but when it occurs it tends to push the diaphragm upward (cephalad), further restricting lung expansion.

Finally, and somewhat speculatively, severe heart failure could compromise respiratory muscle function (diaphragm, intercostals), on the basis of impaired oxygen delivery. O_2 delivery is the product of muscle blood flow and arterial [O_2], and both are reduced during severe heart failure. To the extent that it occurs with advanced heart failure, it could contribute to muscle fatigue, especially if there is concurrent obstructive pulmonary disease, which increases the work of breathing.

PULMONARY BLOOD FLOW

With increasingly severe heart failure, total cardiac output may fall. In an otherwise normal subject, a fall in cardiac output (e.g., from blood loss) would lead to pulmonary arterial hypotension and inadequate or even the lack of perfusion of the lung apices. With left heart failure, however, pulmonary arterial and venous pressures rise rather than fall. This situation opposes the normal gravitationally based reduction in blood flow progressively up the lung and serves to more evenly distribute pulmonary blood flow than in health. The physiologic advantage is minimal, however, because, as explained earlier, the normal apex-to-base gradient in blood flow hardly perturbs gas exchange. The fall in cardiac output exerts its effects on lung function mostly in another way—by reducing venous [O_2] in blood returning to the lungs (discussed below).

The distribution of pulmonary blood flow can be altered locally during left heart failure by perivascular edema fluid accumulation reducing the cross-sectional area and thus the blood flow in affected pulmonary blood vessels. It is particularly likely at the lung bases due to the gravitational preponderance of fluid extravasation; it is accentuated by the loss of lung volume caused by reduced compliance. Together these changes explain an otherwise curious observation on blood flow distribution in heart failure: a zone of lower (rather than higher) blood flow at the lung bases compared to the region above the base.[18]

Hypoxic pulmonary vasoconstriction is a phenomenon in which there is constriction of small pulmonary arterial smooth muscle in response to reduced local ventilation and thus also alveolar PO_2, reducing local blood flow and tending to restore therefore the balance between local ventilation and blood flow.[19] When the pulmonary vasculature is distended by the high pressures described above, such compensatory effects may be somewhat less effective; how important hypoxic vasoconstriction is during heart failure is not clear, but systemic vasodilators such as nitroprusside clearly dilate blood vessels in areas of low PO_2.[20]

PULMONARY TRANSVASCULAR FLUID BALANCE

The most important consequence of left heart failure on the lungs is the increase in net fluid movement from the microvasculature into the alveolar interstitium, perivascular regions, and eventually the alveolar spaces. Water and protein normally move from capillaries through the peribronchial lymphatic system centrally to the hilum and back to the superior vena cava, and the conductance of this system is sufficient to prevent fluid accumulation in any of the above-mentioned lung regions. However, elevation of left ventricular diastolic filling pressures mandates similar elevation of pulmonary venous, microvascular, and pulmonary arterial pressures. At microvascular pressures of about 20 mmHg, transvascular fluid flux begins to outstrip lymph drainage capacity (Fig. 17-2), and interstitial edema develops in the alveolar wall (Fig. 17-4) and around conducting airways and pulmonary arteries (Fig. 17-3). It is believed that compression of conducting airways by peribronchial fluid accumulation may cause rhonchi (wheezing) due to turbulent airflow and thus give rise to what is described as "cardiac asthma." Additional mechanisms for wheezing may be present, however. Thus stimulation of myelinated sensory fibers in the vagus nerve produced by venous congestion or peribronchial fluid accumulation can lead to reflex bronchoconstriction and contribute to the syndrome of cardiac asthma.[13] Not until microvascular pressures increase above 25 mmHg or more does the alveolar epithelium transmit fluid into the alveoli. This event is likely associated with direct microvascular damage from the high pressure, causing cell leakage into alveoli.[4] Supporting evidence is the pink tinge of expectorated sputum, which is due to small numbers of red blood cells.

Lymph drainage is potentially compromised if right heart failure coexists with left-sided insufficiency, as right heart failure gives rise to increased systemic venous pressures, which work to oppose lymph movement from the pulmonary lymphatics into the superior vena cava. Pulmonary fluid accumulation is therefore accentuated in the presence of biventricular failure.

Although gravitational forces suggest that edema would collect preferentially in dependent lung regions, the elevation of both pulmonary arterial and venous pressures serves to make the distribution of edema less nonuniform than expected. The several well known radiologic changes in the lung fields during heart failure (prominence of upper zone blood vessels, alveolar opacities, Kerley lines) can be explained by the vascular pressure changes from normal and the consequent fluid accumulation. Clinical signs, rales in particular, can be explained by the opening and closing of small peripheral airways (containing edema fluid) with each breath. Severely impaired cardiac function can elevate venous pressures to the point of generating pleural space fluid accumulation. Such effusions are generally transudative, suggesting conformation to Starling's equation of fluid balance rather than microvascular and tissue damage resulting in an exudate.

PULMONARY GAS EXCHANGE

The combination of physiologic changes described above often lead to substantial abnormalities in pulmonary gas exchange. Local ventilation in edematous regions is typically greatly reduced, often to zero. Alveolar interstitial edema (reducing local compliance) and peribronchial edema (increasing local airways resistance) disturb the distribution of ventilation; and alveolar flooding with edema fluid creates unventilated areas (i.e., shunts). Not uncommonly, substantial fractions of the cardiac output (often 20–30 percent) still perfuse such poorly ventilated or unventilated regions, causing considerable reduction in arterial PO_2. Failure to hyperventilate would also cause arterial PCO_2 to rise somewhat; but because of the different characteristics of O_2 and CO_2 transport in blood, arterial PCO_2 would not rise by more than about 5 mmHg even when the arterial PO_2 falls by 50–60 mmHg. This small rise can be easily compensated by a minor degree of hyperventilation. The beneficial effect of this hyperventilation on arterial PO_2 would be minimal owing to the particular, nonlinear shape of the O_2-hemoglobin dissociation curve.[21] Typically, patients with heart failure (but no primary lung disease) increase ventilation more than is required to maintain normocapnia. Arterial PCO_2 values in the range of 30–35 mmHg are common and unequivocally indicate hyperventilation. Under such conditions, arterial PO_2 may be improved somewhat, but considerable residual hypoxemia is the rule (PO_2 is often in the neighborhood of 60 mmHg) because the shunts and poorly ventilated regions are still present despite overbreathing.

A particular facet of left heart failure that contributes to the severity of hypoxemia is reduced cardiac output. To maintain O_2 consumption by the various tissues in the face of a fall in cardiac output, O_2 extraction from arterial blood must increase, thereby lowering venous O_2 levels. Consequently, blood shunted past flooded alveoli in the lungs—and reflecting this reduced venous $[O_2]$—mixes with oxygenated blood coming from less affected alveoli. This more severe venous admixture leads to greater arterial hypoxemia than would have been the case had cardiac output and venous PO_2 remained normal. As a result, arterial hypoxemia reflects not only the extent of pulmonary edema but also any reduction in cardiac output; the relative contribution of the two can be difficult to identify.

Depending on individual factors, such as the extent of edema and the strength of the hypoxic pulmonary vasoconstrictor response (which can vary among patients), blood flow is reduced in poorly ventilated or unventilated alveoli. Although it somewhat attenuates the magnitude of the gas exchange defect, it never completely compensates for edema; and it has the negative effect of forcing a further increase in pulmonary artery pressure. This increase is due to the increase in total pulmonary vascular resistance, which can only worsen right ventricular function.

As a therapeutic approach to heart failure, afterload reduction with vasodilators such as nitroprusside can effectively reduce vascular pressures. Cardiac output is then significantly augmented so PO_2 in venous blood rises again toward normal. This situation would be expected to improve arterial oxygenation according to the above principles by lessening the effective venous admixture. In practice, however, little or no improvement in arterial PO_2 is seen after drugs such as nitroprusside. The reason is that, in addition to reducing systemic vascular pressures, these drugs dilate the pulmonary circulation. This dilation appears to occur preferentially in the previously most vasoconstricted areas—those that are poorly ventilated or unventilated and thus the most hypoxic. Hence blood flow through these areas increases markedly, and the fractional shunt therefore increases. The benefit of a higher venous PO_2 is offset by a larger shunt fraction; and arterial PO_2 is often unchanged from that prior to administering the drug. Note, however, that even with no change in arterial O_2 levels the increase in cardiac output means that systemic O_2 delivery to the organs is increased. This increase is generally considered beneficial, and the lack of arterial oxygenation responses are described to give pathophysiologic insight, not to argue against the use of vasodilators.

CONTROL OF BREATHING

As indicated above, most patients in heart failure hyperventilate chronically. Severe hypoxemia (arterial PO_2 below 50–60 mmHg) may be one stimulus, but it is generally agreed that additional factors must be present. Discovery of J receptors, thought to be in the alveolar wall and to be innervated by vagal nonmyelinated fibers, fire in response to distortion, congestion, and edema independently of PO_2 and are thought to play a role in hyperventilation.[11] More recently, myelinated vagal fibers emanating from so-called rapidly adapting receptors in the proximal (larger) airways have been shown to respond in a sustained fashion to peribronchial fluid accumulation in experimental animals.[13] The results are hyperventilation and an increase in bronchomotor tone (which may contribute to bronchoconstriction and the syndrome of cardiac asthma). These drives appear to be substantial as they support chronic hyperventilation and hypocapnia over long periods despite the intrinsic ventilatory inhibition provided by hypocapnia itself.

These neuronal reflexes, from several sites within the lungs, certainly can account for the dyspnea, wheezing, and hyperventilation of heart failure; but the evidence is derived mostly from animal studies. It is difficult to define their role in human heart failure with precision. Current thought is that the rapidly adapting airway receptors respond early (and in mild heart failure to peribronchial edema and venous congestion), prior to frank alveolar edema. J receptors appear unresponsive to simple venous congestion but probably augment the ventilatory response over the longer term with more severe heart failure when edema becomes marked at the alveolar level.[15]

THE HEART AND LUNG DISEASE

A large number of primary pulmonary diseases have the potential to affect cardiac function. It can be through long-term, slowly progressive disease or acutely with tumultuous, severe lung disease. The basic pathophysiologic mechanism is common to all of the lung diseases, acute or chronic, and revolves around pulmonary artery pressure elevation (due to the lung disease), which, according to severity and duration, elevates right ventricular afterload and work. As a result, the right heart hypertrophies and eventually may fail. As a part of the process, right ventricular enlargement and higher pressures can combine to restrict left ventricular function. If this happens, left ventricular filling pressures may rise and be reflected in elevated pulmonary venous pressures. In this way, pulmonary artery pressure may have to increase further, and it is possible for a vicious circle to arise.

These principles are common to most lung diseases, although the details vary with disease. The ensuing sections briefly summarize the major contributing factors to heart failure during common lung diseases and highlight the mechanisms responsible for pulmonary hypertension in each (Table 17-1).

Chronic Obstructive Pulmonary Disease

Chronic obstructive pulmonary disease (COPD) is a disease complex characterized by two distinct but usually coexistent pathologic processes: alveolar emphysema and chronic inflammation in the conducting airways.[22] Emphysema destroys alveolar walls and the capillaries within them slowly, usually over

Table 17-1. Causes of Pulmonary Hypertension in Lung Disease

Disease States	Mechanisms								
	Vasoactive Mediator Release	Vascular Destruction	Medial/Intimal Thickening	Vascular Distortion	Capillary Stretch/Compression	Loss of Radial Traction	Intravascular Thrombo-Embolism	Hypoxic Pulmonary Vasoconstriction	↑ [Hb]
COPD	−	+	+	+	+	+	−	+	+
Asthma	(+)	−	−	(+)	−	−	−	+	−
Chronic interstitial lung disease	−	+	(+)	+	−	−	−	+	+
ARDS (early phase)	(+)	−	−	−	+	−	+	+	−
Pulmonary vascular diseases	(+)	−	+	−	−	−	+	(+)	−
HAPE	(+)	−	−	−	−	−	−	+	−

Abbreviations: COPD, chronic obstructive pulmonary disease; ARDS, adult respiratory distress syndrome; HAPE, high altitude pulmonary edema; [Hb], hemoglobin concentration.

Parentheses indicate a speculative but likely role. Table as a whole indicates most common findings; individual patients may present differently.

a period of years. The process is based on protease-antiprotease imbalance.[23] Because the airways run through and are directly attached to the elastic alveolar parenchyma, alveolar wall destruction during emphysema reduces radial traction on airways and blood vessels, permitting reductions in their cross-sectional area, which in turn increases resistance to flow of blood and gas.[16]

Alveolar wall breakdown further affects the lungs by increasing lung compliance, resulting in an increase in lung volumes; this increase can stretch alveolar walls, compressing alveolar capillaries and increasing their resistance. The lack of radial airway traction causes dynamic compression of small airways during expiration, keeping alveolar pressures abnormally high, further impeding the pulmonary circulation (much as does therapeutic application of positive end-expiratory pressure in patients on assisted ventilation). Chronic airway inflammation is a chemical insult also continuing over years and often complicated by superimposed viral and bacterial infective episodes. Over time, this bronchitis causes mucous gland hyperplasia, airway mucosal edema and thickening, excess mucus secretion into the airway lumen, anatomic distortion of airway segments, and malfunction of the mucociliary clearance system in the airways. As a result, affected airways are obstructed and have a greatly reduced ability to allow ventilation of the alveoli they supply. Areas of reduced ventilation are therefore common, and the alveoli they supply are hypoxic as a result, promoting local hypoxic vasoconstriction. There is also evidence of pulmonary vascular medial and intimal thickening, which likely contributes to pulmonary hypertension.[24–27] Finally, secondary polycythemia can occur in COPD patients owing to tissue hypoxia and erythropoietin release.

Factors that increase pulmonary vascular resistance in COPD and thus cause pulmonary hypertension are evidently several.[28,29]

1. Reduced microvascular number from emphysematous alveolar wall destruction
2. Loss of radial traction on pulmonary arteries from emphysema
3. Compression/stretch of alveolar capillaries due to hyperinflation
4. Hypoxic pulmonary vasoconstriction in poorly ventilated areas
5. Vascular distortion from the pathologic processes in COPD
6. Medial and intimal thickening of pulmonary arteries
7. Increased blood viscosity in those patients with high hemoglobin concentration

Clinically, the more hypoxic patients who tend to develop hypercapnia, sometimes referred to as "type B,"[30] are more prone to pulmonary hypertension and right heart failure than their less hypoxemic hyperventilating "type A" counterparts. Episodes of peripheral edema and weight gain typically accompany infective exacerbations in COPD and are evidence of decompensating right heart function.

Cardiac function in such patients may well be compromised by two additional factors compounding the effects of pulmonary hypertension: COPD is accompanied by arterial hypoxemia, sometimes severe, which reduces O_2 delivery to an already overburdened right ventricle. Second, COPD is caused by cigarette smoking in most patients. Cigarette smoking per se increases the risk of coronary artery disease, potentially limiting blood flow to the myocardium. O_2 delivery is compromised therefore by limitations to both arterial O_2 concentration and coronary artery flow, yet O_2 demand is elevated owing to pulmonary hypertension.

The above makes it all the more surprising that right heart failure is not as frequent as might be expected. Although more common in the type B patient as a chronic complication, it tends to be a near-terminal, end-stage event in the type A COPD patient. Note, however, that even in the absence of any clinical evidence of right heart failure in such patients, their pulmonary artery pressure responses to even light exercise are excessive.[31] This is true even if resting pulmonary artery pressures are within normal limits. The message of Figure 17-1 is worth keeping in mind: For vessel destruction to significantly raise pulmonary artery pressures, a large fraction of the circulation must be affected.

Asthma

Asthma is a disease of excessive immunologic and inflammatory response of the airways to one or more of a variety of stimuli. The results are obstruction in potentially all airways from the bronchi to the smallest bronchioles, reducing local ventilation. The alveoli per se are normal (in the absence of complications such as pneumonia). The mechanisms of obstruction are smooth muscle contraction, airway wall thickening from inflammation, and excessive, tenacious, mucus plugging of the airways. This plugging can be extensive, resulting in marked hypoxemia and hypoxic pulmonary vasoconstriction. As a result, a degree of pulmonary hypertension can develop. Although right heart failure can occur with asthma, it is uncommon, despite arterial hypoxemia and pulmonary hypertension. This is probably because (1) there is no vascular destruction, (2) most asthmatic patients are relatively young with intrinsically good cardiac and coronary artery function, and (3) asthma is typically periodic with remissions interrupting exacerbations that, if well managed, can be short. Thus the load on the right ventricle is not as severe or continuous as in COPD patients. The presence of right heart failure in asthma is therefore evidence of the extreme severity of the disease process.

Interstitial Lung Disease

The development of right heart failure in individuals with interstitial lung disease is not generally as well recognized as in those with COPD, but it is equally devastating and commonly a cause of death. Interstitial lung disease is here considered to be the end result of any of more than 100 inflammatory processes of various causes: infections, immunologic, toxic, and idiopathic.[32] Despite recognizable variations in acute inflammatory pathology, there is a final common pathway of interstitial fibrosis at the alveolar level. Aggressive deposition of collagen occurs, destroying alveoli and their capillaries, severely distorting the remaining blood vessels as the connective tissue strands change length, and creating noncompliant alveoli that are therefore poorly ventilated if at all. Lung volumes are reduced, but radial traction on large airways and blood vessels is, if anything, greater than normal, preventing their collapse and facilitating gas and blood flow. Small vessels buried deep in thick fibrous alveolar wall remnants act as shunts, not permitting O_2 exchange. Local hypoxia results from the poorly or unventilated areas, contributing to pulmonary hypertension through hypoxic vasoconstriction. Finally, secondary polycythemia can develop in these patients owing to chronic arterial hypoxemia.

Although the detailed pathology is different from that in COPD, pulmonary hypertension develops for many of the same reasons.

1. Reduced capillary number due to alveolar wall destruction
2. Hypoxic pulmonary vasoconstriction in poorly ventilated areas
3. Vascular distortion from the scarring process of collagen deposition
4. Increased blood viscosity when the hemoglobin concentration is elevated

Because progression of the interstitial fibrosis is commonly rapid, so too can be the development of right heart failure. Unlike patients with COPD, most patients with interstitial fibrosis develop right heart failure as the disease advances.

Adult Respiratory Distress Syndrome

Adult respiratory distress syndrome (ARDS) is a complex disease state of acute, diffuse lung damage (to previously normal lungs) usually resulting in severe respiratory failure, multiorgan dysfunction, and a high incidence of fatal outcome. Many causes exist, the most common being severe pulmonary or systemic viral or bacterial infections, severe trauma, and major surgery. Irrespective of the primary causes, the basic pathologic responses are clinically similar and involve widespread inflammation at the alveolar level. There is alveolar wall edema and much fluid and cell debris filling substantial numbers of alveoli. This acute state, if survived, can resolve completely or progress to a diffuse fibrotic lung disease. Right ventricular function can be compromised during the acute stages for several reasons. Metabolic rate and cardiac output are usually and persistently elevated to about twice resting levels, with metabolic acidosis frequently present as well. Because of the extent of the disease, alveolar filling and collapse cause substantial hypoxic vasoconstriction and vascular distortion. Although their role is speculative, a host of vasoactive inflammatory cytokines are present and may contribute to vascular smooth muscle contraction and thus pulmonary hypertension.

Physical vascular obstruction due to local small vessel thrombosis is common and further elevates vascular resistance, as may emboli from systemic venous sites. The aggressive ventilatory strategies used to maintain oxygenation result in overdistension of the more normal alveoli, which increases their capillaries' vascular resistance due to vessel compression and stretch. Such ventilatory patterns also reduce cardiac output and may increase O_2 demand for a heart already working substantially harder than normal. Finally, cardiac function may be perturbed by the cellular damaging processes of ARDS itself.

Thus with this syndrome the cardiac work requirement is increased, cardiac function may be compromised by the disease process, and several pulmonary mechanical factors increase pulmonary vascular resistance. One should not be surprised, especially in the older patient with a smoking history, to see evidence of right ventricular dysfunction and even failure develop in association with ARDS.

Pulmonary Vascular Diseases

Pulmonary thromboembolic disease from distant venous thrombotic sites is a common disease complex in susceptible patients (those who are inactive, are hypercoagulable, or have some coexistent vascular inflammatory or traumatic process). Primary pulmonary hypertension is a much less common but also potentially fatal disease of the pulmonary vasculature.[33] Pulmonary hypertension, often severe, results from vascular obstruction, which in turn is due to anatomic vascular occlusion by emboli (or to lumen reduction by vessel wall hypertrophy in primary pulmonary hypertension). With acute thromboembolism, there may be additional factors that further increase vascular pressures: vasoactive cytokines released presumably due to endothelial damage from emboli. Just which factors are important will be difficult to establish in human disease.

Severe vascular obstruction can cause right heart failure quickly, reducing cardiac output and thus coronary artery blood flow. Arterial hypoxemia, caused by mismatching of ventilation, and blood flow in the lungs due to the emboli, explains the occasional myocardial ischemic chest pain pattern seen in some patients with emboli. This pain must of course be differentiated from the more classic pleuritic chest pain due to pleural inflammation caused by a peripheral embolic event.

It is well worth again remembering the tremendous vascular reserve of the normal human lung (Fig. 17-1): Pulmonary artery pressure may increase by only 5–10 mmHg when fully half of the vasculature is obstructed.[5] The basis of this, as explained earlier, is the potential for both recruitment of unperfused capillaries and distension of the remainder, permitting large reductions in pulmonary vascular resistance as pressures rise. Thus when pulmonary vascular pressures are clearly elevated, the degree of vascular obstruction must be substantial.

High Altitude Pulmonary Edema

High altitude pulmonary edema (HAPE), a unique, uncommon syndrome, is one of patchy pulmonary edema developing at high altitude in the absence of specific causes, such as coronary insufficiency/left heart failure, or pulmonary infectious or inflammatory agents.[34] The cause is hypoxia, and the cure is restoration of normoxia. The syndrome is more likely to occur when altitude ascent is too rapid and if vigorous exercise is performed early on arrival at that altitude. Left ventricular failure as the primary cause is excluded by normal ventricular filling pressures as inferred from pulmonary arterial wedge pressure recordings. Susceptible patients studied after complete recovery as a group, show an exaggerated pulmonary vasoconstrictor response to hypoxia.[35] Data suggest elevated left ventricular filling pressures during exercise (but not at rest).[36] Whereas the former may have a genetic basis, high wedge pressures may reflect normal extremes of left ventricular stiffness or may be the result of pulmonary hypertension and its effects on the right ventricle impeding left ventricular function through ventricular interdependence.

Consequently, it remains uncertain if HAPE is purely a problem of the hypoxic vasoconstrictor response or contains an element of abnormal left ventricular performance that requires high filling pressures, which cause pulmonary microvascular hypertension and hence edema. A role for the left ventricle is suggested by the observation that left ventricular filling pressures in HAPE-susceptible subjects are elevated to the same degree in normoxia as in hypoxia.[36] It is clear, however, that as HAPE occurs within hours of reaching the altitude the erythrocytosis of altitude, which takes days to weeks to become established, cannot be a contributing factor.

REFERENCES

1. Weibel ER: Morphometry of Human Lung. Springer-Verlag, Berlin, 1963
2. West JB: Ventilation/Blood Flow and Gas Exchange. 5th Ed. Blackwell Scientific, Oxford, 1990
3. Harris P, Heath D: The Human Pulmonary Circulation. Its Form and Function in Health and Disease. E&S Livingstone, Edinburgh, 1962
4. West JB, Mathieu-Costello O: Strength of the pulmonary blood-gas barrier. Respir Physiol 1992;88:141
5. Wilson III JE, Pierce AK, Johnson RL Jr et al: Hypoxemia in pulmonary embolism. A clinical study. J Clin Invest 1971;50:481
6. Guyton AC: Textbook of Medical Physiology. 8th Ed. WB Saunders, Philadelphia, 1991
7. Guyton AC, Lindsey AW: Effect of elevated left atrial pressure and decreased plasma protein concentration on the development of pulmonary edema. Circ Res 1959;7:649
8. Meyer EC: Acute and chronic clearance of lung fluids, proteins, and cells. p. 277. In Staub NC (ed): Lung Water and Solute Exchange. Vol. 7. Marcel Dekker, New York, 1978
9. Low FN: Lung interstitium: development, morphology, fluid content. p. 17. In Staub NC (ed): Lung Water and Solute Exchange. Vol. 7. Marcel Dekker, New York, 1978
10. Staub NC: Pathophysiology of pulmonary edema. p. 719. In Staub NC, Taylor AE (eds): Edema. Lippincott-Raven, Philadelphia, 1984

11. Paintal AS: Mechanism of stimulation of type J pulmonary receptors. J Physiol (Lond) 1969;203:511

12. Sellick H, Widdicombe JG: The activity of lung irritant receptors during pneumothorax, hyperpnoea and pulmonary vascular congestion. J Physiol (Lond) 1969;203:359

13. Ravi K, Kappagoda CT: Reflex effects of pulmonary venous congestion. Role of vagal afferents. NIPS 1990;5:95

14. Paterson DJ: Potassium and ventilation in exercise. J Appl Physiol 1992;72:811

15. Coleridge HM, Coleridge JCG: Pulmonary reflexes. Neural mechanisms of pulmonary defense. Annu Rev Physiol 1994;56:69

16. West JB: Pulmonary Pathophysiology. The Essentials. 3rd Ed. Williams & Wilkins, Baltimore, 1987

17. Hubmayr RD, Rodarte JR: Cellular effects and physiologic responses. Lung mechanics. p. 79. In Cherniack NS (ed): Chronic Obstructive Pulmonary Disease. WB Saunders, Philadelphia, 1991

18. Hughes JMB: Distribution of pulmonary blood flow. p. 1135. In Crystal RG, West JB, Barnes PJ, Cherniack NS, Weibel ER (eds): The Lung: Scientific Foundations. Vol. 1. Lippincott-Raven, Philadelphia, 1991

19. Rodman DM, Voelkel NF: Regulation of vascular tone. p. 1105. In Crystal RA, West JB, Barnes PJ, Cherniack NS, Weibel ER (eds): The Lung. Scientific Foundations. Vol. 1. Lippincott-Raven, Philadelphia, 1991

20. Bencowitz HZ, LeWinter MM, Wagner PD: Effect of sodium nitroprusside on ventilation/perfusion mismatching in heart failure. J Am Coll Cardiol 1984;4:918

21. West JB: Ventilation/perfusion inequality and overall gas exchange in computer models of the lung. Respir Physiol 1969;7:88

22. Thurlbeck WM: Pathology of chronic airflow obstruction. p. 3. In Cherniack NS (ed): Chronic Obstructive Pulmonary Disease. WB Saunders, Philadelphia, 1991

23. Hoidal JR, McCusker KT, Marshall BC, Rao NV: Oxidative damage and COPD. p. 44. In Cherniack NS (ed): Chronic Obstructive Pulmonary Disease. WB Saunders, Philadelphia, 1991

24. Lamb D: Pathology of COPD. p. 497 In Brewis RAL, Gibson GJ, Geddes DM (eds): Respiratory Medicine. Baillière Tindall, London, 1990

25. Wilkinson M, Langhorn CA, Heath D, Barer GR, Howard P: A pathophysiological study of 10 cases of hypoxic cor pulmonale. Q J Med 1988;66:65

26. Wright JL, Lawson L, Paré PD et al: The structure and function of pulmonary vasculature in mild chronic obstructive pulmonary disease. The effect of oxygen on exercise. Am Rev Respir Dis 1983;128:702

27. Magee F, Wright JL, Wiggs BR, Paré PD, Hogg JC: Pulmonary vascular structure and function in chronic obstructive pulmonary disease. Thorax 1988;43:183

28. MacNee W: Pathophysiology of cor pulmonale in chronic obstructive pulmonary disease. Part one. Am J Respir Crit Care Med 1994;150:833

29. MacNee W: Pathophysiology of cor pulmonale in chronic obstructive pulmonary disease. Part two. Am J Respir Crit Care Med 1994;150:1158

30. Burrows B, Fletcher CM, Heard BE et al: The emphysematous and bronchial types of chronic airways obstruction. A clinicopathological study of patients in London and Chicago. Lancet 1966;1:830

31. Szidon JP: The effect of COPD on pulmonary circulation. p. 101. In Cherniack NS (ed): Chronic Obstrictive Pulmonary Disease. WB Saunders, Philadelphia, 1991

32. Fishman AP: Pulmonary Diseases and Disorders. 2nd Ed. McGraw-Hill, New York, 1988

33. Voelkel N, Reeves JT: Primary pulmonary hypertension. p. 573. In Moser KM (ed): Pulmonary Vascular Diseases. Vol. 14. Marcel Dekker, New York, 1979

34. Ward MP, Milledge JS, West JB: High altitude pulmonary edema (HAPE). p. 383. In: High Altitude Medicine and Physiology. University of Pennsylvania Press, Philadelphia, 1989

35. Hultgren HN, Grover RF, Hartley LH: Abnormal circulatory responses to high altitude in subjects with a previous history of high altitude pulmonary edema. Circulation 1971;44:759

36. Wagner PD, Eldridge MW, Podolsky A et al: Elevated wedge pressure in HAPE-susceptible subjects during exercise. pp. 251–264. In Sutton JR, Houston CS, Coates G (eds): Hypoxia and the Brain. Queen City Printers, Burlington, Vermont, 1995

18 Syndrome of Cardiac Cachexia

Stefan D. Anker
Andrew J. S. Coats

Cachexia is a severe complication of several chronic diseases, including cancer, acquired immunodeficiency syndrome (AIDS), thyrotoxicosis, and rheumatoid arthritis. It has long been recognized that significant weight loss and wasting are also important features of severe chronic heart failure (CHF), dating back 2300 years to the time of classical Greece and the school of medicine of Hippocrates (about 460–370 BC) on the island of Cos: "The flesh is consumed and becomes water . . . the shoulders, clavicles, chest and thighs melt away. This illness is fatal . . . ."[1] In 1785 Withering wrote of a patient with dropsy: "his countenance was pale, his pulse quick and feeble, his body greatly emaciated, except his belly, which was very large."[2]

Although the syndrome of cardiac cachexia is well recognized by clinicians, little research into the pathophysiology of cardiac cachexia has been carried out. One major problem is the lack of an objective, widely accepted definition of cachexia. Research concerning CHF has focused on the peripheral changes that complicate it. Loss of strength and muscle atrophy, decreased oxidative capacity, and structural changes in skeletal muscle have been described. These patients fatigue more easily than healthy controls. The nutritive blood flow to the skeletal muscle is reduced in CHF, attributable to altered vasomotor tone, diminished responses to vasodilators, or increased circulating levels of vasoconstrictors. Most of these results were gained studying CHF populations that included cachectic as well as noncachectic CHF patients, so the relative importance of the atrophic state to the genesis of these changes remains unknown (see Ch. 16.

DEFINITION OF CARDIAC CACHEXIA

There is still no accepted definition of cachexia. Several approaches are possible. Body fat estimation and anthropometric measurements (skinfold thickness, arm muscle circumference), calculations of predicted percent ideal mass matched for sex, age, and height (usually using data of the Metropolitan Life Insurance Tables from 1959[3] or the Build Study from 1979[4]), and scores including serum albumin concentrations, cell-mediated immunity changes, weight/height index or body mass index (weight/height^2), and the history of weight loss have been used. In one study patients were classified as "malnourished" when the body fat content was less than 22 percent in women and less than 15 percent for men or when the individual was less than 90 percent of ideal weight.[5] Other groups have defined CHF patients prospectively as "cachectic" when the body fat content was less than 29 percent (females) or less than 27 percent (males),[6] or when the weight was less than 85 percent of ideal body weight[7] or even less than 80 percent.[8] It is also possible to characterize the lean tissue by studying urinary creatinine excretion rates, skeletal muscle protein turnover using labeled amino acids, bioelectrical impedance, or total body potassium content. Skeletal muscle size can be directly estimated by means of magnetic resonance imaging (MRI), computed tomography (CT), or body densiometry; but for few of these methods is there an accepted threshold defined as cachectic.

The development of the cachectic state in CHF is a process that can only be proved by an unintentional documented weight loss measured in a nonedematous state. Including weight loss as a criterion excludes patients who are constitutionally underweight. Until an accepted definition is established, "clinical cardiac cachexia" is likely to refer to severe symptomatic loss of lean body mass.

In patients with CHF of at least 6 months duration without signs of other primary cachectic states (e.g., cancer, thyroid disease, or severe liver disease), the following two major criteria should be fulfilled: (1) documented unintentional nonedematous weight loss of at least 5 kg; and (2) a body mass index (BMI) of less than 24 kg/m^2. The body mass index (weight/height^2) represents lean tissue and fat tissue,[9] which is useful in CHF patients, as cardiac cachectic patients suffer from a loss of muscle (i.e., protein reserves) and fat (i.e., energy reserves). The criterion of a BMI of less than 24 also excludes previously obese patients who could have lost weight intentionally. The introduction of a third criterion (i.e., less than 85 percent of ideal weight) may identify a more "severe" level of cardiac cachexia.

It has been suggested that a documented loss of at least 10 percent of lean tissue should be used as the major criterion to define cardiac cachexia[10]; the disadvantage of this criterion is that not all cardiologists have access to facilities that allow prospective measurements of lean body mass. Any of these definitions remains to some degree arbitrary. An important goal of future studies on cardiac cachexia is to define criteria that allow reliable detection of cardiac cachexia in its early stages.

EPIDEMIOLOGY

There is no comprehensive study on the epidemiology of cardiac cachexia. Studies on CHF suggest that with an increasing proportion of elderly people in the population CHF increases in frequency, reaching a prevalence of up to 30 percent in the over-80-year-olds.[11] It has been shown that up to 50 percent of CHF patients are to some degree malnourished.[5] In our CHF clinic, as many as 15 percent of the patients develop cachexia during the course of their heart disease. The loss of lean tissue predicts the prognosis for cancer and AIDS.[12] It has been found that it is incompatible with life to lose more than 40 percent

of lean tissue.[13] The natural and perioperative morbidity and mortality of patients with cardiac cachexia is increased compared to that of non-cachectic CHF patients.[8,14] This unfavorable subgroup prognosis may largely contribute to the overall adverse prognosis of CHF. Most cachectic CHF patients are over 40 years old, have had CHF for at least 5 years, and are New York Heart Association (NYHA) functional classes III and IV. The NYHA class, however, does not correlate well with disease morbidity or mortality in cardiac cachexia.[15] Nevertheless, cardiac cachexia may also occur during childhood related to malnutrition or malabsorption diseases (i.e., kwashiorkor or marasmus).

PATHOGENESIS AND PATHOPHYSIOLOGY

Historically, three mechanisms were thought to be responsible for the development of cardiac cachexia; (1) malabsorption and metabolic malfunction; (2) dietary deficiency; and (3) loss of nutrients via the urinary or digestive tracts. Pittman and Cohen were in 1964 the first to analyze extensively the pathogenesis of the syndrome of cardiac cachexia.[16] In general, they thought that the development of cellular hypoxia was the leading pathogenic factor, causing less efficient intermediary metabolism, which in turn produced increased catabolism (protein loss) and reduced anabolism. Additionally, they suggested that anorexia and an increased basal metabolic rate were closely related and possibly in part the result of a lack of oxygen.

Anorexia can be related to heart failure via intestinal edema, which causes nausea, a protein-losing gastroenteropathy, or both. Additionally, anorexia may be iatrogenic, as a side effect of digitalis use, sodium-restricted diets, and some angiotensin-converting enzyme (ACE) inhibitors. To test this hypothesis, in 1977 Buchanan and colleagues performed a study in 11 cachectic patients (NYHA class IV, mitral valve disease, pre- and postoperative assessment).[17] Most commonly, they found marked anorexia (reversible) to be the cause of the cachectic state. Neither malabsorption (D-xylose absorption test) nor cellular hypoxia (assessed by lactate and pyruvate concentration) was of importance in their patients.

Simple starvation and anorexia in otherwise healthy persons can lead preferentially to a loss of fat tissue. A study in 27 CHF patients (mean weight 21 percent lower than normal) in 1979[18] failed to show fat tissue loss but documented an average total body potassium decrease of 35 percent (measure of lean tissue independent of body water content). Another study[19] demonstrated increased resting metabolic rates in CHF patients compared to controls. The resting metabolic rates have been shown to correlate with increasing concentrations of catecholamines.[20] Because of these strikingly different views Ansari stated in his 1987 review[21] that it appeared unlikely that a single physical or biochemical disorder causes cardiac cachexia.

Physical inactivity and deconditioning have been suggested to be important to the muscle atrophy observed in many CHF patients,[22] but recent histologic evidence suggests that the atrophy in states of reduced activity is significantly different from the atrophy observed with CHF.[23,24] Therefore it seems unlikely that physical inactivity is of great importance to the genesis of cardiac cachexia.

BIOCHEMICAL BASIS OF CACHEXIA

As early as the 1930s it was suggested that an unexplained pyrogen as a product of anaerobic metabolism may exist in cases of fever associated with heart failure.[25] Could low grade fever, increased basal metabolic rate, local hypoxia, and anorexia be related by common factors? Several immunologic interactions at the cellular level might be involved in the development of cardiac cachexia. In 1990 it was reported by Levine and colleagues that tumor necrosis factor α (TNFα) is increased in patients in cardiac cachexia,[7] which was subsequently confirmed by others.[6,26] TNFα is one of the key cytokines important to the development of catabolism together with interleukin 1 (IL-1), IL-6, interferon γ, and transforming growth factor β. Two studies failed to show increased levels of IL-1 or IL-6 in CHF patients,[27,28] but we were able to demonstrate increased levels of IL-1 and IL-6 in cachectic versus noncachectic patients with CHF (unpublished data). Multiple factors increase or decrease the effects of TNFα. In animal experiments it has been shown that skeletal muscle cachexia occurs when TNFα-producing tumor cells are implanted in skeletal muscle; and TNFα-producing cells in the brain caused profound anorexia.[29] These results show that (1) the site of the production and action of TNFα modifies its effect and (2) increased levels of TNFα may indeed play a causative role in the genesis of cachexia.

No reported data show different immune activation status in CHF due to ischemic or dilated cardiomyopathy, so the initial stimulus triggering the immune activation seems to lie in changes due to the abnormalities of heart failure itself. The following TNFα-stimulating processes are known.

1. When the peripheral blood flow is reduced in CHF it certainly could produce local ischemic and hypoxic states, causing macrophage stimulation. Indeed the maximal vasodilating capacity in patients with CHF (i.e., their peak leg blood flow measured by means of plethysmography) is inversely related to the plasma levels of TNFα.[30]
2. Prostaglandin E_2 has been found to be increased in patients with severe CHF[31] and can stimulate the release of TNFα.[32]
3. The failing human heart can produce TNFα.[33]

The TNFα has many biologic actions in endothelial cells, including rearrangement of the cytoskeleton, increased permeability to albumin and water, enhanced expression of activation antigens, induction of surface procoagulant activity, and IL-1 release.[34] TNFα is known to reduce constitutive nitric oxide (NO) synthase mRNA in vascular endothelial cells.[35] These actions could impair endothelial function. Therefore the observed inverse relation between maximal peripheral blood flow and TNFα levels in CHF patients (regardless of disease etiology and functional status[30]) could reflect the detrimental action of long-term increases in TNFα. It is also known that TNFα can induce NO production via inducible NO synthase (iNOS), therefore contributing to vasodilation.[36] These phenomena could be explained by differing short-term (activation of iNOS) and long-term (inhibition of the constitutive NO synthase) effects of TNFα.[30,37]

The TNFα has been shown to be increased in cachectic CHF patients prospectively defined, but TNFα levels in noncachectic CHF patients and healthy controls were similar[38] (Table 18-1). The immune activation was accompanied by increased human growth hormone, aldosterone, and plasma renin activity, whereas the levels of insulin (a strong anabolic factor) were found to be reduced in cachectic CHF patients compared to noncachectic patients, although the two groups showed similar degrees of insulin resistance (unpublished data). In addition to muscle and fat tissue loss, we demonstrated reduced total bone mass and bone density in cachectic CHF patients, which was correlated to the overall degree of atrophy (percentage ideal body weight) and increased catabolic factors (TNFα and cortisol).[39] Therefore it is concluded that the development of cardiac cachexia is closely related to immune activation and neurohormonal dysfunction caused by the pathophysiologic changes of heart failure. These changes cause increased catabolism and reduced anabolism

Table 18-1. Plasma Hormones and TNFα in Cachectic and Noncachectic CHF Patients and Healthy Controls

Substance Measured	cCHF (n = 16)	ncCHF (n = 37)	Con (n = 16)	P Value cCHF vs. ncCHF	P Value cCHF vs. Con	P Value ncCHF vs. Con
TNFα (pg/ml)	15.3 ± 3.1	6.9 ± 0.8	7.0 ± 0.7	0.0009	0.014	NS
hGH (ng/ml)	3.8 ± 1.6	0.9 ± 0.3	1.1 ± 0.4	0.012	0.11	NS
PRA (ng/ml/h)	17.0 ± 3.7	9.2 ± 2.2	7.9 ± 0.2	0.063	0.0002	0.021
Aldost (pmol/L)	1039 ± 227	552 ± 77	279 ± 42	0.013	0.003	0.028
IGF-1 (nmol/L)	137 ± 13	149 ± 9	148 ± 11	NS	NS	NS

TNFα, tumor necrosis factor α; hGH, human growth hormone; PRA, plasma renin activity; Aldost, aldosterone; IGF-1: insulin-like growth factor-1; C, cachectic; nc, noncachectic; Con, controls.

and may partially explain the anorexia observed in some patients.

DIAGNOSIS

In addition to the routine investigative procedures recommended for patients with CHF, an important part of diagnosing cardiac cachexia is recognition of the cachectic process, which should be not problematic. The detection of cardiac cachexia in a CHF patient means that this patient is at increased risk of death. Because of these prognostic implications we emphasize the importance of a carefully documented *weight history* (weight taken regularly in a nonedematous state) for all CHF patients who are under a follow-up regimen. It is an easy and worthwhile task. It is additionally important to document the weight changes during in-hospital stays in discharge letters, along with assessments of lean and ideal body weight.

Obvious weight changes are often accompanied by signs of severe heart failure (hyponatremia and increased catecholamines, aldosterone, plasma renin activity, and creatinine), chronic inflammation (slightly increased C-reactive protein and erythrocyte sedimentation rate), malnutrition (decreased serum transferrin and serum triglyceride), and other nonspecific signs (lymphopenia and cutaneous anergy) and more rarely hypoalbuminemia and total hypoproteinemia are found.

Cardiac cachectic patients can have biventricular heart failure, and a predominant right ventricular component is thought to be more common in these patients.[40] Interestingly, increased right atrial pressure was the only independent predictor of malnutrition in 24 of 48 investigated patients with severe congestive heart failure.[5] In this study the cardiac index and pulmonary capillary wedge pressure had been similar in malnourished and well nourished patients.

Additional laboratory procedures are necessary to evaluate heart failure in cachectic patients (electrocardiogram, echocardiogram, nuclear scan, radiograph). They should be used simultaneously to exclude cancer and evaluate the organic changes related to heart failure and wasting (e.g., chest radiograph and ultrasonography of the abdomen). It is recommended that body composition be assessed in those with cardiac cachexia by means of dual energy x-ray absorptiometry (DEXA), as it allows simultaneous measurement of lean, fat, and bone tissue. It is an excellent follow-up tool, as it is fast and reasonably inexpensive, provides accurate information, and exposes the patient to only a minimal amount of radiation.

The relevance of serial assessments of plasma hormones such as insulin, human growth hormone, and IGF-1, is unknown, but the prognostic value of other hormones, such as plasma catecholamines and endothelin-1,[41] have been demonstrated. Two immunologic factors have already been demonstrated to be of independent prognostic value for patient survival. Elevated levels of soluble intercellular adhesion molecule-1 (sICAM-1), above 230 ng/ml, predicted patient mortality ($P = 0.001$),[41] as did plasma concentrations of soluble vascular cell adhesion molecule-1 above 830 ng/ml.[42] In the later study (86 CHF patients) increased TNFα levels also predicted mortality during this 2-year follow-up but was not of independent predictive value. Dutka and colleagues[26] found that TNFα had no predictive value in their clinically stable CHF patients, but only two of nine patients in the follow-up were malnourished here. We found TNFα levels in 16 cachectic CHF patients to be correlated to the total amount of documented weight loss ($r = 0.79$, $P < 0.001$[38]).

THERAPEUTIC MANAGEMENT

There are several therapeutic strategies for management of cardiac cachexia. Basically, the nutritional status must be improved, the lean tissue must be increased, and anticytokine therapy may prove feasible. Except for pre- and postoperative nutritional support of cardiac cachectic patients, there are no controlled studies for the outcome of the various therapeutic strategies in these patients.

Nutritional Support

Although increased nutritional support might increase the oxidative demands of the body, it was shown that it is safe in cardiac cachectic patients and can lead to an increased amount of lean tissue.[43] In stable CHF patients with no signs of severe malnutrition nutritional support alone had no significant effect on the clinical status of heart failure.[44] This strategy is of great importance during the pre- and postoperative phases when surgery must be performed. Immediate postoperative intravenous hyperalimentation alone did not improve survival in one study,[14] whereas a study of the factors associated with operative mortality due to mitral or tricuspid disease revealed that patients with preoperative support (5–8 weeks duration, intravenously up to 1200 kcal/day) was associated with a mortality of 17 percent compared with 57 percent for those without nutritional support ($P < 0.05$[8]). Other authors[14] have suggested providing 40–50 kcal/m^2 body surface per hour, including protein (1.5–2.0 g/kg per hour), and restricting the supplementation to 2 g sodium per day and 1000–1500 ml/day using high density continuous feeding. In any case (especially for stable, ambulant cachectic patients) the consultation of dietitians could be helpful. In view of the side effect of anorexia, digitalis should be used carefully and levels monitored frequently. Also some ACE inhibitors (especially captopril) can impair taste and exacerberate anorexia.

Exercise

Reduced peripheral blood flow, metabolic abnormalities, and atrophy of skeletal muscle, which contribute to exertional fatigue in CHF, can be reversed by exercise rehabilitation training and result in increased exercise capacity and anaerobic threshold.[45,46] We have found that moderate exercise training could safely be applied to NYHA class I–III cachectic CHF patients. It can certainly increase the status of daily physical activity. We have demonstrated that peak leg blood flow, rather than muscle size and strength, is the best predictor of exercise capacity in cardiac cachectic patients, whereas strength and age are the best predictors in noncachectic patients.[47] Whether it has implications for rehabilitation therapy (e.g., the use of physiotherapeutic procedures to increase peripheral perfusion before beginning any exercise program) has not yet been studied.

Drugs

For sepsis and rheumatoid arthritis nonspecific drugs (corticosteroids, pentoxifylline, hydralazine sulfate) and specific drugs (monoclonal antibodies or soluble receptors against TNFα and IL-1 receptor antagonists) have been shown to reduce cytokine activity and partly inhibit their biologic effects. Most interestingly, fish oil (n-3 polyunsaturated fatty acids) has been shown to reduce TNFα and IL-1 in healthy volunteers (also with documented reduction of prostaglandin E$_2$[48]) and patients with rheumatic disease (with low levels of leukotriene B$_4$ documented[49]). The mode of action could be via the inhibition of arachidonic pathways.[48]

In cachectic CHF patients specific anticytokine therapy has not yet been studied. In animal experiments of sepsis the administration of soluble TNFα receptors improved hemodynamic performance and could reduce cytokine induction.[50] Increased levels of these soluble TNFα receptors have been found in CHF patients with advanced heart failure,[51,52] and they relate to disease severity.[28,52] As these soluble receptors can neutralize the effects of TNFα, it seems interesting to suggest testing the effects of these antibodies and soluble receptors in cardiac cachectic patients. There are no animal studies in this area reported to date, however, and one study showed that CHF patients with high levels of soluble TNFα receptors had a markedly increased 30-day mortality.[52] Whether these receptors play a causative role, are only a highly sensitive marker of disease severity, or are perhaps not even high enough in these patients with fatal outcome is not clear.

Many physiologic and humoral alterations have been described in patients with severe CHF and cardiac cachexia, and many more may be discovered soon. Changing one or two cytokines by any therapeutic approach may be a major step in the right direction, but it seems doubtful that it can cure the cachectic syndrome. Extending the scope of the neurohormonal hypothesis,[53] we regard cardiac cachexia as a neurohormonal disease with an imbalance of catabolism and anabolism as well as changed immune-activating and immune-suppressing conditions.

We regard this area of heart research as one of the most interesting, and it requires a joint effort from cardiologists, endocrinologists, and immunologists. The aim of current research is to address cachexia directly and specifically. Enhancing the prognosis of individuals with cardiac cachexia or even reversing the cachectic process will have significant influence on the quality of life of many patients and may improve the long-term prognosis of CHF overall.

REFERENCES

1. Katz AM, Katz PB: Diseases of heart in works of Hippocrates. Br Heart J 1962;24:257–264
2. Aronson JK: An Account of the Foxglove and Its Medical Uses pp. 11–100. Oxford University Press, London, 1985
3. New Weight Standards for Men and Women. Statistical Bulletin. Metropolitan Life Insurance Company, New York, 1959
4. Build Study, 1979. Society of Actuaries and Association of Life Insurance Medical Directors of America. Recording and Statistical Corporation, Philadelphia, 1980
5. Carr JG, Stevenson LW, Walden JA, Heber D: Prevalence and hemodynamic correlates of malnutrition in severe congestive heart failure secondary to ischemic or ideopathic dilated cardiomyopathy. Am J Cardiol 1989;63:709–713
6. McMurray J, Abdullah I, Dargie HJ, Shapiro D: Increased concentrations of tumor necrosis factor in "cachectic" patients with severe chronic heart failure. Br Heart J 1991;66:356–358
7. Levine B, Kalman J, Mayer L, Fillit HM, Packer M: Elevated circulating levels of tumor necrosis factor in severe chronic heart failure. N Engl J Med 1990;323: 236–241
8. Otaki M: Surgical treatment of patients with cardiac cachexia. An analysis of factors affecting operative mortality. Chest 1994;105:1347–1351
9. Garn SM, Leonard WR, Hawthorne VM: Three limitations of the body mass index. Am J Clin Nutr 1986; 44:996–997
10. Freeman LM, Roubenoff R: The nutrition implications of cardiac cachexia. Nutr Rev 1994;52:340–347
11. Kannel WB, Belanger AJ: Epidemiology of heart failure. Am Heart J 1991;121:951–957
12. Kotler DP, Tiermey AR, Wang J, Pierson RN: Magnitude of body cell mass depletion and the timing of death from wasting in AIDS. Am J Clin Nutr 1989;50: 444–447
13. Roubenoff R, Kehayias JJ: The meaning and measurement of lean body mass. Nutr Rev 1991;49:163–175
14. Abel RM, Fischer J, Buckley MJ, Barnett GO, Austen WG: Malnutrition in cardiac surgical patients. Arch Surg 1976;111:45–50
15. Blackburn GL, Gibbons GW, Bothe A et al: Nutritional support in cardiac cachexia. J Thoracic Cardiovasc Surg 1977;73:489–495
16. Pittman JG, Cohen P: The pathogenesis of cardiac cachexia. N Engl J Med 1964;271:403–409
17. Buchanan N, Keen RD, Kingsley R et al: Gastrointestinal absorption studies in cardiac cachexia. Intensive Care Med 1977;3:89–91
18. Thomas RD, Silverton NP, Burkinshaw L, Morgan DB: Potassium depletion and tissue loss in chronic heart disease. Lancet 1979;2:9–11
19. Poehlmann ET, Scheffers J, Gottlieb SS, Fisher ML, Vaitekevicius P: Increased resting metabolic rate in patients with congestive heart failure. Ann Intern Med 1994;121:860–862
20. Poehlman ET, Danforth E: Endurance training increases metabolic rate and norepinephrine appearance rate in older individuals. Am J Physiol 1991;261: E233–E239
21. Ansari A: Syndromes of cardiac cachexia and the cachectic heart. Current perspectives. Prog Cardiovasc Dis 1987;30:45–60
22. Mancini DM, Walter G, Reichek N et al: Contribution of skeletal muscle atrophy to exercise intolerance and altered muscle metabolism in heart failure. Circulation 1992;85:1364–1373
23. Vescovo G, Facchin L, Tenderini P et al: A new micromethod for assessing myosin heavy chains composition in skeletal muscle needle biopsies. Differences between chronic heart failure and diffuse muscle atrophy [abstract] Eur Heart J, suppl. 1995;16:357
24. Simioni A, Long CS, Yue P, Dudley GA, Massie BM: Heart failure in rats causes changes in skeletal muscle phenotype and gene expression unrelated to locomotor activity [abstract]. Circulation, suppl. I 1995;92:259
25. Cohn AE, Steele JM: Unexplained fever in heart failure. J Clin Invest 1934;13:853–868
26. Dutka DP, Elborn JS, Delamere F, Shale DJ, Morris GK: Tumor necrosis factor α in severe congestive cardiac failure. Br Heart J 1993;70:141–143
27. Katz SD, Rao R, Berman JW et al: Pathophysiological correlates of increased serum tumor necrosis factor in patients with congestive heart failure. Circulation 1994;90:12–16
28. Nozaki N, Yamaguchi S, Nakamura H, Takahashi K, Tomoike H: Two types of soluble tumor necrosis factor (TNF) receptors are increased in relation to severity in heart failure [abstract]. Circulation, suppl. I 1994; 90:381
29. Tracey KJ, Morgello S, Koplin B et al: Metabolic effects of cachectin/tumor necrosis factor are modified by site of production. Cachectin/tumor necrosis factor-secreting tumor in skeletal muscle induces chronic cachexia, while implantation in brain induces predominantly acute anorexia. J Clin Invest 1989;86:2014–2024
30. Anker SD, Swan JW, Felton C et al: TNF-α as predictor of peak leg blood flow in chronic heart failure [abstract]. Circulation, suppl. I, 1995;92:430
31. Dzau VJ, Packer M, Lilly LS et al: Prostaglandins in severe congestive heart failure. Relation to activation of the renin-angiotensin system and hyponatremia. N Engl J Med 1984;310:347–352
32. Renz H, Gong J-H, Schmidt A, Nain M, Gemsa D: Release of tumor necrosis factor-α from macrophages. Enhancement and suppression are dose-dependently regulated by prostaglandin E_2 and cyclic nucleotides. J Immunol 1988;141:2388–2393
33. Doyama K, Fujiwara H, Fukumoto M et al: Expression of tumor necrosis factor is augmented in right atrium

of human failing hearts [abstract]. Circulation, suppl. I 1994;90:547

34. Tracey KJ, Cerami A: Tumor necrosis factor, other cytokines and disease. Annu Rev Cell Biol 1994;10: 317–343

35. Yoshizumi M, Perella MA, Burnett JCJ, Lee M-E: Tumor necrosis factor downregulates an endothelial nitric oxide synthase mRNA by shortening its half-life. Circ Res 1993;733:205–209

36. Kilbourn RG, Gross SS, Jubran A et al: N^G-methyl-L-arginine inhibits tumor necrosis factor-induced hypotension. Implications for the involvement of nitric oxide. Proc Natl Acad Sci USA 1990;87:3629–3632

37. Tedgui A, Bernard C: Cytokines and vascular reactivity. Heart Failure 1995;11:159–165

38. Anker SD, Volterrani M, Swan JW et al: Hormonal changes in cardiac cachexia [abstract]. Eur Heart J, suppl. 1995;16:359

39. Anker SD, Chua TP, Harrington D et al: Bone loss in cardiac cachectic CHF patients [abstract]. J Am Coll Cardiol (in press)

40. Braunwald E: Clinical manifestation of heart failure. p. 499. In: Heart Disease. A Textbook of Cardiovascular Medicine. Vol. 1. WB Saunders, Philadelphia, 1984

41. Tsutamoto T, Hisanaga T, Fukai D et al: Prognostic value of plasma soluble intercellular adhesion molecule-1 and endothelin-1 concentration in patients with chronic congestive heart failure. Am J Cardiol 1995; 76:803–808

42. Tsutamoto T, Hisanaga T, Maeda K, Maeda Y, Wada A: Plasma soluble vascular cell adhesion molecule-1 and tumor necrosis factor-α levels as markers of prognosis in patients with congestive heart failure [abstract]. Circulation, suppl. 1 1995;92:331

43. Heymsfield SB, Casper K: Congestive heart failure. Clinical management by use of continuous nasoenteric feeding. Am J Clin Nutr 1989;50:539–544

44. Broqvist M, Arnqvist H, Dahlström U et al: Nutritional assessment and muscle energy metabolism in severe congestive heart failure. Effects of long-term dietary supplementation. Eur Heart J 1994;15: 1641–1650

45. Coats AJS, Adamopoulos S, Meyer TE, Conway J, Sleight P: Effects of physical training in chronic heart failure. Lancet 1990;335:63–66

46. Coats AJS, Adamopoulos S, Radaelli A et al: Controlled trial of physical training in chronic heart failure. Circulation 1992;85:2119–2131

47. Anker SD, Volterrani M, Chua TP et al: Peak blood flow as a predictor of exercise capacity in cardiac cachexia. Eur Heart J, suppl. 1995;16:356

48. Endres S, Ghorbani R, Kelley V et al: The effect of dietary supplementation with n-3 polyunsaturated fatty acids on the synthesis of interleukin-1 and tumor necrosis factor by mononuclear cells. N Engl J Med 1989;320:265–271

49. Kremer JM, Jubiz W, Michalek A et al: Fish-oil fatty acid supplementation in active rheumatoid arthritis. A double-blinded, controlled, crossover study. Ann Intern Med 1987;106:497–503

50. Van Zee KJ, Kohno T, Fischer E et al: Tumor necrosis factor soluble receptors circulate during experimental and clinical inflammation and can protect against excessive tumor necrosis factor-α. Proc Natl Acad Sci USA 1992;89:4845–4849

51. Smith JJ, Shapiro L, Dolan NA et al: Cytokine antagonists circulate in the blood of patients with advanced congestive heart failure [abstract]. J Am Coll Cardiol 1993;21:268

52. Ferrari R, Bachetti T, Confortini R et al: Tumor necrosis factor soluble receptors in patients with various degrees of congestive heart failure. Circulation 1995; 92:1479–1486

53. Packer M: The neurohormonal hypothesis. A theory to explain the mechanism of disease progression in heart failure. J Am Coll Cardiol 1992;20:248–254

19 History, Definition, and Classification of Heart Failure

Philip A. Poole-Wilson

Since the 1970s the treatment of chronic heart failure has been transformed, resulting in major benefit to patients. This advance has been the consequence of better understanding of the pathophysiology, new techniques for the investigation of patients, the introduction of new drugs, and cardiac transplantation. The traditional treatment of heart failure with digoxin and diuretics has been replaced by diuretics, angiotensin-converting enzyme (ACE) inhibitors, and drugs directed against the origins of heart failure, such as aspirin or lipid-lowering agents. With modern diuretics the alleviation of symptoms, elimination of edema, and prevention of fluid overload is relatively straightforward. Newer objectives are optimization of the quality of life, avoidance of hospital admission, prevention of the progression of damage to the myocardium, and prolongation of life. New therapies are emerging, such as β-blockers, intermittent positive inotropes, angiotensin receptor inhibitors, specific hormone and cytokine inhibitors, ventricular assist devices, gene therapy, and transplantation.

HISTORY

Heart failure, angina, and the pulse were known in the ancient Egyptian and early Greek civilizations.[1-3] Cardiac glycosides were probably used in India several centuries BC.[4] Hippocrates described cardiac cachexia most vividly: "The flesh is consumed and becomes water, . . . the shoulders, clavicles, chest and thighs melt away."[5] Reports of the benefits of foxglove exist in the Roman literature.[6] It is inconceivable that the intelligent observers and philosophers of the ancient and Latin world were not aware of what is now called heart failure. Other than pragmatic treatment and the immediately obvious physical signs, such as a fast pulse, prominent venous pulsations in the neck, and fluid retention with a swollen abdomen and peripheral edema, no progress on the understanding of the nature of heart failure could be made until Harvey described the circulation in 1628.[7] The clinical features of "right-sided heart failure" were reported a century later in 1728.[8] The diagnosis of heart failure must have portended early death; many patients had untreatable valve disease or infectious endocarditis. Nursing such patients must have been as unpleasant as the nature of the death. No cardiologist could deny the benefits that accrued from subsequent scientific and technologic advances outside the field of medicine but which in later years for the first time allowed the physician to investigate the physiology of heart failure. The key scientific advances, which affected cardiology and the understanding of heart failure, were the discovery of x-rays,[9] the electrocardiogram,[10] the cardiac catheter,[11-13] an understanding of cardiac and circulatory physiology,[14-17] and clinical application of this new medical knowledge.[18]

Effective pharmaceutical treatments have been available for several centuries. Some of them are unattractive by modern standards, such as blood letting, the use of leeches, and Southey's tubes. The benefit and appropriate clinical use of cardiac glycosides extracted from *Digitalis purpurea* were described by Withering in 1785.[19] Withering portrayed terminal heart failure in unmistakable terms: "His countenance was pale, his pulse quick and feeble, his body greatly emaciated, except his belly, which was very large." Hering used nitrates in 1853 to treat heart failure, the first use of a vasodilator. Brunton later in 1867 described the use of amyl nitrate to treat angina and showed that the effects of amyl nitrate were similar to loss of blood.[20] The diuretic effects of sulfonamides were first reported in 1920,[21] the circulatory effects of mercurial diuretics in heart failure in 1949,[22] and the effects of thiazide diuretics for the treatment of heart failure in 1958.[23,24] Key studies and trials with vasodilator agents were reported in 1956[25] and 1986,[26] respectively. ACE inhibitors were shown to be of benefit in terms of mortality in patients with heart failure for the first time in 1987.[27] A large trial of digoxin, showing no effect on overall mortality, was reported in 1996.

DEFINITIONS

When a phrase is used in medicine as often as "heart failure," the expectation is that the term is well understood and capable of definition. Yet controversy has, it seems, always surrounded the use of the phrase partly because advances in physiology have rendered earlier definitions inadequate and partly because of the way in which the term is used by the clinical scientist and by the physician. The physician uses the phrase in a practical sense to convey information about an individual patient. Provided teaching in medical schools is similar, all doctors have a similar understanding and response to the phrase. This function is useful indeed, but the phrase in that context is being used in an entirely pragmatic manner. The clinical scientist and epidemiologist inevitably demand a more robust approach to use of the term.

A practical and entirely pragmatic definition of heart failure is that heart failure is a clinical syndrome (readily diagnosed by doctors) caused by an abnormality of the heart and recognized by a characteristic pattern of hemodynamic, renal, neural, and hormonal responses (Table 19-1).[28,29] This definition requires an abnormality of the heart to be present and states that much of the clinical picture is a consequence of the response of the body to the malfunction of the heart. The definition is compatible with common usage of the phrase. A shorter, possibly more limited, definition is ventricular dysfunction with symptoms.

Some early definitions of heart failure are shown in Table 19-1.[18,28,30–35] Most are totally unsatisfactory because emphasis is placed on one or another physiologic or biochemical feature of heart failure.

Table 19-1. Heart Failure: Some Definitions

"A condition in which the heart fails to discharge its contents adequately"—*Thomas Lewis, 1993*

"A state in which the heart fails to maintain an adequate circulation for the needs of the body despite a satisfactory filling pressure"—*Paul Wood, 1950*

"A pathophysiological state in which an abnormality of cardiac function is responsible for the failure of the heart to pump blood at a rate commensurate with the requirements of the metabolising tissues"—*Eugene Braunwald, 1980*

"Heart failure is the state of any heart disease in which, despite adequate ventricular filling, the heart's output is decreased or in which the heart is unable to pump blood at a rate adequate for satisfying the requirements of the tissues with function parameters remaining within normal limits"—*H. Denolin, H. Kuhn, H.P. Krayenbuehl, F. Loogen, A. Reale, 1983*

"A clinical syndrome caused by an abnormality of the heart and recognized by a characteristic pattern of haemodynamic, renal, neural and hormonal responses"—*Philip A Poole-Wilson, 1985*

" . . . syndrome . . . which arises when the heart is chronically unable to maintain an appropriate blood pressure without support"—*Peter Harris, Br Heart J, 1987*

"A syndrome in which cardiac dysfunction is associated with reduced exercise tolerance, a high incidence of ventricular arrhythmias and shortened life expectancy"—*Jay N. Cohn, 1988*

"Abnormal function of the heart causing a limitation of exercise capacity" *or* "Ventricular dysfunction with symptoms—*Anonymous and pragmatic*

"Symptoms of heart failure, objective evidence of cardiac dysfunction and response to treatment directed towards heart failure"—*Task Force of the ESC, 1995*

The symptoms of heart failure occur or predominate on exercise so definitions based on observations at rest are inevitably flawed. With modern treatment the classic physical signs of overt heart failure may be absent at rest. Emphasis should not be placed on the ventricular filling pressure, as it may be normal at rest, can be manipulated by diuretics, varies from moment to moment, and in chronic heart failure is poorly related to symptoms.[36,37] The symptoms and clinical signs of heart failure after treatment are subtle. The reason the filling pressure was originally considered to be crucial was because the relation between the cardiac output and filling pressure had been described by Starling and was regarded at that time as a sensitive marker of myocardial dysfunction. The phrases "discharge its contents adequately," "adequate circulation for the needs of the body," or "requirements of the metabolizing tissues" refer to concepts that cannot easily be tested. The limiting metabolic substrate of most tissues in the body is oxygen. The oxygen content of blood in the femoral vein at peak exercise during heart failure is almost nil. The total body oxygen consumption of patients with heart failure at rest or at low workloads is identical to that of normal persons and is reduced only toward the end of exercise when anaerobic metabolism is activated. Even at peak exercise the reduction of oxygen consumption, compared to that of a normal person exercising at the same workload, is only a small proportion of the total oxygen consumption at that workload because theoretical considerations and experimental data show that the ability of anaerobic metabolism to generate high energy phosphates within skeletal muscle cells is limited when compared to aerobic metabolism.

A helpful distinction can be made between patients who have heart failure according to the above definition and those who have only ventricular dysfunction without symptoms, without evidence of sodium and water retention, and on no treatment. The prognosis of asymptomatic patients is more favorable, and these patients sometimes provide the lie to the aphorism "a big heart is a bad heart." In general, prognosis is related to three features of heart failure: the size of the heart (related to the ejection fraction), the ability of the heart to function as a pump (related to the maximum body oxygen consumption on exercise), and the body's response to heart failure in terms of metabolism (activation of hormones and cytokines, reflected in a low plasma sodium concentration).

A special problem arises in epidemiologic studies of heart failure where a practical definition is essential. The differences that exist in the estimates of the prevalence and incidence of heart failure in epidemiologic studies can largely be accounted for by variability in diagnosis related to definition. Patients should have documented evidence of an abnormality of the heart, symptoms or signs of heart failure on at least one occasion, and preferably be on treatment or have responded to treatment.[35] These criteria mistakenly exclude a few patients with early heart failure but allow a more accurate identification of patients than if only physical signs and a history are used.[38-40] The identification of an abnormality of the heart by imaging techniques is not always clear-cut because most global measurements, such as end-diastolic dimension or ejection fraction, are distributed normally in the population, and many techniques do not take sufficient account of regional dyskinesia.

Many adjectives have been used to modify the description of heart failure, including high and low output cardiac failure, forward and backward failure,

right and left heart failure, congestive heart failure, systolic and diastolic heart failure, and acute and chronic heart failure. For practical purposes patients can be classified using three categories: acute heart failure (pulmonary edema), circulatory collapse, and chronic heart failure.

Chronic heart failure should not be regarded as a steady-state condition, as the function of the heart and the interaction of the heart and circulation vary with time. Many patients with chronic heart failure develop acute exacerbations that are not always due to identifiable causes, such as arrhythmias, ischemic episodes, failure to take medicines, pulmonary embolus, dietary indiscretion, lung infection, or concurrent illness. The clinical entity whereby patients spontaneously recover and relapse with chronic heart failure can be called undulating heart failure and is not yet fully understood. The terms "right" and "left" heart failure are widely used terms that convey helpful clinical information between doctors but are otherwise misleading, as the commonest cause of "right" heart failure is failure of the left ventricle. In so-called high output cardiac failure the primary abnormality is not one of ventricular dysfunction; the increased cardiac function is a response to systemic metabolic or circulatory changes. These conditions, such as nephritis, Paget's disease, arteriovenous shunts, thyrotoxicosis, pregnancy, anemia, and beri-beri, are perhaps best regarded as conditions of salt and water retention rather than heart failure.

Forward and Backward Failure

The terms forward and backward failure have been used for more than 150 years. Hope[41] in 1832 argued that failure of the ventricle to emit blood resulted in accumulation of blood in the atria, increased pressure, and lung congestion. Certainly in acute conditions that is a valid hypothesis, although with treated chronic heart failure dyspnea is not well related to the left atrial pressure.[37,42] The alternative view of forward failure was strongly put by Sir James McKenzie,[43] who contended that the sensation of fatigue and exhaustion were the consequence of inadequate tissue perfusion. Because the circulation is contained within the body, a reduced cardiac output is entirely compatible with a simultaneously elevated venous pressure. The clinical syndrome of chronic heart failure (increased venous pressure, edema) observed by the physician is dominated by the consequences of salt and water retention.[44] This retention of fluid is a consequence of abnormal function in the kidney. A fall of blood pressure[45] (forward failure) and a rise of venous pressure[46] (backward failure) lead to sodium retention. Despite the decreased blood flow, the glomerular filtration rate is maintained as a result of greater constriction of the efferent arteries compared to the afferent arteries in the glomeruli. Filtration fraction is increased. A consequence is that the osmotic pressure of blood reaching the renal tubules is higher and contributes to retention of sodium in the distal tubule. An increased aldosterone and other hormonal changes also stimulate tubular sodium reabsorption. With severe heart failure renal blood flow is markedly reduced, the glomerular filtration rate falls, and the plasma urea and creatinine may be increased. If the renin-angiotensin system is greatly activated by the use of high doses of diuretics for severe heart failure, the addition of ACE inhibitors can cause a further reduction of the glomerular filtration rate and an increase in plasma urea despite increased blood flow. This chain of events occurs because angiotensin II has a greater effect on the efferent artery than the afferent artery. A preferential reduction of resistance in the afferent artery leads to a fall in the pressures that determine the glomerular filtration rate. Under these circumstances the filtration fraction eventually falls. The renal effects of mild heart failure are not well characterized.[47] The decreased total blood flow may be small, even negligible. Intrarenal redistribution of blood flow may contribute to the early retention of sodium. Alternatively, sodium retention may be explained by activation of neurohumoral systems.[48,49]

Systolic or Diastolic Heart Failure

The mechanism by which the cardiac output increases on exercise during heart failure varies according to the cause of the failure.[50] With dilated cardiomyopathy the end-diastolic volume changes hardly at all (ejection fraction increases), whereas with coronary heart disease the end-diastolic volume enlarges (ejection fraction unchanged). These volume changes are compatible with the idea that with dilated cardiomyopathy the end-diastolic volume is maximal, whereas in some patients with heart failure due to ischemic heart disease the volume at end-diastole is submaximal. Diastole can be divided into four periods: isovolumic relaxation, early filling, late filling, and atrial contraction. Abnormalities of any diastolic event may affect the end-diastolic volume of the heart depending on the heart rate.

A distinction can be made with difficulty between systolic and diastolic heart failure.[51,52] In patients with diastolic heart failure, the stroke volume would be greater if filling during diastole had been more complete. In some conditions, such as hypertrophic obstructive cardiomyopathy, following valve replacement for aortic stenosis, hypertensive heart disease with hypertrophy, and angina pectoris, relaxation may be incomplete at end-diastole particularly if a tachycardia is present. Diastolic heart failure should be suspected in patients with the symptoms of heart failure, normal size hearts and hypertrophy, or myocardial ischemia and in the elderly. Even under these circumstances a systolic abnormality may be evident on exercise. In the presence of ischemic heart disease the key abnormality may not be incomplete relaxation of myocytes (affecting primarily isovolumic relaxation and rapid filling during early diastole) but, rather, incoordinate relaxation of different regions of the ventricle (affecting the later passive phase of ventricular filling). The evidence that diastolic function is a major factor limiting the maximal function of dilated hearts is not compelling.

The diagnosis of systolic or diastolic heart failure has therapeutic implications. Patients with diastolic heart failure, especially those with small hearts and angina or breathlessness as limiting symptoms in the presence of myocardial ischemia or hypertrophy, may benefit from nitrates, vasodilator drugs, or β-blockers. Endocardial ischemia is reduced, compliance increased, and diastolic filling enhanced. In general, the prognosis is better than for systolic heart failure.[53]

Diastolic heart failure occurs in up to 50 percent of patients with heart failure in the community; but among patients admitted to hospital with heart failure, diastolic heart failure is rare (less than 10 percent). There are at least two reasons. The symptoms of diastolic heart failure may be less marked, and heart failure is a disease of old age, when diastolic heart failure is more common.

EVOLUTIONARY ORIGINS OF HEART FAILURE

Harris has argued that the syndrome of heart failure reflects the body response when the heart is unable to maintain the blood pressure long term.[33,54] The reflex, renal, and hormonal response to hypovolemia, hemorrhage, and exercise are similar to the response to heart failure, particularly in terms of activation of the neurohormonal system. The sequelae of coronary heart disease that occur in middle-age to old-age patients during the last decade of the twentieth century elicit a body response that was developed during evolution for an entirely different purpose: to be able to stand erect and respond rapidly to either a threat or an opportunity of obtaining sustenance.

These ideas can be extended to explain current ideas on the origin of symptoms of heart failure and the role of skeletal muscle. A key problem is the nature of the signal that gives rise to activation of the neural and hormonal systems. It cannot be the baroreceptor system because this system adapts quickly to change, and complete inhibition of the system does not result in heart failure. More probably chemoreceptors or ergoreceptors in skeletal muscle initiate the body's response. The purpose of maintaining a blood pressure is not merely to perfuse the brain but also to allow sufficient blood to reach exercising muscle so as to sustain physical activity. Skeletal muscle atrophy is a common feature of heart failure and, particularly, worsening heart failure. Thus for a given workload any muscle must perform greater work. Activation of ergoreceptors could then initiate and maintain the syndrome of heart failure. This concept has been called the "muscle hypothesis."[55]

SPIRALS OF HEART FAILURE

Several models of the mechanism by which heart failure progresses have been suggested. Six spirals of progression are depicted in Figure 19-1. The simplest is that the increased afterload resulting from vasoconstriction as a result of hormonal activation leads to greater stress on the myocardium and causes further damage. This hypothesis is hardly tenable in the face of the disappointing results from trials of vasodilators.[26,56] Fluid retention is an attractive hypothesis that explains easily the benefit to be gained from ACE inhibitors in contrast to vasodilators. A popular argument is that these drugs are beneficial in part because they reduce the future incidence of myocardial infarction.[57–59] Much of the progression of heart failure may be attributable to progression of coronary heart disease, with the commonest cause, myocardial damage, leading to heart failure. More recent hypotheses have focused on remodeling of the myocardium, apoptosis, and cell loss due to activation of free radicals or cytokines. The muscle hypothesis[55] provides a mechanism for activation of the neural and hormonal mechanisms in heart failure.

CAUSES OF HEART FAILURE

The causes of heart failure have traditionally been classified by disease process. Once arrhythmias, valve disease, pericardial disease, and congenital heart disease have been excluded, the cause of heart failure resides in the myocardium (Table 19-2). Myocardial disease is traditionally divided into disease related to coronary events subsequent to atheromatous lesions in the wall of the major coronary arteries. The abnormal myocardial function in the presence of coronary heart disease is described by a myriad of other words, such as stunned,[60] hibernating,[61] preconditioned,[62] fibrotic, mummified, or simply damaged. Stuttering ischemia[63] and chronic ischemia are other terms occasionally used.

A different way to consider heart failure is shown

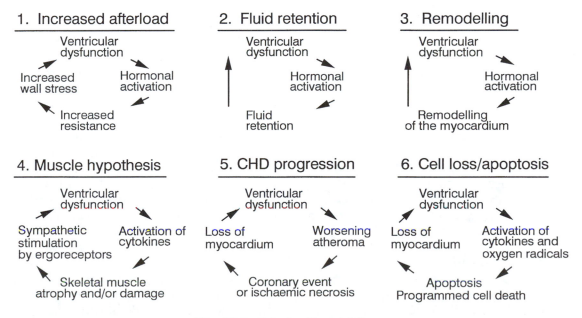

Fig. 19-1. Spirals of heart failure.

Table 19-2. Causes of Heart Failure

General causes
  Arrhythmias
  Valve disease
  Pericardial disease
  Congenital heart disease
  Myocardial disease
Myocardial disease
  Coronary artery disease
  Cardiomyopathy
      Dilated (DCM)
          Specific
          Idiopathic
      Hypertrophic (HCM)
      Restrictive
  Hypertension
  Drugs
      β-Blockers
      Calcium antagonists
      Antiarrhythmic drugs

Table 19-3. Underlying Causes of Chronic Heart Failure Due to the Myocardium[a]

Loss of muscle

Incoordinate contraction and abnormal timing of contraction

Extracellular
    Fibrosis, altered extracellular architecture, shape and size of ventricle
    Slippage of cells, fiber orientation

Cellular
    Change of cell structure: hypertrophy, ?hyperplasia, ?addition of sarcomeres
    Change of cell function: systolic, diastolic, or both

    Calcium release, uptake, or both
    Receptor down-regulation
    Reduced cAMP
    Sarcoplasmic reticulum dysfunction
    Reduced number of ion channels or pumps

    Response of contractile proteins to calcium
    Altered contractile proteins (isoforms)
    Altered phosphorylation of contractile proteins
    ?Energy-deficient state

---

[a] Many of these factors combine to cause systolic or diastolic failure. Diastolic heart failure is common in the presence of hypertrophy, fibrosis, or ischemia.

---

in Table 19-3. Here the emphasis is not on a disease process but on the mechanism responsible for the loss of function. Loss of cells and incoordinate contraction are the commonest abnormalities in coronary heart disease. Once these two entities have been excluded, heart failure is attributable to an abnormality of the extracellular structures or to the function of the myocyte itself. In the cell there can exist structural abnormalities or loss of function due to the control mechanisms for calcium or the response of the contractile proteins to calcium.[64]

DEFINITION OF DILATED CARDIOMYOPATHY AND OTHER TERMS

Cardiomyopathies were originally defined as heart muscle diseases of unknown cause. They were traditionally classified into three types: hypertrophic, restrictive, and dilated (formerly congestive).[65] The three varieties were distinguished by physiologic, anatomic, and clinical features. By far the commonest cardiomyopathy is dilated cardiomyopathy. Dilated cardiomyopathy was defined in the following terms. "The condition is recognised by dilatation of the left or right ventricle, or both ventricles. Dilatation often becomes severe and is invariably accompanied by hypertrophy. Systolic ventricular function is impaired. Congestive heart failure may or may not supervene. Presentation with disturbances of ventricular or atrial rhythm is common and death may

occur at any stage."[66] Heart muscle disease known to be associated with a medical condition was called specific heart muscle disease.

Advances in biology and common parlance have played havoc with the definition of cardiomyopathy.[65–68] A large number of cardiomyopathies now have a known cause. The cardiomyopathies have come to be regarded as diseases of the myocardium leading to abnormal cardiac function in the absence of coronary heart disease, hypertension, congenital anatomic distortion, and valve or pericardial disease. The coronary arteries must be entirely normal as assessed by coronary angiography. If any aspect of coronary heart disease is confused with cardiomyopathy, the phrase "dilated cardiomyopathy" merely indicates a large heart, a rather unhelpful piece of jargon. Dilated cardiomyopathies are classified as either specific cardiomyopathies (denoting that a cause is recognized) or idiopathic dilated cardiomyopathies (when the cause is unknown).

Hypertrophic cardiomyopathy is a heart condition characterized by a hypertrophied, nondilated left or right ventricle (or both) in the absence of a cardiac or systemic cause. Another name is hypertrophic obstructive cardiomyopathy, used when there is a demonstrable outflow gradient. Another phenotype is characterized by hypertrophy dominantly in the sep-

Table 19-4. Causes of Dilated
Cardiomyopathy

Familial cardiomyopathies

Genetic cardiomyopathies

Infectious causes
    Viruses and HIV
    Rickettsia
    Bacteria
    Mycobacteria
    Fungus
    Parasites

Toxins and poisons
    Ethanol
    Cocaine
    Metals
    Carbon dioxide or hypoxia

Drugs
    Chemotherapeutic agents
    Antiviral agents

Metabolic disorders
    Nutritional deficiencies and endocrine diseases

Collagen disorders

Autoimmune cardiomyopathies

Peripartum cardiomyopathy

Neuromuscular disorders

Table 19-5. Causes of Restrictive
Cardiomyopathies

Associated with fibrosis
    Diastolic dysfunction
        Elderly
        Hypertrophy
        Ischemia
        Scleroderma

Infiltrative disorders
    Amyloidosis
    Sarcoid disease
    Inborn errors of metabolism
    Neoplasia

Storage disorders
    Hemochromatosis and hemosiderosis
    Fabry disease
    Glycogen storage disease

Endomyocardial disorders
    Endomyocardial fibrosis
    Hypereosinophilic syndrome
    Carcinoid
    Metastases
    Radiation damage

tal region of the myocardium (ASH: asymmetric septal hypertrophy). Restrictive cardiomyopathy is characterized by a stiff ventricle that is not greatly enlarged; the hallmark is abnormal diastolic filling of the ventricle. Dilated cardiomyopathy is characterized by an enlarged ventricle (left ventricle internal end-diastolic dimension of more than 2.7 m^2 body surface area) and ejection fraction of less than 45 percent or M-mode fractional shortening of less than 30 percent.[68,69] A brief list of the causes of dilated and restrictive cardiomyopathies are shown in Table 19-4 and 19-5. More detailed information is available in other chapters.

A major problem exists with the use of such a definition in epidemiologic studies. There is a distribution of ventricular size in the population. Rigid criteria based on size alone inevitably includes persons at the extreme range of normal. There is a danger that a presumed pathologic state, dilated cardiomyopathy, becomes synonymous with a large heart; a small group of persons with hearts exceeding the normal range would be incorrectly diagnosed as having a disease, dilated cardiomyopathy. Other evidence of heart failure is necessary.

REFERENCES

1. Dalla Volte S: A short historical survey of heart failure. Clin Invest 1993;71:S167–S176
2. Horine EF: An epitome of ancient pulse lore. Bull Hist Med 1941;10:209–249
3. Leibowitz JO: Antiquity and the Middle Ages. In: The History of Coronary Heart Disease. pp. 15–48. William Clowes, London, 1970
4. Sharma JN: Cardiovascular system and its diseases in the ancient Indian literature. Indian J Dis 1986;9:32
5. Katz AM, Katz PB: Diseases of the heart in works of Hippocrates. Br Heart J 1962;24:257–264
6. Moore DA: William Withering and digitalis. BMJ 1985;290:324
7. Harvey W: De Motu Cordis. Willaim Fitzer, Frankfurt, (translated as Movement of the Heart and Blood in Animals by KJF, 1628
8. Lancisi JM: De Motu Cordis et Aneurysmatibus. Salvioni, Rome, 1728
9. Rontgen W: Eine neue Art von Strahlen. Verlaufige Mitteilung. Sitzungsberichte Physik Med Ges Wurzburg 1895;132–141
10. Einthoven W: Ueber dei Form des menschlichen Elektrokardiogramms. Arch Ges Physiol 1895;60:101–123
11. Forssman W: Die Sondierung des rechten Herzens. Klin Wochenschr 1929;8:2085
12. Cournand AF, Riley RL, Breed ES, Baldwin EF, Richards DW: Measurement of cardiac output in man using the technique of catheterisation of the right auricle. J Clin Invest 1945;24:106–116
13. Cournand A, Ranges HA: Catheterisation of the right auricle in man. Proc Soc Exp Biol 1941;46:462

14. Fick A: Ueber die Messung des Blutquantums in den Herzventrikeln. Sitzungsberichte Physik Med Ges Wurzburg 1870; July 9

15. Frank O: Zur Dynamik des Herzmuskels. Z Biol 1895; 32:370–437

16. Starling EH: On the absorption of fluids from the connective tissue spaces. J Physiol (Lond) 1896;19: 312–326

17. Ringer S: A further contribution regarding the influence of the different constituents of the blood on the contraction of the heart. J Physiol (Lond) 1883;4:29–42

18. Lewis T: Diseases of the Heart. Macmillan, London, 1933

19. Withering W: An Account of the Foxglove, and Some of its Medical Uses: With Practical Remarks on Dropsy, and Other Diseases. Robinson, London, 1785

20. Brunton TL: On the use of nitrate of amyl in angina pectoris. Lancet 1867;2:97–98

21. Saxl R, Heilig R: Uber die Diuretische Wirkung von Novasurol-und Anderen. Quecksilberinjektionen. Wien Klin Wochenschr 1920;33:943–944

22. Pugh LGC, Wyndham CL: The circulatory effects of mercurial diuretics in congestive heart failure. Clin Sci 1949;8:11–19

23. Novello FC, Sprague JM: Benzothiadiazine dioxides as novel diuretics. J Am Chem Soc 1957;79:2028–2029

24. Slater JDH, Nabarro JDN: Clinical experience with chlorothiazide. Lancet 1958;1:124–126

25. Judson WE, Hollander W, Wilkins RW: The effects of intravenous Apresoline (hydralazine) on cardiovascular and renal function in patients with and without congestive heart failure. Circulation 1956;13:644–674

26. Cohn JN, Archibald DG, Ziesche S et al: Effect of vasodilator therapy on mortality in chronic congestive heart failure. Results of a Veterans Administration Cooperative Study. N Engl J Med 1986;314:1547–1552

27. CONSENSUS Trial Study Group: Effects of enalapril on mortality in severe congestive heart failure. Results of the Cooperative North Scandinavian Enalapril Survival Study (CONSENSUS). The CONSENSUS Trial Study Group. N Engl J Med 1987;316:1429–1435

28. Poole-Wilson PA: Heart failure. Med Interne 1985;2: 866–871

29. Poole-Wilson PA: Diseases of the Heart. WB Saunders, London, 1996

30. Wood P: Diseases of the Heart and Circulation. Eyre & Spottiswoode, London, 1950

31. Braunwald E: Heart disease. In: A Textbook of Cardiovascular Medicine. WB Saunders, Philadelphia, 1980

32. Denolin H, Kuhn H, Krayenbuehl HP, Loogen F, Reale A: The definition of heart failure. Eur Heart J 1983; 4:445–448

33. Harris P: Congestive cardiac failure. Central role of the arterial blood pressure. Br Heart J 1987;58: 190–203

34. Cohn J: Is neurohormonal activation deleterious to the long term outcome of patients with congestive heart failure? J Am Coll Cardiol 1988;12:547–548

35. Task Force on Heart Failure of the European Society of Cardiology: Guidelines for the diagnosis of heart failure. Eur Heart J 1995;16:741–751

36. Lipkin DP, Canepa-Anson R, Stephens MR, Poole-Wilson PA: Factors determining symptoms in heart failure. Comparison of fast and slow exercise tests. Br Heart J 1986;55:439–445

37. Lipkin DP, Poole-Wilson PA: Symptoms limiting exercise in chronic heart failure [editorial]. BMJ 1986;292: 1030–1031

38. Remes J, Miettinen H, Reunanen A, Pyorala K: Validity of clinical diagnosis of heart failure in primary health care. Eur Heart J 1991;12:315–321

39. Dunselman PH, Kuntze CE, van-Bruggen A et al: Value of New York Heart Association classification, radionuclide ventriculography, and cardiopulmonary exercise tests for selection of patients for congestive heart failure studies. Am Heart J 1988;116:1475–1482

40. Marantz PR, Tobin JN, Wassertheil-Smoller S et al: The relationship between left ventricular systolic function and congestive heart failure diagnosed by clinical criteria. Circulation 1988;77:607–612

41. Hope JA: Treatise on the Diseases of the Heart and Great Vessels. William Kidd, London, 1832

42. Poole-Wilson PA: Relation of pathophysiologic mechanisms to outcome in heart failure. J Am Coll Cardiol, suppl. 4 1993;22:22–29

43. McKenzie J: Diseases of the Heart. Oxford Medical Publications, Oxford; 1913

44. Anand IS, Ferrari R, Kalra GS et al: Edema of cardiac origin. Studies of body water and sodium, renal function, hemodynamic indexes, and plasma hormones in untreated congestive cardiac failure. Circulation 1989; 80:299–305

45. Merrill AJ: Edema and decreased renal blood flow in patients with chronic congestive heart failure. Evidence of "forward failure" as a primary cause of edema. J Clin Invest 1946;25:389–400

46. Firth JD, Raine AE, Ledingham JG: Raised venous pressure. A direct cause of renal sodium retention in oedema? Lancet 1988;1:1033–1035

47. Francis GS: Sodium and water excretion in heart failure. Efficacy of treatment has surpassed knowledge of pathophysiology. Ann Intern Med 1986;105:272–274

48. Bayliss J, Norell M, Canepa-Anson R, Sutton G, Poole-Wilson P: Untreated heart failure. Clinical and neuroendocrine effects of introducing diuretics. Br Heart J 1987;57:17–22

49. Remes J, Tikkanen I, Fyhrquist F, Pyorala K: Neuroendocrine activity in untreated heart failure. Br Heart J 1991;65:249–255

50. Shen WF, Roubin GS, Hirasawa K et al: Left ventricular volume and ejection fraction response to exercise in chronic congestive heart failure. Difference between dilated cardiomyopathy and previous myocardial infarction. Am J Cardiol 1985;55:1027–1031

51. Brutsaert DL, Sys SU: Relaxation and diastole of the heart. Physiol Rev 1989;69:1228–1315

52. Brutsaert DL, Sys SU, Gillebert TC: Diastolic failure. Pathophysiology and therapeutic implications. J Am Coll Cardiol 1993;22:318–325

53. Brogan WC, Hillis LD, Flores ED, Lange RA: The natural history of isolated left ventricular diastolic dysfunction. Am J Med 1992;92:627–30

54. Harris P: Evolution and the cardiac patient. Cardiovasc Res 1983;17:313–319, 373–378, 437–445

55. Coats AJS, Clark AL, Piepoli M, Volterrani M, Poole-Wilson PA: Symptoms and quality of life in heart failure. The muscle hypothesis. Br Heart J 1994;72:36–39

56. Cohn JN, Johnson G, Ziesche S et al: A comparison of enalapril with hydralazine-isosorbide dinitrate in the treatment of chronic congestive heart failure. N Engl J Med 1991;325:302–310

57. Yusuf S, Pepine CJ, Garces C et al: Effect of enalapril

on myocardial infarction and unstable angina in patients with low ejection fractions. Lancet 1992;340: 1173–1178

58. Ganley CJ, Hung HMJ, Temple R: More on the survival and ventricular enlargement trial. N Engl J Med 1993;329:1204–1205

59. Pfeffer M, Braunwald E, Moye LA et al: Effect of captopril on mortality and morbidity in patients with left ventricular dysfunction after myocardial infarction. Results of the Survival and Ventricular Enlargement Trial. N Engl J Med 1992;327:669–677

60. Bolli RL: Myocardial "stunning" in man. Circulation 1992;86:1671–1691

61. Rahimtoola SH: A perspective on the ghree large multicenter randomized clinical trials of coronary bypass surgery for chronic stable angina. Circulation, suppl. V 1985;72:123–135

62. Murry CE, Jennings RB, Reimer KA: Preconditioning with ischemia. A delay of lethal cell injury in ischemic myocardium. Circulation 1986;74:1124–1136

63. Poole-Wilson PA: Angina—pathological mechanisms, clinical expression and treatment. Postgrad Med J, suppl 3 1983;59:11–21

64. Davies CH, Harding SE, Poole-Wilson PA: Cellular mechanisms of contraciledysfunction in human heart failure. Eur Heart J 1996;17:189–198

65. Goodwin JF, Oakley CM: The cardiomyopathies. Br Heart J 1972;34:545–552

66. Report of the WHO/ISFC Task Force on the definition and classification of cardiomyopathies. Br Heart J 1980;44:672–673

67. WHO Techinical Report Series: Cardiomyopathies. Report of a WHO Expert Committee. Technical Report Series 697. WHO, Geneva, 1984

68. Keren A, Popp RL: Assignment of patients into the classification of cardiomyopathies. Circulation 1992; 86:1622–1633

69. Manolio TA, Baughman KL, Rodeheffer R et al: Prevalence and etiology of idiopathic dilated cardiomyopathy (Summary of a National Heart, Lung, and Blood Institute Workshop). Am J Cardiol 1992;69: 1458–1466

20 Epidemiology of Heart Failure in the United States

William B. Kannel

Over the past decade cardiac failure has become a major public health problem in cardiovascular medicine in the United States.[1,2] It is estimated that about 4 million Americans have heart failure with 400,000 new cases occurring each year.[1,2] It was listed as the cause of death for 37,400 in 1988, a gross underestimate of its impact as a force of mortality because it was noted as a contributing cause in another 200,000 deaths.[3,4] Data from the National Hospital Discharge Survey in the United States indicates a rising number of hospital admissions for congestive heart failure (CHF).[5]

It is estimated that heart failure afflicts 1.5 percent of the adult U.S. population and is a major cause of disability and morbidity. It is now one of the most common reasons for hospitalization of the elderly.[6] It is a major contributor to the cost of health care in the United States with an $8 billion expenditure for the care of such patients annually.[1]

Epidemiologic data can provide a relatively undistorted population-based insight into the prevalence, incidence, secular trends, and modifiable predisposing cardiac conditions and risk factors for cardiac failure. These data can be obtained from the Framingham Study based on four decades of biennial surveillance of a cohort of 5209 subjects.

PREVALENCE AND INCIDENCE

Comparison of the prevalence and incidence of cardiac failure in different parts of the world is hampered because of the different diagnostic criteria used, nonuniform methods of case ascertainment, variations in hospital admission practices, and different survey methods. Mortality data, autopsy studies, and clinical estimates of morbidity do not readily translate into general population rates of prevalence and incidence of cardiac failure.

Based on the National Health and Nutrition Survey it was estimated that 1 million to 2 million people in the United States under age 75 years and excluding persons in institutions have cardiac failure.[7] When persons over age 65 and those institutionalized are included, the estimated range is closer to 2 million to 3 million.[7] The prevalence is reported to rise from 1 percent in those ages 25–54 years to 4.5 percent at ages 65–74 years.[7] In the Framingham Study the prevalence of cardiac failure rose stepwise from 0.8 percent at age 50–59 to 9.1 percent at ages 80–89 years (Table 20-1), approximately doubling with each decade of age. These estimates are not too different from those derived from the national survey.

Table 20-1. Prevalence of Cardiac Failure by Age: 34-Year Follow-Up, Framingham Study, Men and Women Combined

Age (years)	Person Bienniums	Bienniums with CHF	Combined Prevalence (%)
50–59	20,520	166	0.8
60–69	19,298	451	2.3
70–79	8,994	438	4.9
80–89	2,084	190	9.1

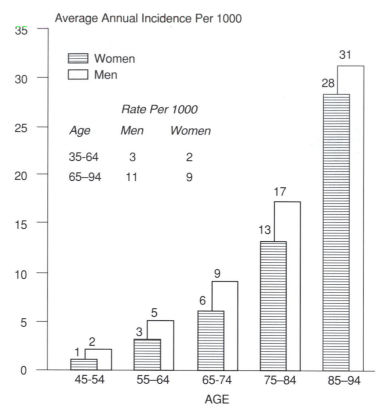

Fig. 20-1. Incidence of cardiac failure by age and sex: 36-year follow-up, Framingham Study.

In the Framingham Study the incidence of cardiac failure also doubled with each decade of age with only a modest male predominance (Fig. 20-1). Extrapolation of the average annual incidence of cardiac failure from the Framingham Study to the population of the United States yields an estimate of 465,000 new events each year.[8]

Morbidity associated with heart failure is substantial, with 60–70 percent of patients having repeated recurrences within 6 years. It is also associated with a fourfold increased risk of a stroke.[9] Recurrences of failure occur at 12–20 times the general population rate and strokes at 4–7 times the rate of persons the same age.[9]

ETIOLOGY

It is difficult to accurately delineate the major etiologies of CHF as a percentage of the total from clinical data because of selection bias introduced by referral patterns and access to medical care. Population-based data, although less biased, seldom can provide accurate or valid estimates of less common causes of cardiac failure, such as the cardiomyopathies. Also,

there is usually clustering of the various possible etiologies such as coronary disease, hypertension, and diabetes.

Coronary disease appears to account for 25–49 percent of the cardiac failure in the general population depending on age and sex, but a substantial proportion also have coexistent hypertension. In the Framingham Study coronary heart disease (CHD), hypertension, and diabetes, singly or in combination, predominate as etiologies for heart failure.[9] About 40 percent of heart failure in men and women in the Framingham Study was attributable to a combination of CHD and hypertension. In addition, 19 percent of failure in men and 7 percent in women was due to CHD in isolation, so that more than half of the cardiac failures had CHD as a major contributing cause (Fig. 20-2). Some 30–37 percent of CHF was attributable to hypertension alone in men and women, respectively. Hypertension alone or in combination with CHD was responsible for about 70 percent of the cardiac failure.[9] Only 7 percent of cardiac failure could not be attributed to CHD, hypertension, or valve disease, suggesting that the cardiomyopathies are uncommon in the general population, in contrast to data derived from clinical studies.

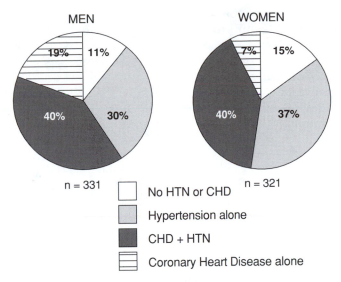

Fig. 20-2. Prevalence of coronary heart disease (CHD) and hypertension (HTN) alone and in combination among Framingham Heart Study subjects with congestive heart failure, by gender.

SURVIVAL

Relatively limited epidemiologic data are available regarding prognostic outlook of cardiac failure and secular changes in survival after its onset in a population-based setting. The Framingham Study cohort was investigated to ascertain the prognosis of heart failure in an unselected population sample in relation to age, sex, cause, and calendar year of first diagnosis of the condition.[10] Median survival after the onset of heart failure was only 1.7 years for men and 3.2 years for women. The 5-year survival rate was only 25 percent in men and 38 percent in women. Survival was better among women than men even after adjustment for age. Mortality increased 27 percent per decade of advancing age in men and 61 percent each decade of age in women. Adjusting for age, no significant change in the prognosis of cardiac fail-

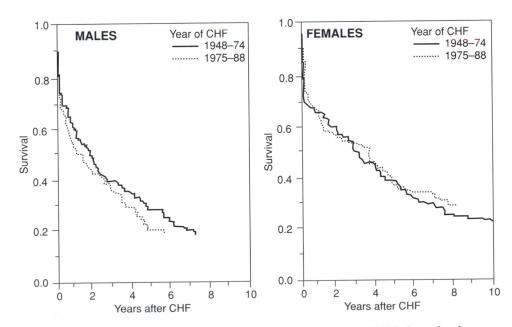

Fig. 20-3. Age-adjusted survival rates after congestive heart failure (CHF) by calendar year of first diagnosis of CHF, for male and female subjects developing CHF during the calendar years 1948–1988. (From Ho et al.,[10] with permission.)

ure over four decades of surveillance of the cohort was noted[10] (Fig. 20-3). There was no significant difference in median survival among the various etiologies for cardiac failure. Thus advances in the treatment of coronary disease, hypertension, and valvular disease during the four decades of observation did not result in substantial improvement in survival in this unselected population sample.

SECULAR TRENDS

Despite rapidly declining cardiovascular mortality rates in the United States, CHF has been cited as the nation's most rapidly growing cardiovascular problem.[1,2] Using uniform case ascertainment and diagnostic criteria in the Framingham Study, there has been no increase in incidence over the years; nor has there been a decline (Table 20-2). The health care burden attributable to CHF is expected to grow substantially, however, based on clinical and demographic trends. An aging population and improvements in survival after myocardial infarction because of thrombolysis and revascularization is likely to fuel an increase in incidence.

National statistics on trends in mortality attributable to cardiac failure are difficult to interpret. Heart failure is seldom coded as the underlying cause of death on death certificates even though the patient died as a result of cardiac failure. Hence heart failure is listed more commonly as a contributing cause of death than an underlying cause. National data, as a consequence, attribute only 5.4 percent of cardiac deaths to heart failure,[8] which makes an analysis of secular trends in cardiac failure mortality difficult. Taken at face value it appears that death rates for cardiac failure increased from 1968 to 1979 in the United States but have reversed beginning in 1988.[8]

Table 20-2. Secular Trends in the Prevalence of Cardiac Failure 1966–1984: Framingham Study Subjects Ages 65–84 Years

Calendar Years	Age-adjusted Prevalence (%)	
	Men	Women
1966–1970	4.6	3.7
1971–1973	5.7	4.3
1975–1977	3.9	3.8
1979–1981	3.5	4.0
1983–1985	4.8	4.0
1987–1989	5.0	4.0
Trend	$P = 0.68$	$P = 0.58$

Table 20-3. Changes in Prevalence of Preexisting Conditions Among CHF Cases: Ages 50–89 in the Framingham Cohort and Framingham Offspring Study 1950–1987

Risk Factor	Age-adjusted Change Per Calendar Decade	
	Men	Women
Coronary heart disease	+41	+25
Diabetes mellitus	+21	+24
Hypertension	−10	−27
ECG-LVH	−23	−33
Valvular heart disease	−45	−32

Abbreviations: ECG-LVH, electrocardiographically diagnosed left ventricular hypertrophy.
(From Kannel et al.,[9] with permission.)

Cardiac failure hospitalization trends suggest an increasing prevalence of heart failure. Rates of hospitalization for heart failure have been rising steadily, especially for those over age 65 years.[4–6] However, this may not reflect the true trends in incidence and prevalence of heart failure because of variable hospital admission practices over time. Taken at face value there is a suggestion of a fourfold increase in admissions to the hospital for cardiac failure since 1971.[8,9,11]

An examination of secular trends in the etiologies for cardiac failure in the general population based on Framingham Study data indicates that coronary disease and diabetes are increasingly responsible for failure in recent years, and hypertension and valvular disease are diminishing as causes (Table 20-3).

CORONARY HEART DISEASE

Ischemic heart disease is an increasingly common cause of cardiac failure in the United States in general and in the Framingham Study in particular.[9] Currently, overt CHD appears to be responsible for more than half the CHF in the general population.[9] In the Framingham Study CHD that deteriorates to the stage of cardiac failure is usually accompanied by hypertension. It is believed by some that chronic stable angina that has not followed a myocardial infarction seldom results in cardiac failure.[12] However, connective tissue changes have been noted in the heart during early ischemia, and repeated episodes of myocardial ischemia could result in alteration of the cellular structure and collagen matrix of the

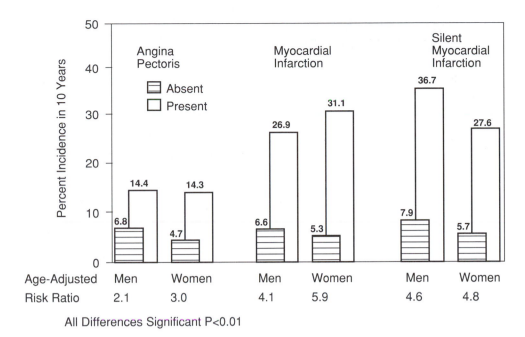

Fig. 20-4. Risk of cardiac failure by clinical manifestations of coronary heart disease, 30-year follow-up of Framingham Study subjects, 35–94 years of age.

heart.[12] In any event, persons in the Framingham Study with uncomplicated angina pectoris have about a twofold increased risk of CHF compared to persons the same age in the general population (Fig. 20-4). Persons who have documented myocardial infarctions have twice the risk of those with uncomplicated angina pectoris (Fig. 20-4). About one-third of myocardial infarctions that occur in the general population are silent and unrecognized. It is of interest that the occurrence of cardiac failure in persons with such infarctions is just as great as in those with symptomatic recognized infarctions (Fig. 20-4).

Myocardial function following a myocardial infarction (MI) is dependent on the extent of hemodynamic derangement, myocyte loss, and adverse remodeling. Hence it is not surprising that non-Q-wave MIs have only half the risk of Q-wave MIs over both the short term and long term.

HYPERTENSION

Hypertension is a major contributor to heart failure in the general population because it is so highly prevalent and because it also predisposes to the cardiac conditions that cause the heart to fail, such as coronary disease, valvar deformity, and left ventricular hypertrophy (LVH). Overall, it increases the risk of

cardiac failure threefold (Fig. 20-5). About 75 percent of cardiac failure is associated with hypertension with or without the conditions associated with it.

The risk of hypertension-induced cardiac failure increases with the degree to which the blood pressure is elevated and whether the hypertension is predominantly systolic or diastolic in character (Table 20-4). The isolated systolic hypertension, which is the dominant variety in the elderly, is a powerful contributor to cardiac failure. Comparison of the impacts of the various components of blood pressure on the incidence of cardiac failure gives no hint of a greater impact of diastolic pressure. In women the systolic pressure appears most important; in men pulse pressure appears to rival the impact of systolic pressure (Table 20-4).

The appearance of the various sequelae of hypertension greatly increases the hazard of cardiac failure imposed by hypertension. A myocardial infarction escalates the risk sixfold, and LVH, valvar disease, and diabetes increase it threefold.

LEFT VENTRICULAR HYPERTROPHY

Hypertrophy of the heart is a common feature of the evolution of hypertension, aortic stenosis, and CHD deteriorating to heart failure. A pressure overload

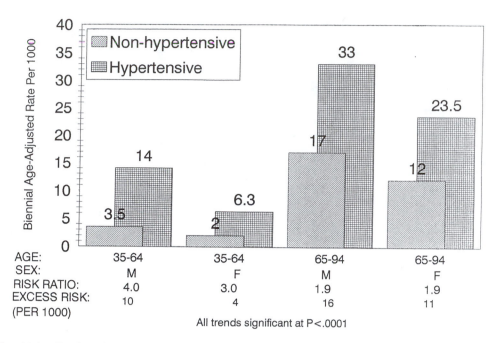

Fig. 20-5. Cardiac failure by hypertensive status, 36-year follow-up to Framingham Study.

rather consistently induces concentric hypertrophy of the heart and increased muscle mass. The risk of cardiac failure increases with the left ventricular muscle mass, with no clear indication where physiologic compensatory hypertrophy leaves off and pathologic hypertrophy ensues. Ventricular hypertrophy at the microscopic level is comprised of enlarged myoctyes, increased collagen matrix, and major internal derangement of the heart muscle. In any event, LVH, whether diagnosed by roentgenogram, electrocardiogram (ECG), or echocardiogram, is associated with a greatly increased risk of cardiac failure. Those with both ECG and anatomic indications of hypertrophy are at greater risk than those with either alone (Table 20-5).

If the stimulus to hypertrophy can be removed before there has been major disturbance to the cytoskeleton of the heart and pronounced reduction in myocardial contractile function has occurred, the process may be reversible. Reduction in the severity of ECG-recognized LVH (ECG-LVH) in the Framingham Study has been found to be associated with improvement in the risk of cardiovascular events.[13]

Electrocardiographic evidence of LVH was noted before the diagnosis of heart failure in 17 percent of men and 18 percent of women. Those who developed ECG-LVH were at a 15-fold increased risk of cardiac failure. LVH was associated with an increased incidence of cardiac failure even after adjusting for the influence of the often associated hypertension.[14]

Table 20-4. Risk of Cardiac Failure by Blood Pressure Components:
34-Year Follow-Up, Framingham Study

| Blood pressure parameters | Q_5Q_1 risk ratio | | | |
| | 35–64 Years | | 65–94 Years | |
	Men	Women	Men	Women
Systolic blood pressure	3.1***	4.4***	1.8***	2.4***
Diastolic blood pressure	1.4*	2.9**	1.6**	1.2*
Mean arterial blood pressure	2.6***	3.9***	2.1***	1.6**
Pulse pressure	3.4***	3.0***	2.3***	2.2***

Q_5Q_1, comparison of rates in fifth versus first quintile of blood pressure parameter.
* $P<0.05$
** $P<0.01$
*** $P<0.001$

Table 20-5. Risk of Cardiac Failure by ECG and Roentgenographic Evidence of Left Ventricular Hypertrophy: 32-Year Follow-Up, Framingham Study

	Age-adjusted Biennial Rate Per 1000			
	Age 35–64		Age 65–94	
ECG-LVH	LVH Absent[a]	LVH Present[a]	LVH Absent[a]	LVH Present[a]
Men				
Absent	3	16	14	56
Present	11	126	102	135
Women				
Absent	2	17	12	21
Present	16	83	89	85

[a] Determined by radiography.

Subjects who also had anatomic evidence of LVH on the chest roentgenogram and echocardiogram had a further escalation of risk of heart failure.

INDICATORS OF DETERIORATING FUNCTION

A low vital capacity or one that is falling is often a sign of deteriorating cardiac function. It appears to be a cost-effective way to detect persons who are at high risk of cardiac failure because of diastolic dysfunction. A reduced vital capacity was found in the Framingham Study to substantially increase the risk of persons with coronary disease or LVH developing heart failure. In persons with these predisposing conditions the risk of cardiac failure varies over a threefold range depending on the vital capacity (Fig. 20-6). Those with a low vital capacity (under 2–3 liters in women and men, respectively) had a further two- to threefold escalation of risk.

As the heart function deteriorates there is an attempt to maintain the cardiac output by increasing the heart rate. An increased heart rate at rest was found to be an independent contributor to the risk of cardiac failure in persons with hypertension in the Framingham Study. Risk of failure increased with the heart rate in a continuous graded fashion (Fig. 20-7).

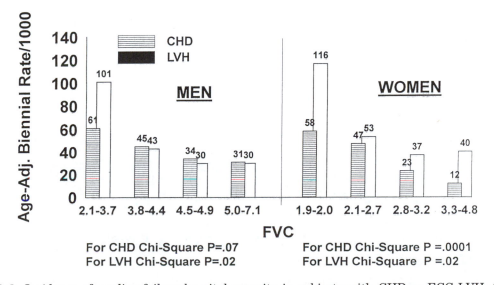

For CHD Chi-Square P=.07
For LVH Chi-Square P=.02

For CHD Chi-Square P =.0001
For LVH Chi-Square P =.02

Fig. 20-6. Incidence of cardiac failure by vital capacity in subjects with CHD or ECG-LVH: 38-year follow-up to Framingham Study in patients 50 to 92 years.

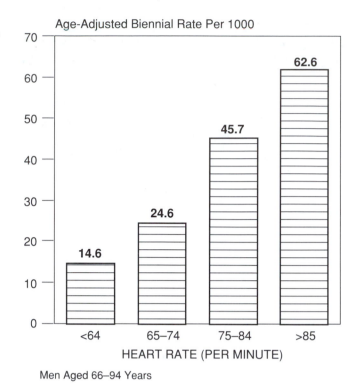

Fig. 20-7. Risk of cardiac failure in definite hypertension by heart rate in men 55–94 years of age from the Framingham Study.

IDENTIFYING HIGH RISK CANDIDATES

In persons with coronary disease, hypertension, or damaged cardiac valves the risk of developing cardiac failure varies over a wide range depending on the associated burden of cardiovascular risk factors (Fig. 20-8). This assessment can be made from ordinary office procedure.[14] A CHF risk profile can be formulated from ingredients such as the systolic blood pressure, diabetic status, Body Mass Index (BMI), ECG-LVH, radiographically recognized car-

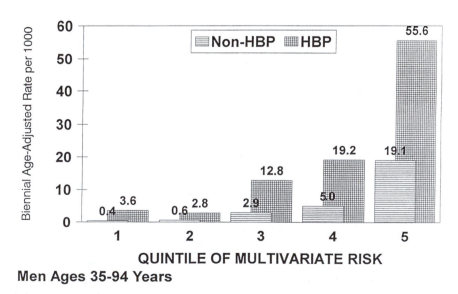

Fig. 20-8. Risk of cardiac failure by quintile of multivariate risk by hypertensive status in men 35–94 years of age; 32-year follow-up to Framingham Study.

diac enlargement, and age in persons with coronary disease, hypertension, or heart murmurs. About 60–65 percent of CHF events in the Framingham Study occurred in those in the upper decile of multivariate risk. These high risk candidates for failure are worthy of noninvasive but expensive investigation for evidence of impaired ventricular function. It is advisable because there is now convincing evidence that preventive measures implemented in asymptomatic persons with impaired left ventricular function can delay cardiac failure.[15,16] A multivariate risk profile can be used as a means to detect persons who are highly likely to have left ventricular dysfunction when subjected to echocardiographic examination.

NEED AND PROSPECTS FOR PREVENTION

Heart failure is a lethal end-stage of cardiovascular disease. Once the heart has used up its reserve capacity, survival is curtailed to the same extent as for cancer. When overt cardiac failure was clinically manifest, median survival in the Framingham Study was only 1.7 years for men and 3.2 years for women, the death often occurring suddenly in persons who appear to be in stable condition. Recent declines in death rates from cardiac disease have not been accompanied by a similar decline in the incidence of cardiac failure.

A substantial reduction in heart failure incidence requires prevention of the cardiac disease that is responsible and early detection and correction of presymptomatic left ventricular dysfunction and the risk factors that predispose to its occurrence. These major contributors to the occurrence of cardiac failure have been identified, many of which are correctable; and high risk candidates for cardiac failure can now be cost-effectively targeted for noninvasive tests for left ventricular dysfunction and treatment to delay failure. Investigations indicate that treatment of left ventricular dysfunction prior to symptoms can delay the onset of overt heart failure and prolong life.[15,16]

From a preventive standpoint we must redefine the entity of cardiac failure in terms of impaired cardiac function rather than overt symptoms and signs. When dealing with the problem of heart failure the goal of therapy must be shifted from relief of symptoms to improvement of left ventricular function and prolongation of survival. We must more clearly determine the optimal therapies for correcting and preventing left ventricular hypertrophy and dysfunction and demonstrate the efficacy of such therapies for preventing cardiac failure and prolonging life. More research is needed on ways to minimize the dysrhythmias and sudden deaths that characterize the mortality of cardiac failure. We also need better insights into the determinants of symptoms in cardiac failure that correlate so poorly with current measures of cardiac function. We must come to regard the onset of overt heart failure as a medical failure and not as the first indication for treatment.

Acknowledgment

This study was supported by NIH grants NO1-HV-92922 and NO1-HV-52971 and the Visiting Scientist Program.

REFERENCES

1. NHLBI Report of the Task Force on Research in Heart Failure. US Department of Health and Human Services. PHS-NIH, Bethesda, 1994
2. Massie BM, Packer M: Congestive heart failure: current controversies and future prospects. Am J Cardiol 1990;66:429–430
3. National Center for Health Statistics: Vital Statistics of the United States, 1988. Vol. II. Mortality, Part A. DHHS Publication. (PHS) 91–101. USPHS, Washington, DC, 1991
4. Gillum RF: Heart failure in the United States 1970–1985. Am Heart J 1987;113:1043–1045
5. Graves EJ: Detailed diagnoses and procedures; National Hospital Discharge Survey, 1989. Vital Health Stat [13] 1991 (108)
6. Ghali JK, Cooper R, Ford E: Trends in hospitalization rates for heart failure in the United States, 1973–1986. Evidence for increasing population prevalence. Arch Intern Med 1990;150:769–773
7. Schocken DD, Arrieta MI, Leaverton PE: Prevalence and mortality rate of congestive heart failure in the United States. J Am Coll Cardiol 1992;20:301–306
8. National Heart Lung and Blood Institute: Morbidity and Mortality Chartbook on Cardiovascular, Lung and Blood Disease, 1990. NHLBI, Bethesda, 1992
9. Kannel WB, Ho K, Thom T: Changing epidemiologic features of cardiac failure. Br Heart J, suppl. 1994;72: 3–9
10. Ho KKL, Anderson KM, Kannel WB, Grossman W, Levy D: Survival after the onset of congestive heart failure in Framingham Study subjects. Circulation 1993;88:107–715
11. Ranofsky AL: In-patient utilization of short-stay hospitals by diagnosis. Vital Health Stat 1974; (HRA)75–1767
12. Swan HJC: Can heart failure be prevented, delayed or reversed? Am Heart J 1990;120:1540–1546
13. Levy D, Salomon M, D'Agostino RB, Belanger AJ, Kannel WB: Prognostic implications of baseline ECG fea-

tures and their serial changes in subjects with left ventricular hypertrophy. Circulation 1994;90:1786–1793

14. Ho KKL, Pinsky JL, Kannel WB, Levy D: The epidemiology of heart failure. The Framingham Study. J Am Coll Cardiol, suppl. A 1993;4A:6–13

15. Pfeffer MA, Braunwald E, Moye LA et al: Effect of captopril on mortality and morbidity in patients with left ventricular dysfunction after myocardial infarction. Results of the survival and ventricular enlargement trial. N Engl J Med 1992;327:669–677

16. SOLVD Investigators: Effect of enalopril on mortality and the development of heart failure in asymptomatic patients with reduced left ventricular ejection fractions. N Engl J Med 1992;327:685–691

21 Epidemiology of Heart Failure in Europe

George C. Sutton
Martin R. Cowie

There are a number of widespread beliefs concerning the epidemiology of heart failure. It is thought that the condition has a high and rising incidence and a high prevalence, especially in the elderly. It is also thought that although associated with a high mortality rate recent advances in treatment have resulted in improved survival. Hospitalization rates for heart failure are substantial and probably rising, and all these trends imply a considerable economic burden from heart failure on the health care system of all countries. In Europe the dominant etiology of heart failure is thought to be ischemic heart disease due to coronary atheroma.

These beliefs are widely accepted, but there is a paucity of epidemiologic information to support them in Europe and other parts of the world. Population-based studies are rare. With an increasing scope for the treatment of heart failure with pharmacologic agents and surgical procedures including cardiac transplantation, there has been increased focus on the problems of heart failure in recent years, and more epidemiologic work is currently in progress. This chapter concentrates on the published information concerning the incidence, prevalence, etiology, hospitalization rate, prognosis, and economic burden of heart failure in Europe.

DEFINITION OF HEART FAILURE

There is no universally agreed definition of heart failure. A group of cardiologists in Europe in 1983 produced the following definition: "Heart failure is the state of any heart disease in which, despite adequate ventricular filling, the heart's output is decreased or in which the heart is unable to pump blood at a rate adequate for satisfying the requirements of the tissues with function parameters remaining within normal limits."[1] Such a physiologic definition is impractical for clinical and epidemiologic work. Clinically, heart failure is a syndrome that develops as a consequence of heart disease and is characterized by certain symptoms and physical signs. The clinical features are the result of circulatory and neurohormonal responses to the underlying cardiac abnormality. The key symptoms are breathlessness and fatigue, and the characteristic findings on physical examination are fluid retention (pulmonary edema or peripheral edema with an elevated jugular venous pressure) and physical signs characteristic of the underlying cardiac abnormality.

In cases of heart failure due to left ventricular myocardial disease, it is conventional to classify cases on a functional basis as due to systolic or diastolic dysfunction. Such a classification may be too simplistic, as most patients exhibit both systolic and diastolic dysfunction, with "pure" cases being in a minority. However, attempts at such a classification of patients with heart failure highlight the importance of the use of noninvasive and invasive diagnostic techniques to provide insight into the function of the left ventricle. Noninvasive techniques include Doppler echocardiography, nuclear ventriculography, and magnetic resonance imaging; invasive techniques—cardiac catheterization and cardiac biopsy—also provide information. It is important to recognize that although a patient may have evidence of heart disease (e.g., left ventricular dysfunction) it does not necessarily follow that the patient has the clinical syndrome of heart failure. There is no single test that enables the clinician to say that the individual patient with heart disease has "heart failure."

These difficulties of defining heart failure and the absence of a "gold standard" for the diagnosis result in considerable variation in the diagnosis of heart failure in the few epidemiologic studies that have been carried out. Most published population studies use one of several scoring systems that combine certain symptoms, physical examination, and investigatory findings; and if an individual scores more than a predetermined number he or she is considered to have heart failure. Such a scoring system was used for the first time in the Framingham Heart Study in the United States[2] and the same criteria were used in a population-based study in Finland.[3] The scoring system used in the Gothenburg studies[4,5] was different; it was designed to detect less severe cases of heart failure than the Framingham criteria but may have resulted in more individuals without heart failure being misclassified as having heart failure. Comparison between such studies is fraught with difficulty because of the different methodologies and case definitions employed. A similar problem exists for comparison between the studies in general practice in Europe published to date.

The widely recognized need for consistent criteria to diagnose and assess heart failure in clinical practice and epidemiologic research has been recognized by the Task Force on Heart Failure of the European Society of Cardiology, which has published guidelines for the diagnosis of heart failure.[6] To satisfy the Task Force's definition of heart failure, both symptoms and objective evidence of cardiac dysfunction must be present, with reversibility of symptoms on appropriate treatment considered desirable. Echocardiography was recommended as the most practical tool to demonstrate cardiac dysfunction. Only recently has echocardiography been employed in population-based research, and previously used scoring systems for heart failure did not include the results of imaging of the heart other than by chest radiography.

PREVALENCE AND INCIDENCE

Studies of the prevalence of heart failure in Europe have included monitoring general practitioners, data collection from medical records, analysis of drug prescription data, and direct questioning and examination of individuals within the general population. A survey of general practitioner consultations was conducted throughout the United Kingdom during 1991–1992.[7] In this survey involving 60 practices (and a population of just over 500,000), the diagnosis of heart failure by the general practitioner was accepted at face value. The value of such information is likely to be poor, as it has been established that the accuracy of the diagnosis in primary health care is low when compared to assessments by a cardiologist or echocardiography.[8,9]

Another general practitioner-based study was reported from two areas in The Netherlands during the early 1990s.[10,11] The general practitioners involved in these studies were given some guidance as to the evidence required for the diagnosis of heart failure, and information that became available from investigation and hospital referral was used to improve the quality of the data. The prevalence of heart failure in the whole population was found to be of the same order as that found in the U.K. survey: around 12 cases per 1000 population, with an exponential rise with age from 5 per 1000 in those aged 45–64 years to 90–160 per 1000 in those aged over 75 years.

A prevalence study reviewing the medical records of 30,204 patients in three general practices in north and west London[12] yielded a crude prevalence rate of 3.8 cases per 1000 in the population, rising from 0.6 cases per 1000 in those aged under 65 years to 28.0 per 1000 in those over 65 years old. The diagnosis of heart failure depended on the presence of heart disease with fluid retention demonstrated by (1) pulmonary edema on chest radiograph, (2) finding peripheral edema with an elevated venous pressure on examination, or (3) the presence of dyspnea that improves on taking diuretics and relapses on discontinuing treatment. The patients were identified by all those taking diuretics in the three general practices. A study using similar methodology in two general practices in Liverpool, U.K., (total patient population 17,400) yielded a crude prevalence of 15 cases per 1000 population, with a prevalence of 80 cases per 1000 in those over 65 years old.[13] This higher prevalence than the one in North and West London might be explained by including less definite cases than those in the London area. Alternatively the survey in the London area failed to find all patients who were receiving diuretics.

A study in Denmark in one urban general practice was performed using a postal questionnaire to 963 patients aged over 40 years followed up by examination of case records, telephone interview, and physical examination.[13] Mild heart failure was considered present if a patient had a history of heart disease and was either breathless on exertion or was on treatment with digoxin, diuretics, or angiotensin-converting enzyme (ACE) inhibitors. Severe heart failure was considered present if both breathlessness on exertion and use of such medication was associated with a history of cardiac disease. Using these criteria the prevalence of heart failure ("mild" or "severe") rose from 0.2 percent in those aged 40–49 years to 26 percent in those over 70 years of age. Such a case definition is likely to overdiagnose heart failure.

A study in Nottinghamshire (U.K.), analyzing prescription data in the county, suggested a prevalence of heart failure of 1.0–1.6 percent in the overall population, rising from 0.1 percent in those aged 30–39 years, to 0.55 percent in those aged 50–59 years, to 4.2 percent in those aged 70–79 years.[15] These figures were derived from acquiring the total amount of diuretic prescribed in the county and sampling the notes of some of the patients being prescribed diuretics to determine the proportion receiving diuretics for heart failure. Further extrapolation using the mean daily dose prescribed for heart failure produced the prevalence figures cited.

Several population-based studies have been reported. The Gothenburg Study of 50-year-old men followed over a 17-year period used a staging method for defining congestive heart failure (CHF).[4] Stage 0 had no dyspnea, no cardiac disease, and no treatment for heart failure; stage 1 had cardiac disease but no dyspnea or treatment; stage 2 had cardiac disease and dyspnea (but no treatment); stage 3 had cardiac disease, dyspnea, and treatment; and stage 4 included men who died during the follow-up period. "Manifest" CHF was considered present in stages 2–4, whereas "latent" CHF was present in stage 1. "Latent" CHF prevalence rose from 0.4 percent at age 50 to 10.3 percent at age 67. The average annual incidence rate was calculated at 0.46 percent for "latent" heart failure in the overall age range 50–67 years and 0.55 percent for "manifest" heart failure.

The incidence of heart failure has been assessed in eastern Finland by a population-based surveillance study.[3] Four rural communities (total population 37,600, of whom 11,000 were 45–74 years old) were studied over a 2-year period, and all those who developed heart failure were identified by general practitioner referral to a special cardiology clinic. A total of 88 patients were referred to the clinic, and another 25 possible cases were identified from hospital-based records, making a total of 113 patients (51 men, 62 women). The diagnosis of heart failure was based either on the Boston criteria,[16] which use a weighted scoring system dependent on symptoms, signs, and chest radiographic criteria, or the Framingham criteria.[2] Of the 113 possible subjects, 51 had "definite" and 24 "possible" heart failure; 38 were "unlikely" to have heart failure using the Boston criteria. The crude annual incidence of "definite" or "possible" heart failure was 0.4 percent in men and 0.3 percent in women aged 45–74 years, with slightly lower figures using the Framingham criteria. Thus two different epidemiologic methods (reexamining individuals within a cohort and a population-based surveillance system) have yielded similar incidence rates in men.

The incidence of heart failure has also been assessed in a population-based surveillance study in Hillingdon district, West London.[16] In 6 months, 61 new cases of heart failure were identified within a population of 155,000 with an incidence rate rising from 0.02 percent per annum in those aged 45-55 years to 1.2 percent per annum in those aged 85 and over. The diagnosis of heart failure was based on the criteria proposed by the Task Force on Heart Failure of the European Society of Cardiology,[6] and involved echocardiography to confirm the underlying cardiac abnormality.

A study in northern Italy examined a sample of 2254 subjects aged over 64 years in one geographic area with a participation rate of 73 percent.[18] The diagnosis of heart failure was based solely on a questionnaire asking the individual if either the general practitioner or the hospital cardiologist had previously made a diagnosis of heart failure and if the patient had received digoxin. If the answer was "yes" to both questions, the diagnosis of heart failure was accepted. Using these rather lax criteria, the prevalence of heart failure rose from 3.6 percent (aged 65–69 years) to 11.1 percent (75–79 years) and 14.1 percent (85+ years).

It is likely that any variation in the incidence or prevalence of heart failure reported in these few European studies reflects differences in methodology rather than genuine differences in the various countries.

ETIOLOGY

Any disease process that affects the heart and impairs its function can result in heart failure. Thus the proportionate etiology of heart failure reflects the distribution of the various forms of heart disease in a particular community. Coronary heart disease is likely to be the dominant etiology of heart failure in the developed world, whereas rheumatic heart disease and nutritional and infective heart disease may be more common in developing countries. The importance of hypertension as an etiology of heart failure may be changing with time owing to earlier detection and treatment of hypertension reducing the development of heart failure in hypertensive heart disease, although there is no information in Europe to support this view. The role of hypertension in the development of heart failure may be underestimated, as patients who present with heart failure may be normotensive at the time and on subsequent follow-up. It may have been that hypertension, never recorded in the past, had played an important part in producing abnormal pathophysiology of the heart.

In the population-based Finnish study,[3] 41 (80 percent) of 51 "definite" incident cases of heart failure had coronary artery disease, hypertension or both. Of the 31 with coronary artery disease (defined as those with previous myocardial infarction or those who fulfilled the Rose criteria[19] or Whitehall electrocardiographic criteria[20], 18 (58 percent) also had hypertension (blood pressure of $^{160}/_{95}$ mmHg or higher had been measured at rest or the patient had been receiving antihypertensive medication). Ten individuals had hypertension without evidence of coronary artery disease.

The accuracy of determining the etiology of heart failure obviously varies depending on the diagnostic criteria used. The conventional criteria for diagnosing coronary artery disease in an individual include a documented myocardial infarction, a history of angina supported by evidence of reversible myocardial ischemia, or positive coronary arteriography. Hypertension can be diagnosed if there are records of the patient's blood pressure over many years (with or without intervening treatment). Using such diagnostic criteria, a hospital-based study in north and west London showed that 41 percent of patients with heart failure had coronary artery disease, and in only 6 percent was hypertension thought to be the main etiology of the heart failure.[21] Many patients with coronary artery disease, however, have coexistent hypertension; and in certain cases it is difficult to determine which is the most important etiologic factor. This study illustrates the difficulties of establishing a precise etiology for heart failure in that the etiology was uncertain in 36 percent. A predominantly elderly population is unlikely to have detailed (e.g., coronary arteriographic) investigation of heart failure; the medical background may be poorly documented, and simple noninvasive investigations (e.g., echocardiography) do not provide precise etiologic information. The importance of atrial fibrillation in precipitating, or even being the sole abnormality in the development of, heart failure in an aging heart lacking myocytes must be recognized.

In an analysis of the hospital records of patients admitted because of heart failure in western Sweden (2711 patients), coronary artery disease was present in 40 percent, and hypertension was found in 17 percent (diastolic blood pressure over 105 mmHg on three occasions within 4 weeks).[22] Among 179 patients with heart failure in eight Norwegian hospitals 59 percent had ischemic heart disease as the etiology and 14 percent had hypertension.

Information from clinical trials may be misleading when related to the overall population of patients with heart failure because of the highly selected nature of patients who enter clinical trials. Thus an overview of published series[23] showing 50 percent of patients having ischemic heart disease but only 4 percent hypertension as the etiology of heart failure cannot be regarded as representative of the total population of patients with heart failure. In the Framingham Heart Study, coronary heart disease was considered to be present in 59 percent of men and 48 percent of women who developed heart failure, although these percentages included patients who also had hypertension or valvar heart disease.[24] Hypertension as a sole etiologic factor accounted for 21 percent of men and 26 percent of women,[25] but its importance in the Framingham cohort appears to be decreasing.[24]

HOSPITALIZATION RATES

Information on heart failure based on hospital admission data suffers from the inaccuracy of the diagnostic coding of hospital records and variations in the need for admission as judged by different doctors in different countries. The accuracy of diagnostic coding in the United Kingdom has risen in recent years with the development of audit and in the United States with the development of diagnostic related groups (DRGs), which determine reimbursement for medical care.

Examination of the Scottish hospital inpatient statistics between 1980 and 1990[27] showed an increase of almost 60 percent (from 1.3 per 1000 to 2.1 per 1000 population per annum) in the number of hospital discharges for the primary diagnosis of heart failure. A similar study in Dutch hospitals between 1980 and 1992 showed an increase of 69 percent.[28] In Gothenburg[29] there has been an 80 percent increase of hospital discharges for men with heart failure between 1970 and 1985 and a 130 percent increase for women over the same period. A high readmission rate is characteristic of patients with heart failure: A hospital survey in The Netherlands during 1991–1992[28] showed that 16 percent of patients were readmitted with heart failure within 6 months of their first admission. If only hospital discharges, rather than individual patients, are considered, the size of the problem of heart failure may be exaggerated.

Heart failure is responsible for some 5 percent of all admissions to general medicine and care of the elderly wards in a district general hospital in Britain.[21] It accounts for almost 7 percent of all general medical discharges in Scottish hospitals.[27] The mean duration for stay in general medical beds in Scottish hospitals was 11 days.[27]

ECONOMIC COST OF HEART FAILURE

The economic burden of heart failure has been calculated to consume approximately 1 percent of the national health care budgets of countries in Europe.[30–33] To make meaningful calculations, accurate information is required on the prevalence of heart failure, the number of general practitioner consultations and outpatient consultations in hospitals, the number of hospital admissions, the number and use of investigations, the amount of inpatient and outpatient treatment prescriptions, and the amount of surgical treatment. One also needs to know the cost of each of these items. The cost to the National Health Service in the United Kingdom during 1990–1991 was estimated to be £358 million, with hospitalization accounting for 60 percent of this cost.[33]

PROGNOSIS

Information on the prognosis of treated heart failure (untreated heart failure is necessarily unknown) may be obtained from population-based studies, hospital series, or the placebo arm of heart failure clinical trails. The latter cannot be representative of the total population with heart failure because the patients are highly selected, and hospital series tend to reflect the prognosis for patients who have severe heart failure. Population-based information would reflect the outlook for all levels of severity of heart failure, but few data are available for Europe.

In the Gothenburg study of men born in 1913,[29] the 5-year mortality rate for men with "manifest" CHF was 26 percent, compared with 10 percent for "latent" CHF and 8 percent for men without CHF. In the Framingham Heart Study, incident cases had a median survival of 1.66 years in men and 3.17 years in women, with a 5-year survival of 25 percent in men and 38 percent in women.[26] If mortality within the first 90 days of the development of heart failure is excluded (as would be the case in patients enrolled in clinical trials of heart failure), the median survival increases to 3.2 years in men and 5.4 years in women.[26] The marked difference between the survival of individuals with heart failure in the Gothenburg and Framingham studies strongly suggests that the criteria used in the Framingham Study identify more severe heart failure than the criteria employed in the Gothenburg study.

The hospital series in Europe provide information from England, Sweden, and Denmark. In a hospital in northwest London, the inpatient mortality was 30 percent and the 1 year mortality 44 percent.[21] This figure is much higher than that cited from hospital activity analysis elsewhere in the United Kingdom[27] but is likely to be more accurate because the accuracy of coding the diagnosis of heart failure in routine hospital data is poor. In western Sweden the 5-year survival rate from hospital admissions was 50 percent.[22] The 1-year mortality for 190 patients under 76 years old admitted to hospital in Denmark was 21 percent, but patients with myocardial infarction and malignant disease were excluded.[34]

It might be expected that there has been an improvement in prognosis of heart failure in recent years with the use of ACE inhibitors and surgical procedures such as cardiac transplantation. No data are available in Europe to confirm or refute this suggestion, but there is nothing to suggest such a change in Framingham,[35] although it may be too early to be noticed. It is of concern that ACE inhibitors are not being used in routine clinical practice in all patients who would benefit from this therapy.[36]

CONCLUSIONS

It is obvious that available information on the epidemiology of heart failure in Europe is limited. Such information as there is suffers from the lack of a uniform definition for heart failure and lack of accuracy of the diagnosis. Any attempt at making comparisons among countries is difficult because of the lack of standardization of available information.

It is possible, however, to show that heart failure has a substantial incidence and prevalence, and that these numbers rise with age. The condition is associated with a high use of hospital care. The economic burden of heart failure is high for these reasons. The dominant etiology in Europe is coronary heart disease. The prognosis for hospitalized patients is poor. There are no data to suggest that the population prognosis is improving or that the number of new cases is increasing either because of improved survival from acute myocardial infarction or the increasing age of the population.

In Europe there is an urgent need to establish a generally accepted definition of heart failure for use in clinical practice and trials and for population-based research. Such a definition must be capable of distinguishing populations with heart failure of different severity and defining the diagnostic criteria for establishing a given etiology. Population-based studies could then be undertaken to establish the incidence, proportionate etiology, and prognosis in various subgroups. Such studies carried out in European countries would highlight fundamental aspects of health care on a comparative basis.

REFERENCES

1. Denolin H, Kuhn H, Krayenbuehl HP, Loogen F, Reale A: The definition of heart failure. Eur Heart J 1983; 4:445
2. McKee PA, Castelli WP, McNamara PM, Kannel WB: The natural history of congestive heart failure: the Framingham Study. N Engl J Med 1971;285:1441
3. Remes, J, Reunanen A, Aromaa A, Pyorala K: Incidence of heart failure in eastern Finland. A population-based surveillance study. Eur Heart J 1992;13: 588
4. Eriksson H, Svardsudd K, Larsson B et al: Risk factors for heart failure in the general population. The study of men born in 1913. Eur Heart J 1989;10:647
5. Landahl S, Svanborg A, Astrand K: Heart volume and the prevalence of certain common cardiovascular disorders at 70 and 75 years of age. Eur Heart J 1984;5: 326
6. Task Force on Heart Failure of the European Society of Cardiology: Guidelines for the diagnosis of heart failure. Eur Heart J 1995;16:741
7. Royal College of General Practitioners, Office of Population Census and Survey, and Department of Health and Social Security: Morbidity Statistics from General Practice: Fourth National Study, 1991–92. HMSO, London, 1995
8. Remes J, Miettinen H, Reunanen A, Pyorala K: Validity of clinical diagnosis of heart failure in primary health care. Eur Heart J 1991;12:315
9. Wheeldon NM, MacDonald TM, Flucker CJ et al: Echocardiography in chronic heart failure in the community. Q J Med 1993;86:17
10. Lamberts H, Brouwer HJ, Mohrs J: Reason for Encounter and Episode and Process Oriented Standard Output from the Transition Project. Parts 1 and 2. Department of General Practice, Amsterdam, 1993
11. Van de Lisdonk EH, Van den Bosch WJHM, Huygen FJA, Lagro-Jansen ALM: Diseases in General Practice [in Dutch]. Bunge, Utrecht, 1990
12. Parameshwar J, Shackell MM, Richardson A, Poole-Wilson PA, Sutton GC: Prevalence of heart failure in three general practices in north west London. Br J Gen Pract 1992;42:287
13. Mair FS, Crowley TS, Bundred PE. Prevalence, aetiology and management of heart failure in general practice. Br J Gen Pract 1996;46:77
14. Wendelboe O, Hansen JF: Prevalence of mild and severe congestive heart failure in the community. In: Heart Failure '95, Meeting of the Task Force on Heart Failure of the European Society of Cardiology, April 1995, Amsterdam
15. Clarke KW, Gray D, Hampton JR: The prevalence of heart failure estimated from prescription data. Br Heart J, suppl. 1994;71:33
16. Carlson KJ, Lee DC-S, Goroll AH, Leahy M, Johnson RA: An analysis of physicians' reasons for prescribing long-term digitalis therapy in outpatients. J Chronic Dis 1985;38:733–739
17. Cowie MR, Penston H, Wood DA et al: A population-based survey of the incidence of heart failure. Heart, suppl. 1 1996;75:38
18. Ambrosio GB, Riva L, Casiglia E: Prevalence of congestive heart failure (CHF) in elderly. A survey from a population in Veneto region. Acta Cardiol 1994; 49:324
19. Rose GA, Blackburn H, Gillum RF, Prineas RJ: Cardiovascular Survey Methods. 2nd Ed. World Health Organization, Geneva, 1982
20. Reid DD, Brett GZ, Hamilton PJS: Cardiorespiratory disease in diabetics among middle-aged civil servants. A study of screening and intervention. Lancet 1974;1: 469
21. Parameshwar J, Poole-Wilson PA, Sutton GC: Heart failure in a district general hospital. JR Coll Phys Lond 1992;26:139
22. Andersson B, Waagstein F: Spectrum and outcome of congestive heart failure in a hospitalized population. Am Heart J 1993;126:632
23. Klemsdal TO, Mangschau A: Heart failure in Norwegian hospital departments. Prevalence, diagnostic and therapeutic aspects [in Norwegian]. Tidsskr Nor Laegeforen 1994;114:2473
24. Teerlink JR, Goldhaber SZ, Pfeffer MA: An overview of contemporary etiologies of congestive heart failure. Am Heart J 1991;121:1852
25. Kannel WB, Ho K, Thom T: Changing epidemiological features of cardiac failure. Br Heart J, suppl. 1994;72: 3
26. Ho KK, Anderson KM, Kannel WB, Grossman W, Levy D: Survival after the onset of congestive heart failure in Framingham Heart Study subjects. Circulation 1993;88:107
27. McMurray J, McDonagh T, Morrison CE, Dargie HJ: Trends in hospitalization for heart failure in Scotland 1980–1990. Eur Heart J 1993;14:1158
28. Reitsma JB, Mosterd A, Koster RW et al: Increase in the number of admissions due to heart failure in Dutch hospitals in the period 1980–1992 [in Dutch]. Ned Tijdschr Geneeskd 1994;138:866
29. Eriksson H, Wilhelmsen L, Caidahl K, Svardsudd K: Epidemiology and prognosis of heart failure. Z Kardiol, suppl. 8 1991;80:1
30. Eriksson H: Heart failure. A growing public health problem. J Intern Med 1995;237:135
31. Dinkel R, Buchner K, Holtz J: Chronic heart failure. Socioeconomic relevance in the Federal Republic of Germany [in German]. Munch Med Wochenschr 1989; 131:686
32. Koopmanschap MA, van Roijen L, Bonneux L: Costs of Diseases in The Netherlands. Report of the

Department of Public Health and Social Medicine and the Institute for Medical Technology Assessment [in Dutch]. Erasmus University, Rotterdam, 1992

33. McMurray J, Hart W, Rhodes G: An evaluation of the economic cost of heart failure to the National Health Service in the United Kingdom. Br J Med Econ 1993; 6:99

34. Madsen BK, Hansen JF, Stokholm KH et al: Chronic congestive heart failure. Description and survival of 190 consecutive patients with a diagnosis of chronic congestive heart failure based on clinical signs and symptoms. Eur Heart J 1994;15:303

35. Ho KK, Pinsky JL, Kannel WB, Levy D: The epidemiology of heart failure. The Framingham Study. J Am Coll Cardiol 1993;22:6A

36. Clarke KW, Gray D, Hampton JR: Evidence of inadequate investigation and treatment of patients with heart failure. Br Heart J 1994;71:584

22 | Syndrome of Chronic Heart Failure: Origin of Symptoms

Andrew J. S. Coats

Chronic heart failure is a syndrome, not a diagnosis. The term refers to the clinical pattern in which left ventricular impairment produces a constellation of secondary changes in other organs, leading to symptoms and exercise limitation. With modern drug therapy, including the angiotensin-converting enzyme (ACE) inhibitors and diuretics, the symptoms that limit exercise bear little correlation to conventional measures of left ventricular function or central hemodynamics.[1] The most common symptoms are fatigue and dyspnea. With acute heart failure the classic pathophysiologic explanation for the genesis of dyspnea is increased pulmonary wedge pressures and the development of pulmonary edema; and inadequate peripheral blood flow due to poor cardiac output is usually cited as the explanation for fatigue. More recent investigations, as described in other chapters in this book, attest to the importance of abnormalities in peripheral blood flow and skeletal muscle for the genesis of the symptoms limiting exercise in the syndrome of chronic heart failure (CHF).

It is now evident, in addition, that changes in the periphery may be partly responsible for the maintenance of sympathoexcitation and other neurohormonal activation in CHF and therefore may play a role in the progression of the syndrome.[2] This chapter reviews some of the abnormalities that can occur secondarily in extracardiac systems during heart failure and explains how they may contribute to exercise limitation and be harmful during the progression of the syndrome.

Heart failure covers a complex range of clinical situations. Several of the more important are reviewed in other chapters, including valvar disease, the cardiomyopathies, the myocarditis diseases, diastolic, and restrictive heart disease, and heart failure during pregnancy and in the pediatric population. This chapter concentrates on the disorders seen with chronic well treated systolic heart failure in adults. It does not cover the pathophysiology of acute cardiac decompensation, which is discussed in Chapter 36.

PATHOPHYSIOLOGY OF CHRONIC HEART FAILURE

Cardiac Pathophysiology

STRUCTURAL CHANGES

Structural changes in the heart are of paramount importance for generating the clinical disorder. Alterations can be seen at macroscopic and microscopic levels and are covered in detail in Section I of this textbook. The clinical picture of systolic heart failure includes enlargement of the left ventricular cavity usually with a change of shape, to a more spherical contour. This change can occur relatively rapidly after a myocardial infarction via a passive process of stretching of the infarcted territory (infarct expansion) or more slowly by a process termed "remodeling." The remodeled and enlarged ventricle has increased stress on the myocardial wall, which may worsen myocardial ischemia. The latter has important implications for myocardial functional performance and energetics, described in more detail in Section I.

Cardiac enlargement has long been known to be

an adverse prognostic sign, even when estimated crudely as the cardiothoracic diameter on the chest radiograph.[3] More precise measurements of the internal dimensions of the left ventricle by echocardiography have confirmed the prognostic value of cardiac enlargement. Cardiac enlargement is also incorporated into the information derived from calculating the ejection fraction by radionuclide ventriculography, long known to be a useful clinical and prognostic measure in CHF.[4]

Prevention of the late remodeling process was the theory behind the use of ACE inhibitors given early after myocardial infarction.[5] These agents have been shown to reduce the ventricular enlargement that occurs in some patients after a large myocardial infarction, and this mechanism may, at least in part, contribute to the reduction in mortality seen in the postinfarct setting for these agents.[6]

The failing heart also shows alterations in cardiac structure at microscopic and ultrastructural levels (reviewed in Section I). There is an increase in the collagen content of the extracellular matrix, a process thought to be related in part to increased wall stress and in part to neurohormonal activation, particularly aldosterone. These changes are important for progression of the syndrome and for the generation of symptoms and cardiac output limitation. Increased ventricular collagen content reduces ventricular wall distensibility and may affect the efficiency with which active restorative forces can assist the diastolic filling process. As a result, this microscopic structural change may help explain the frequent coexistence of systolic and diastolic dysfunction of the enlarging ventricle during CHF.

Enlargement of the ventricle is associated with thinning of the ventricular wall, which must involve a realignment of the intercellular attachments between individual myocytes. This process, wherein there is continual breaking and reforming of cell-to-cell junctions to allow remodeling, has been termed "cell slippage," although exactly how it occurs has not been established. Improvements in our understanding of this process may help explain how effective therapies work and how we can improve these treatments. They may explain why some treatments aimed specifically at the heart during heart failure are effective, whereas historically most that have had this purpose behind their development have not proved successful in practice.

FUNCTIONAL ABNORMALITIES OF THE MYOCARDIUM

The description of an objective measurement of systolic function in intact humans has proved difficult. In simplest terms the left ventricle is a pump that generates both pressure and flow. It has a theoretic operating range from a pure pressure generator to a pure flow generator, although it always functions as a mixed pump. The function of this pump can be described in terms of the kinetic and potential energy it imparts to the blood ejected at each beat or in terms of the average power output of the circulation (flow × mean pressure drop, described as cardiac power output) assuming the left ventricle is the only significant power source in the circulation.[7]

Cardiac power output is well preserved at rest, even with severe heart failure. The maximal reserve of cardiac power output is reduced, however, and it can be studied during either maximal exercise or inotropic stimulation of the heart. Low maximal power output during inotropic stimulation is a poor prognostic sign.[8] Cardiac power output is a global measure, however, and tells us little of the mechanisms responsible. Ventricular filling or emptying or wasted myocardial power such as with aortic stenosis may be the predominant cause; and therapeutic interventions differ depending on the circumstances.

Attempts have been made therefore to define the components of ventricular function in order to explain the nature of reduced overall circulatory function. The difficulty lies in trying to separate the interacting components. There is no method that can measure the pure inotropic or diastolic (or "lusitropic") function of the myocardium of the heart independent of reflex control systems and the loading conditions of the circulation in the intact human. Attempts are described in Section I and in Chapter 25. Even studies of isolated myocytes from patients with heart failure have led to differing conclusions about the relevant importance of inotropic dysfunction of the myocyte versus abnormalities in cardiac dysfunction due to the environment or cellular connections of the myocytes. Extrapolating these data to the intact patient with neurohormonal and reflex system abnormalities and altered ventricular loading conditions is orders of magnitude more complex, and attempts to do so may prove misleading or even futile. The alternative is to study the function of the integrated system and devise treatments based on the abnormalities detected by this approach.

GLOBAL CARDIAC FUNCTION

Systole can be defined clinically, as the ejection phase between mitral valve closure and aortic valve closure, or in terms of ventricular dynamics as the phase of contraction of the myocytes within the ventricle. These two definitions do not coincide, as there is a period of isovolumic contraction at the onset of ventricular systole during which myocyte contraction generates a pressure increase within the ventricle and a conformational change in its shape but during which no blood is ejected. Similarly, during the latter phase of ventricular ejection the blood is flowing out of the left ventricle passively, and the myocardial elements may be already relaxing. These considerations are reviewed in greater detail in Chapter 25.

Systolic dysfunction can be documented by abnormalities of the pressure or flow-generating properties of the left ventricle or by measurements of ventricular wall function. Useful hemodynamic measurements include the peak rate of pressure rise within the ventricle (positive dP/dt max), filling pressures [e.g., left ventricular end-diastolic pressure (LVEDP) or pulmonary capillary wedge pressures], and measurements of ventricular volumes (by echocardiography, radionuclide ventriculography, or other imaging modalities: see specific chapters). Although not a direct measure of ventricular performance, the ejection fraction (fractional emptying of the ventricle with each beat) carries information about ventricular volumes and global ventricular function. The left ventricular ejection fraction has proved to be the most convenient global summary of systolic function when clinically evaluating the CHF patient.

Diastolic dysfunction of the heart, covered in more detail in Chapter 25, can be quantified by a variety of measurements—hemodynamic, echocardiographic, radionuclear, ventriculographic—but overall objective measurements of diastolic function are more problematic than those of systolic function; no single global summary measurement is acceptable for routine clinical and research use. The most commonly employed are the rate of constant of isovolumic relaxation of the ventricle during early diastole (tau), the early/late peak filling velocity ratio (E/A) across the mitral valve on Doppler echocardiography, and the peak rate of ventricular filling on radionuclear gated acquisition (MUGA) scans (in end-diastolic volumes per second). None of these parameters is independent of the loading conditions of the ventricle, atrioventricular delay, or heart rate, or the effect of systolic dysfunction. Pure diastolic dysfunction is rare, as indeed is pure systolic dysfunction, as the two are almost inseparably interdependent. One can speak, however, of cases where the heart failure is predominantly due to systolic or diastolic impairment of the ventricle. The simplest distinction is via the size of the end-diastolic volume; if it is large, systolic dysfunction is likely to be the major abnormality; if small, there is a diastolic problem. This differentiation is important because of differing effects of treatment, in particular vasodilators, which may be less

useful for diastolic dysfunction because of the requirement for high ventricular filling pressures in this condition.

CIRCULATORY FUNCTION

Integrated function of the heart and blood vessels involves delivery of oxygen and elimination of carbon dioxide and other metabolic products of metabolism at a rate sufficient for resting or stressed metabolism, without excessively high filling pressures. Historically, cardiac output was measured, but it proved to be a poor discriminator between degrees of heart failure. In fact, during progressive exercise in heart failure the cardiac output may be near normal until the patient ceases exercise. Blood pressure, heart rate, peripheral vascular resistance, and ventricular filling pressures are important central hemodynamic parameters, but like cardiac output they only poorly describe the degree of limitation in a patient with CHF.

Noncardiac Pathophysiology

Although initiated by ventricular dysfunction, CHF as a clinical syndrome includes many characteristic pathophysiologic changes in other organ systems. The cause of many of the disparate organ pathologies that develop are poorly understood, as are the mechanisms by which these pathologies are corrected, often after some delay, by effective therapies. The genesis of the classic symptoms and the exercise limitation of patients with CHF may depend more on these changes than on a derangement of central hemodynamics.

PERIPHERAL MICROVASCULATURE

Changes occur in the microvasculature in many organ systems and may contribute to the organ underperfusion seen with this syndrome and are particularly important for renal, hepatic, and pulmonary vascular impairment.[9,10] Structural changes in the microvasculature are subtle and remain poorly evaluated. We know more about the importance of functional endothelial deficiencies, such as impaired endothelial-dependent vasodilation and exaggerated endothelial vasoconstrictor activity.[11] These subjects are discussed in greater detail in Chapters 12 and 13. Therapeutically, little has developed to address these systems specifically, although endothelin receptor antagonists are under evaluation.

LARGE-ARTERY FUNCTION

Large-artery function is abnormal during heart failure owing to a combination of high sympathetic tone, increased activity of the local renin-angiotensin system within the arterial wall, and a high prevalence of atherosclerotic arterial disease in this population.[12] These changes decrease the compliance of the central aorta and large conduit arteries and reduce the efficiency of ventriculoaortic coupling. The net effect is increased impedance to ventricular output, which further worsens global cardiovascular function while at the same time increasing myocardial wall stress and oxygen consumption, possibly reducing effective myocardial blood flow. Direct-acting vasodilators do not specifically address these alterations, and other, more specific therapeutic interventions have not been developed; hence practical applications of our knowledge about these large-artery changes remain elusive.

AUTONOMIC AND NEUROENDOCRINE SYSTEMS

Many neuroendocrine systems are activated during chronic heart failure.[13] Many of them evolved, in a teleologic sense, as a way of compensating for blood or fluid loss or sodium depletion; but during heart failure, although initially helping to support the circulation, continuous activation may be harmful.[14] Such systems include the renin-angiotensin-aldosterone system, sympathetic nervous system, vasopressin system, and the counteracting cardiac natriuretic peptide systems. Simultaneous with neuroendocrine activation there is a reduction in vasodilator influences and vagal tone, which when maintained chronically may be harmful. Adverse consequences have been described, such as organ hypoperfusion, myocardial toxicity, and increased susceptibility to ventricular arrhythmias. These neurohormonal systems are so important to the development of the CHF syndrome that many experts consider neuroendocrine activation to be an essential part of the recognition of the syndrome and an equally essential target of therapeutic strategies to improve the syndrome. Several components of the neuroendocrine systems and the autonomic nervous system are addressed in specific chapters in Section II of this book, and only aspects relevant to the integrated pathophysiology of the CHF syndrome are briefly reviewed here.

RENIN-ANGIOTENSIN-ALDOSTERONE SYSTEM

With untreated heart failure there is mild activation of the renin system, which is dramatically augmented by the first use of diuretics for treatment of the heart failure.[15] After that there is a reasonable relation between the severity of the heart failure and further increases in circulating renin and angiotensin II levels. The components of the circulating renin-angiotensin system exist in tissue sites as well, and these local tissue systems are probably activated in the heart, kidney, brain, and blood vessel walls. Their role and effects in health and in the progression of heart failure are unknown, but some of the beneficial effects of ACE inhibition (described in other Sections) stress how important these systems may be to the syndrome of CHF.

The effects of activation of local systems in the kidney can cause either preservation or reduction of the glomerular filtration rate depending on whether the glomeruli are already dependent on angiotensin II-mediated efferent arteriolar constriction to maintain an adequate filtration pressure in Bowman's capsule. Such a dependence can be seen with bilateral renal artery stenosis. In the heart local increases in angiotensin II can cause coronary vasoconstriction and toxic effects on the myocytes, and in the periphery local angiotensin activation can contribute to vasoconstriction and abnormal large-artery function.

AUTONOMIC NERVOUS SYSTEM

The autonomic nervous system, an important component of heart failure physiology, is dealt with extensively in Chapter 14, to which the reader is referred. The persistent overactivity of sympathetic discharge and the concomitant reduction in vagal tone are seen early in the progression of heart failure due to mild asymptomatic left ventricular dysfunction and are enhanced by the administration of diuretics. Our understanding of these systems and their importance to the syndrome is limited by the lack of clear methods of quantitation, so we are often left with indirect estimates, such as circulating levels of plasma norepinephrine, as an indirect estimate of the highly complex regional sympathetic nerve discharge pattern in a patient with heart failure.

There is no clear mechanism for either activation of the sympathetic system during mild heart failure or its persistence and increase during the chronic syndrome. Understanding of the sympathoexcitation of CHF requires an appreciation of the excitatory and inhibitory inputs to the sympathetic nervous system.[16] These inputs are predominantly the cardiopulmonary reflex systems, arterial baroreflex, low pressure receptor systems, and arterial and central chemoreflexes. Most attention has been devoted to chronic loss of an inhibitory input from the arterial baroreflex. With asymptomatic left ventricular dysfunction or mild heart failure, no perceptible change in blood pressure occurs at a stage when sympathetic activation commences; even complete denervation of the baroreceptors does not lead to such persistent sympathoexcitation as is seen with CHF. Hence the baroreflex system alone does not seem to explain the persistent sympathoexcitation. Two other candidate reflex systems are excitatory, and both are overactive during heart failure: the skeletal muscle ergoreceptor system[17] and the arterial chemoreflex system.[18] Both the ergoreflex and the chemoreflex cause sympathetic activation and may be abnormal throughout the progression of CHF, as discussed below.

Analysis of heart rate variability has identified characteristic harmonic oscillations in cardiovascular parameters, the relative oscillatory power of which shows promise for estimating sympathovagal balance. The pattern during heart failure is abnormal with a dramatic reduction in total heart rate variability and a selective loss of the higher frequency (predominantly vagally mediated) rhythm characteristic of respiratory sinus arrhythmia and relative preservation of low frequency and very low frequency rhythms. The latter have their genesis more in the action of the sympathetic system (low frequency) and renin-angiotensin or chemoreflex system (very low frequency).[19] Analysis of total heart rate variability and, in particular, individual frequency components has shown that the pattern seen with heart failure is one associated with high risk for the development of unstable ventricular arrhythmias and cardiac sudden death, although why this should be the case is not certain.

With chronic sympathetic activation there is a depletion of myocardial catecholamine stores and down-regulation of β-$_1$-receptors on the myocardium. There is also decoupling of receptors from the postreceptor response, all of which lead to a loss of myocardial response to increased sympathetic drive. Clinically, it manifests as chronotropic incompetence, loss of response to sympathomimetic stimulation, and further impaired exercise tolerance. Specific treatments are few, but there has been some improvement after β-blockade, ACE inhibition, and even short-duration, intermittent sympathomimetic stimulation.[20] This topic is discussed in greater detail in Chapter 9.

NATRIURETIC PEPTIDE SYSTEMS

The atria and ventricles contain granulated cells that release peptides, atrial natriuretic peptide (ANP or ANF), brain natriuretic peptide (BNP), and C-type natriuretic peptide (CNP) in response to stretch or volume distension. These peptides are weak natriuretic agents that also relax the peripheral vasculature and thereby mildly oppose the actions of the sympathetic and renin-angiotensin systems. The levels of these hormones reflect the degree of cardiac enlargement, but they appear to be too weak as vasodilators or natriuretic agents in their own right to be useful therapeutically. They may have an interesting role in the detection of ventricular enlargement if the blood levels reliably reflect ventricular or atrial wall stress.

OTHER HORMONAL SYSTEMS

Vasopressin (antidiuretic hormone, or ADH), a hormone released from the posterior pituitary gland, has a role in free water handling by the distal convoluted tubule in its passage through the hypertonic renal medulla and has a direct vasoconstrictor effect on the peripheral systemic resistance vessels. It is found in elevated plasma concentrations in patients with CHF, but its importance to the pathophysiology of the syndrome remains uncertain.

Abnormalities have been described in several other hormonal systems during CHF, but the significance of these changes is uncertain. Thyroid hormone handling in the cells is deranged, with an increase in reverse T_3 similar to that seen with the "sick euthyroid syndrome." Plasma insulin levels are increased during heart failure, whether of ischemic, valvar, or idiopathic etiology; and the increases are associated with decreased sensitivity to the glucose transport effects of insulin. Alterations in sex hormones and growth factors are seen with advanced cardiac cachexia, leading to a loss of anabolic function (or resistance to their effects) and activation of catabolic systems. The reader is referred to Chapter 18 for further discussion and below for the importance of skeletal muscle wasting to the progression of the CHF syndrome.

KIDNEY

The kidney is of major importance during heart failure for understanding the development of the syndrome and for correct management of the afflicted patient. The importance of fluid and electrolyte balance is discussed in Chapter 11, and the interactions between renal and cardiac disease are discussed in Chapter 10. Only the aspects of particular relevance to the progression of the CHF syndrome are reviewed here.

The kidney is only partly a passive organ responding to neuroendocrine activation outside its control; it is also an active endocrine and autocrine organ that responds to the reduced renal perfusion pressure during heart failure. The juxtaglomerular apparatus adjacent to the distal convoluted tubule senses the reduction in the rate of delivery of sodium to the distal tubule and releases renin in response. This action is an important part of the activation of the circulating renin-angiotensin system described above. The homeostatic role of this system is that blood flow is diverted to the kidney, the glomerular filtration rate (GFR) is increased, and there is increased active reabsorption of sodium. Angiotensin II has additional effect on thirst and possibly salt hunger, which completes the response, ensuring an increase in salt and water intake.

The components of the renin-angiotensin system also exist within the kidney, and there can be local autocrine activation, which can have important effects on intrarenal hemodynamics. These effects may either increase or decrease the GFR depending on the level of renal perfusion pressure and other factors operating on the kidney, such as the renal sympathetic nerves and circulating vasoactive factors.

KALLIKREIN-KININ SYSTEM

The second autocrine system of the kidney, the kallikrein-kinin system, is less well studied because of the short-half life of some of its active components and the difficulty isolating how and where they are operative. In simplest terms, the kinin system appears to be complementary to the renin-angiotensin system, causing vasodilatation, whereas the latter causes vasoconstriction. It is also thought to be involved in the control of renal tubular function, but its precise role in heart failure and the effects of ACE inhibitors (which also block the enzyme that breaks down bradykinin) are unknown.

LUNGS AND RESPIRATORY SYSTEM

Despite the frequency of dyspnea as the central complaint of a patient with heart failure, relatively little is known of the role of the lung and the abnormalities of ventilatory control in symptom generation during CHF. With acute heart failure, changes within the lung are profound and easily explain much of the acute respiratory distress of the syndrome; this subject is dealt with in greater detail in Chapter 17.

Few changes are detected in the lung histology of well diuresed and nonedematous CHF patients. The changes of pulmonary siderosis seen with chronic untreated mitral stenosis are not seen with well treated CHF. Even pulmonary venous pressures may be normal if diuretic treatment is effective. The question of lung function in CHF remains controversial. Some authors report a reduction in oxygen-diffusing capacity, suggesting an alveolar-arterial block to oxygen transfer,[21] whereas others find oxygen transfer to be nonlimiting and that arterial oxygen desaturation during exercise is rare with otherwise uncomplicated CHF.[22] Similarly, although intermittent, nonasthmatic bronchial constriction has been reported by some authors and even made a target for therapeutic intervention[23]; in a detailed evaluation of well diuresed patients we could find no excessive bronchoconstriction or bronchial reactivity over that seen in a carefully matched control group. There is also an oft-reported increase in deadspace ventilation, thought by some to account for the exaggerated ventilatory response to exercise by patients with CHF[24]; but there is no anatomic substrate for this explanation, and it may be a functional abnormality related to abnormal ventilatory control rather than a primary defect in the lung or pulmonary circulation.

One pathophysiologic change that can lead to respiratory distress is an alteration in the volume, structure, strength, and fatigability of the respiratory musculature. Early muscle deoxygenation, respiratory muscle fatigue, and histologic changes have been described,[25,26] and they may contribute to the sensation of dyspnea. Whether these abnormalities can explain the excessive ventilatory response to exercise remains unknown. Whatever the cause, the increased ventilatory response to exercise appears to be an important abnormality in CHF, with a close correlation to objective measures of exercise intolerance.[27]

VENTILATORY CONTROL

The mechanisms of normal respiratory control during exercise are not fully understood, nor are the mechanisms underlying the abnormal respiratory response seen with CHF. Patients with heart failure, even in the absence of pulmonary edema, have an increased ventilatory response to exercise while maintaining normal arterial blood gas tensions.[22] They show reduced maximal oxygen consumption, early dependence on anaerobic metabolism, and an increased ventilatory equivalent for carbon dioxide even at low work levels. The latter feature can be best appreciated by the plot of minute ventilation (V_E) against CO_2 production (VCO_2) during progressive exercise: the V_E/VCO_2 slope.[28] The relation is approximately linear for most subjects at least until near-maximal exercise, but its slope is significantly (up to three-fold) steeper throughout both aerobic and anaerobic levels of exercise in patients with CHF, and its steepness correlates closely with the reduction of maximal oxygen consumption. There are deviations from linearity in more severe heart failure cases.[29]

Although often thought to be due to ventilation-perfusion mismatch within the lung, causing excessive but noncontributory ventilation,[30] there are flaws in this argument. The ventilatory compensation is excessive, with arterial blood gases being normal or even supernormal during CHF,[31] so whatever is causing the hyperventilation cannot be sensing abnormalities in arterial blood gases. An alternative explanation is that there is enhanced sensitivity of ventilatory control mechanisms to progressive exercise during CHF. Two reflexes with enhanced gain in CHF patients are the arterial chemoreceptors and the muscle ergoreflex system.[17,18] Either reflex abnormality could explain increased ventilation and abnormal sensitivity to dyspnea during exercise. The ergoreflex system senses the metabolic state of exercising skeletal muscle and reflexly increases ventilation. It is sensed by small work-sensitive afferents and carried by small myelinated or unmyelinated nerve fibers.[32] These fibers are histologically inseparable from pain fiber afferents, and it is possible that they serve a sensory as well as a reflex function, perhaps mediating to some extent both the sensation of fatigue and the exaggerated ventilatory and cardiovascular reflex responses to exercise. Overactivity of these fibers and the resultant reflex responses has been described for CHF.[17]

Other overactive ventilatory control systems in CHF are the arterial and central chemoreflex systems.[18] We have described augmentation of peripheral hypoxic and central CO_2 sensitivity in CHF patients.[18] These alterations could explain the heightened ventilatory responses and could lead to excessive sympathoexcitation. The cause of the heightened chemosensitivity itself remains undetermined, but it is possible that there is central augmentation of the handling of chemoreflex inputs.

SLEEP-APNEA SYNDROME

Detailed sleep physiology studies have revealed that dips in oxygen saturation in CHF patients, often to below 80–85 percent, are not uncommon[33] despite the relative rarity of exercise-induced desaturation, mentioned above. These episodes coincide with episodes of apnea and often follow episodes of relative hyperventilation.[34] The episodes are followed by semiarousal from sleep and hyperventilation, which may awaken and frighten the sleeping partner. The pattern is reminiscent of the Cheyne-Stokes respiratory pattern, which is well recognized in severe heart failure.

The mechanisms of both abnormalities of respiratory rhythm are incompletely understood, but their detection in CHF during sleep suggest that the ventilatory control is abnormal, rather than it being a structural obstructive sleep apnea seen in obese patients with sleep disorders. The central abnormality may be an alteration in the central sensitivity to carbon dioxide, so oscillating levels of the respiratory drive and hence arterial oxygen saturation develop.

A possibly related finding is that patients with CHF exhibit reduced total and high frequency heart rate variability but a relatively enhanced variability of heart rate at very low frequencies (< 0.01 Hz, or 1 cycle every 100 seconds), a specific rhythm we have shown to be related to hypoxic chemosensitivity and that can be abolished by supplemental oxygen. Several features of this very low frequency rhythm suggest that chemoreflex activity may play a role in its genesis. First, the rhythm is particularly prominent during heart failure, where circulation time is long. Second, it has a frequency similar to that of the more obvious rhythm of Cheyne-Stokes breathing. Third, the chemoreflex loop has sufficient delay characteristics and sufficient interactions with the baroreflexes and control of heart rate for a harmonic of oscillatory arterial gas concentrations to set up a similar harmonic oscillation in respiration, which would then entrain the heart rate via an effect of the baroreflex. Lastly, similar rhythms are particularly prominent in pulmonary arterial pressure tracing during heart failure.[35] Thus it may be that periodic sleep apnea, very low frequency rhythms of heart rate variability, and Cheyne-Stokes respiration may be reflections of harmonic oscillations of chemoreflex–baroreflex interactions, a finding of particular importance given that it would lead to nocturnal surges of chemoreflex-induced sympathoexcitation coinciding with profound arterial deoxygenation, a potent mix that would allow opportunistic ventricular arrhythmias to develop. The promising reports of nocturnal oxygen supplementation and of nasal positive-pressure ventilation for treatment of CHF may support this contention.[36]

RESPIRATORY MUSCLE FUNCTION

Respiratory muscle is abnormal in CHF. Early muscle deoxygenation, respiratory muscle fatigue, and histologic changes have been described[25,26] and may contribute to the sensation of dyspnea. Whether these abnormalities can explain the excessive ventilatory response to exercise seen frequently in CHF patients remains unknown. Whatever the cause, the increased ventilatory response to exercise appears to be an important abnormality in CHF, with a close correlation to objective measures of exercise intolerance.[27]

SKELETAL MUSCLE

Patients with CHF can have markedly reduced exercise tolerance and evidence of early muscular lactate release despite normal skeletal muscle blood flow.[37] An inherent defect in skeletal muscle metabolism independent of blood flow has been described in association with this condition[38] along with many reports of abnormalities in histology, mitochondrial structure and function, oxidative enzymes, and a shift in fiber type distributions.[39] Metabolic abnormalities have also been described, including early dependence on anaerobic metabolism, excessive early depletion of high energy phosphate bonds, and excessive early intramuscular acidification.[38] Biopsy studies have confirmed defects in oxidative and lipolytic enzymes, succinate dehydrogenase and citrate synthetase, and β-hydroxyacyl dehydrogenase.[39] Muscle also has abnormal gross function, showing in particular early fatigability and reduced maximal strength.[40] These changes are described in detail in Chapter 16. What is reviewed here is the contribution of skeletal muscle pathophysiology to the symptoms and possibly the progression of the CHF syndrome.

MUSCLE ERGOREFLEX EFFECTS

The muscle ergoreflex system is a system of small, free receptor endings within skeletal muscle that connect to group III and IV small myelinated or unmyelinated fibers that travel in the lateral spinothalamic tract to the brain stem. This receptor/reflex system contributes to the reflex cardiovascular responses that support and augment the early circulatory adjustments to the onset of muscular exercise, such as a vasoconstrictor sympathetic output to non-exercising muscle vascular beds. It has long been known that this system can mediate the sympathoexcitatory and vasoconstrictor responses to exercise,[32] but they also play a role in generating and maintaining the early ventilatory responses. We have demonstrated the importance of this system to ventilatory control in normal subjects and in patients with CHF. Furthermore, we have demonstrated a dramatically enhanced dependence on this system during heart failure, possibly explaining the exaggerated ventilatory response during heart failure.[17]

The abnormalities of muscle in this syndrome means that there is an early and exaggerated build-up of metabolites within the muscle, which could then stimulate the ergoreceptors and explain the heightened reflex responses. The potential importance of this reflex lies in its multiple effects. With chronic and repetitive recruitment of this exaggerated reflex there could be persistent and progressive sympathetic activation and persistently adverse loading conditions due to a diverse and persistent vasoconstrictor drive. Thus like the renin-angiotensin-aldosterone system, the muscle ergoreflex system could contribute to the progression of the syndrome by its dual effects on the load on the heart and the level of harmful neuroendocrine activation. It has been proposed that skeletal muscle abnormalities during heart failure contribute to a vicious cycle of deterioration, coined the "muscle hypothesis."[2]

The cause and most appropriate management of these muscle changes are uncertain. Physical inactivity is likely to play a role in some cases, along with activation of catabolic processes, loss of normal anabolic function (e.g., insulin resistance),[41] elevated levels of tumor necrosis factor α, and excessive norepinephrine levels.[42] Anorexia and intestinal malabsorption may also play a role in some patients.

We have demonstrated in the rat coronary artery ligation model of heart failure by use magnetic resonance spectroscopy that some of the metabolic disturbances of peripheral muscle (early high energy phosphate bond depletion and early acidification) can be completely avoided by regular exercise training commencing 6 weeks after the myocardial infarction.[43] In humans with CHF we have demonstrated partial correction of these muscle abnormalities by exercise training.[44]

HEMATOLOGIC SYSTEM

An increased arterial hemoglobin content has been described as an adaptive response during heart failure, possibly secondary to chronic tissue hypoxia, via an increase in erythropoietin production. It is doubtful if the increase in hemoglobin is important for increasing oxygen delivery. Any excessive increase also increases the hematocrit to a level where whole blood viscosity increases, reducing net tissue perfusion by increasing the resistance to blood flow. Hepatic dysfunction can reduce clotting factor production, leading to autoanticoagulation. Reduced peripheral blood flow and habitually reduced exercise could predispose patients to venous thromboses, so the interactions of these conflicting complications could lead either to bleeding or to thromboembolic events. The use of aspirin or formal anticoagulation is common in CHF patients. The white blood cell count may be mildly elevated during heart failure as part of a generalized but poorly understood immune activation in this syndrome.

LIVER AND GASTROINTESTINAL TRACT

During heart failure the liver can be affected by increased venous back-pressure, an impaired arterial supply, and the metabolic complications of the syndrome. It can also be affected by the underlying process that leads to the heart failure (e.g., alcohol excess or hemochromatosis). The most common hepatic abnormality seen with CHF is congestion due to high right atrial pressure. Persistent venous engorgement can result in a noticeable increase in hepatic size, local tenderness, and minor derangements in liver function, varying from the common modest increases in transaminase levels to profound hepatic dysfunction, including loss of clotting factor production and impaired hepatic metabolism of drugs or alcohol. In more severe cases nausea and right hypochondrial discomfort develop, and in severe cases jaundice, impaired albumin and clotting factor production, and malabsorption of fats may result. The nausea and malabsorption can worsen the catabolic state of the patient and can contribute to the wasting seen with cardiac cachexia.

Intestinal malabsorption and bacterial overgrowth are common in those with severe heart failure when the intestinal mucosa becomes congested. Cardiac valvar abnormalities are also associated with a high rate of intestinal angiodysplasia, which can lead to recurrent blood loss, a considerable management problem for a patient who requires anticoagulation. These intestinal complications may be important in the genesis of cardiac cachexia, as reviewed in Chapter 18. The combination of intestinal edema, sluggish blood flow, and intestinal overgrowth allows endotoxic stimulation of lipopolysaccharide, which can set in motion a cascade of cytokine release, including tumor necrosis factor, which may itself be associated with muscle wasting, impaired endothelial-dependent blood flow, and an adverse prognosis. Like many systems in this complex syndrome, the integrated whole is far more complex than the isolated and apparently independent components.

Sypmtoms of Chronic Heart Failure

DYSPNEA VERSUS FATIGUE

The two cardinal symptoms of CHF are dyspnea and fatigue, and the classic physiologic explanation for their genesis describes different processes for each. It has long been taught that the dyspnea results primarily as a manifestation of "backward" heart failure (i.e., increased ventricular filling pressures). This theory was based on the pathophysiology of acute heart failure, where increased left ventricular end-diastolic pressure as a result of systolic impairment produces an increase in left atrial and pulmonary venous pressures, which in turn eventually leads to pulmonary edema. Even before fluid extravasation into the alveoli occurs, the increased pulmonary venous pressures can increase the stiffness of the alveolar wall and can reduce the effective area for gas exchange. It might also increase the resistance to airflow in the small bronchioles, although experimental evidence of this phenomenon is sparse. A hallmark of this theoretic construct is that pulmonary arterial or wedge pressures should increase, and this increase generates the sensation of dyspnea at a fairly reproducible level of wedge pressure.

Numerous lines of evidence argue against this theory. The limiting symptom during progressive exercise in an individual can be altered by changes in the details of the exercise test.[45] The use of a rapidly incremental exercise load leads more frequently to dyspnea, whereas a slower workload leads to fatigue. There appears to be no substantial difference in the level of pulmonary arterial and wedge pressures achieved, but the limiting symptom differs.[2,46] Second, studies of 24-hour ambulatory pulmonary arterial pressure monitoring in patients with chronic heart failure showed no significant relation between the levels of pulmonary arterial pressures achieved by various forms of exercise and the symptoms reported by the patients at the time.[47] In fact, the highest levels of pulmonary arterial pressure were seen during supine rest, when the patients were comfortable. Lastly, we have compared the physiologic and clinical characteristics of patients limited by fatigue to those limited by dyspnea on a standard incremental cardiopulmonary exercise test.[48] There were no significant differences in the clinical, hemodynamic, or functional characteristics between the two groups, leading us to propose that the pathophysiologic processes generating dyspnea may have more in common with those generating muscle fatigue that we had previously imagined. Two alternatives have been discussed: (1) The same receptors that carry the sensation of muscular fatigue could also carry the sensory input perceived as dyspnea; or (2) The patients are experiencing an unpleasant sensation that is different from the conventional fatigue or dyspnea perceived by a normal subject. This idea might help explain why, with deterioration during heart failure, fatigue and dyspnea often worsen simultaneously and why, with improvement, they similarly disappear together: They may represent the same underlying pathophysiologic abnormality.

FATIGUE

Drexler and I have reviewed the pathophysiologic mechanisms underlying the genesis of muscular fatigue during CHF.[49] Impaired muscular blood flow, deficient endothelial function, and disordered skeletal muscle structure and function play an important role. Fatigue within skeletal muscle depends on excessive build-up of metabolic products (including potassium, adenosine, lactate, and acid) within the extracellular space. This build-up has two effects. (1) It contributes to objective fatigue of the muscle itself and neurophysiologic fatigue of the neuromuscular apparatus; and (2) it leads to the perception of fatigue by the cortex. The sensory endings that carry this sensation have not been characterized, but it is possible that they are similar or indeed identical to the receptors that carry the afferent part of the muscle ergoreflex described above.

It is not difficult to understand why the CHF patient develops muscular fatigue. The extensive range of structural and functional abnormalities described for CHF could all produce early muscular fatigue. In addition, there may be a heightened sensory mechanism to carry the sensation of this muscular distress to the cortex. What is of interest is how this theory fits with what we know about objective limitation to exercise. We have known for years that objective measures of cardiac output—left ventricular ejection fraction or central hemodynamics—correlate poorly with exercise tolerance in well treated patients with CHF. In contrast, several groups have reported strong correlations between exercise intolerance and objective independent measures of muscle function, such as those derived from magnetic resonance spectroscopy studies of in vivo metabolism[50] or structural measures of skeletal muscle bulk or maximal quadriceps strength, which predominantly reflects the bulk of the leg muscle.[51] In addition, the delayed improvement in exercise capacity after vasodilator,[52] positive inotropic, or even cardiac transplant therapy suggests that a structural abnormality is being overcome; and muscle changes leading to muscular fatigue are prime candidates for this limiting factor.[53]

DYSPNEA

Dyspnea is poorly understood in normal subjects despite our understanding its associations and features. It has been studied in chronic lung disease, and there remains little consensus as to the primary cause of dyspnea in this setting.[54] It is likely that several candidate physiologic processes can be invoked, including the sensation of abnormal blood gases sensed via a chemoreceptor afferent input, a perception of the effort of ventilation, a mismatch between the desired level of ventilation and that achieved, and a feeling of difficult or restricted airflow arising from within the lung. Despite many reviews, even less is known about the processes operative in the genesis of the dyspnea associated with heart diseases, with the exception of the simple case of acute heart failure with pulmonary edema described above.

There is a good correlation between the level of achieved ventilation during progressive exercise and the perception of dyspnea associated with that level of exercise effort. This correlation has led cardiologists to consider the control of ventilation during exercise as an objective measurement that tells us something about the pathophysiology of ventilatory control and the symptoms limiting the patents with CHF.

A normal subject during progressive exercise below the level of anaerobic threshold increases the level of minute ventilation in proportion to the increasing rate of carbon dioxide production (the V_E/VCO_2 slope described above). The increased V_E/VCO_2 slope seen wtih CHF is closely correlated with objective limitation to exercise and appears to be a good surrogate for the pathophysiologic processes causing dyspnea. Furthermore, in the presence of normal blood gases during exercise this increased slope suggests relative hyperventilation during exercise rather than an appropriate response to abnormalities of lung function, where we would expect some residual error signal and mild hypoxemia or hypercapnia on exercise. If anything, the opposite is seen: almost supernormal blood gases in patients with CHF.

This finding led us to search for alternative ventilatory stimuli that may be exaggerated in CHF. We have described two candidate control systems as having an increased gain: the muscle ergoreflex system (whose ventilatory component we have demonstrated in CHF[17]) and hypoxic chemosensitivity and central CO_2 chemosensitivity.[18] Either could lead to an exaggerated ventilatory response to exercise in CHF patients. Of interest is the finding that both these reflex systems, in addition, are potent stimuli for activation of the sympathetic nervous system, so they may help explain the persistent sympathoexcitation that is so much a part of the syndrome of CHF.

Exercise Limitation

NORMAL SUBJECTS

In normal subjects exercise is usually possible until maximal cardiac output is achieved, at which time a further increase in workload produces extra CO_2 but no increase in O_2 uptake.[55] This condition is termed maximal oxygen uptake (VO_2max). At 85–95 percent VO_2max the anaerobic threshold is reached, where skeletal muscle begins to depend on anaerobic metabolism for the continued production of adenosine triphosphate (ATP). Despite much use of this quantity, it is doubtful that a distinct transition point from aerobic to anaerobic metabolism occurs; more likely there is a gradual transition in different muscle groups at different stages during progressive exercise.[31]

EXERCISE CAPACITY DURING CHRONIC HEART FAILURE

In well treated patients with CHF who have no residual pulmonary congestion, exercise proceeds along normal lines with little difference in submaximal cardiac output but with an exaggerated ventilatory response even at low level exercise.[31] Most patients with CHF fail to achieve their VO_2max, and it has been shown that in contrast to normal subjects the addition of arm exercise to a patient already performing maximal leg exercise leads to a further increase in the rate of O_2 uptake.[56] Hence O_2 delivery—and by extrapolation cardiac output—was not maximal during the maximal leg exercise test in the CHF patients. The limitation to exercise therefore appears to be peripheral: Either the vasculature is unable to accept an adequate blood flow or the exercising muscle is unable to take up or metabolize O_2 efficiently. Both defects are present in patients with CHF, as discussed earlier.

Wilson et al. described a subset of patients in whom exercise was clearly limited by skeletal muscle metabolic inefficiency despite nonlimiting cardiac output and normal leg blood flow responses.[37] Distinguishing the effects of limiting blood flow from skeletal muscle limitation may to some extent be artificial, as the process of skeletal muscle wasting characteristic of CHF reduces the vascular conductance of the limb, leading to an apparently increased vascular resistance even with no change in endothelial function or vascular resistance tone. Although this situation does not reduce the potential importance of endothelial, vasodilatory, and large-vessel functional defects, it does highlight the importance of the pathologic skeletal muscle of this condition.

IMPLICATIONS FOR TREATMENT OF CHF

Effective therapies for exercise tolerance and prognostic benefit have been established for heart failure. Foremost among them is the use of ACE inhibitors. The mechanisms underlying the reduction in mortality rate and the improved tolerance to exercise are unknown, but reduction of persistent and exaggerated neuroendocrine activation appears important at least for the former. There are some suggestions that peripheral actions are necessary for improved exercise tolerance. The increase in exercise tolerance with ACE inhibition is delayed and is closely related to improvements in skeletal muscle blood flow.[57] In the future we may look to therapeutic approaches for improving symptoms and exercise capacity that are different from those designed to enhance survival.

EXERCISE TRAINING PRESCRIPTIONS

Exercise training in carefully selected patients with stable, mild to moderate CHF can increase exercise capacity and lessen dyspnea and fatigue.[58] Such improvement has been shown for asymptomatic left ventricular dysfunction[59–61] and mild to moderate CHF[62,63] with no consistent effect on left ventricular ejection fraction, either beneficial or detrimental. Most of the beneficial effects seem to depend on training-induced adaptations in the periphery.[64] This subject is further reviewed in Chapter 41.

CORRECTING PATHOPHYSIOLOGY

In normal subjects training is known to be able to increase endothelial, large-vessel, and resistance-vessel function.[65] During heart failure exercise training can reduce peripheral vascular resistance and increase skeletal muscle blood flow[63] and endothelial function.

Partial corrections of skeletal muscle abnormalities have been demonstrated after training in heart failure patients.[43,44,66,67] Single-limb and whole-body training can improve histology, mitochondrial structure,[68] oxidative enzymes, and metabolic function. Training, particularly with a resistive training component, has the potential to stabilize or reverse skeletal muscle wasting, although as yet this practice has not been adequately evaluated. These improvements may explain the reduction in muscular fatigue seen after training.

Specific respiratory muscle training has been reported for CHF patients that leads to improved exercise tolerance.[69] It may have a particular role of alleviating dyspnea in these patients.

Training has also been shown to alleviate some of the abnormalities of neuro-hormonal overactivity, including a reduction in norepinephrine spillover, an increase in the vagal high frequency component of heart rate variability, and a relative diminution in the more sympathetically mediated low frequency component.[70] These changes are all consistent with what is known of training effects in normal subjects, although the mechanisms, even in normal subjects, have not been fully established. Given the absence of effects on central hemodynamics and the prominence of peripheral training effects, it is possible that these autonomic training effects are secondary to skeletal muscle or peripheral vascular training effects. In this regard the finding that single-limb training has been shown to reduce the overactivity of the skeletal muscle ergoreflex[17] has important implications. It could explain the removal of a major sympathoexcitatory influence as well as removing a stimulus to the exaggerated ventilatory response to exercise.

CONCLUSIONS

The symptoms limiting exercise performance in CHF patients appear to be related to alterations in the physiology of the periphery: skeletal muscle, endothelium, regional blood flow, and reflex cardiopulmonary control systems. These alterations may set in motion a vicious cycle of deterioration, involving catabolic activation and reflex neurohormonal overactivity, that may lead to progressive disease severity. Understanding the complex pathophysiology of the syndrome of CHF may allow us to develop novel therapeutic strategies for this complex but common condition.

REFERENCES

1. Franciosa JA, Park M, Levine TB: Lack of correlation between exercise capacity and indexes of resting left ventricular performance in heart failure. Am J Cardiol 1981;47:33–39
2. Coats AJS, Clark AL, Piepoli M, Volterrani M, Poole-Wilson PA: Symptoms and quality of life in heart failure. The muscle hypothesis. Br Heart J, suppl. 1994; 72:36–39
3. Parameshwar J, Keegan J, Sparrow J, Sutton GC, Poole-Wilson PA: Predictors of prognosis in severe chronic heart failure. Am Heart J 1992;123:421–426
4. Saxon LA, Stevenson WG, Middlekauff HR et al: Predicting death from progressive heart failure secondary to ischemic or idiopathic dilated cardiomyopathy. Am J Cardiol 1993;72:62–65
5. Pfeffer MA, Pfeffer JM, Lamas GA: Development and prevention of congestive heart failure following myocardial infarction. Circulation, suppl. 14 1993;87:120–125
6. Pfeffer MA, Braunwald E, Moye LA et al: Effect of captopril on mortality and morbidity in patients with left ventricular dysfunction after myocardial infarction. Results of the survival and ventricular enlargement trial. The SAVE Investigators. N Engl J Med 1992;327:669–677
7. Tan LB, Murray RG, Littler WA: An analytical method to separate inotropic and vasodilatory drug effects in patients with heart failure. Cardiovasc Res 1987;21:625–630
8. Tan LB: Evaluation of cardiac dysfunction, cardiac reserve and inotropic response. Postgrad Med J, suppl. 1 1991;67:10–20
9. Wallerson DC, Devereux RB: Reproducibility of echocardiographic left ventricular measurements. Hypertension, suppl. II 1987;9:6–18
10. Drexler H, Hayoz D, Munzel T et al: Endothelial dysfunction in chronic heart failure. Experimental and clinical studies. Arzneimittelforschung 1994;44:455–458
11. Treasure CB, Alexander RW: The dysfunctional endothelium in heart failure. J Am Coll Cardiol 1993;22:129A–134A
12. O'Rourke M: Arterial stiffness, systolic blood pressure, and logical treatment of arterial hypertension. Hypertension 1990;15:339–347
13. Packer M, Lee WH, Kessler PD et al: Role of neurohormonal mechanisms in determining survival in patients with severe chronic heart failure. Circulation, suppl. IV 1987;75:80–92
14. Harris P: Congestive cardiac failure: central role of the arterial blood pressure. Br Heart J 1987;58:190–203
15. Anand IS, Ferrari R, Kalra GS et al: Edema of cardiac origin. Studies of body water and sodium, renal function, hemodynamic indexes, and plasma hormones in untreated congestive cardiac failure. Circulation 1989;80:299–305
16. Floras JS: Clinical aspects of sympathetic activation and parasympathetic withdrawal in heart failure. J Am Coll Cardiol 1993;22:72A–84A
17. Piepoli M, Clark AL, Volterrani M et al: Contribution of muscle afferents to the hemodynamic, autonomic, and ventilatory responses to exercise in patients with chronic heart failure. Effects of physical training. Circulation 1996;93:940–952
18. Chua TP, Clark AL, Amadi AA, Coats AJS: Relation between chemosensitivity and the ventilatory response to exercise in chronic heart failure. J Am Coll Cardiol 1996;27:650–657
19. Saul JP, Arai Y, Berger RD et al: Assessment of autonomic regulation in chronic congestive heart failure by heart rate spectral analysis. Am J Cardiol 1988;61:1292–1299
20. Adamopoulos S, Piepoli M, Qiang F et al: Effects of pulsed β-stimulant therapy on β-adrenoceptors and chronotropic responsiveness in chronic heart failure. Lancet 1995;345:344–349
21. Puri S, Baker BL, Dutka DP et al: Reduced alveolar-capillary membrane diffusing capacity in chronic heart failure. Its pathophysiological relevance and relationship to exercise performance. Circulation 1995;91:2769–2774
22. Clark AL, Coats AJ: Usefulness of arterial blood gas estimations during exercise in patients with chronic heart failure. Br Heart J 1994;71:528–530
23. Cabanes LR, Weber SN, Matran R et al: Bronchial hyperresponsiveness to methacholine in patients with impaired left ventricular function. N Engl J Med 1989;320:1317–1322
24. Sullivan MJ, Higginbotham MB, Cobb FR: Increased exercise ventilation in patients with chronic heart fail-

ure. Intact ventilatory control despite hemodynamic and pulmonary abnormalities. Circulation 1988;77: 552–559

25. Mancini DM, Ferraro N, Nazzaro D, Chance B, Wilson JR: Respiratory muscle deoxygenation during exercise in patients with heart failure demonstrated with near-infrared spectroscopy. J Am Coll Cardiol 1991;18: 492–498

26. Mancini DM, Henson D, LaManca J, Levine S: Evidence of reduced respiratory muscle endurance in patients with heart failure. J Am Coll Cardiol 1994;24: 972–981

27. Buller NP, Poole-Wilson PA: Mechanism of the increased ventilatory response to exercise in patients with chronic heart failure. Br Heart J 1990;63: 281–283

28. Clark AL, Poole Wilson PA, Coats AJ: Relation between ventilation and carbon dioxide production in patients with chronic heart failure. J Am Coll Cardiol 1992;20:1326–1332

29. Clark AL, Poole-Wilson PA, Coats AJS: Relation between ventilation and carbon dioxide production in patients with chronic heart failure. J Am Coll Cardiol 1992;20:1326–1332

30. Sullivan MJ, Higginbotham MB, Cobb FR: Increased exercise ventilation in patients with chronic heart failure. Intact ventilatory control despite hemodynamic and pulmonary abnormalities. Circulation 1988;77: 552–559

31. Clark A, Coats A: The mechanisms underlying the increased ventilatory response to exercise in chronic stable heart failure. Eur Heart J 1992;13:1698–1708

32. Abboud FM, Heistad DD, Mark AL, Schmid PG: Reflex control of the peripheral circulation. Prog Cardiovasc Dis 1976;18:371–403

33. Bradley TD, Takasaki Y, Orr D et al: Sleep apnea in patients with left ventricular dysfunction. Beneficial effects of nasal CPAP. Prog Clin Biol Res 1990;345: 363–368

34. Naughton M, Benard D, Tam A, Rutherford R, Bradley TD: Role of hyperventilation in the pathogenesis of central sleep apneas in patients with congestive heart failure. Am Rev Respir Dis 1993;148:330–338

35. Gibbs JS, Sanderson W, Smith LD et al: Low frequency oscillations in pulmonary arterial pressure in chronic heart failure. Cardioscience 1993;4:31–39

36. Naughton MT, Benard DC, Rutherford R, Bradley TD: Effect of continuous positive airway pressure on central sleep apnea and nocturnal PCO_2 in heart failure. Am J Respir Crit Care Med 1994;150:1598–1604

37. Wilson JR, Mancini DM, Dunkman WB: Exertional fatigue due to skeletal muscle dysfunction in patients with heart failure. Circulation 1993;87:470–475

38. Massie BM, Conway M, Rajagopalan B et al: Skeletal muscle metabolism during exercise under ischemic conditions in congestive heart failure. Evidence for abnormalities unrelated to blood flow. Circulation 1988; 78:320–326

39. Sullivan MJ, Green HJ, Cobb FR: Skeletal muscle biochemistry and histology in ambulatory patients with long-term heart failure. Circulation 1990;81:518–527

40. Buller NP, Jones D, Poole-Wilson PA: Direct measurement of skeletal muscle fatigue in patients with chronic heart failure. Br Heart J 1991;65:20–24

41. Swan JW, Walton C, Godsland IF et al: Insulin resis-

tance in chronic heart failure. Eur Heart J 1994;15: 1528–1532

42. Anker SD, Volterrani M, Swan J et al: Hormonal changes in cardiac cachexia. Circulation, suppl. I 1995; 92:206–207

43. Brunotte F, Thompson CH, Adamopoulos S et al: Rat skeletal muscle metabolism in experimental heart failure. Effects of physical training. Acta Physiol Scand 1995;154:439–447

44. Adamopoulos S, Coats AJ, Brunotte F et al: Physical training improves skeletal muscle metabolism in patients with chronic heart failure. J Am Coll Cardiol 1993;21:1101–1106

45. Lipkin DP, Canepa Anson R, Stephens MR, Poole-Wilson PA: Factors determining symptoms in heart failure. Comparison of fast and slow exercise tests. Br Heart J 1986;55:439–445

46. Lipkin DP, Poole-Wilson PA: Symptoms limiting exercise in chronic heart failure. BMJ 1986;292:1030–1031

47. Gibbs JSR, Keegan J, Wright C, Fox KM, Poole-Wilson PA: Pulmonary artery pressure changes during exercise and daily activities in chronic heart failure. J Am Coll Cardiol 1990;15:52–61

48. Clark AL, Sparrow JL, Coats AJS: Muscle fatigue and dyspnoea in chronic heart failure. Two sides of the same coin? Eur Heart J 1995;16:49–52

49. Drexler H, Coats AJS: Explaining fatigue in congestive heart failure. Annu Rev Med 1996;47:241–256

50. Mancini DM, Coyle E, Coggan A et al: Contribution of intrinsic skeletal muscle changes to ^{31}P NMR skeletal muscle metabolic abnormalities in patients with chronic heart failure. Circulation 1989;80:1338–1346

51. Volterrani M, Clark AL, Ludman PF et al: Determinants of exercise capacity in chronic heart failure. Eur Heart J 1994;15:801–809

52. Franciosa JA, Goldsmith SR, Cohn JN: Contrasting immediate and long-term effects of isosorbide dinitrate on exercise capacity in congestive heart failure. Am J Med 1980;69:559–566

53. Sinoway L, Minotti JR, Davis D et al: Delayed reversal of impaired vasodilatation in congestive heart failure after heart transplantation. Am J Cardiol 1988;61: 1076–1079

54. Adams L, Guz A: Dyspnea on exertion. pp. 449–494. In Whipp BJ, Wasserman K (eds): Exercise. Pulmonary Physiology and Pathophysiology. Marcel Dekker, New York, 1991

55. Clausen JP: Circulatory adjustments to dynamic exercise and effect of physical training in normal subjects and in patients with coronary artery disease. Prog Cardiovasc Dis 1976;18:459–495

56. Jondeau G, Katz SD, Zohman L et al: Active skeletal muscle mass and cardiopulmonary reserve. Failure to attain peak aerobic capacity during maximal bicycle exercise in patients with severe congestive heart failure. Circulation 1992;86:1351–1356

57. Drexler H, Banhardt U, Meinertz T et al: Contrasting peripheral short-term and long-term effects of converting enzyme inhibition in patients with congestive heart failure. A double-blind, placebo-controlled trial. Circulation 1989;79:491–502

58. Coats AJS: Exercise rehabilitation in chronic heart failure. J Am Coll Cardiol, suppl. A 1993;22:172–177

59. Williams RS: Exercise training of patients with ventricular dysfunction and heart failure. Cardiovasc Clin 1985;15:218–231

60. Letac B, Cribier A, Desplanches JF: A study of left ventricular function in coronary patients before and after physical training. Circulation 1977;56:375–378
61. Conn EH, Williams RS, Wallace AG: Exercise responses before and after physical conditioning in patients with severely depressed left ventricular function. Am J Cardiol 1982;49:296–300
62. Sullivan MJ, Higginbotham MB, Cobb FR: Exercise training in patients with chronic heart failure delays ventilatory anaerobic threshold and improves submaximal exercise performance. Circulation 1989;79:324–329
63. Sullivan MJ, Higginbotham MB, Cobb FR: Exercise training in patients with severe left ventricular dysfunction. Hemodynamic and metabolic effects. Circulation 1988;78:506–515
64. Koch M, Douard H, Broustet JP: The benefit of graded physical exercise in chronic heart failure. Chest 1992;101:231S–235S
65. McAllister RM: Endothelial-mediated control of coronary and skeletal muscle blood flow during exercise. Introduction. Med Sci Sports Exerc 1995;27:1122–1124
66. Minotti JR, Johnson EC, Hudson TH et al: Skeletal muscle response to exercise training in congestive heart failure. J Clin Invest 1990;86:751–758
67. Stratton JR, Dunn JF, Adamopoulos S et al: Training partially reverses skeletal muscle metabolic abnormalities during exercise in heart failure. J Appl Physiol 1994;76:1575–1582
68. Hambrecht R, Niebauer J, Fiehn E et al: Physical training in patients with stable chronic heart failure. Effects on cardiorespiratory fitness and ultrastructural abnormalities of leg muscles. J Am Coll Cardiol 1995;25:1239–1249
69. Mancini DM, Henson D, La Manca J, Donchez L, Levine S: Benefit of selective respiratory muscle training on exercise capacity in patients with chronic congestive heart failure. Circulation 1995;91:320–329
70. Coats AJ, Adamopoulos S, Radaelli A et al: Controlled trial of physical training in chronic heart failure. Exercise performance, hemodynamics, ventilation, and autonomic function. Circulation 1992;85:2119–2131

23 Valvular Heart Disease

Rodney H. Stables
Paul J. Oldershaw

The proposition of a diagnosis of heart failure or ventricular dysfunction should prompt a careful consideration of etiology. Assessment of heart valve function is vital in this respect, not least because an otherwise irreversible decline in ventricular function can, in some instances, be delayed or prevented with appropriate medical therapy or surgical intervention. A high index of suspicion is required as valvular problems can underlie presentations across the spectrum of circulatory disturbance: acute or chronic disease, forward or backward failure, left or right ventricular syndromes, systolic or diastolic dysfunction, high or low output states.

Clinical assessment of these patients can be demanding. Valvular problems often coexist with other pathologies, usually affecting the myocardium. Characterization of these abnormalities and assessment of their relative influences on symptoms and prognosis is often problematic. Furthermore, some valvular abnormalities are a secondary manifestation of ventricular dysfunction rather than its cause.

With chronic valvular disease, patients can remain essentially asymptomatic over many years, and the optimum timing of a surgical intervention is sometimes difficult to determine. Operative mortality in elective cases can be as high as 5–10 percent, and up to 60 percent of patients with a prosthetic valve experience some complication within 7 years from the date of operation. The desire to avoid premature surgery must be balanced against the concern that the myocardium may sustain irreversible damage that adversely affects future surgical risk and the patient's eventual physical capacity.

A full description of the clinical syndromes of valvular heart disease can be found in standard cardiology texts. The account herein focuses on valvular pathology as a cause or consequence of ventricular dysfunction with symptoms. Most valvular pathology affects initially and predominantly the left side of the heart; isolated right ventricular dysfunction is rare. Primary abnormalities of the tricuspid and pulmonary valves can present in this way but are not examined in this chapter.

AORTIC STENOSIS

Etiology and Pathology

With the decline in rheumatic fever, most cases of valvular aortic stenosis (AS) now have a degenerative or congenital etiology[1] (Table 23-1), and this lesion has emerged as that most commonly encountered in adult cardiology practices. The valve cusps are involved in most cases with supravalvular and subvalvular stenosis recognized but uncommon. Calcification of the valve and its annulus tends to occur with long-standing disease, regardless of etiology.

The term congenital aortic stenosis is reserved for cases when there is demonstrable limitation of flow at, or soon after, birth. The definition excludes congenitally abnormal valves, with no initial hemodynamic impact, that undergo calcific degeneration later in life. Some 1–2 percent of the population are affected in this way with a marked male predomi-

Table 23-1. Relative Frequencies of the Causes of Adult Valvular Aortic Stenosis

Cause	Frequency - (%)
Rheumatic	
Isolated aortic lesion	2
Associated mitral disease	15
Congenital/Degenerative	
Bicuspid	56
Tricuspid	12
Other/unknown	15

(From Davies,[1] with permission.)

nance. As many as one-third remain asymptomatic with another one-third developing either predominantly valvular stenosis or regurgitation, respectively.[2] Most of the affected valves are bicuspid; and when the morphology is tricuspid, the cusps may be of unequal size and with varying degrees of commissural fusion.

Pathophysiology

The cross-sectional area of a normal aortic valve orifice is 2.6–3.5 cm.[23] As the disease process reduces this orifice to around 1.0 cm^2 a pressure gradient begins to develop across the valve. Systemic arterial pressure is maintained and regulated by normal baroreceptor mechanisms and remains at near-normal values in all but advanced cases. The pressure gradient is developed and maintained with an increase in left ventricular systolic pressure. Blood flow is related to the square root of the pressure gradient, and hence substantial pressure gradients can be required to support cardiac output.

Left ventricular hypertrophy ensues as a secondary phenomenon. In general, the extent of hypertrophy mirrors the severity of the stenosis, though some individual variation is noted. Left ventricular cavity dimensions remain normal until late in the natural history of the disease.

In well compensated AS, the hypertrophied left ventricle can maintain normal wall stress.[4] This parameter is a major determinant of cardiac work, and hence the cardiac output and other indices of contractility can appear normal. The ventricle begins to fail when the compensatory hypertrophy can no longer prevent a rise in left ventricular wall stress and the chamber dilates. Reduced wall thickness and an increase in cavity dimension accelerate the problem, as wall stress is related to these indices, simply stated by the Laplace relation for a spherical object:

$$\text{Wall stress} = \frac{\text{pressure} \times \text{dimension}}{4 \times \text{wall thickness}}$$

Deterioration of the clinical condition can then be rapid. With a reduced cardiac output the measured gradient across the valve can fall to levels as low as 20–30 mmHg, potentially confusing diagnostic assessment.

This progression to ventricular dysfunction and overt heart failure usually occurs with increasing afterload as the natural history of the valve lesion develops. An additional, often unrecognized factor of reduced myocardial contractility may also be involved. Chronic pressure overload can directly compromise myocardial function; and with long-standing severe hypertrophy, subendocardial ischemia and interstitial fibrosis may develop.[5] In one study 60 percent of patients with aortic stenosis, evaluated at a tertiary referral center, demonstrated fibrosis on endomyocardial biopsy; and the extent of fibrosis correlated strongly with the ejection fraction, peak valve gradient, symptoms, and mortality.[6]

Abnormalities in diastolic function are evident even with well compensated disease. Wall hypertrophy results in changes in compliance and chamber geometry that compromise left ventricular filling. The normal, synchronous, and brisk relaxation of the ventricular wall that occurs during early diastole can be lost,[7] and late fibrosis can further affect myocardial stiffness. These changes seem to be an important factor in the development of impaired exercise tolerance, the most prominent symptom.[8]

Diastolic dysfunction is associated with a slow early phase of transmitral flow, and atrial systole may make a substantial contribution to ventricular filling. In such cases a large "a" wave is usually seen on left atrial and ventricular pressure tracings, and there is a reversal of the normal e/a ratio on mitral inflow Doppler recordings. The onset of atrial fibrillation with loss of coordinated atrial contraction can markedly compromise cardiac function.

Clinical Presentation

Heart failure develops relatively late in the natural history of the condition, and the untreated prognosis for this group is poor with a mean life expectancy of less than 2 years. Although mild breathlessness is sometimes noted at first presentation, prominence of this symptom and the presence of paroxysmal nocturnal dyspnea or other features of left ventricular failure tend to be late manifestations. It is worth remembering that aortic stenosis can present as intractable cardiac failure with no evidence of a murmur or other supporting physical signs, and the diagnosis should be considered in all patients with cardiac failure of unknown etiology.[9]

In the compensated state the mean left atrial pressure is usually normal, though the a wave may be exaggerated. As failure develops, the pulmonary pressures rise, reflected by right ventricular systolic pressures. In a small proportion of cases inappropriate pulmonary vasoconstriction can result in significant pulmonary hypertension, though moderate elevation is the rule. Elevation of right ventricular end-diastolic pressures and signs of congestive cardiac failure are not seen until late in the clinical course and indicate a markedly poor prognosis.

Investigations and Treatment

All cases of aortic stenosis presenting with overt ventricular dysfunction should be considered for aortic valve replacement, as the untreated prognosis is otherwise uniformly poor. Echocardiography allows characterization of valve morphology and can usually exclude subvalvular and supravalvular stenosis and hypertrophic cardiomyopathy. Left ventricular function, cavity size, and wall thickness can be assessed; and Doppler studies can estimate the velocity of blood flow in the outflow tract and hence the pressure gradient over the stenosed valve. This gradient can fall as ventricular performance declines and is often a poor index of severity in late disease.

Cardiac catheterization allows direct measurement of the pressure gradient, usually achieved with retrograde passage of a catheter into the left ventricle across the stenosed valve. Transseptal puncture or direct left ventricular puncture are alternative approaches. With impaired left ventricular function there is merit in calculating the aortic valve area, using the Gorlin formula, from the pressure tracings and measurements of cardiac output. If catheterization is performed, the state of the coronary arteries can be assessed with selective angiography.

There is no real role for medical therapy in this condition as both preload and afterload reduction can be detrimental and in some cases catastrophic. Atrial arrhythmias are relatively rare, even with advanced aortic stenosis; and this finding should prompt a consideration of coexisting mitral valve disease. In these cases restoration of sinus rhythm and hence transmitral atrial transport can be of great value and should be considered.

Balloon valvoplasty was originally employed for treatment of pulmonary stenosis. It has a role in the management of neonatal and pediatric aortic valve disease when a pliable valve can be split, improving symptoms and postponing the need for surgical intervention until later in life. Its application in adults with advanced calcific disease has produced disappointing long-term results. An initial improvement in gradient and cardiac output is often observed, though the individual response is variable. These early gains are probably due to the fracture of calcified nodules,[10] though some stretching of the aortic valve ring may also occur. The value of the approach is limited by two main factors. Dangerous immediate procedural complications, including myocardial perforation, infarction, and severe aortic regurgitation, complicate up to 6 percent of cases.[11] A more gradual restenotic process also occurs as calcified lesions reform during the 3–6 months following a procedure. Balloon dilatation has not been able to match the results of valve replacement surgery, and its use tends now to be reserved for palliative therapy in inoperable cases or as a bridge to definitive surgery.

Aortic valve replacement remains the treatment of choice. Patients with established cardiac failure do benefit from surgical intervention, though an irreversible decline in myocardial performance is a feature of late disease and operative mortality in these patients is correspondingly high. There is as yet no reliable method for assessing the likely response to afterload reduction with valve replacement; and because the untreated prognosis is so poor, all patients should at least be considered candidates for operative management.

AORTIC REGURGITATION

Etiology and Pathology

Aortic regurgitation is a commonly encountered valvular lesion with wide-ranging etiology (Table 23-2). The incidence of rheumatic disease has fallen and in the West now accounts for only some 25 percent of cases.[1] Coexisting stenosis and involvement of the mitral valve is the rule in these cases. Noninflammatory aortic root dilatation is the next most prevalent etiology. Most of these cases are idiopathic, though conditions involving the defective synthesis of tissue structural components are often encountered, including Marfan and Ehlers-Danlos syndromes and osteogenesis imperfecta. There is no evidence of inflammation, but there is destruction of the muscular and elastic layers in the media, often isolated to discrete patchy areas. As a result, the aortic root dilates. Concentric dilatation leads to failure of cusp fusion, whereas eccentric expansion can create a picture of

Table 23-2. Prominent Causes of Aortic Regurgitation

Cusp abnormality (perforation or area reduction)
    Bacterial endocarditis
    Rheumatic disease
    Rheumatoid disease
Aortic root distension
    Ankylosing spondylitis
    Nonspecific urethritis
    Nonspecific aortitis
    Rheumatoid disease
    Syphilis
Loss of commissural support
    Fallot-type ventricular septal defect
    Aortic dissection
Aortic root dilatation
    Inflammatory aortitis (including syphilis)
    Familial
    Idiopathic
    Connective tissue disorders

(From Davies,[1] with permission.)

isolated cusp prolapse. The valve cusps can themselves be affected by the disease process and show thickening and rolling of their edges.

Inflammatory aortitis is another important etiology, previously dominated by syphilitic infection. Before World War II the spirochete accounted for some 20 percent of all cases of aortic regurgitation, but such cases are now rare. Rheumatoid arthritis ankylosing spondylitis, Reiter syndrome, and giant cell arteritis are other causes, producing fibrosis that distorts the aortic root and can extend to involve the atrioventricular ring.

Dissecting aortic aneurysm can compromise the integrity of the aortic valve with prolapse of a valve cusp (often the right) and the intimal flap into the left ventricle. The demonstration of aortic regurgitation in patients with acute dissection is an indication for urgent surgical repair or aortic root replacement.

Finally, aortic regurgitation can be caused or worsened by infective endocarditis occurring on an abnormal valve. Although stenotic or regurgitant disease may already have been present, asymptomatic bicuspid or apparently normal valves can also be affected particularly with virulent organisms such as *Staphylococcus aureus*. Rupture or perforation of a valve cusp can result in acute, severe regurgitation.

Pathophysiology

The abnormal movement of blood from the aorta to the left ventricle during diastole imposes an additional volume load on this chamber. With mild or slowly progressive disease, compensatory changes occur with left ventricular dilatation and hypertrophy. Cavity enlargement permits an increased stroke volume that maintains the ejection fraction and cardiac output, and patients can remain asymptomatic for many years.

An increase in heart rate is often noted with moderate or severe regurgitation. The duration of systole is largely unaffected by heart rate variation; hence the diastolic period and time available for regurgitation proportionately shorten with an increasing heart rate. Such changes can make a useful contribution to chronic compensation and provide some protection from developing symptoms on exercise during early disease.

Left ventricular hypertrophy helps to normalize the increase in wall stress that would otherwise result from chamber enlargement, and in most cases it has a beneficial effect on compensatory adaptation. Abnormalities in diastolic function are well described, however, even before the development of heart failure[12]; and although fibrosis and ischemia may be involved, muscle hypertrophy seems central to these changes. It is important to note that with well compensated, chronic aortic regurgitation the left ventricle remains compliant and can accommodate large volumes at relatively low diastolic pressures. This phenomenon seems critical to the adaptive process, but its mechanism is poorly understood.

With acute aortic regurgitation, volume loading of an unprepared and hence poorly compliant ventricle can result in a dramatic, rapid rise in left ventricular diastolic pressures, which can approach 60–70 mmHg. Backward transmission of this pressure results in the development of acute pulmonary edema. Severe regurgitant flow causes the left ventricular pressure to rise sharply during early diastole. This pressure profile causes the mitral valve to close early during diastole as left atrial pressure is soon exceeded. Furthermore, as the pressure difference between the aorta and ventricle equalizes early during diastole, the duration of regurgitant flow can be short and a classic early diastolic murmur may be soft or absent.

Clinical Presentation

Acute aortic regurgitation is usually caused by infective endocarditis, with perforation or rupture of a cusp; or it may result from aortic dissection or cardiac trauma. It presents as a low output state with acute left ventricular failure. Severe dyspnea, orthopnea, and paroxysmal nocturnal dyspnea are prominent symptoms. The patient may have cold peripheries with central and peripheral cyanosis. There is often a sinus tachycardia and low systolic blood pressure with normal pulse pressure. The classic early diastolic murmur may be soft or absent, as markedly elevated left ventricular diastolic pressure shortens the duration of regurgitant blood flow. A loud third heart sound is often heard.

Patients with chronic aortic regurgitation may remain asymptomatic for years and tend to present at midlife and later. Some notice a vigorous apex beat or prominent peripheral arterial pulsation, particularly on exercise. Beyond this picture, the classic first symptoms of dyspnea and tiredness on exercise develop when compensatory mechanisms can no longer prevent an exercise-induced rise in end-diastolic pressure and limitation of maximal cardiac output. With further disease, progression to frank left heart failure ensues; and during the later stages of the natural history, congestive cardiac failure develops.

Angina pectoris can occur with pure aortic regurgitation, but this presentation is rare in the absence of other obstructive coronary artery disease. With syphilitic aortitis the primary disease process can cause nonatherosclerotic aortoostial stenosis.

Clinical Assessment

The physical signs of aortic regurgitation are well described in standard cardiology texts. With moderate disease they tend to be prominent, and a clinical diagnosis is usually secure. Infective endocarditis is an important, dangerous condition and should be considered at diagnosis in all cases.

Echocardiography with Doppler examination is particularly useful for assessing aortic regurgitation. It can distinguish the handful of clinical conditions that often confuse the initial diagnosis, including pulmonary regurgitation, patent ductus arteriosus, high ventricular septal defect with aortic valve cusp prolapse, and a ruptured sinus of Valsalva.

Cardiac catheterization is mainly of value in cases when there is doubt about the severity of the regurgitation or when other pathology, particularly mitral valve disease, complicates the clinical picture. Pressure recordings in patients with advanced disease reveal an elevated end-diastolic pressure that may exceed the left atrial pressure by mid to late diastole. This situation can cause premature closure of the mitral valve (best seen at echocardiography) and in some cases diastolic mitral regurgitation. Left ventriculography defines cavity size and wall motion abnormalities, and aortography allows semiquantitative assessment of the degree of regurgitation. Selective injection of the coronary arteries should be performed in all patients with anginal symptoms.

Once a patient has become symptomatic, the deterioration of ventricular function, and hence the prognostic outlook, can be rapid. These patients should be considered for definitive therapy with valve replacement without delay. The management of asymptomatic patients presents a more difficult clinical problem principally when timing the aortic valve replacement. Operative mortality in elective cases can be as high as 5 percent, and up to 60 percent of patients with a prosthetic valve may experience some complication within 7 years from the date of operation. The desire to avoid premature surgery must be balanced against the concern that as the ventricle undergoes compensatory dilatation it may sustain irreversible damage that adversely affects future surgical risk and the patient's eventual physical capacity. The natural history of left ventricular dysfunction and the impact of valve replacement surgery on these processes are not well characterized, and clinical uncertainty remains.

Echocardiographic studies of left ventricular dimensions and wall movement have assumed a primary role in the follow-up of patients with aortic regurgitation. Although exact criteria have not been framed, if the left ventricular end-systolic dimension exceeds 55 mm on M-mode examination the prognosis may be poor following valve replacement. Changes in cavity dimensions are often taken as a signal for more intensive assessment. In the first instance it may involve simply repeat assessment at more frequent intervals, followed if indicated by cardiac catheterization.

The search for a reliable index for assessment of chronic aortic regurgitation continues. The effects of exercise on left ventricular function, usually assessed by radionuclide ventriculography, have been used to unmask early abnormalities.[14] The full clinical significance of these changes is not fully characterized, but this method does seem to correctly identify otherwise silent dysfunction. Indeed the detection of impaired exercise tolerance has been shown to be a useful adjunct to several other indices and may independently predict a poor prognosis.[15]

Interpretation of "ejection phase" indices of left ventricular performance, such as the ejection fraction, may be complicated, as changes can be induced by variations in preload and afterload. A reduction in ejection fraction can be precipitated by either a deterioration in left ventricular function or an increase in the extent of the regurgitation. Nevertheless, it has been shown that measurements of the ejection fraction (EF) can predict long-term survival, particularly if reduced ventricular function (EF < 45 percent) has been present for some time or is associated with reduced exercise tolerance.[15] The use of end-systolic pressure/volume or stress/strain indices may be of more value, as they are independent of loading.[16]

Nuclear magnetic spectroscopy has been used to study changes in cellular biochemistry that may indicate declining myocardial function in patients with aortic valve disease. Patients with heart failure were found to have marked changes in the relative proportions of high energy phosphates with a reduced phosphocreatine/adenosine triphosphate ratio.[17] Prospective studies to evaluate this noninvasive screening method are in progress.

Treatment

When symptoms first develop, relief can be obtained with diuretic therapy. Vasodilators lower systemic vascular resistance and reduce the severity of aortic regurgitation. Anginal symptoms should not be treated with β-blockers because with a reduced heart rate the diastolic interval and hence the period of regurgitation are prolonged. Medical therapy can provide useful symptomatic relief but should not delay consideration of definitive surgical treatment for these patients.

MITRAL REGURGITATION

Etiology and Pathology

The causes of mitral regurgitation are summarized in Table 23-3. In the developed world most cases are nonrheumatic in origin,[18] with ischemic and degenerative etiologies prominent. Mild mitral regurgitation is a surprisingly common finding in patients undergoing surgery for ischemic heart disease[19] and is usually of no clinical significance.

Acute papillary muscle rupture complicates fewer than 1 percent of acute cases of myocardial infarction but produces dramatic, severe symptoms of left ventricular failure. Surgical intervention is usually required to avoid an otherwise adverse prognosis. Ischemic papillary muscle dysfunction is more common, though it now seems clear that abnormalities of ventricular wall function below one or both of the papillary muscles is a feature of this condition.[20]

Mitral valve prolapse is the commonest manifestation of mitral valve disease and involves prolapse of one or both of the valve cusps toward the left atrium during systole. Although usually idiopathic, the syndrome can be a feature of the connective tissue disorders. Hemodynamically significant regurgitation is rare, though infective endocarditis can occur on a

Table 23-3. Prominent Causes of Mitral Regurgitation

Rheumatic heart disease
  Valve cusp scarring, thickening, and retraction
  Chordae involvement with shortening
  Valve ring may be dilated
Ischemic heart disease
  Papillary muscle rupture in acute myocardial infarction
  Papillary muscle ischemic dysfunction
Functional regurgitation
  Secondary to left ventricular cavity dilatation
Mitral valve prolapse
  Idiopathic
  Connective tissue disorders
Chordal rupture
  Spontaneous/traumatic
  Floppy degenerative valve (prolapse)
  Infective endocarditis
Infective endocarditis
  Chordal rupture
  Cusp perforation
  Papillary muscle damage
Annulus calcification
  Degenerative change in the elderly
  Renal failure, secondary hyperparathyroidism
Hypertrophic cardiomyopathy
Congenital
  Cleft leaflet
  Chordae and papillary muscle abnormalities

(Data from Davies.[1])

prolapsing valve and cause additional disruption. The normal pathology involves myxomatous degeneration of not only the valve cusps but also the annulus and chordae. Progressive stretching of these structures can lead to a condition described as "floppy valve" with prominent regurgitation. Chordal rupture often complicates this picture and can precipitate a dramatic deterioration in symptoms.

Chordal rupture can also occur in otherwise normal patients and is another important cause of mitral regurgitation. It is more common in men and is a condition of midlife or later.[21] There is no established link between rupture and ischemic heart disease. Calcification of the mitral valve annulus is another degenerative condition, this time more common in elderly women. The secondary hyperparathyroidism of chronic failure is the most prominent of a number of associated conditions, including diabetes mellitus, mitral valve prolapse, and hypertrophic cardiomyopathy. Significant regurgitation is rare and is thought to occur with loss of annulus contraction, which is seen during systole and helps to maintain valve competence.

Pathophysiology

The effects of acute and chronic presentations are different and are discussed separately. With an acute onset there is an initial, marked rise in left atrial pressure, as this chamber, with normal dimensions and compliance, cannot cope with the additional volume load. This rise results in an elevated left ventricular preload, initially stimulating myocardial contractility. A proportion of the ventricular output is vented into the low pressure atrium rather than into the aorta (against the resistance of systemic pressures). As a result there is also an effective reduction in afterload. Ejection fraction and stroke volume both increase, and the cardiac output is maintained at an elevated heart rate, stimulated by reflex changes in response to blood pressure and cardiac output fluctuations. When the regurgitation is severe, these compensatory mechanisms are inadequate and cardiac output falls. The elevated left atrial pressure, often augmented by a significant "v" wave of ventricular systole, is transmitted to the pulmonary circulation, and pulmonary edema can develop.

The clinical situation any given patient may be subject to fluctuation. For example, if afterload is increased with a rise in peripheral vascular resistance, the severity of the regurgitation worsens; and, conversely, measures to reduce afterload are beneficial. As the left atrial pressure rises, the extent of regurgitation may vary in either direction. Increased filling pressures can reduce the pressure gradient between the left ventricle and atrium and limit backflow; or with marked increases in left ventricular end-diastolic pressures, ventricular dilatation can augment the regurgitant jet. Acute ischemia may be present as primary causation, or it may be secondary to hemodynamic perturbations and can cause marked fluctuations in the clinical picture.

When regurgitation develops more gradually, adaptive mechanisms allow cardiac output to be maintained with only moderate increases in intracardiac pressures, and severe regurgitation can be tolerated with minimal symptoms. Chronic volume overload tends to increase the end-diastolic volume of the ventricular cavity, whereas end-systolic dimensions remain essentially normal. Stroke volume is augmented, but increased compliance allows this additional volume load to be tolerated at near-normal end-diastolic pressures. Hence pulmonary congestion does not develop. Dilatation of the left atrial cavity can also help in this regard but is more common with a rheumatic etiology.

Left ventricular hypertrophy also develops. An increase in wall thickness helps normalize any increase in wall stress induced by cavity dilatation, and an increased muscle mass can augment the force of contraction.

Left ventricular performance is near-normal during the initial stages of the natural history; but if the regurgitation is severe and long-standing, left ventricular performance eventually deteriorates. The onset of this decline can prove difficult to detect, as the regurgitation provides a low impedance runoff into the left atrium. This runoff effectively reduces afterload, and hence ejection phase indices can remain normal despite myocardial deterioration. By the time the ejection fraction begins to fall, ventricular performance is often so poor the patient does not derive benefit from surgical intervention.

Clinical Presentation

With acute mitral regurgitation the presenting symptoms and signs are of acute left heart failure superimposed on any resulting from the primary etiology (e.g., acute myocardial infarction). In the most florid cases there is immediate cardiovascular collapse, poor peripheral perfusion, and florid pulmonary edema. In other cases symptoms develop gradually over 2–3 days and then signs of congestive cardiac failure may also be present.

In contrast, chronic regurgitation may be asymptomatic over many years. Breathlessness on exertion and fatigue are often the initial complaints. Congestive failure is a late finding. Abrupt deterioration is sometimes precipitated by another factor, for example the onset of atrial fibrillation, myocardial ischemia, or infective endocarditis. Exercise almost always causes exacerbation of symptoms: The duration of systole does not significantly shorten with an increasing heart rate, and hence the advantages of a reduced period for regurgitation, seen with aortic regurgitation, are not realized.

Treatment

In all cases the etiology must be defined and treated as appropriate. Conditions such as anemia, rhythm disturbance, thyrotoxicosis, and myocardial ischemia can adversely affect the clinical state and should be identified and treated if active.

When regurgitation is secondary to a dilated, poorly contracting left ventricle, the outlook is poor. Although medical therapy can provide some palliation, progressive heart failure and early demise are the rule. Surgical treatment has little to offer this group.

Medical therapy with diuretics and vasodilators or angiotensin-converting enzyme (ACE) inhibitors can provide excellent symptomatic relief. Digoxin may be added, especially if the patient is in atrial fibrillation. The outlook for medically treated patients with mild regurgitation is good, with up to 80 percent 5-year survival in some series. Left ventricular enlargement and a reduced ejection fraction predict a poor prognosis and the need for surgical intervention with valve repair or replacement.

Echocardiographic examination is the most practical tool for routine follow-up and permits characterization of ventricular cavity size and, to some extent, function. A variety of techniques to quantify the extent of regurgitation have been proposed, but none has gained widespread acceptance. Cardiac catheterization may not be essential in patients with a clear clinical diagnosis and a satisfactory echocardiographic examination, but it does allow examination of the coronary arteries.

In cases of acute, severe mitral regurgitation (e.g., papillary muscle rupture with acute myocardial infarction), immediate surgery is indicated. Sometimes moderate or severe regurgitation can present in a subacute fashion some days or weeks after a completed infarction. The prognosis in this group tends to be poor, and surgical intervention is usually indicated.

MITRAL STENOSIS

Etiology and Pathology

In the developed world the decline of rheumatic fever has resulted in dramatic changes in the incidence of individual valvular lesions, with a marked reduction in the burden of rheumatic mitral stenosis. In contrast, this lesion is still an important cause of morbidity and mortality in other parts of the globe and has a marked impact on both right and left ventricular function. Acquired mitral stenosis is almost always rheumatic in origin, though a viral etiology has been proposed in a few cases.[22] Scarring of the cusps results in thickening, shortening, and deformity; and these changes also affect the chordae tendineae. Late calcification is the norm. Stenotic lesions arise when cusp fusion occurs with relative preservation of the leaflets. Shortening of the subvalvular apparatus and less complete cusp fusion leads to retraction of the valve leaflets toward the left ventricular cavity, and some degree of mitral regurgitation usually results. Mixed lesions are common. Rheumatic scarring of the mitral valve ring can interfere with the

muscular systolic contraction at its circumference that helps to secure valve competence and can exacerbate regurgitation.

Pathophysiology

The normal mitral valve area is in the range of 4–6 cm.[2] As the disease process reduces this area below a critical threshold, hemodynamic disturbance and clinical symptoms manifest. With mild to moderate stenosis, at a valve area of around 1.5 cm^2, the left atrial pressure (LAP) at rest may be normal but rises on exercise when a pressure gradient is required to maintain forward transmitral flow. As the stenosis becomes more severe a consistently elevated LAP becomes the norm, and pulmonary hypertension with compensatory vascular changes develop.

For patients in sinus rhythm, left atrial contraction comes to play a significant part in support of ventricular filling and hence cardiac output. The left atrium usually hypertrophies in response to this challenge. The loss of atrial contraction with the onset of atrial fibrillation can have a dramatic effect on cardiac output (with up to a 20 percent reduction) and is usually associated with marked symptomatic deterioration.

Left ventricular performance is usually abnormal with prominent diastolic dysfunction. Systolic problems are also described and can be grouped into regional and global abnormalities. Regional wall motion abnormalities may be related to tethering of part of the ventricular wall by subvalvular fibrosis or to the effects of right ventricular overload affecting left ventricular performance.[23]

A global reduction in systolic function is sometimes noted and has been attributed to the effects of the rheumatic process on the myocardium and to myocardial atrophy resulting from reduced left ventricular work.[24] Measures of ventricular performance, particularly ejection phase indices (e.g., the ejection fraction) are often abnormal but may be influenced by the abnormal loading conditions that are usually present. Correction of the preload and afterload burdens often results in normalization of these ventricular indices. Abnormalities of systolic function are, in most cases, not significant and rarely present a clinical problem following valve surgery.

In contrast, diastolic dysfunction is universal. The normal pattern of transmitral flow (with early, mid, and late phases) is lost, and diastolic filling proceeds at a near-uniform rate. The normal, coordinated ventricular relaxation that accommodates early rapid filling is lost, and outward wall motion becomes asynchronous. The reasons for this change are complex and not well characterized.

Pulmonary hypertension is characteristic and results initially from passive backward transmission of elevated left atrial pressures. Chronic pulmonary venous hypertension results in pulmonary arteriolar constriction and, if prolonged, obliterative changes in the pulmonary arterial vessels. Thrombosis in situ or thromboembolic events can further increase pulmonary vascular resistance. The lung parenchyma is often also affected, resulting in reduced lung volumes, impaired gas transfer, and increased lung stiffness.

Pulmonary hypertension leads to right ventricular hypertrophy, which initially maintains cardiac output. Eventually the chamber fails with dilatation, often associated with functional tricuspid regurgitation.

Clinical Presentation

Dyspnea on exertion is the most frequent presenting symptom. Orthopnea and paroxysmal nocturnal dyspnea are late features, and episodes of acute pulmonary edema are rare in the absence of a precipitating factor such as new atrial fibrillation, pregnancy, or an intravenous fluid load. Fatigue and cough are prominent symptoms, and hemoptysis occurs in some 10 percent of cases.

Investigations and Treatment

Detailed assessment is undertaken with ultrasound imaging and cardiac catheterization. Two-dimensional echocardiographic imaging and Doppler examination can now provide a thorough preoperative assessment, and catheterization may not be required, unless there is need to assess the state of the coronary arteries.

With mitral stenosis, medical management has an important role in controlling symptoms of mild disease and preparing patients with more severe disease for operative intervention. Restoration and maintenance of sinus rhythm can bring great benefits; or if atrial fibrillation is established, the ventricular rate should be controlled with digoxin or another antiarrhythmic drug. Systemic anticoagulation offers some protection against the common, potentially devastating complication of systemic embolization and should be initiated in most patients. Diuretics can provide some measure of symptomatic relief of mild or moderate disease.

Definitive therapy involves the relief of obstruction with some form of intervention. Surgical options, include open and closed valvotomy and the current management of choice, mitral valve replacement. Balloon dilatation of the mitral valve is now available as a less invasive approach to the management of some patients with mitral stenosis. Evaluation of this technique and its long-term outcome is ongoing, but it seems to provide an effective, safe alternative for patients who might otherwise have undergone a closed valvotomy procedure or in whom there is a strong contraindication to surgical intervention.

REFERENCES

1. Davies MJ: Pathology of Cardiac Valves. Butterworth, London, 1980
2. Fengolio JJJ, McAllister HAJ, DeCastro CM et al: Congenital bicuspid aortic valve after age 20. Am J Cardiol 1977;39:164–169
3. McMillan IKR: Aortic stenosis. A postmortem cinephotographic study of valve action. Br Heart J 1955;17:56
4. Grossman W, Jones D, McLaurin LP: Wall stress and patterns of hypertrophy in the human left ventricle. J Clin Invest 1975;56:56–65
5. Hess OM, Schneider J, Koch R et al: Diastolic function and myocardial structure in patients with myocardial hypertrophy. Special reference to normalised viscoelastic data. Circulation 1981;63:360–371
6. Oldershaw PJ, Brooksby IAB, Davies MJ et al: Correlations of fibrosis in endomyocardial biopsies from patients with aortic valve disease. Br Heart J 1980;44:609–611
7. Hui WKK, Gibso DG: The dynamic of rapid left ventricular filling in AMN. p. 735. In: Advances in Cardiology. Karger, Basel, 1985
8. Oldershaw PJ, Dawkins KD, Ward DE, Gibson DG: Diastolic mechanisms of impaired exercise tolerance in aortic valve disease. Br Heart J 1983;49:568–573
9. Morgan JD, Hall RJC: Occult aortic stenosis as a cause of intractable heart failure. BMJ 1979;1:784–787
10. Safian RD, Mandell VS, Thurer RE et al: Postmortem and intraoperative balloon valvuloplasty of calcific aortic stenosis in elderly patients. Mechanisms of successful dilatation. J Am Coll Cardiol 1987;9:655
11. Isner JA: Acute catastrophic complications of balloon aortic valvuloplasty. J Am Coll Cardiol 1991;17:1436
12. Lavine SJ, Follansbee WP, Shreiner DP et al: Pattern of left ventricular diastolic filling in chronic aortic regurgitation. A gated blood pool assessment. J Am Coll Cardiol 1985;55:127–132
13. Henry WL, Bonow RO, Rosing DR, Epstein SE: Observations on the optimum time for operative intervention for aortic regurgitation. Circulation 1980;61:484
14. Greenberg B, Massie D, Thomas D et al: Association between the exercise ejection fraction response and systolic wall stress in patients with chronic aortic insufficiency. Circulation 1985;71:458–465
15. Bonow RO, Picone AL, McIntosh CL et al: Survival and functional results after valve replacement for aortic regurgitation from 1976–1983. Impact of pre-operative left ventricular function. Circulation 1985;72:1244–1256
16. Osbakken M, Bove AA, Spann JF: Left ventricular

function in chronic aortic regurgitation with reference to end-systolic pressure, volume and stress relations. Am J Cardiol 1981;47:193

17. Conway MA, Allis J, Outwerkerk R et al: Detection of low phosphocreatine to ATP ratio in failing hypertrophied human myocardium by P magnetic resonance spectroscopy. Lancet 1991;338:973–975

18. Selzer A, Katayama F: Mitral regurgitation. Clinical patterns, pathophysiology and natural history. Medicine (Baltimore) 1972;51:337–366

19. Gahl K, Sutton R, Pearson M et al: Mitral regurgitation in coronary heart disease. Br Heart J 1977;39:13

20. Godley RW, Wann LS, Rogers EW et al: Incomplete mitral leaflet closure in patients with papillary muscle dysfunction. Circulation 1981;63:565–571

21. Howe J, Strachan BW: Case reports. Aortic regurgitation as a manifestation of giant cell arteritis. Br Heart J 1978;40:1052

22. Ward C, Ward AM: Virus antigen demonstrated in valvular heart disease. Lancet 1974;755–756

23. Curry GC, Elliot LP, Ramsey HW: Quantitative left ventricular angiographic findings in mitral stenosis. Am J Cardiol 1972;29:621–627

24. Dodge HT, Kennedy JW, Peterson JL: Quantitative angiographic methods in the evaluation of valvular heart disease. Prog Cardiovasc Dis 1973;16:1

24 Hypertension and Cardiac Hypertrophy

Bodo Schwartzkopff
Bodo E. Strauer

Arterial hypertension is an important risk factor for cardio-, reno-, cerebro-, and peripheral vascular complications, which account for more than 50 percent of the total mortality of the industrialized population. In the Framingham Study, hypertension and coronary disease were the predominant causes of heart failure and accounted for more than 80 percent of all clinical events.[1] Coronary disease has been identified as the most important cause of systolic dysfunction.[2,3] A major risk factor for coronary artery disease is arterial hypertension. Furthermore, 40 percent of patients with heart failure have normal systolic function but diastolic dysfunction that is mainly associated with hypertension.[4] Arterial hypertension is the most common cause of left ventricular pressure overload that induces left ventricular hypertrophy. Left ventricular hypertrophy predisposes to diastolic and later to systolic heart failure, malignant arrhythmias, and sudden death.[1,5,6]

A distinction must be made between (1) the degree of hypertension and the extent, localization, and severity of the resulting myocardial hypertrophy (myocardial factor); (2) the activation of the nonmyocytic cells (interstitial factor); and (3) the concomitant coronary manifestations (coronary factor)[7] (Fig. 24-1). In hypertension these three factors may develop independently, but in the presence of severe, prolonged cardiac involvement the ventricular and coronary mechanisms almost invariably interact, and each propagates heart failure. Independent from its etiology, the prognosis of heart failure is poor,[1–4] and

therapeutic approaches do not basically reverse its dramatic course. Thus early diagnosis and adequate treatment of hypertensive heart disease and its determining factors should make an important contribution to alleviating this situation.

CLINICAL, EPIDEMIOLOGIC, AND PROGNOSTIC DATA

Development of Left Ventricular Hypertrophy

Left ventricular hypertrophy (LVH) represents the general structural mechanism of adaptation of the heart to a chronic pressure load on the ventricle. This mechanism of adaptation enables the left ventricle to eject a normal stroke volume into the periphery despite an excessively elevated systolic pressure in the left ventricle. According to Linzbach, compensatory growth of the heart may be regarded as harmonious up to a left ventricular weight of 250 g.[8] Compensated hypertrophy due to high blood pressure is characterized by a thickened ventricular wall and septum, normal or reduced ventricular volume (high mass/volume ratio), and an extended left ventricular outflow tract.[7,9]

A number of important factors determine the development of hypertrophy, including the extent and duration of the left ventricular systolic pressure load, age and gender, whole blood viscosity, catecholamines, sodium intake, humoral influences, body

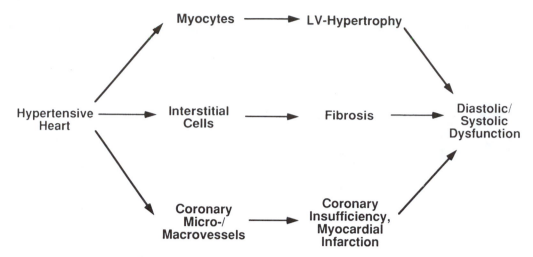

Fig. 24-1. Involvement and remodeling of myocardial structure (myocyte, interstitium, vessels) in hypertensive heart disease.

mass, cardiac rate and contractility, and genetic factors.[10–14] The 30-year average systolic blood pressure was found to be a better predictor of left ventricular mass and wall thickness than is the current resting blood pressure. Both current and long-term systolic blood pressures are better predictors than current and long-term values for diastolic blood pressure.[10] The association with exaggerated exercise systolic blood pressure response and the occurrence of LVH in healthy, normotensive individuals was reported to be confounded by age, resting systolic blood pressure, and body mass. Therefore the biologic significance of this relation has been questioned.[15]

Absolute ventricular mass may further increase as the cardiac manifestations of hypertension (coronary disease, ventricular dilation) become more marked.

Epidemiologic Data

Left ventricular hypertrophy detected by electrocardiography (ECG) and echocardiography has been shown to be an independent predictor of subsequent cardiovascular mortality and morbidity.[16] In the Framingham Heart Study[17] the prevalence of ECG-LVH has been found to be 2.9 percent for men and 1.5 percent for women. ECG sensitivity for LVH was low (6.9 percent), whereas specificity reached 98.8 percent.

The sensitivity of echocardiography is much higher, and LVH has been reported to be a common finding, with a prevalence of 15–20 percent in an adult population.[18] The Framingham Heart Study, applying the Penn Convention, revealed LVH was associated with a left ventricular mass of more than 143 g/m (131 g/m^2) for men and 102 g/m (100 g/m^2)

for women.[16,17,18] Nevertheless, even lesser values can mean LVH for the individual patient, as regression of the left ventricular mass can be observed in some patients after normalization of blood pressure under antihypertensive medication.

Arterial hypertension is the most frequent cause of LVH, though the correlation between left ventricular load and the extent of hypertrophy is loose. The incidence of LVH in hypertensive patients is reported to be 23–48 percent in comparison with normotensive subjects, whose incidence is 0–10 percent.[18,19]

LVH and Prognosis

Left ventricular mass is an important risk factor in cardiovascular disease. The first evidence was reported from ECG data of the Framingham Study. ECG-LVH conferred a six- to eightfold excess risk of cardiovascular death, but the incidence of cardiovascular events depended mainly on repolarization abnormalities included in left ventricular mass criteria.[1,17] Thus the influence of silent coronary disease cannot be ruled out, even though a direct link between LVH voltage criteria and prognosis was reported.[20]

Echocardiography delivered important information about the relation between left ventricular mass and prognosis. It has been shown that LVH was combined with an increased risk of all causes of cardiovascular morbidity and mortality.[13,16] This association was independent and persisted after adjustment for age, systolic blood pressure, obesity, and cholesterol concentrations and was not dependent on any associated lesions of the coronary arteries.[16,21,22] Levy et al.[16] reported about cardiovascular morbidity and mortality in respect to left ventricular muscle mass, where the association was continuous, without threshold. The echocardiographic evidence for each 50 g/m increment in the left ventricular mass index corrected by height was associated with a risk factor-adjusted relative risk of 1.49 for men and 1.57 for women. Regarding hypertensive patients, the prognosis was significantly worsened when LVH was present compared with those without LVH.[23]

In addition to the quantitative evaluation of left ventricular mass, other information related to left ventricular geometry may add to the prediction of outcome.[23,24] Koren et al.[23] reported a threefold increased risk for cardiovascular complications in patients with concentric LVH compared to those with normal geometry. This risk was even higher than with eccentric hypertrophy. Even concentric remodeling of the left ventricle with a left ventricular mass below the hypertrophy criteria may be associated with an increased risk.

These findings support the concept that the hypertensive heart suffers pathologic remodeling from the beginning. Hypertension involves all compartments of the heart, as well as myocytes, interstitium, and macro- and microvessels. Pathologic alterations in one or more compartments could be the keystone for the development of heart failure (Fig. 24-1).

MYOCARDIAL STRUCTURE IN HYPERTENSIVE HEART DISEASE

Hypertrophy of Myocytes

Myocytes occupy 70 percent or more of the myocardial mass, whereas their number accounts for only 25 percent of all the cells in the myocardium.[25] When systolic tension is continuously or intermittently elevated above normal, the heart quickly adapts to the augmented load by an increase in ventricular mass. This increase in ventricular mass is mainly caused by an enlargement in myocyte cross-sectional area.[25] Hypertrophy of myocytes is a function of the tension they generate and sustain during systole.[26,27] Although the principal mechanism that links mechanical work to protein synthesis is unknown, during the initial phase of myocyte hypertrophy new myosin and actin isoforms appear at different times[27,28] and new sarcomeres align in parallel, causing thickening of the myocytes and consequently of the ventricular wall.[25] This process of wall thickening reduces the physical stress on the single cell exerted by the pressure generated by systole of the left ventricle.[29,30] Quantitative ultrastructural investigations revealed a normal or slightly reduced mitochondria/myofibril

ratio, mainly caused by an alignment of new sarcomere.[31,32] At this stage, isovolumetric contractility indices, as well as isometric and isotonic contractility indices of isolated papillary muscle, are normal.[33,34] Thus left ventricular myocytic hypertrophy is an adaptive, appropriate response to increased left ventricular pressure from the standpoint of wall stress regulation.

The number of myocytes does not change until a critical weight is reached. Linzbach[8] reported hyperplasia of myocytes in human hearts that exceed a left ventricular weight of more than 250–300 g. He pointed out that such an increase in mass must be regarded as pathologic. However, it remains unclear by which mechanism the transition from the hypertrophied heart to the dilated and failing heart is brought about. Even though the critical heart weight is not exceeded, ultrastructural studies revealed degenerative changes in the myocytes with a decrease of myofibrils, increase of mitochondria, abnormal Z strips, and increases in myelin figures, lipid droplets, and lipofuscin during heart failure.[32] Molecular changes of the proteins, synthesized in the myocytes, may play an important part in the progression of adaptive hypertrophy to heart failure. During myocardial hypertrophy, isoforms of fetal contractile proteins, such as β-myosin heavy chain, β-troponin, and skeletal actin, are expressed.[27,35] Myocardial hypertrophy therefore is not merely a quantitative augmentation of normal contractile protein production; it reflects reexpression of an early developmental stage of myocardium; the ability of the myocardium to generate new contractile proteins is therefore eventually exhausted, terminating cardiac function.[27]

Additionally, the increase in myocytic size may reduce oxygen diffusion and substrate supply, reducing intercellular energy generation. A loss of cardiomyocytes, mainly in the subendocardium, and the appearance of scars were reported the late stage of left ventricular hypertrophy due to experimental arterial hypertension.[36] Slippage and remodeling of the myocytes in the ventricular wall follows, leading to ventricular dilatation with wall thinning. At the stage of ventricular dilatation, isovolumetric contractility is impaired, as are the isometric and isotonic contractility indices of isolated papillary muscles in spontaneously hypertensive rats and other experimental models of slowly developing arterial hypertension.[30,33,34,37]

Coronary Microvessels

Intramural coronary vessels with a luminal diameter of less than 100 μm mainly control coronary blood flow and are regarded as resistance vessels.[38] These vessels constitute more than 70 percent of the intramural arterial tree, and a loss in branches (rarefaction) or inadequate growth in relation to hypertrophy of myocytes may diminish oxygen and substrate delivery.[39] Furthermore, structural alterations of the vessel wall have been discussed for years[40] in regard to increased vascular resistance. One explanation entails remodeling of the arteriolar wall with a reduced lumen at unchanged wall mass.[41] Thus the components of the wall are rearranged, but there is no absolute augmentation of the material. Another possible explanation is true vascular hypertrophy by thickening of the arteriolar wall due to an increase in the number or size (or both) of components of the vessel wall, as reported for intramyocardial arteries in spontaneously hypertensive rats.[42]

In hypertensive patients, Opherk et al.[43] found no structural qualitative abnormalities. On the other hand, van Hoeven and Factor[44] reported thickened walls and reduced lumens of arterial vessels in endomyocardial biopsy specimens of 23 of 27 hypertensives with angina pectoris. In right septal endomyocardial biopsies of 30 patients with arterial hypertension and angina pectoris in the absence of coronary macroangiopathy, we observed wall thickening of intramyocardial arterioles, compared to that of 10 heart donors with no evidence of heart disease.[45] Even in hypertensive individuals without LVH, thickening of the intramyocardial arteriolar wall was observed (Plate 24-1). Therefore it has been assumed that vascular hypertrophy is controlled independently from ventricular hypertrophy[45,46] and may be an early manifestation of hypertensive heart disease.

The arteriolar wall consists mainly of smooth muscle cells and, to a small extent, extracellular matrix. Medial hypertrophy can be caused by hypertrophy or hyperplasia of smooth muscle cells, edema, and increased contents of collagens and other matrix components (i.e., elastin).[41,45–50] Other features include intimal hyalinization and endothelial hyperplasia.[48] Vascular growth may be induced by many factors. Shear stress and mechanical stretch are reported to induce vascular growth.[47] Furthermore, hormonal stimulation and growth factors are involved[49,50] that may act in endocrine, paracrine, and autocrine ways. The renin-angiotensin system, in particular, modulates the growth of vascular smooth muscle cells and reinforces the process of hypertensive cardiac remodeling via angiotensin II-mediated induction of proto-oncogenes and growth factors.[49] Other growth factors, such as platelet-derived growth factor and epidermal growth factor, have been found to modulate medial hypertrophy by smooth muscle cell hypertrophy or hyperplasia.[50]

Structural alterations of the intramural arteriolar tree may predispose or even induce myocardial ischemia. Wall hypertrophy at a small lumen is associated with reduced distensibility and consecutively impairs vascular conductance. Furthermore, an increased wall/lumen ratio may predispose to microvascular vessel closures, as every contraction of the thickened vessel wall leads to ever-greater lumen reduction.[51] Thus limited coronary reserve and microvascular spasms could be the consequences of vascular hypertrophy (Plate 24-1).

Another vascular factor associated potentially with LVH is the loss or inadequate growth of capillary pathways leading to an increase in the distance between capillaries, thereby limiting oxygen diffusion in the myocardium.[39]

Myocardial Fibrosis

The interstitium of the myocardium contains fibrillar connective tissue, which consists mainly of type I and III collagen.[52] The fibrillar collagen network is an essential element for maintaining the structural integrity and architecture of the myocardium during systole and diastole, delivering the stress developed by sarcomeres to the ventricular cavity, and distributing diastolic filling stress throughout the ventricle so at least adjacent myocytes are at equivalent levels of stretch. An abnormal increase of collagen (e.g., fibrosis) and its inelastic properties are responsible for increased myocardial stiffness.[52] In human hearts with pressure overload, as reported for hypertension and aortic stenosis, there is an increase in collagen, leading to a reactive fibrosis next to the ventricular myocytes[53–56] (Fig. 24-2). Caulfield[57] has identified

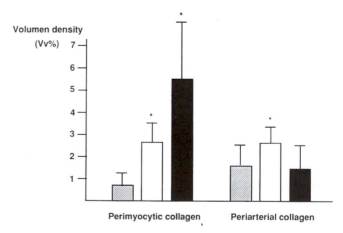

Fig. 24-2. Increased content of perimyocytic collagen in human hypertensive hearts (*open bars*) and hearts with aortic stenosis (*closed bars*); periarterial collagen content is increased only in hypertensive hearts, not in aortic stenosis or controls (scattered bars). *$P \leq 0.05$. (Adapted from Schwartzkopff et al.,[56] with permission.)

that this reactive perimyocytic fibrosis is caused by an increased thickness of perimysial and endomysial collagenous fibers that surround groups of myocytes, muscle bundles, and individual myocytes. Furthermore, collagen accumulation appears around intramyocardial coronary arteries and arterioles.

In a quantitative morphometric study of autopsied hearts and in biopsy specimens from hypertensives, we observed a marked increase of periarteriolar fibrosis.[46,56] This perivascular fibrosis was found in the left hypertensive ventricle as well as in the right, non-pressure-overloaded ventricle. In contrast, no perivascular fibrosis was observed with valvular aortic stenosis.[56]

It appears therefore that with hypertension perivascular interstitium is especially activated, independent from myocyte hypertrophy. Whereas reactive fibrosis, surrounding myocytes, may impair their ability to be stretched and therefore correlates with abnormal diastolic function of the left ventricle, perivascular fibrosis may impair coronary vasodilator capacity and induce further deterioration of the coronary microcirculation. After a prolonged period of hypertension, parenchymal cell injury and loss of myocytes occurs, which leads to replacement or reparative fibrosis when microscopic scarring is present secondary to myocytic necrosis.[36] Causative for this cell loss may be the adverse remodeling and hypertrophy of intramyocardial coronary arteries leading to acute or chronic myocardial ischemia.[36,46,51,56] Furthermore, myocytes embedded in collagen were also reported to degenerate.[52]

The mechanism involved in mediating collagen accumulation leading to fibrosis is not fully understood. A proliferation of fibroblasts—responsible for the generation of collagen,[58] augmentation of local fibroblast activity, or both—or reduced local collagenolysis are discussed[52] as being causative for reactive fibrosis. Myocardial and vascular wall stress may be a primary stimulus for fibroblasts, and ischemia was found to be a stimulus for reactive and reparative fibrosis.[59] Studies indicate that myocardial fibrosis may also be produced by chronically elevated growth hormones, such as circulating mineralocorticoids.[52] An increased renin-angiotensin-aldosterone system (RAAS) is especially regarded as an important cause of reactive fibrosis. Humoral and tissue-bound activation of the RAAS was reported in pressure-loaded hearts,[60] which might be more relevant to the development of fibrosis than pressure alone.

Thus the combined involvement of myocytes, intramyocardial vasculature, and connective tissue characterizes the structural changes in hypertensive heart disease. Hypertensive cardiac remodeling reflects the fundamental reorganization of the heart at the level of the (1) myocytes, (2) extracellular matrix, and (3) vasculature that goes far beyond LVH in terms of increased mass.

LEFT VENTRICULAR SYSTOLIC AND DIASTOLIC FUNCTION IN HYPERTENSIVE HEART DISEASE

Compensated Status

Left ventricular wall thickness increases as a result of myocardial cell hypertrophy. As a consequence, the relation between left ventricular wall thickness and left ventricular radius (i.e., wall thickness/radius ratio) is augmented because the left ventricular end-diastolic diameter remains unchanged or is even reduced. The wall-thickening process reduces the physical force (i.e., stress exerted on the individual cells in the myocardial structure) by the pressure generated during systole in the left ventricle.[29,30] With concentric LVH, systolic wall stress remains constant. Because systolic wall stress, which reflects the left ventricular afterload, is the main determinant of left ventricular systolic function and myocardial oxygen consumption, systolic pump function and oxygen consumption per unit weight of myocardium are normal.[9] The isovolumetric contractility indices at this stage are normal, as are the isotonic contractility indices of isolated papillary muscles in experimental models of slowly developing hypertension[33,34,37] (Fig. 24-3).

Although in this early form of LVH the systolic pump function (measured by the ejection fraction) is not reduced,[7] impaired diastolic filling of the left ventricle is mainly caused by LVH if coronary macroangiopathy is ruled out.[61–63] Mere thickening of the wall due to the increased size of myocytes reduces left ventricular distensibility or compliance without there necessarily being any change in the elastic material properties of the myocardium.[29,30] The pressure–volume curve of the left ventricle is shifted upward and leftward. Disturbances of relaxation may precede the geometric component of diastolic ventricular dysfunction. Fouad-Tarazi[61] described a reduced filling rate of the left ventricle in hypertensive patients prior to deterioration of the systolic indices. Inouye et al.[64] observed a decline in radionuclide-determined early diastolic peak filling rate (PFR) even in the absence of LVH. These observations in humans confirm experimental findings indicating that an increase in afterload at the beginning of ejection lowers the left ventricular relaxation capacity.[65]

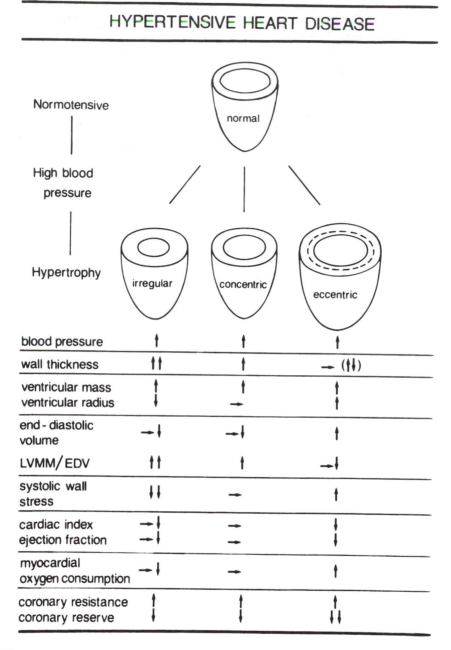

Fig. 24-3. Three possible forms of hypertrophy in the hypertensive heart (irregular, concentric, eccentric). The three forms of hypertrophy may follow both primary (normal-irregular, normal-concentric, normal-eccentric) and a consecutive (normal-irregular-eccentric, normal-concentric-eccentric) course of development. →, normal; ↑, elevated; ↓, decreased; LVMM/EDV, mass/volume ratio. (Adapted from Strauer et al.,[24] with permission.)

Additionally, in some hypertensive subjects remodeling of the extracellular matrix may be an early finding of hypertensive heart disease. An increased content of collagen has been found in right septal endomyocardial biopsy specimens from hypertensive patients even without LVH, indicating alteration of the interstitium even before LVH appears.[45] An increase in myocardial stiffness along with progressive interstitial fibrosis moves the pressure–volume curve upward and leftward. The integral of abnormal relaxation, ventricular and myocardial stiffness, explains why patients with arterial hypertension complain of exertional dyspnea and have a pathologic increase in pulmonary artery pressure under exercise despite well preserved systolic pump function[29,30,65] (Fig. 24-3).

Manifestation of Systolic and Diastolic Heart Failure

After prolonged exposure to high blood pressure, left ventricular dilatation occurs.[8,62] Progressive heart failure is accompanied by activation of the sympathoadrenergic system and the RAAS, which accelerates the process of functional and structural remodeling, leading to further deterioration. The ultimate cause of structural dilatation of the left ventricle, which is accompanied by loss and slippage of myocytes, is unclear.[8,27,52] A disturbance in collagen cross-linking may play a key role in this process.[52] As a result of an alteration in left ventricular geometry, such as wall thinning corresponding to an increase in the left ventricular diameter, afterloading of the left ventricle increases owing to an increase in systolic wall stress.[7,9,29,30] The left ventricular ejection fraction simultaneously drops with a parallel increase in systolic wall stress. At this stage, isovolumetric contractility is also impaired, as are the isometric and isotonic contractility indices of isolated papillary muscles in spontaneously hypertensive rats and other experimental models of slowly developing arterial hypertension.[33,34,37]

At this stage, diastolic function is characterized by a shift to the right and a steep change in the pressure–volume curve owing to a marked increase in myocardial stiffness.[29,30] The change enables the heart to handle large stroke volumes at low pressures over a wide range of volumes. When a certain volume is exceeded, however, a sharp, large rise in ventricular pressure occurs. The reduction in left ventricular pump function is similarly associated with an increase in systolic wall stress (e.g., afterload due to structural ventricular dilatation), a decline in intrinsic myocardial contractility, and a decrease in the elastic properties of the myocardium due to progressive interstitial fibrosis. This pattern clearly demonstrates the close relation between diastolic and systolic function. Extensive alterations in the functional and structural composition of this elastic network of contractile and noncontractile components are reflected in corresponding changes in systolic and diastolic function.[52] Dysfunction of the left ventricle in hypertension is at first diastolic and later systolic.

FUNCTIONAL IMPAIRMENT OF CORONARY CIRCULATION

Patients with arterial hypertension often have angina pectoris, fluctuant ST segment depression on the ECG, and a positive exercise tolerance test even if their epicardial coronary arteries appear anatomically normal.[7,43,67–69] Determining the coronary reserve allows evaluation of the functional impairment of coronary regulatory capacity and, as a consequence, evaluation of microvascular angina.[70]

The coronary reserve is frequently impaired in hypertensive patients. Maximal coronary blood flow after administration of dipyridamole is reduced by 30–50 percent, and the minimal coronary resistance is accordingly elevated. Coronary reserve (the ratio between resting coronary resistance and coronary resistance observed at maximal vasodilatation following dipyridamole administration) is likewise reduced relative to that seen in normotensive individuals[7,70,71] (Fig. 24-4).

Myocardial hypertrophy (myocardial component) may contribute owing to extravascular compressive forces that elevate the extravascular component of coronary resistance. The myocardial component of coronary resistance reflects forces that appear during the myocardial contraction–relaxation process. Perimyocytic and periarteriolar fibrosis may reduce reserve by increasing the myocardial component of coronary resistance due to alteration of the elastic properties of the myocardium. Extravascular compressive forces include elevated end-diastolic pressure, which can lead to compression from the outer surface. We did not observe a significant correlation between elevated end-diastolic pressure and minimal coronary resistance after dipyridamole in hypertensive subjects. Therefore end-diastolic pressure is not the important factor for impaired coronary conductance in hypertensive heart disease.[67,71] Coronary reserve can be metabolically impaired as the wall stress per unit weight is increased, leading to increased oxygen consumption. Thus enhanced coronary blood flow under basal conditions can exhaust the coronary reserve. At least in concentric LVH without chamber enlargement, both myocardial oxygen consumption and coronary blood flow per 100 g of myocardium are unchanged owing to normal systolic wall stress levels.[7] In LVH with chamber enlargement, coronary flow reserve is reduced owing to increased oxygen consumption and increased coronary blood flow per 100 g of myocardium as a consequence of the high afterload of wall stress even at rest (Figs. 24-3 and 24-5).

With moderately severe LVH the reduction in coronary flow reserve exceeds the estimated amount owing to increased left ventricular muscle mass.[71] Moreover, an impaired vasodilator reserve was reported in hypertensive patients without LVH.[67] These findings indicate that structural and functional alterations of coronary resistance vessels (vascular component) are important to the impairment

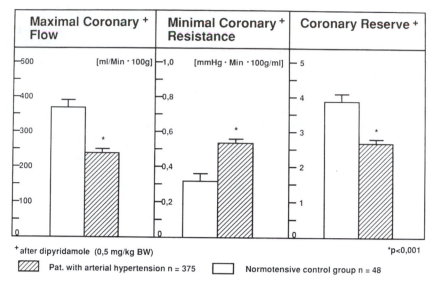

Fig. 24-4. Impairment of coronary reserve with reduced maximal coronary blood flow and increased coronary resistance after dipyridamole (0.5 mg/kg body weight) in hypertensive patients compared with normotensive controls.

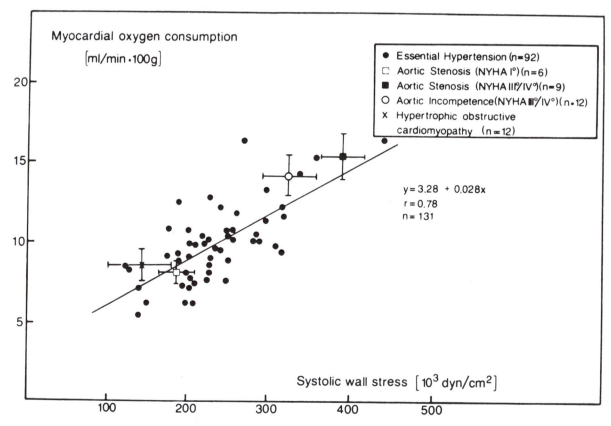

Fig. 24-5. Relation between systolic wall stress and myocardial oxygen consumption. Myocardial oxygen consumption (MVO_2) is increased with increasing systolic wall stress ($y = 03.28 + 0.028x$; $r = 0.78$, $n = 138$). (Adapted from Strauer,[9] with permission.)

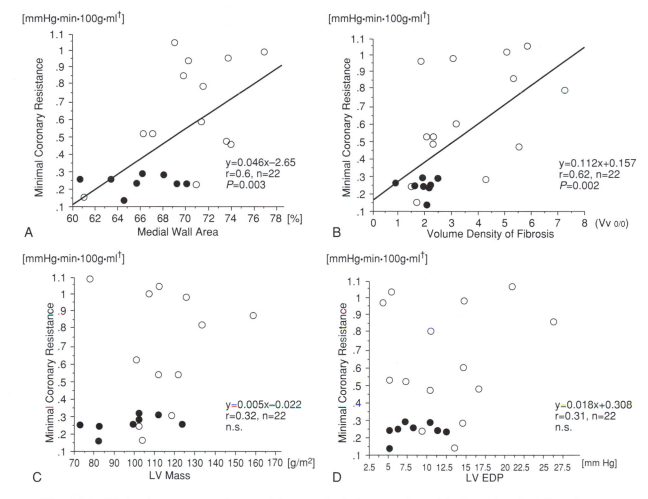

Fig. 24-6. Minimal coronary resistance (pharmacologic intervention with dipyridamole 0.5 mg/kg was significantly associated with (**A**) a higher percent medial wall thickness of arterioles and (**B**) increased content of myocardial collagen (fibrosis), but not with the end-diastolic pressure (LVEDP) or (**C**) mass. (**D**) left ventricular (LV) *Open circles*, normotensives; *closed circles*, hypertensive patients. (Adapted from Schwartzkopff et al.,[46] with permission.)

of coronary vasodilator reserve. Vascular remodeling of coronary arterioles (diameter < 100 μm) includes wall thickening and an increased wall/lumen ratio in hypertensive subjects with microvascular angina compared with that in normotensive subjects.[46] Furthermore, there was a significant correlation between the percentage of medial wall resistance vessels with diameters in the range 10–30 μm and minimal coronary resistance to dipyridamole as an index of overall coronary conductance capacity[46] (Fig. 24-6).

According to Folkow's theory,[72] structural changes to the resistance vessels such as vascular smooth muscle hypertrophy are the result of hypertensive tissue perfusion. On the one hand, medial hypertrophy can be regarded as a protective reaction against hyperperfusion in the hypertensive state; on the other hand, the same wall thickening leads to reduced vasodilator capacity and therefore to limited

coronary blood flow under increased demand. Because intramural arterioles contribute more to the arteriovenous pressure drop than capillaries, medial wall thickening of intramural resistance arteries must be considered the most relevant vascular mechanism contributing to the impaired coronary flow reserve in arterial hypertension.[38,46]

ENDOTHELIUM IN HYPERTENSIVE HEART DISEASE

In addition to structural factors that may contribute to the impairment in coronary reserve in LVH, attenuations in endothelium-mediated control of coronary resistance vessels may also exist. Endothelial cells enzymatically synthesize the endothelium-derived relaxing factor, nitric oxide, from L-arginine concentrations high enough to cause vasodilatation.[73] Baseline endothelial nitric oxide production can be stimulated by bradykinin, acetylcholine, or physical forces such as shear stress. Impaired endothelium-dependent coronary vasodilatation in response to acetylcholine has been observed in patients with essential hypertension and angiographically smooth coronary arteries.[74,75] This finding is consistent with an alteration of the endothelium-dependent reserve flow system in human hypertension. Enhanced activity of endothelium-derived vasoconstricting factors, such as endothelin, may be an alternative mechanism.[73] Furthermore, the interaction of vascular hypertrophy and endothial dysfunction, in terms of absolute or relative diminished vasodilating factors or in terms of a preponderance of vasoconstricting factors, might be the key mechanism leading to angina pectoris and the clinical signs of myocardial ischemia.

VENTRICULAR ARRHYTHMIAS IN HYPERTENSION

A statistically higher incidence of ventricular premature beats and ventricular arrhythmias during ambulatory monitoring was reported in hypertensive patients with ECG-determined LVH than either hypertensive patients without LVH or normotensive subjects.[76-78] Data from the Framingham Study suggest that the presence of asymptomatic complex or frequent ventricular arrhythmias is associated with higher mortality in patients with LVH.[79] Most studies are limited, as the coronary artery disease might have been the major risk factor for cardiac events. The direct relation between ventricular arrhythmias and the occurrence of cardiac events in hypertensive patients with LVH was investigated by Zehender et al.[80] in a 3-year follow-up study performed in 150 hypertensive patients with LVH without manifest coronary artery disease. Arrhythmias were frequent, but they were especially frequent during asymptomatic ST segment depressions. Moreover, transient ST segment abnormalities during daily activities were independent predictors of cardiac events during follow-up, in contrast to repetitive ventricular arrhythmias. The interaction of transient myocardial ischemia and repetitive ventricular arrhythmias was suspected to be the link for fatal arrhythmias.

The mechanisms causing ventricular arrhythmia in patients with hypertension are far from uniform and are still puzzling. Atrial fibrillation and flutter may follow elevated end-diastolic pressure, causing an increased burden to and stretching of the left atrium. Ventricular arrhythmias may be of multiple etiologies. Anatomic factors such as enlarged myocytes, multiple intercalated discs, and areas of fibrosis have been proved to facilitate intercellular conduction and thus produce areas of reentry mechanisms. Mechanical factors such as the stretching of isolated myocardial cells have been shown to lower electric threshold amplitude and therefore increase automaticity. Subendocardial ischemia and medial hypertrophy of the coronary arteries, impeding homogeneous impulse propagation throughout the myocardium, contribute to an increased proarrhythmogenic risk.[5,6,77-80] Thus tissue anisotropy, ventricular dysfunction, and myocardial ischemia may facilitate reentrant circuits, increased triggering activity, and a lowered fibrillation threshold.

THERAPEUTIC CONSIDERATIONS

Normalization of elevated blood pressure is an important therapeutic aim. Several studies have shown that morbidity and mortality from stroke, heart failure, hypertensive encephalopathy, renal failure, and aortic dissection can be reduced by antihypertensive therapy, weight reduction, and restricted salt intake.[81-85] Up to now, the results of treatment of heart failure and prevention of coronary complications in hypertension are still far from satisfying. Therefore, in addition to reducing blood pressure, prevention and repair of hypertensive organ damage should be the major therapeutic goals.

Reversal of LVH

Reduction in load is regarded as an important factor for reversal of LVH.[86-92] During treatment with enalapril,[89] calcium channel blockers,[90] prazosin and clonidine,[91] and β-blockers[92] the reduction in blood pressure was paralleled by regression of the left ventricular mass. Overall, however, the correlation is loose, and a normalized blood pressure is not necessarily associated with a normalized left ventricular mass.[86,87]

A meta-analysis reported 109 studies comprising 2357 patients (28% previously untreated) with an average age of 49 years (range 30–71 years and a mean follow-up of 2.6–17.5 months for different types of treatment.[86] It was found that ACE inhibitors, β-blockers, and calcium antagonists reduced the left ventricular mass by reversing wall hypertrophy, and that ACE inhibitors had the most pronounced effect[86] (Fig. 24-7). Conversely, diuretics reduced the left ventricular mass mainly by reducing the left ventricular volume.

Another meta-analysis[87] revealed that combination therapy, either as dual therapy (thiazide plus methyldopa, ACE inhibitor, dihydropyridine, α-blocker, or β-blocker; or β-blocker plus thiazide, ACE

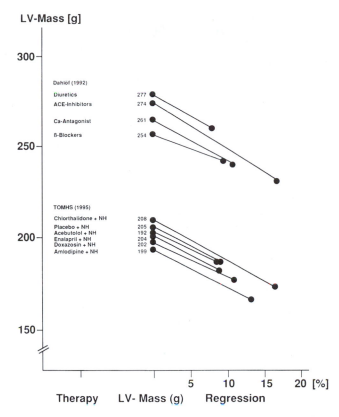

Fig. 24-7. Results from the meta-analysis of Dahlöf et al.[86] and from the TOMHS study[88] in regard to reversal of left ventricular mass under antihypertensive treatment. In the meta-analysis ACE inhibitors achieved the best reversal, whereas in the TOMHS study significant differences in change existed after 1 year of therapy for amlodipine versus acebutolol and placebo, and for chlorthalidone versus acebutolol, enalapril, and placebo plus nutritional hygiene (NH).

inhibitor, or calcium blocker) or triple therapy (diuretics plus calcium blocker plus ACE inhibitor or β-blocker), achieved the best reversal of LVH. The change in left ventricular mass by combination therapy was followed by monotherapy with an ACE inhibitor and then calcium antagonists.[87]

These meta-analyses revealed a large variance in the change of the left ventricular mass for each type of treatment in the various studies. Differences in patient characteristics (e.g., age; pretreatment; duration and severity of hypertension; extent, form, and structural remodeling due to LVH) and in the pharmacologic efficacy of subclasses and the duration and dosage of the drug may be important factors that influence the regression of LVH.

A double-blind, placebo-controlled studies was performed to elucidate the effects of different pharmacologic treatments. The TOMHS study[88] reported five antihypertensive monotherapies (acebutolol, amlodipine, chlorthalidone, doxazosin, enalapril) plus nutritional and hygienic intervention (weight reduction, dietary sodium) compared with placebo plus nutritional and hygienic intervention in 844 mildly hypertensive participants. Only 7–22 percent of hypertensives in each group had LVH. All groups showed a significant decrease (10–15 percent) in the left ventricular mass, which appeared at 3 months and continued for 4 years. Weight loss and reduction of dietary sodium was effective as pharmacologic treatment plus nutritional hygienic intervention in reducing the echocardiographically determined left ventricular mass. The addition of diuretic (chlorthalidone) had a modest additional effect on reducing the left ventricular mass and showed the most reduction in left ventricular end-diastolic diameter. Significant differences in the change existed after 1 year of therapy for amlodipine versus acebutolol and placebo and for chlorthalidone versus acebutolol, enalapril, and placebo. After 4 years of treatment the reversal of the left ventricular mass was in the same range for each medication. Note that hypertensives with mild hypertension and mild LVH were investigated in this study, so applying these data to patients with moderate to severe hypertension and marked LVH must be done with caution. Up to now the influence of the extent of LVH and remodeling on the success of treatment is not clear.

Repair of Extracellular Matrix

The disproportional increase in collagen content during hypertensive heart disease and its resulting deleterious consequences on systolic and especially diastolic function, as well as on the coronary microcirculation, make regression of fibrosis a clinical desideratum. In patients with arterial hypertension and heart failure, myocardial fibrosis was found to be associated at least in part by an activated RAAS.[52] Reversal of reactive fibrosis is called cardioreparation. In experimental studies it has been established that reactive fibrosis can be regressed by chronic ACE inhibition combined with a reduction in myocardial stiffness.[93] Furthermore, calcium antagonists and aldosterone antagonists were found to reverse myocardial fibrosis.[94,95] In animal experiments cardioreparation and cardioprotection (the preventive action of treatment on myocardial fibrosis) have been described for antialdosterone even in doses that do not lower blood pressure significantly.[95] In hypertensive patients we showed that after long-term antihypertensive and antiproliferative therapy with the ACE inhibitor enalapril regression of interstitial reactive fibrosis, including collagen type I and collagen type III, was achieved.[66] Diez et al.,[96] who administered antihypertensive therapy with lisinopril, reported reversal of LVH, decreased serum procollagen types I and III, and an improvement in Doppler echocardiographic determined diastolic function.

Restitution of Coronary Microcirculation

Although it has been shown that LVH can be reversed by suitable antihypertensive agents, information regarding their ability to repair the coronary microcirculation is still required for humans. In spontaneously hypertensive rats, it is known that coronary reserve is enhanced after hydralazine administration without a concomitant regression of LVH,[97] whereas administration of the calcium antagonist felodipine leads to reversal of medial hypertrophy in coronary resistance vessels.[98] ACE inhibition with lisinopril has been shown to improve coronary reserve along with reversal of both medial hypertrophy and myocardial fibrosis in spontaneously hypertensive rats.[93] These experimental findings obtained using genetically determined hypertensive rats should be extrapolated with caution to humans.

The first evidence for restoration of the coronary microcirculation was reported in an open therapy study comparing the effect of calcium antagonists, ACE inhibitions, and β-blockers on the coronary reserve, determined by the argon method.[99–101] In hypertensive patients with microvascular angina pectoris, evidence of myocardial ischemia during the exercise tolerance test or thallium scan, and normal epicardial arteries, long-term therapy (9–12 months) with the ACE inhibitor enalapril, the calcium antagonist diltiazem, and the β-blocker bisoprolol was investigated. During antihypertensive therapy systolic and diastolic blood pressure was in the normotensive range in all three treatment groups. The left ventricular muscle mass decreased in all three groups similarly, by about 8–10 percent. Minimal coronary resistance as the reciprocal parameter of coronary conductance decreased in the bisoprolol group by 11 percent (not significant), in the diltiazem group by 41 percent (significant), and in the enalapril group by 22 percent (significant), accompanied by an increase in coronary reserve (Fig. 24-8).

Possible structural mechanisms that lead to improvement in coronary reserve are regression of myocardial hypertrophy and fibrosis, a decrease in medial thickening, an increase in capillary density, and a decrease in perivascular fibrosis. Concomitant with reversal of hypertrophy and blood pressure reduction are a decrease in the myocardial component of coronary resistance. Consequently, it is difficult to differentiate between the influence of the myocardial factors (e.g., hypertrophy and fibrosis) and the vascular factors (e.g., medial wall thickening and capillary density) on the coronary flow reserve. An antiproliferative effect of ACE inhibitors on the vessel wall has been found in experimental studies,[49,50,93] that could explain disproportionate increase of coronary reserve compared with regression in LVH. Furthermore, investigation of peripheral resistance arteries gave evidence for different efficiency on vascular hypertrophy in essential hypertensive patients. Treatment for 1 year with the ACE inhibitor cilazapril corrected in part the functional and structural abnormalities in subcutaneous resistance arteries of men, whereas the β-blocker atenolol had no effect on vascular structure and function.[102]

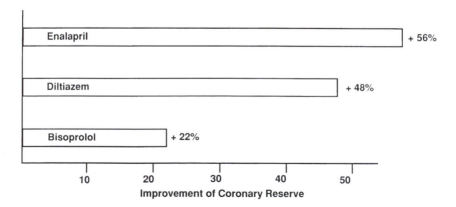

Fig. 24-8. Improvement of coronary reserve after antihypertensive medication with bisoprolol, diltiazem, and enalapril. (Data from Motz and colleagues.[99–101,110])

Treatment Strategies

DIURETICS, VASODILATORS, SYMPATHOLYTIC DRUGS

In addition to blood pressure reduction, humoral factors may influence the effect of LVH reversal. Catecholamines and angiotensin II have been identified as growth cofactors for LVH; they reinforce the growth response and remodeling of the left ventricle due to increased fiber stretching as a consequence of the increased systolic pressure load.[60] Thus antihypertensive substances that stimulate the sympathoadrenergic system or the RAAS, such as diuretics (thiazide) and arterial vasodilators (hydralazine, minoxidil), seem to have less impact on left ventricular wall thickness and myocardial structure (Table 24-1). Otherwise sympatholytic therapy (clonidine, methyldopa) was found to be effective in reversing LVH, particularly in combination with diuretics.[91] Furthermore, diuretics have no beneficial influence on ventricular arrhythmias in hypertensive patients with LVH.[103] High density lipoproteins may be reduced and glucose tolerance diminished, which may influence coronary sclerosis. Hypomagnesemia, hyponatremia, and hypokalemia may be induced, which can exacerbate ventricular arrhythmias.[5,6] In patients with hypertensive heart failure, monotherapy with diuretics is not preferred because they cause further activation of the RAAS and the sympathoadrenergic system. Thus combination therapy is sensible when it consists of a diuretic, digitalis, and an ACE inhibitor to treat hypertensive systolic heart failure.[2,3,104]

α-ADRENERGIC RECEPTOR–BLOCKERS

α-blockers (prazosin, doxazosin) reduce LVH. These drugs favorably influence hemodynamics and lipid metabolism. Their value in cardioreparation and heart failure is not completely known.

ALDOSTERONE ANTAGONISTS

Aldosterone antagonists are effective in reversing myocardial fibrosis.[95] However, the required dosage is not sufficient to lower blood pressure satisfactorily in humans in most cases, and treatment is frequently associated with side effects.

β-BLOCKERS

The effect of treatment with β-adrenergic blockers on LVH may be influenced by their intrinsic sympathomimetic activity. β-Blockers without intrinsic activity (e.g., atenolol) may be more effective than those with intrinsic activity (e.g., acebutolol).[105] On the other hand, Schulman et al.[106] reported that atenolol, unlike the calcium antagonist verapamil, failed to achieve left ventricular mass regression in elderly patients. At the present time there is no clear and convincing explanation for the observation that β-blockers reverse LVH in some patients but not in others.[92,106] It is possible that β-blockers act on the hypertrophied myocardium only indirectly by reducing the pressure load and peak systolic wall stress via shifting the peak systolic pressure to later in the auxotonic phase of contraction. A direct myocardial

Table 24-1. Therapeutic Strategies for Various Cardiac Abnormalities

Abnormality	ACE inhibitors	β-Blockers	Calcium channel blockers	Diuretics	Vaso-dilators	α-Blockers	Sympa-tholytic drugs
High blood pressure	+	+	+	+	+	+	+
LV hypertrophy							
Myocyte	+	+	+	(+)	−	+	+
Fibrosis	+	−	+	−	?		?
VSMC	+	?	+	−	?		?
Heart failure	+	+	!	(+)	+	(+)	−
Extrasystole	−	+	+	−	−	−	−
AV conduction	−	!	!	−	−	−	!
Atherosclerosis							
Schemia	+	+	+	?	−	?	?
Dyslipidemia	−	!	−	!	−	+	?
Diabetes mellitus	(+)	!	−	!	−	−	−

Abbreviations: LV, left ventricular; VSMC, vascular smooth muscle cell; AV, atrioventricular; ACE, angiotensin-converting enzyme.

+, positive influence; −, no influence; !, may ameliorate; ?, unknown.

effect is unlikely because norepinephrine-mediated growth of isolated myocytes can only be prevented by blockade of α-1 receptors.[107] Thus their effect on cardioreparation of the coronary microcirculation might be determined by blood pressure reduction alone. For ischemic syndromes of coronary artery disease, β-blockers are effective, though metabolic syndromes such as diabetes and hyperlipoproteinemia may be ill affected by these drugs. Ventricular arrhythmias in hypertensive hypertrophy were found to be reduced by β-blocker.[103] Acute application of β-blockers to patients with heart failure may aggravate their pump function, whereas long-term treatment was found to have a beneficial effect on the survival of patients with nonischemic dilative cardiomyopathy.[108]

CALCIUM ANTAGONISTS

Calcium antagonists seem to reverse LVH primarily through their antihypertensive action and by lack of undesirable stimulation of the RAAS when given long term. Thus in addition to reversal of LVH, cardioreparation of the interstitium and the microvessel can be anticipated.[103,110]

Under diltiazem a reduction of ventricular arrhythmias was reported in patients with hypertension as early as after 4 weeks of treatment.[103] Reduced numbers of premature ventricular complexes were found after reversal of LVH by calcium antagonists.[78] Their influence on coronary artery disease is not yet clear. Besides the beneficial effect on myocardial ischemia in patients with coronary artery disease, a trend towards an improved prognosis after myocardial infarction was reported under verapamil.[109] Futhermore, metabolic syndromes are not influenced by calcium antagonists. On the other hand, a population-based case-control study reported an increased risk of myocardial infarction in hypertensive patients with the use of short-acting calcium channel blockers, especially dihydopyridines of the first generation in high dose.[111] For short-acting dihydropyridines, a reflex increase in sympathetic activity was discussed, that could theoreticallly produce plaque-rupture. As ongoing large-scale clinical trials are not yet finally reported, the relevance of these findings is still open as well as the indication of calcium antagonists in heart failure.

ACE INHIBITORS

The ACE inhibitors are potent in reversing LVH because they support the physical unloading of the left ventricle by virtue of inhibiting the growth cofactor angiotensin II. Lipid metabolism is not influenced, but glucose tolerance can be improved. Otherwise, no direct antiischemic effects on coronary artery disease or primary antiarrhythmic effects could demonstrated.[103] Effective cardioreparation and cardioprotection, as well as restitution of coronary microcirculation, are beneficial effects of ACE inhibitors in hypertensive heart disease.[66,102,110] A beneficial effect on survival in patients with heart failure of various causes has been demonstrated in several studies.[2,3,104]

ACKNOWLEDGMENT

This work was supported by a grant from the Deutsche Forschungsgemeinschaft, SFB 242, Germany.

REFERENCES

1. Kannel WB, Belanger AJ: Epidemiology of heart failure. Am Heart J 1991;121:951–957
2. SOLVD Investigators: Effect of enalapril on mortality and development of heart failure in asymptomatic patients with reduced left ventricular ejection fraction. N Engl J Med 1992;327:685–691
3. Pfeffer MA, Braunwald E, Moyé A et al: Effect of captopril on mortality and morbidity in patients with left ventricular dysfunction after myocardial infarction. Results of the Survival and Ventricular Enlargement Trial. N Engl J Med 1992;327:669–677
4. Soufer R, Wohlgelernter D, Vita NA et al: Intact systolic function in clinical congestive heart failure. Am J Cardiol 1985;55:1032–1036
5. McLenachan JM, Henderson A, Morris KL, Dargie HJ: Ventricular arrhythmias in patients with hypertensive LVH. N Engl J Med 1987;317:787–792
6. Borhani NO: Left ventricular hypertrophy, arrhythmias and sudden death in systemic hypertension. Am J Cardiol, suppl. I 1987;60:13–18
7. Strauer BE: Ventricular function and coronary hemodynamics in hypertensive heart disease. Am J Cardiol 1979;44:999–1006
8. Linzbach AJ: Heart failure from the point of view of quantitative anatomy. Am J Cardiol 1960;5:370–382
9. Strauer BE: Myocardial oxygen consumption in chronic heart disease. Role of wall stress, hypertrophy and coronary reserve. Am J Cardiol 1979;44:999–1006
10. Lauer MS, Anderson KM, Levy D: Influence of contemporary versus 30-year blood pressure levels on the left ventricular mass and geometry. J Am Coll Cardiol 1991;19:130–134
11. Devereux RB, de Simone G, Ganau A, Koren MJ, Roman MJ: Left ventricular hypertrophy associated with hypertrophy associated with hypertension and its relevance as a risk factor for complications. J Cardiovasc Pharmacol, suppl. 2 1993;21:38–44
12. Lauer MS, Anderson KM, Levy D: Separate and joint influences of obesity and mild hypertension on left ventricular mass and geometry. The Framingham Heart Study. J Am Coll Cardiol 1992;19:130–134

13. Ganau A, Devereux RB, Roman MJ et al: Patterns of left ventricular hypertrophy and geometric remodelling in essential hypertension. J Am Coll Cardiol 1992;19:1550–1558

14. Arnett DK, Rantaharju P, Crow R et al: Black-white differences in electrocardiographic left ventricular mass and its association with blood pressure (the ARIC Study). Am J Cardiol 1994;74:247–252

15. Lauer MS, Levy D, Anderson KM, Plehn YF: Is there a relationship between exercise systolic blood pressure response and left ventricular mass? Ann Intern Med 1992;116:203–210

16. Levy D, Garrison RJ, Savage DD, Kannel WB, Castelli WP: Prognostic implications of echocardiographically determined left ventricular mass in the Framingham Heart Study. N Engl J Med 1990;322:1561–1566

17. Levy D, Labib SB, Anderson KM et al: Determinants of sensitivity and specificity of electrocardiography criteria for left ventricular hypertrophy. Circulation 1990;81:815–820

18. Savage DD, Garrison RJ, Kannel WB et al: The spectrum of left ventricular hypertrophy in a general population sample. The Framingham Study. Circulation, suppl. I 1987;75:26–33

19. Dahlöf B: Factors involved in the pathogenesis of hypertensive cardiovascular hypertrophy. A review. Drugs, suppl. 5 1988;35:6–26

20. Rautaharju PM, Lacroix AZ, Savage DD: Electrographic estimate of left ventricular mass versus radiographic cardiac size and the risk of cardiovascular disease mortality in the epidemiologic follow-up study of the FNHANES. Am J Cardiol 1988;62:59–66

21. Cooper RS, Simmons BE: Left ventricular hypertrophy is associated with worse survival independent of ventricular function and of number of coronary arteries severely narrowed. Am J Cardiol 1990;65:441–445

22. Casale PN, Devereux RB, Milner M: Value of echocardiographic measurement of left ventricular mass in predicting cardiovascular morbid events in hypertensive men. Ann Intern Med 1986;105:173–178

23. Koren MJ, Devereux RB, Casale PN, Savage DD, Laragh JH: Relation of left ventricular mass and geometry to morbidity and mortality in uncomplicated essential hypertension. Ann Intern Med 1991;114:345–352

24. Strauer BE: Coronary hemodynamics in hypertensive heart disease. Am J Med 1988;84:45–54

25. Anversa P, Ricci R, Olivetti G: Quantitative structural analysis of the myocardium during physiologic growth and induced cardiac hypertrophy. A review. J Am Coll Cardiol 1986;7:1140–1149

26. Weber KT, Clark WA, Janicki JS, Shroff SG: Physiologic versus pathologic hypertrophy and the pressure-overloaded myocardium. J Cardiovasc Pharmacol, suppl. 6 1987;10:37–49

27. Katz A: Cardiomyopathy of overload. A major determinant of prognosis in congestive heart failure. N Engl J Med 1990;322:100–110

28. Swynghedauw B: Remodelling of the heart in response to chronic mechanical overload. Eur Heart J 1989;10:935–943

29. Ford EF: Heart size. Circ Res 1985;39:297–303

30. Grossman W, Jones D, McLaurin LP: Wall stress and patterns of hypertrophy in the human left ventricle. J Clin Invest 1975;56:56–64

31. Anversa P, Load AV, Giacomelli F, Wiener Z: Absolute morphometric study of myocardial hypertension. II. Ultrastructure of myocytes and interstitium. Lab Invest 1978;38:597–609

32. Frenzel H, Schwartzkopff B, Rettig B, Vogelsang H: Morphologic criteria of progression and regression of cardiac hypertrophy. J Cardiovasc Pharmacol, suppl. 6 1987;10:20–28

33. Spann JF, Buccino RA, Sonnenblick EH, Braunwald E: Contractile state of cardiac muscle obtained from cats with experimentally produced ventricular hypertrophy and heart failure. Circ Res 1967;21:341–348

34. Bürger SB, Strauer BE: Left ventricular hypertrophy in chronic pressure load due to spontaneous essential hypertension. I. Left ventricular function, left ventricular geometry and wall stress. pp. 13–35. In: Strauer BE (ed): The Heart in Hypertension. Springer-Verlag, Berlin, 1981

35. Nadal-Ginard B, Mahdavi V: Molecular mechanisms of cardiac gene expression. pp. 65–80. In: Grobecker H, Heusch G, Strauer BE (eds): Angiotensin and the Heart. Springer-Verlag, New York, 1993

36. Capasso JM, Palackal T, Olivetti G, Anversa P: Left ventricular failure—induced by long-term hypertension in rats. Circ Res 1990;66:1400–1412

37. Bürger SB, Strauer BE: Left ventricular hypertrophy in chronic pressure load due to spontaneous essential hypertension. II. Contractility of the isolated left ventricular myocardium and left ventricular stiffness. pp. 37–52. In: Strauer BE (ed): The Heart in Hypertension. Springer-Verlag, Berlin, 1981

38. Tillmanns H, Steinhausen M, Leinberger H, Thederau H, Kübler W: Pressure measurement in the terminal vascular bed of the epimyocardium of rats and cats. Circ Res 1981;49:1202–1211

39. Tomanek RJ, Schalk KA, Marcus ML, Harrison DG: Coronary angiogenesis during long-term hypertrophy and left ventricular hypertrophy in dogs. Circ Res 1989;65:352–359

40. Kathke N: Die Veränderungen der Koronararterienzweige des Myokards bei Hypertonie. Beitr Pathol Anat 1955;115:405–418

41. Mulvany MJ: Vascular growth in hypertension. J Cardiovasc Pharmacol 1992;22:7–11

42. Amann K, Gharehbagli H, Stephan S, Mall G: Hypertrophy and hyperplasia of smooth muscle cells of small intramyocardial arteries in spontaneously hypertensive rats. Hypertension 1995;25:124–131

43. Opherk D, Mall G, Zebe H et al: Reduction of coronary reserve. A mechanism for angina pectoris in patients with arterial hypertension and normal coronary arteries. Circulation 1984;69:1–7

44. Van Hoeven KH, Factor S: Endomyocardial biopsy diagnosis of small vessel disease. A clinicopathologic study. Int J Cardiol 1990;26:103–110

45. Schwartzkopff B, Motz W, Knauer S, Frenzel H, Strauer BE: Morphometric investigations of intramyocardial arterioles in right septal endomyocardial biopsy of patients with arterial hypertension and left ventricular hypertrophy. J Cardiovasc Pharmacol, suppl. 1 1992;20:12–17

46. Schwartzkopff B, Motz W, Frenzel H et al: Structural and functional alterations of the intramyocardial coronary arterioles in patients with arterial hypertension. Circulation 1993;88:993–1003

47. Hudlicka O, Brown M, Egginton S: Angiogenesis in

skeletal and cardiac muscle. Physiol Rev 1992;72:369–417

48. Moritz AR, Oldt MR: Arteriolar sclerosis in hypertensive and non-hypertensive individuals. Am J Pathol 1937;13:679–728

49. Dzau VJ, Gibbons GH, Cooke JP, Omoigui N: Vascular biology and medicine in the 1990's. Scope, concepts, potentials and perspectives. Circulation 1993;87:705–719

50. Scott-Burden T, Resink TJ, Baur U, Bürgin M, Bühler FR: Epidermal growth factor responsiveness in smooth muscle cells from hypertensive and normotensive rats. Hypertension 1989;13:295–304

51. James JN: Morphologic characteristics and functional significance of focal fibromuscular dysplasia of small coronary arteries. Am J Cardiol 1990;65:12G–22G

52. Weber KT, Sun Y, Guarda E: Structural remodeling in hypertensive heart disease and the role of hormones. Hypertension 1994;23:869–877

53. Huysman JAN, Vliegen HW, Van der Laarse A, Eulderink F: Changes in nonmyocyte tissue composition associated with pressure overload of hypertrophic human hearts. Pathol Res Pract 1989;184:577–581

54. Anderson KR, Sutton GSTJ, Lie JT: Histopathological types of cardiac fibrosis in myocardial disease. J Pathol 1979;128:79–85

55. Cheitlin MD, Rubinowitz M, McAllister H et al: The distribution of fibrosis in the left ventricle in congenital aortic stenosis and coarctation of the aorta. Circulation 1980;62:823–830

56. Schwartzkopff B, Frenzel H, Dieckerhoff J et al: Morphometric investigation of human myocardium in arterial hypertension and valvular aortic stenosis. Eur Heart J, suppl. D 1992;13:17–20

57. Caulfield JB: Alterations in cardiac collagen with hypertrophy. pp. 49–57. In Tarazi RC, Dunbar JB (eds): Perspectives in Cardiovascular Research. Vol. 8. Lippincott-Raven, Philadelphia, 1983

58. Eghbali M, Blumenfeld OO, Seifter S et al: Localization of types I, III, and IV collagen mRNAs in rat heart cells by in situ hybridization. J Mol Cell Cardiol 1989;21:103–113

59. Weber KT: Cardiac interstitium in health and disease. Remodelling of the fibrillar collagen matrix. J Am Coll Cardiol 1989;13:1637–1652

60. Schunkert H, Dzau VJ, Tang SS et al: Increased rat cardiac angiotensin converting enzyme, activity and mRNA expression in pressure overload left ventricular hypertrophy. J Clin Invest 1990;86:1913–1920

61. Fouad-Tarazi FM: Left ventricular diastolic dysfunction and cardiovascular regulation in hypertension. Am J Med 1989;87:425–445

62. Serizawa T, Mirsky J, Carabello BA, Grossman W: Diastolic myocardial stiffness in gradually developing left ventricular hypertrophy in dog. Am J Physiol 1982;242:H633–H637

63. Iriarte U, Murga N, Sagastagoitia D: Congestive heart failure from left ventricular diastolic dysfunction in systemic hypertension. Am J Cardiol 1993;71:308–312

64. Inouye I, Massie B, Loge D et al: Abnormal left ventricular filling. An early finding in mild to moderate systemic hypertension. Am J Cardiol 1984;53:120–126

65. Brutsaert DL, Sys SU, Gillebert TH: Diastolic failure. Pathophysiology and therapeutic implications. J Am Coll Cardiol 1993;22:318–325

66. Schwartzkopff B, Motz W, Strauer BE: Repair of human myocardial structure by chronic treatment with ACE-inhibitors in hypertensive heart disease [abstract]. Circulation, suppl. I 1994;90:343

67. Brush JE, Cannon RO III, Schenke WH et al: Angina due to coronary microvascular disease in hypertensive patients without left ventricular hypertrophy. N Engl J Med 1988;319:1302–1307

68. Houghton JL, Frenk MJ, Carr AA, von Dohlen TW, Presant LM: Relations among impaired coronary flow reserve, left ventricular hypertrophy and thallium perfusion defects in hypertensive patients without obstructive coronary artery disease. J Am Coll Cardiol 1990;15:43–51

69. Scheler S, Motz W, Strauer BE: Mechanism of angina pectoris in patients with systemic hypertension and normal epicardial coronary arteries by angiogram. Am J Cardiol 1994;73:478–482

70. Cannon RO III: The coronary microcirculation in heart disease. Hypertrophic cardiomyopathy, hypertension and microvascular angina. Coronary Artery Dis 1992;3:555–563

71. Vogt M, Motz W, Schwartzkopff B, Strauer BE: 1990: Coronary microangiopathy and cardiac hypertrophy. Eur Heart J, suppl. B 1990;11:133–138

72. Folkow B: The fourth Volhard Lecture. Cardiovascular structural adaption. Its role in the initiation and maintenance of primary hypertension. Clin Sci Mol Med 1975;48:205–211

73. Lüscher TF, Wenzel RR, Noll G: Local regulation of the coronary circulation in health and disease. Role of nitric oxide and endothelin. Eur Heart J, suppl. C 1995;16:51–58

74. Motz W, Vogt M, Rabenau O et al: Evidence of endothelial dysfunction in coronary resistance vessels in patients with angina pectoris and normal coronary angiograms. Am J Cardiol 1991;68:996–1003

75. Panza JA, Garcia CE, Kilcoyne CM et al: Impaired endothelium-dependent vasodilation in patients with essential hypertension. Evidence for a generalized endothelial abnormality [abstract]. J Am Coll Cardiol 1994;23:274A

76. Levy D, Anderson K, Savage D et al: Risk of ventricular arrhythmias in LVH. The Framingham Study. Am J Cardiol 1987;60:560–565

77. McLenachan JM, Dargie HJ: Ventricular arrhythmias in hypertensive LVH. Relationship to coronary artery disease, left ventricular dysfunction and myocardial fibrosis. Am J Hypertens 1990;3:735–740

78. Messerli FH, Nunez BD, Nunez MM et al: Hypertension and sudden death: Disparate effects of calcium entry blockers and diuretic therapy on cardiac dysrhythmias. Arch Intern Med 1989;149:1263–1267

79. Bikkina M, Larson MG, Levy D: Asymptomatic ventricular arrhythmias and mortality risk in subjects with left ventricular hypertrophy. J Am Coll Cardiol 1993;22:1111–1116

80. Zehender M, Meinertz T, Hohnloser S et al: Prevalence of circadian variations and spontaneous variability of cardiac disorders and ECG changes suggestive of myocardial ischemia in systemic arterial hypertension. Circulation 1992;85:1808–1815

81. MacMahon S, Peto R, Cutler J et al: Blood pressure, stroke and coronary heart disease. Part 1. Lancet 1990;335:765–774

82. Hypertension Detection and Follow-up Program Cooperative Group: Persistence of reduction in blood

pressure and mortality of participants in the hypertension detection and follow-up program. JAMA 1988;259:2113–2122

83. Lewis CE, Liebson PR: Treatment of mild hypertension study. JAMA 1993;270:713–724

84. Dahlöf B, Lindholm LH, Hansson L et al: Morbidity and mortality in the Swedish trial in old patients with hypertension (STOP-Hypertension.) Lancet 1991;338:1281–1285

85. Hypertension Prevention Trial: Three-year effects of dietary changes on blood pressure. Arch Intern Med 1990;150:153–162

86. Dahlöf B, Pennert K, Hansson L: Reversal of left ventricular hypertrophy in hypertensive patients. A metaanalysis of 109 treatment studies. Am J Hypertens 1992;5:95–110

87. Cruickshank JM, Lewis J, Moore V, Dodd C: Reversibility of left ventricular hypertrophy by differing types of antihypertensive therapy. J Hum Hypertens 1992;6:85–90

88. Liebson PR, Grandis GA, Dianzumba S et al: Comparison of five antihypertensive monotherapies and placebo for change in left ventricular mass in patients receiving nutritional-hygeinic therapy in the treatment of mild hypertension study (TOMHS). Circulation 1995;91:698–706

89. Nakashima Y, Fouad FM, Tarazi RC: Regression of left ventricular hypertrophy from systemic hypertension by enalapril. Am J Cardiol 1984;53:1044–1049

90. Strauer BE, Mahmoud MA, Mayer F, Bohn F, Motz W: Reversal of left ventricular hypertrophy and improvement of cardiac function in man by nifedipine. Eur Heart J, suppl. F 1984;5:53–60

91. Strauer BE, Bayer F, Brecht HM, Motz W: The influence of sympathetic nervous activity on regression of cardiac hypertrophy. J Hypertens Suppl 4 1985;3:39–44

92. Dunn FG, Ventura HO, Messerli FH et al: Time course of regression on left ventricular hypertrophy in hypertensive patients treated with atenolol. Circulation 1987;76:254–258

93. Brilla CG, Janicki JS, Weber KT: Cardioreparative effects of lisinopril in rats with genetic hypertension and left ventricular hypertrophy. Circulation 1991;83:1771–1779

94. Motz W, Strauer BE: Left ventricular function and collagen content after regression of hypertensive hypertrophy. Hypertension 1989;13:43–56

95. Brilla CG, Matsutara LS, Weber KT: Anti-aldosterone treatment and the prevention of myocardial fibrosis in primary and secondary hyperaldosteronism. J Moll Cell Cardiol 1993;25:563–575

96. Diez J, Laviades C, Mayor G, Gil MJ, Monreal I: Increased serum concentrations of procollagen peptides in essential hypertension. Relation to cardiac alterations. Circulation 1995;91:1450–1456

97. Anderson PG, Bishop SB, Digernen SB: Vascular remodeling and improvement of coronary reserve after hydralazine treatment in spontaneously hypertensive rats. Circ Res 1989;64:1127–1136

98. Eisenlohr H, Schmiebusch H, Strauer BE: Regression of media hypertrophy in hypertensive coronary resistance vessels by antihypertensive therapy [abstract]. Circulation, suppl. II 1988;78:169

99. Motz W, Vogt M, Scheler S et al: Prophylaxe mit gefäßaktiven Substanzen. Z Kardiol, suppl. 4 1992;81:199–204

100. Vogt M, Motz W, Pölitz B, Scheler S, Strauer BE: Improvement of coronary reserve by chronic treatment with ACE inhibitors [abstract]. Circulation, suppl. III 1991;84:136

101. Motz W, Vogt M, Scheler S, Schwartzkopff B, Strauer BE: Verbesserung der Koronarreserve nach Hypertrophie-regression durch antihypertensive Therapie mit einem Beta-Rezeptorenblocker. Dtsch Med Wochenschr 1993;118:540–553

102. Schiffrin EL, Deng LY, Larochelle P: Effects of a β-blocker or a converting enzyme inhibitor on resistance arteries in essential hypertension. Hypertension 1994;23:83–91

103. Papademetriou V, Narayan P, Kokkinos P: Effects of diltiazem, metoprolol, enalapril and hydrochlorothiazide on frequency of ventricular premature complexes. Am J Cardiol 1994;73:242–246

104. SOLVD Investigators: Effect of enalapril on survival in patients with reduced left ventricular ejection fraction and congestive heart failure. N Engl J Med 1991;325:293–302

105. Sau F, Seguro C, Merano G, Cherchi A: Atenolol but not acebutolol reverses left ventricular hypertrophy secondary to arterial hypertension [abstract]. J Am Coll Cardiol, suppl. 1986;7:186

106. Schulman SP, Weiss JL, Becker LC et al: The effects of antihypertensive therapy on left ventricular mass in elderly patients. N Engl J Med 1990;322:1350–1356

107. Simpson P: Norepinephrine stimulated hypertrophy of cultured rat myocardial cell is an alpha-1-adrenergic response. J Clin Invest 1983;72:732–738

108. Waagstein F, Bristow MR, Swedberg K et al: Beneficial effects of metoprolol in idiopathic dilated cardiomyopathy. Lancet 1993;342:1441–1446

109. Danish Study Group: The Danish Verapamil Infarction Trial II-DAVIT III. Effect of verapamil on mortality and major events after acute myocardial infarction. Am J Cardiol 1990;66:779–785

110. Motz W, Vogt M, Scheler S, Strauer BE: Pharmacotherapeutic effects of antihypertensive agents on myocardium and coronary arteries in hypertension. Eur Heart J, suppl. D 1992;13:100–106

111. Psaty BM, Heckbert SR, Koepsell TD et al: The risk of myocardial infarction associated with antihypertensive drug therapies. JAMA 1995;274:620–625

25 Diastolic Heart Failure

Derek Gibson

Diastolic heart failure is suspected when limitation of exercise tolerance, pulmonary congestion, or fluid retention are too severe to be explained by the extent of systolic ventricular disease. If the diagnosis is not simply to be one of exclusion, diastolic function should be systematically investigated and abnormalities compatible with the clinical picture demonstrated. In the literature, the idea of diastolic heart failure has been developed almost exclusively with respect to the left ventricle, so it is with this aspect that the current chapter is concerned.[1]

Ventricular diastolic function differs from that of systole in several important ways. It is much more dependent on age, so values that are normal in the elderly would be frankly abnormal in the young.[2,3] Most measurements of diastolic function depend critically on ventricular loading conditions, which are likely to be abnormal in patients with clinical heart failure. In addition, the most effective means of treating such patients do not affect diastolic function directly but modify loading conditions. Relations between them and intrinsic disease must always be considered when such measurements are being interpreted.[4,5] Finally diastolic function is greatly influenced by events during activation and systole. Thus a disturbance whose most obvious manifestations occur during diastole may have its origin much easier in the cardiac cycle.

There is no general agreement as to what constitutes diastolic disease, though "increased resistance to ventricular filling" has been proposed as a simple definition of its effects.[6] If this were indeed the case, diastolic disease ought to be readily quantifiable in individual patients. Though resistance to flow across a valve or circulation is clearly defined and has unambiguous physical dimensions, "resistance" to filling has neither. Indeed, there is no simple definition of diastolic disease. In this chapter normal mechanisms as they occur in humans are described and potential disturbances in disease identified. Valvar disease and pathologic conditions of the pericardium are not considered. However, the extent to which any particular abnormality of diastolic function, especially when measured at rest, contributes to impaired exercise tolerance or reduced prognosis in many cases remains uncertain. Although there are few studies in which diastolic mechanisms limiting exercise tolerance have been definitively identified, it is usually possible to identify those in whom the presumption is strong.

PHASES OF DIASTOLE

The terminology established by Wiggers for describing the phases of diastole is used here.[7] Isovolumic relaxation is assumed to start with aortic valve closure and to end with mitral valve opening and the onset of atrioventricular flow. Normal ventricular filling has a normal early diastolic phase, a mid-diastolic period of diastasis, followed by atrial systole.

ISOVOLUMIC RELAXATION

Events during isovolumic relaxation are of considerable importance in determining diastolic function. Its onset, aortic valve closure, can be unambiguously timed from cusp apposition (on M-mode studies),

339

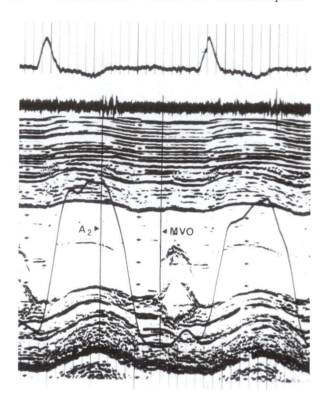

Fig. 25-1. Abnormally prolonged isovolumic relaxation (to 280 ms) due to ventricular disease. Note that during isovolumic relaxation there has been a striking increase in left ventricular transverse dimension indicating that in the absence of filling the cavity shape must have changed. A2, aortic valve closure; MVO, mitral valve opening. These two events are marked by the two vertical lines.

which coincides with A2, the onset of the first high frequency component of the aortic component of the second heart sound on the phonocardiogram, as well as with the end of the aortic flow signal and the leading edge of the aortic closure artifact seen on pulsed-wave Doppler. The end of isovolumic relaxation is less well defined, as mitral valve opening and the onset of detectable flow are not synchronous in normal individuals or in patients with heart disease. Mitral cusp separation, defined from an M-mode echocardiogram, characteristically precedes the onset of flow, as determined by pulsed-wave Doppler with the sample volume at mitral tip level. This interval is normally 25 ms, but it may be 50 ms in patients with left ventricular hypertrophy and 100 ms or more in patients with coronary artery disease.

In normal adults, left ventricular isovolumic relaxation time measured by M-mode echocardiography is 60 ± 10 ms and by Doppler is 85 ± 15 ms. It increases with age, the values in the elderly being approximately double those in children.[4] It correlates positively and weakly with the heart rate. With left ventricular disease, two opposing processes can

be identified. The first is prolongation by the disease process itself, a situation seen with hypertension, diabetes, coronary artery disease, or cardiomyopathy. Such prolongation has many causes, which are analyzed in more detail in a later section and may be striking (Fig. 25-1). The second is shortening by an elevated left ventricular filling pressure, to 0–10 ms when end-diastolic pressure is around 30 mmHg (Fig. 25-2). Negative values (i.e., when the mitral valve opens before the aortic valve closes) are some-

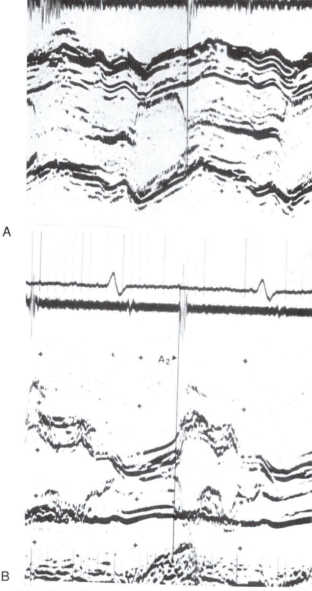

Fig. 25-2. Short isovolumic relaxation time from a patient with a high left atrial pressure. **(A)** Aortic echogram. The timing of aortic cusp closure corresponds with A2 on the phonocardiogram. **(B)** Mitral cusp separation precedes A2.

times seen when the left atrial V wave is even higher. This effect of filling pressure counteracts prolongation by ventricular disease. Aortic diastolic pressure has little effect on the isovolumic relaxation time, probably because the aortic pressure is dropping much more rapidly at the time of aortic closure than at the time of mitral opening. These interrelations illustrate how changes in loading conditions can interact with the effects of disease. Isovolumic relaxation time therefore is not a measure of relaxation. A normal isovolumic relaxation time does not therefore exclude a major abnormality of the relaxation process when the filling pressure is elevated. Measurements of isovolumic relaxation time can, however, give useful information. When prolonged to 90 ms or more it is likely that relaxation is abnormal and the filling pressure is low, whereas if it is abnormally short, the left atrial pressure is almost certainly increased.

Quantification of Changes in Left Ventricular Relaxation

The major change in relaxation with left ventricular disease is a change in the time course of the decline in wall tension, so the rate of decline is reduced and the duration of the period over which it takes place is increased. It is difficult to study this process directly in intact humans, so indirect measures must be used. Of these measures the most commonly used is the high fidelity left ventricular pressure. When cavity dimension and wall thickness are constant, changes in left ventricular wall tension are directly reflected in changes in cavity pressure. The time course of the left ventricular pressure has been assessed noninvasively, with considerable accuracy, from the trace of functional mitral regurgitation detected by continuous-wave Doppler echocardiography. Experimental and clinical evidence suggests that peak values can be estimated at least semiquantitatively[9,10] and that time intervals agree between the two within 5 ms.[11] Although values derived in this way might theoretically be affected by left atrial pressure, it does not appear to have been a problem in published accounts. This noninvasive approach has greatly extended the use that can be made of abnormalities in the time course of the pressure decrease when characterizing disturbances of diastole.

The peak rate of fall of pressure (peak negative dP/dt) is derived by simple differentiation of the output of a micromanometer. It is largely determined by the peak systolic pressure.[12] Independent of this situation, the rate of fall is reduced during pacing-induced ischemia. Low values are also seen in patients with coronary artery disease and severe left ventricular hypertrophy.[13] However, any value it may have in detecting diastolic disease is limited by its sensitivity to loading conditions.

An alternative approach has been to accept this load dependence and assume that the rate of left ventricular pressure fall is exponential from the time of its peak value (peak dP/dt) until mitral valve opening,[14,15] which implies that the rate of fall is directly proportional to instantaneous pressure. The reciprocal of the constant of proportionality in this relation is identical with the time constant of pressure fall (T), sometimes referred to as the time constant of relaxation. Although there is no theoretic basis for the pressure fall within the ventricle being exponential, predicted and observed values in normal individuals agree well enough. In experimental animals, T is largely independent of the peak left ventricular pressure, stroke volume, heart rate, and peak systolic shortening rate. In humans, T increases with advancing age and shortens with tachycardia due to atrial pacing. It falls strikingly with exercise in normal subjects to a much greater extent than would be expected from any increase in arterial pressure.[16] T is most conveniently calculated from a plot of dP/dt against instantaneous pressure. If the pressure fall is truly exponential, it is a straight line, of slope 1/T. The normal value for T is 55 ± 12 ms. There is usually a negative pressure intercept, implying that the baseline for the exponential fall is not zero. In normal subjects it has a mean value of -25 ± 9 mmHg, suggesting that the equilibrium pressure is strikingly subatmospheric. Its exact physical significance is not clear, and no great clinical importance has been attached to it.

The time constant of pressure fall is frequently prolonged in patients with coronary artery disease, hypertrophic cardiomyopathy, or severe secondary left ventricular hypertrophy.[17,18] In an isolated muscle fiber the rate of tension decline reflects the termination of the active state and thus the rate of uptake of calcium into the sarcoplasmic reticulum. The effects of calcium depend on the availability of adenosine triphosphate (ATP), largely glycolytic in origin. It is thus possible to classify interventions of potential benefit when treating patients with ventricular disease in terms of their effect on these variables. Experience treating impaired systolic function has demonstrated that extrapolation from effects seen in single cells to the ventricle as a whole, particularly in the presence of disease, is fraught with difficulty. Even in the normal subject the time course of ventricular pressure fall deviates from an exponential; and in the presence of disease, such as hypertrophic cardiomyopathy, these changes may be substantial. When the filling pressure is high, the isovolumic relaxation time is short and may even be zero, so the mitral valve has opened before the pressure curve has approximated to exponential. Even more important is the problem of regional disturbances of function: These disturbances may represent differences in the time of onset of tension decline, its rate, and its extent.[19] Taken together, these factors reduce the rate of pressure fall, though there is no reason to suppose that their resultant effect causes the time course to conform to a single exponential. Even if time constants can be contrived, therefore, it is doubtful that they have any physical significance.

Regional Left Ventricular Wall Motion

Although the volume of the ventricle may remain constant during isovolumic relaxation, its shape may change. Such change occurs even in normal subjects, and it was for this reason that the original term, "isometric" relaxation, was abandoned. In addition, it has been demonstrated by magnetic resonance imaging (MRI) myocardial tagging that these small changes in cavity dimension are accompanied by reversal during isovolumic relaxation of systolic rotation (torsion) around the long axis and shearing between endocardial and epicardial muscle layers.[20]

Although the extent of myocardial torsion and shearing are often reduced in the presence of disease, changes in cavity shape may be much more striking than in normal individuals.[21,22] They can be demonstrated by a variety of imaging techniques, including contrast or radionuclide angiography,[23,24] and by echocardiography, either M-mode[25] or cross-sectional.[26] They are seen in patients with left ventricular hypertrophy and, in particular, those with coronary artery disease. Early after acute myocardial infarction, abnormal inward motion, implying abnormal persistence of myocardial tension, occurs in the region supplied by the occluded coronary artery.[27] Similar changes occur with balloon inflation during coronary angioplasty. However, wall motion during isovolumic relaxation is incoordinate at rest in approximately 50 percent of patients with chronic, stable angina severe enough to merit coronary arteriography.[22]

There are many causes of incoordination. Abnormal ventricular activation leads to regional delay in the onset, and therefore the termination, of contrac-

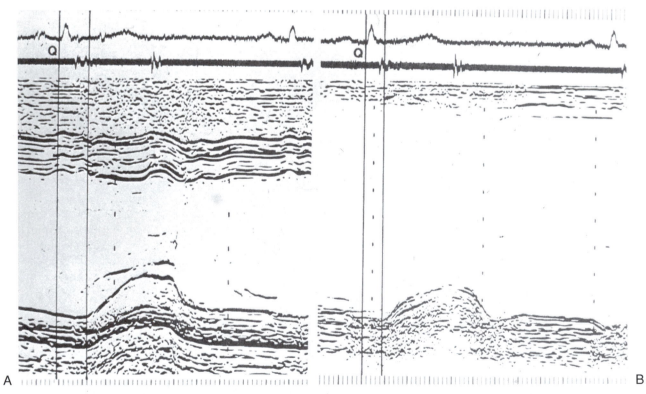

Fig. 25-3. **(A)** Normal transverse M-mode echocardiogram of the left ventricular cavity. **(B)** Normal long axis echocardiogram of the left ventricle. Vertical lines represent the onset of the Q wave of the ECG and the onset of systolic shortening, that of the long axis preceding that of the minor axis. Note that, in both, the peak shortening corresponds with the second sound.

tion. Regional differences in systolic stress may predispose to local differences in the time of onset and rate of tension decline.[28] Severe pulmonary hypertension may cause striking prolongation of the pressure decline on the right side of the heart, interfering with isovolumic relaxation on the left.[29] Whatever the primary cause of the incoordination, the rate of pressure decline is reduced, and isovolumic relaxation time is prolonged.

Incoordination represents a significant departure from the normal pattern of regional ventricular function. It was recognized by William Harvey that circumferential and longitudinally directed fibers normally move synchronously.[30] The function of circumferential fibers has been studied in great detail, whereas longitudinal function has received less attention. In instrumented animals, small differences in the relative timing of motion in the two directions causes minor changes in cavity shape during the two isovolumic periods.[31] The same applies in normal humans, with a minor change toward a more spherical cavity during both isovolumic periods. In general, normal longitudinal left ventricular shortening is synchronous with circumferential function (Fig. 25-3), and neither changes significantly during isovolumic relaxation. The effects of intermittent left bundle branch block on long axis function are shown in Figure 25-4. With normal activation, long axis function is also normal, with peak shortening coinciding with aortic valve closure. When bundle block develops, it shortens abnormally by 2–3 mm during isovolumic relaxation. This effect is consistent. All that is necessary for its appearance is loss of the septal Q wave on the electrocardiogram (ECG).[32] The effect of left bundle branch block on the overall time course of left ventricular contraction is to increase it by 100–150 ms. The ejection time itself is unaffected, but both contraction and relaxation times are in-

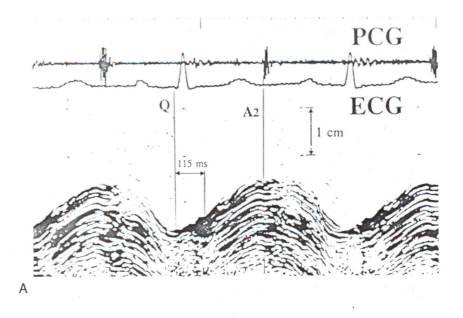

A

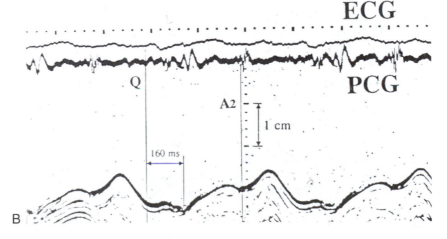

Fig. 25-4. Effect of intermittent left bundle branch block on left ventricular long axis function. **(A)** Normal activation. **(B)** Left bundle branch block. Note that with normal activation the peak shortening corresponds with the second sound. With left bundle branch block the onset of systolic shortening is delayed 115–160 ms after the Q wave of the ECG, and that striking further shortening (5 mm) occurs after the second sound.

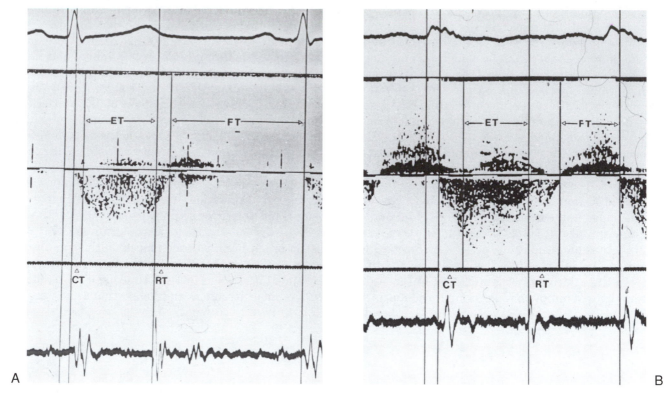

Fig. 25-5. Effect of ventricular activation sequence on the time course of functional mitral regurgitation in dilated cardiomyopathy. **(A)** Normal activation. **(B)** Left bundle branch block. Note that contraction and relaxation times are greatly prolonged with left bundle branch block compared to normal. CT, contraction time from the onset of mitral regurgitation to that of ejection; RT, relaxation time, from end-ejection (A2) to the end of regurgitation; ET, ejection time; FT, filling time.

creased by approximately equal amounts (50–75 ms), with a corresponding drop in peak rates of pressure change (Fig. 25-5).[33] Thus the regional asynchrony demonstrated by M-mode studies is reflected in major changes in overall function.

Regional disturbances within the myocardium during isovolumic relaxation are often accompanied by detectable flow within the left ventricular cavity. Two distinct patterns are seen. The first, which is directed from base to apex, is associated with a small end-systolic cavity size and occurs in normal subjects as well as patients with left ventricular hypertrophy[34] (Fig. 25-6). It starts during late ejection, usually reaches its peak at or close to aortic valve closure, and then decelerates throughout the period of isovolumic relaxation. It can be demonstrated by pulsed-wave or color M-mode echocardiography. The second type, directed from apex to base, is much commoner in coronary artery disease and is a sign of major regional asynchrony.[35] Acceleration and deceleration phases both occur during isovolumic relaxation. Peak velocities are in the range of 40–60 cm/s, and a column length of 3–4 cm is often involved, so

the calculated pressure drop along the column of blood may be in excess of 10 mmHg.

Significance of Abnormalities of Isovolumic Relaxation

The extent to which abnormalities of isovolumic relaxation are mechanisms rather than markers of disease is still not clear. Most do not arise primarily during isovolumic relaxation but are the result of disturbances earlier in the cardiac cycle on the left or possibly in the right ventricle. Their interpretation, and if appropriate their treatment, should therefore be based on defining the primary abnormality, not its secondary effects during relaxation. The significance of normal reversal in myocardial torsion and shear during this period is still unclear; they may be associated either with facilitating a rapid fall in ventricular pressure or in maintaining cavity dimensions constant as myocardial properties are rapidly changing. An abnormally short isovolumic relaxation time strongly suggests an elevated left atrial pressure (Fig. 25-7). Incoordinate wall motion during

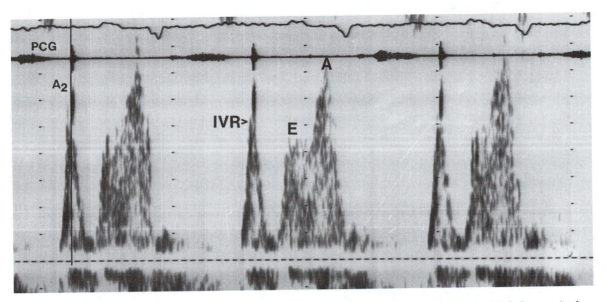

Fig. 25-6. Pulsed-wave Doppler recording of intraventricular flow (IVR) in a patient with left ventricular hypertrophy. Note that the flow signal starts before A2 and decelerates during isovolumic relaxation. This phase is followed by normal E and A waves. A2, aortic component of the second heart sound. Velocity calibration = 10 cm/s.

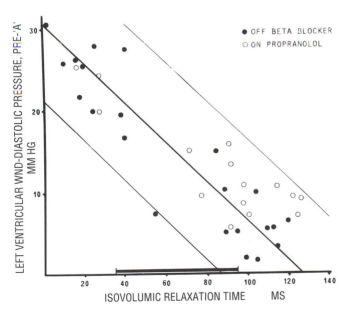

Fig. 25-7. Relation between left ventricular end-diastolic pressure and isovolumic relaxation time (A2 to mitral cusp separation) in a group of patients with coronary artery disease. The 95 percent confidence limits of normal (35–95 ms) are indicated. Note that in individuals when the isovolumic relaxation time is abnormally short, the end-diastolic pressure is always elevated. Conversely, when end-diastolic pressure is normal, the isovolumic relaxation time is often increased.

isovolumic relaxation leads to practical problems when defining end-systole. The timing of the onset of diastole may differ by up to 100 ms in different regions of the myocardium. Analysis of regional wall motion, based on comparison of "end-diastolic" and "end-systolic" cavity outlines, is ambiguous in approximately half of patients with clinically significant coronary artery disease, with corresponding effects on the apparent pattern of regional wall motion displayed by this technique.[36] In the same way, the presence of intracavitary flow clearly demonstrates that pressure gradients can exist within the ventricular cavity during isovolumic relaxation, so pressure measured at a single point with a micromanometer is not necessarily unique. This is particularly the case when relaxation is asynchronous. Regional wall motion and associated changes in wall thickness during isovolumic relaxation fundamentally affect the relation between wall stress and cavity pressure. When they occur, therefore, it can no longer be assumed that the time course of changes in wall stress can be derived from changes in pressure.

Normal rapid filling depends critically on the mechanisms of isovolumic relaxation being intact. With left ventricular hypertrophy, coronary artery disease, and disturbances of ventricular activation, prolongation of isovolumic relaxation correlates strongly with a reduction in peak early diastolic filling velocity.[37] The extent to which these resting abnormalities correlate with impairment of exercise tolerance has been little studied.

Measurements of the isovolumic relaxation time may thus be useful when analyzing disturbances in patients with diastolic heart failure. An abnormally short time indicates an elevated left atrial pressure, itself documented as being associated with reduced exercise tolerance.[38,39] Abnormal prolongation of the isovolumic relaxation time represents a wasted period in the cardiac cycle when the ventricle is neither ejecting or filling. In patients with left ventricular hypertrophy and prolonged resting isovolumic relaxation time, as the RR interval decreases with exercise the isovolumic relaxation time becomes abnormally short, again suggesting elevation of left atrial pressure. Conversely, intracoronary infusion of nitroprusside in patients without heart disease hastens the onset of relaxation by approximately 20 ms without significantly altering T.[40] In those with left ventricular hypertrophy, intracoronary enalaprilat reduces the time constant of the pressure fall.[41] Additional studies are needed to determine how relaxation disturbances that are present at rest are modified during exercise and if these drug effects contribute in any way to the improved effort tolerance demonstrated in clinical trials.

RAPID VENTRICULAR FILLING

Volume Changes

The first direct measurement of ventricular volume changes during early diastole were made by contrast angiography, the cavity size being estimated on successive frames. Hammermeister and Warbasse[42] confirmed that the pattern of filling in humans was similar to that described experimentally more than half a century earlier by Henderson et al.[43] The peak rate of inflow occurs early during diastole, reaching a peak value of 500–700 ml/s (Fig. 25-8). The corresponding values normalized to end-diastolic volume (measured by radionuclide angiography) are 3.1–3.3/s in the young, falling to 2.5/s1 or less in the elderly.[2] The filling rate is greatly increased on exercise.[44] The peak filling rate occurs 150–170 ms after the time of minimum counts from the nuclear time–activity curve; the corresponding interval determined angiographically from mitral valve opening to peak rate is less, at 60 ms.[45] The difference probably reflects the uncertain relation between the time of minimum counts and mitral valve opening. The filling fraction, the proportion of the stroke volume to enter the ventricle during the first third of diastole, has a mean value of 47 ± 15 percent at rest.[46]

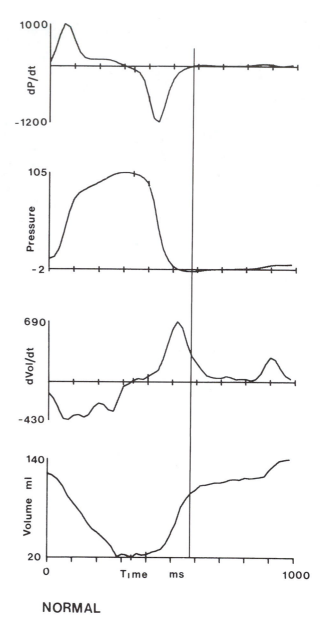

NORMAL

Fig. 25-8. Normal changes in left ventricular pressure and volume as assessed by contrast angiography. From the top: rate of change of ventricular pressure, ventricular pressure, rate of change of volume, and ventricular cavity volume. Vertical line represents the time of minimum left ventricular diastolic pressure.

Ventricular Inflow Velocity

Blood velocity during ventricular filling can readily be measured by pulsed-wave Doppler studies from the apex, with the sample volume at the level of the tips of the mitral leaflets. A flow signal is first detectable at this level of the inflow tract 20–30 ms after the mitral leaflets separate (Fig. 25-9). Peak early diastolic (E wave) filling velocity in young adults is in the range of 80–100 cm/s, falling with age.[47] The

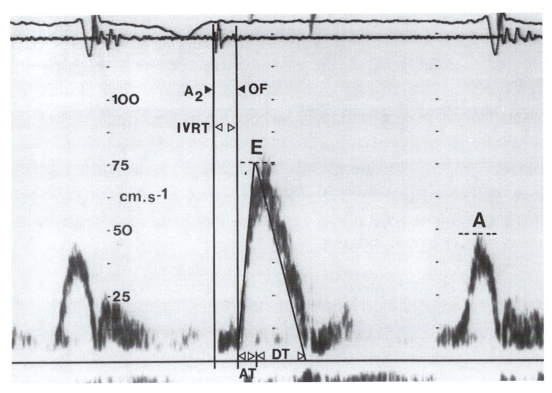

Fig. 25-9. Normal transmitral flow velocities measured by pulsed-wave Doppler echocardiography, showing early diastolic (E) and atrial (A) waves. The interval from aortic valve closure (A2) on the phonocardiogram to the onset of filling (OF) represents the Doppler-isovolumic relaxation time (IVRT). The interval from the onset of flow to peak velocity represents the acceleration time (AT) and from the peak until the end of the E wave the deceleration time (DT).

peak value occurs 100–150 ms after the onset of flow, the interval being referred to as the acceleration time. The corresponding value, from the time of peak velocity to the end of the E wave, extrapolated to zero if necessary, is referred to as the deceleration time and is normally in the range of 150–250 ms.

When the heart rate is slow, the form of the flow velocity trace is similar to that of the rate of volume increase. After the E wave, inflow velocities are low during diastasis, until the onset of atrial systole (A wave) (Fig. 25-9). Peak atrial velocity is normally in the range of one-half to two-thirds that of the E wave, although this value increases with advancing age. Doppler inflow records are quantified by measuring either the peak E and A wave velocities or the corresponding time integrals. This exercise usually presents no problem when the heart rate is low. However, with increasing tachycardia diastasis shortens, and the A wave becomes superimposed on the declining E wave, increasing its apparent amplitude. This situation leads to ambiguity when assessing atrial activity by Doppler echocardiography.[48] The usual practice is to measure A wave amplitude with respect to the baseline of zero velocity, regardless of its relation to the E wave. However, because atrial activity

is best defined as the difference between the flow velocity curve in its presence and its absence, it seems more logical to use the extrapolated termination of the E wave as the baseline for measuring A wave height and the flow velocity integral. The difference is an important one, as measurement above zero flow suggests that left atrial activity increases with increasing heart rate, whereas measurement above the extrapolated E wave does not. As long as the question remains unsettled, the method used in individual studies should be explicitly stated.

The relation between instantaneous atrioventricular pressure difference and flow has been widely studied in the literature. Blood, like any other matter, moves because it is acted on by a force. Newton's second law of motion states that the rate of change of velocity (i.e., the acceleration) is proportional to the impressed force and takes place in the direction in which it acts. In a fluid a force is expressed as a pressure gradient with the physical dimensions of millimeters of mercury per centimeter. It should be noted that the term "gradient" is commonly used by cardiologists to express what is more properly termed a "difference," as it does not take any account of the distance between the two points at which measurements are made. Acceleration of 1g requires a pressure gradient of somewhat less than 1 mmHg/cm along the direction of flow. The velocity (V) at any instant is given by the product of acceleration (a) and the time over which it has acted (t) (V = at). Peak blood flow velocity therefore depends not only on the pressure gradient but on the time over which the pressure gradient has acted. Conditions during normal early diastolic filling are complex, as the pressure gradient itself varies continuously as atrial and ventricular pressures approach one another. Furthermore, at any instant there may also be spatial variation, which constitutes a pressure field. It is thus an oversimplification to speak of a unique "atrial" or "ventricular" pressure during this period. During early diastole blood accelerates from the base toward the apex of the ventricle, which implies that the pressure at the base must be higher than that at the apex. If the pressure were uniform throughout the ventricle, flow would not occur. Such pressure differences have been detected experimentally using double microtip catheters and are of the order of 2–3 mmHg when the sensors are separated by 2 cm.[49]

These considerations stress how incomplete are single pressure measurements as evidence of loading conditions during periods of rapid changes in blood velocity. Peak blood velocity is not uniquely determined by the difference between single pressures determined within the atrium and ventricle from micromanometers placed an unspecified vertical and horizontal distance apart. It is even less satisfactory to rely on a single pressure, such as that in the atrium or wedge, or to invoke some "driving pressure" corresponding to that in the ventricle at the time of presumed mitral valve opening. An alternative approach is to invert the problem and use the blood itself as an accelerometer. Local velocities and accelerations plus the column length can be measured by pulsed-wave Doppler studies or MRI; and hence local pressure gradients can be estimated. Changes in the pattern of left ventricular inflow are frequently used as evidence of diastolic ventricular disease. However, as in normal individuals, blood flow from atrium to ventricle still depends only on the forces acting on it and thus on the pressure field. Diastolic disease does not directly affect filling velocities—only indirectly by modifying atrioventricular pressure gradients.

Left Ventricular Wall Motion During Filling

The normal left ventricular cavity becomes more spherical as it fills. This change allows the incoming stroke volume to be accommodated with less myocardial distension; its loss would cause cavity stiffness

to increase even in the absence of any change in the properties of the myocardium itself. Cavity shape changes almost exclusively during early rapid filling and remains constant for the remainder of diastole, including atrial systole. It is brought about by a greater proportional increase in the minor axis during systole (25–40 percent) compared to that in the longitudinal axis (10–15 percent).

The mechanisms by which the two dimensions change are also different. The long axis runs from the fibrous apex to the fibrous skeleton at the base of the heart, so it increases simply because longitudinally directed fibers lengthen.[50] These fibers are situated in the subendocardial and subepicardial regions of the left ventricular wall and include the papillary muscles. Minor axis shortening depends largely on thickening of the free ventricular wall, and its extent (25–40 percent) is much greater than that of a normal sarcomere. Free wall thickening depends on shortening of the long axis and of circumferentially arranged fibers. The same must therefore apply to minor axis lengthening during diastole, which is again the result of coordinate longitudinal and circumferential shortening.[51] Measurements in humans by directed M-mode echocardiography correspond closely to those obtained from implanted ultrasonic crystals in experimental animals.

Wall Thickness Changes

Left ventricular wall thickness was first estimated in vivo in humans by contrast angiography as the distance between the epicardial border of the heart shadow and the outer edge of the ventricular cavity opacified by dye. This method is subject to error, and much more satisfactory estimates can be obtained by echocardiography or MRI, which allow myocardium and pericardium to be distinguished. Wall thickness increases during isovolumic relaxation by 1–2 mm, reaching its maximum value at the time of mitral valve opening.[52] The early diastolic thinning rate is high, approximately 11 ± 2 cm/s, a value considerably greater than the rate of increase of wall thickness during ejection. This period of rapid thinning ends at approximately the same time as the period of rapid filling. The septum does not show rapid thinning, whereas in the free wall its extent and velocity are both maximum at midcavity level. Thickness does not change at all during atrial systole.

Pressure Changes During Rapid Filling

Left ventricular filling is assumed to begin at the time the left ventricular pressure falls below that in the left atrium (i.e., at the time of pressure crossover).[53] This analysis is based on the idea of unique atrial and ventricular pressures, which cannot be assumed to apply. Pressure crossover represents the onset of a force directed from atrium to ventricle. It can therefore be timed precisely from the onset of diastolic blood flow. It can readily be measured by color M-mode echocardiography and has been shown to propagate into the ventricle with a normal velocity of 100 cm/s.

The greater part of early diastolic filling of the left ventricle occurs as ventricular pressure is falling[54] (Fig. 25-9). Even at rest this component accounts for 55 ± 16 percent of the stroke volume, and on exercise this proportion is much higher. Extrapolation of the exponential of pressure decline suggests that even in normal individuals significant myocardial tension may still be present during early filling. The phenomenon has been termed incomplete relaxation. In open chest dogs, it can be detected for a period of three times T after minimum peak dp/dt. Incomplete relaxation has not been definitively identified in normal humans. Related to incomplete relaxation is the idea of diastolic tone, which refers to sustained active tension developed by myofibrils, rather than simple slowing of relaxation.[55]

Ventricular pressure negative to atmospheric pressure early during diastole is referred to as ventricular suction.[56] Strikingly negative ventricular pressures can be demonstrated experimentally when ventricular inflow is occluded: Nikolic et al.[57] reported values as low as -18 mmHg for normal beats and -25 mmHg for postextrasystolic beats. Subatmospheric values have been reported in humans at the time of balloon inflation during the course of mitral valvoplasty and to a lesser extent with uncorrected mitral stenosis.[58] Diastolic suction cannot be demonstrated when inflow is unrestricted. The zero for diastolic pressure measurement is not well defined, as there is much evidence to suggest that physiologic tissue pressure is negative to atmospheric pressure. Diastolic suction arises when muscle fibers are shortened by active tension during systole to less than an equilibrium length, determined probably by their connective tissue matrix. When the active state has declined, therefore, compressive forces are stored within the myocardium, which have the effect of restoring it to its equilibrium length.[59] The smaller the end-systolic volume, the greater are the restoring forces. The more completely the ventricle empties, therefore, whether from increased contractility or reduced peripheral resistance, the greater is their effect on early diastolic inflow. Forces are vectorial quantities and thus have direction as well as magnitude. Restoring forces need not be directed parallel to the ventricular long axis. Indeed, using pulsed-wave Doppler mapping, the pressure differences needed to explain normal early diastolic filling can be reconstructed from the observed acceleration of blood passing into the ventricle. In normal humans the total pressure drop is only 2–3 mmHg, which does not suggest a major effect of such axial restoring forces. A high volume filling rate with a low atrioventricular pressure difference is achieved when the column of blood entering the ventricle is short, with a large cross-sectional area.[60] The rapid disappearance of blood from the jet as it passes into the ventricle suggests that if restoring forces do have a role in normal subjects they may act in a direction perpendicular to transmitral flow (i.e., parallel to the ventricular minor axis). It is possible that restoring forces are closely related to rapid thinning of the myocardium during early diastole. This process is normally tightly coupled to rapid filling of the ventricle; but if relaxation is incoordinate, they may become dissociated so that rapid thinning is complete before filling starts (Fig. 25-10). The extent of rapid thinning varies topographically within the ventricle: It is most obvious along the free wall at midcavity level and is not shown by the septum at all. Although it is possible that loss of restoring forces may lead to disturbed early diastolic filling, this possibility has yet to be proved.

Left Ventricular Filling Time

At normal resting heart rates the left ventricular filling time may account for considerably more than half the total cardiac cycle. However, as the heart rate increases, this proportion rapidly falls because the relative duration of systole is maintained at the expense of diastole. Ventricular filling time, measured as the time the mitral valve is open, falls with increasing heart rate, reaching a plateau of 90–100 ms at a heart rate of 160/bpm in normal subjects aged 20–30 years[61] (Fig. 25-11). With a stroke volume of 100 ml, this implies a mean filling rate of 1 L/s. Mechanisms underlying normal rapid filling during exercise have not been studied in detail. The end-systolic cavity size is likely to decrease owing to the positive inotropic effect of catecholamines and decreased peripheral resistance. This state, in turn, increases the restoring forces; and the atrioventricular pressure drops even in the absence of an increase in left atrial pressure.

ABNORMAL LEFT VENTRICULAR FILLING

Left Ventricular Hypertrophy

The pattern of left ventricular filling may be abnormal in patients with left ventricular hypertrophy, whether primary or secondary,[62–64] even though sys-

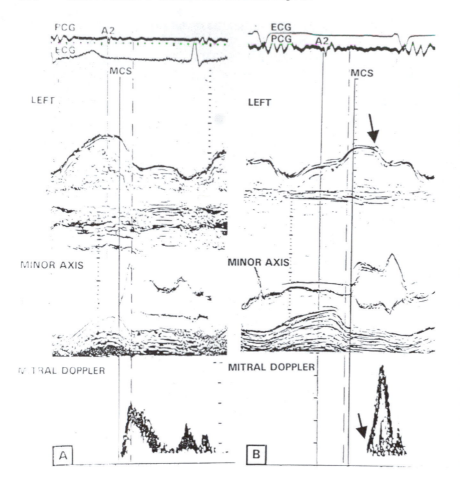

Fig. 25-10. Composite M-mode and Doppler display of the effects of incoordinate relaxation on left ventricular filling pattern. **(Left panel)** Normal. **(Right panel)** Incoordinate relaxation right. From the top: ECG, phonocardiogram, LV long-axis M-mode echocardiogram; LV minor-axis M-mode echocardiogram with mitral valve cusps, and transmitral Doppler recording. *Solid vertical lines* represent A2 and mitral cusp separation; *dotted vertical line* represents the end of rapid posterior LV wall thinning. Note that in the normal pattern the E wave is inscribed during the period of posterior left ventricular wall thinning, and that mitral cusp separation precedes the onset of transmitral flow by 20–30 ms. Note also that when relaxation is incoordinate there is striking shortening of the long axis after A2, and that during this period there is no detectable flow across the mitral valve, although the transverse ventricular dimension increases and the mitral valve cusps separate. In fact, ventricular filling occurs only with left atrial systole.

tolic function appears well preserved. This pattern was originally suspected from the presence of a slow *y* descent on the left atrial pressure trace and a reduced closure rate of the mitral valve as shown on M-mode echocardiography. Both these measurements are multifactorial, however, and neither is now considered to give a valid estimate of the ventricular filling rate.

A reduced peak filing rate was found in a small number of cases studied angiographically; but a larger series subsequently showed that the mean filling rate was normal, although the scatter was increased. Peak filling rate correlates negatively with isovolumic relaxation time, so that when isovolumic relaxation time is prolonged the filling rate is low. Nuclear angiography has confirmed these findings and has demonstrated an increase in the time to peak filling along with a reduction in filling fraction.[65]

On pulsed-wave Doppler echocardiography, the commonest disturbance seen with left ventricular hypertrophy is a reduced early diastolic velocity with an increase in that during atrial systole, so the E/A ratio falls.[66] Wide scatter is seen, however, so that in some patients, particularly young ones, the pattern of mitral flow velocity may be normal and in others the atrial velocities low or absent altogether.

M-mode echocardiography shows a similar spread of values.

The peak rates of increase of the transverse dimension and posterior wall thinning are usually reduced. Incoordinate wall motion during isovolumic relaxation can be detected in approximately half of all patients with severe hypertrophy, primary or secondary.[63] Diastolic disturbances may become functionally significant on exercise, as a short filling time cannot be achieved in patients with left ventricular hypertrophy when the heart rate is rapid. Instead, the minimum value reached is 200 ms, double the normal value, which occurs at the expense of abbreviating both ejection and isovolumic relaxation times.[61]

A similar reduction in resting peak left ventricular filling rate occurs in the absence of hypertrophy and is seen in diabetics, particularly those with microvascular complications.[67] These changes also occur in a variety of connective tissue disorders, such as ankylosing spondylitis and psoriatic arthropathy.[68] The effects of coronary artery disease, diabetes, and hypertrophy are additive, so in combination they give rise to particularly severe diastolic dysfunction. This situation is a common basis for diastolic heart failure.

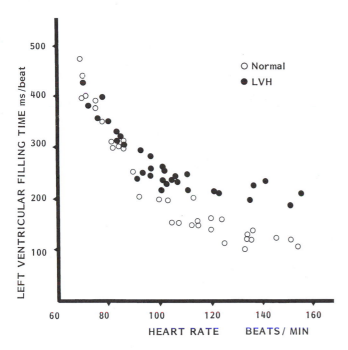

Fig. 25-11. Relation between left ventricular filling time and heart rate in normal subjects *(closed symbols)* and patients with left ventricular hypertrophy *(open symbols)*. Note that in normals the filling time decreases to 100 ms with increasing heart rate, but that in patients it does not fall below 200 ms. (From Oldershaw et al.,[61] with permission.)

Dilated Cardiomyopathy

The left ventricular filling pattern is highly variable in dilated cardiomyopathy, whether idiopathic or ischemic. The early diastolic E wave is often dominant, so the record is indistinguishable from normal, particularly when the filling pressure is high.[5] It is associated with a normal or short isovolumic relaxation time, functional mitral regurgitation, and a third heart sound, whose onset coincides with the timing of the peak E wave velocity.[69] Because it is widely assumed that left ventricular diastolic function can be assessed from the Doppler transmitral flow velocity pattern, the combination of normal E and A waves with what is evidently an abnormal ventricle is reconciled only by the unsatisfactory expedient of referring to such a filling pattern as "pseudonormalized." Early diastolic filling may become so preponderant that no A wave is apparent at all, suggesting that the ventricle is effectively not distensible at end-diastole. Alternatively, ventricular filling may occur entirely during atrial systole.[70] This pattern is associated with low or normal left atrial pressures and a prolonged isovolumic relaxation time. It is characteristically seen during treatment with an ACE inhibitor. Finally, with sinus tachycardia the resting filling time may be so short that only a single filling peak is seen consisting of superimposed E and A waves, often accompanied by a summation gallop sound (Fig. 25-12). Such patients frequently have advanced disturbances of activation with a greatly increased QRS duration, associated with prolongation of functional mitral regurgitation to 600 ms or more.[71] Because this duration is effectively fixed, the filling time is reduced to 200 ms or less when the heart rate is only 80 bpm.

Restrictive Cardiomyopathy

"Restrictive cardiomyopathy" covers an ill-defined group of disorders in which filling is limited by increased ventricular stiffness during mid and late diastole. Amyloid infiltration is present in about half of these cases[72]; it is uncommon to identify a clear cause in the remainder. Peak inflow velocity during early diastole is often normal, but its duration is short, so acceleration and deceleration times are reduced, reflecting the combined effects of increased myocardial stiffness and a high left atrial pressure.[73] Blood flow acceleration and deceleration rates are therefore increased, implying a corresponding increase in early diastolic pressure gradients. A third sound is thus common. Restrictive filling does not therefore represent a specific diagnosis, as patients with dilated cardiomyopathy or severe hypertrophy may show restrictive features. Regardless of the underlying etiology, these features regress when the left atrial pressure falls. A restrictive filling pattern should therefore be regarded the result of a combination of diastolic disease and a high filling pressure.

Coronary Artery Disease

Rapid ventricular filling may be abnormal during acute ischemia or chronic coronary artery disease. Angina—whether induced by increased oxygen demand with atrial pacing or by reduced delivery, as during balloon angioplasty—characteristically prolongs the time constant of left ventricular fall.[74,75] Changes in filling velocity and the E/A ratio are inconsistent and depend on the balance between the rate and coordination of tension decline and loading conditions. A similar variable diastolic response is seen after acute myocardial infarction, with strikingly incoordinate wall motion, a high filling pressure, and no consistent change in ventricular filling pattern.[27]

Similar variability is seen with chronic coronary artery disease. Early diastolic filling rates are fre-

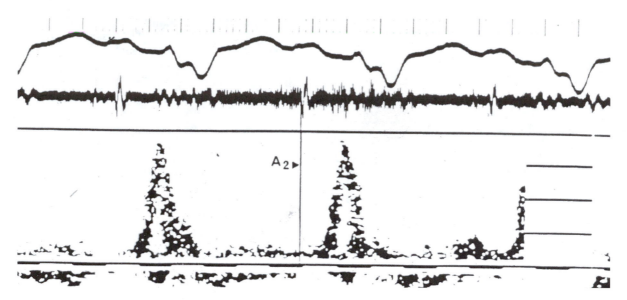

Fig. 25-12. Pulsed-wave Doppler trace of a summation filling pattern from a patient with dilated cardiomyopathy and functional mitral regurgitation. Note that the normal E and A waves are lost, and that total filling time is reduced to 130 ms. Calibration: time markers 100 ms, vertical 1 KHz frequency shift.

quently low, whether expressed in absolute units or normalized to end-diastolic volume.[54,76,77] At the same time, the early diastolic period of rapid filling may be prolonged, so diastasis is shortened or lost. The filling fraction is thus reduced; and on radionuclide angiography, the time interval from minimum counts to peak inflow rate is increased. A reduced filling rate correlates most closely with prolongation and incoordination during isovolumic relaxation. The incidence of such abnormalities, whether at rest or during exercise, is too low to make them reliable noninvasive markers for the diagnosis in individual cases. Coronary artery disease and hypertension can coexist in individuals and have additive effects on the increase in left atrial pressure that occurs with exercise.[78]

MECHANISMS AND CLINICAL SIGNIFICANCE OF RAPID FILLING

Ventricular diastolic disease does not influence rapid filling directly but only insofar as it modifies atrio-ventricular pressure gradients. Because these pressure gradients vary continuously throughout the period of filling and show spatial variation along the left ventricular inflow tract, their definition in intact humans remains a technical challenge. It is still not possible therefore to dissociate the effects of ventricular disease from those of abnormal loading conditions. Nevertheless, a number of processes can be recognized. Events during isovolumic relaxation con-

sistently influence rapid filling. If isovolumic relaxation is prolonged or there is significant incoordination during this period, the early diastolic filling velocity is reduced and the deceleration time prolonged. Characteristic relations are shown in Figure 25-13. The effects of age are similar: The isovolumic

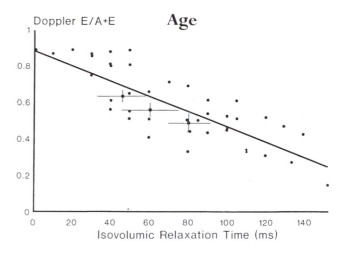

Fig. 25-13. Relation between isovolumic relaxation time (A2 to mitral cusp separation) and transmitral Doppler filling pattern, expressed as E/(A + E). Individual points represent values from patients with dilated cardiomyopathy. The shorter the duration of isovolumic relaxation time, the more prominent is the E wave. The three populations (mean and 1 standard deviation) represent normals with mean ages of 21, 40, and 65 years. As age increases, the isovolumic relaxation time increases and the E wave becomes less prominent. Note that this relation is effectively the same for patients and normals.

relaxation time increases as the E wave velocity falls. The combination of the duration of isovolumic relaxation time and the extent of incoordinate wall motion during this period accounts for most of the variance in the E/A ratio. If both are normal, the E wave velocity is also normal, regardless of whether ventricular disease is present. The left ventricular isovolumic relaxation time itself is multifactorial and strongly affected by events during activation and systole; it is also subject to potential interference from the right ventricle. Exactly the same considerations therefore apply to early diastolic filling velocity, where the effects are superimposed on those of loading conditions and primary diastolic disease. Clearly, therefore, the diastolic filling pattern cannot be used to give information about any one of these factors unless the effects of the remainder have either been eliminated or allowed for. It is thus unfortunate that a large literature has accumulated suggesting that diastolic disease can be confirmed or excluded on the basis of measurements of filling pattern alone.

Ventricular Long Axis

Motion of the left ventricular long axis and pulmonary venous flow, to which it is closely related, give further information that is useful for interpreting alterations in rapid filling.[79] Motion of the mitral ring toward the apex during ventricular systole results in external work being done on the left atrium, increasing its capacity. It is this movement that is responsible for the normal x descent on the atrial pressure pulse and for blood flow from the pulmonary veins into the left atrium during ventricular systole. During early diastole the ring moves backward toward the atrium at a time when blood is accelerating from atrium to ventricle as the result of a positive atrioventricular pressure gradient. This backward ring motion cannot therefore be passive and is likely to be the result of elastic forces in the atrial wall stored from the previous ventricular systole. It thus represents a ventricular restoring force whose anatomic basis is outside the ventricle. Finally, as the result of ring motion, blood that was within the atrium at the start of early diastole finds itself within the ventricle during diastasis. The same events recur during atrial systole. Together this effect of the ring moving around the blood accounts for 10–15 percent of the stroke volume on the left side of the heart and more than 20 percent on the right. Because the blood does not move with respect to a transducer on the chest wall or esophagus, it is not detected by Doppler echocardiography. These long axis interactions thus have major effects on blood flow from the pulmonary veins

and on the pressure–volume relations of the atrium, so their loss might be expected to have significant effects on ventricular filling.

Long axis function is frequently disturbed in patients with left ventricular disease. With restrictive physiology the systolic shortening amplitude is characteristically reduced, even though the cavity size is normal.[80] Free wall thickening is thus depressed and fractional shortening low. During early diastole the onset of long axis lengthening is delayed, whereas a high left atrial pressure causes ventricular filling to start early, before the onset of long axis relaxation. This effect and the impaired ventricular shape changes resulting from reduced minor axis shortening and reduced systolic interaction between the long axis and the left atrium are all likely to impair early diastolic function independent of the passive elastic properties of the myocardium itself. In patients with uncomplicated left ventricular hypertrophy, peak early diastolic long axis lengthening rates are characteristically reduced. More significantly, long axis function, being subtended by subendocardial muscle fibers, is particularly likely to become incoordinate with ventricular disease of any sort. Persistent long axis shortening during isovolumic relaxation, whether due to ischemia or abnormal activation, combines with an increase in the minor axis to change the cavity shape even though the volume remains constant. Abnormal long axis shortening may persist until the onset of atrial systole, suppressing early diastolic filling altogether. An example of these highly disturbed interrelations is given in Figure 25-10.[70] These findings are characteristic of patients in whom the filling pressure is low.

Pulmonary Venous Flow

The pulmonary venous flow pulse has three components. Forward flow occurs during ventricular systole and during early diastole when it is synchronous with rapid filling of the ventricle; whereas back wave flow may be detected during atrial systole. Pulmonary venous flow is multifactorial. It is sensitive to pericardial and pleural pressures and to the pressure in the left atrium.[81,82]

Changes in atrial dynamics resulting from altered ventricular diastolic function and long axis changes are also likely to be important. Nevertheless, useful information has been obtained. When ventricular end-diastolic compliance is reduced, the deceleration time of the early diastolic component of pulmonary flow parallels that of the transmitral E wave. Semiquantitative estimates of left atrial pressure can be obtained from the time integral of the systolic component, normalized for heart rate. The extent to which these changes reflect atrial pressure as distinct from ventricular systolic function, to which it is likely to be closely related, has yet to be determined. Pulmonary venous flow is clearly one step removed from ventricular diastolic function, so it seems useful to consider it in association with atrioventricular ring motion, which has a major effect on the properties of the atria.

Relation of Disturbed Rapid Filling to Diastolic Heart Failure

Abnormalities of rapid filling, such as an isolated E wave or a reduced deceleration time, are excellent markers of an elevated left atrial pressure or a restrictive ventricular filling pattern and thus make a positive contribution to the diagnosis of diastolic heart failure. A strong inverse correlation between the mean left atrial pressure and exercise tolerance as assessed by maximal oxygen consumption has been demonstrated. In addition, the E/A ration also correlates negatively with exercise tolerance. Conversely, increasing prominence of the A wave is compatible with an adequate response to treatment. In a patient with abnormal ventricular relaxation and a dominant A wave, the loss of atrial function due to the onset of atrial fibrillation causes prompt reversion to early diastolic filling. Relaxation abnormalities are overridden, but only at the expense of a high left atrial pressure. A short left ventricular filling time in patients with dilated cardiomyopathy as the result of disturbed activation prolonging systole is also likely to limit stroke volume. In such cases, simple right ventricular pacing consistently shortens the duration of the functional mitral regurgitation and increases the filling time at a constant heart rate. This situation has been confirmed by the consistent improvement in exercise tolerance and maximal oxygen consumption, both short and long term, brought about by pacing.[83]

The prognosis may be associated with an early diastolic filling pattern. In patients with dilated cardiomyopathy, a dominant E wave has been found to be a marker of poor prognosis in some[84,85] but not all[39] studies. The same applies to the presence of a third heart sound, which is likely to be associated with dominant early (E wave) rather than later (A wave) filling. The variability of the filling pattern with loading conditions and, in particular, with treatment, seems to limit its value as a marker of prognosis. It is not certain, for example, whether the reversal of the E/A ratio induced by treatment with an ACE inhibitor should be regarded as a confounding factor

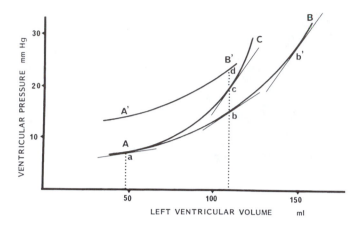

Fig. 25-14. Pressure–volume relation in humans. *AB* represents a normal passive pressure–volume curve, and *AC* is that from a ventricle with increased stiffness. *A'B'* represents the effect of upward displacement of *AB*. The slopes of the pressure–volume curves (i.e., stiffness values) are shown as the tangents at *a, b, b'* and *c*.

or if it directly reflects, and perhaps even quantifies, the known improvement in exercise tolerance and prognosis brought about by these agents. Intraventricular conduction delay prolongs the isovolumic relaxation time and reduces E wave amplitude, even though it is a major marker of poor prognosis.[86] This point illustrates the multifactorial basis of diastolic filling patterns and thus their limitations as indices of prognosis in individual patients.

PASSIVE VENTRICULAR STIFFNESS

Ventricular Chamber Stiffness

The period of passive ventricular stiffness is that during which pressure and volume increase together. It starts from the time of minimum ventricular pressure, usually after that of peak inflow blood flow velocity, and ends with the onset of atrial systole. When the heart rate is slow, only 10–20 percent of the total stroke volume enters the ventricle during this time and even less does so during exercise. If pressure and volume do increase together, the slope of the pressure–volume curve represents the stiffness of the ventricle. Stiffness is given by the ratio dP/dV, where P is cavity pressure and V is cavity volume. It thus represents the pressure increase that occurs with unit increase in volume and has the physical dimensions of millimeters of mercury per cubic centimeter (Fig. 25-14). The reciprocal of stiffness, dV/dP, is referred to as compliance.[87] These definitions mean that the relative values of stiffness for two ventricles are proportional to their volumes; this effect can be allowed for by considering not an absolute but a relative increment in volume, dV/V, defining volume stiffness as V·dP/dV, and volume compliance as 1/V·dV/dP.

The normal left ventricular pressure curve is not linear but becomes steeper (i.e., cavity stiffness increases) as filling proceeds. This change is reflected in a corresponding increase in slope at any point. In the normal subject there is often an approximately linear relation between cavity pressure and dP/dV, whose slope is referred to as the stiffness constant, with the physical dimensions of cubic centimeters. A linear relation between pressure and stiffness implies an exponential relation between pressure and volume of the form:

$$P = ke^a + b$$

where a corresponds to the stiffness constant, and b and k are empiric constants. There is no theoretic reason why the pressure–volume curve should be exponential. In many patients, particularly those with ventricular disease, it clearly is not. In one series, even the undemanding criterion that stiffness should increase continuously even if not linearly, with pressure was met in only one-fourth of subjects.[88] A logarithmic curve may give a better fit than an exponential curve in normal subjects but not consistently so in those with disease. Any continuous curve can, of course, be fitted to any required degree of precision with a polynomial of high enough order. This approach has also been applied to the pressure–volume curve, but no physical significance can be attached to the coefficients of the various power terms.

Because stiffness varies throughout diastole, the pressure or the time during the cardiac cycle that a measurement is made must be specified. To do so it is necessary to know the unstressed volume (i.e., the volume at zero transmural pressure). This parameter cannot be determined in the beating heart. The stiffness constant, whose existence depends on assuming an exponential pressure–volume relation, cannot be a direct measure of stiffness, either from its derivation or from its units (cm^3). Rather, it states how cavity stiffness depends on pressure. A ventricle in which pressure and volume are linearly related (i.e., one that obeys Hooke's law) would have a stiffness constant of zero, however steep the pressure–volume relation itself. The physical significance of measurements of cavity stiffness is thus not clear, although they have been widely undertaken in the past. Their scatter is wide, with considerable overlap between normal and abnormal ventricles.[89,90]

Possible relations between cavity stiffness and end-diastolic pressure are summarized in Figure 25-

14. The normal pressure volume curve is represented by AB. The stiffness at any point (e.g., a or b) is represented by the tangent at that point. Clearly the stiffness is greater at b than at a. The curve AC is that of a ventricle with a higher stiffness constant than AB. Though the stiffness at a is the same for both, that at c, although at the same volume, is higher than at b. However, if the volume of ventricle AB were to be increased (e.g., by a fluid load), the stiffness would increase to the value at b′, which is similar to that at c. Below A, the stiffness of the ventricle represented by AB at any given volume is greater than that represented by AC, although its stiffness constant is less. Clearly, therefore, the stiffness constant is not a measure of stiffness.

With ischemia, the curve AB may be displaced upward to that represented by A′B′[91,92] (Fig. 25-15). The reverse may occur with acute administration of vasodilators[93] or a β-blocker.[94] This process is referred to, as parallel shift, or less happily, as a change in ventricular distensibility. Despite the elevation of ventricular diastolic pressure at any given volume, the slope of the curve (i.e., its stiffness at A′ and B′) is the same as that at A and B, respectively. Whatever its mechanism, therefore, this upward parallel shift in the curve does not alter cavity stiffness. It follows that stiffness cannot be assessed from

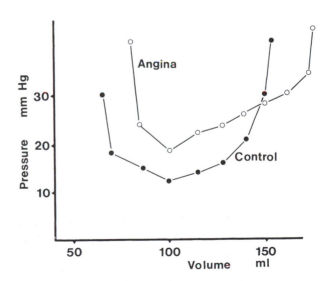

Fig. 25-15. Left ventricular pressure–volume relation in a patient with coronary artery disease, measured from simultaneous cavity pressure and contrast angiograms under control conditions and during pacing-induced angina. Note that with angina the end-systolic and end-diastolic cavity dimensions increase, and the curve itself moves upward. Its slope, representing cavity stiffness, does not change significantly.

single pairs of measurements of end-diastolic pressure and volume, as was suggested some years ago.

Clinical Importance of Abnormal Pressure–Volume Relations

Because so small a proportion of the stroke volume enters the left ventricle during the period of the cardiac cycle when passive stiffness can be measured, it might be argued that its measurement is of little clinical relevance at rest and of almost none on exercise. Certainly such measurements do not constitute a sensitive or specific marker of ventricular disease. Increased passive stiffness, however, does play a significant role in the pathophysiology of restrictive ventricular disease because, although the stroke volume may be normal or low, ventricular filling pressures are disproportionately elevated, contributing to symptoms and reflex changes. In addition, any increment in stroke volume with atrial systole is lost. A second significant area in which left ventricular diastolic pressure–volume relations may be useful for understanding human disease arises from the possibility of their upward or downward shift. These effects are large, with diastolic pressure changing by up to 10–15 mmHg at constant volume, though the ventricular filling rate, T, and pleural pressure are usually unaltered. Parallel shifts in right ventricular diastolic pressure sometimes but not always occur. The underlying mechanism remains uncertain, although disturbances in the rate or extent of relaxation have been invoked.[91] Other possibilities include pericardial restraint associated with a change in right ventricular volume.[95] The increase in diastolic distensibility that occurs with intracoronary infusion of nitroprusside[40] or enalaprilat[41] cannot be explained on this basis and suggests that intrinsic changes in left ventricular properties are possible. Although their mechanism is not clear, these shifts in the pressure–volume relation go some way to explaining therapeutically significant effects of drugs or other maneuvers on ventricular diastolic pressure in patients with disease. Paradoxically, they also provide strong evidence against considering the ventricle as a passive elastic structure at any time during diastole.

Effects of Pericardial Restraint

True transmural ventricular diastolic pressures are not usually measured in humans; some external reference point is used instead, such as midchest or atmospheric pressure. A change in pericardial pressure could therefore alter the measured ventricular pressure without altering the transmural pressure difference or the properties of the myocardium itself. The possibility thus arises that shifts in the diastolic pressure volume curve are in fact due to alterations in pericardial pressure with no change in the ventricle.[96–98] The pericardium is inextensible in the short term, so if the volume of any of its contents were to increase there would be a corresponding rise in its pressure. The right or left ventricle might be involved. Thus blood volume expansion in the dog causes upward displacement of the pressure–volume curve only when the pericardium is intact. Whether a similar mechanism applies in humans is less certain.

The exact nature of pericardial interference with ventricular filling is complex. There may be an increase in the hydrostatic pressure within the pericardium, particularly if an effusion is present, whose pressure can readily be measured with a simple manometric system. A pericardial effusion under pressure would increase the measured ventricular pressures throughout diastole, although a parallel upward shift would occur only if the pressure within the pericardial space did not change despite the volume of its contents increasing. Alternatively, pericardial restraint may operate only when the ventricular volume reaches a certain level late during diastole, which would cause an abrupt late diastolic increase in measured ventricular cavity stiffness, not a parallel upward shift of the pressure–volume curve. In addition, although the pericardium might restrain minor axis lengthening, it is not clear how it would interfere with motion of the long axis toward the left atrium. Indeed, increased long axis motion is a conspicuous feature of clinically significant pericardial constriction.

In humans the evidence for pericardial involvement is not clear. During the immediate postoperative period, changes in right atrial pressure are largely reflected in those of the pericardium.[99,100] With pacing-induced angina, however, changes in right ventricular pressure are significantly less than those on the left.[95] In postoperative patients, ventricular surface pressure can be measured by a solid-state manometer left in situ at the time of surgery: Acute dimension changes of up to 10 percent induced by handgrip or nitroglycerin administration do not cause appreciable alteration in pericardial pressure.[101] The possibility of restriction by a normal pericardium arises when cardiac size increases rapidly owing to disease, such as may occur with myocarditis or acute valvar regurgitation, thus increasing the apparent severity of the diastolic component of the condition. Although pericardial constraint sometimes alters the ventricular pressure–volume relations, particularly after cardiac surgery or with acute ventricular dilatation, it does not appear to be the only mechanism by which these changes come about in human disease.

Alteration in Right Ventricular Volume

Changes in right ventricular volume and pressure modify left ventricular diastolic properties and vice versa. In dogs an increase in right ventricular pressure, whether by fluid loading or increasing resistance to ejection, is associated with upward displacement of the left ventricular pressure–volume curve. Similar effects may be seen in humans, mediated via the epicardium or the interventricular septum. Distortion of the left ventricular cavity by the right ventricle can readily be demonstrated by cross-sectional echocardiography when the right ventricular systolic pressure is elevated.

Coronary Perfusion Pressure and Ventricular Diastolic Function

Changes in coronary artery perfusion pressure represent another mechanism that might potentially affect left ventricular pressure–volume relations.[102] Such changes are minimal within the physiologic range of 50–110 mmHg. Perfusion pressures higher than this level may influence diastolic pressure–volume relations, particularly in the presence of additional myocardial injury. Similar effects occur when the right atrial pressure is elevated, leading to a coronary venous "erectile" effect.[103] Whether these mechanisms underlie the acute changes in left atrial pressure that occur with hypertensive crises or contribute to the beneficial actions of a diuretic in patients with venous congestion remains to be demonstrated.

Of probably greater significance is the reverse effect: that of elevated ventricular diastolic pressures or short filling time on the dynamics of coronary flow. This potentially important field has scarcely been explored in the clinical literature. Clearly, though, an increase in left atrial pressure may maintain early diastolic left ventricular filling velocities in the presence of diastolic disease, but at the same time reduces the pressure drop from aortic to ventricular diastolic pressure that supports coronary flow. If end-diastolic pressure is high and aortic pressure normal or low, this value may well drop below 40 mmHg, the lowest level at which autoregulation occurs. Similarly, if ventricular filling time is greatly shortened by prolonged systolic tension development, that available for coronary flow is also significantly reduced. Examples of relations between trans-

mitral and coronary flow velocity patterns measured by transesophageal echocardiography are shown in Fig. 25-16.

Ventricular Cavity Shape

A final mechanism by which the ventricular pressure–volume relation might be altered is a change in cavity shape.[104,105] If the shape is allowed to vary, the volume can increase as the ventricle assumes a more spherical configuration without distension of the myocardium. Such a volume increase would thus be expected to occur with less increase in pressure than would have been the case had shape remained constant. Changes in cavity shape are prominent in the normal heart, its configuration becoming less spherical during ejection and reverting during early diastolic filling. Shape changes do not occur during atrial systole. These alterations are often lost during disease; with chronic coronary artery disease, they may disappear before any fall in ejection fraction.

Problems Associated with Assessing Ventricular Compliance

The many factors potentially affecting ventricular pressure–volume relations make it clear that it is not possible to measure passive stiffness in the same way as the ejection fraction. Unstressed volume (i.e., the volume in equilibrium) with zero transmural pressure cannot be measured in the beating heart. It is not possible to compare measurements among patients, as stiffness depends on volume, and comparable volumes cannot be identified. A volume of 150 ml, for instance, may be that at end-systole in one patient, end-diastole in another, and not achieved during diastole at all in a third. It is frequently stated in the literature that reduced early diastolic filling rate with a prominent A wave indicates increased cavity stiffness.[106] However, stiffness is rate of change of volume with pressure, and the filling rate is the rate of change of volume with time; time and pressure are clearly different entities, and it is not helpful to equate them. Furthermore, rapid filling occurs mainly as the ventricular pressure is falling. Unless pressure and volume move in the same direction, compliance does not even exist. Insofar as any relation exists between cavity stiffness and the filling pattern, reduced compliance is associated with increased E wave prominence.[107] Finally, it is possible to estimate myocardial stress–strain relations with a view to determining myocardial elastic modulus. To do this in any realistic way requires complex calculations, and the results have proved to be of little clinical relevance.

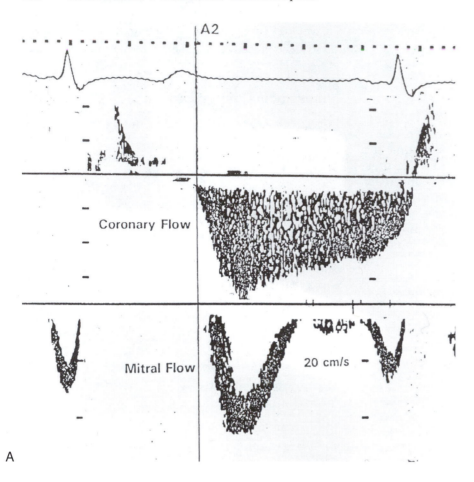

A

Fig. 25-16. Relation between proximal LAD coronary flow and transmitral flow velocities, determined by intraoperative transesophageal echocardiography. **(A)** Normal filling pattern. Note that peak diastolic coronary flow velocity is 70 cm/s, and high values are maintained throughout diastole. *(Figure continues.)*

ATRIAL SYSTOLE

Left atrial systole accounts for 20–30 percent of the normal resting stroke volume, but in the presence of disease this proportion may approach 100 percent. The mechanics of left atrial contraction differ fundamentally from those of the left ventricle.[108] The main muscle bundles are the interatrial band, arranged circumferentially around the atrial base, and the septoatrial bundle, arranged longitudinally. The main support for mechanical movement of both atrial is the rim of the oval fossa. The left atrial wall thickness ranges from 3 to 5 mm, though it may be increased with disease. Because the left atrium is fixed to mediastinal structures superiorly and laterally, atrial contraction has the effect of elevating the left atrioventricular (AV) ring, to which the longitudinal fibers are attached, and approximating the posterior wall of the aorta to the posterior wall. As a result, the increase in ventricular volume during left atrial systole is asymmetric, with a preferential increase in the left ventricular long axis as the AV ring moves toward the atrium. As during early diastole, motion of the AV ring has the additional effect of including blood within the ventricle undetectable by Doppler echocardiography.

The peak rate of increase of the ventricular volume during atrial systole is in the range of 200–300 ml/s, and peak blood flow velocity is 40–60 cm/s. The relative proportion of the stroke volume accounted for by atrial systole increases with age, so the E/A ratio falls from well above 1.0 in young adults to values of 0.5 or less in the elderly.

The proportion of the stroke volume entering the ventricle with atrial systole varies widely in the presence of disease. The E/A ratio is easy to measure using pulsed-wave Doppler echocardiography. It is multifactorial in origin, depending not only on the diastolic properties of the left ventricle but on atrial pressure and the force of left atrial contraction. An increase in the proportion of the stroke volume entering the left ventricle with atrial systole is nearly always associated with striking prolongation of the isovolumic relaxation time, often with incoordinate wall motion. Total suppression of early diastolic filling is not uncommon in patients with dilated cardiomyopathy who have responded well to treatment with an ACE inhibitor. This abnormality, though striking, should not therefore be regarded as a potential cause of diastolic heart failure but, rather, a mark of its successful treatment. Indeed, its presence appears fundamental to the modified relation that develops

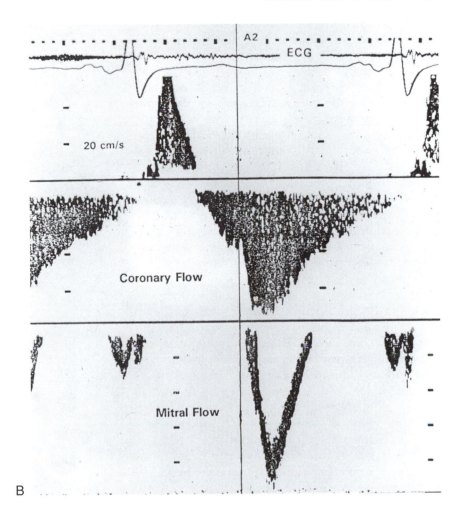

Fig. 25-16. *(Continued)* **(B)** Restrictive left ventricular filling pattern with reduced transmitral A wave. Note that coronary flow velocities decline strikingly during late diastole. **B**

between the heart and the circulation with successful preload and afterload reduction. Similar findings are seen with successful physical conditioning. The nature of the underlying changes, which take several weeks or months to occur and contrast strikingly with the effects of acute unloading, is still unclear. By contrast, in a few patients in sinus rhythm, no flow at all can be detected across the mitral valve during atrial systole, usually a marker of low end-diastolic ventricular compliance. This lack of flow is associated with an absence of long axis motion during atrial systole[80] and thus is a significant finding in patients with presumed diastolic failure.

To confirm the diagnosis, it is necessary to obtain evidence of mechanical atrial contraction. The most satisfactory method here is to record a pressure A wave from the atrium, either directly from the cavity itself or indirectly using a wedge pressure or an apex cardiogram. In addition, it is usually possible to demonstrate retrograde flow in the pulmonary veins. This condition must be distinguished from left atrial mechanical failure, which is common for the first 24–48 hours after DC shock. However, prolonged me-

chanical failure of the left atrium has been documented in patients with amyloid disease, where it may represent amyloid infiltration,[109] and with less severe restrictive disease.[110] The question obviously arises as to how often partial loss of atrial mechanical function may be present; an answer to this question must await the development of satisfactory methods of assessing atrial function in vivo.

CONCLUSION

Disturbances in left ventricular diastolic function are common in patients with the clinical syndrome of heart failure. Diastolic function is multifactorial, and interpreting any individual abnormality is possible only when the effects of age and loading conditions have been taken into account. Furthermore, many of these disturbances, though manifesting during diastole, have their origin earlier in the cardiac cycle, being caused by abnormalities of systolic function or activation.

In an individual patient, isovolumic relaxation

should be studied first. If isovolumic relaxation time, measured from A2 to mitral cusp separation, is less than 20 ms, the left atrial pressure is likely to be increased, regardless of age or any other abnormalities that may be present. Any significant dimension change in either the minor axis or the long axis during isovolumic relaxation can be taken as evidence of incoordination. Its origin is likely to arise earlier in the cardiac cycle, with abnormal activation or systolic function of either ventricle. An abnormally prolonged isovolumic relaxation time, seen by M-mode echocardiography to 80 ms or more or by Doppler studies to 100 ms or more, is likely to be accompanied by a reduction in E wave amplitude and an increase in the relative A wave. A fourth sound may be audible. In the setting of known ventricular disease, this combination of findings strongly suggests normal filling pressures.

Diastolic disease with significant symptoms is frequently present in patients with ventricular hypertrophy, coronary artery disease, diabetes, or any combination thereof. Conversely, remarkable ventricular incoordination is often found in patients who have responded well to medical treatment with diuretics and ACE inhibitors. A short isovolumic relaxation time (M-mode) combined with a dominant E wave and a short deceleration time indicates a high left atrial pressure and restrictive physiology and is one of the commonest causes of "diastolic heart failure." Its presence is independent of cavity size. It can often be recognized clinically from a loud third heart sound. Functional mitral regurgitation is often present whose downslope delays the onset of forward mitral flow.

Reduced A wave amplitude may represent further evidence of reduced end-diastolic ventricular compliance, provided that some other manifestation of atrial contraction can be recognized, such as retrograde flow in the pulmonary veins or an increase in the pressure A wave. In the absence of such evidence, a small A wave is likely to indicate atrial mechanical failure. Examination of diastolic function may thus give useful information about the nature of ventricular disease in an individual patient and can be used to follow treatment. More information is needed, however, as to the extent to which these abnormalities contribute to symptoms and impairment of prognosis, and even more as to their basic nature to allow more effective means of treatment to be devised.

REFERENCES

1. Dougherty AH, Naccarelli GV, Gray EL, Hicks CH, Goldstein RA: Congestive heart failure with normal systolic function. Am J Cardiol 1984;54:778–782
2. Miller TR, Grossman SJ, Schectman KB et al: Left ventricular diastolic filling and its association with age. Am J Cardiol 1986;58:531–535
3. Bryg RJ, Williams GA, Labovitz AJ: Effect of aging on left ventricular diastolic filling in normal subjects. Am J Cardiol 1987;59:971–974
4. Mattheos M, Oldershaw P, Sacchetti R, Shapiro E, Gibson DG: Relation of isovolumic relaxation time to left ventricular end-diastolic pressure and third heart sound. Br Heart J 1982;47:253–260
5. Appleton CP, Hatle LK, Popp RL: Relation of transmitral flow velocity to left ventricular diastolic function. New insights from a combined hemodynamic and Doppler echocardiographic study. J Am Coll Cardiol 1988;12:426–440
6. Grossman W: Diastolic dysfunction and congestive heart failure. Circulation, suppl. III 1990;81:1–7
7. Wiggers CJ: Studies on the duration of the consecutive phases of the cardiac cycle. I. The duration of the consecutive phases of the cardiac cycle and criteria for their precise determination. Am J Physiol 1921; 56:415–438
8. Lee CH, Vancheri F, Josen MS, Gibson DG: Discrepancies in the measurement of isovolumic relaxation time. A study comparing M mode and Doppler echocardiography. Br Heart J 1990;64:214–218
9. Chen C, Rodriguez L, Levine RA, Weyman AE, Thomas JD: Noninvasive measurement of the time constant of left ventricular relaxation using the continuous wave velocity profile of mitral regurgitation. Circulation 1992;86:272–278
10. Chung N, Nishimura RA, Holmes DR, Tajik AJ: Measurement of left ventricular dP/dt by simultaneous Doppler echocardiography and cardiac catheterization. J Am Soc Echocardiogr 1992;5:147–152
11. Xiao HB, Jin XY, Gibson DG: Doppler reconstruction of left ventricular pressure from functional mitral regurgitation. Potential importance of varying orifice geometry. Br Heart J 1995;73:53–60
12. Cohn PF, Liedtke AJ, Serur J, Sonnenblick EH, Urschel CW: Maximal rate of pressure fall (peak negative dP/dt) during ventricular relaxation. Cardiovasc Res 1972;6:263–267
13. McLaurin LP, Rolett EL, Grossman W: Impaired left ventricular relaxation during pacing-induced ischemia. Am J Cardiol 1973;32:751–757
14. Weiss JL, Fredericksen JW, Weisfeldt ML: Hemodynamic determinants of the time-course of fall in canine left ventricular pressure. J Clin Invest 1976;58: 751–760
15. Thompson DS, Waldron CB, Coltart DJ, Jenkins BS, Webb-Peploe MM: Estimation of time constant of left ventricular relaxation. Br Heart J 1983;49:250–258
16. Nonogi H, Hess O, Ritter M, Krayenbuehl HP: Diastolic properties of the normal left ventricle during supine exercise. Br Heart J 1988;60:30–38
17. Thompson DS, Wilmshurst P, Juul SM et al: Pressure-derived indices of left ventricular isovolumic relaxation in patients with hypertrophic cardiomyopathy. Br Heart J 1983;49:259–267
18. Thompson DS, Waldron CB, Juul SM et al: Analysis of left ventricular pressure during isovolumic relaxation in coronary artery disease. Circulation 1982;65: 690–697
19. Ruttley MS, Adams DF, Cohn PF, Abrams HL: Shape and volume changes during "isovolumetric relaxa-

tion" in normal and asynergic ventricles. Circulation 1974;50:306–316

20. Rademakers FE, Rogersw WJ, Guier WH et al: Relation of regional cross-fiber shortening to wall thickening in the intact heart. Three-dimensional analysis by NMR tagging. Circulation 1994;89:1174–1182

21. Gaasch WH, Blaustein AS, Bing OHL: Asynchronous (segmental early) relaxation of the left ventricle. J Am Coll Cardiol 1985;5:891–897

22. Gibson DG, Prewitt TA, Brown DJ: Analysis of left ventricular wall movement during isovolumic relaxation and its relation to coronary artery disease. Br Heart J 1976;38:1010–1019

23. Upton MT, Rerych SK, Newman GE et al: Detecting abnormalities in left ventricular function during exercise before angina and ST depression. Circulation 1980;62:341–349

24. Bonow RO: Regional left ventricular nonuniformity. Effect on left ventricular diastolic function in ischemic heart disease, hypertrophic cardiomyopathy, and the normal heart. Circulation, suppl. III 1990; 81:54–65

25. Upton MT, Gibson DG, Brown DJ. Echocardiographic assessment of abnormal left ventricular relaxation in man. Br Heart J 1976;38:1001–1009

26. Kondo H, Masuyama T, Ishihara K et al: Digital subtraction high frame-rate echocardiography in detecting delayed onset of regional left ventricular relaxation in ischemic heart disease. Circulation 1995;91:304–312

27. Gibson D, Mehmel H, Schwarz F, Li K, Kubler W: Asynchronous left ventricular wall motion early after coronary thrombosis. Br Heart J 1986;55:4–13

28. Brutsaert DL, Housmans PR, Goethals MA: Dual control of relaxation. Its role in the ventricular function in the mammalian heart. Circ Res 1980;47: 637–652

29. Stojnic BB, Brecker SJD, Xiao HB et al: Left ventricular filling characteristics in pulmonary hypertension. A new mode of ventricular interaction. Br Heart J 1992;68:16–20

30. Harvey W: The Movement of the Heart and Blood. pp. 124–125. Blackwell, Oxford, 1976

31. Jones CJH, Raposo L, Gibson DG: Functional importance of the long axis dynamics of the human left ventricle. Br Heart J 1990;63:215–220

32. Xiao HB, Gibson DG: Absent septal q wave. A marker of the effects of abnormal activation on left ventricular diastolic function. Br Heart J 1994;72:45–51

33. Xiao HB, Lee CH, Gibson DG: Effect of left bundle branch block on diastolic function in dilated cardiomyopathy. Br Heart J 1991;66:443–447

34. Sasson Z, Hatle L, Appleton CP et al: Intraventricular flow during isovolumic relaxation. Description and characterization by Doppler echocardiography. J Am Coll Cardiol 1987;10:539–546

35. Tanaka Y, Sanada J, Odachi M: Assessment of reversed isovolumic relaxation flow in patients with old myocardial infarct. Jpn J Med Ultrasonics 1991;18: 138–143

36. Marier DL, Gibson DG: Limitations of two frame method for displaying regional left ventricular wall motion in man. Br Heart J 1980;44:555–559

37. Brecker SJD, Lee CH, Gibson DG: Relation of left ventricular isovolumic relaxation time and incoordination to transmitral Doppler filling patterns. Br Heart J 1992;68:567–573

38. Yuasa F, Sumimoto T, Takeuchi M et al: Effects of left ventricular diastolic dysfunction on exercise capacity three to six weeks after acute myocardial infarction in men. Am J Cardiol 1995;74:14–17

39. Rihal CS, Nishimura RA, Hatle L, Bailey KR, Tajik AJ: Systolic and diastolic dysfunction in patients with clinical diagnosis of dilated cardiomyopathy. Relation to symptoms and prognosis. Circulation 1994; 90:2772–2779

40. Paulus W, Vantrimpont PJ, Shah AJ: Acute effects of nitric oxide on left ventricular relaxation and diastolic distensibility in humans. Assessment by bicoronary sodium nitroprusside infusion. Circulation 1994;89:2070–2078

41. Haber HL, Powers ER, Gimple LW et al: Intracoronary angiotensin-converting enzyme inhibition improves diastolic function in patients with hypertensive left ventricular hypertrophy. Circulation 1994; 89:2616–2625

42. Hammermeister KE, Warbasse JR: The rate of change of left ventricular volume in man. II. Diastolic events in health and disease. Circulation 1974;49: 739–747

43. Henderson Y, Scarbrough MM, Chillingworth FP: The volume curve of the ventricles of the mammalian heart, and the significance of this curve in respect to the mechanics of the heart-beat and the filling of the ventricles. Am J Physiol 1906;16:325–367

44. Bonow RO, Kent KM, Rosing DR et al: Improved left ventricular diastolic filling in patients with coronary artery disease after percutaneous transluminal coronary angioplasty. Circulation 1983;66:1159–1167

45. Iskandrian AS, Hakki AH, DePace NL, Manno B, Segal BL: Evaluation of left ventricular function by radionuclide angiography during exercise in normal subjects and in patients with chronic coronary artery disease. J Am Coll Cardiol 1983;1:1518–1529

46. Reduto LA, Wickemeyer WJ, Young JB et al: Left ventricular diastolic performance at rest and during exercise in patients with coronary artery disease. Assessment with first pass radionuclide angiography. Circulation 1981;63:1228–1237

47. Nishimura RA, Abel MD, Hatle LK, Tajik AJ: Assessment of diastolic function of the heart. Background and current applications of Doppler echocardiography. Part II. Clinical studies. Mayo Clin Proc 1989; 64:181–204

48. Iliceto S, D'Ambrosio G, Marangelli V, Di Biase M, Rizzon P: Echo-Doppler evaluation of the effects of heart rate increments on left atrial pump function in normal human subjects. Eur Heart J 1991;12: 345–351

49. Courtois M, Kovacs SJ, Ludbrook PA: Transmitral pressure–flow velocity relations. Importance of regional pressure gradients in the left ventricle during diastole. Circulation 1988;78:661–671

50. Greenbaum RA, Ho SY, Gibson DG, Becker AE, Anderson RH: Left ventricular fibre architecture in man. Br Heart J 1981;45:248–263

51. Dumesnil JG, Shoucri RM, Laurenceau JL, Turcot J: A mathematical model of the dynamic geometry of the intact left ventricle and its application to clinical data. Circulation 1979;59:1024–1034

52. Traill TA, Gibson DG, Brown DJ: Study of left ven

tricular wall thickness and dimension changes using echocardiography. Br Heart J 1978;40:162–169

53. Tsakiris AG, Gordon DA, Padiyar R, Frechette D: Relation of mitral valve opening and closure to left atrial and ventricular pressures in the intact dog. Am J Physiol 1978;234:146H–151H

54. Fioretti P, Brower RW, Meester GT, Serruys PW: Interaction of left ventricular relaxation and filling during early diastole in human subjects. Am J Cardiol 1980;46:197–203

55. Weisfeldt ML, Weiss JL, Frederiksen JT, Yin FCP: Quantification of incomplete left ventricular relaxation. Relationship to the time constant for isovolumic pressure fall. Eur Heart J, suppl. A 1980;1:119–129

56. Katz LN: The role played by the ventricular relaxation process in filling the ventricle. Am J Physiol 1930;95:542–553

57. Nikolic SN, Yellin EL, Tamura T, Frater RWM: Effect of early diastolic loading on myocardial relaxation in the intact canine left ventricle. Circ Res 1990;66:1217–1226

58. Sabbah HN, Anbe DT, Stein PD: Negative intraventricular diastolic pressure in patients with mitral stenosis. Evidence of left ventricular diastolic suction. Am J Cardiol 1980;45:562–566

59. Nikolic S, Yellin EL, Tamura K et al: Passive properties of canine left ventricle. Diastolic stiffness and restoring forces. Circ Res 1988;62:1210–1222

60. Fujimoto S, Parker KH, Xiao HB, Inge KSK, Gibson DG: Early diastolic left ventricular inflow pressures in normal subjects and patients with dilated cardiomyopathy. Reconstruction from pulsed Doppler echocardiography. Br Heart J 1995;74:419–425

61. Oldershaw PJ, Dawkins KD, Ward DE, Gibson DG: Effect of exercise on left ventricular filling in left ventricular hypertrophy. Br Heart J 1983;49:568–573

62. Sanderson JE, Gibson DG, Brown DJ, Goodwin JF: Left ventricular filling in hypertrophic cardiomyopathy. An angiographic study. Br Heart J 1977;39:661–670

63. Sanderson JE, Traill TA, St John Sutton MG et al: Left ventricular relaxation and filling in hypertrophic cardiomyopathy. An echocardiographic study. Br Heart J 1978;40:596–601

64. Fouad FM, Slominski MJ, Tarazi RC: Left ventricular diastolic function in hypertension. Relation to left ventricular mass and systolic function. J Am Coll Cardiol 1984;3:1500–1506

65. Bonow RO, Leon MB, Rosing DR et al: Effects of verapamil and propranolol on left ventricular systolic function and diastolic filling in patients with coronary artery disease. Radionuclide angiographic studies at rest and during exercise. Circulation 1982;65:1337–1350

66. Ohkushi H, Asai M, Ishito T: Left ventricular diastolic filling patterns in hypertrophic cardiomyopathy and myocardial infarction. Studies by pulsed Doppler echocardiography and multigate blood pool scans. J Cardiogr 1984;14:95–114

67. Shapiro LM, Leatherdale BA, Coyne ME, Fletcher RF, Mackinnon J: Prospective study of heart disease in untreated maturity onset diabetics. Br Heart J 1980;44:342–348

68. Brewerton DA, Goddard DH, Moore RB et al: The myocardium in ankylosing spondylitis. Lancet 1987;2:995–998

69. Vancheri F, Gibson D: Relation of third and fourth heart sounds to blood velocity during left ventricular filling. Br Heart J 1989;61:144–148

70. Henein M, Gibson DG: Suppression of left ventricular early diastolic filling by long axis asynchrony. Br Heart J 1995;73:151–157

71. Ng KSK, Gibson DG: Impairment of diastolic function by shortened filling period in severe left ventricular disease. Br Heart J 1989;62:246–252

72. Hatle LK, Appleton CP, Popp RL: Differentiation of constrictive pericarditis and restrictive cardiomyopathy by Doppler echocardiography. Circulation 1989;79:357–370

73. Appleton CP, Hatle LK, Popp RL: Demonstration of restrictive physiology by Doppler echocardiography. J Am Coll Cardiol 1988;11:757–768

74. Iliceto S, Amico A, Marangelli V, D'Ambrosio G, Rizzon P: Doppler echocardiographic evaluation of the effect of atrial pacing-induced ischemia on left ventricular filling in patients with coronary artery disease. J Am Coll Cardiol 1988;11:53–61

75. Carroll JD, Hess OM, Hirzel HO, Krayenbuehl HP: Exercise induced ischemia. The influence of altered relaxation on early diastolic pressures. Circulation 1983;67:521–528

76. Yamagishi T, Ozaki T, Kumada T et al: Asynchronous left ventricular diastolic filling in patients with isolated disease of the left anterior descending coronary artery. Assessment with radionuclide ventriculography. Circulation 1984;69:933–942

77. Hui WKK, Gibson DG: Mechanisms of reduced left ventricular filling rate in coronary artery disease. Br Heart J 1983;50:362–371

78. Sobue T, Yokata M, Iwase M, Ishihara H: Influence of left ventricular hypertrophy on left ventricular function during dynamic exercise in the presence or absence of coronary disease. J Am Coll Cardiol 1995;25:91–98

79. Keren G, Sonnenblick EH, LeJemtel TH: Mitral anulus motion. Relation to pulmonary venous and transmitral flows in normal subjects and patients with dilated cardiomyopathy. Circulation 1988;78:621–629

80. Henein MY, Gibson DG: Abnormal subendocardial function in restrictive left ventricular disease. Br Heart J 1994;72:237–242

81. Nishimura RA, Abel MD, Hatle LK, Tajik AJ: Relation of pulmonary vein to mitral flow by transesophageal Doppler echocardiography. Circulation 1990;81:1488–1497

82. Nishimura RA, Abdel MD, Hatle LK, Tajik AJ: Relation of pulmonary vein to mitral flow velocities by transesophageal Doppler echocardiography. Effects of different loading conditions. Circulation 1990;81:1488–1497

83. Brecker SJ, Kelly PA, Chua TP, Gibson DG: Effects of permanent dual chamber pacing in end-stage dilated cardiomyopathy [abstract]. Circulation, suppl. I 1995;92:724

84. Shen WF, Tribouilly C, Rey J-L, et al: Prognostic significance of Doppler derived ventricular filling variables in dilated cardiomyopathy. Am Heart J 1992;124:1524–1533

85. Pinamonti B, Lenarda A, Sinagra G, Camerini F: Restrictive left ventricular filling pattern in dilated cardiomyopathy assessed by Doppler echocardiography. Clinical, echocardiographic and hemodynamic corre-

lations and prognostic implications. J Am Coll Cardiol 1993;22:808–815

86. Unverforth DV, Marorien RD, Moeschberger ML et al: Factors influencing the one year mortality of dilated cardiomyopathy. Am J Cardiol 1984;54: 147–152

87. Mirsky I: Assessment of passive elastic stiffness of cardiac muscle. Mathematical concepts, physiologic and clinical considerations, direction of future research. Prog Cardiovasc Dis 1976;18:277–308

88. Yettram AL, Grewal BS, Gibson DG, Dawson JR: Relation between intraventricular pressure and volume in diastole. Br Heart J 1990;64:304–308

89. Diamond G, Forrester JS: Effect of coronary artery disease and acute myocardial infarction on left ventricular compliance in man. Circulation 1972;45: 11–19

90. Fester A, Samet P: Passive elasticity of the human left ventricle. The "parallel elastic element." Circulation 1974;50:609–618

91. Sasayama S, Nonogi H, Miyazaki S et al: Changes in diastolic properties of the regional myocardium during pacing-induced ischemia in human subjects. J Am Coll Cardiol 1985;5:599–606

92. Gilbert JC, Glantz SA: Determinants of left ventricular filling and of the diastolic pressure–volume relation. Circ Res 1989;64:827–852

93. Ludbrook PA, Teifenbrunn AJ, Reed FR, Sobel BE: Acute hemodynamic responses to sublingual nifedipine. Dependence on left ventricular function. Circulation 1982;65:489–498

94. Coltart DJ, Alderman EL, Robison SC, Harrison DC: Effect of propranolol on left ventricular function, sequential wall motion and diastolic pressure–volume relation in man. Br Heart J 1975;37:357–364

95. Ludbrook PA, Byrne JD, MacKnight RC: Influence of right ventricular hemodynamics on left ventricular diastolic pressure–volume relations in man. Circulation 1979;59:21–31

96. Tyberg JV, Misbach GA, Galnyz SA, Moores WY, Parmley WW: A mechanism for shifts in the diastolic, left ventricular, pressure–volume curve. The role of the pericardium. Eur J Cardiol, suppl. 1978;7: 163–175

97. Smiseth OA, Frais MA, Kingma I, Smith ER, Tyberg JV: Assessment of pericardial constraint in dogs. Circulation 1985;71:158–164

98. Smiseth OA, Refsum H, Junemann M et al: Ventricular diastolic pressure–volume shifts during acute ischemic left ventricular failure in dogs. J Am Coll Cardiol 1984;3:966–977

99. Hamilton DR, Dani RS, Semlacher RA et al: Right atrial and right ventricular transmural pressures in dogs and humans. Effects of the pericardium. Circulation 1994;90:2492–2500

100. Boltwood CM, Skulsky A, Drinkwater DC Jr et al: Intraoperative measurement of pericardial restraint. Role in ventricular diastolic mechanics. J Am Coll Cardiol 1986;8:1289–1297

101. Oldershaw PJ, Shapiro E, Mattheos M, St John Sutton MG, Gibson D: Independence of changes in left ventricular diastolic properties of pericardial pressure. Br Heart J 1982;48:125–129

102. Salisbury PF, Holmes U, Arnold G, Lochner W: The influence of coronary artery pressure and coronary flow upon myocardial elasticity. Circ Res 1960;8: 794–802

103. Vogel WM, Briggs LL, Apstein CS: Separation of inherent diastole myocardial fiber tension and coronary vascular "erectile" contributions to wall stiffness of rabbit hearts damaged by ischemia, hypoxia, calcium paradox and reperfusion. J Mol Cell Cardiol 1985;17:57–68

104. Burton AC: The importance of the size and shape of the heart. Am Heart J 1957;54:801–800

105. Gould KL, Lipscomb K, Hamilton GW, Kennedy JW: Relation of left ventricular shape, function and wall stress in man. Am J Cardiol 1974;34:627–634

106. Danford DA, Huhta JC, Murphy DJ: Doppler echocardiographic approaches to ventricular diastolic function. Echocardiography 1986;3:33–40

107. Stoddard MF, Pearson AC, Kern MJ et al: Left ventricular diastolic function. Comparison of pulsed Doppler echocardiographic and hemodynamic indices in subjects with and without coronary artery disease. J Am Coll Cardiol 1989;13:327–336

108. Wang K, Ho SY, Gibson DG, Anderson RH: Architecture of atrial musculature in humans. Br Heart J 1995;73:559–565

109. Dubrey S, Pollak A, Skinner M, Falk RH: Atrial thrombi occurring during sinus rhythm in cardiac amyloidosis. Evidence for atrial electromechanical dissociation. Br Heart J 1995;7:541–544

110. Wang K, Gibson DG: Noninvasive detection of left atrial mechanical failure in patients with left ventricular disease. Br Heart J 1995;74:536–540

26 Heart Failure During Pregnancy

Celia M. Oakley

Young women with heart disease usually try to live normal lives, which includes raising a family. Most of these patients do well if they are in New York Heart Association (NYHA) symptomatic classes I or II before pregnancy, though there are exceptions. Patients with mitral stenosis may develop heart failure during pregnancy despite having been asymptomatic before it; and patients with pulmonary hypertension, solitary or associated with congenital heart disease, face high risk and may suffer permanent deterioration due to progression of their pulmonary vascular disease during pregnancy.

Cardiovascular problems may first develop during pregnancy in previously fit women, or preexisting heart disease may be exacerbated by complications that arise during pregnancy. Some of the preexisting cardiac disorders that may give rise to heart failure during pregnancy are listed in Table 26-1 under group headings, together with causes of heart failure that may result from or be a complication of pregnancy. Interactions are frequent. For example, the coagulopathy of pregnancy may increase the risk of left atrial thrombus formation and embolism in mitral stenosis; the risk of aortic or coronary artery dissection is likely to be increased in patients with Marfan syndrome who become pregnant; and peripartum cardiomyopathy sometimes represents activation of previously latent dilated cardiomyopathy in a genetically susceptible individual.

In general, heart disease tends to get worse, and women with any sort of heart disease who are ever going to have children should be advised to have them early and to complete their families before the disease advances or they need prosthetic valve re-placement. This advice does not apply of course if a corrective procedure can be carried out.

CIRCULATORY CHANGES DURING NORMAL PREGNANCY

The cardiac output increases by 30–50 percent during normal pregnancy, and this increase is already well established by the time the pregnancy is first recognized, well before the end of the first trimester.[1] It is associated with a similar increase in circulating blood volume consequent on prostaglandin-induced relaxation of vascular smooth muscle. There is a greater increase in plasma volume than in red-blood cell volume, the disparity giving rise to the physiologic anemia of pregnancy.[2] Most of the increase in cardiac output is achieved by an increase in stroke volume with only a small increase in heart rate of about 10 beats per minute (bpm) at rest.[3,4] This remarkable adaptation is analogous to that achieved by athletes only after hard training. Left ventricular mass and end-diastolic volume increase, as do the contractile indices calculated from echocardiographic scanning.[5] The increase in cardiac output reaches near peak half-way through pregnancy with only a slight increase thereafter. During the third trimester of pregnancy wide swings in cardiac output and stroke volume occur according to whether the measurement is made in the supine or the lateral position. This difference is because the gravid uterus compresses the inferior vena cava, obstructing venous return from the legs.[6] This effective brake on venous return from the lower segment was used to

Table 26-1. Heart Failure
During Pregnancy: Etiology

Due to preexisting disease
    Hypertension
    Congenital
    Valvar
    Marfan syndrome
    Cardiomyopathy
    Coronary disease
Arising in or exacerbated by pregnancy
    Eclampsia and preeclampsia
    Pulmonary hypertension
    Embolism
        Pulmonary
        Coronary
    Dissection
        Aortic
        Coronary
    Peripartum cardiomyopathy
    Myocardial infarction

good effect by obstetricians in the past who put their patients with mitral stenosis to bed during the last trimester of pregnancy, where rest and posture effectively kept the heart rate and left atrial pressure down and the patient out of pulmonary edema.

The amount of increase in the circulating blood volume and cardiac output correlates with the size and weight of the products of conception.[7] The load is therefore greater in a multiple pregnancy, as is the risk of heart failure with heart disease.

The circulatory changes during labor and delivery are modified by the mode of delivery and by the analgesia and anesthesia chosen.[8,9] Increases in stroke volume occur with each uterine contraction during labor; the blood pressure rises, and during the second stage up to half a liter of blood may be expelled into the maternal circulation with each contraction. During the puerperium cardiac output remains high, even up to 30 percent above the predelivery level, particularly if there has been no blood loss. Restoration of normal blood volume, cardiac output, and extracellular fluid to normal levels takes 4–6 weeks.

Epidural anesthesia is popular but, as used for cesarean delivery, is associated with major circulatory changes.[9] The opiate venous infusion usually given to allay anxiety causes venodilatation and a reduction in venous return to the heart. The hemodynamic changes associated with the blockade necessary for surgical delivery reduces systemic vascular resistance and blood pressure. There is a fall in venous pressure and shift of blood out of the thorax. This change may be well tolerated and even helpful in the presence of mitral stenosis but lethal with primary

pulmonary hypertension, where maintenance of stroke volume and blood pressure are dependent on the right ventricular filling pressure and high systemic vascular resistance. Equally, the patient with Eisenmenger syndrome is subject to a brisk fall in arterial oxygen saturation if the balance between systemic and pulmonary vascular resistance is changed in favor of an increase in right-to-left shunting.

Cardiac patients with marginal cardiovascular reserve are best delivered by cesarean section under general anesthesia, which provides freedom from anxiety and pain, reduction in metabolic demand through complete rest, together with optimal oxygenation; it can be conducted with maximal stability of blood pressure, heart rate, volemia, and distribution of blood volume. Continuous electrocardiography (ECG) and pulse oximetry are standard, but a Swan-Ganz catheter is only rarely necessary. Placement of a temporary pacemaker for delivery may be wise for certain patients: for example, those with corrected transposition of the great arteries at risk of developing heart block or Ebstein's anomaly with risk of atrial flutter and 1:1 conduction down an accessory pathway. The latter patients may need overdrive pacing or DC reversion.

The use of antibiotic prophylaxis for cardiac patients is discretionary. Normal delivery is associated with only low rates of bacteremia with a variety of organisms. Infective endocarditis is a low risk and has rarely been reported.[10] Despite this fact, most physicians choose to give antibiotics to patients with artificial valves or a history of endocarditis.

CONGENITAL HEART DISEASE

Most patients with uncorrected simple defects do well with no risk of heart failure, including atrial septal defect, restrictive ventricular septal defects, and pulmonary stenosis. Patients with previous radical correction of tetralogy of Fallot in general also do well despite the variable presence of some residual pulmonary stenosis, pulmonary regurgitation, ventricular septal defect, impaired right ventricular function, tricuspid regurgitation, or any combination. Although the latter may develop congestive features during pregnancy, problems are rare.[11] Ventricular arrhythmias have been identified as a cause of late death in these patients, particularly in those who were operated on after early childhood; but they have not been encountered in our patients during pregnancy.

Patients with more complex surgically palliated congenital heart disease may wish to become pregnant, including patients with valve-bearing conduits, as after Rastelli repair or single ventricle circulations after the Fontan procedure. Patients with Rastelli conduits may do well during pregnancy unless they have outgrown the conduit and developed severe outflow obstruction. After the Fontan procedure and its many variations, adults tend to have high venous filling pressures with marked chronic leg edema and low cardiac output. Although pregnancy may be successful, these patients are at high risk of fetal loss and always endure a considerable increase in congestive features. Those with right atrial-pulmonary artery conduits who are dependent on right atrial contraction may suffer a precipitous fall in output and blood pressure if right atrial function is lost through the onset of atrial flutter or fibrillation.

Patients with uncorrected cyanotic congenital heart disease who have a low pulmonary artery pressure such as cyanotic Ebstein's anomaly or complex pulmonary stenosis (e.g., uncorrected tetralogy of Fallot[12] or complex pulmonary atresias or transpositions[13] often tolerate pregnancy remarkably well even though arterial oxygen saturation tends to fall throughout pregnancy with an increase in an already elevated hematocrit. They face the risk of venous thrombosis and paradoxical embolism. Fetal growth is impaired in cyanotic mothers and requires careful monitoring during pregnancy, with delivery of the baby as soon as fetal growth seems to have seriously slowed or stopped. Most patients with a resting arterial oxygen saturation of 85 percent or more manage to produce a live child, although it is likely to be born prematurely and be small for dates. The placentas are oversized and often infarcted, resembling those in mothers resident at high altitudes. The quality of maternal arterial blood oxygenation should be optimized by bed rest and 60 percent oxygen, which may be needed continuously throughout the middle and later parts of pregnancy. Arterial oxygen should be monitored by continuous pulse oximetry and fetal growth by frequent ultrasonography. Prophylactic subcutaneous heparin should be given to the mother as soon as the need for bed rest is established.[14]

Aortic Stenosis

Congenital aortic valve stenosis due to some variety of bicuspid valve is up to five times more common in men than in women; but being a common condition, it is seen not infrequently during pregnancy. Asymptomatic patients with mild or moderate valve stenosis have no difficulty. Aortic valve stenosis, however, is a progressive condition during childhood and ado-

lescence due to differential growth and early degenerative changes, so the history of a previous successful pregnancy without problems is not necessarily reassuring. Most of these young patients have good left ventricular systolic function and a progressive increase in left ventricular systolic pressure and Doppler velocity shown on echocardiography if they succeed in raising the stroke volume in a normal fashion. The development of angina and shortness of breath is frequently associated with a resting tachycardia indicative of failure to achieve the higher stroke volume, and the tachycardia may cause a critical reduction in coronary blood flow. Tachycardia may lead to further loss of stroke volume because of slow left ventricular filling, and systolic failure may quickly supervene with fatal results.

Balloon aortic valvoplasty should be considered in any patient with severe aortic valve stenosis who develops evidence of commencing trouble during pregnancy,[15,16] although the results are not always good and there is a risk of inducing free aortic regurgitation. Patients who have already had an open aortic valvotomy or balloon valvotomy during childhood may not receive further relief from repeat ballooning (although it may be attempted), and such patients require aortic valve replacement. If possible, this procedure should be delayed until the baby is viable; patients may respond well to bed rest with administration of oxygen and a β-blocker to slow the heart rate and improve coronary blood flow and left ventricular filling. Cautious additional use of nitrates may reduce pulmonary congestion without loss of output in patients with a high left ventricular filling pressure. Placement of a Swan-Ganz catheter may be necessary to guide therapy. The baby should be delivered by cesarean section under general anesthesia before aortic valve replacement because the risk of fetal loss during induction of anesthesia or cardiopulmonary bypass in such circumstances is still close to 50 percent.

Discrete subaortic stenosis may also be encountered during pregnancy and addressed in the same way. These patients are more likely to have impaired left ventricular function, particularly if they have had previous surgery, and there may be associated mitral regurgitation compounding the problem. Others resemble hypertrophic cardiomyopathy with gross wall thickening, small left ventricular cavities, and diastolic dysfunction.

Pulmonary Hypertension

Pulmonary hypertension, whether "solitary" as in primary pulmonary hypertension or associated with congenital heart disease and right-to-left shunting in the Eisenmenger syndrome, carries high risk. The risk is so high that patients should be advised against pregnancy. Moreover, because pulmonary vascular disease is incurable, sterilization should be recommended.[14,17–19]

Patients with primary hypertension may be diagnosed for the first time during pregnancy. A few may have a family history of the condition or autoimmune disease, particularly systemic lupus erythematosus (SLE) or one of the "overlap" syndromes. Pulmonary hypertension is an exception among "cardiac" diseases in being associated with risk of permanent deterioration during pregnancy. In some patients dyspnea or syncope may first develop during pregnancy, with the condition rapidly progressing to right ventricular failure. Patients with primary pulmonary hypertension who are first recognized too late for therapeutic abortion or who refuse it should be rested in hospital, given nifedipine and oxygen, and delivered by cesarean section under general anesthesia with careful attention to maintaining venous filling pressure, systemic vasoconstriction, heart rate, and volemia. They are not at risk from pulmonary edema, so administration of fluid and restoration of blood loss should be generous. They should be maintained in the intensive therapy unit (ITU) for close monitoring postoperatively. Subcutaneous heparin should be used in hospital before delivery and long-term warfarin started postpartum.

It has long been known that, if patients with the Eisenmenger syndrome become pregnant and insist on continuing, they face a high risk of dying.[16] The risk is more than 50 percent in patients with the Eisenmenger complex (ventricular septal defect) and slightly less for patients with patent ductus, atrial septal defects, or a combination. If the resting arterial oxygen saturation is less than 85 percent there is a high chance of spontaneous abortion; but with maximum care many babies reach viability and can be saved. Most of the maternal deaths occur during the first postpartum week.[14,17–19]

Patients with the Eisenmenger syndrome who have refused sterilization or termination and insist on continuing with the pregnancy should, with their partners, have been made well aware that they face these high risks. They should be admitted to hospital by the 20th week of pregnancy or earlier if resting oxygen saturation falls, hematocrit rises, or symptoms increase. They need to be kept in bed with continuous 60 percent oxygen to maximize arterial saturation and continuous pulse oximetry with subcutaneous heparin to prevent venous thrombosis. As soon as fetal growth falters, the child should be delivered by cesarean section under general anesthesia and the mother maintained in the ITU with care-

ful monitoring continued. Mobilization should be gradual. Despite these measures, sudden death is usual. The precipitating cause appears to be a sudden tilting of the balance between systemic and pulmonary vascular resistance in favor of right-to-left shunting. This tilt may be due to a systemic vasodilator response in neurocardiogenic syncope. Intravenous atropine and phenylephrine would be appropriate, as patients who are being monitored at the time show a brisk drop in the oximeter reading with bradycardia rapidly followed by ventricular fibrillation. The postmortem examination provides no further explanation, and pulmonary embolism is conspicuously absent.

Ebstein's Anomaly

Mild ventricular displacement of elements of the tricuspid valve is not uncommon, revealed only by echocardiography and associated with good right ventricular function and an absence of cyanosis. Such patients do well during pregnancy, although they may be troubled by supraventricular tachycardias associated with right-sided preexcitation.[20] If attacks are prolonged and drug treatment is required, the choice may be difficult. β-Blocking drugs are safe during pregnancy; and even if they do not prevent attacks, they may slow the rate. Other antiarrhythmic drugs are not approved for use during pregnancy, but administration of amiodarone may be unavoidable to prevent prolonged attacks of tachycardia, which may precipitate right ventricular failure and jeopardize the fetus. There is also the risk of tachycardia triggering atrial flutter, which can be associated with 1:1 conduction down the accessory pathway at rates of 300 per minute. If that happens, prompt DC reversion is required, which can be carried out safely during pregnancy.

Patients with Ebstein's anomaly who are cyanotic usually have an elevated venous pressure and right-sided failure. They face the risk of paradoxical embolism, worsening failure, falling arterial saturations during pregnancy, and impaired fetal growth. They tend to do badly.

CARDIOMYOPATHY

Hypertrophic Cardiomyopathy

In general, hypertrophic cardiomyopathy (HOCM) is well tolerated during pregnancy.[21,22] The main hemodynamic abnormality of this disorder is the small size of the left ventricular cavity, limiting stroke volume, and impaired diastolic relaxation, advancing later to a restrictive filling pattern with absence of late filling. It seems that during pregnancy the heart in HOCM (with or without outflow gradient) responds favorably to the hormonal changes by an increase in cavity size and stroke volume. β-Blockers are given only to patients who need to avoid tachycardia in order to preserve left ventricular filling and optimize coronary blood flow (systolic retropulsion of blood up the left anterior descending coronary artery has been shown in HOCM with outflow gradients, as is seen with aortic stenosis). Patients who have bursts of ventricular tachycardia on Holter monitoring or who have developed recurrent atrial fibrillation are usually treated with amiodarone, and it may not be wise to stop the amiodarone if pregnancy is contemplated or arises. Amiodarone is not licensed for use during pregnancy, but personal experience has indicated it to be benign. Neonatal hypothyroidism has been described,[23,24] but it does not appear to be teratogenic.

Some patients with HOCM have high left atrial pressures that may rise further during pregnancy; and in a few patients it may be impossible to avoid the use of a diuretic. Vaginal delivery is usually well tolerated, but the risk of a rise in left atrial pressure immediately after delivery should be appreciated, especially if there has been little blood loss. A small dose of intravenous furosemide or bumetanide may be needed, and the patient should be sat up promptly after delivery.

Patients with HOCM should of course appreciate the genetic risks, although it does not usually discourage them from wanting to raise a family. Genetic testing can be carried out in the newborn in families with identified mutations for parents who desire it.

Peripartum Cardiomyopathy

Peripartum cardiomyopathy is the term used to describe a dilated cardiomyopathy that is temporally related to pregnancy and parturition. It is loosely defined as heart failure that develops during the last month of pregnancy or the first 3 to 6 months postpartum in women who had not previously been known to have heart disease.[25] Most are seen within a few days or weeks of delivery. The worst cases develop severe heart failure with an explosive onset within a few days of the birth. Milder cases may present up to 6 months later.[26]

The disorder is rare, but the true prevalence is unknown because mild cases may not be diagnosed. A patient presenting with a peripartum cardiomyopathy may have had subclinical left ventricular dys-

function before the pregnancy, and the causal relation of the pregnancy has thus been argued even though it is usually clear that the pregnancy precipitated the heart failure. Cardiac biopsies usually show evidence of myocarditis when carried out during the acute illness.[27] During pregnancy a decrease in cell-mediated immunity occurs that prevents rejection of the fetus but increases maternal susceptibility to viral infections. Because peripartum cardiomyopathy usually develops postpartum, it makes viral infection seem less likely. Certainly other features of viral infection are notably absent. Dilated cardiomyopathy (unrelated to pregnancy) is often familial, with other cases either overt or occult discovered in about 20 percent of members. In this context some patients with peripartum cardiomyopathy give a family history of dilated cardiomyopathy.[28] It seems likely that patients with peripartum cardiomyopathy have a genetic propensity to develop dilated cardiomyopathy. It is now regarded as an immunologically based disease, and in these predisposed subjects pregnancy may be the trigger. Longer-term follow-up and family and genetic studies are needed for patients with peripartum cardiomyopathy.

Individual experience of peripartum cardiomyopathy tends to be sparse because the disorder is rare. The literature is vast and does not enlighten. Early series almost certainly included a heterogeneous mix of conditions, and recent publications contain more speculation than information. The disorder seems to be more frequent in association with multiple births, but the higher blood volume and extracellular fluid volume associated with multiple pregnancy may simply increase the severity of the clinical presentation. The high prevalence of postpartum heart failure reported among the Hausa women of northern Nigeria is quite different and attributable to traditional practices, with fluid overload caused by excessive salt intake from eating "kanwa." The high salt intake is associated with overheating from lying on a hot mud bed. The women suffer a high output heart failure that usually resolves after withdrawing the inciting factors.[29]

Severe cases of peripartum cardiomyopathy present with biventricular failure and dilated poorly contracting ventricles. Echocardiography rapidly enables other conditions, such as β_2-agonist-induced pulmonary edema, amniotic fluid embolism, pulmonary embolism, or previously undiagnosed valve disease, to be excluded (Table 26-2). The patients are fluid overloaded with hypotension, tachycardia, and a third heart sound gallop; but except in the worst cases, they have a well preserved cardiac output. Ventricular tachycardia and sudden death may

Table 26-2. Differential Diagnosis of Peripartum Cardiomyopathy

Toxemia
Pulmonary embolism
Amniotic fluid embolism
Myocardial infarction
Ritodrine-induced pulmonary-edema
Adult respiratory distress syndrome
Undetected valvular heart disease

occur. Peripheral embolism is occasionally a presenting feature associated with intraventricular thrombosis.[25]

The impact of acute myocarditis is sometimes rather focal, and the ECG may suggest acute myocardial infarction. Because myocardial infarction (usually resulting from coronary dissection) can also complicate pregnancy and because of the need for early cardiac biopsy, left and right heart catheterization and coronary angiography should be carried out urgently.

The most severe cases may need intubation, ventilation, Swan-Ganz catheter monitoring, and intravenous inotropes. Less severe cases are treated with digoxin, angiotensin-converting enzyme (ACE) inhibitors, diuretics, and warfarin. Ventricular arrhythmias are common and may precipitate cardiogenic shock. DC reversion, overdrive pacing, and antiarrhythmic drugs may tide the patient over the crisis.

In the worst cases seemingly at high risk of a fatal outcome, there may be nail biting for a few days when cardiac transplantation seems to offer the only way forward. Against this measure, however, is the high chance of major improvement if the acute stage is survived. This is also true of acute myocarditis that occurs outside of pregnancy.

Patients with peripartum cardiomyopathy sometimes recover from profound failure with mitral regurgitation and gross cardiomegaly and revert to near-normal function within a few months. Even the worst cases must show some early improvement if the patient is to survive. Sometimes it is rapid, but in other cases there is little further progress over many weeks or months. Rarely, improvement is not detected for 1 year or even 2 years following the onset, although return to normal or near-normal function is still possible in these patients. Ventricular function should be monitored by serial echocardiography.

Treatment with an ACE inhibitor should probably be continued long term for as long as left ventricular function remains abnormal. Because myocytolysis is usually prominent on biopsy sections, and there may be large tracts of dead myocytes, it is clear that some measure of cardiovascular reserve has been lost even in patients who seem to recover completely. Healing with fibrosis may lead to subsequent ventricular arrhythmias.

Because cardiac biopsy usually shows myocarditis and there is no reason to believe that it is of infective origin, there is a strong case for immunosuppression. Prednisolone is given in a starting daily dose of 1.5 mg/kg plus azothiaprine as a steroid sparer in a daily dose of 1 mg/kg. This regimen is undertaken for 4–6 weeks in patients who improve rapidly but longer for more slowly resolving cases. Some guidance may be obtained from repeat biopsy, but sampling errors may confuse the issue; multiple biopsies from different right ventricular sites are desirable. There is no advantage from biopsying the left ventricle, as it seems to carry greater risk of perforation.

Peripartum cardiomyopathy may recur in subsequent pregnancies but not necessarily. It is usually wise to advise against additional pregnancies in patients who exhibit incomplete recovery of ventricular function and to wait 3–5 years before another pregnancy even for patients who have apparently recovered fully.

Cardiomyopathy

There is little experience of patients with previously diagnosed dilated cardiomyopathy during subsequent pregnancy. Most women treated for this condition are advised against pregnancy, and most are middle aged or older. Women with dilated cardiomyopathy of mild severity may go through pregnancy under cardiologic supervision without trouble, which may be related to special care they get, particularly with regard to admission before birth for rest, low salt intake, avoidance of fluid overload, and early institution of ACE inhibitors after delivery. ACE inhibitors are contraindicated during pregnancy because of adverse effects on fetal renal function and oligohydramnios.

Restrictive Cardiomyopathy

Restrictive cardiomyopathy is rare and frequently familial. Pregnancy may be relatively well tolerated because of rapid ventricular filling and the ability to compensate for a low stroke volume by tachycardia. Exacerbation of congestive features can be expected. No immunologic mechanism is invoked for these cases, and no postpartum exacerbation is expected.

VALVULAR HEART DISEASE

Rheumatic fever is still common in South Asia, parts of the Middle East, and Central and South America. The incidence has fallen as dramatically in many parts of the Far East as it has in the West,[30] although there have been small "epidemics" with recrudescence of rheumatic fever reported from the United States during the last few years.[31] Mitral stenosis and rheumatic heart disease in the young is virtually confined to the immigrant population in the United Kingdom.

In medically unmonitored populations mitral stenosis is frequently first diagnosed during pregnancy. In the United Kingdom these young women may be newly resident and previously asymptomatic or only mildly short of breath. Shortness of breath and pulmonary edema can develop rapidly during pregnancy. It is caused by sinus tachycardia without change in rhythm and even without any antecedent precipitating infection or anemia, although these conditions may have contributed. The tachycardia may have been precipitated by anxiety or exertion, but reducing the time for left atrial emptying causes the left atrial pressure to rise and stroke volume to fall, giving rise to a reflex increase in rate, which further exacerbates the rise in left atrial pressure and fall in stroke volume with still more rise in heart rate. Such a vicious circle can lead to pulmonary edema within hours or less of the onset of shortness of breath.

For emergencies, upright posture, reassurance, a β-blocker,[32] and a small dose of intravenous diuretic can relieve the situation. Most of these patients have pliable noncalcified stenosed valves, without chordal fusion or regurgitation, that are suitable for balloon mitral valvotomy. The Inoue balloon has shortened the time required for the procedure to about 1.5 hours, thereby reducing irradiation risks. The results are usually excellent in this age group.[33]

The balloon technique has largely obviated the need for closed mitral valvotomy. This operation has become unfamiliar to surgeons trained in the West, but it is safe, inexpensive, and effective; and it costs less than the Inoue balloon in developing countries where surgical skills in closed mitral valvotomy remain well practiced.

If neither facility is available or the valve is unsuitable for valvotomy, patients can be maintained free from pulmonary congestion by use of a β-adrenergic blocking drug given in sufficient doses to maintain the heart rate below 90 bpm until open mitral valvotomy or replacement can be carried out after delivery of the baby. Few patients in this age group are in

atrial fibrillation, which of course should be treated with digoxin.

Patients with rheumatic mitral regurgitation or multivalve rheumatic disease without severe stenosis, but perhaps with mitral, aortic, and tricuspid regurgitation, may fare much better during pregnancy despite even gross cardiomegaly and a high jugular venous pressure. Regurgitant valve disease is tolerated far better during pregnancy than stenotic valve disease. If left ventricular filling is rapid, pulmonary edema is unlikely, and tachycardia is better tolerated than in mitral stenosis. Moreover, the peripheral vasodilatation associated with pregnancy is beneficial in tilting the balance toward forward flow rather than regurgitant flow.

Mitral Leaflet Prolapse and Floppy Mitral Valves

Mitral regurgitation is in general well tolerated during pregnancy because of systemic vasodilatation, and no additional vasodilator need be prescribed. If the regurgitation is severe and the valve is reparable (as it usually is with nonrheumatic mitral regurgitation), the valve should be repaired before pregnancy is undertaken.

Patients with Prosthetic Valves

Patients who are going to need prosthetic valves should, whenever possible, complete their families before the valve(s) is inserted. Patients with mechanical valve prostheses require continuation of meticulous anticoagulation throughout pregnancy because the hypercoagulable state induced by pregnancy increases the risk of valve thrombosis and thromboembolism.[34,35]

Controversy continues regarding a change to heparin or continuation of warfarin or other coumarin anticoagulant during pregnancy. Warfarin is safe and effective for the mother but carries a small risk of inducing a fetal embryopathy (caused by fetal vitamin K deficiency) when given between the sixth and ninth weeks and a continuing risk of causing fetal cerebral hemorrhage. The latter occurs because of fetal overdosage due to the immature liver and reduced fetal production of procoagulants together with the inability of these large molecules to pass to the fetal side from the maternal side. The baby is variably but inevitably overanticoagulated, and the risk of fetal damage is related to the maternal dose requirement. It has been suggested that if the maternal daily requirement of warfarin is less than 5 mg the fetal risk is minimal.[36] Conversely, a few women require doses in excess of 10 mg per day and are probably at heightened risk of fetal damage, although no figures exist to confirm this possibility. The overall risk of embryopathy, regardless of the maternal warfarin dose, has been estimated to be 3–4 percent.[35] Most damaged fetuses are aborted early, and the number of damaged liveborn babies is small, although there seems to be a small increased risk of stillbirth in warfarin-treated patients. Although heparin has never been shown to be safe or effective in preventing arterial thromboembolism,[34] it has been suggested that patients should take heparin throughout the pregnancy, at least during the first trimester, or even starting before conception. No controlled randomized trials have ever been carried out for the obvious reasons of small numbers and different styles, sites, and sizes of artificial valves; but the literature suggests that both prosthetic valve thrombosis and maternal bleeding are more likely with heparin than with warfarin anticoagulation during pregnancy.[34] Heparin is a drug with a powerful effect, a narrow therapeutic index, a short half-life, and a need to be given parenterally. Moreover, there is no unanimity about the target level of anticoagulation or the test to be used, figures for the activated partial thromboplastin time (APTT) of 1.5–2.5 being variously suggested. If patients are at home it is difficult for them to check the APTT midway between the 12-hourly dosage as advised or to attend hospital frequently enough for the dose of heparin to be adjusted according to increasing need as the pregnancy advances. Continuous intravenous heparin for patients with mechanical prostheses[37] is impractical and brings the added risk of septicemia and endocarditis.

On the basis of data from case series and retrospective questionnaires it is suggested that warfarin be continued throughout pregnancy with the possible exception of patients with unusually high dose requirement. The patient should be fully informed of the increased risks to both her and her baby if she transfers to heparin. Similarly, the usual advice that the patient should be admitted to hospital for the last 2 weeks of pregnancy in order to receive intravenous heparin and await spontaneous labor can probably be improved by elective cesarean section at 38 weeks. This measure avoids the risks of heparin, minimizes the risk to these precious babies, and can be associated with the shortest possible time off warfarin for the mother.

The risk of prosthetic valve thrombosis is increased during pregnancy in women on heparin anticoagulation and may be slightly increased for patients on oral anticoagulant treatment unless the latter is meticulous.[38] Valve thrombosis, unlike mechanical valve strut fracture with release of the occluder, usually develops gradually and mimics the physical signs of combined stenosis and regurgitation of the valve. This picture arises because the occluder usually sticks in a half-open/half-closed position. Prosthetic clicks disappear to be replaced by stenotic and regurgitant murmurs. Embolism does not always occur. The diagnosis is easily made. In contrast, patients with strut fraction have a sudden disaster and should be sent to the nearest major cardiac center and straight to the operating room without delay for investigation. Patients with valve thrombosis present with a more gradual onset of increasing shortness of breath culminating in heart failure and have telltale physical signs; the clinical diagnosis can readily be confirmed on echocardiography. Fluoroscopy, less readily available now than it used to be, can be used to show outlet strut fracture of a Bjork-Shiley valve or diminished opening if the valve has thrombosed.

Fibrinolytic treatment can be effective, particularly in the case of tricuspid prosthetic thrombosis when it is the treatment of choice. It has been used during pregnancy without compromising the fetus, though there is risk of retroplacental hemorrhage. Thrombolytic therapy for left-sided prosthetic valve thrombosis carried a 9.5 percent risk of cerebral embolism and of irreversible neurologic damage in 4.4 percent in a review of 173 cases, but the alternative is emergency surgery.[39]

Bioprostheses avoid the need for anticoagulant treatment of women who are in sinus rhythm but carry the serious disadvantage of accelerated deterioration during pregnancy. This situation may necessitate emergency valve re-replacement or an elective second valve replacement while the children are still young. Re-replacement carries appreciable and individually unpredictable risk (> 10 percent in a recent series).[40] Although bioprostheses usually deteriorate gradually, emergencies with pulmonary edema may occur caused by sudden tearing of the valve. Emergency operations made necessary by the sudden onset of profound heart failure carry high risk to both mother and baby.

MARFAN SYNDROME

Fifty percent of aortic dissections in women under age 50 years occur during pregnancy, most often during the third trimester or during labor.[41] Most of these women are hypertensive, some have Marfan syndrome, and others have annuloaortic ectasia without Marfan phenotype.[42]

Women with cardiovascular abnormality associated with the Marfan syndrome tend to do badly during pregnancy. It is a hazardous combination because of the risk of aortic dissection, reduced maternal prognosis, and genetic transmission of the defect to 50 percent of the offspring. Some patients with floppy mitral valves but without aortic root dilatation have no trouble during pregnancy, and some patients who already have a dilated aortic root survive pregnancy despite a high risk of aortic dissection, rupture of a dilated root or increase in mitral or aortic regurgitation with heart failure. The family history is important, as the disorder tends to run true. Some families have a history of aortic dissection despite minimal aortic root dilatation. If the family history is poor in respect to early cardiovascular deaths, counseling against pregnancy must be considered. Prenatal diagnosis is now possible.

If a patient with Marfan syndrome and cardiovascular features of the disease elects to accept the risks of pregnancy, a β-adrenergic blocking drug should be continued throughout the pregnancy unless there is significant aortic regurgitation, in which case prolonging the diastolic interval for regurgitation may be inadvisable. Patients with Marfan syndrome who have previously undergone aortic root replacement with a valve-bearing conduit or who have had an interposition aortic graft with resuspension of their own aortic valve have gone through pregnancy without problems but not without risk.

Patients with Marfan syndrome may ultimately develop myocardial failure even after successful correction of mitral or aortic regurgitation. It may possibly be associated with dilatation of an enfeebled fibrous skeleton of the heart. Such patients come to resemble patients with a dilated cardiomyopathy.

PULMONARY EMBOLISM

Pulmonary embolism may occur during pregnancy or more often postpartum, particularly after surgical delivery. It is particularly liable to complicate diabetic pregnancy and cesarean birth in diabetics. It may complicate other heart disease in the mother or, more often, occurs out of the blue in a previously fit individual.

Pulmonary embolism during pregnancy is unexpected and frequently missed. The patient develops shortness of breath that may be attributed to the pregnancy or panic. The patient may have syncope or develop pleuritic pain or hemoptysis. Major or massive pulmonary embolism may be associated with collapse, right ventricular dilatation, and low output failure. Tachypnea and hyperpnea are usually striking unless the patient has collapsed and there is a third heart sound gallop. The venous pressure, although elevated, may be difficult to see because of strenuous respiratory efforts or the need for the patient to lie supine because of hypotension. In the hyperacute situation the ECG and chest radiograph may look relatively normal, and the quickest confirmation comes from echocardiography, which immediately allows the dilated, almost immobile right ventricle to be identified in dramatic contrast to a small vigorously contracting left ventricle. Sometimes coils of thrombus are seen in the right atrium. In such cases and in any patient with sudden onset of shortness of breath and right ventricular overload, the patient should be taken immediately to the cardiac catheterization laboratory (or, in its absence, to the radiology department), a catheter introduced from an arm vein into the pulmonary artery, and contrast injected. This maneuver allows the position of emboli to be identified so the catheter can be advanced to break them up. When the material moves further down the pulmonary tree, the right ventricle is immediately unloaded, cardiac output increases, and blood pressure rises.[43] Injecting streptokinase after this mechanical dispersion is unnecessary because endogenous fibrinolytic activity in the lungs is intense and rapidly completes the process of thrombus dissolution.

Subsequent anticoagulant treatment is obligatory with warfarin (INR 2.0) or subcutaneous heparin (APTT 1.5). Complete resolution is the rule. Perfusion lung scans should not be repeated during pregnancy but should be checked after delivery. Doppler echocardiography provides information on the restoration of right ventricular function and pressure.

Leg vein stasis should be minimized by avoiding the supine position and selecting a semiprone posture for sleep. Placement of an intracaval filtration umbrella is not recommended.

Postpartum pulmonary embolism is treated with heparin followed by oral anticoagulants for 3 months.

MYOCARDIAL INFARCTION

Coronary disease is rare during pregnancy. When myocardial infarction occurs it is usually due to acute events in previously nonatheromatous coronary arteries, although coronary atheromatous disease in the presence of severe familial hypercholesterolemia or diabetes may cause angina or myocardial infarction during pregnancy. Because all the conditions that can give rise to myocardial infarction and heart failure during pregnancy are rare, there can be no consensus regarding management. Its incidence has been estimated to be about 1 in 10,000 pregnancies.

Myocardial infarction during pregnancy usually develops without preceding angina. The most frequent underlying mechanism is probably coronary artery dissection, but numerous other contributory pathogenic factors peculiar to or aggravated by pregnancy may be incriminated in the development of coronary artery occlusion (Table 26-3).

Dissection of the aorta is well recognized during pregnancy, but dissection may also occur in a coronary artery and lead to myocardial infarction. The dissection is nearly always in the left anterior descending coronary artery, and there is a high risk of sudden death. Spontaneous coronary artery dissection can also lead to severe chest pain or angina at rest without progressing to infarction. In a review of 134 cases of spontaneous coronary dissections, Kearney et al. found that more than two-thirds occurred in women, and one-third of the women were either pregnant or puerperal.[44] The cause may be weakening of the integument resulting from hormonal influences on vessel wall collagen synthesis, which may be depressed during pregnancy.

Ergot derivatives used for control of uterine hemorrhage or for termination of pregnancy[45,46] may cause acute chest pain followed by myocardial infarc-

tion, as in one of our patients. These vasoconstrictor agents can cause spasm of coronary arteries with endothelial breeches, attracting platelet aggregation and subsequent clot formation. Bromocriptine, another ergot derivative, has also been reported to cause spasm and infarction while being used to suppress lactation.[47]

Infarction due to metastases from choriocarcinoma and during curettage for hydatidiform mole are among the many reported causes of myocardial infarction complicating pregnancy.[48,49] Other causes suggested when there has been no obvious culprit include spontaneous coronary artery spasm and thrombosis and associated maternal preeclampsia, hypertension, and possible vasospasm triggered by renin release from the chorion.

Myocardial infarction is well recognized as a complication of polyarteritis nodosa, SLE, the antiphospholipid syndrome, and old Kawasaki disease.[50,51] It has been described in a patient with Still's disease who developed an infarct 12 weeks after delivery; in this patient coronary angiography 9 days after the event showed a thrombus in the coronary artery.[52]

Myocardial infarction in young drug abusers is being reported with increasing frequency and includes a pregnant woman who developed myocardial infarction temporally related to the use of "crack" cocaine.[53] Because of its increasing prevalence, cocaine use should be considered in any young patient with a sudden coronary event.

Other causes include coronary embolism from prosthetic valves, infective endocarditis, or mitral stenosis. A patient of ours, a 19-year-old immigrant Asian woman with tight mitral stenosis in sinus rhythm, developed acute posterobasal infarction attributable to coronary embolism when only 8 weeks pregnant. The coronary arteries were normal angiographically. After treatment for acute pulmonary congestion, the mitral stenosis was successfully relieved. Since then she has had two additional uneventful pregnancies and remains in sinus rhythm. Coronary embolism is well described as a complication of infective endocarditis, and myocardial infarction has been described during pregnancy in patients with prosthetic, aortic, or mitral valves. Myocardial infarction occurring during pregnancy in women with premature atherosclerotic disease, being less exotic, is probably underrepresented in the literature, accounting for only 9 of 70 cases reviewed by Hankins et al.[54]

Two-thirds of reported myocardial infarcts occurred during the third trimester perhaps because hemodynamic stress, changes in collagen, and hypercoagulability are all greatest late in pregnancy. Nearly all reported cases of infarction during preg-

Table 26-3. Myocardial Infarction During Pregnancy

Causes predisposed to or peculiar to pregnancy
  Coronary artery
    Dissection
    Spasm
    Thrombosis
  Drug-induced
    Ergotamine
    Prostaglandins
    Bromocriptine
  Preeclampsia
  Embolism from placenta

Causes coincidental to pregnancy
  Coronary atheroma
    Hypercholesterolemia
    Diabetes
  Coronary arteritis
    Polyarteritis nodosum
    Systemic lupus erythematosus
    Antiphospholipid syndrome
    Old Kawasaki disease
  Coronary embolism
    From prosthetic valve
    In mitral stenosis
    Left atrial myxoma
    Infective endocarditis
    Paradoxical
  Cocaine abuse

nancy and the postpartum period involve the anterior wall. This predilection for the anterior wall is probably due to the left anterior descending artery being most at risk from coronary dissection and possibly also from coronary embolism, the two most frequent causes of infarction at this time.

Total creatine kinase (CK) and CKMB isoenzyme levels are significantly elevated immediately postpartum owing to enzyme release from the uterus. Hence the diagnosis should be confirmed from ECG changes and elevation of other cardiac enzymes.[55]

Reports of coronary angiograms after myocardial infarction during pregnancy have usually stated that they appeared normal. This error is almost certainly because only a few such infarcts have been so investigated and these only late after the event. Coronary dissections might already have healed, an occlusive thrombus might have spontaneously lysed, or coronary spasm may have resolved. When abnormalities have been recognized, they were dissections or thrombi usually in the anterior descending artery. Normal coronary arteries were found at angiography in 74 patients after myocardial infarction by Raymond et al. who reported that 32 were women; and of these women 11 were either peripartum or on oral contraceptives or estrogens.[56] Smoking and altered hormonal state were the only risk factors identified.

The literature reviews have reported a mortality of 25–50 percent; but these reports were not recent, and the patients were not treated in a modern way. The mortality was found to be highest when the infarct occurred late, especially if it occurred during delivery or the early postpartum period.

Pregnancy is only a relative contraindication to the use of thrombolytic agents, and their use may be justified for large anterior infarcts. We have used streptokinase during pregnancy without problems; but because coronary dissection may be worsened by thrombolytic therapy, the mechanism of the infarct should, whenever possible, be clarified by immediate coronary angiography. A lytic agent can then be delivered locally if a thrombus is found, thereby minimizing the dose required and maximizing efficacy. Primary angioplasty should not be entertained, as most of these coronary thromboses occur in previously normal arteries. Infarction resulting from coronary artery spasm may be treated by intracoronary vasodilators but is not likely to benefit from thrombolytics unless local thrombosis has resulted. Thrombus in the false lumen of a dissection can compress the true lumen, causing obstruction; successful use of intracoronary streptokinase has been reported for iatrogenic coronary dissection. It may be possible to seal off a small dissection by stenting; but for major dissections threatening the entire anterior descend-

ing territory, urgent coronary bypass is indicated despite the risk to the fetus. Both percutaneous angioplasty and coronary artery bypass grafting have been performed safely during pregnancy. β-Blockers should be started as soon as possible after the infarct to reduce the risk of arrhythmias, limit infarct size, and reduce the risk of cardiac rupture. ACE inhibitors are relatively contraindicated but should be given if there has been major infarction. Management of arrhythmias is largely the same as for nonpregnant patients, and DC cardioversion can be carried out safely without fetal risk.

In the event of ventricular fibrillation during the latter part of pregnancy, the uterus causes significant aorta caval compression and should be displaced laterally during resuscitation. In the event of failure of resuscitative measures, emergency cesarean section should be carried out within 15 minutes.

Every effort should be made to maintain the pregnancy until the infarct has healed. β-Blockers should be continued during delivery to reduce myocardial oxygen demand. Cesarean section is performed if there is any doubt about a speedy delivery or if the left ventricle is compromised.

HYPERTENSION AND TOXEMIA

Toxemia of pregnancy (gestational hypertension) is a multisystem vascular disorder of unknown origin arising late during pregnancy or immediately after delivery. It is characterized by a rise in blood pressure, peripheral edema, and proteinuria (preeclampsia). In its more severe form, seizures and encephalopathy may occur (eclampsia). It is most common in primigravidas with a family history of toxemia. It should be distinguished from essential and renal hypertension, although each may be complicated by eclampsia.[57,58]

The onset is most often heralded by rapid weight gain followed by edema. The edema typically involves the face and hands, which appear puffy, and not just the feet, where edema is common during normal pregnancy. The onset is usually after the 32nd week of pregnancy but is sometimes earlier in patients with preexisting renal disease.[59] Toxemia is rare during the first trimester; but when it occurs it is usually associated with a hydatidiform mole. Apart from the rise in blood pressure, the cardiac examination is usually normal, although in severe cases left ventricular failure and pulmonary edema may develop. Preexisting essential hypertension is usually but not always present during the first trimester and is associated with a gradual rather than a rapid gain in weight and edema; the blood pressure, although higher, is better tolerated. Moreover, essential hypertension persists after delivery, whereas the manifestations of preeclampsia including the elevated blood pressure usually resolve immediately with delivery. Only rarely is toxemia observed during the postpartum period.

The development of toxemia is associated with an unexplained increase in the usually wide open peripheral vascular resistance. It results in reduced utero/placental perfusion, fetal hypoxia, and intrauterine starvation.[60,61]

A major difficulty in the diagnosis and management of hypertensive disorders during pregnancy is a lack of agreement on definition and classification.

1. Chronic hypertension is blood pressure above 140/90 mmHg during the first trimester.
2. Pregnancy-induced hypertension is an increase in systolic blood pressure by 30 mmHg or in diastolic blood pressure by 15 mmHg above the first trimester level.
3. Preeclampsia is the appearance of edema, proteinuria of more than 0.5 g in 24 hours, plus a rise in blood pressure above 140/90 mmHg usually after the 24th week of pregnancy.
4. Eclampsia is the development of fits, disseminated intravascular coagulation, hypertensive crisis, renal failure, and coma.
5. Chronic hypertension with superimposed preeclampsia is blood pressure elevation more than 30/15 mmHg above the usual level.

Whatever the classification, pregnant women with proteinuria plus hypertension are at much greater risk than those with high blood pressure alone. The most definitive approach to differentiation between the groups is renal biopsy, but this invasive procedure carries a high risk of hemorrhage. The diagnostic finding on renal biopsy is renal glomeruloepitheliosis.

One cause for the diagnostic confusion is the fall in peripheral vascular resistance and blood pressure early in pregnancy followed by a rise toward prepregnancy levels during the third trimester. A patient with undetected chronic hypertension could present during early pregnancy with a normal blood pressure only to be misdiagnosed as having preeclampsia when the blood pressure rises during the third trimester. This situation is particularly likely if the blood pressure elevation is accompanied by some edema, even though it is seen in 80 percent of normal pregnancies.[62]

Although methyldopa has the track safety record, the drug of choice for the treatment of severe hypertension during pregnancy including hypertensive heart failure may be labetolol.[63] Though predominantly a β-adrenergic blocking drug, it also has α-blocking properties and induces vasodilatation, which is particularly beneficial for the uteroplacental vasculature. Diuretics are best avoided during pregnancy and are indicated only for the treatment of hypertension complicated by heart failure and for hypervolemic secondary hypertension. Both labetolol and diuretics pass the placental barrier.

REFERENCES

1. Robson SC, Hunter S, Boys RJ, Dunlop W: Serial study of factors influencing changes in cardiac output during human pregnancy. Am J Physiol 1989;25b: H1060–H1050
2. Lung CJ, Donovan JC: Blood volume during pregnancy. Significance of plasma and red cell volume. Am J Obstet Gynecol 1967;98:393
3. Knuttgen HG, Emerson K Jr: Physiological response to pregnancy at rest and during exercise. J Appl Physiol 1974;36:549
4. Katz R, Karliner JS, Resnik R: Effects of a natural volume overload state (pregnancy) on left ventricular performance in normal human subjects. Circulation 1978;58:434
5. Rubler S, Damani M, Pinter ER: Cardiac size and performance during pregnancy estimated with echocardiography. Am J Cardiol 1977;40:534
6. Lees MM, Taylor SH, Scott DB et al: A study of cardiac output at rest throughout pregnancy. J Obstet Gynaecol Br Commonw 1967;74:319
7. Robson SC, Hunter S, Boys RJ, Dunlop W: Hemodynamic changes during twin pregnancy. A Doppler and M-mode echocardiographic study. Am J Obstet Gynecol 1989;161:1273–1278
8. Robson SC, Boys RJ, Hunter S, Dunlop W: Maternal hemodynamics after normal delivery and delivery complicated by postpartum haemorrhage. Obstet Gynecol 1989;74:234–239
9. Robson S, Hunter S, Boys R, Dunlop W, Bryson M: Changes in cardiac output during epidural anaesthesia for caesarean section. Anaesthesia 1989;44:465–479
10. Sugrue D, Blake S, Troy P et al: Antibiotic prophylaxis against infective endocarditis after normal delivery—is it necessary? Br Heart J 1980;44:499
11. Singh H, Bolton PJ, Oakley CM: Outcome of pregnancy after surgical correction of tetralogy of Fallot. BMJ 1983;285:168
12. Meyer EC, Tulsky AS, Sigmann P, Siber EN: Pregnancy in the presence of tetralogy of Fallot. Am J Cardiol 1984;14:874
13. Stiller RJ, Vintzileos AM, Nochimson DJ et al: Single ventricle in pregnancy. Case report and review of the literature. Obstet Gynecol 1984;64:185
14. Oakley CM: Congenital heart disease in pregnancy. pp. 131–144. In Zipes DP, Rowlands DJ (eds) Lea & Febiger, Philadelphia, 1992
15. McIvor RA: Percutaneous balloon aortic valuloplasty during pregnancy. Int J Cardiol 1991;32:1–4
16. Banning AP, Pearson JF, Hall RJC: Role of balloon dilatation of the aortic valve in pregnant patients with severe aortic stenosis. Br Heart J 1993;70:544–545

17. Morgan-Jones A, Howitt G: Eisenmenger syndrome in pregnancy. BMJ 1965;1:1627
18. Gleicher N, Midwall J, Hochberger D, Jaffin H: Eisenmenger's syndrome in pregnancy. Obstet Gynecol Surv 1979;34:721–741
19. Spinnato JA, Kraynak BJ, Cooper MW: Eisenmenger's syndrome in pregnancy. N Engl J Med 1981;304:1215
20. Waickman LA, Skorton DJ, Varner MW, Ehmke DA, Goplerud CP: Ebstein's anomaly and pregnancy. Am J Cardiol 1984;53:357
21. Oakley GDG, McGarry K, Limb DC, Oakley CM: Management of pregnancy in patients with hypertrophic cardiomyopathy. BMJ 1979;37:305–312
22. Shah DM, Sundderji SG: Hypertrophic cardiomyopathy in pregnancy. Report of the maternal mortality and revision of the literature. Obstet Gynecol Surv 1985;40:444
23. Laurent M, Betremicux P, Biron Y, Lellelloco A: Neonatal hypothyroidism after treatment by amiodarone during pregnancy. Am J Cardiol 1987;60:142
24. Foster CJ, Love HG: Amiodarone in pregnancy. Case report and review of literature. Int J Cardiol 1988;20:307
25. Julian DG, Szekely P: Peripartum cardiomyopathy. Prog Cardiovasc Dis 1985;27:223
26. Homans DC: Peripartum cardiomyopathy. N Engl J Med 1985;312:1432
27. Midei MG, DeMent SH, Feldman AM et al: Peripartum myocarditis and cardiomyopathy. Circulation 1990;81:922–928
28. Pierce JA, Price BO, Joyce JW: Familial occurrence of postpartal heart failure. Arch Intern Med 1963;111:651
29. Sanderson JE, Adesanya CO, Anjorin FI, Parry EHO: Postpartum cardiac failure. Heart failure due to volume overload? Am Heart J 1979;97:613
30. Sanderson JE, Woo KS: Rheumatic fever and rheumatic heart disease. Declining but not gone. Int J Cardiol 1994;43:231–232
31. Ayoub EM: Resurgence of rheumatic fever in the United States. The clinical picture of preventable disease. Postgrad Med J 1992;92:133–136
32. Narasimhan C, Joseph G, Singh TC: Propranolol for pulmonary oedema in mitral stenosis. Int J Cardiol 1994;44:178–179
33. Cohen JM, Glower DD, Harrison JK et al: Comparison of balloon valvuloplasty with operative treatment for mitral stenosis. Ann Thorac Surg 1993;56:1254–1262
34. Oakley CM: Anticoagulants in pregnancy. Br Heart J 1995;74:107–111
35. Sbarouni E, Oakley CM: Outcome of pregnancy in women with valve prostheses. Br Heart J 1994;71:196–201
36. Cotrufo M, de Luca TSL, Calabro R, Mastrogiovanni G, Lama D: Coumarin anticoagulation during pregnancy in patients with mechanical valve prostheses. Eur J Cardiol Surg 1991;5:300–305
37. Hanania G, Thomas D, Michel PL et al: Pregnancy in patients with valvular prostheses. Retrospective cooperative study in France (155 cases). Arch Mal Coeur Vaiss 1994;87:429–437
38. Renzulli A, De Luca L, Caruso A et al: Acute thrombosis of prosthetic valves. A multivariate analysis of the risk factors for a life threatening event. Eur J Cardiothorac Surg 1992;6:412–421
39. Birdi I, Angelini GD, Bryan AJ: Thrombolytic therapy for left sided prosthetic heart valve thrombosis. J Heart Valve Dis 1995;4:154–159
40. Mazzucco A, Milan A, Mazzaro E, Bortolotti U: Reoperation in patients with a bioprosthesis in the mitral position. Indications and early results. J Heart Valve Dis 1993;2:646–648
41. Katz NM, Collea JV, Moront MG, MacKenzie RD, Wallace RB: Aortic dissections during pregnancy. Am J Cardiol 1984;54:699
42. Eagles KA, De Sanctis RW: Diseases of the aorta. In Braunwald E (ed): Heart Disease. Saunders, Philadelphia, 1992
43. Brady AJB, Crake T, Oakley CM: Percutaneous catheter fragmentation and distal dispersion of proximal pulmonary embolism. Lancet 1991;338:1186–1189
44. Kearney P, Singh H, Hutter J et al: Spontaneous coronary artery d issection. A report of three cases and review of the literature. Postgrad Med J 1993;69:940–945
45. Liao JK, Cockrill BA, Yurchak PM: Acute myocardial infarction after ergonovine administration for uterine bleeding. Am J Cardiol 1991;68:823–824
46. Fjiwara Y, Yamanaka O, Nakamura T, Yokoi H, Yamaguchi H: Acute myocardial infarction induced by ergonovine administration for artificially induced abortion. Jpn Heart J 1993;34:803–808
47. Iffy L, TenHove W, Frisoli G: Acute myocardial infarction in the puerperium in patients receiving bromocriptine. Am J Obstet Gynecol 1986;155:371–372
48. Akaike A, Ito T, Sada T et al: Myocardial infarction due to metastasis of choriocarcinoma in a 29 year old woman. Jpn Circ J 1977;41:1257–1263
49. Asada M, Nakayama K, Yamaguchi O, Kudo I: A case of myocardial infarction associated with pulmonary edema during curettage for hydatidiform mole. Jpn J Anaesthesiol 1991;40:113–118
50. Nolan TE, Hankins GD: Myocardial infarction in pregnancy. Clin Obstet Gynaecol 1989;32:66–75
51. Rallings P, Exner T, Abraham R: Coronary artery vasculitis and myocardial infarction associated with antiphospholipid antibodies in a pregnant woman. Aust NZ J Med 1989;19:347–350
52. Parry G, Goudevenos J, Williams DO: Coronary thrombosis postpartum in a young woman with Still's disease. Clin Cardiol 1992;15:305–307
53. Liu SS, Forrester RM, Murphy GS, Chen K, Glassenberg R: Anaesthetic management of a parturient with myocardial infarction related to cocaine use. Can J Anaesth 1992;39:858–861
54. Hankins GDV, Wendel GD Jr, Leveno KJ et al: Myocardial infarction during pregnancy. A review. Obstet Gynecol 1985;65:139
55. Leiserowitz GS, Evans AT, Samuels SJ, Oman K, Kost GJ: Creatine kinase and its MB isoenzyme in the third trimester and the peripartum period. J Reprod Med 1992;37:910–916
56. Raymond R, Lynch J, Underwood D, Leatherman J, Razavi M: Myocardial infarction and normal coronary arteriography. A 10 year clinical and risk analysis of 74 patients. J Am Coll Cardiol 1988;11:471–477
57. O'Brien WF: Predicting pre-eclampsia. Obstet Gynecol 1990;75:445
58. Guzick DS, Klein VR, Tyson JE et al: Risk factors for the occurrence of pregnancy-induced hypertension. Clin Exp Hypertens 1987;B6:281
59. Ihle BU, Long P, Oats J: Early onset pre-eclampsia.

Recognition of underlying renal disease. BMJ 1987; 294:79

60. Mabie WC, Ratts TE, Sibai BM: The central haemodynamics of severe preeclampsia. Am J Obstet Gynecol 1989;161:1443

61. Loquet PH, Broughton Pipkin F, Symonds EM, Rubin PC: Influence of raising maternal blood pressure with angiotensin II on utero-placental and feto-placental blood velocity indices in the human. Clin Sci 1990;78: 95

62. Mabie WC, Pernoll ML, Biswas MK: Chronic hypertension in pregnancy. Obstet Gynecol 1986;67:197

63. Nader RP, Redman WG: Antihypertensive drugs in pregnancy. Clin Perinatol 1985;12, 521

27 Hypertrophic Cardiomyopathy

Aman S. Coonar
William J. McKenna

Hypertrophic cardiomyopathy (HCM) was first described more than 120 years ago.[1,2] Sporadic reports followed, for example of a child of 3 months who died after a crying fit and subsequently was found to have had a "diffuse tumor of the lateral wall of the left ventricle."[3] Detailed characterization waited until 1958 when, based on the autopsy findings of nine adolescents and young adults who had died suddenly, Donald Teare at St. George's Hospital, London reported "asymmetrical hypertrophy of the heart."[4]

DEFINITION

Advances in knowledge presaged by new diagnostic tools have been reflected in myriad nomenclature, currently standing at more than 75 titles.[5] The definition in contemporary use remains one of exclusion—"cardiomyopathies are heart muscle diseases of unknown cause"—and is largely reliant on techniques of clinical assessment: Hypertrophic cardiomyopathy is "characterized by disproportionate hypertrophy of the left ventricle and occasionally also of the right ventricle which typically involves the septum more than the free wall but occasionally is concentric. Typically the left ventricular volume is normal or reduced. Systolic gradients are common."[6]

Such a definition is increasingly considered inadequate. It has been based on a pattern of disease seen in selected tertiary centers and reflects the status of the technology available. Advances in determining the molecular basis of the disease, accompanied by improvements in clinical diagnostic methods, have delivered the concept of a broader, often subtle phenotype. The challenge for future definitions is to combine the clinical and molecular facets into classifications useful for diagnosis and treatment.

EPIDEMIOLOGY

Hypertrophic cardiomyopathy has been described in Western, African, and Asian groups. As most investigations have been directed toward affected pedigrees, precise population data are unknown. It is estimated that HCM affects up to 1 in 1000 live births. This figure may rise further with increasing recognition of HCM as a cause of stillbirths and deaths during early childhood,[7] the recognition of unsuspected "latent" disease in adults, especially the elderly,[8,9] and as molecular-genetic screening becomes available as a diagnostic tool. There is also evidence that disease expression may vary among ethnic groups.[10,11]

PATHOLOGY

Macroscopic Appearance

Cardiac hypertrophy (Plate 27-1) is common but varies widely in severity and distribution. Most characteristically the left ventricle is affected with asymmetric hypertrophy predominantly involving the septum, leaving the ventricular cavity small or normal in size.[12] Hypertrophy affecting the left ventricular apex may be more common in Japanese patients.[1,10] Whether this is due to environmental or genetic factors or simply represents different diagnostic criteria or referral patterns is unknown.

Though hypertrophy may occur at any age and without obvious stimulus,[13] it is not often present prior to the adolescent acceleration in growth. In infants and children the disease is usually associated with marked septal hypertrophy, severe biventricular outflow obstruction, progressive cardiac failure, and a poor prognosis.[13-15] Hypertrophy does not usually become more severe after the end of adolescence, when most growth has already been achieved.[16] Overall left ventricular hypertrophy is considerably more severe in young than in old patients, and there is an inverse relation between left ventricular wall thickness and age.[17] If the right ventricle is involved, the pattern tends to be symmetrically concentric and often correlates closely with the degree of left-sided involvement.[18] In addition, in some patients progressive ventricular wall thinning accompanied by cardiac dilatation and systolic failure, occurs.[16,19]

Identification of specific gene mutations causing HCM has also led to the observation that the severity of hypertrophy associated with mutations in the cardiac troponin T gene is less than that associated with mutations in the β-MHC gene.[20] There is some correlation between the severity of the hypertrophy and symptoms and with sudden death. Associated with myocardial hypertrophy is atrial enlargement, thickening of the mitral valve leaflets, patchy fibrosis of the ventricular wall, and a patch of endocardial thickening just below the aortic valve arising from contact with the anterior mitral valve leaflet.

Microscopic Appearance

Disorganization of myocyte ultrastructure, myofibrils, and muscle bundles is accompanied by variable, often marked interstitial fibrosis[21,22] (Plate 27-2). Myocardial cells may be wide, short, and of bizarre shape.[23] The changes may be discontinuous, with foci of disorganized cells scattered among areas of apparently normal hypertrophied muscle cells. Experienced pathologists consider that myocardial disarray affecting more than 5 percent of the sections obtained from the ventricular septum is a sensitive, specific marker for HCM.[24,25] Such histologic abnormalities may also be found at postmortem examination of nonhypertrophied hearts,[26] which may have been associated with largely normal echocardiograms. This again demonstrates our view of a far

broader disease phenotype than previously recognized.

Immunostaining of heart sections from patients with HCM reveals an abnormal distribution of gap junctions, with apparently random expression over the myocyte surface (Plate 27-3). The failure of restriction of gap junctions to the intercalated discs may contribute to electrical instability and abnormal contractile function.

Abnormalities of small intramural coronary arteries are found in the presence of normal epicardial vessels. The abnormal arteries are mainly in the septum and have thickened walls and narrow lumens, largely due to the proliferation of medial or intimal components, or both (particularly smooth muscle cells and collagen). Increased numbers of arteries may be seen within or at margins of areas of fibrosis,[27,28] possibly reflecting a response to a chronic, intermittent ischemic process. Changes consistent with myocardial infarction are also seen[29,30] and may be a substrate for later fibrosis.

It has been reported that histologic changes in skeletal muscle resembling central core disease may be found in HCM due to β-MHC mutations.[31] Central core disease of skeletal muscle is a rare autosomal dominant nonprogressive myopathy characterized by a predominance of type I "slow" fibers and an absence of mitochondria in the center of many type I fibers. Myocyte disarray and disorganization in a pattern similar to that of HCM may also be found in Noonan syndrome[32,33] as may ventricular hypertrophy. Otherwise the diseases are dissimilar. In Noonan syndrome the degree of hypertrophy is usually not severe, the prognosis is different, and linkage to chromosome 12q22-qter has been identified.[34]

Mitral Valve Abnormalities

There is evidence not only of functional mitral valve abnormalities (systolic anterior motion) but also of structural abnormalities.[35-39] The mitral valve of HCM patients may be larger than that of normal persons with a greater contribution from the anterior leaflet. Anomalous insertion of the papillary muscle into the anterior leaflet may cause structural obstruction to flow during systole. There may also be an increased rate of mitral valve prolapse in patients with HCM, though there is some controversy over whether this feature is more frequent than in the general population.[40,41]

PATHOPHYSIOLOGY

A constellation of factors contribute to the pathophysiology of HCM. They are hypertrophy, hyperdynamic function, outflow tract gradients, diastolic dysfunction, mitral valve abnormalities, ischemia, late systolic cardiac failure, arrhythmia, thromboembolism, and abnormal autonomic function.

Hypertrophy

The mechanism inducing hypertrophy is not fully known. It is possible that, arising from mutations in the genes for sarcomeric elements, the aberrant protein products result in abnormal velocity–force relations, with hypertrophy occurring as a secondary rather than a primary response. Hypertrophy contributes to both diastolic and systolic function and is associated with increased metabolic demands and therefore probably ischemia. The factors that cause one pattern or another are unknown.[42] That hypertrophy is only rarely present before puberty suggests that it is partly contingent on the neuroendocrine processes occurring at that time.

Hyperdynamic Function

Most patients have hyperdynamic systolic function with early, rapid, and often nearly complete ventricular emptying. This situation may occur in the absence of hypertrophy and so is not purely a reflection of increased muscle mass. It has been suggested that it is due to abnormalities of myocardial calcium handling.[43,44] Abnormalities of systolic function may act to increase myocardial oxygen consumption, and it may induce or be a manifestation of isoform changes in myocardial structural or metabolic proteins. The chronic effects of an increase in wall stress may contribute to this process.

Outflow Tract Gradient

Approximately 30 percent of patients have resting left ventricular outflow tract gradients.[45–48] Another 25 percent develop an outflow tract gradient following measures that increase contractility (effect of sympathomimetic drugs) or reduce the left ventricular cavity size by reducing afterload (vasodilator) or venous return (venodilators, the Valsalva maneuver, or hypovolemia).[49] Conversely, an increase in afterload (squatting or vasoconstrictor agents) or venous return (filling) or a decrease in myocardial contractility (β-blockers or calcium antagonists) may reduce the outflow gradient. The presence and severity of gradients is labile, and regression may occur. Because it occurs relatively late during systole the gradient does not usually significantly limit stroke volume except when severe.

Factors contributing to the genesis of outflow tract gradients include (1) hyperdynamic left ventricular ejection, producing a high velocity jet and causing a relative fall in outflow tract pressure (Venturi effect) sucking the mitral valve leaflets into it and thus toward the septum (systolic anterior motion)[42,50,51]; (2) hypertrophy of the septum[52,53]; (3) anomalous mitral valve and papillary muscle architecture.[37,53,54]

Diastolic Dysfunction

Studies of left ventricular function have identified abnormalities in relaxation and filling that are present in most (approximately 80 percent) patients with HCM and are independent of the presence or absence of cardiac symptoms or an outflow tract gradient.[55]

The period during which the heart is isovolumetric (end-systole and early diastole) is prolonged, filling is slow, and the proportion of filling volume that results from atrial systole may be increased. Occasionally a pattern is seen similar to that of a restrictive state when early filling is rapid but then is abruptly curtailed.

The mechanism of diastolic dysfunction is unknown but may arise from factors determining the passive elastic properties of the ventricular chamber (severity of hypertrophy, fibrosis, myocyte disarray) and from those affecting the rate and extent of active left ventricular relaxation. Abnormal diastolic function reduces left ventricular filling and so contributes to reduced stroke volume and possibly abnormal compressive effects on the intramural vasculature.

Diastolic dysfunction correlates only poorly with the patient's professed symptomatic status or exercise capacity measured objectively.[56] However, impairment of diastolic left ventricular function is a risk marker for disease-related death.[57,58]

Mitral Regurgitation

Malposition of the mitral valve during midsystole (due to systolic anterior motion of the mitral valve), structural mitral valve abnormalities, and high intraventricular pressures also contribute to mitral regurgitation, which is often present, especially in the presence of an outflow tract gradient.

Myocardial Ischemia

Chest pain is commonly reported with HCM.[59] Resting and exercise electrocardiograms (ECGs) are associated with abnormalities consistent with ischemia,[60] but interpretation is complicated by ventricular hypertrophy. Abnormalities of perfusion are suggested by thallium scans, but correlation between symptoms and changes suggestive of ischemia using these modalities is limited by poor resolution.[60-62] Positron emission tomography is being evaluated and supports the presence of ischemia in patients with HCM.[63,64] Pacing or dipyridamole-induced tachycardia has been shown to cause the development of chest pain accompanied by increased lactate production, as sampled from the coronary sinus in patients with HCM.[60] This point strongly supports a predisposition to ischemia, possibly caused by increased myocardial bulk, abnormal metabolism, or vasculature. The presence of patchy, diffuse fibrosis, as well as changes of myocardial infarction, also support an ischemic process.

Rhythm Disturbance

Abnormalities of myocardial structure, intercellular communication, perfusion, and metabolism contribute to an environment conducive to the development of rhythm disturbances. Patients with HCM have increased rates of paroxysmal supraventricular tachycardia, atrial fibrillation, and reentrant tachyarrhythmia arising from accessory pathways. Ventricular tachycardia and ventricular fibrillation also occur commonly.[65-69]

Modulators of rhythm disturbance may be abnormal autonomic activity and peripheral vascular responses. Several of the clinical features of HCM (e.g., hyperdynamic left ventricular function, atrial and ventricular arrhythmias, and the clinical response to β-blockers) are shared with other disorders characterized by sympathetic overactivity,[70] and in animal models catecholamines induce myocyte hypertrophy.[71] Evidence for autonomic disturbance comes from different avenues. Studies of heart rate variability show loss of diurnal variation[72] with a reduction in the parasympathetic contribution. Investigation of myocardial catecholamine[73] and β-receptor metabolism[63] reveals abnormalities. Peripheral vascular responses have also been found to be abnormal. Frenneaux et al.[74] demonstrated that the systolic blood pressure response during symptom-limited exercise testing was abnormal (i.e., failed to rise more than 20 mmHg or fell from baseline values) in 33 percent. The presence of a pressure-dependent vasodepressor response in patients with HCM may explain the poor tolerance of paroxysmal arrhythmia or sinus tachycardia seen in some patients. In patients with a particular susceptibility, systemic hypotension may also cause a fall in myocardial perfusion pressure with consequent metabolic changes that may trigger ventricular arrhythmia.

Endocarditis

There is an increased risk of infective endocarditis in patients with hypertrophic cardiomyopathy.[75] The areas affected tend to be the mitral valve, the septum at the proposed site of contact with the mitral valve during systolic anterior motion, and the noncoronary cusp of the aortic valve at the septum. Endocarditis may also occur after surgery for myotomy/myectomy, mitral valve replacement, or pacemaker insertion. Antibiotic prophylaxis and dental toilet is advisable in appropriate patients, particularly those with a significant left ventricular outflow tract gradient or valvlar regurgitation.

CLINICAL FEATURES

Presentation

Presentation may be at any age, and the diagnosis is often made during family screening after the sudden death of a close relative. The patient may be asymptomatic or have any combination of symptoms (chest pain, shortness of breath on exertion or at rest, syncope, or palpitation). Occasionally HCM is found at autopsy in a stillborn infant or presents with cardiac failure in an infant (usually fatal).[13-15,59,76] Paroxysmal symptoms and mild impairment of exercise tolerance are common, especially in children. In contrast, approximately 50 percent of consecutive adult patients present with symptoms.[59] Approximately half of the patients experience dyspnea,[59,77] thought to result from elevated left atrial and pulmonary venous pressures consequent on impaired ventricular relaxation and filling. The relation between these parameters and functional capacity is not simple. In one study, there was no relation between maximal exercise capacity and pulmonary capillary wedge pressure, suggesting that as with cardiac failure other mechanisms such as control of muscle energetic and blood flow and a central perception of breathlessness may be important.[78] Approximately half of the patients complain of chest pain that is atypical, exertional, or both.[59,79-82] Atypical pain may have no obvious precipitant or more commonly, may follow exercise or anxiety-induced tachycardia; in the latter case it may persist for several hours after the stress has been removed without evidence of myocardial infarction. Approximately 15 percent of patients have syncopal episodes. In only a few are there findings suggestive of arrhythmia or overt conduction disease.[59] In most patients the mechanism cannot be determined. Contributory factors include infrequent rhythm disturbance, abnormal autonomic and peripheral vascular responses, and impaired hemodynamic performance. The latter is more likely in the presence of marked outflow obstruction and in some series is improved by myotomy/myectomy.[83] Rarely patients present with symptoms attributable to left or right heart failure with paroxysmal nocturnal dyspnea, cough, peripheral edema, or abdominal discomfort associated with hepatomegaly. Thus there is a wide spectrum of clinical features, which may vary from severe cardiac failure during infancy to an incidental finding that may occur at any age.

Physical Examination

In most patients physical examination is unremarkable. Subtle signs may be the only clinical clue to the diagnosis. Most patients have a rapid upstroke arterial pulse, best felt in the carotid area reflecting dynamic left ventricular emptying. In the young it may be difficult to distinguish from normal, whereas in the elderly the normal pulse transmitted from the arteriosclerotic vessel may appear to have a rapid upstroke. Most patients also have a forceful, brief left ventricular cardiac impulse, best appreciated on full expiration with the patient in the left lateral position. This impulse may be preceded by a palpable beat corresponding to forceful left atrial contraction immediately prior to left ventricular systole. One-third of patients demonstrate a prominent "a" wave in the jugular venous pressure wave, reflecting right atrial hypertrophy in response to the diminished right ventricular compliance associated with diastolic abnormalities and right ventricular hypertrophy. The first and second heart sounds are usually normal; and, providing the patient is in sinus rhythm, there may be a loud fourth heart sound.

An ejection systolic murmur is heard in the one-third of patients who have a resting left ventricular (LV) outflow tract gradient. It is best heard at the left sternal border and radiates toward the aortic and mitral areas but not into the neck or axilla. The intensity of this murmur varies with changes in ventricular volume: It can be increased by physiologic or pharmacologic maneuvers that reduce afterload or venous return and decreased by maneuvers that increase afterload and venous return. Occasionally ejection systolic murmurs are associated at their onset with an ejection sound.

Most patients with an LV gradient also have mitral regurgitation, which may be difficult to hear on auscultation. Doppler examination reveals that mitral regurgitation begins 30–40 ms before the onset of the gradient and then continues through the remainder of systole. Radiation of the systolic murmur to the axilla may be the best clue to the presence of mitral regurgitation. Occasionally the mitral regurgitation is moderate to severe, either alone or in the absence of an LV outflow tract gradient; or it may be associated with the development of infective endocarditis. A mid-diastolic rumble may result from increased transmitral flow in patients with severe mitral regurgitation; more commonly it occurs in isolation, reflecting inflow tract turbulence. Early diastolic murmurs of aortic incompetence may develop following surgical myotomy/myectomy or after ineffective endocarditis involving the aortic valve. An ejection systolic murmur in the pulmonary area reflecting right ventricular outflow tract obstruction is also uncommon; if present, it usually reflects severe biventricular hypertrophy and is more commonly heard in the young.[13–15,59]

INVESTIGATIONS

Assessment aims to clarify the diagnosis, characterize the extent of the abnormality, and determine prognosis.

Electrocardiography

Electrocardiographic abnormalities increase with age and disease severity. The 12-lead ECG is normal in 5 percent of symptomatic patients and in 25 percent of asymptomatic patients.[84,85] At diagnosis, 10 percent of patients are in atrial fibrillation, 20 percent have left axis deviation, and 5 percent have a right bundle branch block pattern.[59,85] Most patients have an intraventricular conduction delay; but complete left bundle branch block pattern is rare, though it may develop after surgery or as a late complication. ST segment depression and T wave changes are the commonest abnormalities and are usually associated with voltage changes of left ventricular hypertrophy (LVH), deep S waves in the anterior chest leads V_1–V_3, or both.[85] Occasionally giant negative T waves are seen.[86] Repolarization changes alone or isolated voltage criteria for LVH are unusual. Approximately 20 percent of patients have abnormal Q waves inferiorly (II, III and aVF) or less commonly in leads V_1–V_3.[87,88] Abnormal Q waves on the 12-lead ECG may reflect right ventricular wall thickness and upper anterior septal thickness. The distribution of the PR interval is similar to that seen in the normal population, but occasionally a short PR interval is associated with a slurred upstroke to the QRS complex, similar to that seen in the Wolff-

Parkinson-White (WPW) syndrome. Of great interest has been the report of a single gene locus associated with HCM or WPW (or both) in a single family.[89] P wave abnormalities of left or right atrial overload are common. In summary, there is no ECG characteristic of HCM; but in the presence of a suggestive history the significance of any ECG abnormality becomes correspondingly greater.

In adults rhythm disturbances are common during 48-hour ambulatory ECG monitoring.[69,90–94] Nonsustained ventricular tachycardia is detected in 25–30 percent of adults. Though almost always asymptomatic, its detection represents an approximately seven-fold increase in the risk of sudden death above those who do not manifest this abnormality.[91,95,96] Established atrial fibrillation is detected in 10–15 percent of consecutive patients; another 30 percent have episodes of paroxysmal atrial fibrillation or supraventricular tachycardia.[59,93] Sustained supraventricular arrhythmias (> 30 seconds) are poorly tolerated unless the ventricular response is controlled, and they carry a risk of embolism.[97] In contrast, most children and adolescents are in sinus rhythm, and rhythm disturbances during ambulatory monitoring are uncommon.[76] Development of these arrhythmias is not surprising, as they are related to the partly age-dependent increase in LV end-diastolic pressure and atrial dimension.[13,17,98] The precise etiology of nonsustained ventricular arrhythmias is not known, but it is assumed that the changes described in the section on pathophysiology become worse with age. The occurrence of documented sustained ventricular tachycardia is rare.[68,69] The optimal duration and the method of ECG monitoring to detect asymptomatic but prognostically important ventricular arrhythmia clearly depends on the frequency at which they occur. Ventricular rhythm disturbances have been shown to have marked biologic variability. At the initial evaluation 120 hours of ECG monitoring is needed to ensure a 75 percent chance of not missing nonsustained ventricular tachycardia.[69] The recommendation of 48 hours, possibly repeated more than once, is practiced by many centers and represents a pragmatic compromise.[99]

Two-Dimensional Echocardiography/Doppler Studies

Two-dimensional echocardiography can be used to assess the severity and distribution of hypertrophy. LVH is most commonly asymmetric and localized to the septum and free wall with relative sparing of the posterior wall, although it may be symmetric or have a patchy distribution. In Japan hypertrophy of the apical region is more common.[11,100,101] In the West hypertrophy confined to the apex is rare, although approximately 10 percent of patients have LVH that is maximal in the distal ventricle from the level of the papillary muscles down.[102] Approximately one-third of patients also have hypertrophy of the right ventricular free wall, the severity of which corresponds closely with the severity of LVH.[18] Typically, LV end-systolic and end-diastolic dimensions are reduced, and the left atrial dimension is increased. Ejection fraction and fiber shortening velocity are increased. The LV outflow tract appears narrowed, particularly in the presence of gross upper septal hypertrophy; and right ventricular dimensions are normal. Color Doppler scanning is a sensitive method for detecting LV outflow tract turbulence. Moreover, when combined with continuous-wave Doppler scanning the peak velocity of LV blood flow can be measured and the LV outflow tract gradient calculated.[51,103–105]

Doppler gradients correlate well with those measured invasively. When the calculated outflow-tract gradient is more than 30 mmHg, systolic anterior motion of the mitral valve is usually observed.[106,107] This motion is well demonstrated on M-mode echocardiography as well as on two-dimensional studies. Measurement of the time from the onset of systolic anterior motion (SAM) to the onset of SAM-septal contact and the duration of SAM-septal contact provides another reliable noninvasive measure of the pressure gradient.[107,108]

Early closure or fluttering of the aortic valve leaflets and Doppler evidence of mitral regurgitation are often seen in association with SAM. Contrary to previous reports, SAM is not pathognomonic of HCM and may be found with other conditions associated with LVH and hyperdynamic systolic performance, such as hypertensive heart disease.[109,110] SAM of the posterior mitral valve leaflet has also been observed[38] in up to 10 percent of patients and can contribute to dynamic outflow tract obstruction.

Exercise Testing

Maximal exercise testing is simple, is noninvasive, and provides useful functional and possibly prognostic information. When used in conjunction with respiratory gas analysis, it provides an objective assessment of exercise capacity that can be monitored serially. Maximal oxygen ventilatory capacity is moderately reduced even in patients who claim that their exercise tolerance is unlimited.[78] Continuous blood pressure monitoring reveals that approximately one-third of patients have an abnormal blood pressure response, with drops of 25–150 mmHg from peak values.[74] The mechanism is not fully elucidated but may relate to abnormal peripheral vascular responses to exercise.[111] In most patients such changes are asymptomatic, but preliminary observations suggest that they may be of prognostic significance.[77,99]

Cardiac Catheterization

Cardiac catheterization with hemodynamic measurements and coronary angiography has been largely replaced by two-dimensional echocardiography and Doppler scanning for assessing LV structure and function in patients with HCM. Cardiac catheterization for surgical assessment is indicated in the presence of severe, refractory symptoms. Coronary angiography specifically may be of use in the assessment of chest pain, particularly if accompanied by significant ECG changes or chest pain on exertion, in patients over age 40, or in cases of a family history of premature coronary artery disease.

Typically, the LV end-diastolic, mean left atrial, and mean pulmonary capillary wedge pressures are elevated as a consequence of abnormal diastolic filling and reduced compliance.[84] Cardiac output may be reduced, normal, or occasionally increased.[84] In approximately one-third of patients there is a pressure gradient at rest between the body and the outflow tract of the left ventricle. Such gradients are usually relatively stable but may be labile; intraventricular pressures up to 300 mmHg have been recorded.[112] In a small proportion of patients (< 15 percent) a right ventricular infundibular gradient of more than 10 mmHg may be recorded. Typically right ventricular end-diastolic and mean right atrial pressures are mildly to moderately elevated.

Left ventricular angiography reveals an abnormally shaped ventricle that typically ejects at least 75 percent of its contents in association with mild mitral regurgitation. Papillary muscles may be prominent or malpositioned and obliterate the LV cavity during late systole. Usually the left coronary arteries are large. The left anterior descending and septal perforator arteries may demonstrate phasic narrowing during systole in the absence of fixed obstructive lesions. Such narrowing is not associated with symptoms.[113]

NATURAL HISTORY

The natural history of HCM is one of slow progression of symptoms, gradual deterioration of LV function, and a significant incidence of sudden death occurring at all ages.[59,76,77,96,114,115] Data from tertiary centers indicates an annual mortality rate from sudden death of 2–4 percent; among children and adolescents it is 4–8 percent.[59,77,116,117] Mortality is higher in patients who have recurrent syncope or a family history of multiple sudden deaths from HCM.[14,77,117] Although the mortality data from nonreferral hospitals are lower, the risk of sudden death is still present.[118] Early data suggest that it may be higher in families with particular gene mutations. Autopsy findings now reveal that unsuspected HCM is the most common cause of sudden death in competitive athletes.[119–123]

Symptomatic deterioration is slow and associated with a gradual decline in systolic performance; in most patients the rate of deterioration is not disproportionate to other system changes with age.[8,9,98] Occasionally symptomatic deterioration is associated with myocardial wall thinning and ventricular dilatation, leading to a severe decline in systolic performance and diastolic filling.[19] In these patients the end-diastolic volume increases, but even at end-stage it rarely exceeds "normal" dimensions. It is rare for patients with HCM to develop a dilated ventricle reminiscent of dilated cardiomyopathy, but occasionally a restrictive pattern develops with grossly enlarged atria, signs of right heart failure, and relative preservation of LV systolic performance.

Though there may be a progression of ECG abnormalities, particularly changes suggestive of further ventricular hypertrophy,[115] serial echocardiography does not support this idea.[16] The development of atrial fibrillation has long been considered to be associated with dramatic symptomatic deterioration and to indicate poor prognosis.[124,125] However, a retrospective study found that 5-year survival of those with atrial fibrillation was similar to that of age- and sex-matched patients who remained in sinus rhythm and whose symptomatic status remained stable, provided the ventricular response was controlled and emboli were prevented by anticoagulation.[97] Indeed most patients in whom atrial fibrillation develops have previously had a palpable atrial beat in the absence of a fourth heart sound, reflecting forceful, atrial contraction but minimal atrial systolic contribution to filling volume.

Prognosis

A major problem of management is the identification of high risk patients and prevention of sudden death. In adults nonsustained ventricular tachycardia during ECG monitoring is associated with sudden death and is the best single marker of high risk, with a sensitivity of 69 percent and a specificity of 80 percent.[91,92,99] However, because most patients with ventricular tachycardia do not die suddenly the positive predictive accuracy of ventricular tachycardia is low (22 percent). Thus further risk stratification of this subgroup would be helpful because a policy of aggressive therapy may include patients at relatively low risk.[99] Risk stratification may be improved by implementing the results of ongoing analysis of potentials the prognostic significance of late identified by the signal-averaged ECG, the role of the QT interval, and from a novel technique of ECG fractionation developed by Saumarez.[99] The latter method relies on programmed right ventricular pacing and an assessment of local myocardial electrical activity. Saumarez found that in patients with HCM those who were at most risk of sudden death (history of ventricular fibrillation or family history of sudden death) had increased dispersion of inhomogeneity of intraventricular conduction and thus concluded that it may create the conditions for reentry and arrhythmogenesis. This technique is now undergoing further validation with a larger patient group. In adults no other clinical features are associated with or predictive of sudden death, including symptoms, LV wall thickness, filling pressures or the presence of an LV gradient.[59,126]

Children and adolescents who have experienced recurrent syncope and those who have two or more siblings with HCM who have died suddenly are at increased risk.[77] However, most young patients who die suddenly have not experienced syncope, nor do they have a family history of HCM.[76,77] The young pose problems in terms of both identification and therapy. Most are asymptomatic, and many are athletic; even those at low risk have an annual mortality from sudden death of 4 percent.

It is a difficult decision whether an individual should abandon athletic participation following the diagnosis of HCM; it depends in part on risk stratification and in part on individual wishes. There is limited evidence, which must be interpreted cautiously, that some individuals with HCM can successfully undertake athletic training and remain well.[123] For those with marked hypertrophy, a significant gradient, arrhythmias, or adverse family history, the precautionary recommendation to abstain from competitive sports is important but often imposes a significant limitation on the life style of the child, adolescent, or young adult.[119,120,122,123,127–130] More accurate risk stratification depends on understanding the likely mechanisms of sudden death. One model postulates that hemodynamic deterioration with reduced stroke volume may occur after an arrhythmia[76,131] or with normal stroke volume following a reduction in venous return or systemic vascular resistance. The latter may arise from altered baroreflex control of peripheral blood flow.[74] Outcome is then influenced by the underlying electrical stability of the myocardium, which may correlate with the extent of myocardial disarray, fibrosis, and ischemia. The latter, in turn, may correlate with etiologic mutations in HCM or may be influenced by other disease-modifying genes.

MANAGEMENT

Symptomatic Treatment

There is considerable experience with β-blockers (especially propranolol) and calcium antagonists (especially verapamil)[132–137] for treating chest pain and dyspnea in HCM. They have several potentially beneficial actions that assist in the reduction of myocardial oxygen consumption and blunting the chronotropic response to exercise providing increased filling time at equivalent workloads in those with diastolic dysfunction. Verapamil improves diastolic filling by enhancing relaxation,[134,136,138–140] whereas propranolol acts by increasing compliance.[141] Both drugs have a negative inotropic effect, reducing hyperdynamic systolic function and LV gradients,[133] and are associated with a regression of LV hypertrophy. Verapamil is more likely to be efficacious than β-blockers and is associated with increased exercise duration in two-thirds of patients.[136,139] Exertional chest pain usually responds to propranolol or verapamil, but when refractory high doses may be beneficial (up to propranolol 480 mg daily; and verapamil 720 mg daily).[142,143]

Experience with disopyramide is more limited. In small groups of patients with reduced exercise tolerance and LV outflow tract obstruction, LV gradients and filling pressures have been reported to be reduced and symptoms of angina and dyspnea alleviated.[144]

Propranolol and verapamil are usually well tolerated, and the beneficial effects outweigh the unwanted ones. The side effects of propranolol are not serious; however, the suppressant effect of verapamil on electrical activity may cause problems in patients with occult conduction disease, and its vasodilator and negatively inotropic properties have resulted in acute systolic cardiac failure, with pulmonary edema and death.[145] It is unclear in which patients verapamil should be avoided. To avoid giving verapamil to patients at highest risk—those with increased filling pressures or paroxysmal nocturnal dyspnea or orthopnea—would be to eliminate the patients in greatest need of therapy.[145] In practice, both drugs are effective, but it is safer to use propranolol. If ineffective, verapamil can then be tried, with high risk patients commencing therapy in hospital.

Diltiazem[146] and nifedipine[147] have been assessed in patients with HCM. Early experience with diltiazem shows results similar to those with verapamil. Nifedipine also improves diastolic function by increasing compliance, but the clinical experience has been disappointing and complicated by peripheral vasodilatation.[148] The role of β-blockers with intrinsic symphathomimetic activity in patients with diastolic dysfunction has not been adequately assessed. Dual demand pacing with short atrioventricular delay to alter the sequence of ventricular electrical activation has been advocated; selection of appropriate patients remains to be established.

Surgery

Partial septal resection, mitral valve surgery, and cardiac transplantation are the available interventions. Coronary artery disease occurs in patients with HCM, and bypass grafting may be indicated. There is considerable experience of these options.[149–156]

Left ventricular outflow tract gradient in severely symptomatic patients who are refractory to medical therapy has been treated with surgical excision of part of the upper anterior septum (myotomy/myectomy) via a transaortic approach. Transventricular routes have been tried but are associated with a high incidence of late complications, particularly cardiac failure. Despite considerable experience, the operation carries a perioperative mortality of 5–10 percent,[114,117,151] and patients remain at risk of sudden cardiac death. Successful surgery confers symptomatic and hemodynamic improvement (reduced LV gradient and filling pressures). The optimal patient for myotomy/myectomy has not been identified. Experimental work by Sigwart et al.[157] has shown that nonsurgical myotomy/myectomy may be produced via a controlled septal myocardial infarction produced by instillation of desiccated alcohol into the first septal branch of the left coronary artery. This technique has provided a good outcome in selected patients.

Mitral valve replacement and plication[152,153] has also been used with excellent results in patients with severe mitral regurgitation and those with severe outflow tract gradients. In patients found to have significant coronary artery disease, coronary artery bypass grafting has been performed with good outcome,[158] even when combined with other procedures such as mitral valve replacement or myotomy. Mortality is largely related to the success of associated procedures.[159]

Arrhythmia

Rhythm disturbances are common in HCM, and supraventricular arrhythmias are particularly associated with embolic complications. Once atrial fibrillation is established, treatment with anticoagulants and digoxin with or without verapamil is appropriate. The aim of therapy is to control the ventricular response and prevent emboli. So long as the ventricular response is well controlled, most patients are unaware of the change from sinus rhythm to atrial fibrillation. This lack of awareness is consistent with the loss of forceful atrial contraction (palpable atrial beat), which does not contribute significantly to the filling volume (no fourth heart sound). In those in whom ventricular filling is critically dependent on atrial systole, pharmacologic cardioversion may occur with amiodarone therapy (300 mg daily). If after 6 weeks cardioversion has not occurred, electrical cardioversion is facilitated by the previous amiodarone loading.[97,160–162]

Sustained (> 30 seconds) episodes of paroxysmal atrial fibrillation or supraventricular tachycardia are relatively uncommon but represent a risk of hemodynamic collapse and emboli. Amiodarone in low doses (1000–1400 mg weekly) effectively suppresses such episodes and provides control of the ventricular response should breakthrough occur.[162]

Prevention of Sudden Death

Treatment of adults is facilitated by the detection of nonsustained ventricular tachycardia during ECG monitoring, a relatively sensitive and specific marker of increased risk.[92] Subsequent investigation aims to identify likely initiating mechanisms amenable to treatment: paroxysmal atrial fibrillation: amiodarone; ischemia: verapamil, β-blockers, surgery; clinically sustained ventricular arrhythmia: automatic implantable cardioverter defibrillator; supraventricular arrhythmia associated with rapid atrioventricular conduction: ablation; obstruction: myectomy. Unfortunately, in most adults investigations fail to determine a likely treatable mechanism. The success of low dose amiodarone (1000 mg/week) in preventing sudden cardiac death in patients provides nonspecific but effective therapy in the remainder.[161]

In the young a higher annual mortality from sudden death in the absence of sensitive risk markers makes treatment problematic. As for adults, investigation is performed to identify a treatable mechanism of sudden death, but usually none is found. For the remainder, low dose (by body weight) amiodarone is also recommended. With plasma concentrations of amiodarone of 1.5 mg/L or less, serious side effects are rare, though photosensitivity and sleep disturbance are common and may be troublesome.[162,163] Until practical treatment guidelines are established, young patients with HCM should undergo risk factor assessment at specialist investigation centers.

Transplantation

Transplantation is an uncommon step in the management of patients with HCM. Indications are severe refractory outflow tract obstruction, end-stage systolic cardiac failure, and refractory severe rhythm disturbance.[164,165] Expert assessment in a referral center is required.

MOLECULAR GENETICS OF HCM

The modern technologies of molecular biology are revealing the basis of HCM. Results have been derived from the assessment of persons and families with "idiopathic" HCM and conditions in which cardiac hypertrophy occurs as a component of a disease syndrome.

Cardiac Hypertrophy Associated with Other Diseases

Cardiac hypertrophy may occur as a component of another disease syndrome. Molecular genetic analysis has identified linkage between the syndrome and chromosomal loci in a number of familial disorders (Table 27-1), such as Noonan syndrome, Friedreich's ataxia, neurofibromatosis, aniridia with catalase deficiency, and hereditary spherocytosis. Cardiac hypertrophy resembling HCM is also seen in the Leopard syndrome, Beckwith Wiedemann syndrome, Swyer syndrome, the fetus and infants of diabetic mothers, certain inborn errors of metabolism (carnitine deficiency, Pompe's disease, Forbe's disease, phosphorylase kinase deficiency, fucosidosis, mucolipidosis II), Hurler syndrome, Hurler-Scheie syndrome, Hunter syndrome, and Fabry's disease. Abnormalities of mitochondrial function are also associated with HCM including the MELAS syndrome (myoclonic epilepsy with ragged red fibers),

Table 27-1. Cardiac Hypertrophy as Part of Another Disease or Syndrome

Disease	Chromosome/gene
Noonan syndrome[a]	12q
Friedreich's ataxia[b,c,d]	9q
Neurofibromatosis[e,f]	17q
Aniridia with catalase deficiency[g]	11p
Hereditary spherocytosis[h,i]	14q
Beckwith-Wiedemann	11p
Hurler syndrome	4p, 22q
Hurler-Scheie syndrome	4p, 22q
Hunter syndrome	Xq
Fabry's disease	Xq
MELAS	Mitochondrial
MERRF	Mitochondrial
NADH-coenzyme Q reductase deficiency	Mitochondrial
Cytochrome b deficiency	Mitochondrial
Leopard syndrome	Unknown
Swyer syndrome	
Fetus and infants of diabetic mothers	
Inborn errors of metabolism (carnitine deficiency, Pompe's disease, Forbe's disease, phosphorylase kinase deficiency, fucosidosis type 1, mucolipidosis II)	

[a] Jamieson et al.[34]

[b] Hanauer A, Chery M, Fujita R et al.: The Friedreich ataxia gene is assigned to chromosome 9q13-q21 by mapping of tightly linked markers and shows linkage disequilibrium with D9S15. Am J Hum Genet 1990;46:133–137

[c] Child JS, Perloff JK, Bach PM et al.: Cardiac involvement in Friedreich's ataxia. A clinical study of 75 patients. J Am Coll Cardiol 1986;7:1370–1378

[d] Chamberlain S, Shaw J, Rowland A et al.: Mapping of mutation causing Friedreich's ataxia to human chromosome 9. Nature 1988;334:248–250

[e] Barker D, Wright E, Nguyen K et al.: Gene for von Recklinghausen neurofibromatosis is in the pericentromeric region of chromosome 17. Science 1987;236:1100–1102

[f] Fitzpatrick AP, Emanuel RW: Familial neurofibromatosis and hypertrophic cardiomyopathy. Br Heart J 1988;60:247–251

[g] Gilgenkrantz S, Vigneron C, Gregoire MJ, Pernot C, Raspiller A: Association of del(11)(p15.1p12), aniridia, catalase deficiency, and cardiomyopathy. Am J Med Genet 1982;13:39–49

[h] Kimberling WJ, Taylor RA, Chapman RG, Lubs HA: Linkage and gene localization of hereditary spherocytosis (HS). Blood 1978;52:859–867

[i] Moiseyev VS, Korovina EA, Polotskaya EL, Poliyanskaya IS, Yazdovsky VV: Hypertrophic cardiomyopathy associated with hereditary spherocytosis in three generations of one family [letter]. Lancet 1987;2:853–854

NADH-coenzyme Q reducatase deficiency, and cytochrome b deficiency (histiocytoid cardiomyopathy). Mutations in mitochondrial transfer RNA genes have also been implicated in producing cardiac hypertrophy.

"Idiopathic" Hypertrophic Cardiomyopathy

Early descriptions of hypertrophic cardiomyopathy suggested a familial disorder. As large pedigrees were characterized a Mendelian pattern of inheritance was observed, strongly suggesting abnormalities of single genes. More recently, improved diagnostic techniques have illustrated a much wider range of disease penetrance and expression than previously considered. Despite such advances a definite clinical diagnosis may be difficult, particularly in children in whom prior to the pubertal growth spurt there may be no evidence of cardiac hypertrophy and in athletes in whom the borderline between physiologic and pathologic hypertrophy is not clearly defined. This point is also important because of the high rate of unheralded sudden cardiac deaths that occur in these groups. Clearly identifying molecular markers of disease predisposition and risk would be of benefit clinically and for explaining the pathophysiology of these disorders.

β-Cardiac Myosin Mutations

The identification of a French-Canadian family with 44 affected members and 58 unaffected by HCM permitted linkage analysis. In 1989 DNA locus D14S26 mapped to chromosome 14q[166] was found to cosegregate with the disease. A LOD score of +9.37 was found, suggesting that the odds were greater than two billion to one that the gene responsible for familial HCM was at this site. This region of chromosome 14 included the genes for both the α and β myosin heavy chains (MHC).[167,168] The α isoform is predominantly expressed in cardiac atrium, whereas the β chain is the main isoform within adult ventricle. In 1990 linkage of HCM in some families was established to the cardiac β-MHC.[169] The chromosomal locus 14q11-12 for this disease was designated CMH 1.

Myosin heavy chains constitute the major component of myofibril thick filaments in striated muscle, are intrinsic to muscle contraction, and are present in various isoforms differentially expressed in various tissues and throughout life. Identification of disease linkage to the β-MHC gene led to a search for the causal mutation. During the search a novel restriction fragment length polymorphism was identified in affected members.[170] Analysis revealed an α/β cardiac MHC hybrid gene co-inherited with HCM. It was postulated that this finding arose from an unequal crossover event during meiosis and that it could be the cause of HCM. Subsequently Geisterfer et al.[171] identified a missense mutation in exon 13 that converted arginine to glutamine at residue 403 (Arg403Gln). Further screening by Watkins et al. of the β cardiac myosin heavy-chain genes of probands from 25 unrelated families with familial HCM using a ribonuclease protection assay identified various missense mutations.[172] Evidence favoring the role of them as etiologic mutations came from a cluster of features: that the mutation was co-inherited with the disease and identical mutations were found in pedigrees not affected by the α/β chain hybrid gene.[172,173]

Subsequent investigation has continued to screen for other etiologic mutations in this gene (Table 27-2). The cardiac β-MHC gene is large: 40 exons consisting of more than 23,000 basepairs (bp), although the messenger RNA (mRNA) encoded is only 6000 bp long. Ectopic transcription of mRNA occurs at low levels in other tissues including peripheral blood leukocytes.[174] Mutations may thus be screened for using technologies such as a ribonuclease protection assay. Other mutation detection methods include sequence-specific conformational polymorphism, denaturing gradient gel electrophoresis, or direct sequencing. They permit indirect assessment of putative cardiac protein mutations from a peripheral blood sample. Such techniques have led to the identification of several mutations in the β-MHC gene thought to cause HCM (Table 27-2). Of particular interest has been the apparent difference in prognosis conferred by the various mutations.

Other Genes

The discovery that β-MHC mutations cause HCM suggested that the disease may be due to abnormalities of sarcomeric elements. Linkage analysis led to identification of disease loci on chromosomes 1q3,[187] 15q2,[188] and 1p13-q13.[189] They have been identified as troponin T (CMH2), α tropomyosin (CMH3),[190] and cardiac myosin-binding protein C (CMH4).

Troponin T Mutations

Eight nonconservative mutations have been found in the troponin T gene.[20,190] Six are missense mutations, one is a splice site mutation, and the other is a three—nucleotide deletion (Table 27-3).

Table 27-2. Published Cardiac β-Myosin Heavy-Chain Gene Mutations (Chromosome 14q CMH1) Identified in HCM

Amino acid	Nucleotide	Exon	Charge change	Reference
Arg249Gln	G832A	9	−1	174
Arg403Gln	G1294A	13	−1	172, 175, 176
Arg453Cys	C1443T	14	−1	172
Phe513Cys	T1624G	15	0	177
Gly584Arg	G1836C	16	+1	172
Val606Met	G1902A	16	0	172
Asn615Lys	G1931C	16	+1	178
Gly716Arg	G2232A	19	+1	177
Arg719Trp	C2241T	19	−1	177
Arg723Cys	C2253T	20	−1	179
Leu908Val	C2808G	23	0	175, 180
Glu924Lys	G2856A	23	+2	172
Glu949Lys	G2931A	23	+2	172
Gly741Arg	G741C	20	+1	31
Gly256Glu	G256A	9	−1	31
Arg403Trp	C403T	13	−1	181
Arg403Leu	G403T	13	−1	181
Asp778Gly	A778G	21	0	182
Asn232Ser	A232G	8	0	183
Gly1208Ala	G1208A	13	0	184
Arg403Trp		13		185
Hybrid gene	α/β Hybrid			170
3' Deletion				186

The vertebrate troponin T gene sequence is highly conserved through evolution, and mutations cause structural and charge changes. The 5′ splice site mutation, in particular, would result in a markedly aberrant cardiac troponin T mRNA transcript. The troponin T region involved by the missense mutations (Ile79Asn, Arg92Gln, Phe110Ile, DGlu160, Glu163-Lys) encodes a section, the functional role of which is thought to involve calcium-insensitive binding to α-tropomyosin.[191–193] The other mutations (Intron15→G1A, Glu144Asp, Arg278Cys) could alter the carboxyterminus of troponin T, a region contributing to tropomyosin interaction as well as to inter-

action with troponin I and troponin C. Indeed the latter mutations may interfere with calcium-dependent binding to α-tropomyosin.[194] The cardiac troponin T isoform is not expressed in adult skeletal muscle,[195–197] thus explaining the tissue-specific effects of this mutation.

α-Tropomyosin Mutations

The vertebrate α-tropomyosin gene consists of 15 exons. The striated muscle isoform has been determined and is identical in both cardiac and skeletal

Table 27-3. Published Troponin T Gene (Chromosome 1q3 CMH2) Mutations Identified in HCM

Amino acid	Nucleotide	Exon	Charge change	Reference
Arg92Gln	G287A	9	−1	190
Ile79Asn	T248A	8	0	190
Intron15 Gl → A	G1A (intron)	Intron 15 splice site	NA	190
Phe110Ile	T340A	9	0	20
Glu163Lys	G499A	11	+2	20
Glu244Asp	G744T	14	0	20
ΔGlu160[a]	ΔGAG	11	+1	20

[a] Deletion of three nucleotides corresponding to an entire glutamic acid codon; therefore does not cause a frameshift mutation. (Frameshift mutation is a mutation causing a change in the reading frame in which triplets are translated into protein.)

Table 27-4. Published α-Tropomyosin Gene (Chromosome 15q2CMH3) Mutations Identified in HCM

Amino acid	Nucleotide	Exon	Charge change	Reference
Asp175Asn	G579A	5	+1	190
Glu180Gly	A595G	5	+1	190

muscle. There is a high level of conservation through evolution: Human and rat muscle α-tropomyosin share 99.6% amino acid homology, and there is high identity between human α and β-tropomyosin genes. Thierfelder et al. identified two nonconservative (producing a change in amino acid sequence) missense mutations in exon 5 of the α-tropomyosin gene in two families affected by HCM[190] (Table 27-4). They result in a single amino acid change and accompanying charge change. They are located near the calcium-dependent troponin T binding domain.

α-Tropomyosin is expressed in many cell types, and it may be that exon 5 is of critical importance only in striated muscle, as the troponin complex is not found in nonmuscle tissues. There may be also other cardiac-specific differences in isoforms of α-tropomyosin-associated molecules (i.e., β-myosin, troponin C, troponin I), or other local cardiac factors which limit disease expression to the heart.

Cardiac Myosin Binding Protein C Mutations

Cardiac myosin-binding protein C (MyBP-C) is a component of the sarcomere thick filament, binding myosin and titin; it has both structural and regulatory functions. Two groups have identified mutations in the gene for protein C.[198,199]

Other Loci

Despite the impressive advances in the molecular characterization of the basis for this disease, it appears that at most only 50 percent of HCM is accounted for by identified mutations. Linkage analysis continues, and Macrae has identified a locus at chromosome 7q3 in a family in whom members had familial HCM, WPW syndrome, or both. This finding suggests the presence of a single gene, the mutation of which may cause either disease or both, suggesting a common pathogenesis.[89]

Other chromosomal loci tentatively suggested to co-segregate with HCM are on chromosome 16 (Italian pedigree)[200] and chromosome 18 (Japanese pedigree).[201,202] Screening of Japanese pedigrees suggests that other chromosomal loci may be more important in the etiology of HCM than those identified in pedigrees of European descent.[202]

MOLECULAR PATHOGENESIS

The mutations detected so far have been heterozygous, which results in mutations and their abnormal protein products coexisting with copies of the normal gene and protein in affected persons. The precise mechanism by which disease is produced remains unknown. It is postulated that the mutant protein may act as a "poison peptide" by incorporation into the multimeric sarcomere structure, which subsequently disrupts the structure or function. Alternatively, a mutation may act to functionally deactivate a gene, potentially reducing protein concentrations by 50 percent.

The interaction between the thick and thin filaments of muscle are a dynamic process reliant on energy-dependent changes in the stoichiometry of the relevant molecules. Small changes at one site are capable of large overall changes in molecular conformation and activity. Abnormal conformation or binding properties may therefore seriously affect force generation, relaxation, and molecular stability. Further compensatory mechanisms may act to produce, as secondary phenomena, myocardial disarray, electrical instability, and hypertrophy. Hypertrophy may arise from the induction of oncogenes or other isoforms of the sarcomeric contractile proteins as has been seen in models of secondary hypertrophy.[203,204]

The splice donor mutation in cardiac troponin T may act as a null allele. The human mutation is analogous to a 5' splice donor site mutation in intron 7 of the *Drosophila* flight muscle troponin T, resulting in the mutant fly upheld2.[205] It results in a truncated polypeptide product. Homozygous upheld2 flies have no troponin T in their flight muscles and have virtually no thin filaments. Heterozygote flies, analogous to the human situation, have disrupted myofibrillar architecture with a disordered architecture of thick and thin filaments in the outer half of each myofibril.[206,207] It is predicted that the effect of this splice site mutation is to produce an aberrant shortened mRNA transcript and resultant polyprotein product.

GENOTYPE AND PHENOTYPE CORRELATIONS

Only a small number of pedigrees and mutations have been identified. Considerable further assessment is required to determine the prognostic significance of a given mutation and how it may be influenced by modifying genetic or environmental factors, for example by interaction with the renin-angiotensin system.

β-Cardiac MHC

Various mutations within the β-cardiac MHC gene appeared to correlate with significantly different rates of survival among affected persons[172,175,177] but have not been shown to correlate convincingly with differences in morphologic features of the disease.[206] In particular, the mutations Arg403Gln, Arg453Gln, and Arg719Trp have been associated with a significantly worse prognosis and have been described as "malignant."[172]

α-Tropomyosin

In contrast, in HCM due to α-tropomyosin mutations, significantly less cardiac hypertrophy was associated with the Glu180Gly than with Asp175Asn, though it was not of prognostic significance, and the life expectancy of patients with either mutation was similar.[188,190]

Troponin T

In troponin T mutations, analysis of more than 100 persons found that the mutations Ile79Asn, Arg92Gln, DGlu160, and intron 15G1A were associated with a significantly shortened life expectancy, comparable to that seen with "malignant" β-MHC mutations.[20]

The degree of cardiac hypertrophy associated with cardiac troponin T mutations was significantly less than that associated with β-MHC mutations (mean maximal wall thickness 16.7 ± 5.5 mm with cardiac troponin T mutations versus 23.7 ± 7.7 mm with β-MHC mutations). Each cardiac troponin T mutation produced a similar increase in the maximal thickness of the LV wall (range 13.4–19.8 mm). Clinical evaluation of family members of probands identified several genetically affected but otherwise apparently normal relatives (asymptomatic, no detectable signs, normal ECG and echocardiogram). This discovery led to an estimate of gene penetrance as 75 percent in contrast to the higher penetrance associated with β-MHC mutations (95 percent) associated with a comparable malignant phenotype.

The disparity between the severity of the degree of cardiac hypertrophy and prognosis in mutations of the cardiac troponin T gene illustrates the relative shortcomings of diagnosis and risk evaluation based on purely clinical criteria; it is expected that a proportion of apparently unaffected individuals as assessed by current clinical criteria will suffer sudden cardiac death. Their prognosis may be significantly improved by the potential interventions arising from a molecular diagnosis.

Contribution to Familial HCM by Mutations in Known Genes

Pooled data have been analyzed.[20,190] Approximately 30 percent of familial HCM is caused by mutations in the β-cardiac MHC gene, 15 percent by mutations in the cardiac troponin T gene, and less than 3 percent by mutations in the α-tropomyosin gene. Thus 50 percent of apparently familial HCM must be explained by abnormalities in other genes.

CONCLUSION

Hypertrophic cardiomyopathy results in heart failure due to outflow tract gradient, diastolic dysfunction, ischemia, rhythm disturbance, and abnormal autonomic activity. Macroscopic abnormalities are cardiac hypetrophy and mitral valve abnormalities. Histology reveals myocyte disorganization and disarray accompanied by fibrosis. Risk stratification is made difficult by the poor correlation between clinical markers and outcome, particularly in children and athletes, the group with the highest risk of sudden death. The dramatic advance in molecular genetics have revolutionized our concept of the disease, offering both etiologic answers and prognostic risk stratification.

Note Added in Proof

Recognizing the importance of the genetic basis of the disease, a new definition of hypertrophic cardiomyopathy has been published. While continuing to include clinical features as diagnostic features, it now acknowledges the concept of a disease which in most cases is inherited in an autosomal dominant fashion and arises due to mutations in contractile protein genes (WHO/ISFC. Report of 1995 WHO/ISFC Task Force on the definition and classification of cardiomyopathies. Circulation 1996;93:841–842).

Since submission of this chapter, two further genes have been identified. A rare HCM variant which is characterized by midventricular chamber thickening has been identified as being due to mutations in either the essential or regulatory myosin light chains (Poetter KJH, Hassanzadeh S, Master SR. et al: Mutations in either the essential or regulatory light chains are associated with a rare myopathy in human heart and skeletal muscle. Nature Genetics 1996;13(May):63–69). The CMH nomenclature for these genes has not yet been declared. The presence of unlinked HCM families imply the presence of at least one more locus. This has been provisionally designated CMH5. (Hengstenberg JA: CMH5. Human Genetics 1993; 53 [suppl.]).

REFERENCES

1. Liouville H: Retrecissement cardiaque sous aortique. Gas Med Paris 1869;24:161
2. Hallopeau L: Retrecissement ventriculo-aortique. Gas Med Paris 1869;24:683
3. Browne G, Gray G: Lancet 1930;1:915
4. Teare D: Asymmetrical hypertrophy of the heart in young adults. Br Heart J 1958;20:1–8
5. Maron B, Epstein S: Hypertrophic cardiomyopathy. A discussion of nomenclature. Am J Cardiol 1979;43:1242
6. WHO/ISFC: Report of the WHO/IFSC task force on the definition a classification of cardiomyopathies. Br Heart J 1980;44:672–673
7. Maron B: Hypertrophic cardiomyopathy in infants. Clinical features a natural history. Circulation 1982;65:7
8. Lewis JF, Maron BJ: Clinical and morphologic expression of hypertrophic cardiomyopathy in patients>or=65 years of age. Am J Cardiol 1994;73:1105–1111
9. Lewis JF, Maron BJ: Elderly patients with hypertrophic cardiomyopathy. A subset with distinctive left ventricular morphology and progressive clinical course late in life. J Am Coll Cardiol 1989;13:36–45
10. Ando H, Imaizumi T, Urabe Y, Takeshita A, Nakamura M: Apical segmental dysfunction in hypertrophic cardiomyopathy. Subgroup with unique clinical features. J Am Coll Cardiol 1990;16:1579–1588
11. Sakamoto T, Tei C, Murayama M, Ichiyasu H, Hada Y: Giant T wave inversion as a manifestation of asymmetrical apical hypertrophy (AAH) of the left ventricle. Echocardiographic and ultrasono-cardiotomographic study. Jpn Heart J 1976;17:611–629
12. Shapiro LM, McKenna WJ: Distribution of left ventricular hypertrophy in hypertrophic cardiomyopathy. A two-dimensional echocardiographic study. J Am Coll Cardiol 1983;2:437–444
13. Maron BJ, Spirito P, Wesley Y, Arce J: Development and progression of left ventricular hypertrophy in children with hypertrophic cardiomyopathy. N Engl J Med 1986;315:610–614
14. Maron BJ, Henry WL, Clark CE et al: Asymmetric septal hypertrophy in childhood. Circulation 1976;53:9–19
15. Maron BJ, Tajik AJ, Ruttenberg HD et al: Hypertrophic cardiomyopathy in infants. Clinical features and natural history. Circulation 1982;65:7–17
16. Spirito P, Maron BJ: Absence of progression of left ventricular hypertrophy in adult patients with hypertrophic cardiomyopathy. J Am Coll Cardiol 1987;9:1013–1017
17. Spirito P, Maron BJ: Relation between extent of left ventricular hypertrophy and age in hypertrophic cardiomyopathy. J Am Coll Cardiol 1989;13:820–823
18. McKenna WJ, Kleinebenne A, Nihoyannopoulos P, Foale R: Echocardiographic measurement of right ventricular wall thickness in hypertrophic cardiomyopathy. Relation to clinical and prognostic features. J Am Coll Cardiol 1988;11:351–358
19. Spirito P, Maron BJ, Bonow RO, Epstein SE: Occurrence and significance of progressive left ventricular wall thinning and relative cavity dilatation in hypertrophic cardiomyopathy. Am J Cardiol 1987;60:123–129
20. Watkins H, McKenna WJ, Theirfelder L et al: Mutations in the genes for cardiac troponin T and alpha-tropomyosin in hypertrophy cardiomyopathy. N Engl J Med 1995;332:1058–1064
21. Davies MJ: The current status of myocardial disarray in hypertrophic cardiomyopathy [editorial]. Br Heart J 1984;51:361–363
22. Davies MJ, McKenna WJ: Hypertrophic cardiomyopathy. An introduction to pathology and pathogenesis. Br Heart J (in press)
23. Ferrans VJ, Morrow AG, Roberts WC: Myocardial ultrastructure in idiopathic hypertrophic subaortic stenosis. A study of operatively excised left ventricular outlflow tract muscle in 14 patients. Circulation 1972;45:769–792
24. Maron BJ, Sato N, Roberts WC, Edwards JE, Chandra RS: Quantitative analysis of cardiac muscle cell disorganization in the vetricular septum. Comparison of fetuses and infants with and without congenital heart disease and patients with hypertrophic cardiomyopathy. Circulation 1979;60:685–696
25. Maron BJ, Roberts WC: Quantitative analysis of cardiac muscle cell disorganization in the ventricular septum of patients with hypertrophic cardiomyopathy. Circulation 1979;59:689–706
26. McKenna WJ, Steward JT, Nihoyannopoulos P, McGinty F, Davies MJ: Hypertrophic cardiomyopathy without hypertrophy: two families with myocardial disarray in the absence of increased myocardial mass [see comments]. Br Heart J 1990;63:287–290
27. Maron BJ, Wolfson JK, Epstein SE, Roberts WC: Morphologic evidence for "small vessel disease" in patients with hypertrophic cardiomyopathy. Z Kardiol 1987;3:91–100
28. Maron BJ, Wolfson JK, Epstein SE, Roberts WC: Intramural ("small vessel") coronary artery disease in

hypertrophic cardiomyopathy. J Am Coll Cardiol 1986;8:545–557

29. Waller BF, Maron BJ, Epstein SE, Roberts WC: Transmural myocardial infarction in hypertrophic cardiomyopathy. A cause of conversion from left ventricular asymmetry to symmetry and from normal-sized to dilated left ventricular cavity. Chest 1981; 79:461–465

30. Maron BJ, Epstein SE, Roberts WC: Hypertrophic cardiomyopathy and transmural myocardial infarction without significant atherosclerosis of the extramural coronary arteries. Am J Cardiol 1979;43: 1086–1102

31. Fananapazir L, Dalakas MC, Cyran F, Cohn G, Epstein ND: Missense mutations in the beta-myosin heavy-chain gene cause central core disease in hypertrophic cardiomyopathy. Proc Natl Acad Sci USA 1993;90:3993–3997

32. Burch M, Mann JM, Sharland M et al: Myocardial disarray in Noonan syndrome. Br Heart J 1992;68: 586–588

33. Burch M, Sharland M, Shinebourne E et al: Cardiologic abnormalities in Noonan syndrome. Phenotypic diagnosis and echocardiographic assessment of the 118 patients. J Am Coll Cardiol 1993;22:1189–1192

34. Jamieson CR, Van der Burgt I, Brady AF et al: Mapping a gene for Noonan syndrome to the long arm of chromosome 12. Nat Genet 1994;80:357–360

35. Klues HG, Proschan MA, Dollar AL et al: Echocardiographic assessment of mitral valve size in obstructive hypertrophic cardiomyopathy. Anatomic validation from mitral valve specimen. Circulation 1993;88: 548–555

36. Klues HG, Maron BJ, Dollar AL, Roberts WC: Diversity of structural mitral valve alterations in hypertrophic cardiomyopathy. Circulation 1992;85: 1651–1660

37. Klues HG, Roberts WC, Maron BJ: Anomalous insertion of papillary muscle directly into anterior mitral leaflet in hypertrophic cardiomyopathy. Significance in producing left ventricular outflow obstruction. Circulation 1991;84:1188–1197

38. Maron BJ, Harding AM, Spirito P, Roberts WC, Wailer BF: Systolic anterior motion of the posterior mitral leaflet. A previously unrecognized cause of dynamic subaortic obstruction in patients with hypertrophic cardiomyopathy. Circulation 1983;68: 282–293

39. Spirito P, Maron BJ: Patterns of systolic anterior motion of the mitral valve in hypertrophic cardiomyopathy. Assessment by two-dimensional echocardiography. Am J Cardiol 1984;54:1039–1046

40. Panza JA, Maron BJ: Simultaneous occurrence of mitral valve prolapse and systolic anterior motion in hypertrophic cardiomyopathy. Am J Cardiol 1991;67: 404–410

41. Petrone RK, Klues HG, Panza JUA, Peterson EE, Maron BJ: Coexistence of mitral valve prolapse in a consecutive group of 528 patients with hypertrophic cardiomyopathy assessed with echocardiography. J Am Coll Cardiol 1992;20:55–61

42. Maron BJ: Echocardiographic assessment of left ventricular hypertrophy in patients with obstructive or nonobstructive hypertrophic cardiomyopathy. Eur Heart J 1983

43. Schwartz K, Carrier L, Lompre AM, Mercadier JJ,

Boheler KR: Contractile proteins and sarcoplasmic reticulum calcium-ATPase gene expression in the hypertrophied and failing heart. [review]. Basic Res Cardiol 1992;1:285–290

44. Pearce PC, Hawkey C, Symons C, Olsen EG: Role of calcium in the induction of cardiac hypertrophy and myofibrillar disarry. Experimental studies of a possible cause of hypertrophic cardiomyopathy. Br Heart J 1985;54:420–427

45. Maron BJ: New observations on the interrelation of dynamic subaortic obstruction and exercise in hypertrophic cardiomyopathy [editorial; comment]. J Am Coll Cardiol 1992;19:534–535

46. Maron BJ, Epstein SE: Dynamic obstruction to left ventricular outflow. The case for its existence in hypertrophic cardiomyopathy [review]. Z Kardiol 1987; 3:69–77

47. Sugrue DD, McKenna WJ, Dickie S et al: Relation between left ventricular gradient and relative stroke volume ejected in early and late systole in hypertrophic cardiomyopathy. Assessment with radionuclide cineangiography. Br Heart J 1984;52:602–609

48. Ciro E, Maron BJ, Bonow RO, Cannon RO, Epstein SE: Relation between marked changes in left ventricular outflow tract gradient and disease progression in hypertrophic cardiomyopathy. Am J Cardiol 1984; 53:1103–1109

49. Spirito P, Maron BJ: Significance of left ventricular outflow tract cross-sectional area in hypertrophic cardiomyopathy. A two-dimensional echocardiographic assessment. Circulation 1983;67:1100–1108

50. Maron BJ, Gottdiener JS, Roberts WC et al: Left ventricular outflow tract obstruction due to systolic anterior motion of the anterior mitral leaflet in patients with concentric left ventricular hypertrophy. Circulation 1978;57:527–533

51. Maron BJ, Gottdiener JS, Arge J et al: Dynamic subaortic obstruction in hypertrophic cardiomyopathy. Analysis by pulsed Doppler echocardiography. J Am Coll Cardiol 1985;6:1–18

52. Louie EK, Maron BJ: Hypertrophic cardiomyopathy with extreme increase in left ventricular wall thickness. Functional and morphologic features and clinical significance. J Am Coll Cardiol 1986;8:57–65

53. Panza JA, Maris TJ, Maron BJ: Development and determinants of dynamic obstruction to left ventricular outflow in young patients with hypertrophic cardiomyopathy. Circulation 1992;85:1398–1405

54. Klues HG, Roberts WC, Maron BJ: Morphological determinants of echocardiographic patterns of mitral valve systolic anterior motion in obstructive hypertrophic cardiomyopathy. Circulation 1993;87: 1570–1579

55. Maron BJ, Spirito P, Green KJ et al: Noninvasive assesment of left ventricular diastolic function by pulsed Doppler echocardiography in patients with hypertrophic cardiomyopathy. J Am Coll Cardiol 1987;10:733–742

56. Nihoyannopoulos P, Karatasakis G, Frenneaux M, McKenna WJ, Oakley CM: Diastolic function in hypertrophic cardiomyopathy. Relation to exercise capacity [see comments]. J Am Coll Cardiol 1992;19: 536–540

57. Sugrue DD, McKenna WJ: Radionuclide assessment of left ventricular function in hypertrophic cardiomyopathy. Postgrad Med J 1986;62:553–555

58. Chikamori T, Dickie S, Poloniecki JD et al: Prognostic significance of radionuclide-assessed diastolic function in hypertrophic cardiomyopathy. Am J Cardiol 1990;65:478–482

59. McKenna W, Deanfield J, Faruque A et al: Prognosis in hypertrophic cardiomyopathy. Role of age and clinical, electrocardiographic and hemodynamic features. Am J Cardiol 1981;47:532–538

60. Elliott P, Rosano GMC, Giu JS, Kashi JC, Poole-Wilson PA, McKenna WJ: Coronary sinus pH during dipyridamole infusion in patients with angina and hypertrophic cardiomyopathy. [abstract]. J Am Coll Cardiol, suppl. 1995;30A

61. O'Gara PT, Bonow RO, Maron BJ et al: Myocardial perfusion abnormalities in patients with hypertrophic cardiomyopathy. Assessment with thallium-201 emission computed tomography. Circulation 1987;76:1214–1223

62. Rubin KA, Morrison J, Padnick MB et al: Idiopathic hypertrophic subaortic stenosis. Evaluation of anginal symptoms with thallium-201 myocardial imaging. Am J Cardiol 1979;44:1040–1045

63. Choudhury L, Al Ms, French J, Oakley CM, Camici PG: An additional marker for familial hypertrophic cardiomyopathy? Coronary Artery Dis 1993;4:565–567

64. Gould KL: Myocardial metabolism by positron emission tomography in hypertrophic cardiomyopathy [editorial]. J Am Coll Cardiol 1989;13:325–326

65. Slade AK, Saumarez RC, McKenna WJ: The arrhythmogenic substrate—diagnostic and therapeutic implications. Hypertrophic cardiomyopathy. Eur Heart J 1993, suppl. E 1993;14:84–90

66. McKenna WJ, Krikler DM, Goodwin JF: Arrhythmias in dilated and hypertrophic cardiomyopathy [review]. Med Clin North Am 1984;68:983–1000

67. Shakespeare CF, Keeling PJ, Slade AK, McKenna WJ: Arrhythmia hypertrophic cardiomyopathy. Arch Mal Coeur Vaiss 1991;4(31):31–36

68. Alfonso F, Frenneaux MP, McKenna WJ: Clinical sustained uniform ventricular tachycardia in hypertrophic cardiomyopathy. Association with left ventricular apical aneurysm. Br Heart J 1989;61:178–181

69. Mulrow JP, Healy MJ, McKenna WJ: Variability of ventricular arrhythmias in hypertrophic cardiomyopathy and implications for treatment. Am J Cardiol 1986;58:615–618

70. Somerville J, Bonham CR: The heart in lentiginosis Br Heart J 1972;34:58–66

71. Simpson P: Norepinephrine-stimulated hypertrophy of cultured rat myocardial cells is an alpha 1 adrenergic response. J Clin Invest 1983;72:732–738

72. Counihan PJ, Fei L, Bashir Y et al: Assessment of heart rate variability in hypertrophic cardiomyopathy. Association with clinical and prognostic features. Circulation 1993;88;1670–1682

73. Brush JJ, Eisenhofer G, Garty M et al: Cardiac norepinephrine kinetics in hypertrophic cardiomyopathy. Circulation 1989;79:836–844

74. Frenneaux MP, Counihan PJ, Calorio AL, Chikamori T, McKenna WJ: Abnormal blood pressure response during exercise in hypertrophic cardiomyopathy [see comments]. Circulation 1990;82:1995–2002

75. Chagnac A, Rudniki C, Loebel H, Zahavi I: Infectious endocarditis in idiopathic hypertrophic subartic ste-

nosis. Report of three cases and review of the literature. Chest 1982;81:346–349

76. McKenna WJ, Franklin RC, Nihoyannopoulos P, Robinson KC, Deanfield JE: Arrhythmia and prognosis in infants, children and adolescents with hypertrophic cardiomyopathy. J Am Coll Cardiol 1988;11:147–153

77. McKenna WJ, Deanfield JE: Hypertrophic cardiomyopathy. An important cause of sudden death. Arch Dis Child 1984;59:971

78. Frenneaux MP, Porter A, Caforio AL et al: Determinants of exercise capacity in hypertrophic cardiomyopathy. J Am Coll Cardiol 1989;13:1521–1526

79. Cannon R III, Rosing DR, Maron BJ et al: Myocardial ischemia in patient with hypertrophic cardiomyopathy. Contribution of inadequate vasodilator reserve and elevated left ventricular filling pressures. Circulation 1985;71:234–243

80. Cannon R III: Myocardial ischemia in hypertrophic cardiomyopathy. Kardiol 1987;3:101–104

81. Maron BJ, Bonow RO, Cannon R III, Leon MB, Epstein SE: Hypertrophic cardiomyopathy. Interrelations of clinical manifestations, pathophysiology, and therapy (1) [review]. N Engl J Med 1987;316:844–852

82. Maron BJ, Bonow RO, Cannon R III, Leon MB, Epstein SE: Hypertrophic cardiomyopathy. Interrelations of clinical manifestations, pathophysiology, and therapy (2) [review]. N Engl J Med 1987,316:844–852

83. Loogen F, Kuhn H, Gietzen F et al: Clinical course and prognosis of patients with typical and atypical hypertrophic obstructive and with hypertrophic nonobstructive cardiomyopathy. Eur Heart J suppl. 1983;4;145–153

84. Braunwald E, Lambrew C, Rockoff S, Ross J Jr, Morrow A: Idiopathic hypertrophic subaortic stenosis. 1. A description of the disease based upon an analysis of 64 patients. Circulation, suppl. IV 1964;30:3

85. Savage DD, Seides SF, Clark CE et al: Electrocardiographic findings in patients with obstructive and nonobstructive hypertrophic cardiomyopathy. Circulation 1978;58:402–408

86. Alfonso F, Nihoyannopoulos P, Steward J et al: Clinical significance of giant negative T waves in hypertrophic cardiomyopathy [see comments]. J Am Coll Cardiol 1990;15:965–971

87. Lemery R, Kleinebenne A, Nihoyannopoulos P et al: Q waves in hypertrophic cardiomyopathy in relation to the distribution and severity of right and left ventricular hypertrophy [see comments]. J Am Coll Cardiol 1990;16:368–374

88. Maron BJ: Q waves in hypertrophic cardiomyopathy. A reassessment [editorial; comment]. J Am Coll Cardiol 1990;16:375–376

89. Macraw CE et al: Familial hypertrophic cardiomyopathy with Wolff-Parkinson-White syndrome maps to a locus on chromosome 7q3. J Clin Invest 1995;96:1216–1220

90. McKenna WJ, Kleinebenne A: Arrhythmias in hypertrophic cardiomyopathy. Significance and therapeutic consequences [in German]. Herz 1985;10:91–101

91. McKenna WJ, England D, Doi YL et al: Arrhythmia in hypertrophic cardiomyopathy. I. Influence on prognosis. Br Heart J 1981;46:168–172

92. Maron BJ, Savage DD, Wolfson JK, Epstein SE: Prognostic significance of 24 hour ambulatory electrocardiographic monitoring in patients with hy-

pertrophic cardiomyopathy. A prospective study. Am J Cardiol 1981;48:252–257

93. Savage DD, Seides SF, Maron BJ, Myers DJ, Epstein SE: Prevalence of arrhythmias during 24-hour electrocardiographic monitoring and exercise testing in patients with obstructive and nonobstructive hypertrophic cardiomyopathy. Circulation 1979;59:866–875

94. McKenna WJ, Chetty S, Oakley CM, Goodwin JF: Arrhythmia in hypertrophic cardiomyopathy: exercise and 48 hour ambulatory electrocardiographic assessment with and without beta adrenergic blocking therapy. Am J Cardiol 1980;45:1–5

95. McKenna WJ, Sadoul N, Slade AK, Saumarez RC: The prognostic significance of nonsustained ventricular tachycardia in hypertrophic cardiomyopathy (editorial; comment). [review]. Circulation 1994;90:3115–3117

96. McKenna WJ: Arrhythmia and prognosis in hypertrophic cardiomyopathy. Eur Heart J 1983

97. Robinson K, Frenneaux MP, Stockins B et al: Atrial fibrillation in hypertrophic cardiomyopathy: a longitudinal study [see comments]. J Am Coll Cardiol 1990;15(6):1279–1285

98. Hecht GM, Panza JA, Maron BJ: Clinical course of middle-aged asymptomatic patients with hypertrophic cardiomyopathy. Am J Cardiol 1992;69:935–940

99. McKenna WJ, Camm AJ: Sudden death in hypertrophic cardiomyopathy. Assessment of patients at high risk [comment]. Circulation 1989;80:1489–1492

100. Louie EK, Maron BJ: Apical hypertrophic cardiomyopathy. Clinical and two-dimensional echocardiographic assessment. Ann Intern Med 1987;106:663–670

101. Maron BJ, Bonow RO, Seshagiri TN, Roberts WC, Epstein SE: Hypertrophic cardiomyopathy with ventricular septal hypertrophy localized to the apical region of the left ventricle (apical hypertrophic cardiomyopathy). Am J Cardiol 1982;49:1838–1848

102. Shapiro LM, Kleinebenne A, McKenna WJ: The distribution of left ventricular hypertrophy in hypertrophic cardiomyopathy. Comparison to athletes and hypertensives. Eur Heart J 1985;6:967–974

103. Sasson Z, Yock PG, Hatle LK, Alderman EL, Popp RL: Doppler echocardiographic determination of the pressure gradient in hypertrophic cardiomyopathy. J Am Coll Cardiol 1988;11:752–756

104. Yock PG, Hatle L, Popp RL: Patterns and timing of Doppler-detected intracavitary and aortic flow in hypertrophic cardiomyopathy. J Am Coll Cardiol 1986;8:1047–1058

105. Panza JA, Petrone RK, Fananapazir L, Maron BJ: Utility of continuous wave Doppler echocardiography in the noninvasive assessment of left ventricular outflow tract pressure gradient in patients with hypertrophic cardiomyopathy. J Am Coll Cardiol 1992;19:91–99

106. Doi YL, McKenna WJ, Gehrke J, Oakley CM, Goodwin JF: M mode echocardiography in hypertrophic cardiomyopathy. Diagnostic criteria and prediction of obstruction. Am J Cardiol 1980;45:6–14

107. Pollick C, Morgan CD, Gilbert BW, Rakowski H, Wigle ED: Muscular subaortic stenosis. The temporal relationship between systolic anterior motion of the anterior mitral leaflet and the pressure gradient. Circulation 1982;66:1087–1094

108. Wigle ED, Adelman AG, Auger P, Marquis Y: Mitral regurgitation in muscular subaortic stenosis. Am J Cardiol 1969;24:698–706

109. Maron BJ, Gottdiener JS, Perry LW: Specificity of systolic anterior motion of anterior mitral leaflet for hypertrophic cardiomyopathy. Prevalence in large population of patients with other cardiac diseases. Br Heart J 1981;45:206–212

110. Doi YL, McKenna WJ, Oakley CM, Goodwin JF: "Pseudo" systolic anterior motion in patients with hypertensive heart disease. Eur Heart J 1983;4:838–845

111. Counihan PJ, Frenneaux MP, Webb DJ, McKenna WJ: Abnormal vascular responses to supine exercise in hypertrophic cardiomyopathy. Circulation 1991;84:686–696

112. Kimball BP, Bui S, Wigle ED: Acute dose-response effects of intravenous disopyramide in hypertrophic obstructive cardiomyopathy. Am Heart J 1993;125:1691–1697

113. Brugada P, Bar FW, de ZC, Roy D, Green M, Wellens HJ: "Sawfish" systolic narrowing of the left anterior descending coronary artery. An angiographic sign of hypertrophic cardiomyopathy. Circulation 1982;66:800–803

114. Maron BJ, Epstein SE, Morrow AG: Symptomatic status and prognosis of patients after operation for hypertrophic obstructive cardiomyopathy. Efficacy of ventricular septal myotomy and myectomy. Eur Heart J 1983

115. McKenna WJ, Borggrefe M, England D et al: The natural history of left ventricular hypertrophy in hypertrophic cardiomyopathy. An electrocardiographic study. Circulation 1982;66:1233–1240

116. Maron BJ, Roberts WC, Edwards JE et al: Sudden death in patients with hypertrophic cardiomyopathy. Characterization of 26 patients with functional limitation. Am J Cardiol 1978;41:803–810

117. Maron BJ, Merrill WH, Freier PA et al: Long-term clinical course and symptomatic status of patients after operation for hypertrophic subaortic stenosis. Circulation 1978;57:1205–1213

118. Spirito P, Chiarella F, Carratino L et al: Clinical course and prognosis of hypertrophic cardiomyopathy in an outpatient population [see comments] [review]. N Engl J Med 1989;320:749–755

119. Maron BJ, Epstein SE, Roberts WC: Causes of sudden death in competitive athletes [review]. J Am Coll Cardiol 1986;7:204–214

120. Epstein SE, Maron BJ: Sudden death and the competitive athlete. Perspectives on preparticipation screening studies [review]. J Am Coll Cardiol 1986;7:220–230

121. Maron BJ, Epstein SE, Roberts WC: Hypertrophic cardiomyopathy. A common cause of sudden death in the young competitive athlete. Eur Heart J, suppl. 1983;4:135–144

122. Maron BJ, Roberts WC, McAllister HA, Rosing DR, Epstein SE: Sudden death in young athletes. Circulation 1980;62:218–229

123. Maron BJ, Klues HG: Surviving competitive athletics with hypertrophic cardiomyopathy. Am J Cardiol 1994;73:1098–1104

124. Glancy DL, O'Brien KP, Gold HK, Epstein SE: Atrial fibrillation in patients with idiopathic hypertrophic subaortic stenosis. Br Heart J 1970;32:652–659

125. Wigle ED, Sasson Z, Henderson MA et al: Hypertrophic cardiomyopathy. The importance of the site and the extent of hypertrophy; a review. Prog Cardiovasc Dis 1985;28:1–83

126. Maron BJ, Roberts WC, Epstein SE: Sudden death in hypertrophic cardiomyopathy. A profile of 78 patients. Circulation 1982;65:1388–1394

127. Maron BJ, Gaffney FA, Jeresaty RM, McKenna WJ, Miller WW: Cardiovascular abnormalities in the athlete: recommendations regarding eligibility for competition. Task force III: Hypertrophic cardiomyopathy, other myopericardial diseases and mitral valve prolapse. J Am Coll Cardiol 1985;6:1215–1217

128. Maron BJ, Isner JM, McKenna WJ: 26th Bethesda conference: recommendations for determining eligibility for competition in athletes with cardiovascular abnormalities. Task Force 3: Hypertrophic cardiomyopathy, myocarditis and other myopericardial diseases and mitral valve prolapse [review]. Med Sci Sports Exerc, suppl. 1994;26;S261–S267

129. Maron BJ, Pelliccia A, Spirito P: Cardiac disease in young trained athletes. Insights into methods for distinguishing athlete's heart from structural heart disease, with particular emphasis on hypertrophic cardiomyopathy [review]. Circulation 1995; 91:1596–1601

130. Maron BJ: Structural features of the athlete heart as defined by echocardiography [review]. J Am Coll Cardiol 1986;7:190–203

131. McKenna W, Harris L, Deanfield J: Syncope in hypertrophic cardiomyopathy. Br Heart J 1982;47:177–179

132. Rosing DR, Kent KM, Maron BJ, Condit J, Epstein SE: Verapamil therapy. A new approach to pharmacologic treatment of hypertrophic cardiomyopathy. Chest, suppl. 1980;78:239–247

133. Rosing DR, Kent KM, Maron BJ, Epstein SE: Verapamil therapy: a new approach to the pharmacologic treatment of hypertrophic cardiomyopathy. II. Effects on exercise capacity and symptomatic status. Circulation 1979;60:1208–1213

134. Bonow RO, Ostrow HG, Rosing DR et al: Effects of verapamil on left ventricular systolic and diastolic function in patients with hypertrophic cardiomyopathy. Pressure-volume analysis with a nonimaging scintillation probe. Circulation 1983;68:1062–1073

135. Rosing DR, Condit JR, Maron BJ et al: Verapamil therapy: a new approach to the pharmacologic treatment of hypertrophic cardiomyopathy. III. Effects of long-term administration. Am J Cardiol 1981;48: 545–553

136. Bonow RO, Rosing DR, Bacharach SL et al: Effects of verapamil on left ventricular systolic function and diastolic filling in patients with hypertrophic cardiomyopathy. Circulation 1981;64:787–796

137. Bonow RO, Dilsizian V, Rosing DR et al: Verapamil-induced improvement in left ventricular diastolic filling and increased exercise tolerance in patients with hypertrophic cardiomyopathy. Short- and long-term effects. Circulation 1985;72:853–864

138. Hanrath P, Mathey DG, Siegert R, Bleifeld W: Left ventricular relaxation and filling pattern in different forms of left ventricular hypertrophy. An echocardiographic study. Am J Cardiol 1980;45:15–23

139. Lorell BH: Use of calcium channel blockers in hypertrophic cardiomyopathy. Am J Med 1985;78(2B): 43–54

140. Betocchi S, Bono RO, Bacharach SL et al: Isovolumic relaxation period in hypertrophic cardiomyopathy. Assessment by radionuclide angiography. J Am Coll Cardiol 1986;7:74–81

141. Alvares RF, Goodwin JF: Non-invasive assessment of diastolic function in hypertrophic cardiomyopathy on and off beta adrenergic blocking drugs. Br Heart J 1982;48:204–212

142. Frank MJ, Abdulla AM, Canedo MI, Saylors RE: Long-term medical management of hypertrophic obstructive cardiomyopathy. Am J Cardiol 1978;42: 993–1001

143. Kaltenbach M, Hopf R, Keller M: Treatment of hypertrophic obstructive cardiomyopathy with verapamil, a calcium antagonist [in German]. D Med Wochenschr 1976;101:1284–1287

144. Pollick C: Muscular subaortic stenosis. Hemodynamic and clinical improvement after disopyramide. N Engl J Med 1982;307:997–999

145. Epstein SE, Rosing DR: Verapamil. Its potential for causing serious complications in patients with hypertrophic cardiomyopathy. Circulation 1981;64: 437–441

146. Suwa M, Hirota Y, Kawamura K: Improvement in left ventricular diastolic function during intravenous and oral diltiazem therapy in patients with hypertrophic cardiomyopathy. An echocardiographic study. Am J Cardiol 1984;54:1047–1053

147. Paulus WJ, Lorell BH, Craig WE et al: Comparison of the effects of nitroprusside and nifedipine on diastolic properties in patients with hypertrophic cardiomyopathy: altered left ventricular loading or improved muscle inactivation? J Am Coll Cardiol 1983;2: 879–886

148. Betocchi S, Cannon R, Watson RM et al: Effects of sublingual nifedipine on hemodynamics and systolic and diastolic function in patients with hypertrophic cardiomyopathy. Circulation 1985;72:1001–1007

149. McKenna WJ, Goodwin JF: The natural history of hypertrophic cardiomyopathy. [review]. Cur Prob Cardiol 1981;6:1–26

150. Spirito P, Maron BJ, Rosing DR: Morphologic determinants of hemodynamic state after ventricular septal myotomy-myectomy in patients with obstructive hypertrophic cardiomyopathy. M mode and two-dimensional echocardiographic assessment. Circulation 1984;70:984–995

151. Cannon R III, McIntosh CL, Schenke WH et al: Effect of surgical reduction of left ventricular outflow obstruction on hemodynamics, coronary flow, and myocardial metabolism in hypertrophic cardiomyopathy. Circulation 1989;79:766–775

152. McIntosh CL, Greenberg GJ, Maron BJ et al: Clinical and hemodynamic results after mitral valve replacement in patient with obstructive hypertrophic cardiomyopathy. Ann Thorac Surg 1989;47:236–246

153. McIntosh CL, Maron BJ, Cannon R III, Klues HG: Initial results of combined anterior mitral leaflet plication and ventricular septal myotomy-myectomy for relief of left ventricular outflow tract obstruction in patients with hypertrophic cardiomyopathy. Circulation, suppl. 5 1992;86:1160–1167

154. Stone CD, McIntosh CL, Hennein HA, Maron BJ, Clark RE: Operative treatment of pediatric obstructive hypertrophic cardiomyopathy. A 26-year experience. Ann Thorac Surg 1993;56:1308–1313

155. Seiler C, Hess OM, Schoenbeck M et al: Long-term follow-up medical versus surgical therapy for hypertrophic cardiomyopathy. A retrospective study [see comments] [review]. J Am Coll Cardiol 1991;17: 634–642

156. Kirklin JW: The science of cardiac surgery. Eur J Cardiol Thorac Surg 1990;4(2):63–71

157. Sigwart U, Knight C, Buszman P et al: Nonsurgical catheter treatment for hypertrophic obstructive cardiomyopathy [abstract]. Br Heart J, suppl 3 1995;73: 64

158. Gill CC, Duda AM, Kitazume H, Kramer JR, Loop FD: Idiopathic hypertrophic subaortic stenosis and coronary atherosclerosis. Results of coronary artery bypass alone and myectomy combined with coronary artery bypass. J Thorac Cardiovasc Surg 1982;84: 856–860

159. Siegman IL, Maron BJ, Permut LC, McIntosh CL, Clark RE: Results of operation for coexistent obstructive hypertrophic cardiomyopathy and coronary artery disease. J Am Coll Cardiol 1989;13:1527–1533

160. Counihan PJ, McKenna WJ: Low-dose amiodarone for the treatment of arrhythmias in hypertrophic cardiomyopathy [review]. J Clin Pharmacol 1989;29: 436–438

161. McKenna WJ, Oakley CM, Krikler DM, Goodwin JF: Improved survival with amiodarone in patients with hypertrophic cardiomyopathy and ventricular tachycardia. Br Heart J 1985;53:412–416

162. McKenna WJ, Harris L, Rowland E et al: Amiodarone for long-term management of patients with hypertrophic cardiomyopathy. Am J Cardiol 1984;54:802–810

163. Harris L, McKenna WJ, Rowland E et al: Side effects of long-term amiodarone therapy. Circulation 1983; 67:45–51

164. Shirani J, Maron BJ, Cannon R III, Shahin S, Roberts WC: Clinicopathologic features of hypertrophic cardiomyopathy managed by cardiac transplantation. Am J Cardiol 1993;22:489–497

165. Hecht GM, Klues HG, Roberts WC, Maron BJ: Coexistence of sudden cardiac death and end-stage heart failure in familial hypertrophic cardiomyopathy. J Am Coll Cardiol 1993;22:489–497

166. Jarcho JA, McKenna W, Pare JA et al: Mapping a gene for familial hypertrophic cardiomyopathy to chromosome 14q1. N Engl J Med 1989;321: 1372–1378

167. Matsuoka R, Yoshida MC, Kanda N et al: Human cardiac myosin heavy chain gene mapped with chromosome region 14q11.2—q13. Am J Med Genet 1989; 32:279–284

168. Matsuoka R, Chambers A, Kimura M et al: Molecular cloning and chromosomal localization of a gene coding for human cardiac myosin heavy-chain. Am J Med Genet 1988;29:369–376

169. Solomon SD, Geisterfer LA, Vosberg HP et al: A locus for familial hypertrophic cardiomyopathy is closely linked to the cardiac myosin heavy chain genes, CRI-L436, and CRI-L329 on chromosome 14 at q11-q12. Am J Hum Genet 1990;47:389–394

170. Tanigawa G, Jarcho JA, Kass S et al: A molecular basis for familial hypertrophic cardiomyopathy. An alpha/beta cardiac myosin heavy chain hybrid gene. Cell 1990;62:991–998

171. Geisterfer LA, Kass S, Tanigawa G et al: A molecular basis for familial hypertrophic cardiomyopathy. A beta cardiac myosin heavy chain gene missense mutation. Cell 1990;62:999–1006

172. Watkins H, Rosenzweig A, Hwang DS et al: Characteristics and prognostic implications of myosin missense mutations in familial hypertrophic cardiomyopathy [see comments]. N Engl J Med 1992;326: 1108–1114

173. Watkins H, Seidman CE, MacRae C, Seidman JG, McKenna W: Progress in familial hypertrophic cardiomyopathy. Molecular genetic analyses in the original family studied by Teare [review]. Br Heart J 1992;67:34–38

174. Rosenzweig A, Watkins H, Hwang DS et al: Preclinical diagnosis of familial hypertrophic cardiomyopathy by genetic analysis of blood lymphocytes [see comments]. N Engl J Med 1991;325:1753–1760

175. Epstein ND, Cohn GM, Cyran F, Fananapazir L: Differences in clinical expression of hypertrophic cardiomyopathy associated with two distinct mutations in the beta-myosin heavy chain gene: a 908Leu→Val mutation and a 403Arg→Gln mutation [see comments]. Circulation 1992;86:345–352

176. Perryman MB, Yu QT, Marian AJ et al: Expression of a missense mutation in the messenger RNA for beta-myosin heavy chain in myocardial tissue in hypertrophic cardiomyopathy. J Clin Invest 1992;90: 271–277

177. Anan R, Greve G, Thierfelder L et al: Prognostic implications of novel beta cardiac myosin heavy chain gene mutations that cause familial hypertrophic cardiomyopathy [see comments]. J Clin Invest 1994;93: 280–285

178. Nishi H, Kimura A, Harada H, Toshima H, Sasazuki T: Novel missense mutation in cardiac beta myosin heavy chain gene found in a Japanese patient with hypertrophic cardiomyopathy. Biochem Biophys Res Commun 1992;188:379–387

179. Watkins H, Thierfelder L, Hwang DS et al: Sporadic hypertrophic cardiomyopathy due to de novo myosin mutations. J Clin Invest 1992;90:1666–1671

180. Al-Mahdawi S, Chamberlain S, Cleland J et al: Identification of a mutation in the beta cardiac myosin heavy chain gene in a family with hypertrophic cardiomyopathy. Br Heart J 1993;69:136–141

181. Dausse E, Komajda M, Fetler L et al: Familial hypertrophic cardiomyopathy. Microsatellite haplotyping and identification of a hot spot for mutations in the beta-myosin heavy chain gene. J Clin Invest 1993; 92:2807–2813

182. Harada H, Kimura A, Nishi H, Sasazuki T, Toshima H: A missense mutation of cardiac beta-myosin heavy chain gene linked to familial hypertrophic cardiomyopathy in affected Japanese families. Biochem Biophys Res Commun 1992;188:379–387

183. Dufour C, Dausse E, Fetler L et al: Identification of a mutation near a functional site of the beta cardiac myosin heavy chain gene in a family with hypertrophic cardiomyopathy. J Mol Cell Cardiol 1994;26: 1241–1247

184. Perryman MMA, Hejtmancik F, Gooch G, Roberts R: The beta-myosin heavy chain missence mutation in exon 13, a putative defect for HCM is present in only one of 39 families. Circulation, (suppl. 2) 1991;84: 418

185. Moolman JC, Brink PA, Corfield VA: Identification of a new missense mutation at Arg403, a CpG mutation

hotspot, in exon 13 of the beta-myosin heavy chain gene in hypertrophic cardiomyopathy. Hum Mol Genet 1993;2:1731–1732

186. Marian AJ, Yu QT, Mares AJ et al: Detection of a new mutation in the beta-myosin heavy chain gene in an individual with hypertrophic cardiomyopathy. J Clin Invest 1992;90:2156–2165

187. Watkins H, MacRae E, Thierfelder L et al: A disease locus for familial hypertrophic cardiomyopathy maps to chromosome 1q3. Nat Genet 1991;3:333–337

188. Thiefelder L, MacRae C, Watkins H et al: A familial hypertrophic cardiomyopathy locus maps to chromosome 15q2. Proc Acad Sci USA 1993;90:6270–6274

189. Carrier L, Hengstenberg C, Beckmann JS et al: Mapping a novel gene for familial hypertrophic cardiomyopathy to chromosome 11. Nat Genet 1993;4:311–313

190. Thierfelder L, Watkins H, MacRae C et al: Alpha-tropomyosin and cardiac troponin T mutations cause familial hypertrophic cardiomyopathy: a disease of the sarcomere. Cell 1994;77:701–712

191. Pan BS, Gordon AM, Potter JD: Deletion of the first 45 NH_2-terminal residues of rabbit skeletal troponin T strengthens binding of troponin to immobilized tropomyosin. J Biol Chem 1991;266:12432–12438

192. Brisson JR, Golosinska K, Smillie LB, Sykes BD: Interaction of tropomyosin and troponin T. A proton nuclear magnetic resonance study. Biochemistry 1986;25:4548–4555

193. Pearlstone JR, Carpenter MR, Smillie LB: Amino acid sequence of rabbit cardiac troponin T. J Biol Chem 1986;261:16795–16810

194. Ishii Y, Lehrer SS: Two-site attachment of troponin to pyrene-labeled tropomyosin. J Biol Chem 1991;266:6849–6903

195. Anderson PA, Greig A, Mark TM et al: Molecular basis of human cardiac troponin T isoforms expressed in the developing, adult, and failing heart. Circ Res 1995;76:681–686

196. Anderson PA, Malouf NN, Oakley AE, Pagani ED, Allen PD: Troponin T isoform expression in humans. A comparison among normal and failing adult heart, fetal heart, and adult and fetal skeletal muscle. Circ Res 1991;69:1226–1233

197. Malouf NN, McMahon D, Oakley AE, Anderson PA: A cardiac troponin epitope conserved across phyla. J Biol Chem 1992;267:9269–9274

198. Watkins HEA: A mutated cardiac myosin binding protein-C gene on chromosome 11 causes familial hypertrophic cardiomyopathy. Nat Genet 1995;11:435–437

199. Bonne G, Carrier L, Bercovici J et al: Cardiac myosin binding protein C gene splice acceptor site mutation is associated with familial hypertrophic cardiomyopathy. Nat Gene 1995;11:438–440

200. Ferraro M, Scarton G, Ambrosini M: Cosegregation of hypertrophic cardiomyopathy and a fragile site on chromosome 16 in a large Italian family. J Med Genet 1990;27:363–366

201. Hejtmancik JF, Brink PA, Towbin J et al: Localization of gene for familial hypertrophic cardiomyopathy to chromosome 14q1 in a diverse US population. Circulation 1991;69:1024–1034

202. Machida M: Genetic heterogeneity of hypertrophic cardiomyopathy in Japanese [in Japanese]. Hokkaido Igaku Zasshi [Hokkaido J Med Sci] 1994;69:1024–1034

203. Parker TG, Schneider MD: Growth factors, proto-oncogenes, and plasticity of the cardiac phenotype [review]. Annu Rev Physiol 1991;53:179–200

204. Parker TG: Molecular biology of cardiac growth and hypertrophy. [review]. Herz 1993;18(4):245–255

205. Fyrberg E, Fyrberg CC, Beall C, Saville DL: Drosophila melanogaster troponin-T mutations engender three distinct syndromes of myofibrillar abnormalities. J Molec Biol 1990;216(3):657–675

206. Mogami K, Hotta Y: Isolation of Drosophila flightless mutants which affect myofibrillar proteins of indirect flight muscle. Molec Gen Genet 1981;183:409–417

207. Mogami K, Fujita SC, Hotta Y: Identification of Drosophila indirect flight muscle myofibrillar proteins by means of two-dimensional electrophoresis. J Biochem 1982;91:643–650

28 Dilated Cardiomyopathy

Thomas D. Giles

Cardiomyopathy literally means disease of the heart muscle. When assessing heart disease, it is necessary to consider the myocardium separately, and the functional state of the myocardium usually determines patient outcome. Therefore the term *cardiomyopathy* is used to indicate myocardial disease, regardless of the pathophysiologic mechanism (e.g., coronary atherosclerosis).[1] The classification scheme recommended by the World Health Organization restricts use of the term to diseases that primarily involve the myocardium and are of unknown cause.[2] However, because all cardiomyopathies have a cause, in this discussion the term *idiopathic* indicates the diagnosis when no discernible cause of cardiomyopathy is found. Idiopathic cardiomyopathy, then, is not a specific disease entity but a term that reflects the state of knowledge concerning the cause of cardiomyopathy in specific patients.

The *dilated cardiomyopathies* are characterized by a common cardiac remodeling process that ultimately produces increased cardiac ventricular chamber dimensions, normal or decreased ventricular wall thickness, and reduced ventricular systolic function.[3,4] This abnormal remodeling process may be the result of diverse myocardial disease processes, and the characteristics that result from this remodeling process differentiate the dilated from the nondilated cardiomyopathies, which include hypertrophic and restrictive subtypes. For that reason, the classification is useful to both the clinician and the investigator.

As so defined, the dilated cardiomyopathies constitute the largest group of heart diseases responsible for heart failure, the physiologic result of progressive cardiomyopathy (Table 28-1). The left ventricle is almost always involved in the dilated cardiomyopathies from the onset, and the early involvement of both ventricles in the cardiomyopathic process may be an important clue to etiology. In rare instances, the right ventricle is involved initially (e.g., familial right ventricular dysplasia).[5]

Before the term dilated cardiomyopathy can be used with confidence, the cardiac ventricles should be dilated. The clinical stages of the dilated cardiomyopathies are potential, early, and late (advanced). These stages parallel the pathophysiologic processes that begin with the initial insult to the myocardium, followed by progression to clinically detectable myocardial failure. *Potential* dilated cardiomyopathy exists when myocardial disease is not clinically detected but conditions are present that may eventually lead to cardiomyopathy (Table 28-2). At the stage of potential cardiomyopathy, preventive therapeutic measures may be of most benefit. The *early* and *late* (advanced) stages of dilated cardiomyopathy are associated with signs and symptoms of cardiac disease, as well as with extracardiac signs and symptoms of specific diseases that involve the heart. Thus the pathophysiology of dilated cardiomyopathy is a continuum that either begins with the initial myocardial insult(s) or is a chronic process that continues until the heart is large, dilated, and failing.

Table 28-1 lists an etiologic/pathophysiologic classification of the dilated cardiomyopathies. This classification is useful to the clinician in search of a precise cause of a particular patient's heart disease, and the clinician should always consider that a particular cardiomyopathy is pluricausal (i.e., stems from more than one pathophysiologic factor). Because of the difficulty of arriving at a consistent definition of dilated cardiomyopathy, data on its incidence are elusive.

Table 28-1. Etiologic and Pathophysiologic Classes of Dilated Cardiomyopathy

Genetic
  Heredofamilial dilated (congestive) cardiomyopathy
  Sporadic
  Neuromuscular
  Friedreich's disease
  Progressive muscular dystrophy: Duchenne's, limb-girdle, fascioscapulohumeral
  Myotonic dystrophy
  Mitochondrial syndromes
      MELAS syndrome (mitochondrial encephalopathy, lactic acidosis, and stroke-like episodes)
      Kearns-Sayre syndrome
      tRNALeu (UUR) gene mitochondrial point mutation: diabetes mellitus, deafness, and cardiomyopathy
  Barth syndrome (skeletal and cardiomyopathy, short stature, and recurrent neutropenia)
  Najjar syndrome (cardiomyopathy and hypergonadotropic hypogonadism

Ischemic
  Coronary artery disease: arteriosclerosis, vasculitis, microvascular disease (e.g., diabetes mellitus)
Myocarditis, acute and chronic
  Infectious: viral, bacterial, rickettsial, protozoal
Hyperergopathic ("overwork")
  Valvular heart disease: aortic regurgitation, aortic stenosis, mitral regurgitation, "mitral stenosis," endocarditis
  Hypertensive heart disease (postpartal)
  High-output states: beriberi, thyrotoxicosis, severe anemia, arteriovenous fistula, osteitis deformans, Paget's disease, chronic liver disease, pregnancy, hypernephroma
  Incessant tachycardia

Toxic
  Substance abuse
      Alcohol
      Cocaine
      Drugs (anthracyclines)
      Heavy metals
Hypertensive heart disease (postpartal)
Metabolic
  Endocrine: diabetes mellitus, hyperthyroidism, hypothyroidism, hyperparathyroidism, hypoparathyroidism, acromegaly
  Electrolyte disturbances (potassium, phosphate, magnesium)
  Nutritional deficiencies (thiamine, protein-calorie)
  Hemochromatosis
Collagen vascular diseases
  Systemic lupus erythematosus
  Polyarteritis nodosa
  Churg-Strauss
  Progressive systemic sclerosis
  Mixed connective tissue disease
Physical agents
  Extreme cold and heat
  Ionizing radiation
  Electric shock
  Altitude
Immunologically mediated
  Postvaccinal
  Serum sickness
  Urticaria
  Transplant
Idiopathic dilated cardiomyopathy

Nonetheless, it is safe to assume that most patients with overt congestive heart failure have dilated cardiomyopathy. This group of patients with such symptoms, however, represents only the "tip of the iceberg." Correct assessment of patients with dilated cardiomyopathy requires both a general and a specific approach. That is, after determining the potential or real likelihood that cardiomyopathy is present, a search for a specific etiology or clinical syndrome is necessary in order to render proper care to the patient.

GENERAL CLINICAL CONSIDERATIONS

History

A meticulous history remains one of the most valuable tools for detecting the presence of cardiomyopathy and establishing an etiology. The cardiac symptoms of dilated cardiomyopathy have been well described.[6-9] A history of any of the conditions listed in Table 28-1 should raise the possibility of potential or early cardiomyopathy, even in the absence of clear-cut cardiac symptoms. Minimal exertional dyspnea, often referred to by the patient as "being out of shape," and palpitations (atrial fibrillation or ventricular dysrhythmias) are among the earliest symptoms. Approximately 50 percent of patients with dilated cardiomyopathy experience chest discomfort, often typical angina pectoris, even when the etiology is not coronary artery disease. Syncope may be an early event in the clinical course of cardiomyopathy. Palpitations, hemoptysis, pleuritic chest pain, unexplained dyspnea, and other protean manifestations of pulmonary thromboembolism accompany dilated cardiomyopathy. In the late (advanced) stage, the symptoms of heart failure predominate (i.e., marked dyspnea on exertion, fatigue, paroxysmal nocturnal dyspnea, orthopnea, and pulmonary and peripheral dependent edema).

A complete medical inventory often rewards the clinician with a correct diagnosis for patients with dilated cardiomyopathy. In the search for specific clues to the etiology, certain aspects of the history deserve mention. A positive family history of heart disease is becoming more evident as one such clue.[10] The term *heart attack* is often used for illnesses that are not myocardial infarction, and the clinician should try to collect clinical data to determine if a familial basis other than coronary artery disease is responsible for the dilated cardiomyopathy. Old medical records are invaluable for assessing the role of common causes of cardiomyopathy (e.g., atherosclerosis and hypertension) in the family. Substance abuse (alcohol, cocaine) histories are essential to understanding the mechanism of cardiomyopathy in some patients; yet these histories are among the most unreliable. Accurate nutritional histories are also notoriously difficult to obtain, and patients also often forget past viral infections or assign them little significance.

The physical examination of patients with early dilated cardiomyopathy may reveal little or no evidence of heart disease. Resting tachycardia, slight cardiomegaly or a diffuse cardiac apical impulse, increased fourth heart sound, and dysrhythmia are often clues to the presence of early myocardial disease. The presence of a systolic murmur dictates that the patient be examined in both the supine and standing positions and during a Valsalva maneuver. In particular, the clinician should attempt to estimate the severity of valvular heart disease in order to judge the nature and severity of the associated cardiomyopathy. A systolic nonejection click varying in timing, with or without murmurs of mitral insufficiency, may be associated with the presence of cardiomyopathy linked to idiopathic mitral valve prolapse.

Table 28-2. Pathogenetic Factors for Consideration of Potential Cardiomyopathy

---

Substance abuse (alcohol, cocaine)
Coronary artery disease (risk factors, angina, myocardial infarction)
Family history of or conditions associated with dilated cardiomyopathy (e.g., hemochromatosis)
Systemic arterial hypertension
Systemic viral illness
Diabetes mellitus
Cardiotoxin exposure (e.g., anthracyclines)
Malnutrition
Valvular heart disease

The presence of the typical systolic click serves to differentiate mitral valve prolapse due to myxomatous or other connective tissue degeneration of the mitral valve from the mitral insufficiency due to the papillary muscle dysfunction found in many dilated cardiomyopathies.

Physical examination for late or advanced dilated cardiomyopathy usually reveals typical clinical findings. Abnormal distension of the neck veins, denoting systemic venous hypertension, is often present. The A wave of the jugular venous pulse may be increased, and a large CV wave indicates tricuspid insufficiency, often a reflection of right ventricular dilatation. A narrow pulse pressure, produced by slightly increased diastolic blood pressure (100–110 mmHg) and relatively low systolic blood pressure (130–140 mmHg), indicates the compensatory mechanisms that increase peripheral resistance. A wide pulse pressure suggests certain diseases (e.g., systemic arteriovenous fistula, thyrotoxicosis, beriberi, or aortic valvular insufficiency). Pulsus alternans is a valuable sign of left ventricular failure and may be detected by palpating the peripheral arterial pulse or by recording the systemic arterial blood pressure with a sphygmomanometer.

The finding of predominantly right-sided cardiac failure in patients with dilated cardiomyopathy may reflect the presence of pulmonary thromboembolism. The presence of signs of pulmonary hypertension (e.g., loud P2), increased right ventricular fourth or third heart sound location at the sternal edge with a positive Carvallo's sign (i.e., no change or increase in intensity with inspiration) are helpful. The source of the emboli is usually the leg veins, even in the absence of edema, or the pelvic veins; in patients with atrial fibrillation, the source may be the heart.

Some patients with dilated cardiomyopathy present with a *restrictive* or *constrictive* picture. Such is often the case when the etiology involves both the right and left ventricles from the onset of the disease (e.g., hemochromatosis, sarcoidosis). Constrictive pericarditis may be associated with ventricular dilatation and present with a restrictive clinical picture. A history of acute pericarditis and the presence of a pericardial knock may be helpful. Further assistance in diagnosis comes from the chest roentgenogram, echocardiogram, and other imaging procedures.

Electrocardiography, Chest Roentgenography, Echocardiography

The electrocardiogram (ECG), chest roentgenogram, and echocardiogram are essential for complete evaluation of the patient with suspected or known dilated cardiomyopathy. These studies are complementary and offer little hazard to the patient. The ECG of most patients with dilated cardiomyopathy shows some, albeit often subtle, abnormalities.[11] The ST segments and T waves often show the first abnormal changes (e.g., nonspecific and ischemic). Atrial fibrillation and ventricular premature beats are often present. Left bundle branch block is present in as many as 40 percent of patients with dilated cardiomyopathy and precedes the development of clinical heart failure by as long as 22 years.[12] ECG criteria for left ventricular hypertrophy (LVH) are frequent findings.

During the late stage of dilated cardiomyopathy, the ECG is nearly always abnormal. Evidence of LVH, left atrial disease, and atrioventricular and interventricular conduction disturbances are common findings. Nonspecific changes of the ST segment or T waves, atrial fibrillation, and ventricular premature beats are commonly found in all types of cardiomyopathy. ECG changes characteristic of myocardial infarction are also frequent in dilated cardiomyopathy not associated with myocardial infarction.

The chest roentgenogram is useful for determining cardiac enlargement in general and specific chamber enlargement in particular. Additionally, clues to the existence of pulmonary disease may be present, and the chest roentgenogram also may suggest coronary artery disease (calcification), valvular heart disease, and certain congenital malformations. The classic chest roentgenogram of late dilated cardiomyopathy shows a large heart, a relatively small aorta (unless hypertension or coronary atherosclerosis is the etiology), signs of pulmonary arterial and venous hypertension (e.g., increased blood flow to the upper lung zones), and evidence of pulmonary edema (e.g., interstitial edema: Kerley "B" lines), or alveolar edema.

The echocardiogram is often essential for evaluation of a patient with suspected or known dilated cardiomyopathy. In fact, the echocardiogram often establishes the diagnostic category of dilated cardiomyopathy. However, with potential or very early cardiomyopathy, the echocardiogram may not be diagnostic.

In clinically apparent dilated cardiomyopathy, the left ventricular diastolic dimension is increased (usually > 65 mm), and fractional shortening is reduced as recorded from an M-mode echocardiogram.[13,14] The two-dimensional echocardiogram shows an enlarged ventricular cavity and reduced ventricular ejection fraction. Wall thickness is normal or decreased, although the calculated left ventricular mass is increased. Importantly, these echocardiographic findings are in contrast to those associated with the nondilated cardiomyopathies. Moreover, in-

formation concerning cardiac valves, intracardiac tumors, and pericardial disease may also be obtained. Use of the echocardiogram for assessing patients with congestive heart failure is discussed in more detail later in the chapter. Discordance between the degree of right and left ventricular dilatation is also important.[15]

Radionuclide Techniques

Multigated radionuclide angiocardiography using autologous erythrocytes labeled with technetium 99m to detect abnormal left ventricular function (e.g., left ventricular ejection fraction) at rest or with stress and wall motion abnormalities is useful for the initial evaluation of patients with dilated cardiomyopathy.[16] Grossly abnormal left ventricular ejection fraction (< 40 percent) suggests well established disease. Radionuclide techniques also may be used to screen patients with specific disease for the presence of myocardial involvement. The gallium 67 scan has been proposed as a means of differentiating acute inflammatory from noninflammatory cardiomyopathy. Resting thallium imaging is useful for distinguishing patients with primary cardiomyopathy from those with ischemic cardiomyopathy.[17] These radionuclide techniques are discussed in more detail later in this volume.

Cardiac Catheterization and Angiography

Careful histories, thorough physical examinations, and the use of ECGs, chest roentgenograms, and echocardiograms have greatly reduced the need for cardiac catheterization. However, coronary angiography may be necessary to evaluate the coronary arteries, particularly in the patient with heart failure and chest discomfort. Unless contraindicated by compelling clinical evidence, coronary angiography is necessary to exclude myocardial ischemia as a principal etiology. It may then follow that studies to define the presence of viable myocardium must be undertaken (e.g., low-dose dobutamine infusion with echocardiography imaging, delayed thallium 201 uptake, or positron emission scanning).

Endomyocardial Biopsy

The primary diagnostic use of endomyocardial biopsy has been for differentiating among the nondilated, nonhypertrophic cardiomyopathies (e.g., amyloidosis, sarcoidosis).[18,19] The biopsy also has been valuable for following cardiac transplant recipients and detecting early damage in anthracycline cardiomyopathy. Biopsies also have uncovered acute and subacute myocarditis in some patients with cardiomyopathy. As discussed below, these findings may be of value when deciding on treatment.

SPECIFIC CLINICAL SYNDROMES

Genetic Dilated Cardiomyopathies

HEREDOFAMILIAL DILATED CARDIOMYOPATHY

Evidence continues to accumulate that many cases of dilated cardiomyopathy are familial.[18,19] A study of 105 consecutive patients with dilated cardiomyopathy yielded 14 probands with at least one first degree relative with documented disease.[10] Twenty-three relatives (21 percent) were classified as potential carriers. Pedigree analysis was most consistent with polygenic inheritance, which increases the likelihood that environmental factors (e.g., infection, toxins) and autoimmunity play a critical role in pathophysiology. An increased frequency of the angiotensin I converting enzyme (ACE) DD genotype has been found in patients with dilated cardiomyopathy.[20]

NEUROMUSCULAR DISEASES

Dilated cardiomyopathy is a common and important component of a number of neuromuscular diseases. Duchenne's dystrophy, an X-linked progressive dystrophy of proximal muscles, is frequently associated with cardiac involvement, and death usually results from respiratory infection and cardiorespiratory failure.[21] The absence of dystrophin, the protein product of this disease's locus, is responsible for the disease, and specific point mutations at the Xp21 locus of the dystrophin gene have been described.[21] Dilated cardiomyopathy may be the only manifestation of the dystrophin gene mutation in carriers.[22] The frequency of respiratory infections with associated pulmonary infiltrates may mask pulmonary thromboembolism.[23]

Patients with myotonic dystrophy (Steinert's disease) are at risk for a high incidence of sudden death, probably the result of arrhythmia or high degree atrioventricular heart block; symptoms usually appear in patients between the ages of 20 and 50 years. The term *congenital myotonic dystrophy* is applied to patients with severe neuromuscular symptoms at

birth. Patients with the congenital syndrome who are free of overt cardiovascular disease when studied at a mean age of 20 years were demonstrated to have a high incidence (71 percent) of atrioventricular and intraventricular conduction defects; decreased left ventricular systolic function also has been observed.[24]

Limb-girdle muscular dystrophy (Erb's disease) is usually an autosomal recessive condition that may have demonstrable cardiomyopathy. Dilated cardiomyopathy may appear before 30 years of age.[25] Other neuromuscular conditions associated with dilated cardiomyopathy include familial centronuclear myopathy[26]; Kugelberg-Welander syndrome, a proximal spinal muscular atrophy[27]; and nemaline myopathy.[28] Although Friedreich's ataxia, an autosomal recessive form of hereditary spinocerebellar ataxia, is usually associated with hypertrophic cardiomyopathy, dilated cardiomyopathy may occur.[29] The latter does not appear to be merely an advanced state of the hypertrophic form and probably represents a genetically different cardiomyopathy in neuromuscular diseases that are phenotypically indistinguishable.[30]

Barth syndrome is an X-linked recessive condition characterized by skeletal myopathy, cardiomyopathy, short stature, and recurrent neutropenia, but with normal cognitive function.[31] Linkage analysis has localized the mutation that causes Barth syndrome to the Xq28 region.[32]

DILATED CARDIOMYOPATHIES ASSOCIATED WITH MITOCHONDRIAL ABNORMALITIES

A number of diseases of oxidative phosphorylation have been recognized, all resulting from mitochondrial DNA mutations. These diseases present primarily with neuromuscular manifestations and include such disorders as Kearns-Sayre syndrome, chronic ophthalmoplegia, myoclonic epilepsy, ragged red fiber disease, mitochondrial encephalomyopathy, maternally inherited myopathy and cardiomyopathy, and Leber's hereditary optic neuropathy.[33] Using endomyocardial biopsy to look for mitochondrial mutations in patients with dilated cardiomyopathy has not been successful because of the age-related mutations that occur.[34]

Cardiac dysrhythmias and both progressive hypertrophic (maternally inherited myopathy and cardiomyopathy) and dilated (myoclonic epilepsy) cardiomyopathies are important manifestations of all mitochondrial myopathies and may occur at any time; either dilated or hypertrophic cardiomyopathy may occur with mitochondrial encephalomyopathy. The MELAS syndrome—mitochondrial encephalopathy, lactic acidosis, and stroke-like episodes—is associated with cardiomyopathy and generalized microangiopathy. Interestingly, diabetes mellitus is one of the heterogeneous phenotypic features of a mitochondrial DNA point mutation with the tRNA-Leu (UUR) gene.[35] Associated abnormalities include deafness and cardiomyopathy.

Because replicative segregation may produce dramatically different quantities of a mitochondrial DNA mutation within different tissues, such that a single organ such as the heart, skeletal muscle, or brain is affected more than others, clinical disease states may vary from primary neurologic involvement to primary skeletal muscle or cardiac disorder, or even no disease manifestations within a single pedigree.[31] Because of the similarity of age-dependent increases in the frequency of mitochondrial deletions in cardiomyopathic and control hearts, there appears to be no relation to heredofamilial dilated cardiomyopathy.[32]

Ischemic Cardiomyopathy

Ischemic cardiomyopathy is a disease of the heart muscle caused by inadequate perfusion of the myocardium relative to its needs and obstructive changes in the coronary circulation.[36,37] Coronary artery arteriosclerosis is the principal etiology of myocardial ischemia, although any disease process that deprives the myocardium of its normal blood supply may be considered a possible cause. As discussed previously, cardiomyopathy is the underlying mechanism responsible for chronic heart failure, and myocardial ischemia is the most common cause of it in the United States. Thus the concept of an ischemic cardiomyopathy has evolved to describe the spectrum of myocardial disease in these hearts.

Pathogenesis

Cardiomyopathy secondary to ischemia is primarily related to four major mechanisms: permanent myocyte loss (e.g., myocardial infarction), myocardial "stunning," myocardial "hibernation," and remodeling (pathological hypertrophy in remaining nonischemic myocytes secondary to the hyperergopathic state, or overwork; see below). Other factors include ventricular aneurysms, dysrhythmias, and papillary muscle dysfunction, with resultant mitral regurgitation.[38–41] These pathophysiologic mechanisms are described in detail elsewhere in the chapter.

Clinical Presentation

The clinical features of ischemic cardiomyopathy are angina pectoris, myocardial infarction, ventricular aneurysm, heart failure, and sudden death. In particular, angina pectoris should always raise the possibility of ischemic cardiomyopathy, although ischemic cardiomyopathy may be present in patients who did not complain of angina pectoris.[42] For example, patients with diabetes mellitus (see below) may have silent ischemic episodes and infarction. Importantly, ischemic cardiomyopathy associated with overt heart failure is almost always associated with previous myocardial infarction, revealed by the history (64–85 percent) or ECG evidence.[37,43] The physical examination may be normal in early ischemic cardiomyopathy, although during episodes of acute ischemia myocardial dysfunction may develop, associated with dyspnea, an increased S4, apical systolic murmur (papillary muscle dysfunction), arrhythmia, and changes in systemic arterial blood pressure.

The ECG is of particular importance to the diagnosis of ischemic cardiomyopathy. Ischemic ST segment and T wave changes, either at rest or during exercise, may be present during the early stage of the disease, as may transient or persistent arrhythmias. ECG evidence of myocardial infarction is of great value for diagnosing ischemic cardiomyopathy in the patient with heart failure. The presence of abnormal Q waves reflecting myocardial infarction strongly favors ischemic cardiomyopathy over other types of dilated cardiomyopathy. Although other types may be associated with Q waves on the ECG, fewer than 10 percent of patients with idiopathic dilated cardiomyopathy have ECG evidence of myocardial infarction. Left bundle branch block is less common in ischemic than in other types of cardiomyopathies, whereas complete atrioventricular, right bundle branch block, and other fascicular blocks are shared by sarcoid cardiomyopathy and Chagas' cardiomyopathy.

Echocardiograms from patients with ischemic cardiomyopathy resemble those from patients with dilated cardiomyopathy, except that in the former segmental wall motion abnormalities are generally more common. Echocardiographic detection of ventricular aneurysm suggests ischemic cardiomyopathy. The differentiation of ischemic cardiomyopathy from the nonischemic cardiomyopathies by advanced noninvasive testing is discussed elsewhere in this volume. However, when ischemic cardiomyopathy must be detected in order to make a correct therapeutic decision, coronary angiography is necessary. The natural history of patients with ischemic heart disease is complex and depends on many factors. Regardless, when ventricular failure is associated with angina, every effort should be made to determine if the patient is a suitable candidate for revascularization procedures.[44]

Hyperergopathic Cardiomyopathy: Cardiomyopathy of Overwork

Chronic increases in myocardial workload may result in pathologic structural and functional alterations of heart muscle.[45,46] When the major cause of the heart muscle disease is chronic overwork, the entities are referred to as hyperergopathic cardiomyopathies, most of which ultimately produce dilated cardiomyopathy. The hyperergopathic process is important for producing abnormalities in the healthy heart muscle that remains after a focal damaging process (e.g., myocardial infarction).[46] In this situation, the hyperergopathic process is considered part of the remodeling associated with progression of the principal etiology and is not included in this discussion. This subset of diseases does not include this group for clinical diagnostic reasons. Some of the conditions that produce chronic generalized ventricular overwork are listed in Table 28-1.

Cardiomyopathy Associated with Myocarditis

Cardiomyopathy may result from acute or chronic inflammatory responses of the myocardium, many of which are presumed to be infectious in origin. The inflammatory response results in the permanent loss of myocytes, dysfunction of the remaining myocytes, and an increase in myocardial fibrosis. Much attention has focused on classifying myocarditis according to chronologic, morphologic, and etiologic groupings.[47,48] The chronopathologic classification demonstrates how acute myocarditis secondary to viruses, for example, may result in chronic cardiomyopathy with heart failure.

INFECTIOUS CARDIOMYOPATHY

Viral Cardiomyopathy

Viruses are the infectious agents most likely to produce chronic cardiomyopathy and heart failure. The list of viruses known to involve the myocardium is extensive[49,50] (Table 28-3). The coxsackie group of enteroviruses is particularly associated with a high incidence of cardiac involvement. The overall prevalence of myocarditis in patients with suspected viral illness ranges from 2.3 to 5.0 percent.[50] The clinical courses that have been described are similar to those included in the clinicopathologic descriptions for other cardiomyopathies.[50,51] Unfortunately, the association is based primarily on data acquired from acute infections or epidemics. Regardless of the causative virus, viral myocarditis may produce a similar

Table 28-3. Some Viruses That Cause Myocardial Disease in Humans

Coxsackie virus (types B and A)
Poliomyelitis virus
Influenza virus (types A and B)
Human immunodeficiency virus (HIV)
Adenovirus
ECHO virus
Cytomegalovirus
Epstein-Barr virus (infectious mononucleosis)
Rubeola virus
Rubella virus
Mumps virus
Respiratory syncytial virus
Varicella-zoster virus
Rabies virus
Hepatitis virus
Yellow fever virus
Smallpox virus
Lymphocytic choriomeningitis virus
Epidemic hemorrhagic fever virus
Chikunguna fever virus
Dengue virus

gross appearance. Softening and mottling of the ventricular wall may be present, and pericarditis is common. Light microscopic changes that occur early include hypereosinophilic myocytes, interstitial edema, and inflammatory cell infiltrates. Later, loss of striations, clumping of cytoplasm, fragmentation, and eventually dissolution or dropout of myocytes occur.

The mechanism whereby viruses produce myocardial damage is not clear. Direct cytotoxicity is a possibility. Immunologic mechanisms involving macrophages, natural killer cells, T lymphocytes, autoantibodies to various cellular components such as myosin, and membrane calcium channels, and cytokines such as interleukin-1 and tumor necrosis factor may be important.[49,50] Apparently viruses either "hit and run" or produce chronic disease. The incidence of viral myocarditis is difficult to determine because of inadequate methods and facilities for etiologically identifying viral diseases in general; however, in a review of 40,000 necropsies, 1,402 patients had evidence of myocarditis, and 0.38 percent of them had evidence of a viral etiology.[51] Evidence of myocarditis was detected in 5 percent of 417 young adults and middle-aged men who were victims of sudden accidental death[52] and in up to 21 percent of cases of sudden death in children.[49] The precise link between the initial myocarditis and chronic dilated cardiomyopathy is not clear.[53] However, long-term follow-up of patients with acute myocarditis demonstrates that some of them have persistent impairment of left ventricular function.[53,54] Persistence of viral RNA, particularly enteroviral RNA, has been demonstrated in the absence of inflammation and is associated with a poor prognosis.[55] Utilizing polymerase chain reaction (PCR) techniques, investigators have recovered enteroviral (coxsackie) RNA sequences in tissue obtained by endomyocardial biopsy from humans with myocarditis.[56]

Acquired Immunodeficiency Syndrome

Dilated cardiomyopathy associated with congestive heart failure or ECG changes is a relatively common association of acquired immunodeficiency syndrome (AIDS) due to human immunodeficiency virus (HIV). Generally, the cardiomyopathy of AIDS has been attributed to cardiac involvement of opportunistic organisms or neoplasms such as Kaposi's sarcoma or lymphoma.[57] Cardiac toxoplasma was common in one necropsy series of patients with HIV infection; solitary cardiac involvement was not uncommon.[58] HIV can infect cardiac myocytes directly, as demonstrated by the use of DNA hybridization techniques.[59] However, the distribution of infected cells did not correlate well with areas of clinical or histopathologic evidence of disease. Children with symptomatic HIV infection may develop progressive left ventricular dilatation.

Chagas' Disease

Chagas' disease (South American trypanosomiasis) remains a leading cause of death in many areas of Central and South America. Acute, indeterminate, and chronic phases of the disease are apparent, with sudden death occurring during each phase and dilated cardiomyopathy during the chronic phase. Acute Chagas' disease is a severe myocarditis characterized clinically by cardiac enlargement, tachycardia, and nonspecific ECG abnormalities; inflammatory changes occur in the myocardium that may be diffuse and severe, with trypanosomes demonstrable within cardiac myocytes.[60]

On the other hand, the cause of chronic Chagas'-related cardiomyopathy remains unclear. Myocardial fibrosis is commonly observed, and one of the characteristic lesions is focal myocytolysis, which, together with demonstrated dynamic abnormalities of the coronary microcirculation in the experimental model, lends support to a more recently proposed pathophysiologic mechanism: that the chronic phase may result from microcirculatory abnormalities, with transient vascular obstruction followed by reflow,[61] a pathophysiology shared by many forms of ischemic cardiomyopathy. Between 10 and 20 percent of patients with asymptomatic, latent disease eventually progress to the chronic stage of disease; right bundle branch block and ventricular premature beats are the most common ECG findings.

An annual progression rate of 5.5 percent, with an annual mortality rate of 0.7 percent, has been described in a longitudinal study from San Felipe, Brazil.[62] Cardiac failure was responsible for 58 percent of deaths and arrhythmias for another 38 percent. Another report indicates that 50 percent of patients with Chagas' cardiomyopathy and heart failure die within 47 months and that VO_2Max and left ventricular ejection fraction are useful for determining the prognosis.[63] The presence of complete heart block, atrial fibrillation, left bundle branch block, complex ventricular ectopy, or septal fibrosis indicates a poor prognosis. Not surprisingly, the presence of conduction disturbances on the ECG and left ventricular aneurysms correlated with the development of sustained ventricular tachycardia by electrophysiologic testing.[62] Because Chagas' disease may mimic coronary artery disease or idiopathic dilated cardiomyopathy, it may be underdiagnosed, particularly in countries such as the United States.[63]

Lyme Disease

Lyme disease is often associated with cardiac involvement. Conduction abnormalities are common, and ECG abnormalities have been reported in up to 90 percent of cases. Left ventricular enlargement and dysfunction may occur.[64] Cardiac changes generally resolve within 6 months. The organism responsible for Lyme disease, Borrelia burgdorferi, has been cultured from endomyocardial biopsy specimens from a patient with chronic Lyme disease and dilated cardiomyopathy, which suggests that direct cardiac tissue infection is the cause of the cardiomyopathy.[65]

Kawasaki Disease

Kawasaki disease, or mucocutaneous lymph node syndrome, may be associated with myocarditis, and round cell infiltration has been a prominent autopsy finding.[66–69] An infectious etiology is suspected. Mortality is most common during the second stage of the illness, characterized clinically by desquamation of the initial rash and joint involvement; death appears to result from coronary artery aneurysms with occlusion of or invasion into the conduction system.[69] Magnetic resonance imaging may show increased signals from coronary arteries, suggesting stagnant and turbulent blood flow in coronary aneurysms.[70]

Toxic Dilated Cardiomyopathy

SUBSTANCE ABUSE

Alcoholic Cardiomyopathy

Alcoholic cardiomyopathy is a disease of heart muscle caused by the direct toxic effects of ethyl alcohol or its metabolites on cardiac myocytes[71,72]; it has been difficult to produce left ventricular failure in animal models. Only a few human alcoholics develop severe cardiomyopathy, despite the high prevalence of subclinical left ventricular involvement.[73] Yet as many as 21 percent of subjects with excessive alcohol intake are reported to have clinical evidence of heart failure,[74] and 60 to 80 percent of patients with idiopathic dilated cardiomyopathy have abused alcohol.[75,76] Thus although the specific pathophysiologic process by which alcohol affects the heart is not yet defined, the ultimate severity of injury appears to be influenced by genetic, metabolic, and environmental factors.[77,78]

Both autopsy and endomyocardial biopsy specimens from alcoholic cardiomyopathy patients reveal marked mitochondrial swelling, with fragmentation of cristae, swelling of sarcoplasmic reticulum, and destruction of myofibrils.[79] These changes are not specific for alcoholic cardiomyopathy but are similar to those produced in the ethanol-fed rat model,[80,81] implicating ethanol as the etiologic agent in humans. It has been postulated that acetaldehyde, the metabolic product resulting from the action of alcohol dehydrogenase on ethanol, is the direct cardiac toxin, possibly aided by the release of norepinephrine.[82,83] Because the myocardium lacks alcohol dehydrogenase, the mitochondrial enzymes may be critical for metabolism of acetaldehyde.

Latent cardiomyopathy may be detected by the presence of diastolic ventricular dysfunction, quantitated by Doppler echocardiography. Diastolic abnormalities are independent of the duration of alcoholism, the quantity of the most recent exposure to ethanol, and increased left ventricular mass.[84] When compared with healthy controls, asymptomatic alcoholic subjects display a prolonged left ventricular relaxation time, a decreased peak early left ventricular diastolic velocity (E), a slower acceleration of early flow, and a lower peak E/A (atrial emptying) velocity ratio. Furthermore, subclinical left ventricular systolic and diastolic dysfunction commonly occurs in alcoholics.[85]

It is difficult to quantitate the amount of alcohol consumption necessary to produce cardiomyopathy. Daily intakes of more than 10 oz of whiskey, 32 oz of wine, or 64 oz of beer have been reported in patients presenting with alcoholic cardiomyopathy.[86] Clues to alcohol abuse include palimpsests (blackouts), marital discord, business failures, excessive absenteeism, high blood alcohol concentrations while apparently not intoxicated, increased mean corpuscular volume of red blood cells, increased γ-glutamyl transpeptidase, and alcoholic-type T waves on the ECG. The identification of alcohol as a main or contributing cause of cardiomyopathy in a particular patient is

important in that alcoholic cardiomyopathy is one of the reversible forms of heart muscle disease. Data recorded from a longitudinal study have indicated that 91 percent of patients with alcoholic cardiomyopathy who abstain from alcohol after the initial diagnosis are alive at 42 months, compared with 43 percent of those who continue to drink.[87]

Cocaine-Related Disease

The unfortunate and widespread abuse of cocaine has resulted in an increased incidence of myocardial disease. Cocaine produces central and peripheral adrenergic stimulation by inhibiting the presynaptic uptake of catecholamines, thus increasing the postsynaptic concentrations and adrenergic receptor stimulation. Cocaine intoxication has been associated with angina, myocardial infarction, ventricular arrhythmias, left ventricular dysfunction, dilated cardiomyopathy, and myocarditis.[82–92] Acute dilated cardiomyopathy may occur after cocaine use followed by clinical recovery over 2 weeks.[93]

OTHER TOXINS

Causal relations between putative toxic agents and recognized myocardial dysfunction are usually difficult to establish owing to inadequate clinical material and an inability to attribute damage to a particular agent in situations that feature multiple potential toxins or disease processes. Those cardiotoxic agents with adequate experimental or clinical evidence are listed in Table 28-4.[94]

ANTHRACYCLINES

Anthracyclines, such as doxorubicin (Adriamycin) and daunorubicin, which are widely employed in cancer chemotherapy, produce cardiac toxicity, possibly by increasing oxygen-derived free radical generation, platelet-activating factor, prostaglandins, histamine, calcium, and C-13 hydroxy metabolites. The C-13 metabolites are considerably more potent myocardial depressants than are the parent compounds and are inhibitors of ATPases of sarcoplasmic reticulum, mitochondria, and sarcolemma.[95]

A chronic, generally dose-dependent dilated cardiomyopathy has been associated with doxorubicin therapy. Other cardiovascular effects have been atrial and ventricular dysrhythmias, acute hypersensitivity reactions, and myocarditis-pericarditis. The incidence of dilated cardiomyopathy increases from less than 3 percent at cumulative doses under 400 mg/m^2 to nearly 20 percent at dose levels over 700 mg/m^2.[96] Unfortunately, in clinical studies, total cumulative

Table 28-4. Cardiotoxic Agents

Class	Examples
Ethanol	
Antineoplastic agents	Doxorubicin, daunorubicin, ifosfamide, cyclophosphamide, 5-fluorouracil
Vasoactive amines/sympathomimetics	Epinephrine, norepinephrine, isoproterenol, dopamine, ephedrine, salbutamol,[a] terbutaline,[a] amphetamine, methylphenidate, tyramine,[a] propylhexedrine, nicotine, allylamines[a]
Methylxanthines[a]	
Antipsychotics	Phenothiazines, tricyclic antidepressants
Metals	Lithium, barium, bismuth, mercury, cobalt, lead, arsenic, antimony, phosphorus, vanadium,[a] cadmium,[a] niobium,[a] zirconium[a]
Methylsergide	
Antimalarials	Chloroquine, quinine
Emetine[a]	
Heroin	
Vasodilators	Diazoxide,[a] minoxidil,[a] hydralazine[a]
Analgesic/antiinflammatory agents	Acetaminophen, methylsalicylate, colchicine
Hydrocarbons	Kerosene, halogenated hydrocarbons,[a] methylene dianiline
Physical agents	Radiation, hyperthermia, hypothermia, cigarettes (CO)
Peptides	Angiotensin II,[a] eledoisin,[a] myocardial depressant factor,[a] polyamines,[a] venoms, cyclosporin A
Antibiotics	Aminoglycosides,[a] tetracycline,[a] oxacillin, vancomycin, erythromycin,[a] colistin,[a] chloramphenicol,[a] amphotericin B,[a]
Antihypertensive agents	Reserpine,[a] guanethidine[a]
Hypersensitivity reactions	Penicillin, sulfonamides, streptomycin, aminosalicylic acid, phenylbutazone, phenindione, methyldopa

[a] Toxicity demonstrated only in animal models.

doses of doxorubicin that have clinically precipitated congestive heart failure ($75-1095$ mg/m^2) are not distinguishable from those that have not ($30-880$ mg/m^2).

Factors that contribute to the high risk of eventual development of dilated cardiomyopathy and congestive heart failure are a decline of 15 percent or more in radionuclide left ventricular ejection fraction from a normal baseline to 50 percent or less, a high cumulative dose of doxorubicin of more than 450 mg/m^2, and therapy begun with abnormal baseline left ventricular ejection fraction (less than 50 percent). Importantly, clinical congestive heart failure has occurred in 18 percent of such patients within 12 months of discontinuing doxorubicin therapy.[97] The long-term effects of doxorubicin administered during childhood appear to be more deleterious, with 65 percent of patients who had received at least 228 mg/m^2 demonstrating echocardiographically determined increased afterload or decreased contractility. The increased afterload resulted from reduced ventricular wall thickness, not from hypertension or ventricular dilatation.[98]

The use of continuous infusion of doxorubicin, rather than bolus dosing, or the co-administration of antioxidants or free radical scavengers may reduce cardiotoxicity.[99] Congestive heart failure improves in up to 90 percent of patients treated with the conventional modalities of digitalis, diuretics, or vasodilators; and complete return of severe left ventricular dysfunction to normal has been reported.[100]

IFOSFAMIDE

Ifosfamide, a substituted nitrogen mustard compound structurally similar to cyclophosphamide, used with carboplatin-etoposide or lomustine-vinblastine combinations, produced clinical congestive heart failure in 9 of 52 consecutively treated patients.[101] Eight of these patients presented with fulminant pulmonary edema. Most improved with standard therapy for heart failure.

Peripartum Cardiomyopathy

Peripartum (postpartal) cardiomyopathy is a clinical syndrome associated with the postpartal state and characterized by the onset of signs and symptoms of dilated cardiomyopathy 2 to 20 weeks after delivery, together with the absence of cardiomyopathy during pregnancy and of any other apparent etiology.

The association with the postpartal state distinguishes postpartal cardiomyopathy from the idiopathic cardiomyopathy category. Viruses may play a role in the pathophysiology of postpartal cardiomyopathy, and approximately 75 percent of patients in one series had biopsy evidence of myocarditis that occasionally responded to immunosuppressive therapy.[102,103] A careful search should be made for other known causes of cardiomyopathy. For example, a series of patients has been reported who abused cocaine during pregnancy and developed dilated cardiomyopathy and congestive heart failure during the postpartal period.[104]

Cardiomegaly that persists for more than 4 months after diagnosis indicates a poor prognosis, with a 50 percent mortality rate at 6 years.[105] Heart failure recurs during subsequent pregnancies in more than 50 percent of patients.[106,107] The prognosis for postpartal cardiomyopathy is clearly different from that for women of similar age with dilated cardiomyopathy that is not associated with pregnancy, even though the features of the clinical presentation are similar.

Endocrine Cardiomyopathy

DIABETES MELLITUS

Diabetic cardiomyopathy is defined as heart muscle dysfunction not due to coronary atherosclerosis artery disease.[108,109] The etiology of diabetic cardiomyopathy is multifactorial and includes microvascular disease, nonenzymatic glycosylation of proteins, and derangements in cellular metabolism and growth. Diabetes does contribute to the development of atherosclerosis. Over an 18-year observation period, diabetic men, particularly those with insulin-dependent diabetes but without significant coronary atherosclerosis, had a 2.4-fold greater incidence of heart failure than did nondiabetic men; the relative risk for diabetic women was 5.1-fold.[110] At necropsy the hearts of diabetic patients exhibit increased weight, pale appearance, and firmness associated with an increase in myocardial collagen; the capillary basement membranes are thickened, capillary microaneurysms are present, and there is focal myocardial fibrosis and intimal proliferation of small myocardial arterioles, with accumulation of interstitial glycoprotein and collagen.[111] Electron microscopy reveals focal perivascular damage, with loss of contractile myocardial elements and deposition of periodic acid-Schiff-positive material or glycoprotein.[112]

The association of hypertension and diabetes produces a particularly severe cardiomyopathy and cardiac failure.[113] Both experimental and clinical evidence clearly suggest that the coexistence of hypertension and diabetes results in more severe cardiomyopathy than would be expected from either process alone.[114] An autopsy study of 67 subjects with diabetes, hypertension, or both found significantly more clinical and pathologic (fibrosis) heart disease in patients with both hypertension and diabetes than in those with either disease alone.[114]

Approximately 50 percent of asymptomatic diabetic subjects (i.e., those with potential or latent cardiomyopathy) experience a reduction in left ventricular ejection fraction with dynamic exercise.[115,116] However, those diabetic subjects who do experience a drop in ejection fraction with exercise display higher resting ejection fractions and heart rates than do diabetics who have normal exercise responses as well as normal responses to afterload manipulation, normal baseline ventricular contractility as assessed by load- and heart rate-independent end-systolic indices, and normal contractile reserve to dobutamine challenge. Possibly, abnormal exercise responses reflect abnormalities in systemic venous tone rather than in cardiac function.

Asymptomatic diabetic patients may have evidence of diastolic dysfunction. Diabetic adolescents displayed significantly reduced E, E/total area, and peak E/A velocity ratio compared with nondiabetic controls; this finding indicates potential abnormalities of ventricular relaxation or compliance.[117] Short-term glycemic control in diabetic patients without retinopathy markedly decreased diastolic abnormalities but did not improve function in those with retinopathy.[118]

Patients with diabetes are more prone to silent myocardial ischemia and infarction. Treadmill-induced ST segment depression occurred earlier in diabetics than it did in nondiabetics with angina, but the anginal perception threshold in the diabetic group was delayed by a mean of 86 seconds.[119] Prolongation of the anginal perception threshold correlates to the degree of abnormality of tests of autonomic function (heart rate responses to the Valsalva maneuver and deep breathing) and to abnormalities of sensory function (measured by median nerve conduction studies).

HYPERTHYROIDISM

Cardiomyopathy may result from thyroid hormone excess.[120–123] Histologic examination reveals a nonspecific pattern, including foci of lymphocytic and eosinophilic infiltration, mild fibrosis, fatty infiltration, and myofibril hypertrophy. Mitochondrial hypertrophy precedes the development of ventricular muscle hypertrophy. Hypertrophy has been described in animal models[124,125] and in clinically affected patients with no apparent cause other than hyperthyroidism,[126] perhaps resulting from the binding of thyroxine to nuclear receptors,[127,128] with a resultant increase in the rate of protein synthesis. Although enhanced sympathoadrenal activity contributes to the hyperdynamic cardiovascular state in hypertension, β-adrenergic blockade does not return the heart rate to normal, alter the preejection phase or duration of ventricular systole, or decrease myocardial contractility.[129,130] Thus increased ventricular function in hyperthyroidism may represent a primary cardiac effect of thyroid hormone with catecholamine responses that are at best additive, with no evidence of adrenergic hypersensitivity.

The clinical cardiovascular picture is related to the high output circulatory state. Warm extremities, a bounding pulse with a wide pulse pressure, and prominent jugular venous pulsations alert the clinician to the presence of a high output state. There may be accentuation of the first heart sound and an increased pulmonic component of the second heart sound. A third sound was accentuated in 67 percent of patients, and a systolic murmur was present in all cases.[131] Frequently, the murmur is an early, harsh, scratchy (Means-Lerman scratch) sound, crescendo-decrescendo, grade 2 to 4 murmur most commonly present in the pulmonic area or at Erb's point but occasionally at the apex. A mid-diastolic murmur associated with cardiomegaly and myocardial damage was present in 17 percent of patients.

Importantly, physical findings tend to be less prominent in older subjects. Sinus tachycardia, ventricular premature beats, and paroxysmal or sustained atrial fibrillation frequently occur with hyperthyroidism. Approximately 5 percent of clinically euthyroid patients with unexplained atrial fibrillation showed evidence of hyperthyroidism in routine thyroid studies, including thyroid-releasing hormone (TRH) testing.[132] The presence of associated systemic signs and symptoms of hyperthyroidism, as well as specific syndromes associated with hyperthyroidism (e.g., Graves' disease and the acute phase of Hashimoto's thyroiditis) assists the clinician in diagnosing hyperthyroidism with cardiomyopathy. Clinically apparent heart failure is relatively uncommon, perhaps due to early recognition and treatment. Yet of 462 thyrotoxic patients, evidence of cardiac dysfunction was found in 150, and 64 of them had atrial fibrillation, congestive heart failure, or cardiomegaly alone, in the absence of clinical or ECG evidence of associated heart disease.[126]

HYPOTHYROIDISM

The classic findings of myxedema heart do not themselves indicate cardiomyopathy. Congestive heart failure occurring in myxedema is more likely a manifestation of preexisting heart disease. However, abnormalities in cardiac systolic and diastolic performance have been reported in both experimental and human hypothyroidism.[133] Abnormal systolic force may improve with thyroid hormone replacement but does not return to normal levels, suggesting the possibility of persistent myocardial dysfunction. Thyroid hormone replacement may result in reversal of echocardiographic changes: thickening of the intraventricular septum and the right ventricular wall, an increased septal thickness/left ventricular posterior wall thickness ratio, decreased regional wall motion of the right ventricle and interventricular septum, and decreased global function of the left ventricle.[134]

The characteristic features of myxedema heart are cardiomegaly, especially prominent on chest roentgenogram; hypoactive cardiac dynamics; and ECG abnormalities, primarily low voltage of all complexes. Pericardial effusions have been reported in 30 to 78 percent of patients.[135,136] Thyroid hormone replacement should be initiated at low doses and increased slowly, as the heart's ability to respond to increased fluid mobilization from peripheral edema is limited, and left ventricular failure may be precipitated.

ACROMEGALY

Myocardial dysfunction is a major cause of morbidity and mortality in acromegaly and appears to be related to both the severity and duration of growth hormone excess. This excess is the result of autonomously functioning tumors of the anterior pituitary that produce the major clinical manifestations of disproportionate soft tissue and bony overgrowth. Acromegaly is often associated with systemic arterial diastolic hypertension and coronary artery disease.

Cardiovascular disease has been reported to cause up to 24 percent of deaths among acromegalic patients.[137] Cardiac hypertrophy, interstitial fibrosis, small-vessel intramyocardial disease, and a lymphomononuclear cell infiltrate have been described at necropsy.[138] Electron microscopy demonstrates an increase in mitochondrial number, vacuolation of sarcoplasmic reticulum, myofibrillar loss, Z-band remnants, and crenation of nuclear membranes, but with preservation of regular myocardial fiber arrangement.[139] Both concentric[140] and asymmetric septal hypertrophy[141,142] patterns have been reported.

The initial cardiac manifestation of acromegaly is ventricular hypertrophy. Progression through left ventricular dysfunction and dilatation to congestive heart failure may occur. Acromegalic patients with ventricular hypertrophy alone display a hyperkinetic state that has been postulated to play a pathophysiologic role in the development of hypertension.[143] The somatostatin analog octreotide has significantly improved cardiac function in acromegalic patients, including those with overt congestive heart failure.[144]

Metabolic Dilated Cardiomyopathy

HEMOCHROMATOSIS CARDIOMYOPATHY

Hemochromatosis is a systemic disease characterized by excessive iron deposition in multiple organ systems due either to exogenous or endogenous iron overload. Cardiomyopathy results from excessive iron deposition within the myocardium.[145–148] Primary hemochromatosis is a recessive genetic disorder linked to chromosome 6 and associated with HLA antigens, with increased gastrointestinal absorption of iron. Ferritin is an iron-containing protein composed of two subunits (H and L), and in hereditary hemochromatosis a specific heart isoferritin exists (i.e., basic isoferritin with L unit immunoreactivity). Myocardial iron deposition is most prominent in and around contractile elements and less common in the conducting system, in contrast to sarcoidosis and amyloidosis, in which the pathologic process commonly involves the conducting system. The mechanism by which iron produces cellular dysfunction is not yet clear, as fibrosis may not be prominent.

Myocardial iron deposits do not occur until other organs such as the liver, pancreas, and connective tissues are saturated with iron. Thus the extracardiac manifestations are present before the cardiomyopathy develops. Nonetheless, 14 percent of patients with hemochromatosis may present with cardiac symptoms.[148] Sixty-five percent of patients with hemochromatosis have abnormal ECGs, even during the early stages of the disease.[149] The ECG most commonly shows decreased voltage and nonspecific ST segment and T wave changes; Q waves are uncommon. The echocardiogram demonstrates increased systolic and diastolic left ventricular dimensions and left atrial dimensions, with decreased fractional shortening. Stratified echoes from the myocardium, similar to those in amyloidosis, have been reported. In patients with a restrictive pattern, evidence of diastolic dysfunction, with dilated ventricles, may be present. As the severity of cardiomyopathy advances, dilated cardiomyopathy with progressive, biventricular heart failure develops.[150,151]

Before phlebotomy and chelation therapy were available, the survival rate among patients with hemochromatosis was less than 20 percent 5 years after diagnosis. The availability of these treatments has dramatically improved outcome, as demonstrated in one study of thalassemia patients. Only 1 of 17 deferoxamine-compliant patients acquired cardiac disease and died in congestive heart failure compared with a group of 19 noncompliant patients, 12 of whom developed heart failure; 7 of them died.[152] It is important to recognize early disease with preserved left ventricular systolic function, as treatment may reverse the process.[153] Additionally, following bone marrow transplants in thalassemia patients, iron removal may result in substantial cardiac improvement.[154] Endomyocardial biopsy may be diagnostic.

THIAMINE DEFICIENCY (BERIBERI)

Thiamine deficiency, primarily seen in alcoholics, decreases conversion of pyruvate acetyl coenzyme A (CoA) and α-ketoglutarate to succinyl CoA, thereby affecting both anaerobic and aerobic metabolism. A reduction in oxidative phosphorylation occurs, which decreases the availability of the high energy phosphate bonds necessary for metabolic functions.

The thiamine-deficient state may present clinically as dry berberi (polyneuropathy without congestive heart failure) or wet beriberi (polyneuropathy with congestive heart failure).[155–157] The cardiovascular signs and symptoms consist of fatigability, dyspnea, and palpitations. Tachycardia is common, and there are usually increased jugular venous pressure and warm extremities. Cardiomegaly is present, and the circulation is hyperkinetic. Biventricular heart failure is present, and there may be both right and left ventricular gallop rhythms. Treatment should consist of administration of thiamine along with other conventional treatment of heart failure.[158]

CARNITINE DEFICIENCY

Carnitine is a cofactor necessary for the oxidation of fatty acids, a deficiency of which may be associated with a syndrome of progressive skeletal myopathy with lipid vacuoles on muscle biopsy. Carnitine deficiency may produce hypertrophic or dilated cardiomyopathy.[159,160] However, in a report of a family in which four of five children developed cardiomyopathy, three had evidence of endocardial fibroelastosis.[161] One surviving sibling was treated with L-carnitine, 3 g/day orally, and showed improved myocardial function and reduced heart size.[162]

SELENIUM DEFICIENCY (KESHAN DISEASE)

Dilated cardiomyopathy occurs in northeast China in a zone in which the soil has a low selenium content.[163-165] Selenium deficiency is thought to be the cause of this condition (Keshan disease) because of a geographic distribution similar to that of white muscle disease in animals, which is known to be due to selenium deficiency; the decreased selenium content in the hair of patients with Keshan disease; and the efficacy of sodium selenite as a prophylactic. Cardiomyopathy associated with selenium deficiency may be seen in patients who have been maintained on parenteral alimentation for prolonged periods.[166,167] Selenium is an essential trace element in humans and animals, and its only established function in humans is the antioxidant activity of glutathione peroxidase, selenoenzyme.[168]

This cardiomyopathy is manifested by the insidious onset of congestive heart failure or a complication of sudden death or thromboembolic phenomena. The hearts show biventricular enlargement and histologically exhibit edema, nonspecific degenerative changes, mitochondrial swelling, hypercontraction bands, and widespread foci of myocytolysis. Fibrosis may be extensive.

Collagen Vascular (Rheumatic) Diseases

The collagen vascular (rheumatic) diseases are commonly associated with cardiac lesions that may manifest clinically or remain hidden. Although the most common cardiac lesion is pericarditis, myocardial dysfunction may occur in virtually all these disease processes.

SYSTEMIC LUPUS ERYTHEMATOSUS

Cardiac involvement in systemic lupus erythematosus (SLE) primarily affects the pericardium and valves, although in one study 54 percent of patients with SLE demonstrated myocardial dysfunction that manifested as regional or global hypokinesis.[169] The left ventricular ejection fraction may decrease significantly, whereas the interventricular septum and posterior wall thickness and the left ventricular mass increase.[170] Abnormal diastolic function manifested by prolonged isovolumic relaxation time, reduced peak E, increased peak A, reduced E/A, and a low deceleration rate of early diastolic flow velocity (E-F slope) have been reported.[171] The abnormalities correlated with the activity of the disease.

CHURG-STRAUSS SYNDROME

The Churg-Strauss syndrome (allergic granulomatosis and angiitis) is associated with interstitial myocardial eosinophilic inflammation ranging from occasional focal infection to diffuse myocarditis and myocardial fibrosis. Ischemia secondary to vasculitis or from scarring caused by focal inflammation may result in cardiomyopathy.[172] Cardiac failure was described in 47 percent of reported cases in one study and accounted for 48 percent of deaths.[173]

The echocardiogram shows an increase in both left ventricular end-diastolic and end-systolic diameters and a reduced shortening fraction. Severe mitral regurgitation may be present and require valve replacement.[174] Patients demonstrated an increase in mean echo amplitude of the septum and the posterior wall, which suggests the presence of myocardial fibrosis. Steroid therapy may dramatically improve ventricular contractility in the presence of cardiac involvement.[173]

PROGRESSIVE SYSTEMIC SCLEROSIS (SCLERODERMA)

Cardiac disease is a significant cause of mortality among patients with scleroderma. For example, of 300 scleroderma patients entered in a survival study, fewer than 5 percent of the 43 patients with cardiac involvement at entry were alive after 7 years of follow-up, compared with a 35 percent overall 7-year survival rate.[175] Approximately half of the hearts from 52 autopsies demonstrated areas of myocardial fibrosis, consisting of myocardial muscle necrosis with contraction band formation, inflammatory changes, and repair with replacement fibrosis.

The fibrosis and contraction band necrosis were distinctive, differing from those of atherosclerosis because of their lack of anatomic relation to coronary vessels, the absence of hemosiderin, and distinctive involvement of the immediate subendocardium. These lesions were postulated to result from intracardiac Raynaud's phenomenon, producing spasms of small vessels, with consequent myocardial necrosis.[176] Thallium radioisotope scans are frequently abnormal in scleroderma patients, despite the presence of normal epicardial coronary vessels.[177] Captopril treatment has been reported to decrease significantly the number of myocardial perfusion defects and to increase the global thallium score[178] in normotensive scleroderma patients compared with placebo-treated control patients.

RHEUMATOID ARTHRITIS

Myocarditis may occur with rheumatoid arthritis but rarely as a solitary finding; additionally, it usually occurs in the presence of active rheumatoid disease.

Cardiac findings in 100 rheumatoid arthritis patients studied at autopsy included pericarditis in 15 patients, chronic endocarditis in 9, and active myocarditis in 11.[179] The usual lesion is focal or diffuse nonspecific infiltration with lymphocytes, plasma cells, fibroblasts, or histiocytes; granulomas are not common.[180]

Cardiomyopathy Due to Physical Agents

After fatal hyperthermia, myocardial hemorrhage, interstitial edema, and myocytolysis occur.[181,182] With hypothermia, congestive heart failure accounts for major mortality, with focal inflammatory and degenerative myocardial lesions associated with interstitial edema and hypertrophy.[183]

Immunologically Mediated Cardiomyopathy

Systemic anaphylaxis and delayed hypersensitivity reactions may result in myocardial dysfunction.[184–187] Heart failure may occur during chronic hypersensitivity reactions, associated with granulomatous and eosinophilic myocarditis; most of these reactions result from antibiotic administration. Combination antituberculosis therapy, penicillin, methyldopa, phenylbutazone, and phenindione have all produced fatal myocarditis.

Idiopathic Dilated Cardiomyopathy

Idiopathic dilated cardiomyopathy exists when data are too insubstantial to establish or generate suspicion of one or more of the known causes of dilated cardiomyopathy. The annual incidence of idiopathic dilated cardiomyopathy in the United States varies between five and eight cases per 100,000 population.[188] The heterogeneity of idiopathic cardiomyopathy is apparent when clinicians attempt to uncover the natural history of this group of patients.[189] For example, alcohol abuse, myocarditis, and a family history of dilated cardiomyopathy are often ignored as exclusions for defining idiopathic dilated cardiomyopathy. Thus in many ways advanced dilated cardiomyopathy is similar to end-stage renal disease; in both instances a specific etiology may never be determined. However, it is likely that most of the known causes of dilated cardiomyopathy have been described. Four specific etiologies seem particularly likely in most cases of idiopathic dilated cardiomyopathy: genetic (heredofamilial) factors, viral agents, alcohol abuse, and cocaine abuse. Some animal studies have suggested an interaction between viral infection and genetic factors.

The clinical presentation of patients with idiopathic dilated cardiomyopathy is heart failure, and the symptoms are often far advanced at the time of diagnosis. The signs and symptoms are those discussed under General Clinical Considerations at the beginning of this chapter. The natural history of idiopathic dilated cardiomyopathy is difficult to determine, as noted above. Mortality rates are 25 to 30 percent at 1 year and 50 percent at 5 years. Clinical predictors of a poor prognosis include the degree of cardiac enlargement, left ventricular ejection fraction, New York Heart Association functional class, and decreased maximal oxygen consumption of less than 10 to 12 ml/kg body weight. Although ventricular arrhythmias and sudden death are common features of dilated cardiomyopathy, the prognostic importance of ventricular arrhythmias remains unclear.

APPROACH TO THE DIAGNOSIS OF DILATED CARDIOMYOPATHIES

When the physician is first confronted with a patient in whom dilated cardiomyopathy is suspected, the number of diagnostic possibilities is challenging. A systematic approach eliminates much of the confusion and helps lead to correct assessment of the patient (Fig. 28-1).

Asymptomatic Patient

Patients without cardiac symptoms may still have potential (latent) or early cardiomyopathy. As stated above, the diagnosis of potential and early cardiomyopathy depends on the presence of clinical clues to the entities listed in Table 28-1. A careful history and physical examination can detect most of the entities detailed in that list. If cardiomyopathy is suspected, an ECG should be recorded. If ancillary tests are to be performed for cardiac function, the echocardiogram is the most valuable. Two recent clinical trials illustrated the need to detect patients with early ischemic dilated cardiomyopathy (i.e., the SOLVD Prevention Trial[190] and the SAVE trial).[191] These studies indicated that the early treatment of patients, regardless of the presence or absence of symptoms, could slow the progression of the dilated cardiomyopathy and improve mortality and morbidity.

Symptomatic Patient

With early and late (advanced) dilated cardiomyopathy (i.e., when the patient has become symptomatic) the course is clear. In dilated cardiomyopathy with symptoms, the heart is large on physical examination, chest roentgenogram, or echocardiogram. The latter diagnostic tool is of particular importance because reduced ventricular function can be quantitated. Measurement of ventricular cavity dimensions and wall thickness can be used to classify the disease as dilated cardiomyopathy. Other tests on initial assessment should include a complete blood count (CBC) and differential, urinalysis, blood glucose, blood urea nitrogen, creatinine, and electrolytes (sodium, potassium, chloride, calcium, magnesium).

Once a diagnosis of symptomatic dilated cardiomyopathy is made, a specific etiology should be sought. The first priority is to determine if the condition has an etiology for which there is a specific treatment (Table 28-5). It is important to reiterate that more than one etiology for dilated cardiomyopathy may be present in the same patient. The first condition to

be excluded in the United States and Europe is an ischemic etiology secondary to coronary atherosclerosis. Clues to its presence are listed in Table 28-5. If another explanation for the cardiomyopathy is present and no strong clues suggest ischemia, no further testing is necessary. However, if the patient has chest pain, an evaluation for myocardial ischemia is warranted.

Among patients with depressed ventricular function (left ventricular ejection fraction approximately 35 percent), only in those with angina does revascularization definitely appear to improve clinical outcome.[191] Thus in patients with left ventricular ejection fractions of less than 25 percent and limiting angina, it is prudent to perform tests to determine if large areas of reversible ischemia are present, and it may be necessary to perform tests for myocardial viability (e.g., low-dose dobutamine infusion echocardiographic test or positron emission tomography testing) before attempting revascularization. Of course, coronary angiography is ultimately necessary to evaluate all of these patients.

Because alcohol and cocaine abuse is so common,

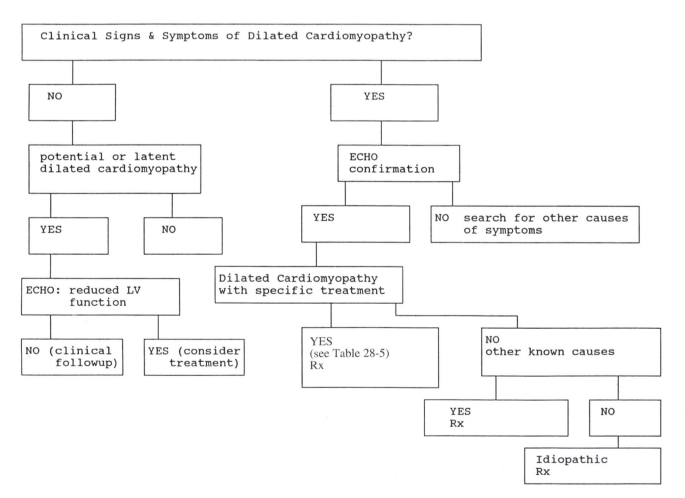

Fig. 28-1. Suggested approach to diagnosis of dilated cardiomyopathy.

Table 28-5. Dilated Cardiomyopathies with Specific Treatment

Specific Cardiomyopathy	Clinical Clues	Specific Treatment
Ischemic (coronary atherosclerosis)	Angina, MI, abnormal Q waves	Revascularization
Alcoholic	Palimpsests, marital or job discord, MCV, GGT, ETOH	Abstinence
Valvular heart disease	Physical examination, echocardiography	Surgery
Hemochromatosis	Diabetes, bronze skin, cirrhosis, increased ferritin	Chelation, phlebotomy
Sarcoid	Clinical features of sarcoidosis	Steroids
Toxoplasmic	AIDS, endomyocardial biopsy, antibodies, S-F	Antibiotics
Mycoplasmic	Pneumonia, cold agglutinins, sputum culture	Antibiotics
Hypocalcemic (hypoparathyroid)	Thyroid surgery, neuromuscular excitability, prolonged Q-T interval	Calcium, parathyroid hormone
Hypophosphatemic	Alcoholism, parenteral hyperalimentation, DKA (recovery phase).	Phosphate
Uremic	BUN, creatinine	Dialysis
Pheochromocytoma	Hypertension, clinical picture, catecholamines	Tumor removal
Hyperthyroidism	Clinical picture, thyroid function tests	Antithyroid drugs, iodine 131, surgery
Carnitine deficiency	Mitochondrial myopathies	Carnitine
Selenium deficiency	Endemic area	Selenium
Arteriovenous fistula	History of trauma, continuous murmur	Surgery

Abbreviations: MI, myocardial infarction; MCV, mean corpuscular volume; GGT, γ-glutamyl transferase; ETOH, ethyl alcohol; S-F, Sabin-Feldman test; DKA, diabetic ketoacidosis; BUN, blood urea nitrogen.

the following tests should be carried out whenever such abuse is suspected: mean corpuscular volume, blood alcohol concentration, urine toxicology screen. If these tests are negative, the following should be done: serum iron and total iron-binding capacity or ferritin, thyroid function tests for hypo- and hyperthyroidism, HIV test, skeletal muscle biopsy, and endomyocardial biopsy, particularly if sarcoid is thought to be present.

REFERENCES

1. Giles TD: A perspective on nosology and incidence of cardiomyopathy. In Giles TD, Sander GE (eds): Cardiomyopathy. PSG Publishing, Littleton, MA, 1988
2. WHO Technical Report Series: Cardiomyopathies. Report of a WHO Expert Committee. p. 7. Technical Report Series 697. WHO, Geneva, 1984
3. Goodwin JF: Cardiac function in primary myocardial disorders. BMJ 1964;1:1527–1533, 1595–1597
4. Abelmann WH, Lorell BH: The challenge of cardiomyopathy. J Am Coll Cardiol 1989;13:1219
5. Miani D, Pinamonti B, Bussani R et al: Right ventricular dysplasia. Clinical and pathological study of two families with left ventricular involvement. Br Heart J 1993;69:151–157
6. Mattingly TW: Clinical features and diagnosis of primary myocardial disease. Part 1. Mod Concepts Cardiovasc Dis 1961;30:677–682
7. Shirey EK, Proudfit WL, Hawk WA: Primary myocardial disease. Correlation with clinical findings, angiographic and biopsy diagnosis. Follow-up of 139 patients. Am Heart J 1980;99:198–207
8. Rahko PS, Orie JE: The clinical presentation and laboratory evaluation of congestive and ischemic cardiomyopathies. Cardiovasc Clin 1988;19:75
9. Stevenson LW, Perloff JK: The dilated cardiomyopathies. Clinical aspects. Cardiol Clin 1988;6:187–218
10. Michels VV, Moll PP, Miller FA et al: The frequency of familial dilated cardiomyopathy in a series of patients with idiopathic dilated cardiomyopathy. N Engl J Med 1992;326:77–82
11. Flowers NC, Horan LG: Electrocardiographic and vectorcardiographic features of myocardial disease. pp. 181–211. In Fowler NO (ed): Myocardial Diseases. Clinical Cardiology Monographs. Grune & Stratton, Orlando, 1973
12. Kuhn H, Breithardt G, Knieriem JH et al: Prognosis and possible presymptomatic manifestations of congestive cardiomyopathy. Postgrad Med J 1978;54:451–459
13. Mintz GS, Kotler MN, Segal BL et al: Echocardiographic features of cardiomyopathy. Cardiovasc Clin 1978;9:125–137
14. Shah PM: Echocardiography in congestive or dilated cardiomyopathy. J Am Soc Echocardiogr 1988;1:20–30

15. Lewis JF, Webber JD, Sutton LL, Chesoni S, Curry CL: Discordance in degree of right and left ventricular dilation in patients with dilated cardiomyopathy. Recognition and clinical implications. J Am Coll Cardiol 1993;21:649–654

16. Pohost GM, Fallon JT, Strauss HW: The role of radionuclide techniques in patients with myocardial disease. Cardiovasc Clin 1979;10:149–163

17. Dunn RF, Uren RF, Sadick N et al: Comparison of thallium-201 scanning in idiopathic dilated cardiomyopathy and severe coronary artery disease. Circulation 1982;66:804–810

18. Zachara E, Caforio AL, Carboni GP et al: Familial aggregation of idiopathic dilated cardiomyopathy. Clinical features and pedigree analysis in 14 families. Br Heart J 1993;69:129–135

19. McKenna WJ: Clinical genetics of dilated cardiomyopathy. Herz 1994;19:91–96

20. Raynolds MV, Bristow MR, Bush EW et al: Angiotensin-converting enzyme DD genotype in patients with ischemic or idiopathic dilated cardiomyopathy. Lancet 1993;342:1073–1075

21. Towbin JA, Hejtmancik JF, Brink P et al: X-Linked dilated cardiomyopathy. Molecular genetic evidence of linkage to the Duchenne muscular dystrophy (dystrophin) gene at the Xp21 locus. Circulation 1993;87:1854–1865

22. Mirabella M, Servidei S, Manfredi G et al: Cardiomyopathy may be the only clinical manifestation in female carriers of Duchenne muscular dystrophy. Neurology 1993;43:2342–2345

23. Riggs T: Cardiomyopathy and pulmonary emboli in terminal Duchenne's muscular dystrophy. Am Heart J 1990;119:690–692

24. Forsberg H, Olofsson BO, Erikkson A, Aanderson S: Cardiac involvement in congenital myotomic dystrophy. Br Heart J 1990;63:119–121

25. Kawashima S, Ulno M, Kondo T et al: Marked cardiac involvement in limb girdle muscular dystrophy. Am J Med Sci 1990;299:411

26. Verhiest W, Brucher JM, Goldeeris P et al: Familial centronuclear myopathy associated with cardiomyopathy. Br Heart J 1976;38:504

27. Kimura S, Yokota H, Tateta K et al: A case of the Kugelberg-Welander syndrome complicated with cardiac lesions. Jpn Heart J 1980;21:417

28. Meier C, Gertsch M, Zimmerman A et al: Nemaline myopathy presenting as cardiomyopathy. N Engl J Med 1983;308:1536

29. Child JS, Perloff JK, Bach PM et al: Cardiac involvement in Friedreich's ataxia. J Am Coll Cardiol 1986;7:1370

30. Alboliras ET, Shub C, Gomez MR et al: Spectrum of cardiac involvement in Friedreich's ataxia. Clinical electrocardiographic and echocardiographic observations. Am J Cardiol 1986;58:518

31. Christodoulou J, McInnes RR, Jay V et al: Barth syndrome. Clinical observations and genetic linkage studies. Am J Med Genet 1994;50:255–264

32. Ades LC, Gedeon AK, Wilson MJ et al: Barth syndrome. Clinical features and confirmation of gene localization to distal Xq28. Am J Med Genet 1993;45:327–334

33. Shoffner JM, Wallace DC: Heart disease and mitochondrial DNA mutations. Heart Dis Stroke 1992;1:235–241

34. Remes AM, Hassinen IE, Ikaheimo MJ et al: Mitochondrial DNA deletions in dilated cardiomyopathy.

A clinical study employing endomyocardial sampling. J Am Coll Cardiol 1994;23:935–942

35. Gerbitz KD, Paprotta A, Jaksch M, Zierz S, Drechsel J: Diabetes mellitus is one of the heterogeneous phenotypic features of a mitochondrial DNA point mutation with the tRNALeu (UUR) gene. FEBS Letter 1993;321:194–196

36. Burch GE, Giles TD, Colcolough HL: Ischemic cardiomyopathy. Am Heart J 1970;79:291

37. Burch GE, Giles TD: Ischemic cardiomyopathy. Diagnostic, pathophysiologic and therapeutic considerations. Cardiovasc Clin 1972;4:203–220

38. Pfeffer MA, Braunwald E: Ventricular remodeling after myocardial infarction. Experimental observations and clinical implications. Circulation 1990;81:1161

39. Braunwald E, Kloner RA: The stunned myocardium. Prolonged, postischemic ventricular dysfunction. Circulation 1982;66:1146

40. Rahimtoola SH: The hibernating myocardium. Am Heart J 1989;117:211

41. Patel B, Kloner RA, Przyklenk K, Braunwald E: Postischemic myocardial "stunning." A clinically relevant phenomenon. Ann Intern Med 1988;108:627

42. Raftery EB, Banks DC, Oram S: Occlusive disease of the coronary arteries presenting as primary congestive cardiomyopathy. Lancet 1969;2:1147–1150

43. Schuster EH, Bulkley BH: Ischemic cardiomyopathy. A clinicopathologic study of fourteen patients. Am Heart J 1980;100:506–512

44. Baker DW, Jones R, Hodges J et al: Management of heart failure. III. The role of revascularization in the treatment of patients with moderate or severe left ventricular systolic dysfunction. JAMA 1994;272:1528–1534

45. Thomas MG, Sander GE, Giles TD: Hyperergopathic cardiomyopathy. pp. 459–484. In Giles TD, Sander GE (eds): Cardiomyopathy. PSG Publishing, Littleton, MA, 1986

46. Katz AM: Cardiomyopathy of overload. A major determinant of prognosis in congestive heart failure. N Engl J Med 1990;322:100–110

47. Lieberman EB, Hutchins GM, Herskowitz A, Rose NR, Baughman KL: Clinicopathologic description of myocarditis. J Am Coll Cardiol 1991;18:1617–1626

48. Waller BF, Slack JD, Orr CD, Adlam JH, Bournique VM: "Flaming," "smoldering" and "burned out." The fireside saga of myocarditis. J Am Coll Cardiol 1991;18:1627–1630

49. Woodruff JF: Viral myocarditis. A review. Am J Pathol 1980;101:427–479

50. Kishimoto C, Kurnick JT, Fallon JT, Crumpacker CS, Abelmann WH: Characteristics of lymphocytes cultured from murine viral myocarditis specimens. A preliminary and technical report. J Am Coll Cardiol 1989;14:799–802

51. Gore I, Saphir O: Myocarditis. A classification of 1402 cases. Am Heart J 1947;34:827–830

52. Stevens PJ, Underwood-Ground KE: Occurrence and significance of myocarditis in trauma. Aerospace Med 1970;41:776–780

53. Richardson PJ, Why HJF: Myocarditis and dilated cardiomyopathy. A pathogenetic link? Heart Failure 1992;8:27–31

54. Quigley PJ, Richardson PJ, Meany BT et al: Long-term follow-up of acute myocarditis. Correlation of

ventricular function and outcome. Eur Heart J, suppl. J 1987;8:39–42

55. Hare JM: The etiologic basis of heart failure. pp. 3.1–3.23. In Braunwald E (ed): Atlas of Heart Disease. Vol. IV: Colucci WS (ed). Heart Failure. Cardiac Function and Dysfunction. Mosby, St Louis, MO, 1995

56. Jin O, Sole MJ, Butany JW et al: Detection of enterovirus RNA in myocardial biopsies from patients with myocarditis and cardiomyopathy using gene amplification by polymerase chain reaction. Circulation 1990;82:8

57. Herskowitz A, Wu T-C, Willoughby SB et al: Myocarditis and cardiotropic viral infection associated with severe left ventricular dysfunction in late-stage infection with human immunodeficiency virus. J Am Coll Cardiol 1994;24:1025–1032

58. Hofman P, Drici MD, Bibelin P, Michiels JF, Thyss A: Prevalence of Toxoplasma myocarditis in patients with the acquired immunodeficiency syndrome. Br Heart J 1993;70:376–381

59. Lipshultz SE, Orav EJ, Sanders SP et al: Cardiac structure and function in children with human immunodeficiency virus infection treated with zidovudine. N Engl J Med 1992;327:1260–1265

60. Mady C, Cardoso RHA, Barretto ACP et al: Survival and predictors of survival in patient with congestive heart failure due to Chagas' cardiomyopathy. Circulation 1994;90:3098–3102

61. Rossi MA: Microvascular changes as a cause of chronic cardiomyopathy in Chagas' disease. Am Heart J 1990;120:233–236

62. De Paola AAV, Horowitz LN, Miyamoto MH et al: Angiographic and electrophysiologic substrates of ventricular tachycardia in chronic Chagasic myocarditis. Am J Cardiol 1990;65:360–363

63. Hagar JM, Rahimtoola SH: Chagas' heart disease in the United States. N Engl J Med 1991;325:763–768

64. Steere AC, Batsford WP, Weinberg M et al: Lyme carditis. Cardiac abnormalities of Lyme disease. Ann Intern Med 1980;93:8–16

65. Stanek G, Klein J, Bittner R, Glogar D: Isolation of Borrelia burgdorferi from the myocardium of a patient with longstanding cardiomyopathy. N Engl J Med 1990;322:249–252

66. Melish ME: Kawasaki syndrome. A new infectious disease? J Infect Dis 1981;143:317–324

67. Fujiwara H, Hamashima Y: Pathology of the heart in Kawasaki disease. Pediatrics 1978;61:100–107

68. Yutani C, Go S, Kamiya T et al: Cardiac biopsy of Kawasaki disease. Arch Pathol Lab Med 1981;105:470–473

69. Fujiwara H, Hamashima Y: Pathology of the heart in Kawasaki disease. Pediatrics 1978;61:100–107

70. Niwa AK, Tashima K, Kawasoe Y et al: Magnetic resonance imaging of myocardial infarction in Kawasaki disease. Am Heart J 1990;119:1293–1302

71. McCall D: Alcohol and the cardiovascular system. Curr Probl Cardiol 1987;12:349–414

72. Kupari M, Suokas A: Effects of ethanol and its metabolites on the heart. pp. 49–60. In Crown K, Batt RD (eds): Human Metabolism of Alcohol. Vol. III. Metabolic and Physiologic Effects of Alcohol. CRC Press, Boca Raton, FL, 1989

73. Hartel G, Louhija A, Konttinen A: Cardiovascular study of 100 chronic alcoholics. Acta Med Scand 1969;185:507–513

74. Schenk KA, Cohen J: The heart in chronic alcoholism. Clinical and pathological findings. Pathol Microbiol 1970;35:96–104

75. Alexander CS: Idiopathic heart disease. 1. Analysis of 100 cases, with special reference to chronic alcoholism. Am J Med 1966;41:213–228

76. Massumi RA, Rios JC, Gooch AS et al: Primary myocardial disease. Report of fifty cases and review of the subject. Circulation 1965;31:19–41

77. Regan TJ: Alcoholic cardiomyopathy. Prog Cardiovasc Dis 1984;28:141–152

78. Moushmoush B, Abi-Mansour P: Alcohol and the heart. The long-term effects of alcohol on the cardiovascular system. Arch Intern Med 1991;151:36–42

79. Alexander CS: Electron microscopic observation in alcoholic heart disease. Br Heart J 1967;29:200–206

80. Segel LD, Rendig SV, Choquet Y et al: Effects of chronic graded ethanol consumption on the metabolism, ultrastructure, and mechanical function of the rat heart. Cardiovasc Res 1975;9:649–663

81. Weishacur R, Sarma JSM, Maruyama Y et al: Reversibility of mitochondrial and contractile changes in the myocardium after cessation of prolonged ethanol intake. Am J Cardiol 1977;40:556–562

82. Schreiber SS, Briden K, Oratz M et al: Ethanol, acetaldehyde and myocardial protein synthesis. J Clin Invest 1972;51:2820–2826

83. James TN, Bear ES: Effect of ethanol and acetaldehyde on the heart. Am Heart J 1967;74:243–255

84. Kupari M, Koskinen P, Suokas A, Ventila M: Left ventricular filling impairment in asymptomatic chronic alcoholics. Am J Cardiol 1990;66:1473–1477

85. Kupari M, Koskinen P: Comparison of the cardiotoxicity of ethanol in women versus men. Am J Cardiol 1992;70:645–649

86. Zambrano SS, Mazzotta JF, Sherman D et al: Cardiac dysfunction in unselected chronic alcoholic patients. Noninvasive screening by systolic time intervals. Am Heart J 1974;87:318–320

87. DeMakis JG, Rahimtoola SH, Sutton GD et al: The natural course of alcoholic cardiomyopathy. Ann Intern Med 1974;80:293–297

88. Isner JM, Estes NAM III, Thompson PD et al: Acute cardiac events temporally related to cocaine use. N Engl J Med 1986;315:1438–1443

89. Karch RA, Billingham ME: The pathology and etiology of cocaine-induced heart disease. Arch Pathol Lab Med 1988;112:225–230

90. Bertolet BD, Freund G, Martin CA et al: Unrecognized left ventricular dysfunction in an apparently healthy cocaine abuse population. Clin Cardiol 1990;13:323–328

91. Virmani R, Robinowitz M, Smialek JE, Smyth DF: Cardiovascular effects of cocaine. An autopsy study of 40 patients. Am Heart J 1988;115:1068–1076

92. Kloner RA, Hale S, Alker K, Rezkalla S: The effects of acute and chronic cocaine use on the heart. Circulation 1992;85:407–419

93. Chokshi SK, Moore R, Pandian NG, Isner JM: Reversible cardiomyopathy associated with cocaine intoxication. Ann Intern Med 1989;111:1039–1040

94. Sander GE: Toxic cardiomyopathy. pp. 255–288. In Giles TD, Sander GE (eds): Cardiomyopathy. PSG Publishing, Littleton, MA, 1988

95. Olson RD, Mushlin PS: Doxorubicin cardiotoxicity. Analysis of prevailing hypotheses. FASEB J 1990;4:3076–3086

96. Von Hoff DD, Layard MW, Basa P et al: Risk factors for doxorubicin-induced congestive heart failure. Ann Intern Med 1979;91:710–717

97. Schwartz RG, McKenzie WB, Alexander J et al: Congestive heart failure and left ventricular dysfunction complicating doxorubicin therapy. Am J Med 1987;82:1109–1118

98. Lipshultz SE, Colan SD, Gelber RD et al: Late cardiac effects of doxorubicin therapy for acute lymphoblastic leukemia in childhood. N Engl J Med 1991;324:808–815

99. Doroshow JH: Doxorubicin-induced cardiac toxicity. N Engl J Med 1991;324:843–845

100. Saini J, Rich MW, Lyss AP: Reversibility of severe left ventricular dysfunction due to doxorubicin cardiotoxicity. Ann Intern Med 1987;106:814–816

101. Quezado ZMN, Wilson WH, Cunnion RE et al: High-dose ifosfamide is associated with severe, reversible cardiac dysfunction. Ann Intern Med 1993;118:31–36

102. Midei MG, Ment SH, Feldman AM, Hutchins GM, Baughman KL: Peripartum myocarditis and cardiomyopathy. Circulation 1990;81:922–928

103. Burch GE, Giles TD: The role of viruses in the production of heart disease. Am J Cardiol 1972;29:231–240

104. Mendelson MA, Chandler J: Postpartum cardiomyopathy associated with maternal cocaine abuse. Am J Cardiol 1992;70:1092–1094

105. Burch GE, Giles TD, Tsui C-Y: Postpartal cardiomyopathy. Cardiovasc Clin 1972;4:269–282

106. Burch GE, McDonald CD, Walsh JJ: The effect of prolonged bed rest on postpartal cardiomyopathy. Am Heart J 1971;81:186–201

107. Meadows WR: Idiopathic myocardial failure in the 1st trimester of pregnancy and the puerperium. Circulation 1957;15:903–914

108. Fein FS, Sonnenblick EH: Clinical diabetic cardiomyopathy. Prog Cardiovasc Dis 1985;27:255–270

109. Starling MR: Does a clinically definable diabetic cardiomyopathy exist? J Am Coll Cardiol 1990;15:1518–1520

110. Kannel WB, Hjortland M, Castelli WP: Role of diabetes in congestive heart failure. The Framingham study. Am J Cardiol 1974;34:29–34

111. Factor SM, Okun EM, Minase T: Capillary microaneurysms in the human diabetic heart. N Engl J Med 1980;302:384–388

112. Regan TJ, Lyons MM, Ahmed SS et al: Evidence for cardiomyopathy in familial diabetes. J Clin Invest 1977;60:885–899

113. Factor SM, Minase T, Sonnnenblick EH: Clinical and morphological features of human hypertensive-diabetic cardiomyopathy. Am Heart J 1980;99:446–458

114. Van Hoeven KH, Factor SM: A comparison of the pathological spectrum of hypertensive, diabetic, and hypertensive-diabetic heart disease. Circulation 1990;82:848–855

115. Borow KM, Jaspan JB, Williams KA et al: Myocardial mechanics in young adult patients with diabetes mellitus. Effects of altered load, inotropic state and dynamic exercise. J Am Coll Cardiol 1990;15:1508–1517

116. Starling MR: Does a clinically definable diabetic cardiomyopathy exist? J Am Coll Cardiol 1990;15:1518–1520

117. Riggs TW, Ttansue D: Doppler echocardiographic evaluation of left ventricular diastolic function in ad-olescents with diabetes mellitus. Am J Cardiol 1990;65:899–902

118. Hiramatsu K, Ohara N, Shigematsu S et al: Left ventricular filling abnormalities in non-insulin-dependent diabetes mellitus and improvement by a short-term glycemic control. Am J Cardiol 1992;70:1185–1189

119. Ambepityia G, Kopelman PG, Ingram D et al: Exertional myocardial ischemia in diabetes. A quantitative analysis of anginal perceptual threshold and the influence of autonomic function. J Am Coll Cardiol 1990;15:72–77

120. Symons C: Thyroid heart disease. Br Heart J 1979;41:257–262

121. Skelton CL: The heart and hyperthyroidism. N Engl J Med 1982;307:1206–1208

122. Klein I, Ojamaa K: Cardiovascular manifestations of endocrine disease. J Clin Endocrinol Metab 1992;75:339–342

123. Zaimis E, Papadaki L, Ash ASF et al: Cardiovascular effects of thyroxine. Cardiovasc Res 1969;3:118–133

124. Sandler G, Wilson GM: The production of cardiac hypertrophy by thyroxine in the rat. Q J Exp Physiol 1959;44:282–289

125. Cohen J, Aroesty JM, Rosenfeld MG: Determinants of thyroxine-induced cardiac hypertrophy in mice. Circ Res 1966;18:388–397

126. Sandler G, Wilson GM: The nature and prognosis of heart disease in thyrotoxicosis. Q J Med 1959;28:347–369

127. Surks MI, Koerner D, Dillman W et al: Limited capacity binding sites for L-triiodothyronine in rat liver nuclei. J Biol Chem 1973;248:7066–7072

128. Samuels HH, Tsai JS, Casanova J et al: In vitro characterization of solubilized nuclear receptors from rat liver and cultured GH_1 cells. J Clin Invest 1974;54:853–865

129. Howitt G, Rowlands DJ, Leung DYT et al: Myocardial contractility and the effects of beta-adrenergic blockade in hypothyroidism and hyperthyroidism. Clin Sci 1968;34:485–495

130. Shapiro S, Steier M, Dimich I: Congestive heart failure in neonatal thyrotoxicosis. Clin Pediatr 1975;14:1155–1156

131. Ueda H, Uozumi Z, Watanabe H et al: Phonocardiographic study of hyperthyroidism. Jpn Heart J 1963;4:509–523

132. Symons C, Myers A, Kingstone D et al: Response to thyrotrophin-releasing hormone in atrial dysrhythmias. Postgrad Med J 1978;54:658–662

133. Lee RT, Plappert M, Sutton SJ: Depressed left ventricular systolic ejection force in hypothyroidism. Am J Cardiol 1990;65:526–527

134. Shenoy MM, Goldman JM: Hypothyroid cardiomyopathy. Echocardiographic documentation of reversibility. Am J Med Sci 1987;294:1–9

135. Kurtzman RS, Otto D, Chepey JJ: Myxedema heart disease. Radiology 1965;84:624–629

136. Hardisty CA, Naik DR, Munro DS: Pericardial effusions in hypothyroidism. Clin Endocrinol-(Oxf) 1980;13:349–354

137. Wright AD, Hill DM, Lowy C et al: Mortality in acromegaly. Q J Med 1970;39:1–16

138. Lie JT, Grossman SJ: Pathology of the heart in acromegaly. Anatomic findings in 27 autopsied patients. Am Heart J 1980;100:41–52

139. Van den Heuvel P, Elbers H, Plokker H, Bruschke A: Myocardial involvement in acromegaly. Int J Cardiol 1984;6:550–553

140. Savage DD, Henry WL, Eastman RC et al: Echocardiographic assessment of cardiac anatomy and function in acromegalic patients. Am J Med 1979;67:823–829

141. Smallridge RC, Rajfer S, Davia J et al: Acromegaly and the heart. Am J Med 1979;66:22–27

142. Csanady M, Gaspar L, Hogye M et al: The heart in acromegaly: an echocardiographic study. Int J Cardiol 1983;2:349–357

143. Thuesen L, Christensen SE, Weeke J, Orskov H, Henningsen P: A hyperkinetic heart in uncomplicated active acromegaly. Explanation of hypertension in acromegalic patients? Acta Endocrinol (Copenh) 1988;233:337–343

144. Chanson, P, Timsit J, Mawquet C et al: Cardiovascular effects of the somatostatin analog octreotide in acromegaly. Ann Intern Med 1990;113:921–925

145. Milder MS, Cook JN, Stray S et al: Idiopathic hemochromatosis. Etiology and clinical significance. Medicine (Baltimore) 1980;59:34–49

146. Buja IM, Roberts WC: Iron in the heart. Etiology and clinical significance. Am J Med 1971;51:209–221

147. James TN: Pathology of the cardiac conduction system in hemochromatosis. N Engl J Med 1964;271:92–94

148. Finch SC, Finch CA: Idiopathic hemochromatosis, an iron storage disease. Medicine (Baltimore) 1955;34:381–430

149. Mattheyses M, Hespel JP, Brissot P et al: La myocardiopathie de l'hemochromatose idiopatique. Arch Mal Coeur 1978;71:371–379

150. Candell-Riera J, Lu L, Seres L et al: Cardiac hemochromatosis: beneficial effects of iron removal therapy. An echocardiographic study. Am J Cardiol 1983;52:824–829

151. Skinner C, Kevmure ACF: Hemochromatosis presenting as congestive cardiomyopathy and responding to venesection. Br Heart J 1973;35:466–468

152. Cecchetti KG, Binda A, Piperno A et al: Cardiac alterations in 36 consecutive patients with idiopathic haemochromatosis. Polygraphic and echocardiographic evaluation. Eur Heart J 12:224–230,1991

153. Wolfe L, Oliveri N, Sallan D et al: Prevention of cardiac disease by subcutaneous deferoxamine in patients with thalassemia major. N Engl J Med 1985;312:1600–1603

154. Mariotti E, Agostini A, Angelucci E, Lucarfelli G, Sgarbi E: Echocardiographic study in ex-thalassemic patients with iron overload, preliminary observation during phlebotomy therapy. Bone Marrow Transplant 1993;12:106–102

155. Weiss S: Occidental beriberi with cardiovascular manifestations. Its relation of thiamine deficiency. JAMA 1940;115:832–839

156. Blankenhorn MA: Occidental beriberi heart disease. JAMA 1946;131:717–726

157. Akbarian M, Uankopoulos NA, Abelmann WH: Hemodynamic studies in beriberi heart disease. Am J Med 1966;41:197

158. Jeffrey FE, Abelmann WH: Recovery of proved Shoshin beriberi. Am J Med 1971;50:123

159. Engel AG, Angelini C: Carnitine deficiency of human skeletal muscle with associated lipid storage myopathy. A new syndrome. Science 1973;173:99

160. DiMauro S, Trevisan C, Hays A: Disorders of lipid metabolism in muscle. Muscle Nerve 190;3:369–388

161. Tripp ME, Katcher ML, Peters HA et al: Systemic carnitine deficiency presenting as familial endocardial fibroelastosis. N Engl J Med 1981;305:385–390

162. Snyder TM, Little BW, Roman-Campos G et al: Successful treatment of familial idiopathic lipid storage myopathy with L-carnitine and modified lipid diet. Neurology 1982;32:1106–1115

163. Chen X, Yang G, Chen J et al: Studies on the relations of selenium and Keshan disease. Biol Trace Element Res 1980;2:91–107

164. Ge K, Xue A, Bai J et al: Keshan disease—an endemic cardiomyopathy in China. Virchows Arch [Pathol Anat] 1983;401:1–15

165. Keshan Disease Research Group of the Chinese Academy of Medical Sciences, Beijing Antiepidemic Station of Sichuan and Antiepidemic Station of Mianning County, Sichuan. Observations on effect of sodium selenite in the prevention of Keshan disease. Chin Med J Engl 1979;92:471–476

166. Johnson RA, Baker SS, Fallon JT et al: An occidental case of cardiomyopathy and selenium deficiency. N Engl J Med 1981;304:1210–1212

167. Fleming CR, Lie JT, McCall JT et al: Selenium deficiency and fatal cardiomyopathy in a patient on home parenteral nutrition. Gastroenterology 1982;83:683–693

168. Lockitch G: Selenium. Clinical significance and analytical concepts. Crit Rev Clin Lab Sci 1989;27:483–541

169. Nihoyannopoulos P, Gomez PM, Joshi J et al: Cardiac abnormalities in systemic lupus erythematosus. Association with raised anticardiolipin antibodies. Circulation 1990;82:369–375

170. Leung WH, Wong KL, Lau C-P et al: Doppler echocardiographic evaluation of left ventricular diastolic function in patients with systemic lupus erythematosus. Am Heart J 1990;120:82–87

171. Crozier IG, Li E, Milne MJ, Nicholls G: Cardiac involvement in systemic lupus erythematosus detected by echocardiography. Am J Cardiol 1990;65:1145–1148

172. Churg J, Strauss L: Allergic granulomatosis. Allergic angiitis, and periarteritis nodosa. Am J Pathol 1951;27:277–301

173. Hasley PB, Follansbee WP, Coulehan JL: Cardiac manifestations of Churg-Strauss syndrome. Report of a case and review of the literature. Am Heart J 1990;120:996–999

174. Morgan JM, Raposo L, Gibson DG: Cardiac involvement in Churg-Strauss syndrome shown by echocardiography. Br Heart J 1989;62:462–466

175. Medsger TA Jr, Masi AT, Rodnan GP et al: Survival with systemic sclerosis (scleroderma). A life table analysis of clinical and demographic factors in 309 patients. Ann Intern Med 1971;75:369–376

176. Bulkley BH, Ridolfi RL, Salyer WR et al: Myocardial lesions of progressive systemic sclerosis. A cause of cardiac dysfunction. Circulation 1976;53:483–490

177. Follansbee WP, Curtiss EL, Medsger TA Jr et al: Physiological abnormalities of cardiac function in progressive sclerosis with diffuse scleroderma. N Engl J Med 1984;310:142–148

178. Kahan A, Devaux JY, Amor B et al: The effect of captopril on thallium 201 myocardial perfusion in systemic sclerosis. Clin Pharmacol Ther 1990;47: 483–489
179. Cruikshank B: Heart lesions in rheumatoid arthritis. J Pathol Bacteriol 1958;76:223–240
180. Kahn SJ, Spodick D: Rheumatoid heart disease. Semin Arthritis Rheum 1972;1:327–337
181. Malamud M, Haymaker W, Custer RP: Heat stroke. A clinicopathologic study of 125 fatal cases. Milit Surg 1946;99:397–449
182. Kew MC, Tucker RBK, Bersohn I et al: The heart in heat stroke. Am Heart J 1969;77:324–335
183. Duguid H, Simpson RG, Stowers JM: Accidental hypothermia. Lancet 1961;2:1213–1219
184. Taliercio CP, Olney BA, Lie JT: Myocarditis related to drug hypersensitivity. Mayo Clin Proc 1985;60: 463–468
185. Delage C, Mullick FG, Irey NS: Myocardial lesions in anaphylaxis. A histochemical study. Arch Pathol 1973;95:185–189
186. MacSearraigh ETM, Patel KM: Cardiomyopathy as a complication of sulphonamide therapy. BMJ 1968; 3:33
187. Sander GE: Toxic cardiomyopathy. pp. 255–288. In Giles TD, Sander GE (eds): Cardiomyopathy. PSG Publishing, Littleton, MA, 1988
188. Dec GW, Fuster V: Idiopathic dilated cardiomyopathy. N Engl J Med 1994;331:1564–1575
189. Redfield MM, Gersh BJ, Bailey KR, Ballard DJ, Rodeheffer RJ: Natural history of idiopathic dilated cardiomyopathy. Effect of referral bias and secular trend. J Am Coll Cardiol 1993;22:1921–1926
190. SOLVD Investigators: Effect of enalapril on mortality and the development of heart failure in asymptomatic patients with reduced left ventricular ejection fractions. N Engl J Med 1992;327:685–691
191. Pfeffer MA, Braunwald E, Moye LA et al: Effect of captopril on mortality and morbidity in patients with left ventricular dysfunction after myocardial infarction. N Engl J Med 1992;327:669–677

29 | Cardiomyopathies and Specific Heart Muscle Diseases

Heinz-Peter Schultheiss
Uwe Kühl

Cardiomyopathies are diseases of the heart characterized by ventricular dysfunction not caused by primary heart disease (e.g., hypertension or congenital, valvar, coronary, arterial, or pericardial abnormalities). They are classified as primary cardiomyopathies if the origin of contractile dysfunction is unknown (dilated cardiomyopathy, hypertrophic cardiomyopathy) and as secondary or specific cardiomyopathies if the heart is affected in association with specific infectious, immunologic, metabolic, neuromuscular, or toxic diseases[1] (Table 29-1).

PATHOGENESIS

The pathogenesis of specific cardiomyopathies is as complex as their etiology. The heart can be affected by a number of diseases and agents. Direct cytopathic effects of viruses and virus-triggered humoral and cellular immune reactions are suggested to impair cardiac function in viral myocarditis. Viral heart disease and other specific cardiomyopathies (e.g., collagen diseases, sarcoidosis, neuromuscular and drug diseases) as well as alcoholic and peripartum cardiomyopathies are discussed in detail later in the chapter. A time-restricted, reversible cardiac dysfunction is seen in association with 10–20 percent of severe viral and bacterial infections. Bacteria (e.g., diphtheria) can cause cardiac dysfunction and arrhythmias owing to a release of toxins that inhibit protein synthesis or metabolism of the cardiac myocyte. However, cardiac involvement is reversible in most of these cases. Irrespective of the metabolic and biochemical injury caused by toxins, secondary immunologic mechanisms may be involved and contribute to myocyte necrosis, development of reactive and reparative fibrosis, and eventually progression of cardiac dysfunction. Rheumatic myocarditis represents an allergic reaction to streptococcal antigens and is discussed in detail elsewhere.

PATHOPHYSIOLOGY

Specific heart muscle diseases are characterized by a variable disturbance of systolic and diastolic cardiac function associated with a normal-sized or dilated left or right ventricle. With respect to the severity of cardiac dysfunction, the disease may present with normal hemodynamic indices or an elevated left ventricular filling pressure resulting in an abnormally high pulmonary artery pressure, an increase of end-diastolic and end-systolic ventricular volumes, an increase in the arteriovenous difference of oxygen saturation, and the development of insufficiency of the atrioventricular valves due to the ventricular enlargement.

Depressed systolic ventricular function is characterized by reduction of the ejection fraction, stroke volume, and cardiac index, resulting in clinical symptoms of congestive heart failure. Elevated catecholamine levels produce tachycardia, increased myocardial contractility, and elevated left ventricular end-diastolic pressure, which results in limited

Table 29-1. Cardiomyopathies

Primary cardiomyopathies
  Dilated cardiomyopathy ("idiopathic")
  Hypertrophic cardiomyopathy
  Familial cardiomyopathy
  Eosinophilic endomyocardial disease
Secondary cardiomyopathies
  Viral myocarditis: picornavirus, arbonvirus, hepatitis A and B, rabies, orthomyxovirus, paramyxovirus, rubella, smallpox, adenovirus, herpes virus, retrovirus (HIV)
  Bacterial myocarditis: rickettsiosis, *Chlamydia*, diphtheria, spirochetosis, *Salmonella paratyphi*, streptococci A-D, staphylococci, *Mycobacterium tuberculosis*
  Parasitization: *Trypanosoma cruzi* (Chagas disease), leishmaniasis, amebiasis, toxoplasmosis
  Collagen disease: rheumatoid arthritis, systemic lupus erythematosus, polyarteritis nodosa, progressive systemic sclerosis, dermatomyositis
  Granulomatosis: sarcoidosis, Wegener's granulomatosis, giant cell arteritis, lymphomatoid granulomatosis
  Metabolic involvement of the heart diabetes mellitus, malnutrition, thiamine deficiency, obesity, thyroid disease, hyperthyroidism, hypothyroidism, carcinoid
  Sensitivity and toxic cardiomyopathies alcohol, radiation, drugs
  Neuromuscular disease muscular dystrophy, myotonic dystrophy, Friedreich's ataxia
  Others amyloidosis, peripartum cardiomyopathy, endocardial fibroelastosis

diastolic coronary blood flow and, consequently, myocardial ischemia. Impaired diastolic relaxation may prolong compression of the intramyocardial vessels and consequently reduce the blood flow to the subendocardial layers. Hence reduced amounts of oxygen are delivered to the muscular tissue, which enhances ventricular stiffness, influencing ventricular contractility. The resulting subendocardial ischemia could lead to myocardial necrosis, fiber replacement, and ultimately decompensation of the left ventricle. This situation induces activation of the neuroendocrine system, resulting in increasing oxygen demand of the myocardium and decreasing coronary perfusion. Thus the progression of heart failure continues.

As is evident, heart failure is the result of several factors on the cellular level. The other main question is the energetic state of the myocardium. It has been discussed whether a depression of mitochondrial function is present with cardiomyopathic heart failure.[2,3] Changes in the creatine kinase system showing low creatine kinase activity, high MB creatine kinase isoenzyme content and activity, and low creatine content in the presence of pressure-overloaded hypertrophy may represent an adaptation toward anaerobic metabolism. In addition, alterations in the isoenzyme pattern of the mitochondrial adenosine diphosphate (ADP) translocator point to an involvement of disturbed myocyte energy metabolism in failing hearts.

DIAGNOSIS AND DIFFERENTIAL DIAGNOSIS

A detailed case history might point to the possible origin of the symptoms (e.g., coronary artery disease), but in most cases it is impossible to differentiate the various forms of heart disease on clinical grounds alone. Physical examination guides attention toward hypertension, valvar heart disease, or pericarditis, or in combination with laboratory examinations toward metabolic or collagen diseases, as a possible cause for cardiac dysfunction. Further information may be gained from electrocardiographic (ECG), echocardiographic, and scintigraphic examinations, and finally from left and right heart catheterization. If the origin of cardiac dysfunction cannot be confirmed with these methods, histologic, immunohistologic, electron microscopic, molecular biologic, and biochemical analysis of endomyocardial biopsy might provide additional information about other infectious, genetic, or systemic diseases affecting the heart (see the specific diseases).

At the cellular level, histologic examination reveals in most cases no specific abnormalities that provide a definitive diagnosis or determination of the etiology of the disease. Myocytic abnormalities (nucleus, mitochondria, contractile proteins), inadequate hypertrophy, myocytic necrosis, interstitial or perivascular fibrosis, and vascular abnormalities may be caused by a variety of infectious, inflammatory, metabolic, toxic, or ischemic processes. Histologic abnormalities only represent the end result of myocardial damage. Immunohistochemically, focal or diffuse cellular infiltrations consisting of lymphocytes, macrophages, or neutrophils and an enhanced expression of various immune markers (e.g., adhesion molecules) confirm the presence of an inflammatory process that might be of pathogenetic importance (see below).

CLINICAL MANIFESTATIONS

Fatigue, atypical chest pain, dyspnea at exertion, palpitations, and newly developed arrhythmias are early symptoms of all forms of primary or secondary cardiomyopathies. During progression of the disease symptoms of left- and right-sided congestive heart failure arise, developing rapidly (hours or days) or gradually (months or even years). Some patients have left ventricular dilatation long before they become symptomatic. In addition to cardiac decompensation caused by reduced myogenic contractility, emboli and arrhythmias (sudden death) might threaten patients and be the first clinical manifestation of the disease.

PHYSICAL EXAMINATION

Left ventricular enlargement with congestive heart failure is noted during the later stages of the disease. Patients present with hypotension and elevated jugular venous pressure. Symptoms of right heart failure mostly develop with the end-stage cardiomyopathies. Systolic heart murmurs of the mitral valve and tricuspid valve regurgitations are due to widening of the valvar rings caused by heart enlargement. Third and fourth heart sounds are commonly noted.

LABORATORY EXAMINATIONS

Cardiomegaly due to ventricular enlargement or pericardial effusions, pulmonary venous hypertension, and pleural effusions are seen on chest roentgenograms in patients with advanced disease. Radiologic findings are confirmed, and primary cardiac disease such as valvular or hypertrophic heart diseases can be excluded echocardiographically. Nonspecific T wave abnormalities and all known forms of arrhythmias and conductive disturbances are common features of early and advanced cardiomyopathies, irrespective of the underlying cause. Although contractility still can be normal at rest, radionucleotide ventriculography may point to a disturbed ventricular function during exercise. By definition, angiography of the large arteries is not helpful.

THERAPY

Heart Failure

Heart failure is first treated according to general guidelines, although known causes demand specific treatment of the underlying disease. Generally, all causes of heart failure should be avoided or at least minimized. Depending on the severity of the cardiac impairment, rest and treatment for fluid and sodium retention have favorable effects. Drug treatment

comprises vasodilators [in particular angiotensin-converting enzyme (ACE) inhibitors or nitrates and hydralazine], diuretics, and digitalis. Depending on the blood pressure, ACE inhibitors should be given in high doses to relieve the cardiac load. β-Blockers have been shown to improve even severe cases of cardiac failure if started at a low dose, which is then increased carefully. Apart from intermittent use of dobutamine in cases of acute developing pump failure and chronic heart failure that do not respond to conventional therapy, there is no indication for long-term treatment with positive inotropic drugs. Whether cyclic adenosine monophosphate (cAMP)-independent, positive inotopic drugs (e.g., vesnarinone, OPC82-12) are of importance in the treatment of severe cardiomyopathies has yet to be established.

Arrhythmias

Supraventricular arrhythmias (inclusing supraventricular and ventricular extra beats) cause problems only for patients with severely impaired cardiac function. Tachyarrhythmias should be prevented with digitalis. Ventricular tachycardia and ventricular runs have been identified as poor prognostic predictors, indicating the possibility of sudden death, and might also be the cause of hemodynamic decompensation if the ventricular runs appear in patients with severe ventricular dysfunction. Most antiarrhythmic drugs have negative inotropic effects and should be used with care to avoid drug-induced cardiac decompensation. Amiodarone may be used if tolerated because of its lack of severe side effects. Alternatively, patients can be provided with an antitachycardial cardioconverter system.

Types of Therapy

ACE INHIBITORS

Compensatory neurohumoral mechanisms are already activated during the early stages of asymptomatic cardiomyopathies with impaired ventricular contractility. These mechanisms are responsible for reorganization of the myocardial matrix (remodeling) and might be partly reversible or prevented by ACE inhibitors if brought into action at an early stage of the disease. Early use of vasodilators reduces mortality even in asymptomatic cases of heart failure, as shown by the SOLVD prevention study.[4,5] To relive the heart of negative hemodynamic effects the ACE inhibitor doses should be titrated as high as tolerated because of the blood pressure. ACE inhibitors are favored over other drugs because other drugs induce regulatory mechanisms of the neurohumoral system that do not favor remodeling of the myocardium and so worsen heart failure in the long term. These drugs (e.g., hydralazine and nitrates) are used only if ACE inhibitors are not tolerated.

DIURETICS

Diuretics alleviate clinical symptoms and thereby the working capacity and quality of life of patients with severe heart failure. To prevent adverse effects of the neuroendocrine system, these drugs should not be used as monotherapy but are combined with ACE inhibitors.

DIGITALIS

Digitalis is another mainstay of basic conventional drug management for patients with severe heart failure. The benefit of digitalis in patients with mild heart failure and with sinus rhythm has not yet been proved by randomized studies. In patients with sinus rhythm but clinical symptoms due to mild heart failure [New York Heart Association (NYHA) class II], various studies (e.g., Radiance study) have supplied evidence for a beneficial effect of digitalis if ACE inhibitors and diuretics were not sufficient for reducing cardiac symptoms.[6]

β-BLOCKERS

β-Blockers, in addition to the above-described baseline therapy, reduce morbidity and mortality. Their effect was shown when metoprolol was administered in addition to these drugs (MDC trial).[7] To avoid worsening the severe cardiac failure by the negative inotropic effect of a β-blocker, the drugs are started on very low doses and titrated up carefully over a period of several weeks.

POSITIVE INOTROPIC DRUGS

End-stage heart failure unresponsive to oral drug management may respond to intermittent intravenous administration of catecholamines (e.g., dobutamine) in relatively low doses ($2-10$ $\mu g \cdot kg^{-1} \cdot min^{-1}$) for 8 hours daily over a period of $12-14$ days. These substances are not suitable for long-time application.

Mechanical Assist Devices

Heart transplantation is the only possible cure for progressive heart failure. Intraaortic balloon pumping may stabilize acute cardiac decompensation for a short period and allow bridge time until an appropriate donor heart is available. Preliminary results have shown that mechanical assist devices can gain several months for the patient before transplantation.

VIRAL HEART DISEASE

Etiology and Pathogenesis

The term "myocarditis" is commonly used in conjunction with acute infectious or hypersensitive inflammation of the heart, although the existence of a chronic form of cardiac inflammation has been demonstrated by clinical and experimental data. In most patients myocarditis is considered a benign condition that recovers completely within several weeks. Those patients who suffer from residual myocardial abnormalities and progress to chronic cardiac dysfunction have a poor predictive outcome. The responsible pathogenetic mechanisms involved and the incidence and exact time course are unknown.

Myocarditis can be caused by a multitude of viruses, but in Western countries enteroviral infections, especially coxsackie B_{1-6} serotypes, are the most frequent to attack the heart[8] (Table 29-1). Nevertheless, in an isolated case the diagnosis of viral myocarditis is difficult. A history in this context or a systemic viral infection does not necessarily mean that a particular organ is affected. Ultimately, after excluding blood contamination, the viral origin of myocarditis can be proved only if the virus is detectible within an altered myocardium. One must keep in mind that myocardial failure can be caused by at least two mechanisms: (1) the infected myocardium can be injured by the direct cytotoxic effect of the virus; or (2) secondary immune responses, triggered by a multitude of agents including viruses, may be responsible for the myocardial impairment. In the first case, a viral infection of the heart or its persistence is required for the development of myocarditis, whereas in the second case a direct attack on the heart by a virus (and its detection later at the time of diagnosis) is not necessary.

Viral infections have been suggested to be a possible precursor of myocarditis and dilated cardiomyopathy.[8] On the other hand, they have been controversial for a long time mostly because virologic methods failed to detect the virus in the myocardium. This situation has changed completely since the development of molecular biologic methods as diagnostic tools for heart diseases. With the application of in situ hybridization or the polymerase chain reaction (PCR), persisting viral RNA could be demonstrated

Table 29-2. Persisting Viral mRNA in Endomyocardial Biopsies of Patients with Proved[a]
Myocarditis or Dilated Cardiomyopathy

Subjects	Slot Blot[b] (Archard et al.[12])	In situ[c] (Kandolff et al.[11])	PCR[c] (Koide et al.[d])	PCR[e] (Pauschinger et al.[f])
Myocarditis	23/96 (24%)	28/69 (41%)	5/9 (56%)	23/42 (55%)
Dilated cardiomyopathy	8/47 (17%)	46/130 (35%)	6/24 (25%)	13/21 (62%)
Controls	0/53 (0%)	2/45 (4%)		0/42 (0%)

[a] Histologically and immunohistologically proved.
[b] Clinically suspected.
[c] Histologically diagnosed.
[d] Koide[36]
[e] Immunohistologically diagnosed.
[f] Pauschinger et al.[37]

in the myocardium of patients with clinically suspected myocarditis and chronic heart failure (dilated cardiomyopathy)[9–12] (Table 29-2). Enteroviral mRNA is detected in all tissues of patients with biopsy-proved acute myocarditis, and nearly 60 percent of biopsy specimens from patients with an immunohistologically proved persisting immune process showed viral RNA persistence. mRNA was found in fewer than 30 percent of immunohistologically negative tissues of patients with clinically suspected acute or chronic viral heart disease. Viral persistence was not seen in any of the analyzed control tissues.

These data, demonstrating enteroviral mRNA in the myocardium over months or even years, corroborate the concept of viral persistence. They also suggest that the infection causes the development of myocarditis, which progresses to chronic heart failure in an unknown percentage of patients with clinically suspected dilated cardiomyopathy. A genetic predisposition must be discussed on the basis of clinical and experimental data. At the moment it is still open whether viral persistence, the virus-induced secondary immune process, or both are responsible for the development and progression of the disease (Fig. 29-1). That (auto)immunologic mechanisms are involved in this process can be assumed owing to a number of observations: the association with immunogenetic markers, the development of organ (heart)-specific autoantibodies, humoral and cellular cytotoxic reactions, and biopsy-proved cellular infil-

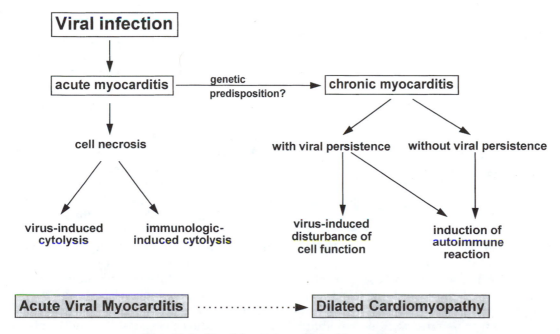

Fig. 29-1. Possible etiology of viral heart disease.

Table 29-3. (Auto)immunologic Mechanisms Involved in the Development and Progression of Viral Heart Disease

Organ-specific autoantibodies
  Sarcolemmal antibodies
    Ca^{2+} channel
    Conexon
    β-Receptor
  Mitochondrial antibodies
    ADP/ATP translocator
    Complex III
  Contractile proteins
    Myosin
Immunoglobulin deposits
Inflammatory cell infiltrates
  Lymphocytes
  Activated macrophages
Expression of histocompatibility antigen classes I and II
Expression of adhesion molecules
Cytotoxic reactions (in vitro)
  Cellular cytotoxicity
  Humoral cytotoxicity
  Complement-dependent cytotoxicity
Reduced natural killer cell activity

trations with enhanced expression of histocompatibility antigens and adhesion molecules[13–16] (Table 29-3).

The often described discrepancy between the histologic findings and clinical symptoms may be due to the localization and severity of the cardiac damage caused by specific pathogens. A focal injury by cellular infiltration or fibrotic replacement of cardiac tissue near the conductive system may cause dramatic clinical consequences by inducing life-threatening brachycardic or tachycardic arrhythmias. A diffuse injury must spread considerably before inducing cardiac enlargement and dysfunction of ventricular contractility.

Clinical Diagnosis

Acute Myocarditis

Except in the early stage, the clinical symptoms of myocarditis vary and bear no relation to the localization and extension of the inflammatory process. After exclusion of other primary heart diseases, the clinical diagnosis is based on the acute onset of chest pain, laboratory changes, conspicious ECG disturbances, arrhythmias, segmental wall motion abnormalities, or pericardial effusions in previously healthy people. In addition, these patients suddenly feel faint and develop reduced working capacity and possibly dyspnea on exertion in association with a recent history of viral infection (within days or weeks).

The ECG commonly shows sinus tachycardia, atrial and ventricular premature complexes, and other arrhythmias of both atrial (supraventricular tachycardia or atrial fibrillation) and ventricular (ventricular tachycardia) origin during ambulatory monitoring. Atrioventricular (AV) conduction disturbances (AV block I–III) and especially abnormalities of ventricular repolarization with deviations (elevation) of the ST segment from the baseline may occur as a result of injury to the conductive system and cardiac muscle. These arrhythmias and ST segment deviations may simulate acute myocardial infarction. Although most of the ECG abnormalities are not specific for myocarditis, fluctuation of ST segments and T waves in conjunction with a specific history of viral infection and corresponding clinical symptoms should direct attention to a possible inflammatory process of the heart.

The mainstay of the echocardiographic diagnosis of acute myocarditis is early detection of segmental wall movement abnormalities, pericardial effusions (perimyocarditis), and occasionally edema of the ventricular walls. Global disturbance of left or right ventricular contractility with AV valve regurgitations due to ventricular enlargement are features of the chronic disease. The importance of echocardiography lies in the rapid, noninvasive exclusion of other specific causes of heart failure (e.g., valvar heart disease, hypertrophic cardiomyopathy).

The chest roentgenogram demonstrates left ventricular enlargement and evidence of pulmonary venous hypertension or congestive heart failure at the end-stage of the disease but normally does not contribute to the diagnosis of the acute disease. The specificity of scintigraphic methods (antimyosin scintigraphy, thallium 201 scintigraphy) must be evaluated for the diagnosis of inflammatory heart disease.

There are no specific laboratory tests for the diagnosis of acute inflammatory heart disease. Common parameters of inflammation are not helpful in most cases because they are influenced by the basic disease. In patients with acute myocarditis with myocytic necrosis, an increase in creatine kinase, its MB isoenzyme, or troponin T levels point to myocytolysis induced by the virus or the virus-triggered secondary immune process. Highest values of enzyme levels are seen on day 2 and normalize after 1 week. Heart autoantibodies are not present during the acute state of the disease but arise in the chronic, immune-mediated processes.

CHRONIC MYOCARDITIS

Although the chronic inflammatory process of the heart does not present with acute laboratory or ECG changes, the clinical presentation does not differ considerably from the acute state of the disease. Symptoms can be moderate. Most patients present with clinical symptoms of advanced left or right ventricular heart failure (or both) in addition to the abovementioned symptoms. Ventricular enlargement and congestive heart failure characterize the progression of the disease. Electrocardiographically, all possible forms of arrhythmias are seen. In addition to cardiac decompensation due to impaired contractility, patients are threatened by bradycardia or, more often, tachycardic arrhythmias (sudden death) and thrombogenic events.

When suggesting the clinical diagnosis of myocarditis one must keep in mind that other heart diseases, especially coronary heart disease and acute myocardial infarction, cause similar clinical symptoms. These life-threatening diseases must be ruled out completely before the diagnosis of viral myocarditis can be taken into consideration. Nevertheless, clinical and laboratory examinations are not specific for cardiac inflammation. This restriction is also true for left heart catheterization, which reveals only secondary causes of myocardial dysfunction. An indubitable diagnosis for specific heart muscle diseases can be obtained only from histologic analysis of cardiac tissue. Myocarditis is a histologic or immunohistologic diagnosis that can be made only by analyzing endomyocardial biopsy specimens. These biopsies should be performed in all cases of unexplained heart failure or life-theatening arrhythmias after excluding other cardiac diseases.

Immunology

During the acute phase of viral invasion and replication, tissue destruction is caused by a direct cytotoxic effect of the responsible virus. The extent of tissue damage and depression of cardiac function at that time depends on the pathogenicity of the infectious agent. This initial phase is followed by a humoral and cellular immune process that might limit further expansion of the destructive process or by itself cause an ongoing injury to the myocardium. The developing immune process is characterized by the appearance of organ-specific autoantibodies, immunoglobulin deposits at the cardiac myocyte cell surface, a humoral or cellular cytotoxic reactivity directed against cardiac myocytes, and cellular infiltration of the myocardium (Table 29-3). The observed picture

of infiltration depends on the pathogenicity of the infectious agent and on the time the specimen is obtained. Immunohistologic analysis of mild cardiac inflammation revealed that activated macrophages might be the first and only indication of the beginning immune process. After a short and variable time lymphocytic infiltrates arise, which in most cases consist of CD4+ helper-inducer cells. A focal infiltration is more commonly seen than a diffuse distribution (Plate 29-1). In rare cases of fulminant myocarditis the diffuse or focal infiltration might involve an enormous percentage of the myocardium (Plate 29-1). The cellular infiltrates of the persistent immune process of chronic myocarditis contain an infiltrate of activated leukocytes, CD4+ and CD8+ lymphocytes, and activated macrophages. The interactions between these immunocompetent cells and the activated vascular endothelium is mandatory for further immune cell activation and infiltration of blood-borne inflammatory cells into inflamed tissues. The enhanced expression of adhesion molecules induced by proinflammatory cytokines, such as interleukin 1α (IL-1α), tumor necrosis factor α (TNFα), and interferon γ (IFNγ), might be a crucial prerequisite for commencement of the immunologic cascade. Cell adhesion molecules provide position-specific information that enables immune cells to selectively adhere and infiltrate impaired tissues.[17–20] Activation of interstitial cells and vascular endothelium is characterized by an enhanced expression of activation markers, histocompatibility antigen classes I and II, and numerous other adhesion molecules (Table 29-4). Additionally, several cytokines, which are responsible for further immune cell activation, leukocyte–endothelial cell interactions, and immune cell recruitment to the areas of inflammation are released from the immunocompetent cells, espe-

---

Table 29-4. Antigens for Immunohistologic Characterization of Inflammatory Cells and Activation State of the Immune Process

Lymphocytes
  CD3: T lymphocytes
  CD4: helper/inducer lymphocytes
  CD8: cytotoxic/suppressor lymphocytes
  CD25: B lymphocytes

Activated cells
  Lymphocytes: CD45-RO, IL-2 receptor, HLA-DR, CD54, CD18, CD7, TIA
  Macrophages: 27E10, HLA-DR, IL-2R
  Inflamed vascular endothelium: HLA-DR, CD54, CD62
  Adhesion molecules: CD18, CD11$_{a-c}$, CD54

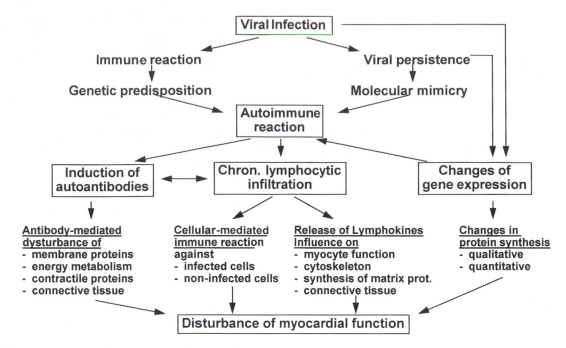

Fig. 29-2. Viral induced immunologic mechanisms causing disturbance of myocardial function.

cially activated macrophages.[21,22] In most patients, virus-induced immunoreactivity leads to a reparative process (fibrosis) in the injured myocardial tissue with disappearance of the described immunologic activity (spontaneous resolution of the inflammatory process). In a limited number of patients, a persisting (auto)immune process develops and may cause progression of the disease (Fig. 29-2).

Histology

Histologic analysis has been considered the gold standard for diagnosing cardiomyopathies. It is certainly true for acute myocarditis, whereas the histologic diagnosis of chronic myocarditis causes difficulties and the results are contradictory.[23,24] According to the Dallas criteria, myocarditis in its acute stage is histologically defined by lymphocytic infiltrates in association with myocytic necrosis.[25] The histologic definition of chronic myocarditis according to the Dallas classification (histologically "borderline and ongoing myocarditis") demands the presence of infiltrating lymphocytes without other histomorphologic signs of myocyte injury or immunohistologic features of a persisting, activated inflammatory process in the first biopsy and the control biopsy. These cellular infiltrates in patients with chronic heart failure, however, are often sparse or focal and therefore might

be missed owing to sampling error (Table 29-5). Moreover, it is difficult to differentiate noninflammatory interstitial cells from infiltrating lymphocytes by light microscopy. This difficulty leads to misinterpretation of interstitial cells as inflammatory lymphocytes and thus to an over- or underestimation of the degree of inflammation. Ultimately, one must keep in mind that infiltrating lymphocytes, especially if not activated, are not necessarily representative of an ongoing immune process that affects the entire myocardium. Those two factors (misinterpretation of interstitial cells and sampling error) are mainly responsible for the low diagnostic yield in the histologic analysis and explain the often reported high interobserver variability.[26,27]

Table 29-5. Problems with Histologic Analysis of Endomyocardial Biopsies

High interobserver variability
    Identification of inflammatory cells
    Differentiation from interstitial cells
    Quantification of lymphocytes
Missing morphologic criteria
Sampling error
    Size of biopsy specimen
    Number of biopsies
    Location of biopsies
Time of biopsy

Immunohistology

Immunohistologic methods have been successfully introduced into the diagnosis of an inflammatory myocardial process.[28-30] In contrast to routine histology, with its difficulty of detecting lymphocytes, cardiac inflammation is immunohistologically characterized by various markers of cell activation and enhanced expression of histocompatibility antigens and adhesion molecules[30,31] (Table 29-4). The sensitivity and specificity of monoclonal antibodies, directed against specific epitopes of immunocompetent cells, allows the unambiguous identification, characterization, and quantification of inflammatory cells infiltrating myocardial tissues. If the number of immunoreactive T lymphocytes is determined by the use of anti-CD2, anti-CD3, anti-CD4, or anti-CD8 antibodies, tissues with a mean number of lymphocytes exceeding 2.0 per high-power field (hpf) (7.0 cells/mm^2) can be considered to have pathologically increased lymphocytic infiltrations because additional markers of immune activation (e.g., enhanced expression of adhesion molecules) are found in more then 90 percent of these cardiac tissues. Control tissues with mean lymphocyte counts of 0.7 ± 0.4 cells/hpf (0-5/mm^2) express these markers in fewer than 30 percent[31] (Table 29-6).

Figures 29-3 and 29-4 compare the results of the histologic and immunohistologic analysis of endomyocardial biopsies from 658 patients with a clinical diagnosis of myocarditis (n = 359) or dilated cardiomyopathy (n = 299). When histologically evaluated, an inflammatory process could be confirmed in only about 3 percent. More reliable results were obtained by immunohistochemical analysis, which showed an activated cardiac inflammation in 327 patients (50 percent) (Figs. 29-3 and 29-4). In the myocarditis group the histologic diagnosis of acute myocarditis was confirmed in 12 patients (3.3 percent). In 24 patients (6.7 percent) the histologic diagnosis was consistent with borderline myocarditis, which does not prove an inflammatory process according to the Dallas classification. Similar results were obtained in the chronic heart failure group, revealing myocarditis in only 1.4 percent and borderline myocarditis in 4.3 percent. Immunohistochemical analysis, however, demonstrated pathologically increased lymphocytic infiltrates and an elevation in expression of histocompatibility antigen classes I or II on interstitial cells or on vascular endothelium in 198 (55 percent) biopsy specimens of patients with clinically suspected myocarditis (Fig. 29-3) and 129 biopsies (45 percent) of patients with suspected dilated cardiomyopathy (Fig. 29-4).

In control tissues and biopsy specimens without lymphocytic infiltrates, only weak immunoreactivity of a few interstitial and endothelial cells is detectable with antibodies to major histocompatibility complex (MHC) class I and II antigens or adhesion molecules of the β1-integrin, immunoglobulin, and selectin families. In biopsy specimens with pathologically increased lymphocytic infiltrates (> 2.0 cells/hpf), however, more than 90 percent of CD3$^+$ samples showed enhanced expression of either class I or II antigens[31] (Table 29-6). Not only the number of stained interstitial cells but also the intensity of staining of each cell in comparison with negative biopsies was increased (Table 29-6). Staining of HLA antigens is also more

Table 29-6. Enhanced HLA and Adhesion Molecule Expression in Immunohistologically Positive and Negative Endomyocardial Biopsies from Patients with Clinically Suspected Myocarditis or Dilated Cardiomyopathy[a]

Antigen	Immunohistologically Positive	Immunohistologically Negative
CD3 (no./hpf)	3.5 ± 2.6	0.7 ± 0.4
HLA-I (%)	52	19
HLA-II (%)	93	26
Integrins (%)	55-89	0-30
Selectins (%)	36-88	<10
Immunoglobulins (%)	36-98	0-30
Lymphokines (%)	10-45	<5

[a] Immunologically positive: more than 2.0 CD3 lymphocytes per high-power field (hpf). Immunologically negative: fewer than 1.5 CD3 lymphocytes per high-power field. A high-power field is ×400.

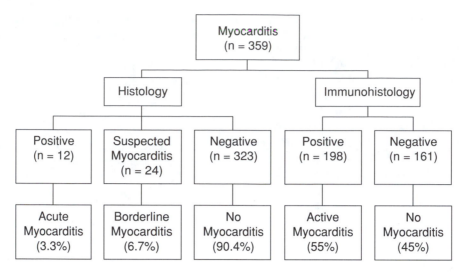

Fig. 29-3. Histologic and immunohistologic analysis of endomyocardial biopsies from patients with clinically suspected myocarditis.

intense on vascular endothelium of immunohistologically positive biopsy specimens. In addition to histocompatibility antigens, cell adhesion molecules are expressed in most of the CD3+ tissues. CD11a/LFA-1, CD11b/Mac-1, CD11c/p150,95 CD49d/VLA-4, and CD29/VLA β-chain of the integrin family can be demonstrated in 55–89 percent. Similarly, members of the immunoglobulin (CD54/ICAM-1, VCAM–1, LFA-3) and selectin (CD26E/ELAM-1, CD62P/GMP140) families are enhanced in 36–98 percent in immunoreactive myocardium. One important feature of the elevated immunoreactivity of the adhesion molecules is that, similar to the MHC antigens, they are up-regulated within the entire biopsy specimen, regardless of the focal or diffuse type of distribution of the lymphocytic infiltration (Plate 29-1). None of the control tissues analyzed showed a significant degree of enhanced expression of these additional immune markers. Activated macrophages were detected in more then 80 percent of CD3+ biopsy specimens (Plate 29-1).

These data confirm impressively that diagnosis of myocarditis can be markedly improved by the use of immunohistologic methods, allowing better characterization of the inflammatory process. A detailed analysis of the various stages of acute and chronic myocarditis allow better understanding of the pathomechanisms involved and improve the management of these patients. Light microscopic analysis of the chronic immune process is hampered by the low sen-

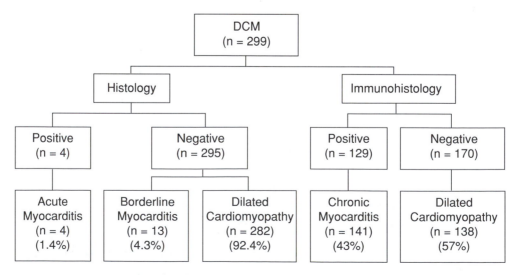

Fig. 29-4. Histologic and immunohistologic analysis of endomyocardial biopsies from patients with clinically suspected dilated cardiomyopathy.

sitivity of histologic staining procedures due to missing specific histologic changes and therefore should not be the only basis of analysis of inflammatory heart disease.

Differential Diagnosis

The combined use of histologic, immunohistologic, and molecular biologic analytic methods allows a detailed differential diagnosis of suspected viral heart disease. As far as acute viral myocarditis is concerned, the Dallas classification has enabled a more standardized assessment of the histologic changes in the myocardium. The clinical benefit, however, is limited by the fact that histologic recording of myocytolysis is possible for only a short time (10–14 days). These specific histologic features are normally no longer present at the time of the biopsy, although most patients present with a typical clinical history of viral myocarditis.

Dilated cardiomyopathy has been regarded the endpoint of various mechanisms that injure the myocardium wherein the harmful agents are unknown. Meanwhile, the combined use of histologic, immunohistologic, and molecular biologic analytic methods allows identification of viral persistence and chronic immunologic processes as a possible cause for heart muscle injury in a considerable number of these patients. Four virus-induced dilated cardiomyopathies can be identified (Fig. 29-5).

1. Postmyocarditic viral heart disease: The clinical presentation is that of dilated cardiomyopathy. Immunohistologically, an inconspicuous endomyocardial biopsy without chronic inflammation is characteristic. Molecular biologic methods do not indicate viral persistence.
2. Chronic viral heart disease: Histologically and immunohistologically, these patients cannot be differentiated from those with postmyocarditic viral heart disease. Viral persistence, however, is diagnosed using in situ hybridization or the polymerase chain reaction.
3. Chronic persistent viral myocarditis: Although histologic findings correspond with those of dilated cardiomyopathy, chronic cardiac inflammation and viral persistence are found by immunohistochemical and molecular biologic analysis.
4. Chronic (auto)immune-mediated myocarditis: Immunohistochemical analysis of endomyocardial biopsy specimens reveal an active inflammatory process within the myocardium in the absence of viral persistence.

The rationale for such an etiologic separation of "dilated cardiomyopathy" into different phases of the disease is a better understanding of the pathomechanism, which might give rise to a more specific treatment strategy. If the developmental process of postmyocarditic heart failure is accelerated by chronic inflammation, viral persistence, or both, the prognosis of patients may depend on whether virus and inflammation persist in the myocardium (Fig. 29-1).

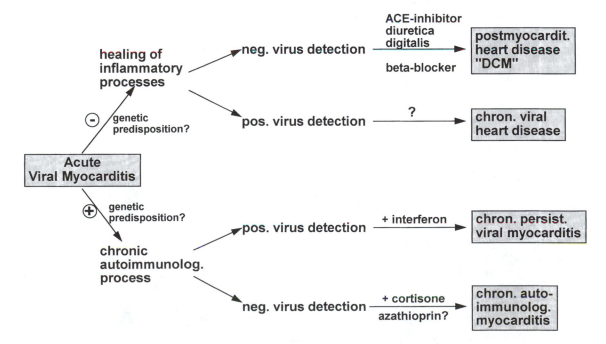

Fig. 29-5. Algorithm showing four types of virus-induced dilated cardiomyopathy.

Differential Therapy

ACUTE MYOCARDITIS

Epidemologic data confirm that in most cases acute viral myocarditis is a benign, self-limiting disease that heals with or without persisting myocardial damage. If myocardial injury causes progressive heart failure, initial therapy follows the above therapeutic guidelines. Progression to pump failure despite bed rest, diuretics, vasodilators, digitalis, and positive inotropic drugs produces an urgent need for an intraaortic ballon pump or finally heart transplantation. Although little is known about the survival rates of these patients, preliminary data point to a worse outcome when compared to other causes of heart transplantation. Stabilization of the hemodynamic situation and a mechanical assist device therefore may help to overcome this critical situation and allow healing of the acute inflammatory process.

The benefit of immunosuppressive treatment is controversial for this acute phase of the disease. Published data including the American Myocarditis Trial[32] were unable to prove any positive or persisting beneficial effects of immunosuppressive therapy. Furthermore, experimental data indicate that immunosuppression causes a fatal outcome if used in animals with acute viral myocarditis presenting with myocyte necrosis because at that phase the replicating virus seems still to be present in the myocardium. The same holds true for nonsteroidal antiinflammatory drugs because the enhanced viral replication and diminished production of interferon caused by these substances result in progression of myocytolysis. The use of other alternative therapeutic agents, such as interferon, monoclonal antibodies, hyperimmune sera, and antiviral drugs, cannot be recommended at this time because of the lack of clinical experience.

CHRONIC MYOCARDITIS

Similar to acute myocarditis, the management of patients with chronic viral heart disease and chronic persistent viral myocarditis is undertaken primarily according to conventional guidelines. Patients with viral persistence may derive benefit from virostatic therapy (e.g., interferon) in future. Clinical studies must first prove such beneficial effects and that the side effects are tolerable before such an therapeutic strategy can be recommended.

In the near future, and in contrast to patients with acute myocarditis, immunosuppression might prove to be an alternative concept of therapy for patients with chronic immune-mediated myocarditis, although published data have questioned this assumption for several reasons. Diagnostic difficulties arising from the clinical or histologic diagnosis used in most of the treatment studies were discussed earlier in the chapter. Moreover, in most of published studies the natural course has not been taken into consideration. At present there is no possibility of estimating whether the immunologically active process will resolve or progress with time; and the resolving myocarditis therefore may be mistaken for positive therapeutic effects, as seen in the American Myocarditis Trial. In that case there was an increase in ventricular contractility due to spontaneous resolution of the inflammatory process, which is often seen during this acute state of the disease and cannot be discriminated from a positive effect of treatment.

A positive response to antiinflammatory treatment is to be expected if an active myocardial inflammation is present at the time of therapy inception. Preliminary results from immunohistologically characterized patients under therapy have shown 83 percent resolution of cardiac inflammation, with a significant reduction in lymphocytic infiltration in parallel with a significant increase in the ejection fraction or stroke volume and a significant decrease in the left ventricular end-diastolic pressure.[33] These data suggest that patients with chronic myocarditis or dilated cardiomyopathy benefit from immunosuppressive therapy if only patients with an immunohistologically defined active inflammatory process are treated. These data can be taken as an indication that, on one hand, a persistent inflammatory process contributes at least in part to the pathogenesis of dilated cardiomyopathy. On the other hand, new diagnostic methods allow selection of patients who can obviously benefit from specific immunosuppression. One must keep in mind, however, that these data are preliminary results from a pilot study, and immunosuppressive therapy cannot be recommended until randomized data have proved its beneficial effects and its safety without doubt.

RHEUMATIC CARDITIS

Most patients who develop carditis do so within the first week(s) of the disease. In most cases patients present with no cardiac symptoms. Heart murmurs due to mitral or aortic regurgitations, congestive heart failure, signs and symptoms of pericarditis, tachycardia, and ECG abnormalities such as ST segment deviations or AV conduction disturbances are seen in severe cases. As a result of rheumatic fever caused by pharyngeal infection due to group A streptococci, all layers of the heart—endocardium, myocardium, pericardium—may be involved.

Neither bacteria nor toxins have been demonstrated in cardiac lesions. Cross-reacting antibodies lead us to expect that autoimmunologic mechanisms may be involved, but this question has not been settled. A family history of rheumatic fever and a concordance of 20 percent in identical twins suggest a genetic predisposition and underline the possible importance of heritable factors for pathogenesis. Endomyocardial biopsy allows a histologic diagnosis when identifying rheumatic granulomas (Aschoff bodies), often accompanied by fibrinoid degeneration of collagen, a characteristic and specific pattern of rheumatic inflammation.

The course of the disease depends on the localization (valves, myocardium) and the severity of the inflammatory process. Chronic heart failure with a markedly dilated heart in most cases cannot be differentiated from other forms of chronic myocarditis when the associated extracardiac features of rheumatic fever are not present. Although most patients recover partially, a few cases of rheumatic carditis are intractable and end fatally after months or even years.

Patients with carditis are treated with glucocorticoids (1 mg/kg bodyweight). Therapy is maintained 2–3 weeks after normalization of the erythrocyte sedimentation rate or of C-reactive protein to prevent a rebound of rheumatic activity. While being tapered off, therapy may be continued with salicylate for additional 2–3 weeks.

COLLAGEN DISEASES

Myocarditis may be present in association with rheumatoid arthritis, but pericarditis is the most common cause, found in about 40 percent of patients with clinically apparent disease. Coronary arteritis with intimal inflammation is involved in about 20 percent and only rarely results in angina pectoris or myocardial infarction.

Cardiac manifestations are found in 55–60 percent of patients with systemic lupus erythematosus (SLE). Pericarditis is the most common cause (80 percent) of clinically apparent SLE. Ventricular enlargement and left or right (10 percent) ventricular heart failure may be present with SLE. Myocarditis, though commonly seen with SLE, in most cases does not result in clinical heart failure. Although coronary arteritis within the scope of a general vasculitis is a common finding in patients with SLE, periarteritis nodosa (cardiac involvement in 55–60 percent) is characterized by a prevailing attack of the coronary arteries and may lead to extensive but scattered myocardial necrosis.

Small vessels are affected in patients suffering from Wegener's granulomatosis and vasculitis due to hypersensitivity. Similarly, a predominant attack of small vessels is seen with scleroderma.

Coronary arteritis or, more generally, vasculitides can be grouped in several categories. One group, encompassing polyarteritis nodosa, allergic angiitis and granulomatosis, and hypersensitivity vasculitis, is characterized by circulating immune complexes that are deposited at the vessel walls, causing vessel necrosis and a pleomorphic cell infiltrate with predominance of polymorphonuclear cells or eosinophils. The permeability of the endothelial layer is thereby increased followed by secretion of various mediators (e.g., histamine, serotonin, or IL-1). Released mediators cause activation of neutrophils, which bind to complement-loaded endothelial cells and destroy the surrounding tissue by releasing lysosomal enzymes (e.g., elastase or collagenases). Free oxygen radicals, released especially from monocytes and neutrophils, further enhance injury of the vascular endothelium and support activation of the inflammatory process. Another vasculitis group comprises a cell-mediated mechanism with typical formation of round cell granulomas (e.g., Wegener's granulomatosis, lymphomatoid granulomatosis, and giant cell arteritis).

Vascular alterations caused by immune processes are an important cause of vasculitis and indirect myocytic injury. Production of proinflammatory cytokines, such as IFNγ, TNFα, and IL-1, increases the expression of histocompatibility antigens I and II or of adhesion molecules (ICAM-1, selectins) on the surface of endothelial cells, interacting with their counterreceptors (LFA-1 or α_1/β_2-integrins) on the surface of circulating monocytes and neutrophils. This interaction promotes further activation and adherence of inflammatory cells to the endothelium, followed by transmigration. Endothelial cell injury due to inflamed cells or locally secreted cytokines results in an inflammatory endothelium with leakage of macromolecules into the interstitium, causing interstitial edema and local tissue inflammation. Cytokine-induced endothelial cell injury is thus responsible for further recruitment of inflammatory cells (neutrophils, lymphocytes, macrophages) at the site of inflammation and may be involved in the progression of vasculitis. Histologic analysis reveals perivascular infiltration, progressive interstitial and perivascular fibrosis, and myocardial scars. Activated vascular endothelium is characterized by enhanced expression of histocompatibility antigen classes I or II and other adhesion molecules immunohistologically.

The clinical symptom of vasculitis is angina pectoris, caused by reduced oxygen delivery to the myocardium. Because of the preferential involvement of small vessels, however, coronary angiography is unhelpful despite typical symptoms except in cases of panarteritis nodosa or allergic angiitis and granulomatosis, where characteristic multiple aneurysms and irregular vessel narrowing are recognized angiographically. Angiography is diagnostic in approximately 80 percent of these cases, but negative results do not exclude the diagnosis. Involvement of small coronary vessels is confirmed by analyzing the coronary reserve, which is significantly reduced in patients with cardiac involvement associated with their collagen disease. Treatment involves symptomatic use of vasodilators in addition to following the general guidelines for the various collagen diseases.

SARCOIDOSIS

Sarcoidosis is a multisystem granulomatous disorder of uncertain etiology in which cardiac involvement has been demonstrated in 13–27 percent of autopsy series; it may also be the major cause of giant cell myocarditis.[34] Common sites of sarcoid granulomas or scars are found in the left ventricular free wall, ventricular septum, and papillary muscle. Scarring or thinning of the ventricular wall may produce cardiac aneurysms. Most frequent functional consequences of these lesions are severe arrhythmias (ventricular tachycardia, complete heart block, or syncope is seen in 20–25 percent of cases) or ventricular enlargement with severely impaired contractility (congestive heart failure 30–40 percent). In one series of 108 patients death was sudden, due to arrhythmias in 67 percent, secondary to progressive heart failure in 23 percent, and due to other or unknown causes in 10 percent.[35] Because of its ability to cause arrhythmias, conduction disturbances, huge cardiac silhouettes, ECG disorders, or chest pain, cardiac sarcoidosis may mimic other cardiac conditions (e.g., acute myocardial infarction or dilated cardiomyopathy). Sarcoid granulomas in the heart respond much better to corticosteroid therapy than sarcoid granulomas located in other organs. Diminution in the frequency of arrhythmias, conduction disturbances, and ECG abnormalities have been reported.[35] Corticoid therapy is given in high doses over a long time.

ALLERGIC MYOCARDITIS

Allergic-toxic cardiomyopathies are most commonly caused by drugs (e.g., methyldopa, D-penicillamine, sulfonamides, phencyclidine, barbiturates, cocaine, tuberculostatic agents, and alcohol). These drugs produce focal or generalized damage to heart muscle.

Histologically, myocytic necrosis is associated with an eosinophilic inflammation. The important clinical symptoms are all forms of arrhythmias and, in rare cases, heart failure. Elimination of the responsible toxin supported by glucocorticoids in high doses is necessary for successful treatment.

PERIPARTUM CARDIOMYOPATHY

Peripartum cardiomyopathy is characterized by unexplained ventricular enlargement and progressive clinical heart failure during the third trimester of pregnancy or the first 6 months after delivery in women previously healthy. It appears to be more common in African women and African Americans than in white women. Several factors, including hypertension or malnutrition, have been implicated as possible causes of peripartum cardiomyopathy. The pathogenesis has not been established.

Hemodynamics differ considerably during pregnancy when compared with healthy, non pregnant individuals. The blood volume increases 50 percent from week 20 to week 30. This change is accompanied by an increased circulation rate and stroke volume, which again normalize at about 6 weeks after delivery. Systolic blood pressure and heart rate increase, and the diastolic blood pressure decreases. Stress induces a further increase in the circulation rate combined with a diminution of the heart rate. These hemodynamic effects might be caused by disturbance of left ventricular function during pregnancy, predisposing eventually, to viral myocarditis. There is, however, only circumstantial evidence that pregnancy and the postpartum state predispose to viral involvement of the heart.

Histologic data have demonstrated inflammation in endomyocardial biopsies of 14 of 18 patients (78 percent). Histologic features of healing/resolved myocarditis are the most common finding on endomyocardial biopsy. These data suggest that immunologic mechanisms contribute to the pathogenesis of the disease. Spontaneous improvement is seen in only 50 percent of cases over a 6-month period. Mortality has been reported to be as high as 50 percent. Most patients, however, clinically respond to immunosuppressive treatment with glucocorticoids and azathioprine.

ALCOHOL-TOXIC CARDIOMYOPATHY

Cardiac contractility and the ejection fraction are reduced by even moderate doses of ethanol. The severity of left ventricular dysfunction is concentration-dependent. Reversible impairment of cardiac function is caused by extensive consumption of alcohol.

Clinically the patient presents with ventricular enlargement similar to that of dilated cardiomyopathy. Histologically, the toxic effect of alcohol is characterized by reduced activity of various enzymes, swelling of mitochondria or the tubular system, myocytic hypertrophy, fragmentation of myofibrils, and interstitial and perivascular fibrosis of the subendocardial layers. All these processes interfere with energy delivery and the contractility of the heart. Chronic alcoholism predisposes to viral infections and the presence of chronic inflammatory infiltrates, and it argues for an immunologic contribution to the pathogenesis and progression of alcohol-toxic cardiomyopathy. The disease, to some extent, resembles virus-induced chronic heart failure.

AMYLOID DISEASE

Perivascular amyloid deposition around the small blood vessels produces a stiff, unyielding myocardium. Although resembling constrictive cardiomyopathy to some extent, the disease has certain specific features. Left ventricular filling is slow throughout diastole, in contrast to the initial rapid and later slow filling found with endomyocardial fibrosis. The absence of the left ventricular third sound is another characteristic of amyloid disease when compared with constrictive pericarditis or restrictive cardiomyopathy.

REFERENCES

1. Report of the 1995 World Health Organization/International Society and Federation of Cardiology Task Force on the definition and classification of cardiomyopathies. Circulation 1996;93:841–842
2. Schulze K, Becker BF, Schauer R, Schultheiss HP: Antibodies to the ADP/ATP carrier—an autoantigen in myocarditis and dilated cardiomyopathy—impair cardiac function. Circulation 1990;81:959–969
3. Schulze K, Becker BF, Schultheiss HP: Antibodies to the ADP/ATP carrier, an autoantigen in myocarditis and dilated cardiomyopathy, penetrate into myocardial cells and disturb energy metabolism in vivo. Circ Res 1989;64:179–192
4. Kjekshus J, Swedberg K, Snapinn S: Effects of enalapril on long-term mortality in severe congestive heart failure. Am J Cardiol 1992;69:103–107
5. Anonymous: Effect of enalapril on survival in patients with reduced left ventricular ejection fraction and congestive heart failure. N Engl J Med 1991;325:293–302
6. Packer M, Gheorgghiade M, Young Jb et al: Withdrawal of digitoxin from patients with chronic heart failure treated with angiotensin-converting-enzyme inhibitors. N Engl J Med 1993;329:1–7
7. Waagstein F, Bristow MR, Swedberg K et al: Beneficial effects of metoprolol in idiopathic dilated cardiomyopathy. Lancet 1993;342:1441–1446
8. Editorials: Dilated cardiomyopathy and enteroviruses. Lancet 1990;336:971–973
9. Bowles NE, Ohlsen EGJ, Richardson PJ, Archard LC: Detection of coxsackie B-virus-specific RNA sequences in myocardial biopsy samples from patients with myocarditis and dilated cardiomyopathy. Lancet 1986;1:1120–1122
10. Grasso M, Arbusti E, Silini E et al: Search for coxsackie B3 RNA in idiopathic dilated cardiomyopathy using gene amplification by polymerase chain reaction. Am J Cardiol 1992;69:658–664
11. Kandolf R, Ameis D, Kirschner P, Canu A, Hofschneider PIH: In situ detection of enteroviral genomes in myocardial cells by nucleic acid hybridization. An approach to the diagnosis of viral heart disease. Proc Natl Acad Sci USA 1985;82:4818–4822
12. Archard LC, Bowles NE, Cunningham L et al: Molecular probes for detection of persisting enterovirus infection of human heart and their prognostic value. Eur Heart J, suppl. D 1991;12:56–59
13. Neu N, Beisel KW, Traysman MD, Rose NR, Craig SW: Autoantibodies specific for cardiac myosin isoform are found in mice susceptible to coxsackie B3-induced myocarditis. J Immunol 1987;138:2488–2492
14. Limas CJ, Goldenberg JF, Limas C: Autoantibodies angainst β-adrenoceptors in human idiopathic dilated cardiomyopathy. Circ Res 1989;64:97–103
15. Schultheiss HP, Ulrich G, Janda I, Kühl U, Morad M: Antibody-mediated enhancement of calcium permeability in cardiac myocytes. J Exp Med 1988;168:2105–2119
16. Wolff P, Kühl U, Schultheiss HP: Laminin distribution and autoantibodies to laminin in dilated cardiomyopathy and myocarditis. Am Heart J 1989;117:1303–1309
17. Dustin ML, Rothlein R, Bhan AK, Dinarello CA, Springer TA: Induction by IL-1 and interferon-gamma. Tissue distribution, biochemistry and function of a natural adherence molecule (ICAM-1). J Immunol 1986;137:245–254
18. Springer TA: Adhesion receptors of the immune system. Review article. Nature 1990;346:425–434
19. Yong K, Khwaja A: Leukocyte cellular adhesion molecules. Blood Rev 1990;4:211–225
20. Mally M, Schaude M: Adhesion molecules are responsible for the communication of cells. Lab Med 1991;15:391–398
21. Satoh M, Tamura G, Segawa I, et al: Expression of cytokine genes and presence of enteroviral genomic RNA in endomyocardial boipsy tissues an myocarditis and dilated cardiomyopathy Virchows Arch 1996;427:503–509
22. Neumann DA, Lane JR, Allen GS, Herskowitz A, Rose NR: Viral myocarditis leading to cardiomyopathy. Do cytokines contribute to pathogenesis? Clin Immunopathol 1993;68:181–190
23. Billingham MB: Acute myocarditis. A diagnostic dilemma. Br Heart J 1987;58:6–8
24. Ohlsen EGJ. The problem of viral heart disease. How often do we miss it? Postgrad Med J 1985;61:479–480
25. Aretz HT: Myocarditis, the Dallas criteria. Hum Pathol 1987;18:619–624
26. Shanes JG, Ghali J, Billingham ME et al: Interobserver variability in the pathologic interpretation of endomyocardial biopsy results. Circulation 1987;75:401–405
27. Hauck AJ, Kearney DL, Edwards WD: Evaluation of

postmortem endomyocardial biopsy specimen from 38 patients with lymphocytic myocarditis. Implication for role of sampling error. Mayo Clin Proc 1989;64: 1235–1245

28. Zee-Cheng CS, Tsai CC, Palmer DC et al: High incidence of myocarditis by endomyocardial biopsy in patients with idiopathic congestive cardiomyopathy. J Am Coll Cardiol 1984;3:63–70

29. Steenbergen C, Kolbeck PC, Wolfe JA et al: Detection of lymphocytes in endomyocardium using immunohistochemical techniques. Relevance to evaluation of endomyocardial biopsies in suspected cases of lymphocytic myocarditis. J Appl Cardiol 1986;1:63–73

30. Kühl U, Noutsias M, Seeberg B et al: Chronic inflammation in the myocardium of patients with clinically suspected dilated cardiomyopathy. J Card Failure 1994;1:13–27

31. Kühl U, Seeberg B, Noutsias M, Schultheiss HP: Immunohistochemical analysis of the chronic inflammatory process in dilated cardiomyopathy: Br Heart J 1995;75:295–300

32. Mason JW, O'Connel JB, Herskowitz A et al: A clinical trial of immunosuppressive therapy for myocarditis. N Engl J Med 1994;321:1061–1068

33. Schultheiss HP, Kühl U, Janda I, Schanwell M, Strauer BB: Immunosuppressive Therapie der Myokarditis. Herz 1992;17:112–121

34. Silvermann KJ, Hutchin GM, Bulkley BH: Cardiac sarcoidosis. A clinicopathologic study of 84 unselected patients with systemic sarcoidosis. Circulation 1978; 58:1204–1211

35. Roberts WC, McAllister HA Jr, Ferrans VJ: Sarcoidosis of the heart. Am J Med 1977;63:86–108

36. Koide H, Kitaura Y, Deguchi H et al: Genomic detection of enteroviruses in the myocardium—studies on animal hearts with Coxsackievirus B3 myocarditis and endomyocardial biopsies from patients with myocarditis and dilated cardiomyopathy. Jpn Circ J 1992; 56:1081–1093

37. Pauschinger M, Preis S, Triesch A, et al: Detection of enteroviral by polymerase chain reaction (PCR) in patients with myocarditis (MC) and dilated cardiomyopathy. Circulation 1994;90:1174

30 Prognostic Factors

Denise D. Hermann
Barry H. Greenberg

The syndrome of heart failure encompasses a multitude of underlying pathologic diagnoses and co-morbidities, as the clinical definition of this common condition does not bespeak etiology. Heart failure is one of the only cardiovascular disorders whose incidence and prevalence are increasing worldwide. The epidemiologic factors related to the development of heart failure are elucidated in detail in earlier sections of this book. In the United States alone the mortality from congestive heart failure increased over the decade between 1980 and 1990 despite considerable advances in medical therapy.[1-3] This trend is attributable in part to the aging of the population and to the success of treatments for hypertension, coronary artery disease, acute myocardial infarction, and valvar heart disease. The most common reason for the development of heart failure in the United States today is ischemic heart disease.[1] Up to 70 percent of the patients included in the large heart failure trials of the late 1980s and early 1990s had systolic dysfunction related to chronic ischemic heart disease. The same increase in the incidence and prevalence of heart failure has been observed in other industrialized areas, such as the Scandinavian countries and Japan, although the relative proportion of etiologic subsets vary.[4-6]

Mortality data from the placebo and treatment groups in the major heart failure trials of the 1980s, such as CONSENSUS, SOLVD, and SAVE, clearly show that the risk of death from heart failure is significantly reduced with angiotensin-converting enzyme (ACE) inhibitor therapy but remains unacceptably high.[3,7-9] In 1995 the overall mortality risk associated with optimally treated heart failure was around 10 percent annually, with a 5-year survival of 50 percent. Interestingly, data from the Framingham study suggest that there has been no significant change in the 5-year survival rate over the past 40 years despite considerable advances in the identification and treatment of ischemic heart disease and hypertension over that period.[10,11] Therefore risk stratification enabling the identification of high risk subsets of patients who might derive a survival benefit from more aggressive medical or surgical therapy, investigational medications, assist devices, or transplantation becomes paramount for improving the prognosis of heart failure. Furthermore, because heart failure has become such a common entity, performing a routine assessment and periodic review of prognostic indicators reinforces the potential lethality of this condition to the patient and practitioner alike. (Table 30-1). This chapter reviews the prognosis of subsets of patients with heart failure based on the underlying etiologic mechanism and acuity, patient demographic factors, and co-morbidities; it also provides an overview for the chapters that follow on evaluative testing to delineate prognostic markers.

Table 30-1. Risk Stratification in Chronic Heart Failure—Variables Influencing Prognosis

Etiology of Heart Failure
Ventricular Dysfunction—Systolic and/or diastolic
Coronary artery disease vs idiopathic dilated cardiomyopathy
Valvular Heart Disease
Unique Etiologies
Myocarditis—Infectious, autoimmune, giant cell
Hypertrophic cardiomyopathy
Toxin-related cardiomyopathy, e.g., alcohol, anthracyclines
Infiltrative diseases, e.g., amyloid, hemachromatosis
Patient Demographics and Co-morbidities
Race
Gender
Age
Co-morbidities: Diabetes, systemic or pulmonary hypertension, sleep apnea, renal, or hepatic dysfunction
Easily Measured Variables
Symptoms—NYHA class, specific activity scale
Ejection fraction—Left and right ventricle
Exercise capacity—$\dot{V}O_2$ max, 6 minute walk distance
Hemodynamics
Serum sodium
Thyroid function
Arrhythmias/ECG antiarrhythmic therapy
Doppler echo–mitral inflow pattern
LV size, volumes, shape, and mass
Research Parameters
Neurohormones–plasma norepinephrine, renin activity, aldosterone, atrial natriuretic factor
Markers of autonomic dysfunction—heart rate variability
Signal-averaged ECG
Endomyocardial biopsy

PROGNOSIS RELATED TO MECHANISM AND ACUITY OF HEART FAILURE

Systolic Ventricular Dysfunction

New-onset acute congestive heart failure due to systolic ventricular dysfunction is classically observed in the setting of a large first myocardial infarction. Even in the apparently uncomplicated patient, mortality risk from myocardial infarction directly correlates with pump function: hemodynamic parameters and cardiac output.[12] As demonstrated by Forrester et al., increased ventricular filling pressures and reduced cardiac output add to the mortality risk of acute infarction.[13] A Swedish study conducted during the late 1980s found heart failure present in 51 percent of 921 patients presenting with an acute myocardial infarction (MI). Mortality at 1 year (including in-hospital deaths) was 24 percent versus 9 percent for patients with and without heart failure, respectively; and it was nearly 50 percent among those with severe heart failure.[14] Excluding patients who die of cardiogenic shock as a complication of acute infarction, an ejection fraction below 40 percent at hospital discharge is a powerful predictor of subsequent mortality, even during this thrombolytic era. An ejection fraction of 30 percent at hospital discharge post-MI carries an approximate 15 percent mortality risk at 1 year.[15] Infarct expansion and ventricular remodeling produce further pressure and volume overload stimuli over the weeks to months following an infarction, leading to late heart failure development or worsening, which in turn adversely affects prognosis.[16,17]

In patients with chronic systolic ventricular dysfunction, the ejection fraction is a powerful prognostic indicator. The mortality risk related to a depressed ejection fraction is substantially increased for each increment of the fraction under 30 percent.[18] Yet even among the population with systolic dysfunction, differences during the clinical course and, perhaps even more importantly, in the response to various therapies are present. Patients with idiopathic dilated cardiomyopathy (IDC) may have a somewhat lower total mortality risk yet higher proportionate risk of sudden death than patients with a similar degree of ventricular dysfunction due to ischemic heart disease (IHD). Although this trend was not demonstrated in the prospective randomized V-HeFT trials,[19] patients with heart failure due to IHD have the worst 5-year survival in Japan (35 percent versus 40 percent for IDC).[6] Moreover, the differential treatment benefit seen in the patient cohorts with IDC in the GESICA (amiodarone), PRAISE (amlodipine), and CIBIS (bisoprolol) trials indicates that the pathophysiologic mechanism may vary depending on etiology, and that these differences may determine the clinical course and the response to treatment.[20–22]

Diastolic Ventricular Dysfunction

Acute heart failure symptoms deriving from predominantly diastolic dysfunction may manifest as flash pulmonary edema, as observed in the setting of acute myocardial ischemia and infarction. More commonly, patients present with the signs and symptoms of heart failure attributed to systolic dysfunction. The key to differentiating between systolic and diastolic dysfunction is preservation of the ejection fraction and the relatively normal heart size in the latter patients. Prognosis in this scenario is determined primarily by the provocative factor (i.e., multivessel coronary artery disease, hypertensive crisis, tachyarrhythmia, or changes in the diastolic properties of the heart).

Diastolic dysfunction producing chronic heart failure symptoms is commonly found in clinical referral practices and can be refractory to treatment. The influence of isolated diastolic heart failure on survival has not been well studied in prospective, controlled clinical trials but is generally thought to be superior to that due to systolic impairment. For example, V-HeFT investigators screened a cohort of patients with clinical heart failure who had an ejection fraction above 45 percent and found only 8 percent annual mortality.[23] More than half of the patients had heart failure related to underlying hypertension. Mortality risk could still be predicted by the exercise VO_2 response, however. Similarly, the 5-year survival after heart failure related to hypertension alone was 80 percent in Japan.[6] However, Setaro reported a 7-year 46 percent mortality and 75 percent combined severe cardiovascular morbidity and mortality for patients with New York Heart Association (NYHA) class III and IV heart failure symptoms yet preserved systolic function.[24] Survival of those with chronic diastolic heart failure may relate more closely to the nature and reversibility of factors inducing the diastolic functional abnormalities. Reduced ventricular chamber compliance and delayed myocardial relaxation each produce an abnormal ventricular diastolic pressure–volume relation and the clinical symptoms of heart failure. Ischemia, hypertension, afterload mismatch, and ventricular hypertrophy are potentially treatable or reversible conditions, whereas the myofibrillar disarray seen with hypertrophic cardiomyopathy and fiber loss with senescence is not. Furthermore, patients with restrictive physiology due to storage, infiltrative, or granulomatous disease, irradiation, or of idiopathic etiology, who typically present with heart failure due to diastolic dysfunction with a normal cardiac output and ejection fraction, can develop ventricular thinning, dilation, and severe systolic functional abnormalities over time. When this situation occurs, the clinical course and prognosis may be worse than that seen in patients with systolic dysfunction alone. In patients with hypertrophic cardiomyopathy in Japan, an increase in the left ventricular systolic dimension/wall thickness ratio was a strong marker for mortality.[25]

Diastolic abnormalities are common with end-stage systolic heart failure; and when severe diastolic and systolic dysfunction coexist, the negative impact on survival is significantly increased.[26,27] For example, when restrictive physiology develops in the setting of chronic systolic heart failure due to extreme ventricular dilatation, pericardial constraint, or intrinsic myocardial lusitropic impairment, the mortality risk is clearly increased.[26–29]

Valvular Heart Disease

After the development of congestive heart failure, the average survival of patients with unoperated critical aortic stenosis is 1.5 years.[30,31] A significant degree of left ventricular dysfunction and hypertrophy related to this pressure overload state may be reversible after aortic valve replacement, although the operative mortality risk increases greatly when there is severe left ventricular dysfunction and reduced cardiac output.[32] Despite normal left ventricular function, severe heart failure symptoms related to hemodynamically critical mitral stenosis protends a 15 percent 5-year survival without surgical intervention, reflecting the mortality associated with severe pulmonary hypertension.[33] The rate of disease development and symptom progression associated with aortic or mitral stenosis varies primarily with the presence or absence of concomitant coronary artery disease and patient demographics.

In contrast, the volume-overloaded ventricle resulting from severe chronic aortic or mitral valve regurgitation has a more finite period for success of operative intervention. Survival with or without valve replacement surgery correlates closely with both the degree of ventricular dilatation and the amount of systolic dysfunction present.[34,35] Although a long latent period exists before symptom development in chronic aortic regurgitation, valve replacement may not improve symptoms or survival after the onset of severe ventricular dysfunction with dilatation and heart failure.[34] However, with earlier, more aggressive use of vasodilator drugs for chronic aortic insufficiency, the clinical course can be altered dramatically.[35,36] Although the natural history of chronic mitral regurgitation is highly variable and etiology-dependent (rheumatic, infectious, or coronary disease), medical treatment results in an approximate 45 percent 5-year survival for the most symptomatic patients.[37]

Unique Etiologies of Heart Failure with Variable Prognoses

The following discussion of survival related to heart failure due to etiologic factors less common than IHD or IDC is limited to diagnoses with unique features or prognostic subsets, as well as those for which controversial therapies exist.

MYOCARDITIS

Grogan and colleagues at the Mayo Clinic confirmed that biopsy-proved lymphocytic myocarditis is uncommon in a referral population, with the Dallas criteria being clearly met in only 28 of 850 biopsies. They found no survival difference in those with acute myocarditis when compared to a cohort of patients with IDC.[38] The 5-year survival rate for each group was approximately 55 percent. However, the median interval from the onset of symptoms to diagnosis was 3.5 months for the patients diagnosed with myocarditis, which likely includes a preponderance of patients with chronic or recrudescent lymphocytic myocarditis and excludes patients with acute, fulminant myocarditis. An additional report from the Massachusetts General Hospital found 18 of 300 (6 percent) of patients referred for evaluation within 6 months of acute-onset dilated cardiomyopathy became asymptomatic with improvement of the ejection fraction to more than 50 percent over a short follow-up period.[39] Symptomatic and resting systolic functional recovery was predicted by the presence of necrosis on biopsy or antimyosin binding on scintigraphy. Significant functional abnormalities were still demonstrable with exercise in these patients, including systolic and diastolic ventricular parameters and reduced aerobic capacity.

Numerous anecdotal reports and small case series suggest that patients with acute, fulminant viral or autoimmune myocarditis may benefit from early steroid or immunosuppressive therapy. Animal studies, typically murine models, have provided conflicting data as to whether the infectious agent or the host immune response causes most of the myocardial cytopathic injury and may not be applicable to humans. Despite the negative results reported in the long-awaited Myocarditis Treatment Trial, this subject remains controversial. Patients with unexplained heart failure were eligible for this National Institutes of Health (NIH)-sponsored, carefully conducted yet referral-dependent trial and were included only if endomyocardial biopsy revealed myocarditis.[40] Recruitment was slow owing to a low disease incidence or a lack of referrals. Subset analysis of patients with acute-onset, fulminant myocarditis was lacking.

Infectious myocarditis of nonviral etiology is rare in immunocompetent adults. An exception may be Chagasic myocarditis in endemic areas of South America, where approximately 10 percent of these patient die during the acute phase. The chronic phase of trypanosomal infection can produce a dilated cardiomyopathy after a latent period of one to two decades, but the proportion of persons developing symptomatic heart failure is fortunately small.[41]

Autopsy series of persons dying from complications of acquired immune deficiency syndrome (AIDS)-related illnesses demonstrate histologic evidence of myocarditis in close to 50 percent of patients; one large series described symptomatic heart failure symptoms preceding death in approximately half of those patients with myocardial involvement.[42] These patients tend to respond as expected to medical heart failure therapy. Treatment with zidovudine (AZT) appears to have little influence on the development or course of cardiac dysfunction. Deaths due to heart failure represent only a small fraction of total deaths due to AIDS, however.

Peripartum cardiomyopathy is presumed to be an autoimmune type of myocarditis and appears to have at least four unique prognostic subsets. Up to half of affected patients demonstrate complete spontaneous recovery within a short time frame (months) and one-third within weeks. For those who do not improve rapidly and have myocarditis documented by biopsy, immunosuppressive therapy appears to significantly improve ventricular function and survival.[43] Patients without early improvement or who have negative biopsies are equally likely to improve or worsen and may require consideration of transplantation.[44] The fourth subset appears to develop a chronic low grade inflammatory myocarditis, and their disease behaves more like IDC in its natural history.

Giant cell myocarditis, of unknown etiology and at the extreme of this spectrum, is uniformly fatal and fortunately rare. Biopsy is the only diagnostic method available. Transplantation seems to be the only viable option.[45]

HYPERTROPHIC CARDIOMYOPATHY

Sudden cardiac death is a well recognized risk in patients with hypertrophic cardiomyopathy, with or without the presence of outflow tract obstruction. Studies from the 1960s estimated this risk at 2–3 percent per year, with higher rates in children and adults to age 35. Maron and Fananapazir reported that the risk of sudden death in patients with hypertrophic cardiomyopathy who have nonsustained ventricular tachycardia on Holter monitoring was nearly 9 percent compared to 1 percent among patients without this finding.[46] Heart failure symptoms were absent or mild in 85 percent of the patients with HCM and sudden death. Also reported by Spirito and Maron, the risk for ventricular tachycardia and sudden death increases directly with the degree of ventricular hypertrophy, even in asymptomatic or mildly symptomatic patients.[47] Most CHF symptoms are attributable to diastolic dysfunction, though certain patients develop systolic dysfunction or ventricular dilation (or both) during later stages. A family history of HCM and sudden death is a marker for poor survival, which correlates with data suggesting that determination of genotype is predictive of patients at higher risk for sudden death.[48] The impact of implantable antitachycardia and defibrillating devices on the natural history of the disease is not yet known.

The hypertensive hypertrophic cardiomyopathy of the elderly, as described by Topol and colleagues, appears to benefit symptomatically more from β-blockers or calcium-channel blockers than from vasodilators.[49] The influence of medical therapy on the natural history of this patient subset has not been studied.

TOXIN-RELATED CARDIOMYOPATHY

Congestive cardiomyopathy due to alcoholism is usually attributed to persons ingesting alcohol on a near-daily basis over a period of years. Despite described benefits on the lipid profile, alcohol ingestion may contribute to or worsen impaired ventricular function from any other cause. It has been estimated that alcohol can be identified as a cardiotoxic risk factor in 20–30 percent of patients with IDC.[50] There may be an undefined genetic predisposition to the development of cardiomyopathy, as (1) women appear to be less susceptible than men and (2) afflicted persons are unlikely to develop cirrhosis. Because the histologic lesion is nonspecific cardiac fibrosis and myocytolysis, the response to medical therapy and prognosis is generally assumed to be similar to that of IDC. Acute cardiotoxicity related to mitochondrial enzyme alterations may be partially or completely reversible with abstinence, though progression of heart failure has been noted to occur despite abstinence. One study of 64 patients with significant ventricular dysfunction attributed to alcohol noted a 9 percent 4-year mortality rate in a subgroup of patients who abstained after diagnosis, compared to a nearly 60 percent mortality rate among those who kept drinking.[51]

Anthracycline cardiotoxicity is dose-related and affects 5–20 percent of patients receiving such agents. Acute or chronic cardiac toxicity with severe heart failure symptoms is uncommon at doses of doxorubicin below 450 mg/m^2, and the incidence increases significantly at doses over 600 mg/m^2. Acute toxicity generally has a fulminant course, a poor response to medical therapy, and usually is fatal within weeks.[52] Prognosis of mild to moderate heart failure relates to the time course of myocardial toxicity and the presence of additional risk factors for myocardial injury, such as concomitant irradiation, preexisting cardiac dysfunction, and hypokalemia. Patients typically respond incompletely to standard agents used for the treatment of chronic systolic heart failure and have a survival curve worse than that seen with IDC.[53] The natural history of patients with chronic heart failure due to anthracycline exposure that has resulted in cure of their malignancy has not been well documented.

INFILTRATIVE DISEASES

Primary or secondary cardiac amyloidosis has a long latent period but a poor actuarial survival after the development of symptoms of heart failure. The response to standard therapy, generally for diastolic dysfunction, is usually suboptimal. Mortality is essentially 100 percent within 2 years of the onset of symptoms.[54] The prognosis is equally poor when severe heart failure occurs in the setting of endomyocardial fibrosis or hemochromatosis.

PROGNOSIS AND PATIENT DEMOGRAPHICS OR CO-MORBIDITIES

Race

In the United States, African Americans have approximately a 1.5- to 2.0-fold higher mortality risk when diagnosed with heart failure than whites.[2] Hypertension and resultant left ventricular hypertrophy are more common in African Americans and represent significant risk factors for the development of heart failure. Although the response to medical treatment of hypertension varies with race, it is unknown whether the response to medical treatment of heart failure also shows racial differences.[55] In the SOLVD registry, which included patients with a hospital discharge diagnosis of heart failure or an ejection fraction of 45 percent or less, the predominant etiology of heart failure was coronary artery disease (69 percent). Although total and cardiovascular mortality was not different between African Americans and whites in this substudy, hospitalization for CHF was twice as frequent among the former.[56] Overall, only 11 percent of the study population was African American, however, illustrating that more definitive data about racial differences in the etiology of heart failure, response to treatment, and prognosis are clearly needed. Socioeconomic factors may also play a role in patient access to medical care, medications, and treatments available and in patient compliance.

Gender

Heart failure is more common in men than women; and the effect of female gender on prognosis is not clear. In general, studies evaluating heart failure have been conducted on predominantly male populations for reasons that include poor recruitment of women or delayed presentation and diagnosis. Women may be more likely than men to develop heart failure after myocardial infarction, although the outcome of interventions when treating IHD (coronary artery bypass grafting, percutaneous transluminal coronary angioplasty) appear to have no gender-related difference in success rates after correcting for body size, age, and co-morbid diseases.[57] The observational SOLVD patient registry included 26 percent female patients. Women had a significantly higher annual risk of heart failure-related mortality (22 percent versus 17 percent) and higher rates of hospitalization for heart failure (33 percent versus 25 percent), though these gender differences were observed in white patients only.[56] The National Health and Nutrition Examination Survey (NHANES) found a lower risk of death among women than men with self-reported CHF.[1] In the Italian Multicenter Cardiomyopathy Study Registry, women (21 percent) with IDC tended to present with a more advanced state of the disease as defined by symptoms and left ventricular dimensions. Survival was not statistically different for women versus men in the same cohort, though a trend toward a poorer outcome was evident.[58] The overall mortality in the study was only 8 percent at 1 year. The Framingham group found that within 2 years of the diagnosis of CHF 37 percent of the men and 38 percent of the women were dead, with approximately 25 percent of the deaths classified as sudden. Interestingly, there was a separation at 6 years of follow-up, with the mortality risk being 82 percent for men compared with 67 percent for women.[10,11] Whether this finding reflects a difference in the natural history of the disease, the underlying etiology, or a gender-dependent response to treatment is uncertain. The SOLVD treatment arm included only 15 percent women and found no difference in survival related to gender in either the placebo or the enalapril group.[8] The currently ongoing BEST study of the β-blocker bucindolol is the first heart failure survival trial to mandate the inclusion of sufficient numbers of women to empower statistically accurate conclusions regarding gender differences in the response to therapy and prognosis related to ischemic versus idiopathic disease. Whether an adequate number of female patients can be enrolled in the BEST trial remains to be seen, as female recruitment in clinical trials has traditionally been poor.

Age

Independent of race and gender, advancing age is an obvious risk factor for mortality due to heart failure. Framingham data delineate that the incidence of heart failure increases twofold with each decade increment of age.[10,11] As reported by the SOLVD registry, the risk for death at 1 year for a person over the age of 64 years with heart failure is 1.5 times that of those under 64 years of age.[56] A relation between chronologic age and survival after heart failure was not demonstrated in the V-HeFT-II study, but patient subgroups may not have been large enough to fully evaluate this factor.[59] Multiple studies demonstrating an age-related increase in both the incidence and prevalence of the disease (linked to the increase in the risk of ischemic heart disease) underscores the magnitude of the problem to be faced by the medical profession as we approach the twenty-first century.[1,2,4,11,60]

Co-morbidities

Many factors are recognized to worsen the prognosis of chronic heart failure, though only two—hypertension and diabetes—have been studied adequately to quantitate their impact. Hypertension increases the risk of developing heart failure by a factor of three.[1,60] In addition, persistent hypertension in the setting of heart failure symptoms warrants aggressive intervention, as peripheral vasoconstriction affects cardiac performance adversely when ventricular dysfunction is present. Diabetes is another significant risk factor for the development of heart failure independent of the risk of developing coronary disease and is at least twice as strong a risk factor among women than among men.[1,61] The combination of hypertension and diabetes increases the risk of developing heart failure by a factor of five. These two diagnoses certainly contribute to the incidence and prevalence of heart failure, yet heart failure mortality data directly attributable to these entities is difficult to analyze given the frequent comorbidities of atherosclerotic disease and stroke.

Diabetic cardiomyopathy as a unique entity was described during the 1970s, but survival data for this specific diagnosis are not available.[62] The syndrome is defined as heart failure in diabetic patients who have no significant valvar heart disease, hypertension, coronary atherosclerotic disease, or other identifiable cause of their cardiomyopathy. Systolic and diastolic abnormalities are common.

Concomitant renal or hepatic dysfunction, which in turn may limit the choice of medication prescribed or blunt the therapeutic response, likely has an impact on prognosis that is not easily elucidated. For example, one might choose to avoid ACE inhibitor administration for heart failure in the setting of severe renal insufficiency not yet requiring chronic dialysis. As evidenced in the V-HeFT trials, patients whose heart failure was treated with the combination of hydralazine and isosorbide (HYD-ISO) rather than ACE inhibitors had a lower survival despite an equivalent clinical response and greater improvement in ejection fraction and exercise capacity.[18,63] The annual mortality risk of systolic heart failure in patients treated with the drug combination HYD-ISO was 13 percent at 1 year and 25 percent at 2 years, compared to 9 and 18 percent, respectively, for patients on enalapril. Patients with NYHA class III or IV CHF refractory to diuretics, inotropes, and vasodilators have a dismal prognosis despite volume and electrolyte control with dialysis or ultrafiltration. Golper pooled the data from more than 60 patients in 11 reports and found a 37 percent 1-year and 15 percent 2-year survival for these patients treated with peritoneal dialysis.[64] The median survival was only 10 months for 35 patients with severe CHF treated with continuous venovenous hemofiltration despite improved hemodynamics.[65]

Pulmonary hypertension of any etiology affects survival by influencing right ventricular function and increasing the risk of arrhythmia. Sleep apnea (hypoxemia on arousal) is a common yet often overlooked contributor to systemic and pulmonary hypertension, right ventricular dysfunction, heightened catecholamine levels, bradyarrhythmias and tachyarrhythmias, and worsened heart failure and quality of life.[66] Treatment of sleep apnea with continuous positive airway pressure may improve the left ventricular ejection fraction and reduce symptoms, although the effect on mortality is not known.[67] The association of sleep apnea and cardiovascular disease is currently being studied in an NIH-sponsored multicenter trial.

EASILY MEASURED PROGNOSTIC VARIABLES FOR CHRONIC HEART FAILURE

As succinctly summarized by Cohn, "heart failure is a multisystem disease involving the heart, peripheral vasculature, kidney, renin-angiotensin system, other circulating hormones, local paracrine and autocrine systems, and metabolic derangements in skeletal muscle."[68] The previous sections have illustrated the complex nature of heart failure and the need to individualize the mortality risk for each patient. It would be naive to seek a single criterion to express either the severity of heart failure or its prognosis. Similarly, it is unwise to assume that inducing a positive change in a single variable may significantly improve a patient's overall prognosis. Although an increase in ejection fraction over time might be thought to have favorable survival implications, the means by which it is achieved is an important consideration, as learned in the PROMISE trial with oral milrinone and in the studies of the unique β-blocker xamoterol.[69,70] With both of these agents there was excess mortality in patients receiving active drug despite increases in ejection fraction. Furthermore, as described below, ventricular ectopy appears to be an independent predictor of subsequent mortality in heart failure patients. Nonetheless, drugs that successfully suppress premature ventricular beats can worsen the prognosis, as illustrated by the CAST trial.[71] This section reviews the parameters identified in major mortality trials of systolic heart failure as strong, independent prognostic variables that are easily measured in clinical practice (Table 30.2).

Symptoms

Symptoms referable to heart failure are important indicators of overall morbidity and mortality, as verified in the important heart failure trials of the late 1980s and early 1990s.[3,7–9] Symptom severity has been evaluated in many ways; the most widely recognized (and criticized) symptom scale is the NYHA functional classification. The less well utilized but more reproducible Specific Activity Scale demonstrates a closer correlation to functional capacity and is much less subjective. Large-scale mortality data are not available.[72] It is clear that with systolic heart failure refractory and severe symptoms correspond to the highest mortality risk, but NYHA class is not at all predictive of the degree of ventricular dysfunction or objective measure of exercise capacity.[18,19,73] Although the presence of severe heart failure symptoms in patients with normal systolic function (i.e.,

Table 30-2. Selected Placebo-Controlled Clinical Heart Failure Trails—Cardiac Mortality

Trial	N	Entry Criteria	IHD (%)	CV Mortality RX (%)	CV Mortality Placebo (%)	Follow-Up Period	Predictive Prognostic Variables(s)
CONSENSUS	253	NYHA IV, Cardiomegaly	73	EN 38	54	1 yr	21% CV mortality risk reduction with ACE-I
SOLVD Prevention	4,228	EF < 0.35 Asymptomatic	83	EN 13	14	4 yr	12% CV mortality risk reduction with ACE-I
SOLVD Treatment	2,569	EF < 0.35 Symptomatic	71	EN 31	36	4 yr	18% CV mortality risk reduction with ACE-I
SAVE	2,231	Post-MI CHF EF ≤ 0.40	100	CAP 17	21	4 yr	21% CV mortality risk reduction with ACE-I
V-HeFT I	642	VO2 < 25 *and* CTR > 0.55 with EF < 0.45 or	44	PR 46 HI 37	41	5 yr	EF, VO2, CRT, CAD, VAr independent mortality risk
V-HeFT II	804	EDD ≥ 2.7 cm/m^{2a}	52	EN 28	HI 34	5 yr	EF, VO2, CTR, VAr, PNE independent mortality risk
PRAISE	1,153	NYHA III or IV EF < 0.30	63	AM 28	33	14.5 mos	35% mortality risk reduction in non-CAD subset only
Metoprolol in Dilated Cardiomyopathy	383	Symptomatic EF < 0.40	0	M 13	20	18 mos	34% "endpoint" risk reduction with β-blocker[b]

Abbreviations: CV, cardiovascular; NYHA, New York Heart Association symptomatology; EN, enalapril; CAP, captopril; ACE-I, angiotensin converting enzyme inhibitor; PR, prazocin; HI, hydralazine-isosorbide dinitrate; EF, ejection fraction; IHD, ischemic heart disease; MI, myocardial infarction; CHF, congestive heart failure; EDD, echocardiographic end-diastolic dimension; CTR, cardiothoracic ratio; VAr, ventricular arrhythmias; PNE, plasma norepinephrine; VO2, maximal oxygen consumption; AM, amlodipine.

[a] VHEFT I and II had the same entry criteria, with three ways to demonstrate cardiac enlargement or dysfunction paired with exercise performance

[b] Excess end-points (death or transplant) in placebo group due entirely to need for transplantation.[7–9,18,22,69,122–124]

severe diastolic abnormalities) may pose a difficult therapeutic dilemma, the long-term prognosis is nonetheless more favorable than if the cause were systolic dysfunction.[6,24,25]

Ejection Fraction

With systolic heart failure the left ventricular ejection fraction (EF) is one of the most powerful independent markers for survival. An EF less than 25 percent represents a major increase in risk compared to an EF more than 35 percent.[18] A reliable measurement of EF is readily available to most practitioners. This allows differentiation of systolic from diastolic dysfunction and should be assessed early during the evaluation of virtually every patient with symptoms of heart failure. Although an important measurement, EF cannot be relied on as a single prognostic indicator for many reasons. First, although quantitation of EF is possible by a multitude of techniques, each has inherent methodologic errors that should be recognized. Furthermore, EF is a descriptor of global ventricular function and may underestimate the degree of ventricular systolic impairment in the setting of severe mitral regurgitation. A serial change in EF may also have prognostic significance, with a decrease in EF of more than 5 percent after 1 year being associated with roughly twice the mortality as an increase of more than 5 percent.[74] Interval changes in EF, however, should be viewed in the context of the intrinsic measurement error. Only those changes that exceed the expected degree of variability should be considered indicative of a true change in ventricular function.

Similarly, a depressed right ventricular EF has proved to be a high risk marker. As measured by radionuclide techniques, a rest or exercise right ventricular EF of more than 35 percent was a more potent predictor of survival of patients with NYHA class III or IV symptoms than was oxygen consumption alone.[75] In contrast to left ventricular function, the right ventricular EF correlates well with exercise capacity as measured by oxygen consumption. Unfortunately, this valuable parameter is not routinely evaluated.

Exercise Capacity

Exercise intolerance, a hallmark symptom of heart failure, is another widely used indicator of outcome.[76] Exercise capacity as measured by maximal oxygen consumption (VO_2) exhibits a random distribution when plotted against the left ventricular EF.[18,73] This nonintuitive observation is often noted in clinical practice and illustrates the complexity of the physiologic response to exercise and the independent prognostic value of these two variables. Interestingly, data exist that diastolic, rather than systolic, dysfunction may play a more important role in limiting exercise capacity and may explain the profound exercise intolerance described for patients with severe diastolic heart failure.[77]

Peak (ideally maximal) exercise oxygen consumption (VO_2max) has been demonstrated to be an objective measurement of functional capacity in heart failure patients and provides an indirect assessment of cardiovascular and pulmonary reserve. For an equal depression of EF, Mancini and colleagues found that a peak VO_2 of less than 14 ml·kg^{-1}·min^{-1} predicts patients with a high (30–50 percent) 1-year mortality compared to patients with preserved exercise capacity (< 10 percent mortality).[78] This range of VO_2 has been confirmed by others as indicative of poor short-term survival; a VO_2max of less than 10 and 14 ml·kg^{-1}·min^{-1} are considered definite and probable indications, respectively, for cardiac transplantation.[79,80]

The 6-minute walk test, though simplistic, still provides valuable prognostic information not attained with treadmill or bicycle stress testing.[81] This modality correlates better with patient symptoms during daily activities. FIRST and other mortality trials of heart failure have found a highly significant correlation of distance walked with survival.[82,83] A total distance walked of less than 305 meters was shown by Bittner et al. to carry an annual mortality risk of 11 percent compared to 4 percent in patients who could walk more than 443 meters.[83] Total distance walked also was a potent predictor of the need for future hospitalization.

Hemodynamics

Although helpful in acute ventricular failure, resting hemodynamic measurements do not correspond well with symptoms, physical examination, or exercise capacity in patients with chronic heart failure, even in those considered appropriate for heart transplantation.[84,85] When resting hemodynamic abnormalities are severely abnormal, however, survival is poor.

Franciosa[86] and others found a higher mortality in patients with chronic heart failure whose left ventricular filling pressure was more than 27 mmHg, the systemic vascular resistance more than 23 Wood units, or the cardiac index less than 2.25 L·min^{-1}·sqm^{-1}. In the FIRST trial, the mean pulmonary artery blood pressure in ambulatory patients with chronic heart failure was the only hemodynamic variable independently associated with a poor outcome.[82]

Serum Sodium

Although a surrogate for the degree of neurohumoral activation and directly affected by medical therapy, the serum sodium concentration is a simple but important marker for poor survival. Serum sodium demonstrates an inverse relation with plasma renin activity and vasopressin concentration. A sodium concentration of 130 mEq/L or less was shown by Lee and Packer to be associated with a survival rate of less than 20 percent at 1 year compared to nearly 50 percent for those with a serum sodium level over 130 mEq/L.[87]

Thyroid Function

Altered thyroid hormone metabolism is common in chronic illness and has likewise been described in association with heart failure. It is well recognized that hypothyroidism and hyperthyroidism can exacerbate underlying heart failure symptoms. The implication of a concomitant "euthyroid sick" state, defined as a low triiodothyronine (T_3) or T_3 index and increased reverse T_3, with normal thyroid-stimulating hormone (TSH) and variable thyroxine (T_4) was evaluated by Hamilton et al.[88] They reported that an increased free T_3 index to reverse T_3 ratio was a stronger predictor of short-term mortality than any other single variable including hemodynamics, serum sodium, and ejection fraction.

Electrocardiography Arrhythmias

Unverferth and colleagues concluded that a left ventricular conduction delay is a significant marker for worsened prognosis in heart failure patients; in fact, it was the strongest predictive parameter in their study.[85] These data were confirmed by a prospective study that noted a strong correlation between arrhythmic events and bundle branch block on baseline electrocardiography (ECG).[86] Given the prevalence of ECG abnormalities in chronic heart failure, however, the utility of these findings may be limited.

Several major clinical trials have demonstrated that the proportionate risk of arrhythmic death is approximately half that of the total cardiac death rate among patients with ventricular dysfunction.[2,84] Furthermore, the risk of sudden death increases with worsening ventricular function. Of note is the observation from available data that sudden death is statistically more common with heart failure due to a nonischemic etiology. The actuarial risk of sudden death in patients awaiting heart transplantation between 1984 and 1992 was 21 percent at a large referral center in southern California and is in keeping with nearly half of the overall expected 40–50 percent annual mortality seen in NYHA class IV patients.[66] These deaths represent combinations of both bradyarrhythmias and tachyarrhythmias, ventricular fibrillation, and asystole. However, since the evaluation of sinus node dysfunction, chronotropic incompetence, and inducible ventricular arrhythmia is not routine in heart failure patients without preexisting symptoms, and the true incidence of these abnormalities as the cause of sudden death is uncertain.

Patients with severe systolic dysfunction have a high incidence of complex ventricular arrhythmias when evaluated by Holter monitoring.[89–92] The Captopril-Digoxin Study Group and the Argentine GESICA investigators demonstrated prospectively that nonsustained ventricular tachycardia is an independent risk factor for sudden death during heart failure, although this finding has not been uniform. The 1-year mortality seen among post-MI patients with nonsustained ventricular tachycardia (NSVT) and an EF under 30 percent is nearly 40 percent compared to 20 percent for those without NSVT; it is approximately 5 percent for patients without NSVT and with an EF over 30 percent.[89,90]

The impact of selected antiarrhythmic drug therapy is controversial in the wake of the CAST study, the results of which imply that the use of an antiarrhythmic drug is in itself an independent marker for mortality![71] In the subset of CAST patients with an EF under 30 percent and clinical heart failure, arrhythmia suppression could be achieved in only half, yet there was a sevenfold increase in the number of life-threatening complications of antiarrhythmic therapy in patients with a depressed EF. An interesting comparison of the effects of empiric low-dose amiodarone administration on survival in heart failure patients is available from the GESICA and STAT CHF Veterans Administration (VA)-sponsored trials.[20,91] The GESICA investigators reported a survival advantage for patients receiving amiodarone,

with sudden death and progressive heart failure mortality risk reductions of 27 and 23 percent, respectfully. The US-based study did not corroborate these data. However, because the proportion of patients with nonischemic cardiomyopathy was more than 60 percent in the Argentine study and less than 30 percent in the VA trial, an etiology-dependent benefit appears implicit but unproved.

The value of electrophysiologic (EP) testing in patients with nonsustained ventricular tachycardia is unclear. In a meta-analysis of 926 patients in 12 studies performed by Kowey et al., only one patient in three had inducible arrhythmia.[93] During follow-up, 7 percent of patients without inducible arrhythmia experienced events compared to 18 percent of those with induced tachycardia. However, because most patients with an inducible arrhythmia were subsequently treated with antiarrhythmic agents, the confounding possibility of proarrhythmia limits the clinical utility of these data. In patients with a history of sustained ventricular tachycardia or prior ventricular fibrillation, the proportion with inducible tachycardia on provocative testing is greater among patients with underlying coronary artery disease than in those with dilated cardiomyopathy. Although EP guided therapy in inducible patients has been shown to reduce the subsequent risk of arrhythmia recurrence and cardiac arrest, although the effects on overall survival are unclear.[93,94] The effects and cost benefit of implantable pacing antitachycardia and cardioverter-defibrillating devices on survival in patients with heart failure are unknown and are being evaluated in several large multicenter trials.[95–97]

The presence of even "benign" or controlled atrial arrhythmias has adverse prognostic implications in the setting of systolic heart failure. Compared to sinus rhythm, atrial fibrillation has been associated with an increased risk of embolic events and sudden death in most studies of heart failure.[98] Investigators reported a V-HeFT trials were a notable exception to this observation but did not include NYHA class IV patients.[99] Prospective studies have failed to demonstrate atrial fibrillation as an independent risk factor.

Doppler Echocardiography

Coexistent diastolic dysfunction with impaired ventricular systolic function worsens survival, as evidenced by studies of mitral inflow velocity by Doppler echocardiography.[26–29] In a carefully performed, prospective study by Xie and colleagues, a restrictive pattern of transmitral inflow was the best single predictor of death over the subsequent 2-year period.[29] A group of 100 patients with an average EF of 26 ± 6 percent were studied; more than 50 percent of the patients had IHD. A mitral inflow E/A ratio greater than 2.0 or an E/A ratio that equaled 2.0 with an E deceleration time of 140 ms or less was their definition of restrictive inflow. This study corroborated earlier data from several smaller studies that evaluated patients with dilated cardiomyopathy. The value of serial change in mitral valve Doppler patterns is unknown.

ADDITIONAL PROGNOSTIC FACTORS: RESEARCH TOOLS

The following variables are potential or proved prognostic indicators that are often used in large referral or research centers. Routine clinical application of these parameters is limited owing to accessibility, expense, technical difficulties, or required expertise for interpretation. Nonetheless, these parameters are often utilized in clinical trials, are well described in the medical literature, and are important to recognize.

Neurohormones

Neuroendocrine activation occurs early in the course of heart failure and directly correlates with mortality.[100–102] Increased plasma norepinephrine levels precedes and predicts the development of heart failure symptoms and death even in patients with asymptomatic ventricular dysfunction.[102] Plasma norepinephrine (NE) elevation corresponds more closely than renin with hemodynamic abnormalities, such as an elevated right atrial or pulmonary capillary wedge pressure, and can predict the degree of survival benefit to be gained by use of ACE inhibitors.[100–103] A plasma NE level of 400–800 ng/ml corresponds to an increased mortality risk; a level over 800 ng/ml predicts a high 1-year mortality risk due to progressive heart failure.[102,103]

The CONSENSUS I investigators were among the first to demonstrate that increased levels of NE, angiotensin II (ANG II), aldosterone, and atrial natriuretic factor correlated significantly with mortality.[104] Unlike most others, this study noted a stronger correlation between mortality and ANG II levels than with NE. This may reflect the influence of the study population which was limited to class IV patients. Furthermore, both neurohormones were reduced by ACE inhibitor therapy, with the greatest reductions seen among patients with the highest pre-treatment values. Because elevation of plasma NE appears to be independent of renin release, both markers have become important variables commonly measured in clinical trials.

In animal models, aldosterone elevation is a more potent stimulus than hypertension or ANG II for fibroblast proliferation and myocardial fibrosis. ACE inhibitor administration reduces both myocyte hypertrophy (mass) and the degree of myocardial fibrosis. In humans ACE inhibitors reduced echocardiographically measured myocardial mass in the SOLVD study and reduced aldosterone levels in the CONSENSUS trial by nearly 60 percent.[100,104,105] An ongoing study adding aldactone to standard therapy for heart failure (RALES) may provide further insight into the relative importance of aldosterone inhibition on survival.

N-terminal proatrial natriuretic factor was analyzed in the CONSENSUS and SAVE trials and was noted to correlate well with patient symptomatology, cardiac index, and left ventricular filling pressure but not with the EF.[106,107] A level exceeding 125 pg/ml was at least as predictive of subsequent mortality as more commonly examined parameters, such as symptoms and the EF.[107]

Given the variability in neurohormonal assays and dependence upon collection times and techniques, the clinical applicability of each of the aforementioned parameters is essentially limited to large investigative centers.

Left Ventricular Dimensions

The placebo group in the radionuclide and contrast ventriculography substudies of the SOLVD trials demonstrated progressive ventricular dilation and increased wall stress and sphericity indices over time.[105,108] Essentially, a large, globular left ventricle has adverse prognostic implications.[108,109] The left ventricular size index as measured by two-dimensional echocardiography was a discriminator of survival, as described by Lee and colleagues.[110] The echocardiographic substudy of SOLVD confirmed that the influence of chamber shape may explain the higher correlation coefficient of ventricular volumes with mortality risk than the more easily measured echocardiographic two-dimensional dimensions.[108] Tischler et al. noted that the dynamic change in left ventricular shape with exercise predicted exercise capacity, though mortality data were lacking.[111]

Survival is also inversely related to increased left ventricular mass. Increased global mass was a better predictor of sudden death in patients with hypertrophic cardiomyopathy than increased septal or free wall mass.[47] Ventricular hypertrophy induced as a compensatory mechanism to impaired function after MI has also been demonstrated to worsen survival, though it can be modulated by ACE inhibition.[9,17,112] The SOLVD investigators also detected a progressive increase in left ventricular mass in patients on placebo compared to a decrease in patients on enalapril.[105,108,112]

Another research tool but easily measured variable related to heart size is the cardiothoracic ratio (CTR). An increased CTR was the third strongest independent marker for mortality in the V-HeFT trials, behind EF and VO_2.[19] Because the anteroposterior chest radiographic cardiac silhouette is predominantly made up of right-sided chambers, this specific but insensitive marker is abnormal in patients with the greatest degree of global cardiac enlargement.

Autonomic Dysfunction

Reduced heart rate variability as documented by power spectral analysis reflects the summation of the autonomic imbalances typically observed during heart failure: excess sympathetic tone, parasympathetic withdrawal, and reduced baroreceptor sensitivity.[113,114] Processing methods vary widely, and interpretation of results requires technical expertise, limiting the widespread applicability of this type of testing. Prognostic data are limited, though heart rate trends correlate significantly with plasma NE levels,[115] and reduced heart rate variability following MI has been noted to have adverse implications.[116] Preservation of the normal diurnal variation of the ventricular response rate in patients with heart failure and chronic atrial fibrillation predicted an improved 12-month survival in an Austrian study.[117]

Signal-Averaged ECG

Following MI, a signal-averaged ECG with absent late potentials has a high negative predictive value for the absence of sustained reentrant ventricular arrhythmias and is associated with a low risk of sudden death.[89,118] The utility of this technique appears to be limited to patients with coronary artery disease whose resting ECG has a relatively normal QRS duration. Yi et al. demonstrated that in patients with IDC an abnormal signal-averaged ECG was able to predict patients with severe heart failure but did not predict sudden death.[119] Furthermore, for patients with a high-risk signal-averaged ECG, programmed

ventricular stimulation provides no incremental prognostic data and has limited applicability in the absence of safe and effective therapy. Patients with heart failure surviving a cardiac arrest who do not have inducible ventricular tachycardia on provocative testing, the risk of recurrent cardiac arrest still exceeds 30 percent over the next 1–3 years.[66,88] Those with inducible ventricular tachycardia have a 15–50 percent chance of recurrent cardiac arrest over a 3-year period despite "directed" antiarrhythmic therapy.

Endomyocardial Biopsy

Patients with ischemic ventricular function have a greater degree of replacement fibrosis and less myocyte hypertrophy than those with dilated cardiomyopathy despite clinically indistinguishable presentations.[120] Those with increased fibrosis and IHD had higher pulmonary artery pressures and lower cardiac indices at presentation, which were assumed to be markers of worsened prognosis. A Japanese study found the degree of histologic intercellular fibrosis was able to predict the response to β-blockade in patients with IDC.[121] The pattern of fibrosis predicted therapeutic efficacy better in peripheral lymphocyte β-receptor concentration. The pattern and degree of fibrosis did not correlate with the EF or left ventricular end-diastolic dimension. Unfortunately, neither of these two studies evaluated the independent correlation of myocardial fibrosis directly with either arrhythmia or mortality risk. Unverferth and colleagues found no relation between the percentage of fibrosis on endomyocardial biopsy specimens and 1-year survival in nonischemic, dilated cardiomyopathy.[85] The overall population exhibited a 35 percent 1-year mortality rate, suggesting a high-risk or end-stage cohort was examined.

CONCLUSION

Congestive heart failure is a common, potentially lethal syndrome that is increasingly prevalent worldwide. Risk stratification of patients is essential in order to identify those patients at the highest risk of death, ideally allowing time to employ more aggressive conventional therapy or more extreme interventions such as investigational drugs, devices, or transplantation. The etiology of the underlying pathophysiologic processes contributing to the development of heart failure, the patients' demographic profile and co-morbid disease(s) contribute to the overall risk of death and require individualized investigation seeking correctable abnormalities.

A minimum database for the purpose of prognostication in every patient with the diagnosis of heart failure should include the assessment of patient symptoms, disease etiology, ejection fraction, exercise capacity, Doppler echocardiography, chest radiography, ECG, and serum sodium assay. Referral to heart failure specialists or cardiomyopathy centers should be prompt for any patient not responding to medical therapy or for whom the etiology is unclear. Finally, it is helpful to realize that a host of disparate parameters serve as independent indicators of mortality. A prognostic index, weighing the relative value of the variables reviewed herein, to enable an individualized annual mortality assessment would be both interesting and useful but would require prospective validation.

REFERENCES

1. Schocken DD, Arrieta MI, Leverton PE, Ross EA: Prevalence and mortality rate of congestive heart failure in the United States. J Am Coll Cardiol 1992; 20:301
2. Massachusetts Medical Society: Mortality from congestive heart failure—United States, 1980–1990. MMWR 1994;43(5):77
3. Konstam MA, Dracup K, Baker DW et al: Heart Failure: Evaluation and Care of Patients with Left Ventricular Systolic Dysfunction. Clinical Practice Guideline No. 11, AHCPR Publication No. 94–0612, June 1994
4. Andersson B, Caidahl K, Waagstein F: Idiopathic dilated cardiomyopathy among Swedish patients with congestive heart failure. Eur Heart J 1995;16:53
5. Andersson B, Waagstein F: Spectrum and outcome of congestive heart failure in a hospitalized population. Am Heart J 1993;126:632
6. Itoh A, Saito M, Haze K et al: Prognosis of patients with congestive heart failure. Its determinants in various heart diseases in Japan. Int Med 1993;31(3): 304
7. CONSENSUS Trial Study Group: Effects of enalapril on mortality in severe congestive heart failure. N Engl J Med 1987;316:1429
8. SOLVD Investigators: Effect of enalapril on survival in patients with reduced left ventricular ejection fractions and congestive heart failure. N Engl J Med 1991;325:293
9. Pfeffer MA, Braunwald E, Moye LA et al: Effect of captopril on mortality and morbidity in patients with left ventricular dysfunction after myocardial infarction. N Engl J Med 1992;327:669
10. McKee PA, Castelli WP, McNamara PM, Kannel WB: The natural history of congestive heart failure. The Framingham study. N Engl J Med 1971;285:1441
11. Ho KK, Pinsky JL, Kannel WB, Levy D: The epidemiology of heart failure. The Framingham study. J Am Coll Cardiol, suppl. A 1993;22:6A
12. Rackley CE, Satler LF, Pearle DL et al: Use of hemodynamic measurements for management of acute myocardial infarction. p. 3. In Rackley CE (ed): Advances in Critical Care Cardiology. FA Davis, Philadelphia, 1986
13. Forrester JS, Diamond G, Chatterjee K, Swan HJC: Medical therapy of acute myocardial infarction by application of hemodynamic subsets. N Engl J Med 1976;295:1356
14. Emanuelsson H, Karlson BW, Herlitz J: Characteristics and prognosis of patients with acute myocardial infarction in relation to occurrence of congestive heart failure. Eur Heart J 1994;15:761
15. Multicenter Postinfarction Research Group: Risk stratification and survival after myocardial infarction. N Engl J Med 1983;309:331
16. Pfeffer MA, Braunwald E: Ventricular remodeling after myocardial infarction. Experimental observations and clinical implications. Circulation 1990;81: 1161
17. Pfeffer MA, Pfeffer JM: Ventricular enlargement and reduced survival after myocardial infarction. Circulation, suppl. IV 1987;75:93
18. Cohn JN, Johnson GR, Shabetai R et al: Ejection fraction, peak exercise oxygen consumption, cardiothoracic ratio, ventricular arrhythmias, and plasma norepinephrine as determinants of prognosis in heart failure. Circulation, suppl. VI 1993;87:5
19. Goldman S, Johnson G, Cohn JN et al: Mechanism of death in heart failure. The vasodilator-heart failure trials. Circulation, suppl. VI 1993;87:24
20. Doval HC, Nul DR, Grancelli HO et al: Randomized trial of low-dose amiodarone in severe congestive heart failure. Lancet 1994;344:493
21. Packer M: PRAISE REF Library ref at binder abstract needed.
22. CIBIS Investigators and Committees: A randomized trial of beta-blockade in heart failure. The cardiac insufficiency bisoprolol study (CIBIS). Circulation 1994;90:1765
23. Cohn JN, Johnson G: Heart failure with normal ejection fraction. The V-HeFT study. Circulation, suppl. III 1990;81:48
24. Setaro JF, Soufer R, Remetz SM, Perlmutter RA, Zaret BL: Long-term outcome in patients with congestive heart failure and intact systolic left ventricular performance. Am J Cardiol 1992;69:1212
25. Hina K, Kusachi S, Iwasaki K et al: Progression of left ventricular enlargement in patients with hypertrophic cardiomyopathy. Incidence and prognostic value. Clin Cardiol 1993;16:403
26. Pinamonti B, Di Lenarda AD, Sinagra G et al: Restrictive left ventricular filling pattern in dilated cardiomyopathy assessed by echocardiography. Clinical, echocardiographic and hemodynamic correlations and prognostic implications. J Am Coll Cardiol 1993; 22:808
27. Werner GS, Schaefer C, Dirks R, Figulla HR, Kreuzer H: Prognostic value of Doppler echocardiographic assessment of left ventricular filling in idiopathic dilated cardiomyopathy. Am J Cardiol 1994;73:792
28. Shen WF, Tribouilloy C, Rey JL et al: Prognostic significance of Doppler-derived left ventricular diastolic filling variables in dilated cardiomyopathy. Am Heart J 1992;124:1524
29. Xie GY, Berk MR, Smith MD, Gurley JC, DeMaria

AN: Prognostic value of Doppler transmitral flow patterns in patients with congestive heart failure. J Am Coll Cardiol 1994;24:132

30. Ross J Jr, Braunwald E: Aortic stenosis. Circulation, suppl. 5 1968;37:67

31. Frank S, Johnson A, Ross J Jr: Natural history of valvular aortic stenosis. Br Heart J 1973;35:41

32. Ross J Jr: Left ventricular function and the timing of surgical treatment in valvular heart disease. Ann Intern Med 1981;94:498

33. Braunwald E: Valvular heart disease. p. 1007. In: Braunwald (ed): Heart Disease. A Textbook of Cardiovascular Medicine. WB Saunders, Philadelphia, 1992

34. Zile MR: Chronic aortic and mitral regurgitation. Choosing the optimal time for surgical correction. Cardiol Clin 1991;9:239

35. Siemienczuk D, Greenberg B, Morris C et al: Chronic aortic insufficiency. Factors associated with progression to aortic valve replacement. Ann Intern Med 1989;110:587

36. Greenberg B, Massie B, Bristow D et al: Long-term vasodilator therapy of chronic aortic insufficiency. A randomized double-blinded, placebo-controlled clinical trial. Circulation 1988;78:92

37. Munoz S, Gallardo J, Diaz-Gorrin JR, Median O: Influence of surgery on the natural history of rheumatic mitral and aortic valve disease. Am J Cardiol 1975; 35:234

38. Grogan M, Redfield MM, Bailey KR et al: Long-term outcome of patients with biopsy-proved myocarditis. Comparison with idiopathic dilated cardiomyopathy. J Am Coll Cardiol 1995;26:804

39. Semigran MJ, Thaik CM, Fifer MA et al: Exercise capacity and systolic and diastolic ventricular function after recovery from acute dilated cardiomyopathy. J Am Coll Cardiol 1994;24:462

40. Mason JW, O'Connell JB, Herskowitz A et al: A clinical trial of immunosuppressive therapy for myocarditis. N Engl J Med 1995;333:269

41. Mady C, Cardisso RH, Barretto AC et al: Survival and predictors of survival in patients with congestive heart failure due to Chagas' cardiomyopathy. Circulation 1994;90:3098

42. Kaul S, Fishbein MC, Siegel RJ: Cardiac manifestations of acquired immune deficiency syndrome. A 1991 update. Am Heart J 1991;122:535

43. Midei MG, DeMent SH, Feldman AM et al: Peripartum myocarditis and cardiomyopathy. Circulation 1990;81:922

44. O'Connell JB, Costanzo-Nordin MR, Subramanian R et al: Peripartum cardiomyopathy. Clinical, hemodynamic, histologic and prognostic characteristics. J Am Coll Cardiol 1986;8:52

45. Cooper LT, Berry GJ, Rizeq M, Schroeder JS: Giant cell myocarditis. J Heart Lung Transplant 1995;14: 394

46. Maron BJ, Fananapazir L: Sudden cardiac death in hypertrophic cardiomyopathy. Circulation, suppl. I 1992;85:57

47. Spirito P, Maron BJ: Relation between extent of left ventricular hypertrophy and occurrence of sudden cardiac death in hypertrophic cardiomyopathy. J Am Coll Cardiol 1990;15:521

48. Vassalli G, Seiler C, Hess OM: Risk stratification in hypertrophic cardiomyopathy. Curr Opin Cardiol 1994;9:330

49. Topol EJ, Traill TA, Fortuin NJ: Hypertensive hypertrophic cardiomyopathy of the elderly. N Engl J Med 1985;312:277

50. Regan TJ: Alcohol and the cardiovascular system. JAMA 1990;264:377

51. Demakis JG, Proskey A, Rahimtoola SH et al: The natural course of alcoholic cardiomyopathy. Ann Intern Med 1974;80:293

52. Hosenpud JD: The cardiomyopathies. p. 196. In: Hosenpud JD, Greenberg BH (eds) Congestive Heart Failure. Pathophysiology, Diagnosis and Comprehensive Approach to Management. Springer-Verlag, New York, 1994

53. Rhoden W, Hasleton P, Brooks N: Anthracyclines and the heart. Br Heart J 1993;70:499

54. Hosenpud JD: Restrictive cardiomyopathy. p. 91. In: Zipes DP, Rowlands DJ (eds) Progress in Cardiology. Lea & Febiger, Philadelphia, 1989

55. Liao Y, Cooper RS, McGee DL, Mensah GA, Ghali JK: The relative effects of left ventricular hypertrophy, coronary artery disease, and ventricular dysfunction on survival black adults. JAMA 1995;273:1592

56. Bourassa MG, Gurne O, Bangdiwala SI et al: Natural history and patterns of current practice in heart failure. J Am Coll Cardiol, suppl. A 1993;22:14

57. Herman MV, Evans MD, Kay RH: Coronary heart disease and ventricular dysfunction in women. p. 198. In: Eaker ED, Packard B, Wenger NK, Clarkson TB, Tyroler HA (eds) Coronary Heart Disease in Women. Proceedings of an NIH Workshop. Haymarket Doyma, New York, 1987

58. DeMaria R, Gavazzi A, Recalcati F et al: Comparison of clinical findings in idiopathic dilated cardiomyopathy in women versus men. Am J Cardiol 1993;72:580

59. Hughes CV, Wong M, Johnson GJ, Cohn JN: Influence of age on mechanisms and prognosis of heart failure. Circulation, suppl. VI 1993;87:111

60. Deedwani PC: Prevalence and prognosis of heart failure. Cardiol Clin 1994;12:1

61. Kannel WB, Hjortland M, Castelli WP: Role of diabetes in congestive heart failure. The Framingham study. Am J Cardiol 1974;34:29

62. Fein FS, Sonnenblick EH: Diabetic cardiomyopathy. Cardiovasc Drugs Ther 1994;8:65

63. Ziesche S, Cobb FR, Cohn JN et al: Hydralazine and isosorbide dinitrate combination improves exercise tolerance in heart failure. Results from V-HeFT I and V-HeFT II. Circulation, suppl. VI 1993;87:56

64. Golper TA: Dialysis and hemofiltration for congestive heart failure. p. 568. In: Hosenpud JD, Greenberg BH (eds) Congestive Heart Failure. Pathophysiology, Diagnosis and Comprehensive Approach to Management. Springer-Verlag, New York, 1994

65. Canaud B, Cristol JP, Klouche K et al: Slow continuous ultrafiltration. A means of unmasking myocardial functional reserve in end-stage cardiac disease. Contrib Nephrol 1991;93:79

66. Stevenson WG, Stevenson LW, Middlekauff HR, Saxon LA: Sudden death prevention in patients with advanced ventricular dysfunction. Circulation 1993; 88:2953

67. Malone S, Liu PP, Holloway R et al: Obstructive sleep apnoea in patients with dilated cardiomyopathy. Ef-

fects of continuous positive airway pressure. Lancet 1991;338:1480

68. Cohn JN: Physiologic variables as markers for symptoms, risk, and interventions in heart failure. Circulation, suppl. VII 1993;87:110

69. Packer M, Carver JR, Rodeheffer RJ et al: Effects of oral milrinone on mortality in severe chronic heart failure. The Promise Study Research Group. N Engl J Med 1991;325:1468

70. Cruickshank JM: The xamoterol experience in the treatment of heart failure. Am J Cardiol 1993;71:61C

71. Hallstrom AL, Pratt CM, Greene HL et al: Relations between heart failure, ejection fraction, arrhythmia suppression and mortality. Analysis of the cardiac arrhythmia suppression trial. J Am Coll Cardiol 1995;25:1250

72. Goldman L, Hashimoto B, Cook EF, Loscalzo A: Comparative reproducibility and validity of systems for assessing cardiovascular functional class. Advantages of a new specific activity scale. Circulation 1981;64:1227

73. Smith RF, Johnson G, Ziesche S et al: Functional capacity in heart failure. Comparison of methods for assessment and their relations to other indexes of heart failure. Circulation, suppl. VI 1993;87:88

74. Cintron G, Johnson G, Francis G et al: Prognostic significance of serial changes in left ventricular ejection fraction in patients with congestive heart failure. Circulation, suppl. VI 1993;87:17

75. DiSalvo TG, Mathier M, Semigran MJ, Dec GW: Preserved right ventricular ejection fraction predicts exercise capacity and survival in advanced heart failure. J Am Coll Cardiol 1995;25:1143

76. Sullivan MJ, Hawthorne MH: Exercise intolerance in patients with chronic heart failure. Prog Cardiovasc Dis 1995;38:1

77. Pouler H, Rousseau MF, van Eyll C et al: Effects of long-term enalapril therapy on left ventricular diastolic properties in patients with depressed ejection fraction. Circulation 1993;88:481

78. Mancini DM, Eisen H, Kussmaul W et al: Value of peak exercise oxygen consumption for optimal timing of cardiac transplantation in ambulatory patients with heart failure. Circulation 1991;83:778

79. Committee on Evaluation and Management of Heart Failure: Guidelines for the evaluation and management of heart failure. Report of the American College of Cardiology/American Heart Association Task Force on Practice Guidelines. J Am Coll Cardiol 1995;26:1376

80. Roul G, Moulichon ME, Bareiss P et al: Exercise peak VO$_2$ determination in chronic heart failure. Is it still of value? Eur Heart J 1994;15:495

81. Lipkin DP, Scriven AJ, Crake T, Poole-Wilson PA: Six minute walking test for assessing exercise capacity in chronic heart failure. BMJ 1986;292:653

82. Sueta CA, Gheorghiade M, Adams KF et al: Safety and efficacy of epoprostenol in patients with severe congestive heart failure. Epoprostenol Multicenter Research Group. Am J Cardiol 1995;75:34A

83. Bittner V, Weiner DH, Yusuf S et al: Prediction of mortality and morbidity with a six-minute walk test in patients with left ventricular dysfunction. JAMA 1993;270:1702

84. Wilson JR, Schwartz S, Sutton MJ et al: Prognosis in severe heart failure. Relation to hemodynamic measurement and ventricular ectopic activity. J Am Coll Cardiol 1983;2:1403

85. Unverferth DV, Magorien RD, Moeschberger ML et al: Factors influencing the one-year mortality of dilated cardiomyopathy. Am J Cardiol 1984;54:147

86. Franciosa JA: Why patients with heart failure die. Hemodynamic and functional determinants of survival. Circulation, suppl. IV 1987;75:20

87. Lee WH, Packer M: Prognostic importance of serum sodium concentration and its modification by converting enzyme inhibition in patients with severe chronic heart failure. Circulation 1986;73:257

88. Hamilton MA, Stevenson LW, Luu M et al: Altered thyroid hormone metabolism in advanced heart failure. J Am Coll Cardiol 1990;16:91

89. Gilman JK, Jalal S, Naccarelli GV: Predicting and preventing sudden death from cardiac causes. Circulation 1994;90:1083

90. Bigger JT: Why patients with congestive heart failure die. Arrhythmias and sudden cardiac death. Circulation, suppl. IV 1987;75:28

91. Singh SN, Fletcher RD, Fisher SG et al: Amiodarone in patients with congestive heart failure and asymptomatic ventricular arrhythmia. N Engl J Med 1995;333:77

92. Just H, Drexler H, Taylor SH et al: Captopril versus digoxin in patients with coronary artery disease and mild heart failure. A prospective, double-blind, placebo-controlled multicenter study. Herz 1993;18(S1):436

93. Kowey PR, Taylor JE, Rials SJ: Does programmed stimulation really help in the evaluation of patients with nonsustained ventricular tachycardia? Results of a meta-analysis. Am Heart J 1992;123:481

94. Constatin L, Martins JB, Kienzle MG et al: Induced sustained ventricular tachycardia in nonischemic dilated cardiomyopathy. Dependence on clinical presentation and response to antiarrhythmic agents. PACE 1989;12:776

95. CABG Patch Trial Investigators and Coordinators: The coronary artery bypass graft (CABG) Patch Trial. Prog Cardiovasc Dis 1993;36:97

96. Baxton AE, Fisher JD, Josephson ME et al: Prevention of sudden death in patients with coronary artery disease. The multicenter unsustained tachycardia trial (MUSTT). Prog Cardiovasc Dis 1993;36:215

97. MADIT Executive Committee: Multicenter automatic defibrillator implantation trail (MADIT). Design and clinical protocol. PACE 1991;14:920

98. Middlekauf HR, Stevenson WG, Stevenson LW: Prognostic significance of atrial fibrillation in advanced heart failure. A study of 390 patients. Circulation 1991;84:40

99. Carson PE, Johnson GR, Dunkman B et al: The influence of atrial fibrillation on prognosis in mild to moderate heart failure. Circulation, suppl. VI 1993;87:102

100. Francis GS, Cohn JN, Johnson G, Rector et al: Plasma norepinephrine, plasma renin activity, and congestive heart failure. Relations to survival and the effects of therapy in V-HeFT II. Circulation, suppl. VI 1993;87:40

101. Remes J, Tikkanen I, Fyhrquist F et al: Neuroendocrine activity in untreated heart failure. Br Heart J 1991;65:249

102. Packer M, Lee WH, Kessler PD et al: Role of neuro-

hormonal mechanisms in determining survival in patients with severe chronic heart failure. Circulation, suppl. IV 1987;75:80

103. Cohn JN, Levine B, Olivari MT et al: Plasma norepinephrine as a guide to prognosis in patients with chronic congestive heart failure. N Engl J Med 1984; 311:819

104. Swedberg K, Eneroth P, Kjekshus J, Wilhelmsen L: Hormones regulating cardiovascular function in patients with severe congestive heart failure and their relation to mortality. Circulation 1990;82:1730

105. Greenberg BH, Quinones MA, Koilpillai C et al: Effects of long-term enalapril therapy on cardiac structure and function in patients with left ventricular dysfunction. Results of the SOLVD echocardiography substudy. Circulation 1995;91:2573

106. Hall C, Rouleau JL, Moye L et al: N-terminal pro-atrial natriuretic factor. An independent predictor of long-term prognosis after myocardial infarction. Circulation 1994;89:1934

107. Gottleib SS, Kukin ML, Ahern D et al: Prognostic importance of atrial natriuretic peptide in patients with chronic heart failure. J Am Coll Cardiol 1989; 13:1534

108. Koilpillai C, Quinones MA, Greenberg B et al: Relation of ventricular size and function to heart failure status and ventricular dysrhythnia in patients with severe left ventricular dysfunction. Am J Cardiol 1996;77:606

109. Wong M, Johnson G, Shabetai R et al: Echocardiographic variables as prognostic indicators and therapeutic monitors in chronic congestive heart failure. Circulation, suppl. VI 1993;87:65

110. Lee TH, Hamilton MA, Stevenson LW et al: Impact of left ventricular cavity size on survival in advanced heart failure. Am J Cardiol 1993;72:672

111. Tischler MD, Niggel J, Borowski DT et al: Relation between left ventricular shape and exercise capacity in patients with left ventricular dysfunction. J Am Coll Cardiol 1993;22:751

112. Swedberg K, Held P, Kjekshus J et al: Effects of the early administration of enalapril on mortality in patients with acute myocardial infarction. N Engl J Med 1992;327:678–684

113. Saul JP, Arai Y, Berger RD et al: Assessment of autonomic regulation in chronic congestive heart failure by heart rate spectral analysis. Am J Cardiol 1988; 61:1292

114. Ferguson DW: Sympathetic mechanisms in heart failure. Pathophysiological and pharmacological implications. Circulation, suppl. VII 1993;87:68

115. Binkley PF, Nunziata E, Haas GJ, Nelson SD, Cody RJ: Parasympathetic withdrawal is an integral component of autonomic imbalance in congestive heart failure. Demonstration in human subjects and verification in a paced canine model of ventricular failure. J Am Coll Cardiol 1991;18:464

116. Kuchar DL, Thorburn CW, Sammel NL: Prediction of serious arrhythmic events after myocardial infarction. Signal averaged electrocardiogram, Holter monitoring and radionuclide ventriculography. J Am Coll Cardiol 1987;9:531

117. Frey B, Heinz G, Binder T et al. Diurnal variation of ventricular response to atrial fibrillation in patients with advanced heart failure. Am Heart J 1995;129: 58

118. Mancini DM, Wong KL, Simson MB: Prognostic value of an abnormal signal-averaged electrocardiogram in patients with non-ischemic congestive cardiomyopathy. Circulation 1993;87:1083

119. Yi G, Keeling PJ, Goldman JF et al: Prognostic significance of spectral turbulence analysis of the signal averaged electrocardiogram in patients with idiopathic dilated cardiomyopathy. Am J Cardiol 1995; 75:494

120. Hare JM, Walford GD, Hruban RH et al: Ischemic cardiomyopathy. Endomyocardial biopsy and ventriculographic evaluation of patients with congestive heart failure, dilated cardiomyopathy and coronary artery disease. J Am Coll Cardiol 1992;20:1318–1325

121. Yamada T, Fukunami M, Ohmori M et al: Which subgroup of patients with dilated cardiomyopathy would benefit from long-term beta-blocker therapy? J Am Coll Cardiol 1993;21:628–633

122. SOLVD Investigators. Effect of enalapril on mortality and the development of heart failure in asymptomatic patients with reduced left ventricular ejection fractions. N Engl J Med 1992;327:685

123. Steffen HM: Amlodipine in heart failure. Initial results of the PRAISE study. Herz, suppl. 2 1995;20:3

124. Waagstein F, Bristow MR, Swedberg K et al: Beneficial effects of metoprolol in ideopathic dilated cardiomyopathy. Lancet 1993;342:1441

31 Role of Exercise Testing

Theresa A. McDonagh
Henry J. Dargie

The syndrome of heart failure is officially defined, in pathophysiologic language, as failure of the heart to pump blood at a rate commensurate with the requirements of the metabolizing tissues or to do so only from an increased filling pressure.[1] This definition alludes to the fact that the central pump responds to the needs of the tissues principally in their requirement for oxygen. Consequently, the hemodynamics of pump malfunction in heart failure are more pronounced on exercise. The cardiac response to exercise therefore is in some ways fundamental to the pathophysiologic dissection of chronic heart failure (CHF).

The clinician requires a more pragmatic approach. In practice "heart failure" is diagnosed when the symptoms of dyspnea and fatigue and signs of fluid retention occur in a patient with demonstrable cardiac dysfunction. That dysfunction is most commonly left ventricular in origin, in particular left ventricular (LV) systolic dysfunction. Moreover, we are now aware that in many cases the syndrome of CHF is the end-stage of progressive deterioration in LV function that may remain asymptomatic for years. Essentially, CHF is symptomatic LV dysfunction (LVD), but it has an occult precursor: asymptomatic LVD.

The cardinal symptoms of CHF—breathlessness and muscle fatigue—occur at least initially on exertion. Therefore exercise testing is as valuable for the clinician as it is for the physiologist for the diagnosis and assessment of this condition.

OXYGEN UPTAKE AND LVD

The best indicator of aerobic capacity, the maximal oxygen uptake ($\dot{V}O_2$ max), measured during incremental cardiopulmonary exercise testing, is reduced in subjects with symptomatic LVD. However, a true maximal oxygen uptake, where the work rate of the subject increases despite a plateau in oxygen consumption, is rarely achieved in heart failure subjects[2] (as they generally stop prior to this point because of muscle fatigue or breathlessness). Hence the peak oxygen uptake is more usually cited. Peak oxygen uptake, similarly reduced in subjects with symptomatic LVD, reflects the severity of symptoms and is reproducible.[3] Of other parameters that can be measured during cardiopulmonary exercise testing, the extrapolated maximum oxygen consumption has been shown to be more reliable than the anaerobic threshold or the ventilation–carbon dioxide slope, and is independent of effort, provided that patients are encouraged to exercise to a point where their respiratory gas exchange ratio exceeds 1.0.[4]

Not only is the peak oxygen uptake reduced in symptomatic LVD, it is also diminished in asymptomatic LVD. Data from the prevention arm of the SOLVD trial show that asymptomatic patients, on no cardiac medication and who had left ventricular ejection fractions of 35 percent or less had a significantly reduced peak $\dot{V}O_2$ compared to controls[5] (Fig. 31-1). Indeed, the mean exercise duration in subjects with ASLVD was 291 seconds, nearly 5 minutes less than normal age- and sex-matched controls.

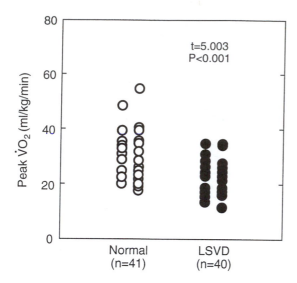

Fig. 31-1. Plot of peak oxygen uptake ($\dot{V}O_2$) reached during maximal graded exercise on a treadmill using a modified Naughton protocol by normal subjects and asymptomatic patients with an LVEF ≤ 35 percent (from the SOLVD prevention study).

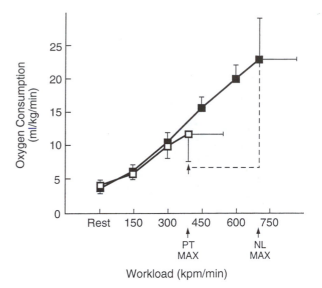

Fig. 31-2. Plot of rest and exercise oxygen consumption in 7 patients (□) and 10 normal (■) subjects. $P < 0.01$ by Student's unpaired t-test. MAX, maximal workload. (From Kitzman et al.,[8] with permission.)

Chronic heart failure can also be caused by diastolic dysfunction, where the left ventricle fails to relax. This disorder is less well studied than systolic dysfunction but is thought to account for 30 to 40 percent of all CHF, becoming increasingly prevalent with advancing age and found more frequently in those with preexisting systemic hypertension.[6,7] Exercise capacity is also reduced with diastolic heart failure. Kitzman and colleagues studied subjects who had at least one episode of symptomatic heart failure whose LV systolic function was preserved. They found that these patients had a diminished peak VO_2 compared to normal controls[8] (Fig. 31-2).

Exercise testing, therefore, appears to be useful for evaluating heart failure, be it symptomatic or asymptomatic or due to systolic or diastolic dysfunction. There are some drawbacks, however, that must be borne in mind when considering its role in the assessment of CHF. They relate to the poor correlation between measures of exercise capacity and other commonly used methods for classifying CHF.

RELATION BETWEEN MEASURES OF EFFORT CAPACITY AND OTHER MARKERS OF CHF

To begin with there is a poor correlation between exercise variables and the New York Heart Association (NYHA) Classification.[9] In addition, there is at best only a weak relation between resting hemodynamic measures of LV function (cardiac index, pulmonary capillary wedge pressure, angiographic ejection fraction) and measures of exercise performance.[10] Finally, there is essentially no relation between commonly used resting echocardiographic methods of determining LV function (LV ejection fraction, LV end-diastolic dimension) and exercise capacity.[3]

The often poor relation between measures of LV function and effort capacity in LVD is hardly surprising, as many factors other than central pump function affect exercise capacity in heart failure subjects. We know that CHF subjects have an abnormal ventilatory response to exercise with an increase in dead-space ventilation.[11] There are also changes in the periphery, with alteration in skeletal muscle biochemistry leading to early acidosis on exercise testing.[12] Effects of secondary physical deconditioning cause changes in skeletal muscle morphology.[13,14] Nutritive flow is impaired and the peripheral vascular resistance increased.[15]

Despite these drawbacks, maximal or peak oxygen uptake measured from an incremental exercise protocol is widely accepted to be the best measure of the severity of CHF. Although resting LV function measurements do not equate with exercise parameters, functional classifications of maximum oxygen uptake do correlate well with exercise hemodynamic measures of LV function. Weber and Janicki have classified heart failure subjects into four categories

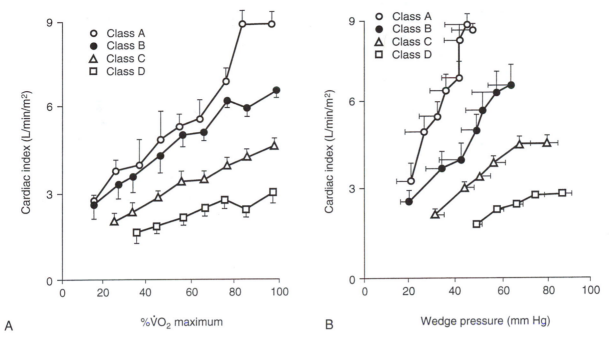

Fig. 31-3. (A) Relation of $\dot{V}O_2$ expressed as a percentage of maximum and cardiac index represented by classes (A to D). See text. Values are ± SEM. **(B)** Relation between resting and exercise cardiac output and pulmonary artery capillary wedge pressure, represented by classes A to D. See text. Values are ± SEM.

based on maximal oxygen uptake[16] (Fig. 31-3). They found that on exercise testing these categories had a good correlation with cardiac index and wedge pressure. The poorest oxygen consumption category had a blunted increase in cardiac index with exercise compared to those with less impairment of aerobic capacity, and the severest group had a higher wedge pressure at peak exercise compared to those groups with superior oxygen uptake. Hence oxygen uptake is useful for grading the severity of CHF.

Exercise testing therefore does have a diagnostic role in evaluating and clarifying symptoms of CHF and grading its severity. It can be done by measuring either maximal (or peak) oxygen uptake or exercise duration, provided that with the exercise protocol used the exercise duration adequately reflects oxygen consumption.

The correlation between exercise duration and oxygen consumption varies among exercise protocols. Figure 31-4 shows oxygen consumption plotted against exercise duration in both normal volunteers and CHF subjects using the standardized exponential exercise protocol (STEEP). It demonstrates a good linear relation between the values for both normals and CHF subjects. Using such a protocol it would be possible to take exercise duration as a surrogate for peak oxygen uptake.[17]

ROLE IN GRADING PROGNOSIS

Exercise testing also has a role in grading the prognosis of heart failure. The poorer survival of CHF subjects who have reduced effort tolerance on exercise testing has been confirmed by some of the larger heart failure treatment trials. In both of the VE Heft trials, with a total of more than 1400 men, maximum oxygen consumption and exercise duration were independent predictors of mortality for up to 5 years of follow-up.[18]

ROLE IN ASSESSING THE ETIOLOGY OF LVD

It must always be remembered that heart failure is not a diagnosis per se but a syndrome consisting of symptoms and signs ultimately attributable to cardiac dysfunction. That dysfunction can, of course be myocardial, valvular, endocardial, or pericardial in origin. The subsequent management depends on the etiology of the CHF. Therefore a cause should always be sought. Exercise testing has an obvious role in the assessment of the main etiologic factor in LVD, ischemic heart disease (IHD).

As well as guiding medical management of ongoing

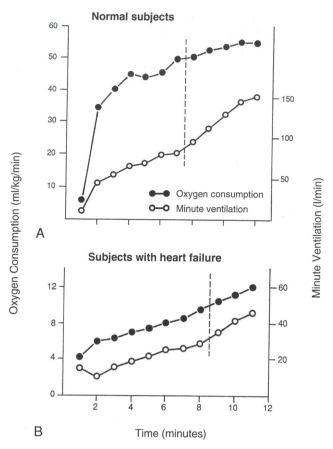

Fig. 31-4. Peak oxygen consumption (●) and minute ventilation (○) in normal subjects (**A**) and CHF subjects (**B**) during a graded maximum exercise test using the STEEP protocol.

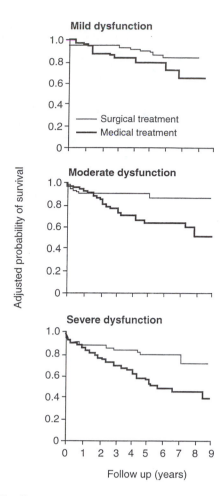

Fig. 31-5. Comparison of survival among patients with mild, moderate, and severe left ventricular dysfunction (left ventricular ejection fraction 38, 32, and 24 percent, respectively) who were treated medically or by coronary artery bypass grafting.

myocardial ischemia, exercise testing is helpful for detecting patients who would benefit from revascularization surgery. Bounous and colleagues demonstrated that in subjects with LVD—whether the LVD is mild, moderate, or severe—who have severe coronary artery disease, there is a survival benefit to be gained from revascularization surgery compared to medical management in over 9 years of follow-up[19] (Fig. 31-5). Other abnormalities discovered on exercise testing, such as arrhythmias, may be amenable to therapy, and exercise testing may be useful for this purpose as well as predicting the likelihood of sudden death.

ROLE IN PREDICTING TRANSPLANTATION

Exercise testing is finding an increasing role in determining the need for and assessing the timing of cardiac transplantation. Roul and colleagues who studied 75 subjects with CHF in NYHA categories II and III, found that those who had a peak oxygen uptake of ≤ 14 ml·kg^{-1}·min have a significantly increased mortality[20] (Fig. 31-6). The figure of 14 ml·kg^{-1}·min has been suggested by Mancini et al. as one at which cardiac transplantation should at least be considered.[21]

Although in this study peak oxygen consumption was the best predictor of mortality, exercise duration also correlated with death. The authors suggested that patients could be followed by exercise duration provided the exercise protocol satisfactorily reflected oxygen consumption.

Other parameters measured during standard exercise testing can also predict a poor outlook. Balk and coworkers followed 109 CHF subjects for whom it was considered too early for cardiac transplantation.[22] They found that failure to increase the systolic blood pressure by at least 20 mmHg on exercise predicted increased mortality and greater risk of clinical

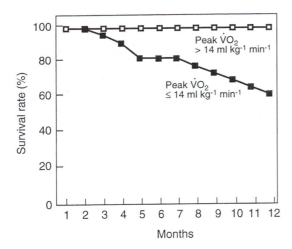

Fig. 31-6. Survival curves: exercise peak $\dot{V}O_2$ threshold value 14 ml·kg^{-1}·min^{-1}.

deterioration. These patients require careful medical supervision and perhaps reversal of the decision to defer transplantation.

ROLE IN ASSESSING RESPONSE TO DRUG THERAPY

One would imagine that exercise testing might be useful for assessing the CHF patient's response to drug therapy. It has proved, however, to be of limited value in individual patients because of the large day-to-day variation in their effort capacity. It has an accepted role in evaluating drug therapy for CHF in clinical trials by measuring functional capacity or peak oxygen consumption as objective markers of CHF severity. Similar problems have been encountered in clinical trials with the large variation in response within the patient population. This subject is clearly huge, but suffice it to say that one of the drawbacks is that improvements in exercise times have not correlated well with improvements in survival. Angiotensin-converting enzyme (ACE) inhibitors have a modest effect on effort capacity but improve survival, whereas some trial drugs that have increased effort capacity have been associated with increased mortality.

PRESCRIPTIVE ROLE OF EXERCISE TESTING

Exercise testing does have some prescriptive role in CHF. We know that secondary physical deconditioning may contribute to altered skeletal muscle function in CHF and that exercise training can reverse some of the abnormalities and increase exercise performance.[23] Exercise testing can distinguish those who can enter an exercise training program safely.

CONCLUSION

Exercise testing is of use for evaluating symptoms of CHF, grading its severity, and predicting prognosis. It is valuable for determining the need and timing of cardiac transplantation, assessing the etiology of LVD, and determining the need for revascularization. It also has a role in judging the safety of prescribed exercise. It is only of limited use in assessing the response to drug therapy in individuals, and it has no role in the assessment of acute heart failure or that secondary to critical obstructive valve disease, where it is contraindicated.

REFERENCES

1. Braunwald E, Grossman W: Clinical aspects of heart failure. p. 444. In Braunwald E (ed): Heart Disease. 4th Ed. WB Saunders, Philadelphia, 1992
2. Lipkin DP, Perrins J, Poole-Wilson PA: Respiratory gas exchange in the assessment of patients with impaired ventricular function. Br Heart J 1985;54: 321–328
3. Weber KT, Wilson JR, Janicki J, Likoff MJ: Exercise testing in the evaluation of the patient with chronic cardiac failure. Am Rev Respir Dis, suppl. 1984;129: 60–62
4. Clark AL, Poole-Wilson PA, Coats AJS: Effects of motivation of the patient on indices of exercise capacity in chronic heart failure. Br Heart J 1994;71:162–165
5. Le Jemtel TH, Chang-seng L, Stewart DK et al: Reduced peak aerobic capacity in ventricular systolic dysfunction. Circulation 1994;90:2757–2760
6. Dougherty AH, Naccarelli GV, Gray EL, Hicks CH, Goldstein RA: Congestive heart failure with normal systolic function. Am J Cardiol 1984;54:778–782
7. Soufer R, Wohlgelertner D, Vita NA et al: Intact systolic left ventricular function in clinical congestive heart failure. Am J Cardiol 1985;55:1032–1036
8. Kitzman DW, Higginbotham MB, Cobb FR, Sheikh KH, Sullivan MJ: Exercise intolerance in patients with heart failure and preserved left ventricular systolic function. Failure of the Frank-Starling mechanism. J Am Coll Cardiol 1991;17:1065–1072
9. Franciosa JA: Functional capacity of patients with chronic left ventricular failure. Relationship of bicycle performance to clinical and haemodynamic characterisation. Am J Med 1979;67:460–466
10. Franciosa JA, Park M, Levine TB: Lack of correlation between exercise capacity and indexes of resting left ventricular performance in heart failure. Am J Cardiol 1981;47:33–39
11. Sullivan MJ, Higginbotham MB, Cobb FR: Increased exercise ventilation in patients with chronic cardiac

failure. Intact ventilatory control despite haemodynamic and pulmonary abnormalities. Circulation 1988;86:552–559

12. Wilson JR, Fink L, Maris J et al: Evaluation of energy metabolism in skeletal muscle of patients with heart failure with gated phosphorus-31 nuclear magnetic resonance. Circulation 1985;71:57–62

13. Mancini DM, Walter G, Reichek N et al: Contribution of skeletal muscle atrophy to exercise intolerance and altered muscle metabolism in heart failure. Circulation 1992;85:1364–1373

14. Wilson JR, Mancini DM, Dunkman B: Exertional fatigue due to intrinsic skeletal muscle dysfunction in patients with heart failure [abstract]. Circulation 1992;86:2045

15. Zelis R, Longhurst J, Capone RJ, Mason DT: A comparison of regional blood flow and oxygen utilisation during dynamic forearm exercise in normal subjects and in patients with congestive cardiac failure. Circulation 1974;50:137–143

16. Weber KT, Janicki JS: Cardiopulmonary exercise testing for evaluation of chronic cardiac failure. Am J Cardiol 1985;55:22A–31A

17. Riley M, Northridge DB, Henderson E et al: The use of an exponential protocol for bicycle and treadmill exercise testing in patients with chronic cardiac failure. Eur Heart J 1992;13:1363–1367

18. Cohn JN, Johnson GR, Shabetai R et al: Ejection fraction, peak exercise oxygen consumption, cardiothoracic ratio, ventricular arrhythmias, and plasma norepinephrine as determinants of prognosis in heart failure. Circulation, suppl. VI 1993;87:5–16

19. Bounous EP, Mark DB, Pollock BG et al: Surgical survival benefits for coronary disease patients with left ventricular dysfunction. Circulation, suppl. I 1988;78:1151–1157

20. Roul G, Moulichin ME, Bareiss P et al: Exercise peak VO_2 determination in chronic cardiac failure. Is it still of value. Eur Heart J 1994;15:495–502

21. Mancini DM, Eisen H, Kussmaul W, Mull R, Edmunds LH: Value of peak oxygen consumption for optimal timing of cardiac transplantation in ambulatory patients with heart failure. Circulation 1991;84:778–786

22. Balk AHMM, Simoons ML, Meeter K et al: Too early for cardiac transplantation—the right decision? Eur Heart J 1992;13:1339–1344

23. Coats AJS, Adamopoulos S, Radaelli A et al: Controlled trial of physical training in chronic heart failure. Exercise performance, haemodynamics, ventilation and autonomic function. Circulation 1992;85:2119–2131

32 Role of Echocardiography in the Diagnosis and Treatment of Cardiomyopathies

Susan E. Wiegers
Ted Plappert
Martin G. St. John Sutton

Echocardiography has been a primary tool in understanding the natural history of the cardiomyopathies and their response to therapeutic interventions. The noninvasive nature of these studies has allowed repeated assessments for serial follow-up, which are impractical with other techniques. A sophisticated understanding of echocardiographic methods is required to appreciate echocardiography's role in the classification of cardiomyopathies. Many advances in this field have been driven by advances in echocardiographic instrumentation and analysis. Were such a reliable, reproducible, and essentially risk-free technique not available, many clinical trials such as SAVE, CONSENSUS, and SOLVD could not have produced such important results.

ECHOCARDIOGRAPHIC ASSESSMENT OF LEFT VENTRICULAR ANATOMY AND FUNCTION

Left Ventricular Mass

One of the first uses of echocardiography was the measurement of left ventricular mass. Figure 32-1 demonstrates the M-mode study of a patient with dilated cardiomyopathy. The standard measurements of the left ventricle during diastole are performed by the "leading edge" method defined by the

American Society of Echocardiography.[1] Left ventricular mass (LVM) is defined by the equation:

$$LVM = 1.04 \, ([LVID + PWT + IVST]^3 - LVID^3) - 14 \text{ g}$$

where LVM is the left ventricular mass, LVID is the left ventricular internal dimension during diastole, PWT is the posterior wall thickness, and IVST is the interventricular septal thickness.[2] Left ventricular mass can be indexed to body surface area and has been shown to correlate with electrocardiographic (ECG) signs of left ventricular hypertrophy.[3,4]

The relation of the posterior wall thickness to the left ventricular internal diameter during diastole defines the four types of left ventricular hypertrophy. Relative wall thickness is given by the equation:

$$RWT = 2 \times PWT/LVID$$

Concentric hypertrophy describes thickening of the walls without dilatation of the cavity and is defined as a relative wall thickness of 45 percent or more. *Eccentric hypertrophy* is accompanied by cavity dilatation, defined as a relative wall thickness of less than 45 percent with a left ventricular diastolic diameter index greater than the normal value (3.2 cm/m^2 for women and 3.1 cm/m^2 for men).[4] *Eccentric nondilated hypertrophy* refers to a relative wall thickness of less than 45 percent with a normal left

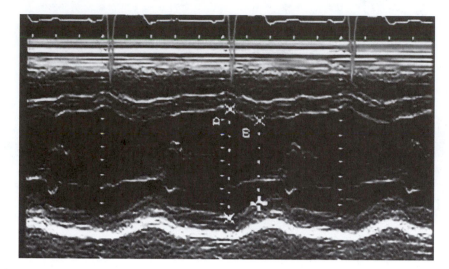

Fig. 32-1. M-mode echocardiogram in the parasternal long axis of a patient with dilated cardiomyopathy. The left ventricular internal dimensions have been measured on-line and have been marked A (diastole) and B (systole). Both dimensions are severely abnormal, consistent with a significantly dilated ventricle and decreased fractional shortening.

ventricular diameter index. The first three categories in particular have been used extensively for defining the response of the left ventricle to volume and pressure overload, although alternate classifications have been suggested.[5] *Disproportionate septal hypertrophy* occurs with a septal wall/posterior wall thickness ratio of 1.3 or more.

Systolic Function

The ability of echocardiography to assess left ventricular function is fundamental to its importance as a diagnostic tool.

LEFT VENTRICULAR VOLUME AND EJECTION FRACTION

Single Plane Methods

The left ventricular ejection fraction was shown to be correlated with the M-mode-derived fractional shortening by:

$$FS = LVIDD - LVIDS/LVIDD$$

where LVIDD is the left ventricular internal diameter during diastole, and LVIDS is the left ventricular internal diameter during systole.[6] The use of fractional shortening as an estimate of left ventricular ejection fraction has been limited by failure to account for asymmetric contraction. In addition, it is difficult to ascertain whether measurements are taken along the largest "minor axis" in dilated and globular hearts.[7,8]

Two-dimensional echocardiography allows a clearer definition of ventricular structure and function, particularly in the asymmetrically contracting ventricle. Fractional area change is similar to the fractional shortening and is defined as:

$$FAC = LVAD - LVAS/LVAD$$

where FAC is the fractional area change, LVAD is the area of the left ventricle in diastole, usually taken in the parasternal short axis at the midpapillary level, and LVAS is the area of the left ventricle during systole (Fig. 32-2). Fractional area change from short-axis views correlates with ejection fraction obtained with nuclear or cine angiography.[9] The disadvantage is that information from only a single view is used. Therefore asymmetrically contracting ventricles cannot be appropriately assessed with this method.

Many schemes developed for cine ventriculograms were applied to two-dimensional images in order to calculate volumes and ejection fractions. These methods rely on constructing a model of the left ventricle from various geometric shapes and summing the calculated volumes. Single plane area–length methods (Fig. 32-3) using an apical view have been shown to correlate with left ventricular cavity volumes determined by cine or nuclear angiography[10,11] as well as anatomically measured volumes.[12]

All of the quantitative assessments of left ventricular volume and ejection fraction have required off-line digitization of echocardiographic images, which

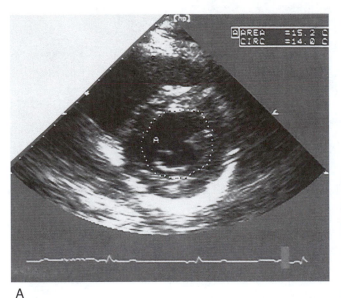
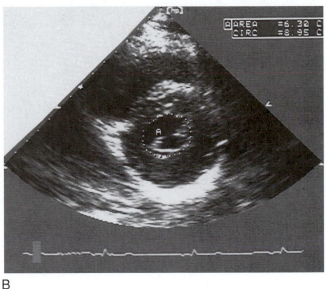

A   B

Fig. 32-2. Two-dimensional echocardiograms of the parasternal short axis have been digitized off-line to obtain the left ventricular area (A) during diastole **(A)** and systole **(B)**. By convention, the papillary muscles have been included in the left ventricular cavity. The fractional area change (FAC) is calculated by the equation: 15.2 cm^2 − 6.3 cm^2 / 15.2 cm^2. It equals 59 percent, a normal value.

is time-consuming, labor-intensive, and requires additional equipment, such as a computer interface. Therefore attempts to base left ventricular volume estimates on axis measurements alone have been reported but are not as reproducible as techniques described below.[9,13] Systolic excursion of the mitral annulus can be correlated with ejection fraction by other techniques.[14,15] Its advantage is that no digitization is required. However, the method assumes that mitral annular motion is parallel to the long axis of the ultrasound beam and is useful only in ventricles without wall motion abnormalities, which limits its application.

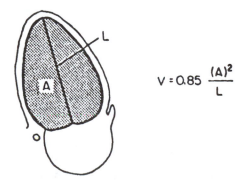

Fig. 32-3. Single-area length method for calculating left ventricular volume (V). The area (A) of the left ventricular cavity is digitized in an apical view, the long axis length (L) is measured as well. (From Schiller,[18] with permission.)

Biplane and Three-Dimensional Methods

The modified Simpson's rule or, more correctly, the summation of disks method requires digitization of two orthogonal apical views and computation off-line of Simpson's algorithm for determination of volumes (Fig. 32-4).[16–19] This is the two-dimensional method recommended by the American Society of Echocardiography. Although the method systematically underestimates cine volumes, the correlation with cine-determined ejection fractions shows improved correlation. The summation of disks method assumes that the imaging planes are orthogonal and is absolutely dependent on detection of the endocardial border and therefore on image quality of the echocardiogram. The off-line digitization should be performed by an experienced observer and the results averaged over several cycles. It has been recommended that serial measurements on a single patient be made by the same person because interobserver variability and beat-to-beat variability can be significant.[20] Intravenous injection of contrast agents, such as sonicated albumin, that pass through the pulmonary circulation have been used to provide enhanced imaging of the endocardial border. This method has not reached widespread clinical use because of the cost and the unpredictable opacification of the left ventricle.[21] The "eyeball" method of visually assessing the left ventricular ejection fraction is still the most widely used in clinical laboratories. Estimates by experienced observers compare favorably with both cine and nuclear ventriculography.[22,23]

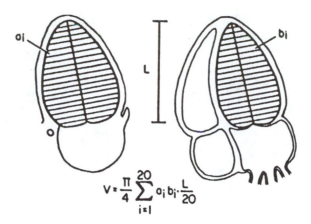

$$V = \frac{\pi}{4} \sum_{i=1}^{20} a_i b_i \cdot \frac{L}{20}$$

Fig. 32-4. Summation of disks method (modified Simpson's rule) for calculation of left ventricular volume (V) based on two nearly orthogonal planes from the apical two- and four-chamber views. Calculation of the volume results from summation of areas from diameters a_i and b_i of 20 equal disks. They are apportioned by dividing the left ventricle's longest length into 20 equal sections. (From Schiller,[18] with permission.)

The development of automated border detection has allowed on-line analysis of left ventricular volume and ejection fraction.[24–26] Commercially available systems process acoustic data and the integrated backscatter characteristics of the reflected ultrasound frequency to differentiate blood from tissue (Plate 32-1). The technique is dependent on acceptable image quality, visualization of 75 percent of the endocardium, and gain settings.[27] A region of interest must be identified by the sonographer. Respiratory motion and vigorous mitral annular apical displacement during systole may move part of the endocardium outside the region of interest during part of the cardiac cycle. Lateral gain control improves endocardial border detection.[25] Volumes calculated with this method underestimate manually digitized areas, predominantly because the papillary muscles are excluded by the automatic border detection but are included in the cavity area by American Society of Echocardiography conventions.[28] Although initial reports found an excellent correlation between cavity areas calculated on-line by automated border detection and those digitized off-line, fractional area change has a poorer correlation.[26] Application of the method to patients with a variety of cardiac diseases resulted in lower correlation coefficients.[29] Although the method is promising, comparison of on-line measurements of ejection fraction with radionuclide angiography[27,30,31] and cine ventriculography[24] show acceptable correlation in normal controls, but patients with regional asynergy are problematic.

Adequate images could be obtained in only 48–75 percent of patients. Automated border detection has been applied to transesophageal images with improvement in the percent of patients with acceptable tracking of the myocardium because of improved image quality. However, correlation with off-line digitized cross-sectional areas has still been modest.[32,33] Demonstration of the true ventricular long axis is not always possible with the transesophageal approach. In addition, this invasive procedure has been demonstrated to increase left ventricular ejection fraction in conscious patients.[34]

Three-dimensional echocardiographic reconstruction[35–38] as well as intracardiac ultrasonography[39] hold promise for future developments. Data suggest that three-dimensional reconstruction of volumes may be more accurate and contain less systematic error than two-dimensional measurements, particularly in ventricles with asymmetric contraction patterns.[36,40]

DOPPLER ASSESSMENTS OF SYSTOLIC FUNCTION

Ejection phase indices, such as ejection fraction, are load-dependent. Therefore a change in ejection fraction may not be due to a change in the intrinsic contractility of the myocardium. Doppler echocardiography can evaluate indices of the isovolumic contraction phase of the cardiac cycle, which may be more representative of the contractile state. The change in left ventricular pressure over time (dP/dt) and the maximum rate of the pressure change (dP/dtmax) classically have been measured during cardiac catheterization. When mitral regurgitation is present, which is frequently the case in cardiomyopathy, continuous-wave Doppler echocardiography measures the instantaneous velocity of mitral regurgitation throughout systole. The velocity spectra can be converted via the modified Bernouilli equation to a measurement of instantaneous pressure gradient change and its change during systole (Fig. 32-5). Assuming any change in left atrial pressure during systole has a negligible effect on this pressure gradient, a plot of left ventricular dP/dt can be generated from the first derivative of the pressure gradient plot.[41,42] Correlation with invasive measurements has been good in both patient[42] and animal[43] studies. Calculation of the mean rate of change in pressure between 4 and 36 mmHg (corresponding to 1 and 3 m/s, respectively) correlates with invasive dP/dt measurements but systematically underestimates dP/dtmax.[43–45] It is well established from hemody-

namic data that dP/dt is sensitive to both preload and heart rate, making it less attractive as a measure of intrinsic contractility.[46,47] Similarly, an abnormal contraction pattern resulting in a prolonged QRS interval reduces peak dP/dt without necessarily effecting a change in contractility.[48] This may limit the use of this technique even in serial studies in the same patient if drugs used for treatment alter QRS duration.

WALL STRESS

Attempts to define load-independent measures of inotropic state have been based on the relation of end-systolic wall stress to the ejection indices of fractional shortening, velocity of circumferential shortening, ejection, fraction, end-systolic fiber length, or end-systolic volume.[49–53] The theoretic basis for the load independence of these measurements is the linear association between end-systolic pressure and end-systolic volume, otherwise known as elastance.[54–57]

End-systolic pressure may be estimated noninvasively by relating brachial systolic and diastolic pressure to the waveform of carotid pulse tracings obtained using applanation tonometry. End-systole is assigned to the dicrotic notch, and the end-systolic pressure is interpolated.[58] Whereas meridional wall stress may be calculated from M-mode and two-dimensional short-axis data, the more physiologically important load, circumferential stress, requires long-axis information.[59] Circumferential stress has been shown to differ from meridional stress in conditions such as aortic stenosis.[60] A normal meridional stress but an increased circumferential end-systolic stress implies excess afterload as the cause for depressed systolic function. On-line pressure–volume relation may be calculated using the technique of automatic border detection to determine left ventricular volume from two-dimensional short-axis areas but requires the measurement of left ventricular pressure or the use of peak systolic pressure.[61,62] Transesophageal echocardiography has been useful for assessing of contractility during cardiac surgery,[63,64] during exercise,[65,66] and with a variety of other conditions.[67,68]

Diastolic Function

Defining diastolic dysfunction is more difficult than assessing systolic function. Diastole results from a complex interaction of active relaxation of the myocardium and passive properties, or compliance of the ventricle. Many measurements and methods have

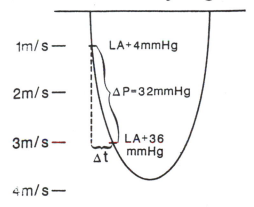

$$LV \quad \frac{\Delta P}{\Delta t} = \frac{32 mmHg}{\Delta t \text{ in sec}}$$

Fig. 32-5. Method of calculating Doppler-derived pressure gradient against time. Time taken for mitral regurgitant velocity signal to rise from 1 to 3 m/s is measured, which would correspond to the change in left ventricular pressure from left atrial (LA) pressure +4 mmHg to LA pressure +36 mmHg. Assuming LA pressure does not change significantly during this time, it amounts to an increase in LV pressure by 32 mmHg. A graph of LV pressure against time can be constructed from the mitral valve velocity profile by similarly applying the modified Bernouilli equation to every point. The slope of this derived function would represent dP/dt at any time during systole. (From Pai et al.,[44] with permission.)

been advocated, but none has gained widespread applicability. The difficulty of reconciling many of these measurements is the result of their differing load and heart rate dependencies.

MITRAL INFLOW PATTERNS

Transmitral Doppler inflow patterns are assessed in most routine clinical studies (Fig. 32-6). By convention, the pattern is recorded at the tips of the mitral valve leaflets. The E wave of the inflow pattern is caused by early passive ventricular filling and is dependent on the pressure gradient between the left atrium and the left ventricle when the mitral valve opens. The A wave is the result of additional flow caused by atrial contraction at the end of ventricular diastole. The E wave/A wave (E/A) ratio can be calculated using peak velocities or velocity time integrals. Measurements can be easily made on-line with good reproducibility.[69] In a normal heart, the E wave velocity–time integral is larger than the A wave velocity–time integral because atrial systole contributes the minor portion of left ventricular filling. However, a complicated relation exists between atrial pressure, ventricular relaxation time, ventricular compliance, systolic function, and the Doppler filling indices.[70,71] An increase in left atrial pressure raises the gradient between atrium and ventricle at mitral valve opening. The resulting E wave velocity is higher, and the acceleration and deceleration slopes increase. Conversely, a decrease in ventricular relaxation (as manifested by an increase in the isovolumic relaxation time constant) results in a lower peak E velocity with slower acceleration and deceleration rates but no significant change in the velocity–time integral.[70,72] The relation is complicated by the fact that an increase in preload causes a higher left atrial pressure and so increases the gradient between the atrium and ventricle. The result is an increase in early filling manifested by a larger velocity–time integral of the E wave. However, systolic dysfunction also raises the left atrial pressure but without a similar increase in gradient or E wave.[73]

The original Doppler pattern found to be related to diastolic dysfunction was E/A reversal in which the atrial contribution to ventricular filling is more significant than early filling (Fig. 32-6B). However, heart rate and PR interval are both inversely associated with the E/A ratio.[74,75] Aging influences Doppler inflow patterns with an increase in the atrial contribution to filling and a decrease in the E/A wave ratio.[75–77] This may be due to an age-related increase in fibrous tissue and resultant decrease in compliance. The left lateral decubitus position can also influence the E/A ratio.[78] These factors along with the

dependence of the E wave height on preload make serial comparisons of diastolic indices problematic. An observed change in parameters may reflect only a difference in heart rate or loading conditions rather than a change in intrinsic diastolic function.

A second Doppler flow pattern of diastolic dysfunction is characterized by a tall E wave with a steep deceleration slope and a small A wave.[79] Restrictive cardiomyopathy with a high left atrial pressure and short isovolumic relaxation time produces this pattern, sometimes referred to as "pseudonormalization" (Fig. 32-6C). This pattern has been demonstrated in ischemic cardiomyopathy[80,81], as well as constrictive pericarditis and restrictive cardiomyopathy.[82] The restrictive pattern of diastolic dysfunction is also associated with more severe systolic dysfunction in dilated cardiomyopathy.[83] With cardiac amyloidosis, early involvement is often accompanied by a typical diastolic dysfunction mitral inflow pattern. However, this pattern evolves to one of restriction as the disease progresses.[84–86] A short mitral deceleration time predicts a poor prognosis in restrictive diseases.[87]

PULMONARY VENOUS FLOW PATTERNS

Figure 32-7 demonstrates the pulmonary venous velocities measured by Doppler echocardiography with concurrent ECG and mitral inflow velocity patterns. Translating velocity patterns into "flow" determinations assumes that the dimensions of the pulmonary veins remain constant throughout the cardiac cycle, which may not be the case.[88] The systolic filling wave corresponds to the x descent in the left atrial pressure tracing and may be the result of atrial relaxation after atrial systole and the "suction" effect achieved by apical descent of the mitral annulus during ventricular contraction. During early ventricular diastole the left atrium serves as an open conduit. The pulmonary venous diastolic wave correlates closely with the E wave of the mitral valve inflow pattern.[89] Normal atrial contraction causes reversal of flow in the pulmonary veins during late diastole. Some studies have shown dependence of the velocity of flow reversal on left ventricular diastolic pressure,[90] but others have not.[89]

An effect of aging similar to the change in mitral valve inflow patterns has been demonstrated on pulmonary venous flow velocity signals. The decrease in the E wave correlates with an increase in the pulmonary venous systolic flow and a decrease in diastolic flow.[77] Conversely, a decrease in pulmonary venous systolic flow velocity may be seen with a high left ventricular diastolic pressure[89] or a high pulmonary capillary wedge pressure.[91] The association of a

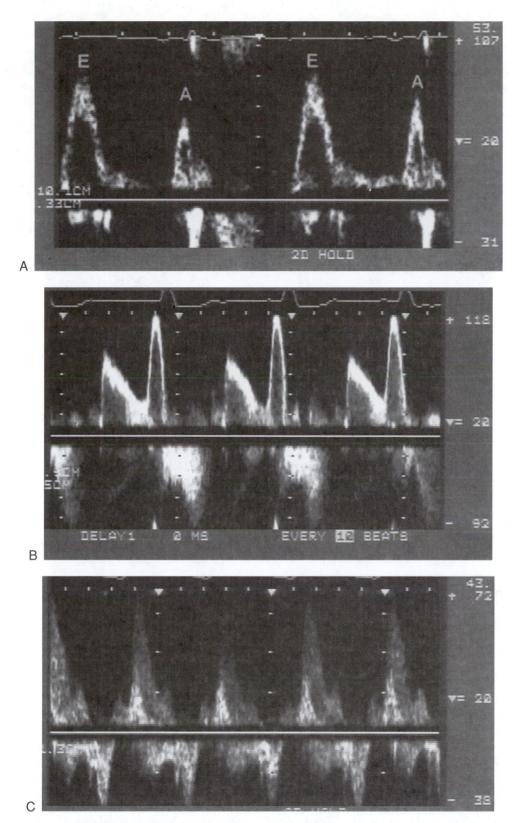

Fig. 32-6. (A) Doppler echocardiogram of mitral valve inflow recorded at the tips of the mitral valve leaflets demonstrates a normal early filling wave (E) and a lower velocity atrial wave (A) from a patient with normal diastolic function. **(B)** Mitral valve inflow pattern from a patient with hypertrophy and abnormal diastolic dysfunction. The E/A ratio is reversed. **(C)** Restrictive type mitral inflow pattern from a patient with amyloidosis. The E wave velocity is high and the deceleration slope steep (arrow). The A wave velocity is less than the E wave, which accounts for the characterization as a "pseudonormalized pattern." With advance amyloid, the A wave may not be discernible because of atrial systolic failure.

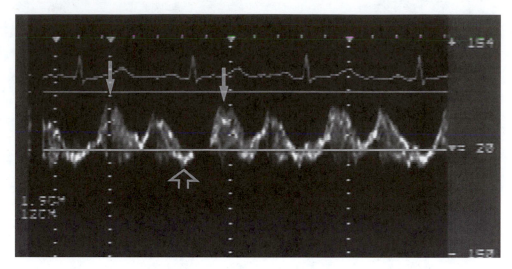

Fig. 32-7. Transesophageal Doppler echocardiogram demonstrating normal pulmonary venous flow from the right upper pulmonary vein. The largest flow occurs during systole (solid arrow). There is a second diastolic filling peak that corresponds to the timing of the E wave during mitral inflow. Brief retrograde flow is noted after atrial systole (open arrow), a normal finding.

pseudonormalized E/A ratio with a decreased systolic flow was seen in all patients with a markedly elevated left ventricular diastolic pressure prior to the A wave but was also seen in a few control patients.[89] Similar to the data obtained in an animal model of mitral inflow patterns, an increase in left atrial pressure due to an increased preload has been shown to result in an increased systolic wave, whereas an increase in left atrial pressure due to ventricular dysfunction is associated with decreased systolic velocity.[92] A blunted systolic wave may also be produced by significant mitral regurgitation.[93]

Similar to mitral valve inflow velocity patterns, comparisons of pulmonary venous patterns between patients or after interventions in a single patient cannot be used as a direct measurement of diastolic function.

OTHER METHODS

The rate of left ventricular posterior wall thinning may be measured directly from M-mode tracings, as can the rate of cavity enlargement. As with other indices, abnormalities have been reported with various disease states that produce diastolic dysfunction but are dependent on loading conditions.[94] Measurement of the time constant of ventricular relaxation can be derived from the left ventricular pressure change during isovolumic relaxation. As can be done for the rise in left ventricular pressure, the fall in ventricular pressure can be derived from the downslope of the mitral regurgitation Doppler velocity profile using the modified Bernoulli equation.[42] The

time constant of ventricular relaxation can be measured from the downslope of the pressure curve but requires knowledge of the left ventricular diastolic pressure and so is difficult to apply clinically.[95] Color M-mode analysis of apical filling patterns has been used to relate diastolic flow propagation[96] and filling patterns with various measures of invasively measured relaxation.[97,98] Similarly, color Doppler M-mode studies may also demonstrate abnormalities in systolic patterns during systolic dysfunction.[99] These methods await clinical validation.

CLASSIFICATION OF CARDIOMYOPATHIES

Identification of the etiology of congestive heart failure is the basis for a rational treatment plan. A substantial number of patients who present with severe congestive heart failure have normal or near-normal left ventricular ejection fractions and are thought to have congestive heart failure on the basis of diastolic dysfunction.[100] Identification of patients with preserved left ventricular function and congestive heart failure can be problematic at the bedside because no clinical variables reliably differentiate this group from those with decreased systolic function[100–103] The fact that prognosis is far better in those with preserved ventricular ejection fraction is a compelling argument for routine echocardiographic assessment of left ventricular function in patients presenting with congestive heart failure.[104] In addition, treatment of asymptomatic patients with decreased

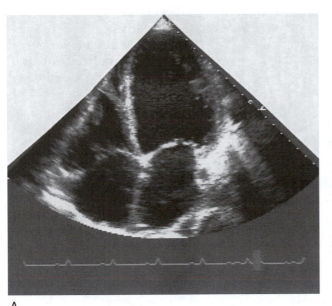
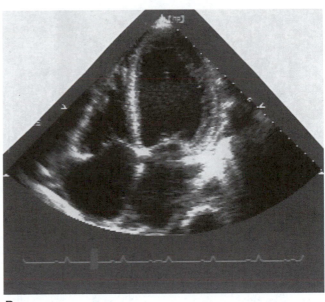

A   B

Fig. 32-8. Apical four-chamber long-axis view of patient with dilated cardiomyopathy. **(A)** During diastole four-chamber dilatation is evident. The left-sided chambers are at the right. **(B)** Corresponding systolic view reveals poor left ventricular function and moderate right ventricular hypokinesis.

left ventricular systolic function can improve long-term survival.[105] Echocardiography has proved an excellent method to diagnose and monitor congestive heart failure. Overzealous limitations on diagnostic testing should not be used as the rationale for withholding this important evaluation.[106]

Dilated Cardiomyopathy

Echocardiographic findings in dilated cardiomyopathy include an enlarged left ventricular cavity, decreased mitral and aortic valve excursion, and decreased systolic function (Fig. 32-8). The presence of right ventricular enlargement and dysfunction is variable but a poor prognostic sign if present.[107] Pulmonary hypertension also predicts a high morbidity and mortality.[108] Echocardiographic assessment of wall motion abnormalities is not a reliable method for distinguishing ischemic cardiomyopathy from the causes of dilated global cardiomyopathies such as idiopathic cardiomyopathy.[109] Regional wall motion abnormalities may be found with idiopathic cardiomyopathy, and global dysfunction may be present with ischemic syndromes. Dobutamine stress echocardiography may be useful for identifying severe coronary artery disease in this patient population,[110] as well as for identifying hibernating or stunned myocardium.[110-114]

Left Ventricular Remodelling

A number of studies have demonstrated an association between the progression of left ventricular remodeling and the progression of congestive heart failure. The compensatory left ventricular hypertrophy and dilatation that follows the development of systolic dysfunction results in a remodeling process that is associated with a poor prognosis. Wall stress rises as the radius of the chamber increases with ventricular dilatation. Hypertrophy of the walls may normalize wall stress for a time, but eventually hypertrophy may not further compensate for the increased volume. Wall stress, a reliable measurement of ventricular afterload, increases, resulting in a further decrease in ejection fraction. The stages and consequences of ventricular remodeling have been well described in several large echocardiographic studies.[115,116]

Ejection fraction and end-systolic volume remain the most reliable prognostic determinants of survival.[117-121] As the left ventricle dilates, it assumes a more spherical shape (Fig. 32-9). That is, the short-axis diameter increases disproportionately to the long axis. A spherical shape has been identified as a poor prognostic sign.[122] In the normal ventricle, meridional stress is higher than circumferential stress. However, as a consequence of the change in shape, they become more nearly equal. A more spherical cavity shape is also associated with functional mitral regurgitation.[123]

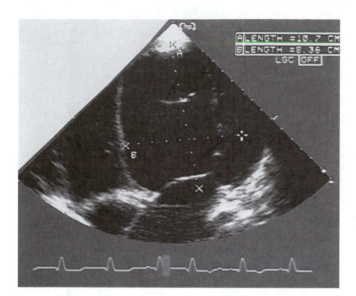

Fig. 32-9. Apical four-chamber long-axis view of end-stage left ventricular dysfunction secondary to idiopathic dilated cardiomyopathy. The ventricle appears to be far more spherical than is normal. The minor axis measurement (B) is approaching the long-axis measurement (A).

A number of echocardiographic variables, including left ventricular end-diastolic size indexed to body surface area, mitral E point septal separation (Fig. 32-10), and the systolic diameter/wall thickness ratio have been found to correlate with survival.[124,125] Other predictors of survival, such as neurohumoral activation, correlate with the severity of left ventricular dysfunction as measured by the ejection fraction, independent of symptoms.[126] Data from the SOLVD echocardiographic substudy demonstrated that improvement in survival in enalapril-treated

patients was associated with an arrest in progressive left ventricular dilatation and increasing mass.[127] Interestingly, initial echocardiographic parameters do not predict survival in children with dilated cardiomyopathy, but lack of improvement at 1–6 months predicts high mortality.[128]

DIASTOLIC FUNCTION

Many studies have noted the association of a pseudo-normalized mitral Doppler velocity pattern with a poor prognosis in dilated cardiomyopathy (Fig. 32-6C).[129–132] The elevated early filling wave results from an elevated left atrial pressure, and the rapid deceleration time reflects a further decrease in left ventricular compliance.[129] A deceleration time under 140 ms identifies a group with a particularly poor prognosis.[131] The development of a short deceleration time correlates with the appearance of an S3 in an animal model.[133] Treatment with vasodilators or inotropic agents increases the atrial contribution to left ventricular filling in animal models[134,135] and clinical studies.[129]

LEFT VENTRICULAR THROMBI

Left ventricular thrombi are identified in as many as 40 percent of patients with dilated cardiomyopathy.[136,137] The positive predictive value of echocardiography is superior to that of cine ventriculography for diagnosing apical thrombi.[138] Thrombi are generally classified as mural or protruding based on their characteristic appearance (Fig. 32-11). Heavy trabeculations are sometimes mistaken for a laminated thrombus. The diagnosis of ventricular thrombus

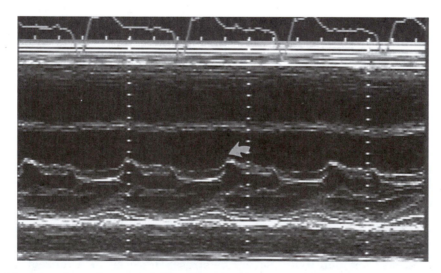

Fig. 32-10. M-mode echocardiogram of the parasternal long axis in a patient with severe dilated cardiomyopathy. There is a decreased mitral valve opening and E point (arrow) to septal separation of more than 2 cm.

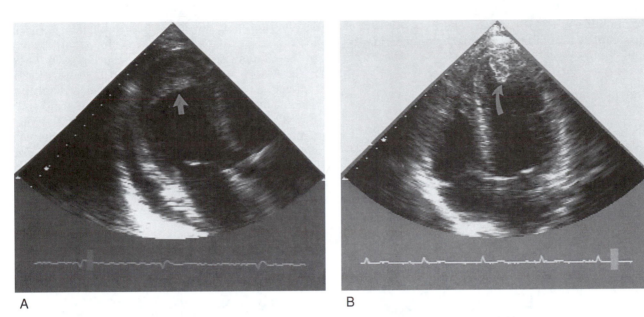

A   B

Fig. 32-11. **(A)** Apical long-axis echocardiogram of a patient with severe ischemic cardiomyopathy. The ventricle is dilated, and there is a large laminated thrombus (arrow) filling the ventricular apex. The thrombus is echo-bright representing calcification. **(B)** Apical four-chamber echocardiogram in a patient with dilated cardiomyopathy. A large apical thrombus (arrow) protrudes into the left ventricular cavity and in real time was mobile.

overlying an area of normal wall motion should be suspected. Studies have also demonstrated apical thrombi in 11–54 percent of patients after an anterior myocardial infarction.[139–143] Low velocity diastolic inflow and systolic outflow measured at the apex correlates with the presence of ventricular thrombi.[144] Mitral regurgitation is inversely correlated with the presence of thrombi perhaps because it would tend to increase the inflow and outflow velocities. Mitral regurgitation carries a negative prognostic value despite its "protective" effect against thrombi.[136] Protrusion of the thrombus into the ven-

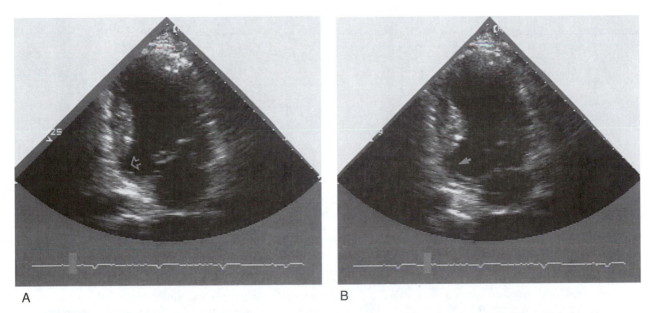

A   B

Fig. 32-12. **(A)** Apical two-chamber long-axis view of a patient with a previous inferior wall infarction. During diastole the inferior wall is thinned (arrow) compared to the other walls. **(B)** During systole the inferior wall at the base (arrow) does not thicken and is dyskinetic. The other walls thicken during systole, although the apex is poorly seen in this reproduction.

tricle, mobility of the thrombus, and hyperkinesia of an adjacent region of myocardium have been identified as factors predicting embolization.[137,141,145,146]

Ischemic Cardiomyopathy

REGIONAL WALL MOTION

Echocardiography is a powerful method for identifying left ventricular wall motion abnormalities (Fig. 32-12), being more sensitive than radionuclide ven-

triculography.[147] Several schemes have been identified for quantitating wall motion abnormalities. Figure 32-13 identifies the nomenclature recommended by the American Society of Echocardiography for the ventricular walls in the standard echocardiographic views. The commonly used wall motion score index (Fig. 32-14) grades each of the 20 segments from 1 to 4 for normal thickening to dyskinesis. Other commonly used models grade 16 myocardial segments. The total score is divided by the number of total segments scored. Although this analysis is usually per-

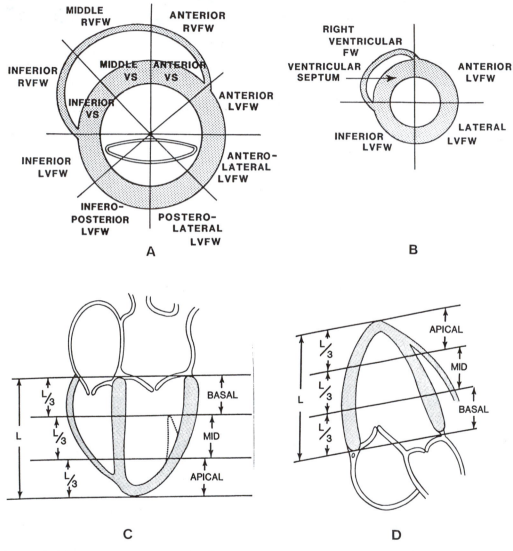

Fig. 32-13. Standard nomenclature for left ventricular walls. **(A)** Short-axis view of the basal region demonstrating the method of subdividing the myocardial walls into segments using a coordinate system consisting of eight lines that are 45 degrees apart. The left ventricular free wall (LVFW) is divided into five segments and the ventricular septum into three segments. The short axis at the midventricular level is divided similarly and is not shown. **(B)** Short-axis view of the apical region demonstrating the method of subdividing the myocardium by four lines 90 degrees apart. The left ventricular free wall is subdivided into three segments, and the septum is one segment. **(C)** Apical four-chamber view demonstrating the method of subdividing the myocardial walls into three regions using the left ventricular papillary muscles as landmarks. **(D)** Apical long-axis view demonstrating the method of subdividing the myocardial walls into three regions of equal length. (From American Society of Echocardiography,[241] with permission.)

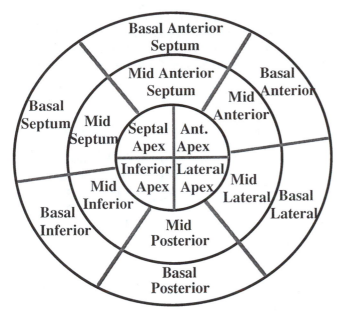

Fig. 32-14. Sixteen segment model used for wall motion score. The outer circle represents the left ventricular walls at the base. The middle circle is the ventricular walls at the midpapillary level. The inner circle represents the apical level.

formed in the short-axis view, three ventricular levels are included, accounting for the entire ventricle. The score correlates with postinfarction prognosis.[148–151] Both early and late prognoses are related to the wall motion score index, which correlates with other measures of infarct size such as enzyme release, ischemic time measured by continuous ST segment monitoring, and pathologic examination.[152–156] The wall motion score index improves in patients undergoing successful thrombolysis or percutaneous transluminal coronary angioplasty (PTCA) during acute myocardial infarction.[157,158] Left ventricular surface mapping[159–161] is an elegant technique for evaluating the increase in ventricular volume, surface area, and infarct size that results from postinfarction remodeling.

VENTRICULAR REMODELING

Infarct extension and expansion account for acute ventricular remodeling after a myocardial infarction.[116,162–164] Once left ventricular dilatation has taken place, further remodeling follows a pattern similar to the progression of dilated cardiomyopathy. The left ventricular remodeling process has been delineated in the rat model.[165] Occlusion of the left anterior descending artery immediately results in a large area of systolic bulging. Over the course of several weeks, the infarcted area thins, and the nonis-

chemic areas undergo compensatory hypertrophy. However, the progressive dilatation due to loss of contractile elements may not be compensated for by the increased wall thickness resulting in a further increase in wall stress. Regional dysfunction develops in the noninfarcted areas, and the ejection fraction falls. A similar process of ventricular remodeling occurs clinically.[162] The left ventricular volume determined by echocardiography predicts volumes at 1 year[151] and is strongly related to survival.[164] The presence of a large aneurysm (Fig. 32-15) predicts the development of congestive heart failure and cardiovascular mortality.[166,167] It is most important to acknowledge that the bedside clinical assessment of left ventricular function after an infarction has low sensitivity (less than 50 percent) for identifying left ventricular ejection fractions of less than 40 percent.[168] This fact argues for an echocardiographic assessment of left ventricular size and function as an important prognostic determination immediately after a myocardial infarction. Endocardial surface area is already above normal values in some patients on presentation with infarction, and continued ventricular enlargement over 1 year of follow-up is common.[169] A decrease in the size of the infarction and the ventricular surface area occurs in a small group of patients predominantly with inferior myocardial infarctions. As could be expected, it is otherwise uncommon.[169,170]

The SAVE trial demonstrated that improvement in prognosis by angiotensin-converting enzyme

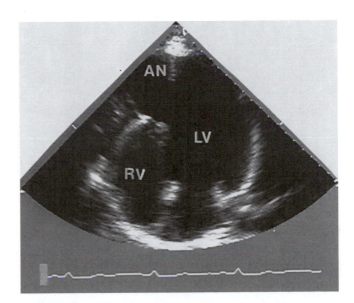

Fig. 32-15. Two-dimensional echocardiogram of apical four-chamber view in a patient with a large apical aneurysm (AN) and a severely dilated left ventricle (LV). The right ventricle (RV) is of normal size but appears diminutive next to the aneurysm.

(ACE) inhibition after a myocardial infarction correlated with an attenuation in left ventricular dilation demonstrated by echocardiography.[171] Other studies continue to focus on attenuation of ventricular dilatation by various interventions.[172]

Abnormalities in echocardiographic indices of diastolic dysfunction accompany left ventricular enlargement during the postinfarction period. In a rat model of infarction, development of a progressively large E wave and rapid deceleration time was associated with progressive systolic dysfunction.[165] Similar to studies in other patient groups, an elevated pulmonary capillary wedge pressure is associated with a high E/A ratio and short deceleration time.[173,174]

Hypertrophic Cardiomyopathy

Hypertrophic cardiomyopathy is characterized by myocardial fiber disarray, associated with thickening of the walls without dilatation of the cavity. The increased stiffness of the walls results in diastolic abnormalities and variably in outflow or midcavity obstruction. The septum is generally more than 1.5 cm thick with a septal/posterior wall thickness ratio of 1.3 or more (Fig. 32-16). Although asymmetric septal hypertrophy (ASH) is the most common finding in hypertrophic cardiomyopathy, other walls may be the predominant site of thickening.[175–177] Apical hypertrophy characterizes the variant most commonly found in Japan.[178] The disease is genetically transmitted as an autosomal dominant trait. However, the echocardiographic findings may not be present during early childhood and have been shown to evolve on serial echocardiographic studies.[179,180]

OUTFLOW OBSTRUCTION

Obstruction to outflow may occur in the outflow tract proximal to the aortic valve or in the midcavity. The presence of obstruction at either level may be inferred by midsystolic aortic valve closure best seen on M-mode examination (Fig. 32-17). The site of obstruction may be discerned using color flow mapping and continuous-wave Doppler echocardiography.[181] The color flow map demonstrates narrowing and turbulence at the level of the obstruction. Continuous-wave Doppler measures an increased velocity at the site of obstruction with the characteristic late-peaking flow pattern (Fig. 32-18). The modified Bernoulli equation is then used to calculate the peak systolic gradient across the obstruction. Care must be taken to exclude the mitral regurgitation jet that often accompanies outflow tract obstruction and that may be misinterpreted as the peak velocity at the obstruction.[182] Maneuvers known to provoke a gradient should be attempted during Doppler interrogation of the outflow tract.

Systolic anterior motion of the mitral valve is present if the obstruction is at the level of the outflow tract (Fig. 32-16). Some controversy exists concerning the mechanism of outflow tract obstruction, the timing and severity of which correlate with systolic anterior motion of the anterior mitral valve leaflet.[183] One hypothesis is that the hyperdynamic contraction associated with high outflow tract velocity generates a venturi force that draws the anterior mitral leaflet into the outflow tract during early systole.[184] Some studies have focused on abnormalities of the mitral valve, its apparatus, and the papillary muscles that allow the valve leaflets to be displaced into the outflow tract during early ejection.[185–187] Anterior and inward displacement of the papillary muscles have been demonstrated by three-dimensional echocardiographic reconstruction in patients with dynamic subvalvar obstruction. This results in less tension on the valve leaflets, allowing them to be more readily displaced into the outflow tract.[188] The cause of midcavitary obstruction appears also to be primarily related to the geometry of the ventricle. Midcavitary gradients can be induce by hypovolemia and inotropes such as dobutamine in susceptible patients. Midcavitary obstruction has also been associated with apical hypertrophy. In some patients api-

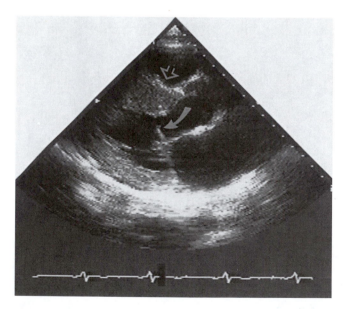

Fig. 32-16. Two-dimensional echocardiogram of the parasternal long-axis view. The septum (open arrow) is severely thickened compared to the posterior wall. Systolic anterior motion (SAM) brings the mitral valve (curved arrow) into the left ventricular outflow tract during systole.

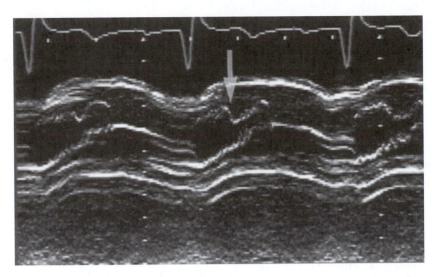

Fig. 32-17. M-mode echocardiogram in the parasternal position through the aortic valve from a patient with obstructive hypertrophic cardiomyopathy. There is early closure of the valve (arrow), which coincides with the timing of maximal outflow obstruction and systolic anterior motion of the mitral valve.

cal hypokinesis develops and can progress to apical aneurysm formation in the absence of coronary artery disease.[189]

DIASTOLIC FUNCTION

Diastolic abnormalities make a significant, and perhaps primary, contribution to the symptom complex in hypertrophic cardiomyopathy.[190,191] Isovolumic relaxation time is increased, and the rate of early filling decreases. The atrial contribution to filling usually increases.[191,192] Diastolic abnormalities have been demonstrated in asymptomatic affected individuals. The degree of abnormality does not correlate with exercise tolerance.[191,193] However, diastolic abnormalities distinguish hypertrophic cardiomyopathy from the hypertrophy in "athletically trained" individuals despite similar wall thickness.[194] Other workers have demonstrated a heterogeneity in diastolic filling patterns from mitral valve annulus to apex, which may relate to temporal nonuniformity in early filling.[192] In some patients with midcavitary obstruction, paradoxical flow from the apex to the base of the ventricle can be recorded and

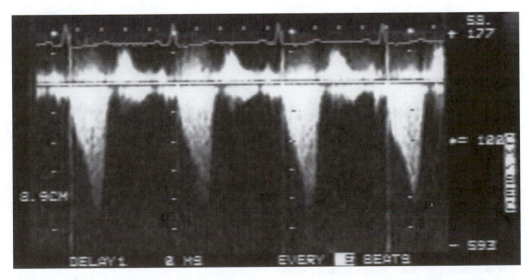

Fig. 32-18. Continuous-wave Doppler velocity recording through the left ventricular outflow tract in a patient with obstructive hypertrophic cardiomyopathy. The characteristic "spade-like" profile peaks during late systole. The peak systolic velocity is approximately 4.2 m/s, which predicts a peak gradient of 71 mmHg across the outflow tract.

may last through 60 percent of diastole.[189,195,196] It has been suggested that this paradoxical flow may be a marker of concealed apical asynergy. Patients with this pattern are at a substantially higher risk of systemic embolization.[189,197]

ULTRASONOGRAPHIC TISSUE CHARACTERIZATION

Because the development of hypertrophic cardiomyopathy is accompanied by disruption of the normal myocyte architecture and an increase in collagen formation, it is not surprising that studies of myocardial tissue characterization can distinguish between hypertrophic and normal myocardium. Integrated backscatter tissue characterization involves analysis of the amplitude of reflected waves or their spatial distribution in a specific region of interest. This difference in myocardial backscatter can be appreciated visually as the increased "speckle" pattern found in hypertrophic cardiomyopathy as well as other diseases with abnormalities of the myocardium.[198,199] Although these techniques reliably distinguish between hypertrophied and normal myocardium, they have been only partially successful in distinguishing pathologic from physiologic hypertrophy.[199–201]

Transthoracic, transesophageal, and epicardial echocardiography have proved useful for monitoring the results of medical therapy,[202] artificial pacing,[203–205] and surgery in the treatment of this disease.[206–209] In addition, it may be lifesaving when determining the cause of unexplained cardiovascular collapse.[210]

Restrictive Cardiomyopathy

The hallmark of restrictive cardiomyopathy is decrease in left ventricular compliance resulting in diastolic abnormalities.[211] The pathogenesis can be infiltration of the myocardium by abnormal deposits such as amyloid or eosinophils, but often no structural abnormality is found.[212,213] Hemachromatosis[214] and glycogen storage diseases[211] may also present with restrictive physiology. Biatrial enlargement is usually present as are increased wall thickness and an abnormal "speckle" pattern. Diastolic abnormalities demonstrated on Doppler flow velocity tracings in restrictive physiology have already been described and include an increase in the early filling wave velocity, a decrease in the atrial filling wave velocity, and a decrease in the deceleration time of the early wave.[79,215] Clinically, it may be difficult to distinguish restrictive cardiomyopathy from constrictive pericarditis, but the difference in respiratory variation in the two conditions may be useful on the Doppler echocardiogram.[82,216,217] Diastolic mitral regurgitation occurs with restrictive disease and rarely with constriction.[82]

AMYLOIDOSIS

Amyloidosis is the most well studied of the restrictive cardiomyopathies. Cardiac involvement can occur with all types of amyloidosis but is most frequent in the primary type (AL amyloid protein). If biopsy of a noncardiac site has diagnosed amyloidosis, cardiac involvement can be inferred without biopsy from the echocardiographic study. Increased wall thickness and echogenicity are both sensitive and specific for the diagnosis in this setting (Fig. 32-19).[218] A marked increase in the spectral pattern is thought to result from scattering of the ultrasound waves by the abnormal amyloid protein fibrils.[219,220] Interatrial septal thickening is frequently seen along with valvar thickening and mild valvar regurgitation. Previously described diastolic filling abnormalities are commonly seen when the wall thickness is increased, but they have also been described in patients as the first sign of cardiac involvement.[86,221] The increased wall thickness and decreased systolic function correlate negatively with survival,[84] as does the development

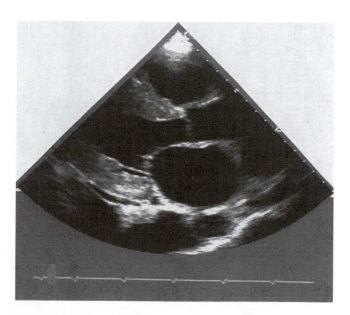

Fig. 32-19. Two-dimensional echocardiogram in the long-axis view demonstrating the thickened and bright walls associated with cardiac amyloidosis. The left ventricular cavity is of normal size despite profound systolic dysfunction. Associated findings include thickening of the mitral and aortic valves, left atrial enlargement, and thickening of the atrial wall. There is a small pericardial effusion evident posteriorly and a larger left pleural effusion.

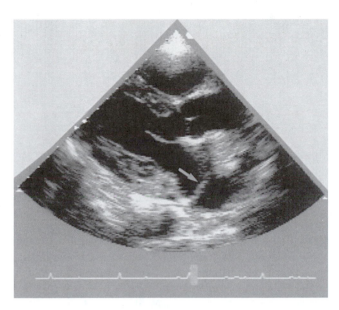

Fig. 32-20. Two-dimensional echocardiogram in parasternal long-axis view demonstrating the prominent atrial anastomosis (arrow) in an orthotopic heart recipient. This prominent anastomosis is normal and not associated with obstruction to flow.

of restrictive Doppler patterns.[222] A mitral deceleration time of less than 150 ms is associated with a 50 percent mortality rate at 1 year.

CARDIAC TRANSPLANTATION

Echocardiography is useful for screening potential transplant donors to detect subclinical cardiac disease or damage and avoid transplantation of hearts with decreased survival potential[223] Most potential transplant donors are intubated or have other conditions associated with inadequate windows for optimal echocardiographic study. In this setting, transesophageal echocardiography is an ideal tool for the assessment of cardiac pathology and may rule out the use of an organ that was otherwise thought to be acceptable.[224] Transesophageal echocardiography is also useful in the operating room during the transplant procedure when abnormalities of the anastomoses and interatrial septum may be promptly repaired.[225,226] Figures 32-20 to 32-23 demonstrate some of the common echocardiographic findings in posttransplant patients.

Many attempts have been made to assess the echocardiographic predictors of acute rejection, as the noninvasive diagnosis of rejection might obviate the need for repeated myocardial biopsy. Left ventricular wall thickening had been suggested as just such a parameter. However, many studies have failed to show a correlation between wall thickening and early mild or moderate rejection.[227–229] Currently, the development of a restrictive mitral inflow pattern is thought to correlate with rejection episodes.[230–232] Evaluation of integrated backscatter tissue characterization is also promising in its ability to diagnose rejection.[233] The persistence of a pericardial effusion may also signal continuing rejection early during the posttransplant period.[230] Transvenous myocardial biopsy may be undertaken via echocardiographic guidance, particularly in the acutely ill patient.[234]

Although mild valvular regurgitation is common after orthotopic transplant, the development of significant tricuspid regurgitation is frequently symptomatic. Tricuspid regurgitation no doubt relates in

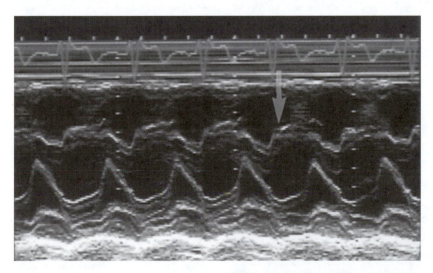

Fig. 32-21. M-mode echocardiogram from the parasternal position. Paradoxical septal motion is apparent and may be prominent (arrow).

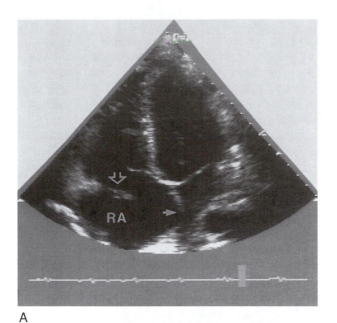

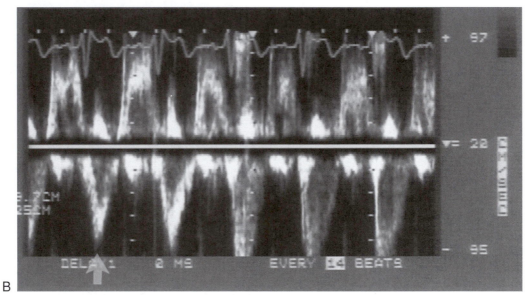

Fig. 32-22. (A) Two-dimensional echocardiogram in the apical four-chamber view in a transplant recipient. The anterior leaflet of the tricuspid valve is flail (open arrow). The right atrium (RA) is severely enlarged, and the interatrial septum bulges to the left (closed arrow). **(B)** Doppler echocardiogram of tricuspid valve flows in the same patient. The sample volume has been placed at the level of the tricuspid valve annulus. The tricuspid valve fails to coapt, resulting in torrential tricuspid regurgitation. The Doppler pattern of the tricuspid regurgitation is laminar (arrow) because there is no impediment to the back-flow.

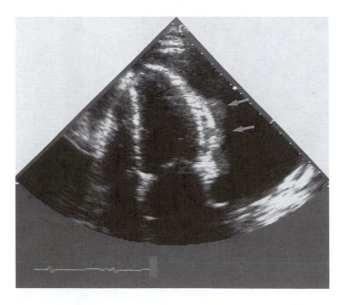

Fig. 32-23. Two-dimensional echocardiogram of the apical four-chamber axis in an orthotopic transplant recipient. There is a large pericardial effusion associated with focal thickening of the pericardium (arrows).

part to the abnormal anatomy after surgical anastomosis of the donor right atrium and resultant distortion of the tricuspid annulus.[235] However, damage to the valve may occur during repeated biopsy attempts.[236,237] Pulmonary hypertension may persist after transplantation contributing to tricuspid valve pathology.[238] Dobutamine stress echocardiographic studies have been useful for screening for the development of coronary artery disease during the long-term posttransplant period.[239,240]

REFERENCES

1. Wyatt H, Haendchen R, Meerbaum S, Corday E: Assessment of quantitative methods for 2-dimensional echocardiography. Am J Cardiol 1983;52:396–401

2. Devereux R, Reichek N: Echocardiographic determination of left ventricular mass in man. Circulation 1977;55:613–618

3. Devereux R, Lutas E, Casale P et al: Standardization of M-mode echocardiographic left ventricular anatomic measurements. J Am Coll Cardiol 1984;4:1222–1230

4. Savage D, Garrison R, Kannel W et al: The spectrum of left ventricular hypertrophy in a general population sample: The Framingham Study. Circulation, suppl. I 1987;75:26–133

5. Huwez FU, Pringle SD, Macfarlane PW: A new classification of left ventricular geometry in patients with cardiac disease based on M-mode echocardiography. Am J Cardiol 1992;70:681–688

6. Fortun N, Hood WJ, Sherman M, Craige E: Determination of left ventricular volumes by ultrasound. Circulation 1971;44:575

7. Abdulla A, Frank M, Canedo M, Stafadourous M: Limitations of echocardiography in the assessment of left ventricular size and function in aortic regurgitation. Circulation 1980;61:148–155

8. Crawford M, Grant D, O'Rourke R, Starling M, Groves B: Accuracy and reproducibility of new M-mode recommendations for measuring left ventricular dimensions. Circulation 1980;66:137

9. Quinones M, Waggoner A, Reduto L et al: A new, simplified and accurate method for determining ejection fraction with two-dimensional echocardiography. Circulation 1981;64:744–753

10. Folland E, Parisi A, Moynihan P et al: Assessment of left ventricular ejection fraction and volumes by real-time, two-dimensional echocardiography. A comparison of cineangiographic and radionuclide techniques. Circulation 1979;60:760–766

11. Gueret P, Meerbaum S, Wyatt H et al: Two-dimensional echocardiographic quantitation of left ventricular volumes and ejection fraction. Importance of accounting for dyssynergy in short-axis reconstruction models. Circulation 1980;62:1308–1318

12. Helak J, Reichek N: Quantitation of human left ventricular mass and volume by two-dimensional echocardiography: in vitro anatomic validation. Circulation 1981;63:1398–1407

13. Tortoledo F, Quinones M, Fernandez G et al: Quantification of left ventricular volumes by two-dimensional echocardiography. A simplified and accurate approach. Circulation 1983;67:579–584

14. Alam M, Hoglund C, Thorstrand C: Longitudinal systolic shortening of the left ventricle. An echocardiographic study in subjects with and without preserved global function. Clin Physiol 1992;12:443–452

15. Pai RG, Bodenheimer MM, Pai SM, Koss JH, Adamick RD: Usefulness of systolic excursion of the mitral annulus as an index of left ventricular systolic function [see comments]. Am J Cardiol 1991;67:222–224

16. Starling M, Crawford M, Sorensen S et al: Comparative accuracy of apical biplane cross-sectional echocardiography and gated equilibrium radionuclide angiography for estimating left ventricular size and performance. Circulation 1981;63:1075–1084

17. Schiller N, Acquatella H, Ports T et al: Left ventricular volume from paired biplane two-dimensional echocardiography. Circulation 1979;60:547–555

18. Schiller N: Two-dimensional echocardiographic determination of left ventricular volume, systolic function, and mass. Circulation, suppl. I 1991;84:280–287

19. Wahr D, Wang Y, Schiller N: Left ventricular volumes determined by two-dimensional echocardiography in a normal adult population. J Am Coll Cardiol 1983;1:863–868

20. Gordon E, Schnittger I, Fitzgerald P, Williams P, Popp R: Reproducibility of left ventricular volumes by two-dimensional echocardiography. J Am Coll Cardiol 1983;2:506–513

21. Crouse LJ, Cheirif J, Hanly DE et al: Opacification and border delineation improvement in patients with suboptimal endocardial border definition in routine echocardiography. Results of the phase III Albunex Multicenter Trial. J Am Coll Cardiol 1993;22:1494–1500

22. Martin RP: Real time ultrasound quantification of ventricular function. Has the eyeball been replaced or will the subjective become objective [editorial; comment]. J Am Coll Cardiol 1992;19:321–323

23. Rich S, Sheikh A, Gallastegui J et al: Determination of left ventricular ejection fraction by visual estimation during real-time two-dimensional echocardiography. Am Heart J 1982;104:603–606

24. Vanoverschelde JL, Hanet C, Wijns W, Detry JM: On-line quantification of left ventricular volumes and ejection fraction by automated backscatter imaging-assisted boundary detection. Comparison with contrast cineventriculography. Am J Cardiol 1994;74:633–635

25. Perez JE, Klein SC, Prater DM et al: Automated, on-line quantification of left ventricular dimensions and function by echocardiography with backscatter imaging and lateral gain compensation. Am J Cardiol 1992;70:1200–1205

26. Perez JE, Waggoner AD, Barzilai B et al: On-line assessment of ventricular function by automatic boundary detection and ultrasonic backscatter imaging. J Am Coll Cardiol 1992;19:313–320

27. Gorcsan J III, Lazar JM, Schulman DS, Follansbee WP: Comparison of left ventricular function by echocardiographic automated border detection and by radionuclide ejection fraction. Am J Cardiol 1993;72:810–815

28. Schiller N, Shah P, Crawford M et al: Recommendations for quantitation of the left ventricle by two-di-

mensional echocardiography. American Society of Echocardiography Committee on Standards, Subcommittee on Quantitation of Two-Dimensional Echocardiograms. J Am Soc Echocardiogr 1989;2: 358–367

29. Herregods MC, Vermylen J, Bynens B, De Geest H, Van de Werf F: On-line quantification of left ventricular function by automatic boundary detection and ultrasonic backscatter imaging. Am J Cardiol 1993;72: 359–362

30. Lindower PD, Rath L, Preslar J et al: Quantification of left ventricular function with an automated border detection system and comparison with radionuclide ventriculography. Am J Cardiol 1994;73:195–199

31. Yvorchuk KJ, Davies RA, Chan KL: Measurement of left ventricular ejection fraction by acoustic quantification and comparison with radionuclide angiography. Am J Cardiol 1994;74:1052–1056

32. Gorcsan J III, Gasior TA, Mandarino WA et al: On-line estimation of changes in left ventricular stroke volume by transesophageal echocardiographic automated border detection in patients undergoing coronary artery bypass grafting. Am J Cardiol 1993;72: 721–727

33. Cahalan MK, Ionescu P, Melton H Jr et al: Automated real-time analysis of intraoperative transesophageal echocardiograms. Anesthesiology 1993; 78:477–485

34. Stoddard MF, Dillon S, Peters G, Kupersmith J: Left ventricular ejection fraction is increased during transesophageal echocardiography in patients with impaired ventricular function. Am Heart J 1992;123: 1005–1010

35. Siu SC, Rivera JM, Guerrero JL et al: Three-dimensional echocardiography. In vivo validation for left ventricular volume and function. Circulation 1993; 88:1715–1723

36. Sapin PM, Schroeder KD, Smith MD, DeMaria AN, King DL: Three-dimensional echocardiographic measurement of left ventricular volume in vitro. Comparison with two-dimensional echocardiography and cineventriculography [see comments]. J Am Coll Cardiol 1993;22:1530–1537

37. Sapin PM, Schroder KM, Gopal AS et al: Comparison of two- and three-dimensional echocardiography with cineventriculography for measurement of left ventricular volume in patients. J Am Coll Cardiol 1994; 24:1054–1063

38. Handschumacher MD, Lethor JP, Siu SC et al: A new integrated system for three-dimensional echocardiographic reconstruction. Development and validation for ventricular volume with application in human subjects. J Am Coll Cardiol 1993;21:743–753

39. Chen C, Guerrero JL, Vazquez de Prada JA et al: Intracardiac ultrasound measurement of volumes and ejection fraction in normal, infarcted, and aneurysmal left ventricles using a 10-MHz ultrasound catheter. Circulation 1994;90:1481–1491

40. Pearlman AS: Measurement of left ventricular volume by three-dimensional echocardiography—present promise and potential problems [editorial; comment]. J Am Coll Cardiol 1993;22:1538–1540

41. Recusani F: Noninvasive assessment of left ventricular function with continuous wave Doppler echocardiography [editorial; comment]. Circulation 1991;83: 2141–2143

42. Chen C, Rodriguez L, Lethor JP et al: Continuous wave Doppler echocardiography for noninvasive assessment of left ventricular dP/dt and relaxation time constant from mitral regurgitant spectra in patients. J Am Coll Cardiol 1994;23:970–976

43. Chen C, Rodriguez L, Guerrero JL et al: Noninvasive estimation of the instantaneous first derivative of left ventricular pressure using continuous-wave Doppler echocardiography [see comments]. Circulation 1991; 83:2101–2110

44. Pai RG, Pai SM, Bodenheimer MM, Adamick RD: Estimation of rate of left ventricular pressure rise by Doppler echocardiography. Its hemodynamic validation. Am Heart J 1993;126:240–242

45. Bargiggia G, Bertucci C, Recusani F et al: A new method of estimation left ventricular dP/dt by continuous wave Doppler-echocardiography. Validation studies at cardiac catheterization. Circulation 1989; 80:1287–1292

46. Quinones M, Gaash W, Alexander J: Influence of acute changes in preload, afterload, contractile state and heart rate on ejection phase and isovolumic indices of myocardial contractility in man. Circulation 1976;63:293–302

47. Peterson K, Skloven D, Ludbrook P, Uther J, Ross J: Comparison of isovolumic and ejection phase indices of myocardial performance in man. Circulation 1974; 49:1088–1101

48. Xiao HB, Brecker SJ, Gibson DG: Effects of abnormal activation on the time course of the left ventricular pressure pulse in dilated cardiomyopathy. Br Heart J 1992;68:403–407

49. Sandor GG, Popov R, De Souza E, Morris S, Johnston B: Rate-corrected mean velocity of fiber shortening-stress at peak systole as a load-independent measure of contractility. Am J Cardiol 1992;69:403–407

50. Reichek N, Wilson J, St. John M et al: Noninvasive determination of left ventricular end-systolic stress. Validation of the method and initial application. Circulation 1982;65:99–108

51. Laskey W, St. John Sutton M, Zeevi G, Hirshfeld J, Reichek N: Left ventricular mechanics in dilated cardiomyopathy. Am J Cardiol 1984;54:620–625

52. Colan S, Borrow K, Nermann A: Left ventricular end-systolic wall stress-velocity of fiber shortening relation. A load independent index of myocardial contractility. J Am Coll Cardiol 1984;4:715–724

53. Borow K, Green L, Grossman W, Braunwald E: Left ventricular end-systolic stress-shortening and stress-length relations in humans. Normal values and sensitivity to ionotropic state. Am J Cardiol 1982;50: 1301–1308

54. Sagawa K, Suga H, Shoukas A, Bakalar K: End-systolic pressure/volume ratio. A new index of ventricular contractility. Am J Cardiol 1977;40:748–753

55. Suga H, Sagawa K, Shoukas A: Load independence of the instantaneous pressure-volume ratio of the canine left ventricle and effects of epinephrine and heart rate on the ratio. Circ Res 1973;32:314–322

56. Suga H, Sagawa K: Instantaneous pressure-volume relationships and their ratio in the excised, supported canine left ventricle. Circ Res 1974;35: 117–126

57. Borow K: An integrated approach to the noninvasive assessment of left ventricular systolic and diastolic performance. pp. 97–154. In St. John Sutton M, Old-

ershaw P (eds): Textbook of Adult and Pediatric Echocardiography and Doppler. Blackwell Scientific, Boston, 1989

58. Colan S, Borow K, Neumann A: Use of the calibrated carotid pulse tracing for calculation of left ventricular pressure and wall stress throughout ejection. Am Heart J 1985;109:1306–1310

59. St. John Sutton M, Plappert T, Hirshfeld J, Reichek N: Assessment of left ventricular mechanics in patients with asymptomatic aortic regurgitation. A two-dimensional echocardiographic study. Circulation 1984;69:259–268

60. Douglas P, Reichek N, Plappert T, Muhammad A, St John Sutton M: Comparison of echocardiographic methods for assessment of left ventricular shortening and wall stress. J Am Coll Cardiol 1987;9:945–951

61. Gorcsan J III, Romand JA, Mandarino WA, Deneault LG, Pinsky MR: Assessment of left ventricular performance by on-line pressure-area relations using echocardiographic automated border detection. J Am Coll Cardiol 1994;23:242–252

62. Davila-Roman VG, Creswell LL, Rosenbloom M, Perez JE: Myocardial contractile state in dogs with chronic mitral regurgitation. Echocardiographic approach to the peak systolic pressure/end-systolic area relationship. Am Heart J 1993;126:155–160

63. O'Kelly BF, Tubau JF, Knight AA et al: Measurement of left ventricular contractility using transesophageal echocardiography in patients undergoing coronary artery bypass grafting. The Study of Perioperative Ischemia (SPI) Research Group. Am Heart J 1991;122:1041–1049

64. Gorcsan J III, Gasior TA, Mandarino WA et al: Assessment of the immediate effects of cardiopulmonary bypass on left ventricular performance by on-line pressure-area relations. Circulation 1994;89: 180–190

65. Kimball TR, Mays WA, Khoury PR, Mallie R, Claytor RP: Echocardiographic determination of left ventricular preload, afterload, and contractility during and after exercise. J Pediatr 1993;122:S89–S94

66. Sullivan J, Hanson P, Rahko PS, Folts JD: Continuous measurement of left ventricular performance during and after maximal isometric deadlift exercise. Circulation 1992;85:1406–1413

67. Lipshultz SE, Colan SD, Gelber RD et al: Late cardiac effects of doxorubicin therapy for acute lymphoblastic leukemia in childhood [see comments]. N Engl J Med 1991;324:808–815

68. De Simone G, Devereux RB, Roman MJ et al: Assessment of left ventricular function by the midwall fractional shortening/end-systolic stress relation in human hypertension. J Am Coll Cardiol 1994;23: 1444–1451 [Erratum in J Am Coll Cardiol 1994;24: 844]

69. Galderisi M, Benjamin EJ, Evans JC et al: Intra- and interobserver reproducibility of Doppler-assessed indexes of left ventricular diastolic function in a population-based study (the Framingham Heart Study). Am J Cardiol 1992;70:1341–1346

70. Thomas JD, Weyman AE: Echocardiographic Doppler evaluation of left ventricular diastolic function. Physics and physiology [review]. Circulation 1991;84: 977–990

71. Marino P, Destro G, Barbieri E, Zardini P: Early left ventricular filling. An approach to its multifactorial nature using a combined hemodynamic-Doppler technique. Am Heart J 1991;122:132–141

72. Brecker SJ, Lee CH, Gibson DG: Relation of left ventricular isovolumic relaxation time and incoordination to transmitral Doppler filling patterns. Br Heart J 1992;68:567–573

73. Yamamoto K, Masuyama T, Tanouchi J et al: Importance of left ventricular minimal pressure as a determinant of transmitral flow velocity pattern in the presence of left ventricular systolic dysfunction. J Am Coll Cardiol 1993;21:662–672

74. Galderisi M, Benjamin EJ, Evans JC et al: Impact of heart rate and PR interval on Doppler indexes of left ventricular diastolic filling in an elderly cohort (the Framingham Heart Study). Am J Cardiol 1993;72: 1183–1187

75. Stewart RA, Joshi J, Alexander N, Nihoyannopoulos P, Oakley CM: Adjustment for the influence of age and heart rate on Doppler measurements of left ventricular filling. Br Heart J 1992;68:608–612

76. Sagie A, Benjamin EJ, Galderisi M et al: Echocardiographic assessment of left ventricular structure and diastolic filling in elderly subjects with borderline isolated systolic hypertension (the Framingham Heart Study). Am J Cardiol 1993;72:662–665

77. Klein AL, Burstow DJ, Tajik AJ et al: Effects of age on left ventricular dimensions and filling dynamics in 117 normal persons. Mayo Clin Proc 1994;69: 212–224

78. Tanabe K, Ishibashi Y, Ohta T et al: Effect of left and right lateral decubitus positions on mitral flow pattern by Doppler echocardiography in congestive heart failure. Am J Cardiol 1993;71:751–753

79. Appleton CP, Hatle LK, Popp RL: Demonstration of restrictive ventricular physiology by Doppler echocardiography. J Am Coll Cardiol 1988;11:757–768

80. Presti C, Walling A, Montemayor I, Campbell J, Crawford M: Influence of exercise-induced myocardial ischemia on the pattern of left ventricular diastolic filling. A Doppler echocardiographic study. J Am Coll Cardiol 1991;18:75–82

81. Gottdiener J: Measuring diastolic function [editorial; comment]. J Am Coll Cardiol 1991;18:83–84

82. Hatle LK, Appleton CP, Popp RL: Differentiation of constrictive pericarditis and restrictive cardiomyopathy by Doppler echocardiography [see comments]. Circulation 1989;79:357–370

83. Himura Y, Kumada T, Kambayashi M et al: Importance of left ventricular systolic function in the assessment of left ventricular diastolic function with Doppler transmitral flow velocity recording [see comments]. J Am Coll Cardiol 1991;18:753–760

84. Cueto-Garcia L, Tajik AJ, Kyle RA et al: Serial echocardiographic observations in patients with primary systemic amyloidosis. An introduction to the concept of early (asymptomatic) amyloid infiltration of the heart. Mayo Clin Proc 1984;59:589–597

85. Cueto-Garcia L, Reeder G, Kyle R et al: Echocardiographic findings in systemic amyloidosis. Spectrum of cardiac involvement and relation to survival. J Am Coll Cardiol 1985;6:737–743

86. Klein AL, Hatle LK, Taliercio CP et al: Serial Doppler echocardiographic follow-up of left ventricular diastolic function in cardiac amyloidosis. J Am Coll Cardiol 1990;16:1135–1141

87. Cetta F, O'Leary PW, Seward JB, Driscoll DJ: Idio-

pathic restrictive cardiomyopathy in childhood. Diagnostic features and clinical course. Mayo Clin Proc 1995;70:634–640

88. Rajagopalan B, Bertram C, Stallard T, Lee G: Blood flow in the pulmonary veins. III. Simultaneous measurements of their dimensions, intravascular pressure and flow. Cardiovasc Res 1979;13:684–692

89. Rossvoll O, Hatle LK: Pulmonary venous flow velocities recorded by transthoracic Doppler ultrasound. Relation to left ventricular diastolic pressures [see comments]. J Am Coll Cardiol 1993;21:1687–1696

90. Nakatani S, Yoshitomi H, Wada K et al: Noninvasive estimation of left ventricular end-diastolic pressure using transthoracic Doppler-determined pulmonary venous atrial flow reversal. Am J Cardiol 1994;73:1017–1018

91. Kuecherer HF, Kusumoto F, Muhiudeen IA, Cahalan MK, Schiller NB: Pulmonary venous flow patterns by transesophageal pulsed Doppler echocardiography. Relation to parameters of left ventricular systolic and diastolic function. Am Heart J 1991;122:1683–1693

92. Hoit BD, Shao Y, Gabel M, Walsh RA: Influence of loading conditions and contractile state on pulmonary venous flow. Validation of Doppler velocimetry. Circulation 1992;86:651–659

93. Castello R, Pearson A, Lenzen P, Labovitz A: Effect of mitral regurgitation on pulmonary venous velocities derived from transesophageal echocardiography color-guided pulsed Doppler imaging. J Am Coll Cardiol 1991;17:1499–1506

94. Colan S, Borow K, Neumann A: Effects of loading conditions and contractile state on LV early diastolic function in normal subjects. Am J Cardiol 1985;55:790–796

95. Nishimura RA, Schwartz RS, Tajik AJ, Holmes D Jr: Noninvasive measurement of rate of left ventricular relaxation by Doppler echocardiography. Validation with simultaneous cardiac catheterization. Circulation 1993;88:146–155

96. Brun P, Tribouilloy C, Duval AM et al: Left ventricular flow propagation during early filling is related to wall relaxation. A color M-mode Doppler analysis. J Am Coll Cardiol 1992;20:420–432

97. Stuggaard M, Risoe C, Halfdan I, Smseth O: Intracavitary filling pattern in the failing left ventricle assessed by color M-mode Doppler echocardiography. J Am Coll Cardiol 1994;24:663–670

98. Yamamoto K, Masuyama T, Tanouchi J et al: Intraventricular dispersion of early diastolic filling. A new marker of left ventricular diastolic dysfunction. Am Heart J 1995;129:291–299

99. Pennestri F, Biasucci LM, Rinelli G et al: Abnormal intraventricular flow patterns in left ventricular dysfunction determined by color Doppler study. Am Heart J 1992;124:966–974

100. Ghali JK, Kadakia S, Cooper RS, Liao YL: Bedside diagnosis of preserved versus impaired left ventricular systolic function in heart failure [see comments]. Am J Cardiol 1991;67:1002–1006

101. Chakko S, Woska D, Martinez H et al: Clinical radiographic, and hemodynamic correlations in chronic congestive heart failure. Conflicting results may lead to inappropriate care. Am J Med 1991;90:353–359

102. Cohn JN, Johnson G: Heart failure with normal ejection fraction. The V-HeFT Study. Veterans Administration Cooperative Study Group. Circulation, suppl. III 1990;81:48–53

103. Ghali JK, Kadakia S, Bhatt A, Cooper R, Liao Y: Survival of heart failure patients with preserved versus impaired systolic function. The prognostic implication of blood pressure. Am Heart J 1992;123:993–997

104. Armstrong PW, Moe GW: Medical advances in the treatment of congestive heart failure [review]. Circulation 1993;88:2941–2952

105. Pitt B: Use of converting enzyme inhibitors in patients with asymptomatic left ventricular dysfunction. J Am Coll Cardiol, suppl. A 1993;22:158–161

106. Clarke KW, Gray D, Hampton JR: Evidence of inadequate investigation and treatment of patients with heart failure. Br Heart J 1994;71:584–587

107. Lewis J, Webber J, Sutton L, Chesoni S, Curry C: Discordance in degree of right and left ventricular dilation in patients with dilated cardiomyopathy. Recognition and clinical implications. J Am Coll Cardiol 1993;21:649–654

108. Abramson S, Burke J, Kelly J et al: Pulmonary hypertension predicts mortality and morbidity in patients with dilated cardiomyopathy. Ann Intern Med 1992;116:888–895

109. Diaz RA, Nihoyannopoulos P, Athanassopoulos G, Oakley CM: Usefulness of echocardiography to differentiate dilated cardiomyopathy from coronary-induced congestive heart failure [see comments]. Am J Cardiol 1991;68:1224–1227

110. Sharp SM, Sawada SG, Segar DS et al: Dobutamine stress echocardiography. Detection of coronary artery disease in patients with dilated cardiomyopathy. J Am Coll Cardiol 1994;24:934–939

111. Cigarroa CG, deFilippi CR, Brickner ME et al: Dobutamine stress echocardiography identifies hibernating myocardium and predicts recovery of left ventricular function after coronary revascularization. Circulation 1993;88:430–436

112. Salustri A, Elhendy A, Garyfallydis P et al: Prediction of improvement of ventricular function after first acute myocardial infarction using low-dose dobutamine stress echocardiography. Am J Cardiol 1994;74:853–856

113. Takeuchi M, Araki M, Nakashima Y, Kuroiwa A: The detection of residual ischemia and stenosis in patients with acute myocardial infarction with dobutamine stress echocardiography. J Am Soc Echocardiogr 1994;7:242–252

114. Tanimoto M, Pai RG, Jintapakorn W, Shah PM: Dobutamine stress echocardiography for the diagnosis and management of coronary artery disease [review]. Clin Cardiol 1995;18:252–260

115. Erlebacher J, Weiss J, Eaton L et al: Late effects of acute infarct dilation on heart size. A two dimensional echocardiographic study. Am J Cardiol 1982;49:1120–1126

116. Erlebacher J, Weiss J, Weisfeldt M, Bulkley B: Early dilation of the infarcted segment in acute transmural myocardial infarction. Role of infarct expansion in acute left ventricular enlargement. J Am Coll Cardiol 1984;4:201–208

117. Diaz RA, Obasohan A, Oakley CM: Prediction of outcome in dilated cardiomyopathy. Br Heart J 1987;58:393–399

118. Hofmann T, Meinertz T, Kasper W et al: Mode of death in idiopathic dilated cardiomyopathy. A multi-

variate analysis of prognostic determinants. Am Heart J 1988;116:1455–1463

119. Keogh AM, Freund J, Baron DW, Hickie JB: Timing of cardiac transplantation in idiopathic dilated cardiomyopathy. Am J Cardiol 1988;61:418–422

120. Olshausen KV, Stienen U, Schwarz F, Kubler W, Meyer J: Long-term prognostic significance of ventricular arrhythmias in idiopathic dilated cardiomyopathy. Am J Cardiol 1988;61:146–151

121. Schwarz F, Mall G, Zebe H et al: Determinants of survival in patients with congestive cardiomyopathy. Quantitative morphologic findings and left ventricular hemodynamics. Circulation 1984;70:923–928

122. Douglas PS, Morrow R, Ioli A, Reichek N: Left ventricular shape, afterload and survival in idiopathic dilated cardiomyopathy. J Am Coll Cardiol 1989;13:311–315

123. Kono T, Sabbah HN, Stein PD, Brymer JF, Khaja F: Left ventricular shape as a determinant of functional mitral regurgitation in patients with severe heart failure secondary to either coronary artery disease or idiopathic dilated cardiomyopathy. Am J Cardiol 1991;68:355–359

124. Lee TH, Hamilton MA et al: Impact of left ventricular cavity size on survival in advanced heart failure. Am J Cardiol 1993;72:672–676

125. Wong M, Johnson G, Shabetai R et al: Echocardiographic variables as prognostic indicators and therapeutic monitors in chronic congestive heart failure. Veterans Affairs cooperative studies V-HeFT I and II. V-HeFT VA Cooperative Studies Group. Circulation, suppl. VI 1993;87:65–70

126. Benedict CR, Johnstone DE, Weiner DH et al: Relation of neurohumoral activation to clinical variables and degree of ventricular dysfunction. A report from the Registry of Studies of Left Ventricular Dysfunction. SOLVD Investigators. J Am Coll Cardiol 1994;23:1410–1420

127. Greenberg B, Quinones MA, Koilpillai C et al: Effects of long-term enalapril therapy on cardiac structure and function in patients with left ventricular dysfunction. Results of the SOLVD echocardiography substudy [see comments]. Circulation 1995;91:2573–2581

128. Lewis AB: Prognostic value of echocardiography in children with idiopathic dilated cardiomyopathy. Am Heart J 1994;128:133–136

129. Shen WF, Tribouilloy C, Rey JL et al: Prognostic significance of Doppler-derived left ventricular diastolic filling variables in dilated cardiomyopathy. Am Heart J 1992;124:1524–1533

130. Werner GS, Schaefer C, Dirks R, Figulla HR, Kreuzer H: Doppler echocardiographic assessment of left ventricular filling in idiopathic dilated cardiomyopathy during a one-year follow-up. Relation to the clinical course of disease. Am Heart J 1993;126:1408–1416

131. Werner GS, Schaefer C, Dirks R, Figulla HR, Kreuzer H: Prognostic value of Doppler echocardiographic assessment of left ventricular filling in idiopathic dilated cardiomyopathy. Am J Cardiol 1994;73:792–798

132. Pinamonti B, DiLenarda A, Sinagra G, Camerini F: Restrictive left ventricular filling pattern in dilated cardiomyopathy assessed by Doppler echocardiography. Clinical, echocardiographic and hemodynamic

correlations and prognostic implications. J Am Coll Cardiol 1993;22:808–815

133. Kono T, Rosman H, Alam M, Stein PD, Sabbah HN: Hemodynamic correlates of the third heart sound during the evolution of chronic heart failure. J Am Coll Cardiol 1993;21:419–423

134. Lavine SJ, Campbell CA, Held AC, Johnson V: Effect of inotropic and vasodilator therapy on left ventricular diastolic filling in dogs with severe left ventricular dysfunction. J Am Coll Cardiol 1990;15:1165–1172

135. Kono T, Sabbah HN, Rosman H et al: Divergent effects of intravenous dobutamine and nitroprusside on left atrial contribution to ventricular filling in dogs with chronic heart failure. Am Heart J 1994;127:874–880

136. Blondheim DS, Jacobs LE, Kotler MN, Costacurta GA, Parry WR: Dilated cardiomyopathy with mitral regurgitation. Decreased survival despite a low frequency of left ventricular thrombus. Am Heart J 1991;122:763–771

137. Falk RH, Foster E, Coats MH: Ventricular thrombi and thromboembolism in dilated cardiomyopathy. A prospective follow-up study. Am Heart J 1992;123:136–142

138. Takamoto T, Kim D, Urie PM et al: Comparative recognition of left ventricular thrombi by echocardiography and cineangiography. B Heart J 1985;53:36–42

139. Keren A, Goldberg S, Gottlieb S et al: Natural history of left ventricular thrombi. Their appearance and resolution in the posthospitalization period of acute myocardial infarction. J Am Coll Cardiol 1990;15:790–800

140. Ciaccheri M, Castelli G, Cecchi F et al: Lack of correlation between intracavitary thrombosis detected by cross sectional echocardiography and systemic emboli in patients with dilated cardiomyopathy. Br Heart J 1989;62:26–29

141. Jugdutt BI, Sivaram CA: Prospective two-dimensional echocardiographic evaluation of left ventricular thrombus and embolism after acute myocardial infarction. J Am Coll Cardiol 1989;13:554–564

142. Spirito P, Bellotti P, Chiarella F et al: Prognostic significance and natural history of left ventricular thrombi in patients with acute anterior myocardial infarction. A two-dimensional echocardiographic study. Circulation 1985;72:774–780

143. Domenicucci S, Bellotti P, Chiarella F, Lupi G, Vecchio C: Spontaneous morphologic changes in left ventricular thrombi. A prospective two-dimensional echocardiographic study. Circulation 1987;75:737–743

144. Maze SS, Kotler MN, Parry WR: Flow characteristics in the dilated left ventricle with thrombus. Qualitative and quantitative Doppler analysis. J Am Coll Cardiol 1989;13:873–881

145. Haugland JM, Asinger RW, Mikell FL, Elsperger J, Hodges M: Embolic potential of left ventricular thrombi detected by two-dimensional echocardiography. Circulation 1984;70:588–598

146. Meltzer RS, Visser CA, Kan G, Roelandt J: Two-dimensional echocardiographic appearance of left ventricular thrombi with systemic emboli after myocardial infarction. Am J Cardiol 1984;53:1511–1513

147. Van Reet R, Quinones M, Poliner L et al: Comparison of two-dimensional echocardiography with gated radionuclide ventriculography in the evaluation of

global and regional left ventricular function in acute myocardial infarction. J Am Coll Cardiol 1984;3: 243–252

148. Cleempoel H, Vainsel H, Dramaix M et al: Limitations on the prognostic value of predischarge data after myocardial infarction. Br Heart J 1988;60: 98–103

149. Kan G, Visser CA, Koolen JJ, Dunning AJ: Short and long term predictive value of admission wall motion score in acute myocardial infarction. A cross sectional echocardiographic study of 345 patients. Br Heart J 1986;56:422–427

150. Shiina A, Tajik AJ, Smith HC, Lengyel M, Seward JB: Prognostic significance of regional wall motion abnormality in patients with prior myocardial infarction. A prospective correlative study of two-dimensional echocardiography and angiography. Mayo Clin Proc 1986;61:254–262

151. Abernethy M, Sharpe N, Smith H, Gamble G: Echocardiographic prediction of left ventricular volume after myocardial infarction. J Am Coll Cardiol 1991; 17:1527–1532

152. Nishimura RA, Tajik AJ, Shub C et al: Role of two-dimensional echocardiography in the prediction of in-hospital complications after acute myocardial infarction. J Am Coll Cardiol 1984;4:1080–1087

153. Nishimura RA, Reeder GS, Miller F Jr et al: Prognostic value of predischarge 2-dimensional echocardiogram after acute myocardial infarction. Am J Cardiol 1984;53:429–432

154. Bhatnagar SK, Moussa MA, Al-Yusuf AR: The role of prehospital discharge two-dimensional echocardiography in determining the prognosis of survivors of first myocardial infarction. Am Heart J 1985;109: 472–477

155. Hasche ET, Fernandes C, Freedman SB, Jeremy RW: Relation between ischemia time, infarct size, and left ventricular function in humans. Circulation 1995;92: 710–719

156. Shen WK, Khandheria BK, Edwards WD et al: Value and limitations of two-dimensional echocardiography in predicting myocardial infarct size. Am J Cardiol 1991;68:1143–1149

157. Otto CM, Stratton JR, Maynard C et al: Echocardiographic evaluation of segmental wall motion early and late after thrombolytic therapy in acute myocardial infarction. The Western Washington Tissue Plasminogen Activator Emergency Room Trial. Am J Cardiol 1990;65:132–138

158. Presti CF, Gentile R, Armstrong WF et al: Improvement in regional wall motion after percutaneous transluminal coronary angioplasty during acute myocardial infarction. Utility of two-dimensional echocardiography. Am Heart J 1988;115:1149–1155

159. Guyer D, Foale R, Gillam L et al: An echocardiographic technique for quantifying and displaying the extent of regional left ventricular dyssynergy. J Am Coll Cardiol 1986;8:830–835

160. Guyer D, Gibson T, Gillam L et al: A new echocardiographic model for quantifying three-dimensional endocardial surface area. J Am Coll Cardiol 1986;8: 819–829

161. Wilkins G, Southern J, Choong C et al: Correlation between echocardiographic endocardial surface mapping of abnormal wall motion and pathologic infarct

size in autopsied hearts. Circulation 1988;77: 978–987

162. Pfeffer M, Braunwald E: Ventricular remodeling after myocardial infarction. Circulation 1990;81: 1161–1172

163. Mann D, Foale R, Gillam L et al: Early natural history of regional left ventricular dysfunction after experimental myocardial infarction. Am Heart J 1988; 115:538–546

164. Eaton L, Weiss J, Bulkley B, Garrison J, Weisfeldt M: Regional cardiac dilatation after acute myocardial infarction. Recognition by two-dimensional echocardiography. N Engl J Med 1979;300:57–62

165. Litwin SE, Katz SE, Morgan JP, Douglas PS: Serial echocardiographic assessment of left ventricular geometry and function after large myocardial infarction in the rat. Circulation 1994;89:345–354

166. Visser C, Kan G, Miltzer R, Koolen J, Dunning A: Incidence, timing and prognostic value of left ventricular aneurysm formation after myocardial infarction. A prospective, serial echocardiographic study of 158 patients. Am J Cardiol 1986;57:729–732

167. Matsumoto M, Watanabe F, Goto A et al: Left ventricular aneurysm and the prediction of left ventricular enlargement studied by two-dimensional echocardiography. Quantitative assessment of aneurysm size in relation to clinical course. Circulation 1985;72: 280–286

168. Choy AM, Darbar D, Lang CC et al: Detection of left ventricular dysfunction after acute myocardial infarction. Comparison of clinical, echocardiographic, and neurohormonal methods. Br Heart J 1994;72: 16–22

169. Picard M, Wilkins G, Ray P, Weyman A: Natural history of left ventricular size and function after acute myocardial infarction. Assessment and prediction by echocardiographic endocardial surface mapping. J Am Coll Cardiol 1990;82:484–494

170. Kumar A, Minagoe S, Chandraratna P: Two-dimensional echocardiographic demonstration of restoration of normal wall motion after acute myocardial infarction. Am J Cardiol 1986;57:1232–1235

171. St. John Sutton MG, Pfeffer MA, Plappert T et al: Quantitative two-dimensional echocardiographic measurements are major predictors of adverse cardiovascular events after acute myocardial infarction. The protective effects of captopril. Circulation 1994; 89:68–75

172. Iliceto S, Scrutinio D, Bruzzi P et al: Effects of L-carnitine administration on left ventricular remodeling after acute anterior myocardial infarction: The CEDIM trial. J Am Coll Cardiol 1995;26:380–387

173. Appleton CP, Galloway JM, Gonzalez MS, Gaballa M, Basnight MA: Estimation of left ventricular filling pressures using two-dimensional and Doppler echocardiography in adult patients with cardiac disease. Additional value of analyzing left atrial size, left atrial ejection fraction and the difference in duration of pulmonary venous and mitral flow velocity at atrial contraction. J Am Coll Cardiol 1993;22:1972–1982

174. Giannuzzi P, Imparato A, Temporelli PL et al: Doppler-derived mitral deceleration time of early filling as a strong predictor of pulmonary capillary wedge pressure in postinfarction patients with left ventricular systolic dysfunction. J Am Coll Cardiol 1994;23: 1630–1637

175. Maron B, Bonow R, Cannon R, Leon M, Epstein S: Hypertrophic Cardiomyopathy. Interrelations of clinical manifestations, pathophysiology, and therapy [second of two parts]. N Engl J Med 1987;316: 844–852

176. Wigle E, Rakowski H: Hypertrophic cardiomyopathy. When do you diagnose midventricular obstruction versus apical cavity obliteration with a small non-obliterated area at the apex of the left ventricle? J Am Coll Cardiol 1992;19:525–526

177. Wigle E, Rakowski H, Kimbal B, Williams W: Hypertrophic cardiomyopathy. Circulation 1995;92: 1680–1692

178. Louie E, Maron B: Apical hypertrophic cardiomyopathy. Clinical and two-dimensional echocardiographic assessment. Ann Intern Med 1987;106:663–670

179. Maron B, Spirito P, Wesley Y, Arce J: Development and progression of left ventricular hypertrophy in children with hypertrophic cardiomyopathy. N Engl J Med 1986;315:610–614

180. Fragola PV, Borzi M, Cannata D: The spectrum of echocardiographic and electrocardiographic abnormalities in nonaffected relatives of patients with hypertrophic cardiomyopathy. A transverse and longitudinal study. Cardiology 1993;83:289–297

181. Schwammenthal E, Block M, Schwartzkopff B et al: Prediction of the site and severity of obstruction in hypertrophic cardiomyopathy by color flow mapping and continuous wave Doppler echocardiography. J Am Coll Cardiol 1992;20:964–972

182. Panza JA, Petrone RK, Fananapazir L, Maron BJ: Utility of continuous wave Doppler echocardiography in the noninvasive assessment of left ventricular outflow tract pressure gradient in patients with hypertrophic cardiomyopathy. J Am Coll Cardiol 1992;19: 91–99

183. Pollick C, Rakowski H, Wigle E: Muscular subaortic stenosis. The quantitative relationship between systolic anterior motion and the pressure gradient. Circulation 1984;69:43–49

184. Lin CS, Chen KS, Lin MC, Fu MC, Tang SM: The relationship between systolic anterior motion of the mitral valve and the left ventricular outflow tract Doppler in hypertrophic cardiomyopathy. Am Heart J 1991;122:1671–1682

185. Sherrid MV, Chu CK, Delia E, Mogtader A, Dwyer E Jr: An echocardiographic study of the fluid mechanics of obstruction in hypertrophic cardiomyopathy. J Am Coll Cardiol 1993;22:816–825

186. Klues HG, Proschan MA, Dollar AL et al: Echocardiographic assessment of mitral valve size in obstructive hypertrophic cardiomyopathy. Anatomic validation from mitral valve specimen. Circulation 1993;88: 548–555

187. Cape EG, Simons D, Jimoh A et al: Chordal geometry determines the shape and extent of systolic anterior mitral motion. In vitro studies. J Am Coll Cardiol 1989;13:1438–1448

188. Jiang L, Levine RA, King ME, Weyman AE: An integrated mechanism for systolic anterior motion of the mitral valve in hypertrophic cardiomyopathy based on echocardiographic observations. Am Heart J 1987; 113:633–644

189. Nakamura T, Matsubara K, Furukawa K et al: Diastolic paradoxic jet flow in patients with hypertrophic cardiomyopathy. Evidence of concealed apical asyn-

190. Yoneda Y, Suwa M, Hanada H, Hirota Y, Kawamura K: Non-invasive detection of left ventricular diastolic dysfunction using M-mode echocardiography to assess left ventricular posterior wall kinetics in hypertrophic cardiomyopathy. Am J Cardiol 1992;70: 1583–1588

191. Maron B, Spirito P, Green K et al: Noninvasive assessment of left ventricular diastolic function by pulsed Doppler echocardiography in patients with hypertrophic cardiomyopathy. J Am Coll Cardiol 1987;10:733–742

192. Losi MA, Betocchi S, Grimaldi M, Spampinato N, Chiariello M: Heterogeneity of left ventricular filling dynamics in hypertrophic cardiomyopathy. Am J Cardiol 1994;73:987–990

193. Nihoyannopoulos P, Karatasakis G, Frenneaux M, McKenna W, Oakley C: Diastolic function in hypertrophic cardiomyopathy. Relation to exercise capacity. J Am Coll Cardiol 1992;19:536–540

194. Lewis AB: Clinical profile and outcome of restrictive cardiomyopathy in children. Am Heart J 1992;123: 1589–1593

195. Seiler C, Jenni R, Krayenbuehl H: Intraventricular blood flow during isovolumetric relaxation and diastole in hypertrophic cardiomyopathy. J Am Soc Echocardiogr 1991;4:247–257

196. Zoghbi W, Haichin R, Quinones M: Mid-cavitary obstruction in apical hypertrophy. Doppler evidence of diastolic interventricular gradient with higher apical pressure. Am Heart J 1988;116:1469–1474

197. Wigle E, Rakowski H: Hypertrophic cardiomyopathy. When do you diagnose midventricular obstruction versus apical cavity obliteration with a small non-obliterated area at the apex of the left ventricle? Am Coll Cardiol 1992;19:525–526

198. Masuyama T, St. Goar F, Tye T et al: Ultrasonic tissue characterization of human hypertrophied hearts in vivo with cardiac cycle-dependent variation in integrated backscatter. Circulation 1989;80:925–934

199. Solomon SD, Kytomaa H, Celi AC et al: Myocardial tissue characterization by autocorrelation of two-dimensional ultrasonic backscatter. J Am Soc Echocardiogr 1994;7:631–640

200. Naito J, Masuyama T, Tanouchi J et al: Analysis of transmural trend of myocardial integrated ultrasound backscatter for differentiation of hypertrophic cardiomyopathy and ventricular hypertrophy due to hypertension. J Am Coll Cardiol 1994;24:517–524

201. Lattanzi F, Di Bello V, Picano E et al: Normal ultrasonic myocardial reflectivity in athletes with increased left ventricular mass. A tissue characterization study. Circulation 1992;85:1828–1834

202. Widimsky P, Ten Cate FJ, Vletter W, van Herwerden L: Potential applications for transesophageal echocardiography in hypertrophic cardiomyopathies. J Am Soc Echocardiogr 1992;5:163–167

203. Jeanrenaud X, Goy JJ, Kappenberger L: Effects of dual-chamber pacing in hypertrophic obstructive cardiomyopathy [see comments]. Lancet 1992;339: 1318–1323

204. Fananapazir L, Cannon R III, Tripodi D, Panza JA: Impact of dual-chamber permanent pacing in patients with obstructive hypertrophic cardiomyopathy with symptoms refractory to verapamil and beta-ad-

renergic blocker therapy. Circulation 1992;85: 2149–2161

205. Fananapazir L, Epstein ND, Curiel RV et al: Long-term results of dual-chamber (DDD) pacing in obstructive hypertrophic cardiomyopathy. Evidence for progressive symptomatic and hemodynamic improvement and reduction of left ventricular hypertrophy. Circulation 1994;90:2731–2742

206. Goldman ME: Hypertrophic cardiomyopathy and intraoperative echocardiography. Too much of a good thing may be dangerous [editorial; comment]. J Am Coll Cardiol 1992;20:53–54

207. Grigg LE, Wigle ED, Williams WG, Daniel LB, Rakowski H: Transesophageal Doppler echocardiography in obstructive hypertrophic cardiomyopathy. Clarification of pathophysiology and importance in intraoperative decision making [see comments]. J Am Coll Cardiol 1992;20:42–52

208. Marwick TH, Stewart WJ, Lever HM et al: Benefits of intraoperative echocardiography in the surgical management of hypertrophic cardiomyopathy. J Am Coll Cardiol 1992;20:1066–1072

209. McIntosh C, Maron B: Current operative treatment of obstructive hypertrophic cardiomyopathy. Circulation 1988;78:487–495

210. Kirschner E, Berger M, Goldberg E: Hypertrophic obstructive cardiomyopathy presenting with profound hypotension. Role of two-dimensional and Doppler echocardiography in diagnosis and management. Chest 1992;101:711–714

211. Klein AL, Oh JK, Miller FA, Seward JB, Tajik AJ: Two-dimensional and Doppler echocardiographic assessment of infiltrative cardiomyopathy. [review]. J Am Soc Echocardiogr 1988;1:48–59

212. Keren A, Billingham ME, Popp RL: Features of mildly dilated congestive cardiomyopathy compared with idiopathic restrictive cardiomyopathy and typical dilated cardiomyopathy. J Am Soc Echocardiogr 1988;1:78–87

213. Siegel RJ, Shah PK, Fishbein MC: Idiopathic restrictive cardiomyopathy. Circulation 1984;70:165–169

214. Olson LJ, Edwards WD, Holmes D, Jr et al: Endomyocardial biopsy in hemochromatosis. Clinicopathologic correlates in six cases. J Am Coll Cardiol 1989; 13:116–120

215. Acquatella H, Rodriguez-Salas LA, Gomez-Mancebo JR: Doppler echocardiography in dilated and restrictive cardiomyopathies [review]. Cardiol Clin 1990;8: 349–367

216. Klein AL, Cohen GI, Pietrolungo JF et al: Differentiation of constrictive pericarditis from restrictive cardiomyopathy by Doppler transesophageal echocardiographic measurements of respiratory variations in pulmonary venous flow. J Am Coll Cardiol 1993;22: 1935–1943

217. Schiavone WA, Calafiore PA, Salcedo EE: Transesophageal Doppler echocardiographic demonstration of pulmonary venous flow velocity in restrictive cardiomyopathy and constrictive pericarditis. Am J Cardiol 1989;63:1286–1288

218. Falk R, Plehn J, Deering T et al: Sensitivity and specificity of the echocardiographic features of cardiac amyloidosis. Am J Cardiol 1987;59:418–422

219. Nicolosi GL, Pavan D, Lestuzzi C et al: Prospective identification of patients with amyloid heart disease by two-dimensional echocardiography. Circulation 1984;70:432–437

220. Pinamonti B, Picano E, Ferdeghini EM et al: Quantitative texture analysis in two-dimensional echocardiography. Application to the diagnosis of myocardial amyloidosis. J Am Coll Cardiol 1989;14:666–671

221. Klein AL, Hatle LK, Burstow DJ et al: Doppler characterization of left ventricular diastolic function in cardiac amyloidosis. J Am Coll Cardiol 1989;13: 1017–1026

222. Klein A, Hatle L, Taliercio C et al: Prognostic significance of Doppler measures of diastolic function in cardiac amyloidosis. A Doppler echocardiography study. Circulation 1991;83:808–816

223. Hauptman P, Gass A, Goldman M: The role of echocardiography in heart transplantation. J Am Soc Echocardiogr 1993;6:496–509

224. Stoddard MF, Longaker RA: The role of transesophageal echocardiography in cardiac donor screening. Am Heart J 1993;125:1676–1681

225. Canivet JL, Defraigne JO, Demoulin JC, Limet R: Mechanical flow obstruction after heart transplantation diagnosed by TEE. Ann Thorac Surg 1994;58: 890–891

226. Polanco G, Jafri SM, Alam M, Levine TB: Transesophageal echocardiographic findings in patients with orthotopic heart transplantation. Chest 1992; 101:599–602

227. Tischler MD, Lee RT, Plappert T et al: Serial assessment of left ventricular function and mass after orthotopic heart transplantation. A 4-year longitudinal study. J Am Coll Cardiol 1992;19:60–66 [erratum in J Am Coll Cardiol 1994;23:281]

228. Mannaerts HF, Balk AH, Simoons ML et al: Changes in left ventricular function and wall thickness in heart transplant recipients and their relation to acute rejection. An assessment by digitised M mode echocardiography. Br Heart J 1992;68:356–364

229. Gill EA, Borrego C, Bray BE et al: Left ventricular mass increases during cardiac allograft vascular rejection. J Am Coll Cardiol 1995;25:922–926

230. Ciliberto GR, Mascarello M, Gronda E et al: Acute rejection after heart transplantation. Noninvasive echocardiographic evaluation. J Am Coll Cardiol 1994;23:1156–1161

231. Simmonds MB, Lythall DA, Slorach C et al: Doppler examination of superior vena caval flow for the detection of acute cardiac rejection. Circulation suppl. II 1992;86:259–266

232. Wilensky RL, Bourdillon PD, O'Donnell JA et al: Restrictive hemodynamic patterns after cardiac transplantation: relationship to histologic signs of rejection. Am Heart J 1991;122:1079–1087

233. Lieback E, Meyer R, Nawrocki M, Bellach J, Hetzer R: Noninvasive diagnosis of cardiac rejection through echocardiographic tissue characterization. Ann Thorac Surg 1994;57:1164–1170

234. Pytlewski G, Georgeson S, Burke J, Jeevanandam V, Pollack PS: Endomyocardial biopsy under transesophageal echocardiographic guidance can be safely performed in the critically ill cardiac transplant recipient. Am J Cardiol 1994;73:1019–1020

235. Rees AP, Milani RV, Lavie CJ, Smart FW, Ventura HO: Valvular regurgitation and right-sided cardiac pressures in heart transplant recipients by complete

Doppler and color flow evaluation [see comments]. Chest 1993;104:82–87

236. Huddleston CB, Rosenbloom M, Goldstein JA, Pasque MK: Biopsy-induced tricuspid regurgitation after cardiac transplantation [see comments]. Ann Thorac Surg 1994;57:832–836

237. Stahl RD, Karwande SV, Olsen SL et al: Tricuspid valve dysfunction in the transplanted heart. Ann Thorac Surg 1995;59:477–480

238. Cladellas M, Oriol A, Caralps JM: Quantitative assessment of valvular function after cardiac transplantation by pulsed Doppler echocardiography. Am J Cardiol 1994;73:1197–1201

239. Ciliberto G, Massa D, Mangiavacchi M et al: High-dose dipyridamole echocardiography test in coronary artery disease after heart transplantation. Eur Heart J 1993;14:48–52

240. Derumeaux G, Redonnet M, Mouton-Schleifer D et al: Dobutamine stress echocardiography in orthotopic heart transplant recipients. VACOMED Research Group. J Am Coll Cardiol 1995;25:1665–1672

241. American Society of Echocardiography: Report of the American Society of Echocardiographic Committee on Nomenclature and Standards. Identification of myocardial wall segments. Presented to the American Society of Echocardiography, Raleigh, NC, 1982

33 Radionuclide Methods

Michael W. Dae
Elias H. Botvinick

Congestive heart failure (CHF) is a complicated clinical syndrome involving a number of pathophysiologic mechanisms. A prerequisite for proper patient management is accurate hemodynamic and physiologic assessment. Radionuclide methods have come to play an important role in providing precise noninvasive measurements of ventricular function, sensitive and specific detection of myocardial viability, and an emerging role in the assessment of neurohormonal influences in CHF.

ASSESSMENT OF VENTRICULAR FUNCTION

There are two scintigraphic methods for evaluating right and left ventricular size and function: first-pass[1-3] and equilibrium[1-3] techniques. In addition to their noninvasive nature, they provide quantitative, reproducible, pathophysiologic evaluation and permit computer analysis with derivation of a variety of useful measurements. Both methods permit accurate serial volume and function measurements, as well as regional and global evaluation of ventricular function.

First-Pass Methodology

The first-pass technique generates data during the first transit of a radionuclide bolus through the central circulation. First-pass evaluation can be per-formed with virtually any pharmaceutical passing through the central circulation. Short-lived, rapidly excreted technetium 99m (^{99m}Tc) diethylenetriamine pentaacetic acid (DTPA) is commonly used. However, for quantitative volume assessment or equilibrium evaluation, a long-lived blood pool marker, such as labeled red blood cells (RBCs), should be used.[4] First-pass quantitation of ventricular size and function depends on principles of the indicator-dilution technique,[5] requiring a compact bolus injection proximal to the mixing chamber and homogeneous mixing of the blood pool indicator.

A sensitive camera or probe[2,3,5] over the central circulation, generally in the 30 degree right anterior oblique projection, follows the bolus through the heart. Its arrival and departure in each chamber produces a low-frequency radioactivity peak. The sequential variations of the cardiac cycle superimpose high-frequency spikes and valleys—proportional to end-diastolic (ED) and end-systolic (ES) volumes, respectively—on the time versus radioactivity curve (Fig. 33-1). These values yield accurate right and left ventricular ejection fractions.[1,3,6] The difference in ED and ES counts (C) is proportional to the stroke volume (SV), which, divided by background-corrected EDC, yields the ejection fraction (EF):

$$EF = EDC - ESC / EDC - background$$

With proper choice of background, these values have been well correlated with invasive methods.[7,8] Subsequent temporal separation permits dynamic evalu-

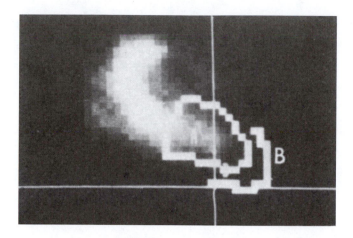

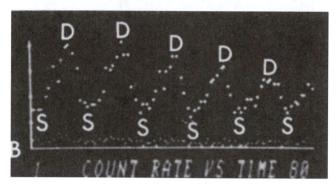

Fig. 33-1. First-pass levophase analysis. **(A)** Levophase of a first-pass radioangiogram. A region of interest has localized the left ventricle. **(B)** High-frequency analysis of the time versus radioactivity data in this region yields the curve shown. Correcting for background, the peaks and valleys may be compared to calculate the left ventricular ejection fraction. (From Botvinick et al.,[64] with permission.)

ation of ventricular wall motion, cardiac output, and ventricular volumes.[1,2,9]

First-pass methodology requires specialized equipment for optimal performance in order to avoid statistical difficulties at low count rates. Multicrystal cameras allow count rates up to 450,000 per second without significant saturation of detector electronics, allowing the injection of higher doses of radioactivity to enhance data density. The high-dose first-pass method becomes less suitable for serial studies, however. Nonetheless, such methods have been applied to the evaluation of changes in ventricular function with dynamic stress,[8,10–12] pharmacologic intervention,[12,13] and in a variety of clinical situations.[14,15]

It would take a count rate five times what is available on first-pass analysis to reduce the statistical error to that generally obtained with equilibrium blood pool studies. Nevertheless, the high-dose first-pass technique compares favorably for ejection fraction determination with equilibrium and selective

ventriculographic methods[1] with an extremely low level of intraobserver and interobserver variability.

Equilibrium Methodology

Equilibrium multiple gated blood pool scintigraphy is the most widely employed scintigraphic method for the evaluation of right and left ventricular size and function.[3,5] Imaging is performed in synchrony with or gated to the surface electrocardiogram (ECG) at equilibrium at least 5 minutes after intravenous administration of the radionuclide with complete mixing of the stable blood pool label. At this time, each volume of blood contains the same amount of radioactivity. There are several methods for labeling the RBCs. Although simply performed in vivo, greater labeling efficiency and stability are offered by the convenient modified in vitro method.[4] From 20 to 25 mCi of ^{99m}Tc pertechnetate (O_4^-) is combined with 10 ml of the patient's blood, previously combined with stannous ions. The labeled cells are then readministered and imaged. In vitro labeling adds efficiency and stability, sometimes necessary in the presence of multiple medications. Radionuclide stability permits repeated imaging in multiple projections without temporal and spatial selectivity of first-pass methods. Resolution of anatomy and wall motion is optimized by acquisition in three projections: anterior; 70 degree left anterior oblique to view the inferior wall; and the "best septal" left anterior oblique projection. The best septal projection distinguishes the two ventricles and is often obtained with a caudal tilt to reduce left atrial overlap. A high-resolution single-crystal camera and a high-resolution or slant-hole collimator is optimally used in adults.

Because equilibrium studies depend on image analysis of a composite sum of serial cardiac cycles, they are always computer-acquired and triggered by, or "gated," to the R wave. The mean length of the RR interval is established prior to acquisition. Frame mode acquisition serially images a predetermined fraction (40 ms or less) of the mean cardiac cycle and is best employed with regular rhythms. In each fraction, temporal interval, or frame, image data are combined to yield a summed picture over 200–600 cycles (Fig. 33-2). The study is terminated when each monitored frame contains sufficient data to permit generation of images with adequate spatial resolution of chamber anatomy and adequate statistical counts analysis. List mode acquisition is employed in the presence of a variable heart rate, such as atrial fibrillation.[3,5] In list mode, sequential counts are acquired in separate memory locations along with accompanying R waves, which enables the data to be

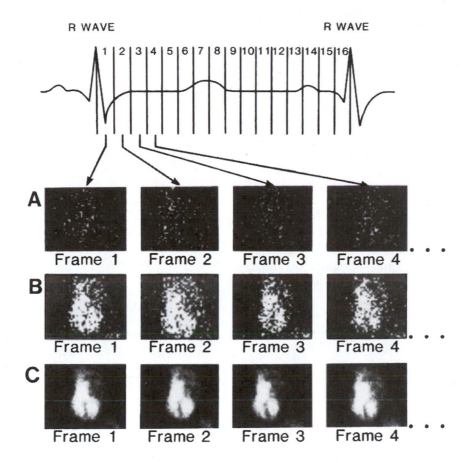

Fig. 33-2. ECG gating of the blood pool images. The computer uses the R wave to signal the start of a new cardic cycle. The cycle here has been divided into 16 equal intervals. Camera counts that occur during the first interval are stored in frame 1 of the computer memory. Those counts occurring during the second interval are stored in frame 2 and so on for all 16 intervals (only the first four frames are illustrated here). Row A demonstrates the contents of the first four computer frames after collecting image data from one cardiac cycle. Because of the low count rate there is not enough statistical information within any frame to form a usable image (750 counts per frame). If image data from additional cardiac cycles are acquired and added to the data already within computer memory, sufficient count statistics eventually are accumulated to produce recognizable images. Row B shows the contents of the first four computer frames after 20 cardiac cycles (15,000 counts per frame). Further accumulation of counts can additionally improve image quality, as demonstrated in row C, which displays the contents of the same four computer frames after collecting counts from 400 cardiac cycles (300,000 counts per frame). (From Botvinick et al.,[22] with permission.)

grouped into more uniform cycle lengths (histogram analysis), with subsequent framing into a a gated study.

It is possible to accurately assess wall motion and calculate ejection fraction using certain classic geometric assumptions. The great advantage of the scintigraphic method lies in the fact that counts within the ventricular region of interest are proportional to volume. Thus in the best septal left anterior oblique projection, background-corrected ESC may be subtracted from EDC and divided by EDC to yield an ejection fraction independent of geometry.[1-3] Ejection fraction, as calculated by this method, demon-

strates extremely low intraobserver and interobserver variability. Background correction is critical.[16] Multiple gated acquisition provides a simple, reproducible, accurate serial assessment of ventricular size and function at rest after infarction[17] and during pharmacologic interventions[18] or exercise.[19,20] Equilibrium time versus radioactivity curves can be employed as well to measure diastolic function. Radionuclide ventriculography can be adapted to study the rapid filling phase of diastole, the time to peak filling, the relative contributions of rapid filling and atrial systole to left ventricular stroke volume,[21] and a variety of other functional parameters.[22] In addition, curves can be assessed serially for relative volume changes or standardized for absolute volume.[23] A number of ventricular edge-detection methods are available to objectify these measurements, but all require occasional observer interventions.[23]

The right ventricular ejection fraction is more accurately assessed using first-pass methodology, largely due to less overlap between the right atrium and right ventricle in the right anterior oblique projection. Yet both first-pass and equilibrium scintigraphic methods are accurate and reproducible and have been useful for the single and serial evaluation of the right ventricular ejection fraction and right ventricular wall motion in the assessment of right ventricular disease[24,25] and in the diagnosis of right ventricular infarction.[25] Calculated right ventricular and left ventricular ejection fractions correlate well with hemodynamic parameters.

Radionuclide studies may provide important information about the etiology of congestive heart failure. The presence of regional wall motion abnormalities or an aneurysm suggest the presence of underlying coronary artery disease as the etiology of heart failure. Alternatively, the presence of global left and right ventricular dilatation and dysfunction suggest an underlying cardiomyopathy. Preserved systolic function with isolated diastolic dysfunction can lead to clinical heart failure and is detectable using radionuclide ventriculography. Studies of ventricular function have provided important prognostic information. The left ventricular ejection fraction (LVEF) is one of the most important determinants of prognosis after myocardial infarction and in patients with chronic stable coronary artery disease.[26,27] Changes in ejection fraction during exercise may offer incremental prognostic information.[27] Radionuclide LVEF is also a powerful predictor of prognosis in patients with heart failure.[28] However, the LVEF has not been shown to be predictive of functional capacity in patients with severe heart failure.[29] DiSalvo et al. showed that the radionuclide right ventricular ejection fraction at rest or exercise predicts both survival and functional capacity as assessed by the peak volume of oxygen consumption (VO_2) during exercise.[30]

ASSESSMENT OF MYOCARDIAL VIABILITY

Most patients with CHF have underlying coronary artery disease,[31] and a significant subset of these patients with ventricular dysfunction and coronary

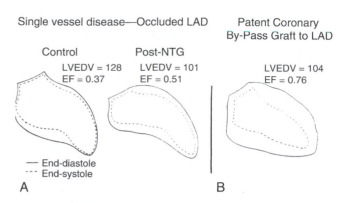

Single vessel disease—Occluded LAD

Patent Coronary By-Pass Graft to LAD

Control Post-NTG

LVEDV = 128 LVEDV = 101
EF = 0.37 EF = 0.51

LVEDV = 104
EF = 0.76

— End-diastole
--- End-systole

A   B

Fig. 33-3. Importance of viability identification. **(A)** Line drawings of diastolic and systolic frames of a left ventriculogram at baseline (control) and after nitroglycerin (NTG). NTG brings improved wall motion, reduced left ventricular end-diastolic volume (LVEOV), and improved ejection fraction (EF). **(B)** At 8 months after subsequent revascularization the wall motion was normal. Prior dysfunction was due to "hibernating" myocardium. The response to NTG is one of several methods to assess viability and the potential restoration of function after revascularization. Most prominent among current methods is the uptake of conventional perfusion agents (e.g., thallium 201) and regional metabolism with PET. (From Rahimtoola,[65] with permission.)

disease may show improved function following revascularization[32] (Fig. 33-3). Identification of dysfunctional but viable myocardium (hibernating myocardium) is of paramount importance to the successful management of patients with CHF, especially if transplantation is being considered as a treatment option. Radionuclide techniques have been useful for identifying patients with a high likelihood of functional improvement after revascularization.

It is clinically important to differentiate viable myocardial regions from those of fixed scar. Functional improvement after revascularization may be expected in dyssynergic myocardial segments related to normal or modestly reduced perfusion or to reversible stress-induced abnormalities after coronary revascularization.[33] Such dysfunctional, but viable, "hibernating" myocardial segments seem to be related to a state of "resting underperfusion and ischemia" and may recover function after revascularization.[32,34,35] In patients with extensive dysfunction at rest, identification of such extensive "hibernation" may indicate the benefit of coronary bypass graft surgery rather than heart transplantation. For this reason, great effort has been spent on the development of radionuclide methods to maximize the detection of myocardial viability.[34,36–40] In this regard, metabolic imaging of [^{18}F]fluorodeoxyglucose (FDG) using positron emission tomography (PET) and perfusion im-

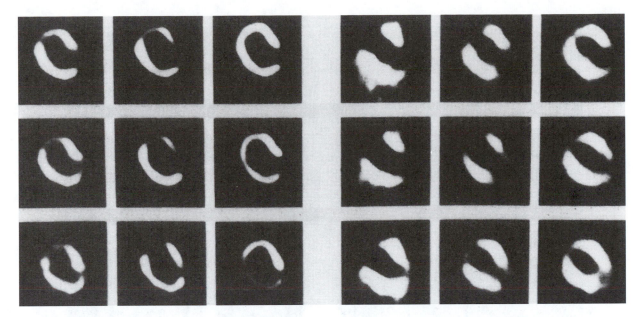

Fig. 33-4. Representative slices from the PET metabolic (FDG) and perfusion (MBF) studies in three subjects with wall motion abnormalities and possible viable, "hibernating" myocardium. The FDG/MBF ratio image attempts to evaluate a relative excess of FDG with a perfusion–metabolism mismatch in a single parametric image: the greater the intensity, the greater the mismatch. These slices are compared with slices from the SPECT exercise (Ex), redistribution (RD), and postreinjection (RI) studies performed in the same patients. Note the improvement in relative perfusion in the RI images compared with the RD images, demonstrating the greater utake of thallium 201 and an expanded ability to identify viable myocardium. Note also the similarity in RI and FDG images, suggesting a similarity of viability-related data in the two studies. (From Bonow et al.,[66] with permission.)

aging using thallium-201 with the reinjection technique provide the best viability assessment.

With PET imaging, a myocardial region with enhanced uptake of FDG relative to reduced perfusion has shown a high likelihood of improved function after revascularization[41] (Fig. 33-4). This FDG–blood flow "mismatch" pattern has emerged as the gold standard for noninvasive detection of hibernating myocardium. Detection of thallium reversibility with either stress or rest imaging is also highly sensitive for predicting improved function after revascularization. However, the absence of reversibility, or a fixed defect, is not highly specific for the absence of an improvement in function following revascularization. The utility of thallium 201 imaging for detecting viable myocardium has been greatly improved by the addition of delayed imaging (usually 24-hour redistribution) and especially by the institution of thallium reinjection following redistribution imaging (Fig. 33-4).[99m]Tc sestamibi uptake, like thallium 201, depends on the presence of viable myocardium. However, sestamibi does not redistribute and is tightly bound to myocytes. This characteristic may lead to underdetection of hibernating myocardium,[42,43] particularly when myocardial segments are ischemic at rest.

ASSESSMENT OF NEUROHORMONAL INFLUENCES

Metaiodobenzylguanidine (MIBG) has been used for several years to assess the function of myocardial sympathetic nerve endings. It has been well established that MIBG is taken up by sympathetic nerves in a manner similar to norepinephrine but is not metabolized[44,45] (Fig. 33-5). Although there is a correlation between tissue norepinephrine and MIBG localization, the distribution of MIBG most closely depicts the distribution of sympathetic neurons with functioning uptake mechanisms. The ability of sympathetic nerve terminals to take up catecholamines is a more sensitive index of nerve function and viability than are measures of catecholamine content.[46] Hence the assessment of MIBG uptake provides an accurate depiction of myocardial sympathetic innervation and allows unique characterization of acute and chronic alterations in regional sympathetic nerve function. Sympathetic nervous system activation and dispersion of regional innervation are two features of nerve function that MIBG imaging seems particularly well suited to detect.

One of the early physiologic responses to counteract depressed myocardial function is activation of a

MIBG

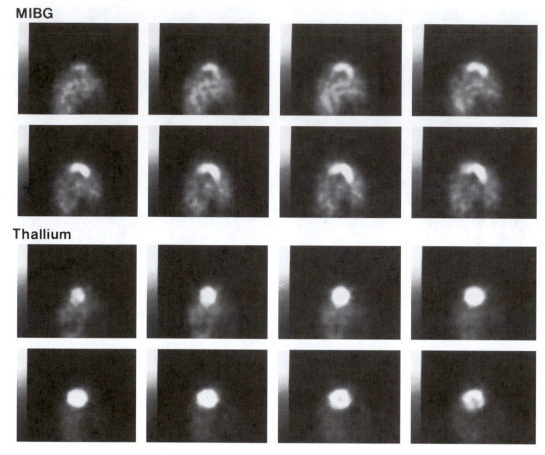

Thallium

Fig. 33-5. Dual isotope emission computed tomograms from a dog with left stellectomy. MIBG images (**top**) show a region of decreased uptake at the posterior left ventricle, whereas the corresponding thallium images (**bottom**) show normal perfusion to this area, indicating regional denervation of the posterior left ventricle. (From Dae et al.,[44] with permission.)

number of neurohumoral systems, such as the renin-angiotensin system, sympathethic nervous system, and arginine-vasopressin system.[47] It is now widely accepted that excessive stimulation of these compensatory systems eventually leads to deterioration of ventricular function and may contribute to sudden cardiac death.[48] Sustained activation of the sympathetic nervous system is thought to play a major role in the etiology of sudden cardiac death.[49] More than 300,000 sudden cardiac deaths occur each year in the United States, accounting for 50 percent of all cardiac-related mortality.[50] Most of these deaths occur in patients with prior healed myocardial infarctions and left ventricular dysfunction.[51] The deaths are thought to originate as ventricular tachycardia, which may degenerate into ventricular fibrillation. In most instances there is no associated evidence for either acute infarction or significant ischemia.[51] Arrhythmia and sudden death are also important features of noncoronary cardiomyopathy

and heart failure. Approximately 40 percent of patients with severe heart failure die suddenly, presumably of arrhythmia.[52]

The incidence of sudden death has been shown to correlate directly with both the extent of myocardial damage after infarction and the presence of complex spontaneous ventricular ectopy.[53,54] In addition, compelling evidence has emerged that implicates the sympathetic nervous system in the genesis of ventricular arrhythmias and sudden death. β-Blocker therapy has been shown to reduce the incidence of total and sudden death in patients with myocardial infarction.[55] β-Blockers have been found to be particularly useful for decreasing the incidence of sudden death in patients with myocardial infarction and left ventricular dysfunction.[56] Elevated plasma catecholamines have been shown to identify patients with heart failure who are also at risk for sudden death.[57] Data showed significantly greater activation of myocardial sympathetic nerves in patients with left ventricular dysfunction and life-threatening ventricular arrhythmias than in age-matched controls with no history of arrhythmia.[49]

Studies suggest that MIBG imaging can play a role in detecting sympathetic nervous system activation. In experimental studies, acute changes in adrenergic nerve activity of the heart have been assessed by measuring the rates of loss of neuronally bound MIBG. Sisson et al.[58] compared rates of loss of norepinephrine (NE) and MIBG in rat and dog hearts. They used yohimbine, an α_2-adrenergic receptor antagonist, to increase the function of the sympathetic nerves, and clonidine, an α_2-agonist, to decrease the activity of the sympathetic nerves. In rat hearts yohimbine induced similar increases in rates of loss of ^{3}H-NE and iodine 125 (^{125}I)-MIBG, and clonidine induced similar decreases in the rates of loss of ^{3}H-NE and ^{125}I-MIBG. Preliminary imaging studies in dog hearts with ^{123}MIBG showed similar responses to yohimbine and clonidine. These results suggest that it may be possible to assess acute changes in efferent sympathetic activity to the heart noninvasively. Although there are no reported studies to date

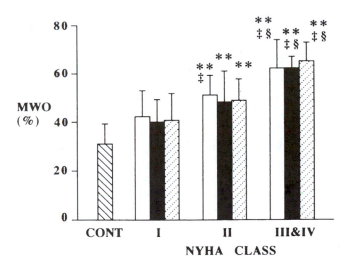

Fig. 33-7. Functional caradiac status [New York Heart Association (NYHA) classification] versus myocardial washout (MWO) of MIBG in each heart failure group. Open bars, dilated cardiomyopathy; solid bars, ischemic cardiomyopathy; dotted bars, valvar disease. **$P < 0.01$ versus control group (CONT); ‡$P < 0.01$ versus functional class I; §$P < 0.01$ versus functional class II. (From Imamura et al.,[62] with permission.)

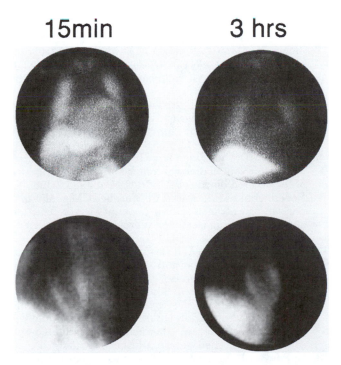

Fig. 33-6. Planar iodine 123 MIBG images from the anterior projection at 15 minutes and 3 hours from a patient with congestive heart failure due to dilated cardiomyopathy (CHF), compared to a control patient (normal). Note the significant washout of MIBG at 3 hours in the patient with congestive heart failure, whereas the control patient shows retention of MIBG. This washout of MIBG likely reflects enhanced activation of myocardial sympathetic nerves.

for human hearts that compare MIBG washout kinetics to generally accepted standards for increased sympathetic tone such as norepinephrine spillover,[59] a number of clinical conditions thought associated with increased sympathetic tone have demonstrated enhanced washout of MIBG (Fig. 33-6). Henderson et al. studied the myocardial distribution and kinetics of MIBG in images obtained from patients with congestive cardiomyopathy compared to normal controls.[60] Patients with congestive cardiomyopathy had a 28 percent washout rate of MIBG from the heart over a period of 15 to 85 minutes following intravenous injection, compared to a washout rate of 6 percent in the controls. The differences were highly significant ($P < 0.001$). Patients with CHF also showed increased heterogeneity of MIBG uptake, likely indicating dispersion of innervation. In a study by Nakajima et al.,[61] patients with various cardiac disorders underwent planar MIBG imaging at 20 minutes and 3 hours after injection. A high washout rate (more than 25 percent) was seen in a number of cases of dilated cardiomyopathy (5/11), hypertrophic cardiomyopathy (9/24), ischemic heart disease (23/34), essential hypertension (5/13), and hypothyroidism (6/13). Mean washout in control patients was 9.6 percent. As demonstrated, enhanced MIBG washout can be seen with a number of diseases. The mechanism in common is most likely activation of the sympathetic nervous system. It can also be seen that not all patients have the same degree of enhanced washout.

There are no reports to date to evaluate the prognostic utility of MIBG washout, although Imamura et al.[62] showed a correlation between MIBG washout and the severity of heart failure as assessed by the New York Heart Association functional classification (Fig. 33-7). Merlet et al.[63] reported the results of a prospective study of a group of 90 patients with congestive heart failure related to idiopathic dilated cardiomyopathy. They assessed MIBG uptake, ejection fraction, cardiothoracic ratio on radiographs, and M-mode echocardiographic data, following the patients up to 27 months. Multivariate life-table analysis showed that MIBG uptake, as assessed by the myocardial/mediastinal count ratio on anterior planar MIBG scans at 4 hours after injection, was the best predictor for survival (Fig. 33-8). The myocardial/mediastinal ratio on delayed MIBG images has been shown to correlate inversely with MIBG washout.[61] These interesting results suggest that there may be a significant role for MIBG imaging when assessing prognosis in patients with heart failure. In addition, there is a possibility that MIBG washout, the myocardial/mediastinal ratio, or both may allow prediction of hemodynamic improvement in response to β-blocker therapy in heart failure patients.[47] More studies involving larger numbers of patients are needed to evaluate the prognostic utility of MIBG uptake and washout kinetics.

REFERENCES

1. Botvinick EH, Glazer H, Shosa D: What is the reliability and utility of scintigraphic methods for the assessment of ventricular function? Cardiovasc Clin 1983; 13:65
2. Botvinick EH, Dae MW, O'Connell W: Blood pool scintigraphy. Cardiol Clin 1989;7:537
3. Johnson L: Radionuclide assessment of ventricular function. Curr Probl Cardiol 1994;19:589
4. Pavel DG, Zimmer AM, Patterson VN: In vivo red blood cell labeling with ^{99m}Tc. A new approach to blood pool visualization. J Nucl Med 1977;18:1035
5. Port SC: Radionuclide angiography. Am J Cardiac Imag 1994;8:240–248
6. Marshall RC, Berger HJ, Cosbin JC et al: Assessment of cardiac performance by quantitative radionuclide angiography. Sequential lift ventricular ejection ratae and regional wall motion. Circulation 1977;56:820
7. Jengo JA, Mena I, Blaufuss A: Evaluation of left ventricular function, ejection fraction and segmental wall motion by single pass radioisostope angiography. Circulation 1978;57:326
8. Jones RH, McEwan P, Newman GE: Accuracy of diagnosis of coronary disease by radionuclide measurement of left ventricular function during rest and exercise. Circulation 1981;64:586
9. Harpen MD, Debulsson RL, Head B et al: Determination of left ventricular volume from first pass kinetics of labeled red blood cells. J Nucl Med 1983;24:98
10. Bodenheimer MM, Banka VS, Fooshee CM et al: Comparison of wall motion and regional ejection fraction at rest and during isometric exercise. J Nucl Med 1979; 20:724
11. Poliner LR, Dehmer GJ, Lewis SE et al: Left ventricular performance in normal subjects. A comparison of the responses to exercise in the upright and supine positions. Circulation 1980;62:528
12. Salel N, Berman D, DeNardo F et al: Radionuclide assessment of nitroglycerin influence on abnormal left ventricular segmental contraction in patients with coronary heart disease. Circulation 1976;53:975
13. DePuey EG, Rozanski A: Pharmacological and other nonexercise alternatives to exercise testing to evaluate myocardial perfusion and left ventricular function with radionuclides. Semin Nucl Med 1991;21:92
14. Port SC: Recent advances in first-pass radionuclide angiography. Cardiol Clin 1994;12:359
15. Berger HJ, Matthay RA, Loke J et al: Assessment of cardiac performance with quantitative radionuclide angiocardiography. Right ventricular ejection fraction with reference to findings in chronic obstructive pulmonary disease. Am J Cardiol 1978;41:897

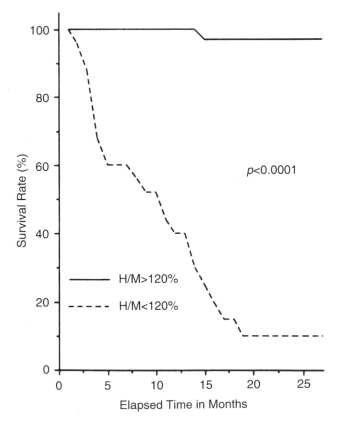

Fig. 33-8. Survival curve, using life-table analysis, with a threshold value of 120 percent for iodine 123 (^{123}I) MIBG heart/mediastinal ratio (H/M). There is a striking difference in survival between patients with H/M lower (dotted line) or higher (unbroken line) than 120 percent ($P < 0.001$). (From Merlet et al.,[63] with permission.)

16. Okada RD, Kirshenbaum HD, Kushner FG et al: Observer variance in the qualitative evaluation of left ventricular wall motion and the quantification of left ventricular ejection fraction using rest and exercise multigated blood pool imaging. Circulation 1980;61:128

17. Nicod P, Corbett JR, Firth BG et al: Prognostic value of resting and submaximal exercise radionuclide ventriculography after acute myocardial infarction in high risk patients with single and multivessel disease. Am J Cardiol 1983;52:32

18. Borer JS, Bacharach SL, Green MV et al: Effect of nitroglycerin on exercise induced abnormalities of left ventricular regional function and efection fraction in coronary artery disease. Circulation 1978;57:314

19. Kent KM, Bonow RO, Rosing DR et al: Improved myocardial function during exercise after successful percutaneous tranluminal coronary angioplastsy. N Engl J Med 1982;306:441

20. Bonow RO, Kent KM, Rosing DR et al: Exercise induced ischemia in mildly symptomatic patients with coronary artery disease and preserved left ventricular function. Identification of subgroups at risk of death during medical therapy. N Engl Med 1984;311:1339

21. Bonow RO: Radionuclide angiographic evaluation of left ventricular diastolic function. Circulation suppl. I 1991;84:208

22. Botvinick EH, Dae MW, O'Connell JW et al: Functional imaging and first harmonic phase analysis of blood pool scintigrams for the evaluation of cardiac contraction and conduction. In Gerson (ed): Cardiac Nuclear Medicine. McGraw-Hill, New York, 1991

23. Links MJ, Becker LC, Shindledecker JG et al: Measurements of absolute left ventricular volume from gated blood pool studies. Circulation 1982;65:82

24. Oldershaw P: Assessment of right ventricular function and its role in clinical practice. Br Heart J 1992;68:12

25. Jain D, Zaret BL: Assessment of right ventricular function. Role of nuclear imaging techniques. Cardiol Clinics 1992;10:23

26. White HD, Norris RM, Brown MA et al: Left ventricular end-systolic volume as the major determinant of survival after recovery from myocardial infarction. Circulation 1987;76:44

27. Lee KL, Pryor DB, Pieper KS et al: Prognostic value of radionuclide angiography in medically treated patients with coronary disease. Circulation 1990;82:1705

28. Cohn J, Johnson GR, Shabetai R et al: Ejection fraction, peak exercise oxygen consumption, cardiothoracic ratio, ventricular arrhythmias, and plasma norepinephrine as determinants of prognosis in heart failure. Circulation, suppl. V 1993;87:15

29. Dell'Italia L, Freeman G, Gaasch W: Cardiac function and functional capacity. Implications for the failing heart. Curr Prob Cardiol 1993;18:711

30. Di Salvo TG, Mathier M, Semigran M, Dec W: Preserved right ventricular ejection fraction predicts exercise capacity and survival in advanced heart failure. J Am Coll Cardiol 1995;25:1143

31. Bonow RO: The hibernating myocardium. Implications for management of congestive heart failure. Am J Cardiol 1995;75:17A

32. Rahimtoola SH: The hibernating myocardium. Am Heart J 1989;117:211–221

33. Dilsizian V, Bonow RO: Current diagnostic techniques of assessing myocardial viability in hibernating and stunned myocardium. Circulation 1993;87:1

34. Bonow RO, Disizian V, Cuocolo A, et al: Identification of viable myocardium in patients with chronic coronary artery disease and left ventricular dysfunction. Comparison of thallium scintigraphy with reinjection and PET imaging with F-18 fluorodeoxyglucose. Circulation 1991;83:26–37

35. Chatterjee KC, Swan HJC, Parmley WW, et al: Influence of direct myocardial revascularization on left ventricular asynergy and function in patients with coronary heart disease. Circulation 1973;47:276–283

36. Gimple LW, Beller GA: Myocardial viability. Assessment by cardiac scintigraphy. Cardiol Clin 1994;12:317–332

37. Iskandrian AS, Schelbert HR (eds): Myocardial viability assessment. J Nucl Med 1994;35:1–58S

38. Dilsizian V, Rocco TP, Freedman NMT et al: Enhanced detection of ischemic but viable myocardium by reinjection of thallium after stress-redistribution imaging. N Engl J Med 1990;323:141–146

39. Dilsizian V, Smeltzer WR, Freedman NMT et al: Thallium reinjection after stress-redistribution imaging. Circulation 1991;83:1247–1255

40. Dilsizian V, Bonow RO: Differential uptake and apparent T1-201 washout after thallium reinjection. Options regarding late redistribution imaging before reinjection or late redistribution imaging after reinjection. Circulation 1992;85:1032–1038

41. Tillisch JH, Brunken R, Marshall R et al: Reversibility of cardiac wall motion abnormalities predicted by positron tomography. N Engl J Med 1986;314:884

42. Maurea S, Cuocolo A, Pace L et al: Left ventricular dysfunction in coronary artery disease. Comparison between rest-redistribution thallium-201 and resting technetium-99m methoxisobutyl isonitrile imaging. J Nucl Cardiol 1994;1:65

43. Sawada SG, Allman KC, Muzik O et al: Positron emission tomography detects evidence of viability in rest technetium-99m sestamibi defects. J Am Coll Cardiol 1994;23:92

44. Dae MW, O'Connell JW, Botvinick EH et al: Scintigraphic assessment of regional cardiac adrenergic innervation. Circulation 1989;79:634–644

45. Sisson JC, Wieland DM, Sherman P et al: Metaiodobenzylguanidine as an index of the adrenergic nervous system integrity and function. J Nucl Med 1987;28:1620–1624

46. Tyce GM: Norepinephrine uptake as an indicator of cardiac reinnervation in dogs. Am J Physiol 1987;235:H289–H294

47. Consensus Trial Study Group: Effects of enalapril on mortality in severe congestive heart failure. N Engl J Med 1986;316:1429–1435

48. Eichhorn E, Hjalmarson A: Beta-blocker treatment for chronic heart failure. Circulation 1994;90:2153–2156

49. Meredith I, Broughton A, Jennings G, Esler M: Evidence of a selective increase in cardiac sympathetic activity in patients with sustained ventricular arrhythmias. N Engl J Med 1991;325:618–624

50. Myerburg R, Kessler K, Castellanos A: Sudden cardiac death—structure, function, and time-dependence of risk. Circulation, suppl. I 1992;85:2–10

51. Hurwitz J, Josephson M: Sudden cardiac death in patients with chronic coronary heart disease. Circulation, suppl. I 1992;85:43–49

52. Francis G: Development of arrhythmias in the patient with congestive heart failure. Pathophysiology, prevalence, and prognosis. Am J Cardiol 1986;57:3B–7B

53. Follansbe W, Michelson E, Morganroth J: Nonsustained ventricular tachycardia in ambulatory patients. Characteristics and association with sudden cardiac death. Ann Intern Med 1980;92:741–752

54. Gang E, Bigger J, Livell F: A model of chronic arrhythmias. The relationship between electrically inducible ventricular tachycardia, ventricular fibrillation threshold, and myocardial infarct size. Am J Cardiol 1982;50:469–477

55. Yusuf S, Peto R, Lewis J, Collins R, Sleight P: Beta-blockade during and after myocardial infarction. An overview of the randomized trials. Prog Cardiovasc Dis 1985;25:335–371

56. Chadda K, Goldstein S, Byington R, Curb J: Effect of propranolol after acute myocardial infarction in patients with congestive heart failure. Circulation 1986; 73:503–510

57. Cohn J, Levine T, Olivari M et al: Plasma norepinephrine as a guide to prognosis in patients with chronic congestive heart failure. N Engl J Med 1984;311: 819–823

58. Sisson J, Bolgas G, Johnson J: Measuring acute changes in adrenergic nerve activity of the heart in the living animal. Am Heart J 1991;121:1119–1123

59. Kingwell B, Thompson J, Kaye D et al: Heart rate spectral analysis, cardiac norepinephrine spillover, and muscle sympathetic nerve activity during human sympathetic nervous activation and failure. Circulation 1994;90:234–240

60. Henderson EB, Kahn JK, Corbett JB et al: Abnormal I-123 metaidobenzylguanidine myocardial washout and distribution may reflect myocardial adrenergic derangement in patients with congestive cardiomyopathy. Circulation 1988;78:1192–1199

61. Nakajima K, Taki J, Tonami N, Hisada K: Decrease 123-I MIBG uptake and increased clearance in various cardiac diseases. Nucl Med Commun 1994;15:317–323

62. Imamura Y, Ando H, Mitsuoka W et al: Iodine-123 metaiodobenzylguanidine images reflect intense myocardial adrenergic nervous activity in congestive heart failure independent of underlying cause. J Am Coll Cardiol 1995;26:1594–1599

63. Merlet P, Valette H, Dubois R et al: Prognostic valve of cardiac metaiodobenzylguanidine imaging in patients with heart failure. J Nucl Med 1992;33:471–477

64. Botvinick EH, Glazer H, Shosa D: What is the reliability and the utility of scintigraphic methods for the assessment of ventricular function? In Rahimtoola S (ed): Controversies in Coronary Artery Disease. p. 65. Davis, Philadelphia, 1981

65. Rahimtoola SA: Coronary bypass surgery for chronic angina. Circulation 1982;65:232

66. Bonow RG, Bacharach LS, Cuocolo A et al: Identification of viable myocardium in patients with chronic coronary disease and left ventricular dysfunction. Comparison of thallium-201 with reinfection and PET imaging with ^{18}F-deoxyglucose. Circulation 1991;83: 26–37

34 Endomyocardial Biopsy

Peter J. Richardson

Most of the patients who require investigation by endomyocardial biopsy have dilated, poorly contracting left ventricles; they suffer from or present with dilated cardiomyopathy. The clinical use of endomyocardial biopsy is dictated by the clinical suspicion that there is underlying heart muscle disease not due to coronary artery disease, hypertension, or valvar heart disease. It is important therefore that prior to a decision to undertake endomyocardial biopsy patients are properly assessed by clinical history and examination and, in most cases, with selective coronary arteriography. Echocardiography has furthermore enabled more accurate identification of patients with dilated poorly contracting hearts and in some cases enables diagnosis of infiltrative conditions such as amyloid or sarcoid.

The technique of endomyocardial biopsy, which was initially pioneered by Konno and Sakakibara, was modified with the development of percutaneous methods of introduction and the Caves Schultz bioptome[1] (Table 34-1). This modification enabled biopsy of the right ventricle using a percutaneous approach through the jugular or subclavian veins in patients requiring biopsy for the assessment of heart transplant rejection. The long sheath technique combined with development of the King's/Cordis biopsy forceps[2] made the femoral route of introduction possible, and both right and left ventricular biopsy could be performed using either the femoral artery or vein.[3] The development of percutaneous techniques thus allowed multiple biopsy procedures to be performed to monitor rejection; and serial investigation in clinical practice had become possible.

Many argue that endomyocardial biopsy, although improving the diagnostic accuracy in the individual patient, does not contribute significantly to treatment decisions or management. There are, however, accepted clinical indications for biopsy.

CLINICAL INDICATIONS

The overriding indication for endomyocardial biopsy is for the diagnosis of suspected heart muscle disease. The major indications include the following.

1. Assessment of heart transplant rejection
2. Diagnosis of myocarditis in a patient presenting with dilated cardiomyopathy
3. Histologic confirmation of a diagnosis of dilated cardiomyopathy
4. Exclusion of infiltrative or inflammatory heart muscle disease
5. Investigation of the patient with restrictive hemodynamics to exclude restrictive cardiomyopathy/constrictive pericarditis
6. Assessment and monitoring of cardiotoxicity (e.g., adriamycin)
7. Diagnosis of arrhythmogenic right ventricular cardiomyopathy
8. Confirmation using molecular techniques of enterovirus infection in the myocardium

CONTRAINDICATIONS

Left ventricular endomyocardial biopsy is contraindicated when there is an intracardiac thrombus, which may be identified by echocardiography or left

Table 34-1. Bioptomes Used for Endomyocardial Biopsy

Bioptome	French Gauge
Caves Schultz	6.5
Cordis	6.0
King's	7.0
Small Konno	8.0
Large Konno	9.0

ventriculography. Right ventricular endomyocardial biopsy should not be performed in patients with septal or other intracardiac defects that might allow paradoxical embolism to occur. It is inadvisable to biopsy patients with bleeding disorders with platelet deficiency, or in whom there is excessive anticoagulation. The two latter situations might promote hemopericardium in the event of perforation. Experience has shown that endomyocardial biopsy is not routinely indicated for evaluation of hypertrophic cardiomyopathy. Restrictive-type hemodynamics, which may be present in these patients, can lead to early tamponade and collapse in the event of cardiac perforation.

TECHNIQUES

Transthoracic needle biopsy of the left ventricle was described by Shirey in 198 patients and there was an unacceptable 8 percent incidence of clinically significant hemopericardium and tamponade. Pleuropulmonary complications may also occur. In contrast, catheter endomyocardial biopsy of the right or left ventricle is usually associated with no greater rate of complications than would be expected with routine cardiac catheterization.

Konno and Sakakibara in 1962 pioneered the technique of endomyocardial biopsy using a catheter forceps. Their instrument, however, had to be introduced by a cutdown route through a vein or an artery. Some technical difficulties were experienced and led to the development by Caves and Schultz of a bioptome predominantly for use with right ventricular biopsy, although subsequently a Stanford left ventricular bioptome was also available. The major design modification included the use of surgical forceps to replace the sliding operating handle. The jaws were modified to consist of one fixed and one mobile cup, which reduced the possibility of mechanical failure. The catheter diameter was reduced from that of the Konno forceps so percutaneous introduction could be performed using the right internal jugular

vein for right ventricular biopsy. The major application of this forceps was for the study of myocardial rejection in the transplanted heart.

The King's/Cordis endomyocardial biopsy forceps was developed by modifying the bronchoscopic biopsy forceps. A small diameter of approximately 7 French gauge enables their percutaneous introduction initially through a short sheath system and subsequently through a long sheath that incorporates a hemostatic valve with the side arm flush, together with a radiopaque nonthrombogenic sheath of 90 cm length. The sheath is suitable for introduction using the Seldinger technique via the right femoral vein or artery.

In most circumstances it is possible to proceed to endomyocardial biopsy at the time of diagnostic cardiac catheterization. It normally prolongs the procedure for no more than 30 minutes. Biventricular endomyocardial biopsy is possible, but diagnostic information is achieved by biopsy of either ventricle. The routes of biopsy are shown in Figure 34-1. The procedure for biopsy of either ventricle is virtually identical. The long sheath system is introduced over a guidewire system. The long sheath system includes a multipurpose catheter for the right ventricle or a standard pigtail catheter for the left ventricle. The ventricle is entered at the appropriate angle and the guidewire removed. The inner catheter is flushed, and pressure measurement verifies the position. The cardiac catheter is removed, with the guiding sheath

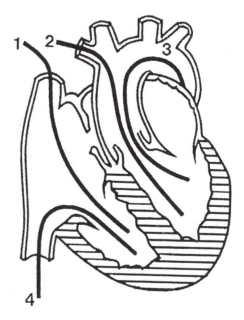

Fig. 34-1. Routes of biopsy. 1, venous, via supraclavicular approach or cutdown median antecubital vein; 2, arterial, via brachial arteriotomy; 3, percutaneous, via femoral artery; 4, percutaneous, via femoral vein.

being positioned under fluoroscopic control within the ventricular cavity. At the time of removal of the catheter it is important that side arm flushing is performed continuously with a heparinized system to obviate clot formation. Another 2000 units of heparin may be given directly down the sheath prior to the biopsy being performed. The long sheath system is monitored continuously on pressure. The bioptome should not be introduced or advanced if there is any suggestion of pressure damping within the system. The latter may be due to the tip of the sheath being against the endomyocardial surface or to clot formation within the sheath. The bioptome is then introduced into the sheath system and advanced to the tip of the sheath, which lies within the ventricular cavity. The bioptome emerges out of the tip of the catheter sheath with the jaws opening as the forceps advance. In the event of the jaws not opening easily, the sheath may need to be withdrawn slightly, as the jaws may be entrapped within trabeculae or chordae. Once the jaws are open they may be advanced against the endomyocardial surface, and the operating handle causes the jaws to close quickly. The whole is then withdrawn rapidly under constant flushing. The sheath position should be rechecked with confirmation of free pressure measurement. The endomyocardial biopsy sample is usually approximately 1 mg wet weight. The procedure may be repeated a number of times to obtain up to six samples. Note that the sheath should be slightly repositioned between each excision to overcome the possibility of the catheter tip returning to the same place in the myocardium for each biopsy.

COMPLICATIONS

Problems encountered during biopsy include occasional *arrhythmias*, but it usually consists of no more than two or three ventricular premature beats at the time of excision. Sustained rhythm changes are rarely if ever encountered. *Damage to the vessel* at the site of entry of the sheath or damage to valves by the forceps is again rare. *Perforation of the myocardium* is usually not a problem provided the biopsy forceps are advanced only when the jaws are widely opened against the end of the myocardial surface. Extreme care should be taken when there is any suggestion of a parchment-thin ventricle. Damage to the myocardium around the site of biopsy seems to be negligible; and in those patients in whom the heart has been examined following biopsy within a matter of days the biopsy site cannot be identified. *Embolization* during biopsy is seen occasionally but in the main is overcome by the liberal use of heparin flushing. Late embolization has not been a problem. In patients with severely dilated ventricles it is essential to establish prior to the procedure that there is no demonstrable intracavity thrombus using echocardiography, ventriculography, or both.

LIMITATIONS OF BIOPSY

One limitation of endomyocardial biopsy is the apparently random sampling of the myocardium. The importance of this point becomes particularly pertinent when there is a focal type of heart muscle disease, such as sarcoidosis or myocarditis. This limitation may be overcome by obtaining biopsy specimens from multiple areas and guiding the bioptome to abnormal tissue. This goal may be achieved by using biplane screening or two-dimensional sector echocardiography.

HISTOPATHOLOGIC DIAGNOSIS

The major application of endomyocardial biopsy is the diagnosis of myocarditis or dilated cardiomyopathy or the exclusion of specific heart muscle diseases. Histologic examination may be able to distinguish groups of patients with differing prognoses who appear on the basis of clinical history and presentation to be indistinguishable. Myocarditis may be present with no other clinical features of a viral infection other than heart failure.

The diagnosis of myocarditis may be classified on the basis of the biopsy findings into active healing or healed phases, the healed phase of myocarditis being histologically indistinguishable from dilated cardiomyopathy.[4] The Dallas criteria were initially developed for histologic diagnosis of acute myocarditis and the subsequent classification of the histologic response to immunosuppressive treatment based on serial biopsy results. To determine the development of a healing or healed phase of myocarditis following initial acute myocarditis, rebiopsy is mandatory. It may be of value in the clinical context if a correlation can be made with alterations in left ventricular function. According to the Dallas criteria, myocarditis is characterized by an inflammatory infiltrate of the myocardium with necrosis or degeneration of adjacent myocytes not typical of the ischemic damage associated with coronary artery disease.[5] On the basis of the first biopsy, the diagnosis of myocarditis may be confirmed, borderline changes may be diagnosed or the diagnosis is excluded. Subsequent biopsy then gives evidence of ongoing myocarditis or resolving or resolved myocarditis. Although a biopsy can confirm the histologic diagnosis of inflammatory heart muscle disease, it does not necessarily provide insight into the diagnosis of the cause. The most important diagnoses that can be made with respect to inflammatory heart disease include sarcoidosis, amyloidosis, borreliosis, and tuberculosis.

In most patients with dilated heart muscle disease in whom myocarditis and specific heart muscle disease have been excluded, the diagnosis is a dilated cardiomyopathy. The histologic features are regularly arranged and attenuated, hypertrophied myocytes with interstitial fibrous replacement. When dilatation of the left ventricle has been of long standing, thickening of the endocardium together with smooth muscle hypertrophy is also seen. Thrombus may be adherent to the endocardial surface. A sparse inflammatory infiltrate is occasionally seen on a biopsy, but the criteria for diagnosis of myocarditis are not fulfilled. In some of these patients evidence of immune activation has been identified.

RELATION BETWEEN MYOCARDITIS AND DILATED CARDIOMYOPATHY DURING HEART FAILURE

Although controversy surrounds the frequency with which myocarditis is diagnosed based on histologic criteria, the biopsy examination must remain the gold standard for the diagnosis of myocarditis. Sensitivity is clearly limited by the frequently focal nature of the inflammatory process. The incidence of myocarditis has varied widely from 3 to 65 percent in various studies. Acute myocarditis defined according to the Dallas criteria has an incidence of approximately 5 percent in our experience. Serial evaluation of these patients even without immunosuppressive therapy has shown that approximately 50 percent spontaneously improve within 6 months even when the initial ejection fraction was less than 30 percent. Those with a biopsy specimen showing the appearances of healing or resolving myocarditis without myocyte necrosis may also improve spontaneously. It has been possible using serial biopsy to document the progression from acute to healing myocarditis and then to dilated cardiomyopathy.[6]

The diagnosis of typical lymphocytic myocarditis is important, but just as important is the identification of giant cell myocarditis. In this group the prognosis is definitely worse. In one series of giant cell myocarditis only 20 percent of patients were alive at follow-up compared with 70 percent of those with a lymphocytic myocarditis. Ventricular arrhythmias

were more frequent in those with giant cell myocarditis, and some of these patients required a permanent pacemaker. Sarcoidosis may be similar to giant cell myocarditis; but its identification by biopsy is important, as cardiac sarcoidosis may respond to immunosuppressive therapy.

Rare forms of heart muscle disease that can be diagnosed by biopsy include endomyocardial fibrosis, which has three stages that are pathologically well documented: myocarditic phase, thrombotic phase, and fibrotic phase. In the myocarditic phase it may be possible to identify degranulated eosinophils in a blood film. Degranulation of the eosinophils is correlated with the release of cationic proteins toxic to the myocardium. This condition can be treated by immunosuppressive therapy. Endocardial fibrosis can be diagnosed in children.

SPECIAL TECHNIQUES APPLICABLE TO BIOPSY TISSUE

Virologic Diagnosis

Many viruses have been implicated in the pathogenesis of myocarditis and dilated cardiomyopathy, but enteroviruses, particularly coxsackie virus B, are most frequently encountered. In clinical practice routine viral serology, including coxsackie B neutralizing antibody titers, may be helpful. A fourfold rise in the neutralizing antibody titer in paired sera is diagnostic. A positive coxsackie B enzyme-linked immunosorbent assay (ELISA) for immunoglobulin M (IgM) may also be helpful for indicating a recent infection. It has been universally accepted that enteroviruses cannot be cultured from myocardial biopsy tissue. It is possible using new cDNA molecular technology, however, to detect enteroviral infection in myocardial biopsy tissue not only during the acute phase of myocarditis but also with healed myocarditis/dilated cardiomyopathy. Enteroviral RNA can be detected in 43 percent of patients with myocarditis during either the acute of the healing phase compared with 41 percent of those with dilated cardiomyopathy and 5 percent of controls.[7] Similar results are obtained using in situ hybridization techniques when the viral RNA is seen to be focally distributed and appears not only in areas where there is histologic evidence of acute inflammation but also in areas of apparently normal myocardium. Enterovirus RNA may persist to the stage of cardiac transplantation and those suffering from end-stage dilated cardiomyopathy. This finding was significantly different from those with end-stage coronary heart disease in whom enterovirus was detectable in only 5 percent.[8] These studies have clearly shown that virus may persist without producing an inflammatory response on the biopsy. It is known that the virus persists in defective mutant form, probably as a result of an aberration of viral RNA synthesis in a nonproductive replication cycle and even in this form may have clinical prognostic significance.[9]

In addition to detection of enteroviral RNA using hybridization techniques, it has been possible using the polymerase chain reaction (PCR) gene amplification technique to detect virus in the small biopsy samples where only low copy numbers of the viral genome are present. In most studies the frequency of virus detection using PCR techniques has been similar to that using hybridization.[10,11]

Analysis of Myocardial Proteins

Alteration in the expression of myocardial proteins—whatever the initial mechanism for the disease process—may lead to altered and impaired function of the heart muscle. Evidence for this type of change in dilated cardiomyopathy comes from studies that have shown abnormal expression of myosin isoforms involving both myosin heavy and light chains in the myocardium. These findings have been interpreted as specific for dilated cardiomyopathy, but it is recognized that other types of cardiac hypertrophy are known to be associated with changes in the expression of myosin and other contractile proteins. It is known that persistent viral infection can interfere with normal gene expression, and it remains to be determined whether the persistence of enteroviral infection in dilated cardiomyopathy can result in modification of specific cell gene expression.

To determine alterations in myocardial gene expression it has been possible to apply two-dimensional polyacrylamide gel electrophoresis, which has sufficient resolution to examine several thousand proteins. The proteins can be separated according to their charge properties in the first dimension and then according to their molecular size in the second dimension. The two-dimensional protein profiles thereby obtained require computerized systems to ensure accurate analysis. Initial studies in this area have shown that a group of up to 20 proteins differ between patients with dilated hearts due to dilated cardiomyopathy and those with end-stage ischemic heart disease.

Myocardial Tissue Enzyme Analysis

The association between excessive alcohol consumption and dilated cardiomyopathy has long been known, and it has been shown that regular consumption of in excess of 80 g of alcohol per day may give rise to impaired heart function indistinguishable from cardiomyopathy. Furthermore, endomyocardial biopsy does not allow distinction of tissue using histopathologic evaluation, as there are no specific changes relating to alcoholic heart muscle disease. Measurement of the activities of several myocardial tissue enzymes, including creatinine phosphokinase (CPK), lactate dehydrogenase (LDH), αHBD (α hydroxy butyric dehydrogenase), and malic dehydrogenase (MDH), were shown to relate to alcohol intake in patients. A subsequent study showed that 38 patients who regularly consumed more than 40 g of alcohol per day exhibited a bimodal distribution of cumulative lifetime alcohol intake. Significantly higher levels of CPK, LDH, and MDH were found in the heavy drinkers compared with those drinking lightly or who were abstinent. Multiple regression analysis was performed to evaluate the relation of consumption, left ventricular ejection fraction, blood pressure, and myocardial enzyme activities, and it was found that the CPK and αHBD levels correlated significantly with both ejection fraction and cumulative lifetime alcoholic intake.[10] LDH, however, correlated only with the cumulative lifetime alcohol intake. These observations appeared to be independent of any effect of blood pressure. It was thought that probably the increase in myocardial enzyme activity in the heavy drinking group were adaptive, and the use of this technique for diagnostic purposes could not be undertaken.

REFERENCES

1. Caves PK, Stinson EB, Billingham ME et al: Percutaneous transvenous endomyocardial biopsy in human heart recipients. Ann Thorac Surg 1973;16:325–336
2. Richardson PJ: King's endomyocardial bioptome. Lancet 1974;1:660–661
3. Brooksby IAB, Swanton RH, Jenkins BS et al: Long sheath technique for introduction of catheter tip manometer or endomyocardial bioptome into left or right heart. Br Heart J 1974;36:908–912
4. Daly K, Richardson PJ, Olsen EGJ et al: Acute myocarditis: role of histological and virological examination in diagnosis and assessment of immunosuppressive treatment. Br Heart J 1984;51:30–35
5. Aretz HT, Billingham ME, Edwards WD et al: Myocarditis. A histologic definition and classification. Am J Cardiovasc Pathol 1986;1:3–14
6. Quigley PJ, Richardson PJ, Meany BT et al: Long-term follow-up of acute myocarditis. Correlation of ventricular function and outcome. Eur Heart J, suppl. J 1987; 8:39–42
7. Bowles NE, Richardson PJ, Olsen EGJ, Archard LC: Detection of coxsackie B virus specific RNA sequences in myocardial biopsy samples from patients with myocarditis and dilated cardiomyopathy. Lancet 1986;1: 1120–1123.
8. Bowles NE, Rose ML, Taylor P et al: Endstage dilated

cardiomyopathy. Persistence of enterovirus RNA in myocardium at cardiac transplantation and lack of immune response. Circulation 1989;80:1128–1136.

9. Why HJF, Meany BT, Richardson PJ et al: Clinical and prognostic significance of detection of enteroviral RNA in the myocardium of patients with myocarditis or dilated cardiomyopathy. Circulation 1994;89:2582–2589

10. Schwaiger A, Umlauft F, Weyrer K et al: Detection of enteroviral ribonucleic acid in myocardial biopsies from patients with idiopathic dilated cardiomyopathy by polymerase chain reaction. Am Heart J 1993;126:406–410

11. Jin O, Sole MJ, Butany JW et al: Detection of enterovirus RNA in myocardial biopsies from patients with myocarditis and dilated cardiomyopathy using gene amplification by polymerase chain reaction. Circulation 1990;82:8–16

35 Magnetic Resonance Imaging, Computed Tomography, and Positron Emission Tomography

Heinrich R. Schelbert

The clinical history and physical examination remain the mainstay in the diagnosis of heart failure. Assessment of the ventricular chamber sizes, systolic wall motion, and myocardial wall thickness together with invasive measurements of left ventricular filling pressures and cardiac output refines the diagnostic workup; parameters obtained with these noninvasive and invasive approaches serve as measures of disease severity and, at the same time, have proved useful for monitoring responses to therapeutic interventions. Although employed less frequently, ultrafast (also referred to as electron beam) computed tomography (cine CT), gated magnetic resonance imaging (MRI), and positron emission tomography (PET) afford an even more comprehensive characterization of the failing heart as well as its anatomy and structure, mechanical function, blood supply, and substrate and high energy phosphate metabolism. To some extent, the diagnostic information obtained with each of the three imaging techniques overlaps and may be complementary. At the same time, each imaging modality offers unique features that can answer specific diagnostic questions. This chapter discusses how each of these sophisticated imaging modalities can contribute to the diagnosis of the failing heart, characterization of disease severity, and elucidation of the primary underlying pathophysiology. Their contribution to monitoring responses to pharmacologic or mechanical interventions is also addressed.

MAGNETIC RESONANCE IMAGING AND SPECTROSCOPY

With its high spatial and ever-increasing temporal resolution, MRI yields three-dimensional images of the human heart's anatomy and structure in exquisite detail. It visualizes both the myocardial tissue and the blood pool. If images are acquired at sampling rates of 40 to 80 ms, patterns of blood flow across the cardiac valves as well as regional and global myocardial wall motion and thickening can be displayed and quantified. With these capabilities MRI serves as a noninvasive tool for characterizing the human heart's mechanical and hemodynamic function in health and disease. MR spectroscopy adds another dimension; it affords measurements of the myocardium's high energy phosphate concentrations and thus provides insights into myocardial metabolism.

Imaging approaches can be broadly categorized into (1) spin echo and (2) cine MR. Spin echo MRI yields three-dimensional images of the myocardium with excellent definition of its endocardial and epicardial edges, although vascular compartments with rapidly flowing blood are "blacked out." Conversely, on cine MRI, with all its currently evolving permutations such as turbo-fast gradient echo imaging or echo planar imaging, flowing blood yields an intensely bright signal. Abnormal or turbulent patterns of blood flow (e.g., that associated with dysfunctional cardiac valves) leads to a reduction or loss of the signal that is readily noted on the images and

Table 35-1. MR Imaging and
Spectroscopy

Left ventricular mass

Ventricular volumes (right and left ventricle)
    End-diastolic volume
    End-systolic volume
    Stroke volume
    Ejection fraction
    Cardiac output

Myocardial wall thickness
    Regional wall thickening

Ventricular time volume curves
    Ejection and filling rates

Valvar regurgitation
    Regurgitant volumes
    Regurgitant fraction

Myocardial perfusion
    Relative distribution
    Semiquantitative estimates
    Coronary stenosis

Myocardial high energy phosphate concentrations

then serves as a means to detect and assess the severity of valvar regurgitation. Although of interest, a detailed description of the technical features of MRI exceeds the scope of this chapter; it is available in the scientific literature. Table 35-1 summarizes the cardiac parameters that can be defined with MRI.

Measurements of Myocardial Mass and Cardiac Volumes

Several investigations have validated measurements of right and left ventricular volumes by spin echo and cine MRI against those by cine ventriculography, echocardiography, and thermodilution measurements of cardiac output and thus of ventricular stroke volumes.[1–5] The accuracy of right ventricular chamber volume measurements has also been confirmed; estimates of right ventricular volumes by

MRI were found to be virtually identical to estimates of left ventricular stroke volumes.[2,5] Furthermore, several clinical investigations have demonstrated the reproducibility of such measurements.[5] For example, the interstudy reproducibility of left ventricular volume and ejection fraction measurements in 11 patients with dilated cardiomyopathy averaged only about 5–6 percent.[6] As expected and as shown in Table 35-2, both left and right ventricular volumes were markedly increased in patients with dilated cardiomyopathy compared to those in normal volunteers, and the left ventricular ejection fraction was markedly decreased.[7]

The high temporal resolution of current cine MR imaging techniques permits the construction of time–volume curves.[8] Ventricular ejection and filling rates can then be derived from these time–volume curves, and afford detailed information on systolic and diastolic function and their interrelations in heart failure patients.[8,9]

As both the endocardial and epicardial borders of the left ventricular myocardium are clearly demarcated on the MR images, the left ventricular wall thickness and myocardial wall thickening can be determined.[10,11] Compared to 10 normal volunteers with average left ventricular masses of 115 ± 10 g at end-diastole and 117 ± 10 g (not significant, or NS) at end-systole, the myocardial mass was found to be markedly increased in patients with dilated cardiomyopathy.[7] It averaged 194 ± 21 g at end-diastole and 202 ± 20 g (NS) at end-systole in 10 dilated cardiomyopathy patients (Table 35-2). Information on regional systolic wall motion and, more importantly, systolic wall thickening was derived from the same gated MR images. In normal volunteers, for example, wall thickening ranged from 35 to 75 percent; it was lowest in the basal portion of the left ventricle and markedly increased toward the left ventricular apex.[7] In 10 patients with dilated cardiomyopathy, however, systolic wall thickening was diminished; moreover, the spatial pattern of wall

Table 35-2. MRI Measurements of Ventricular Mass and Ejection Fraction

Measurement	Normal Volunteers	Idiopathic Dilated Cardiomyopathy Patients
LV mass (g)		
End-diastole	115 ± 10	194 ± 21
End-systole	117 ± 10	202 ± 20
RV end-diastolic volume (ml)	90 ± 7	220 ± 30
RV end-systolic volume (ml)	34 ± 4	173 ± 28
LV ejection fraction (%)	64.3 ± 2.5	23.5 ± 3.1

Abbreviations: LV, left ventricular; RV, right ventricular.
(Data from Buser et al.[7])

thickening differed from that in the normal left ventricle. For example, systolic wall thickening failed to increase in magnitude from the base to the apex in the cardiomyopathy patients.[7,12] If the left ventricular dimensions together with the myocardial wall thickness is known, and as they can be derived from gated MR images, regional wall stresses can readily be calculated from simultaneous measurements of left ventricular pressures.[12] Left ventricular wall stress at peak systole and end-systole were found to be markedly higher in patients with dilated cardiomyopathy than in normal volunteers. Figure 35-1 de-

picts an example of gated MR images from a patient with a markedly enlarged left ventricle.

Mitral regurgitation frequently accompanies the left ventricular enlargement in patients with dilated cardiomyopathy. Several approaches are available for the detection and quantification of the severity of valvar regurgitation. One approach compares the stroke volumes of both ventricles. Normally, these stroke volumes approach unity. In the presence of mitral regurgitation the stroke volume of the left ventricle exceeds that of the right ventricle. The ratio of left to right ventricular stroke volumes then indi-

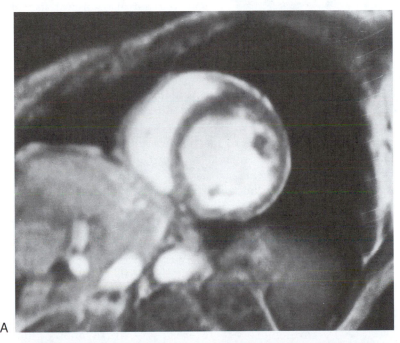

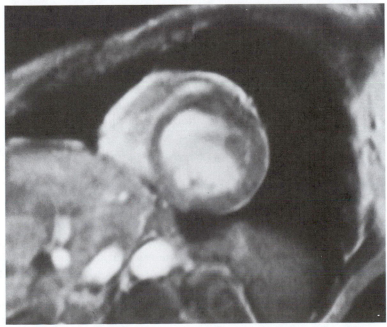

Fig. 35-1. Gated short axis MRI images obtained from a patient with dilated cardiomyopathy. End-diastolic (**A**) and end-systolic (**B**) short axis cut at the mid left ventricular level. Note the marked enlargement of the left and the right ventricular chamber. (Courtesy of C.B. Higgins, M.D., Department of Radiology, University of California at San Francisco.)

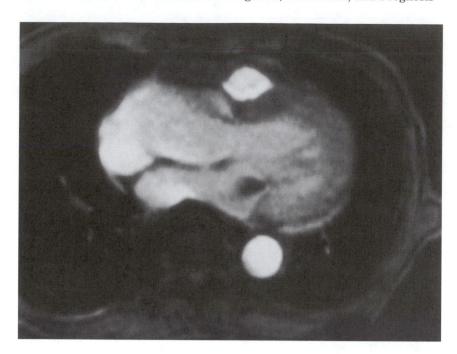

Fig. 35-2. Cine MR (gradient echo) image obtained during systole in a patient with mitral regurgitation. This transaxial image plane demonstrates a signal void emanating from the mitral valve (dark area), which is characteristic for mitral regurgitation. (Courtesy C.B. Higgins, M.D., Department of Radiology, University of California at San Francisco.)

cates the magnitude of the regurgitant volume.[4,13] A second approach takes advantage of the loss of signal in the blood chambers due to abnormal or turbulent flow patterns (Fig. 35-2). Again, the area of an abnormal or loss of signal corresponds to the severity of valvar regurgitation.[13,14] Lastly, a third approach uses velocity-encoded cine MRI.[15] The ventricular inflow and outflow volumes can be estimated by velocity encoding of the ventricular inflow (transmitral valvar flow) and outflow (aortic flow). Their difference again yields estimates of regurgitant volumes. Regurgitant fractions determined with this method in 19 patients and 10 normal volunteers correlated well with those determined by echocardiography.[15] Such measurements thus allow assessment of the presence of mitral regurgitation and its magnitude in patients with dilated cardiomyopathy.

The introduction of MR contrast agents at the same time has opened new possibilities for assessing the relative distribution of myocardial blood flow and for deriving semiquantitative indices of regional blood flow.[16] Although still largely unexplored, this possibility might prove useful for distinguishing between ischemic and idiopathic etiologies accounting for the impairment in left ventricular function and heart failure. Within the same context are current attempts to visualize the normal and abnormal anatomy of the large epicardial coronary arteries with gated MRI.[16] Initial studies have indeed indicated the possibility of detecting coronary stenosis in the major coronary vessels entirely noninvasively by MRI.[17]

Other studies explored the possibility of probing the myocardium's metabolism with MR spectroscopy. Regional measurements of high energy phosphate concentrations and their alterations (e.g., in coronary artery disease) remain limited and problematic, though promising; initial investigations in patients with dilated cardiomyopathies and diffuse myocardial abnormalities, however, have demonstrated distinct alterations in the composition of high energy phosphates. In an early report, phosphorus 31 MR surface coil spectroscopy uncovered an approximately 50 percent reduction in the myocardial phosphocreatine (PCr)/inorganic phosphate (Pi) ratio in an 8-month-old female infant with massive cardiomegaly.[18] Interestingly, intravenous glucose or oral carbohydrate administration was associated with marked improvement in the PCr/Pi ratio. Thus phosphorus MR spectroscopy may also be of use for designing therapeutic strategies in patients with idiopathic dilated cardiomyopathies. In a more recent study in 13 patients with congestive cardiomyopathy, phosphorus 31 MR spectroscopy found normally preserved PCr/β-adenosine triphosphate (ATP) peak ratios. However, the phosphodiesterase (PDE)/PCr and the PDE/β-ATP ratios were significantly elevated in congestive cardiomyopathy patients when compared to those in a group of normal volunteers.[12]

Monitoring Responses to Therapy

As measurements of ventricular volumes and function and of myocardial mass are highly reproducible, MRI appears to be ideally positioned for monitoring the responses to therapeutic interventions. Accurate delineation of changes in global and regional myocar-

Table 35-3. Responses to ACE Inhibitor Treatment for 3 Months in 17 Dilated Cardiomyopathy Patients

Measurement	Before	After	P
LV ejection fraction (%)	29.7 ± 2.2	36.0 ± 2.2	< 0.05
LV end-diastolic volume (ml)	166 ± 14	158 ± 12	NS
LV end-systolic volume (ml)	118 ± 12	106 ± 11	< 0.05
LV mass (g)	235 ± 13	220 ± 12	< 0.05
End-systolic wall stress (dynes·s·cm^{-5})	90 ± 5	64 ± 5	< 0.05
End-systolic stress/volume	0.83 ± 0.05	0.67 ± 0.06	< 0.05

Abbreviations: LV, left ventricular; NS, not significant.
The end-diastolic stress volume ratio serves as a load-independent index of myocardial contractility.
(From Doherty et al.[19] with permission.)

dial function in ischemic cardiomyopathy in response to revascularization seems possible and desirable. Yet such studies remain to be performed.

On the other hand, some information on the response to pharmacologic treatment is available.[19] This study explored the responses of left ventricular function to a 3-month course of angiotensin-converting enzyme (ACE) inhibitor therapy in 17 patients with dilated cardiomyopathy. All patients were in New York Heart Association (NYHA) heart failure class II or III, and all received the ACE inhibitor benazepril hydrochloride. As shown in Table 35-3, after 3 months of benazepril administration the left ventricular ejection fraction had increased by an average of 21 percent. The end-diastolic volume failed to change significantly, although the end-systolic volume declined by an average of 10 percent ($P <$ 0.05). The end-diastolic wall stress decreased by an average of 29 percent, associated with a 6 percent decline in left ventricular mass. The marked (15 percent) decrease in end-systolic pressure appeared to account primarily for the decline in end-systolic wall stress, which implied that the improvement in left ventricular function depended primarily on an afterload reducing effect of the ACE inhibitor. A subsequent study on the same topic[9] reported an improvement in the peak filling rate to end-systolic ratios, but this improvement was confined to patients without significant mitral regurgitation. The authors concluded that ACE inhibitor therapy may favorably affect the left ventricular diastolic function but cautioned that this effect might be obscured or not occur in dilated cardiomyopathy complicated by mitral regurgitation.

X-RAY COMPUTED TOMOGRAPHY

X-ray CT, especially with its ultrafast cine CT version (also referred to as electron beam CT) and the more recently developed spiral cine CT, shares many diagnostic capabilities and features available through cine MRI. As with MRI, these capabilities derive from the high spatial and temporal resolution capabilities of modern x-ray CT and are enhanced by the use of radiopaque contrast agents. The cardiac chambers and vascular structures are selectively visualized with these contrast agents administered intravenously. During their transit through the myocardial circulation, the contrast agents can depict the relative distribution of myocardial blood flow. Placement of regions of interest in the myocardium and cardiac chambers or large vessels permit construction of time–density curves, which can then be used to estimate regional myocardial blood flow or overall ventricular function. As an additional feature, cine CT depicts vascular calcification, which ultimately may prove useful for the detection of vascular and coronary artery disease. Table 35-4 summarizes the measurements and indices available through cine CT.

Measurement of Ventricular Volumes and Function

Because myocardium and blood exhibit similar densities on x-ray films, delineation of the myocardium and the blood pools and visualization of vessel lu-

Table 35-4. Cine Computed Tomography

Left ventricular myocardial mass
Left ventricular myocardial wall thickness and thickening
Systolic wall motion
Ventricular volumes
Ejection fraction
Myocardial perfusion
Vascular calcification

mens requires administration of angiographic contrast agents. Both endocardial and epicardial margins of the left ventricular myocardium are clearly demarcated on the resulting images. Thus the mass of the left ventricular myocardium can be measured.[20,21] Also, the chamber volumes and their changes during the cardiac cycle can be determined from the contiguous tomographic images.[22-25] As such measurements do not rely on geometric assumptions regarding the chamber geometry but are derived from the sum of the product of the areas of the left ventricular chamber (obtained by planimetry or Simpson's rule) and the slice thickness of all image slices encompassing the heart, such estimates appear to be more accurate than those obtained from single or biplanar cine ventriculograms. Time–volume curves can then be constructed and ejection fractions and filling and ejection rates calculated. Stroke volumes can be determined from end-diastolic and end-systolic chamber volumes. Discrepancies between right and left ventricular stroke volumes point to the presence of valvar regurgitation and afford measurements of regurgitant volumes.

As cine CT clearly depicts the left and right ventricular myocardium, cavity dimensions, myocardial wall thickness, and wall thickening can be measured. Combined with pressure measurements, regional and circumferential wall stresses can be estimated, as can compensatory changes in wall thickness in response to increased pressure or volume loads.[22,26]

Potential Applications to Heart Failure Patients

VENTRICULAR REMODELING AFTER ACUTE MYOCARDIAL INFARCTION

Ventricular remodeling can occur after an acute myocardial infarction, ultimately leading to marked impairment of ventricular function and heart failure symptoms. Studies with serial cine CT measurements have in fact examined the long-term effects on biventricular function and biventricular volumes.[27,28] Patients with anterior infarctions exhibited a 15–35 percent increase in right and left ventricular volumes over a 1-year follow-up. This increase was paralleled by an increase in wall stress and a proportionate decline in circumferential shortening as a measure of myocardial contractility.

Another study by the same investigators[27] noted that such remodeling also affects the free right ventricular wall and intraventricular septum. Over a 4 to 5 year period after an acute anterior myocardial

infarction, the length of the intraventricular septum and the right ventricular wall had increased by 13–23 percent accompanied by a 20–29 percent increase in right and left ventricular volumes. Cine CT investigations demonstrated further that the extent of left ventricular remodeling over a 1-year period corresponded to the initial size of the acute myocardial infarction.[29] For example, the size of the initial infarct defined as a percentage of the total left ventricular myocardium correlated inversely with the end-systolic volume and the left ventricular ejection fraction.

LEFT VENTRICULAR FUNCTION IN VALVULAR REGURGITATION

Other studies with cine CT have characterized the left ventricular dynamics in pure aortic regurgitation.[22,30] For example, peak emptying and filling rates in aortic regurgitation significantly exceeded those in normal volunteers. Moreover, other studies by the same investigators[26] concluded that, contrary to the widely held hypothesis of globally and regionally normalized ventricular radius/wall thickness (RT) ratios in compensated aortic regurgitation, such RT ratios were found to be higher than in normal volunteers, suggesting incomplete normalization of wall thickness. Lastly, cine CT has been found useful for characterizing the interrelations between left and right ventricular function.[31]

No specific studies have monitored responses to pharmacologic interventions. However, highly reproducible measurements of ventricular chamber sizes, functional parameters, wall stress, and wall thickness should provide an accurate means for examining responses to pharmacologic interventions in heart failure patients.

POSITRON EMISSION TOMOGRAPHY

Like cine CT and MRI, gated image acquisition with PET permits assessment of regional contractile function.[32,33] Unlike the other two imaging modalities, PET uniquely affords the evaluation, and in particular the nontraumatic quantification, of regional myocardial blood flow and regional myocardial substrate metabolism. This section briefly reviews the major technical features of PET and then discusses how this imaging technique can differentiate ischemic from nonischemic cardiomyopathies. It also defines abnormalities in substrate metabolism and especially how distinct patterns of blood flow and metabolism have proved useful for risk stratification of patients and clinically for deciding on the most advantageous therapeutic approach.

Methodologic Aspects

Although it offers lower spatial resolution than cine CT or MRI, PET exhibits exquisite contrast resolution. It allows measurements of tissue tracer concentrations in the nanomolar to picomolar range. Furthermore, tomographic images of tracer tissue concentrations acquired with PET are free of photon attenuation artifacts, so the images resemble in vivo acquired autoradiographs. Given a temporal resolution in the range of one to several seconds, it is possible to quantify noninvasively rapidly changing concentrations of radiotracer in arterial blood and the myocardium. This information then forms the basis for applying tracer kinetic principles for the quantification of regional rates of blood flow and substrate metabolism.

Rubidium-82 (^{82}Rb) and nitrogen-13 (^{13}N) ammonia are used to examine the relative distribution of myocardial blood flow and static images of the regional myocardial tracer concentrations. For measurements of regional myocardial blood flow in absolute units of milliliters of blood per gram of myocardium per unit of time, either oxygen-15 (^{15}O) water or ^{13}N-ammonia are available.[34–36]

Other positron-emitting tracers offer the exciting possibility of probing specific aspects of the human heart's substrate metabolism. As validated in animal experiments, carbon-11 (^{11}C) acetate yields quantitative information on myocardial oxygen consumption. Once administered intravenously, the compound rapidly accumulates in the myocardium from which it then clears in proportion to the rate of substrate flux through the tricarboxylic acid (TCA) cycle. As the activity of the TCA cycle is closely linked to oxidative phosphorylation, the regional clearance rates of ^{11}C activity from the myocardium then reflect regional rates of oxidative metabolism.[37,38] ^{11}C-labeled palmitate permits assessment of myocardial fatty acid metabolism, though in a more qualitative fashion. Injected intravenously, the myocardium avidly extracts ^{11}C-palmitate. The ^{11}C activity then distributes in proportion to natural, nonlabeled free fatty acid between the slow-turnover endogenous lipid pool and the small, rapid-turnover "oxidative pool" (including β-oxidation, TCA cycle activity, and release of ^{11}C-CO_2 from the myocardium). Consistent with this tracer distribution between at least two functional pools of largely different sizes and turnover rates, ^{11}C activity clears from the myocardium

in a characteristic biexponential fashion. The clearance curve morphology, as defined by the two slopes and the relative sizes of the two clearance curve components, thus reflects the intramyocardial distribution of free fatty acid and its rate of oxidation.[39–41]

Fluorine-18 (^{18}F) 2-fluoro-2-deoxyglucose traces the initial transmembranous exchange in the subsequent hexokinase-mediated phosphorylation of glucose to glucose-6-phosphate. As the tracer label then becomes effectively trapped in the myocardium, images of the myocardial ^{18}F concentrations mirror the regional rates of exogenous glucose utilization. Beyond such qualitative assessments, estimates of the rates of exogenous glucose utilization in absolute units of micromoles of glucose per minute per gram of myocardium can be obtained from rapidly acquired serial images. Both the arterial tracer input function and the myocardial tissue response to it can be determined from regions of interest in the arterial left ventricular blood pool and the myocardium on the serially acquired images. The resulting time–activity curves are then fitted with a well validated tracer compartment model.[42–44]

In addition to static and dynamic (rapid serial) image acquisition (the latter is essential for evaluating oxidative and fatty acid metabolism with ^{11}C-palmitate and ^{11}C-acetate, respectively), image acquisition can also be synchronized with the patient's electrocardiogram. Such gated images then offer the possibility of assessing regional systolic wall motion and wall thickening.[32,45,46]

With dilated cardiomyopathies of ischemic or idiopathic origin, external cardiac work is demonstrated by reduced systolic wall motion and wall thickening (also demonstrated by cine MRI). Contributing factors include increased wall stress, diffuse interstitial fibrosis, or increased connective tissue formation. Hence connective tissue may contribute an excessive fraction of the myocardial wall. It is possible to determine this fraction with PET.

Unlike fibrous tissue, living myocytes are capable of rapidly exchanging water. The total extravascular "myocardial mass" can be measured from transmission images corrected for blood pool activity with ^{11}C- or ^{15}O-labeled carbon monoxide attached to red blood cells.[47] The myocardial fraction capable of rapid water exchange is then assessed with ^{15}O-labeled water. Theoretically, if all constituents of the myocardium exchange water, the water-exchanging volume and the total volume approach unity. If, on the other hand, non-water-exchanging scar tissue is present, the ratio of the water-exchanging mass to the total mass is less than 1.0. This concept has been tested in chronic coronary artery disease patients with prior myocardial infarction, and it might prove

Table 35-5. PET Measurements
of Myocardial Function

Left ventricular volumes and ejection fraction

Regional systolic wall motion and thickening

Myocardial blood flow
  Relative distribution
  Absolute flows $(ml \cdot min^{-1} \cdot g^{-1})$

Substrate metabolism
  Exogenous glucose utilization: relative and absolute $(\mu mol \cdot min^{-1} \cdot g^{-1})$
  Fatty acid uptake and metabolism
  Oxidative metabolism $(\mu mol \cdot min^{-1} \cdot g^{-1})$

Adrenergic neuronal system
  Adrenergic neuron function
  β-Receptor density and affinity

Fractional tissue fibrosis

useful for estimating the extent of connective tissue formation in remote and possibly remodeled myocardium as well as in myocardium of idiopathic dilated cardiomyopathies. Theoretically, it could also be of use in distinguishing between idiopathic and ischemic cardiomyopathy, as in the latter type scar tissue formation is more heterogeneous and is enhanced in discreet regions,[48] in contrast to the diffuse increase in connective tissue in idiopathic dilated cardiomyopathy.

A more detailed description of the technical features of PET exceeds the scope of this chapter. The interested reader is referred to a more extensive review on this subject.[49] Table 35-5 summarizes the measurements available with PET.

Evaluation of Regional Contractile Function

Different from cine CT or gated MRI, which directly display changes in regional wall thickness, estimates of regional myocardial wall thickening are obtained from gated PET images by measuring the changes in regional activity concentrations from diastole to systole. This approach takes advantage of the partial volume effect, which in turn depends on the spatial resolution of the imaging device.[46] As a general principle applicable to all imaging approaches, the observed tissue activity concentration equals the true tissue activity concentration only if the object size (e.g., the myocardial wall thickness) exceeds the effective spatial resolution as defined by the full-width at half-maximum (FWHM) by at least a factor of two. The effective spatial resolution of most current PET systems ranges from 7 to 11 mm compared to a myo-

cardial wall thickness of about 10–12 mm. As the object size decreases, the observed activity concentrations decline nonlinearly as a function of the partial volume effect. Thus even though the true activity concentrations remain constant, the observed tissue concentrations increase from diastole to systole.[45,46] In experimental animals, the change in observed activity concentrations correlated linearly with the systolic increase in myocardial wall thickness as determined by echocardiography.[32] Applied in patients with ischemic cardiomyopathy, systolic wall thickening in normally perfused myocardial regions averaged 78 ± 29 percent.[33] Wall thickening declined progressively with more severe flow reductions. It was 52 ± 30 percent in mildly, hypoperfused and 33 ± 31 percent in severely hypoperfused myocardium. Regions with flow metabolism matches revealed a systolic wall thickening of only 23 ± 24 percent compared to 38 ± 33 percent in mismatch regions. Thus PET permits direct correlation between regional contractile function and regional blood flow or metabolism, especially when used in conjunction with gated imaging of myocardial ^{13}N ammonia or ^{18}F-12-fluoro-2-deoxyglucose uptake.

Differentiation of Ischemic from Nonischemic Cardiomyopathy

In most patients a clinical history points to the specific pathophysiology responsible for the impaired left ventricular function; in some patients, however, identification of the specific cause of ventricular failure poses diagnostic challenges. In other patients again, coronary artery disease may coexist with a myopathic process so the leading cause for the decrease in left ventricular function remains undetermined. Early studies had demonstrated clear differences in the spatial distribution of the initial myocardial ^{11}C-palmitate uptake between normals, patients with idiopathic cardiomyopathy, and patients with ischemic cardiomyopathy.[50] Compared to the homogeneous ^{11}C-palmitate concentrations in normal volunteers the tracer was distributed more heterogeneously in patients with idiopathic dilated cardiomyopathies, most likely reflecting spatially and temporally disparate tissue abnormalities that ultimately result in spotty necrosis. In contrast, there were large confluent regions of reduced ^{11}C-palmitate uptake in patients with ischemic cardiomyopathy. Such regions of reduced or even absent ^{11}C-palmitate accumulation correspond to the distribution of coronary vascular territories and thus probably reflect reductions in fatty acid metabolism as a function of regionally reduced blood flow or, in the presence of myocardial infarction, scar tissue formation.

Resting Perfusion

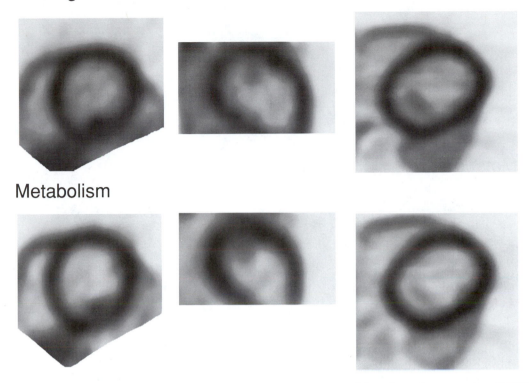

Metabolism

Fig. 35-3. Comparison of the blood flow–metabolism patterns in dilated cardiomyopathy (DCM) and ischemic heart disease (also Figures 35–4 and 35–5). Selected transaxial slices of the myocardial[13]N-ammonia uptake reflect myocardial blood flow (MBF) and the myocardial[18]F-deoxyglucose (FDG) concentrations in the myocardium. Note the marked enlargement of the left ventricular cavity in all three patients. In this patient with dilated cardiomyopathy shown in this figure myocardial blood flow (MBF) and FDG uptake is distributed homogeneously throughout the left ventricular myocardium.

A subsequent study compared the distribution of myocardial blood flow using ^{13}N ammonia and [18]F-12-fluoro-2-deoxyglucose uptake in patients with markedly reduced left ventricular function with or without angiographically documented coronary artery disease.[51] Idiopathic dilated cardiomyopathies exhibited the characteristic left ventricular enlargement with homogeneous blood flow and exogenous glucose utilization as evidenced by the uniform accumulation of both ^{13}N ammonia and [18]F-12-fluoro-2-deoxyglucose (Fig. 35-3). In contrast and similar to the earlier findings with ^{11}C palmitate, ischemic cardiomyopathy characteristically exhibited segmental reductions in blood flow. These reductions again followed the distribution of coronary vascular territories (Fig. 35-4). However, the [18]F-12-fluoro-2-deoxyglucose uptake differed from blood flow (Fig. 35-5). In some patients it paralleled the distribution of blood flow; that is, glucose utilization rates were found to be segmentally decreased in proportion to blood flow. This pattern is subsequently referred to as a blood flow metabolism match and indicates an irreversible loss of contractile function. Other pa-

tients again revealed homogeneous or even enhanced ^{18}F-2-fluoro-2-deoxyglucose uptake in hypoperfused myocardial segments. This disparity is subsequently referred to as "blood flow–metabolism mismatch" and indicates the presence of potentially reversible dysfunction or of myocardial viability (see below).

The blood flow metabolism patterns on PET scans distinguished with 85 percent accuracy between ischemic and nonischemic cardiomyopathies.[51] On the other hand, electrocardiographic criteria such as Q waves, concomitant right ventricular enlargement, and regional rather than diffuse depression of left ventricular wall motion were of limited if any value in distinguishing between the two types of cardiomyopathy.

Idiopathic Dilated Cardiomyopathy

Initial studies with PET have assessed quantitatively regional myocardial blood flow, fatty acid metabolism, and oxidative rates in patients with idiopathic dilated cardiomyopathy.

Resting Perfusion

Metabolism

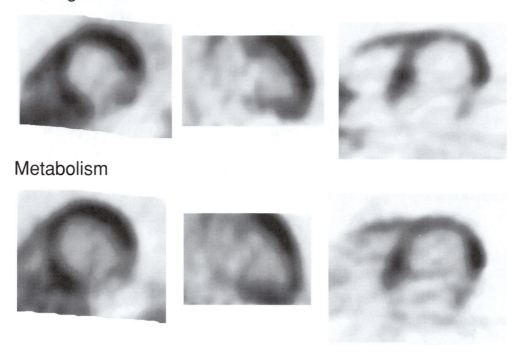

Fig. 35-4. In this patient with ischemic heart disease, myocardial blood flow is decreased in the lateral and inferolateral walls. The ^{18}F-deoxyglucose (FDG) uptake parallels myocardial blood flow; glucose utilization is decreased equally to blood flow in the lateral and inferolateral walls, consistent with the presence of a large blood flow metabolism match.

Resting Perfusion

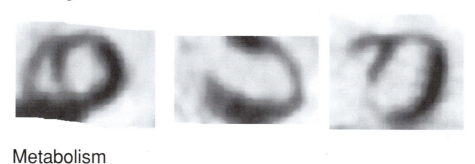

Metabolism

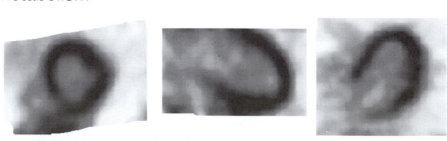

Fig. 35-5. In contrast to the study shown in Figure 35-4, this ischemic heart disease patient revealed reduced blood flow in the anterior wall. Yet glucose utilization is normal or even slightly increased. This pattern represents a "blood flow–metabolism mismatch."

MYOCARDIAL BLOOD FLOW

In normal volunteers, myocardial blood flow closely follows myocardial oxygen demand as defined by the rate–pressure product.[52,53] In view of the marked left ventricular enlargement with a considerable increase in wall stress and active tension development as a major determinant of myocardial oxygen consumption, myocardial blood flow at rest was expected to be elevated in idiopathic dilated cardiomyopathy. Yet in seven idiopathic dilated cardiomyopathy patients, myocardial blood flow at rest averaged 0.88 ± 0.37 ml·min^{-1}·g^{-1} and was similar to that in a group of 16 age-matched normal volunteers.[54] Also, myocardial flow reserve as tested with intravenous dipyridamole averaged 3.5 ± 1.4 and did not differ from that in the normal control group.

In contrast, another study of 22 patients with idiopathic dilated cardiomyopathy and an average left ventricular ejection fraction of 35 ± 8 percent reported modestly reduced blood flow at rest.[55] In response to atrial pacing, blood flow increased less in these patients than in a group of normal volunteers. Moreover, myocardial flow reserve as tested with intravenous dipyridamole was only 2.45 compared to a reserve of 3.49 in the 13 normal controls. There was also an inverse correlation between blood flow at rest and during atrial pacing and left ventricular end-diastolic pressures. Reduction in resting and hyperemic blood flow thus appear to be consistent with abnormalities at the level of the microcirculation or with increased extravascular resistive forces due to the elevated left ventricular wall stress, as also evidenced by the correlation to the end-diastolic left ventricular pressures.

Different from these mildly decreased blood flows were the normal rates of oxidative metabolism, as assessed with ^{11}C-acetate in 10 patients with idiopathic dilated cardiomyopathy and an average left ventricular ejection fraction of only 21 ± 8 percent. Overall, clearance rates were distributed homogeneously throughout the left ventricular myocardium and averaged 0.061 ± 0.006 min^{-1}, which was similar to that in 10 normal volunteers.[56]

A mild, probably not statistically significant increase in oxidative rates, again as determined with ^{11}C-acetate, has been reported in eight patients with idiopathic dilated cardiomyopathy. In this study, k_{mono} averaged 0.064 ± 0.012 min^{-1}, which was slightly higher than the 0.058 ± 0.009 min^{-1} reported previously from the same laboratory for fasting normal volunteers.[57]

In view of the homogeneous blood flow, oxidative metabolism, and exogenous glucose utilization, the observed heterogeneity of myocardial fatty acid metabolism with ^{11}C-palmitate and serial image acquisition is a surprise. Similar to the previously reported heterogeneous ^{11}C-palmitate uptake,[50] there was considerable heterogeneity in regional ^{11}C-palmitate clearance rates in patients with nonischemic cardiomyopathy. This heterogeneity was independent of the underlying pathophysiology. Moreover, manipulation of myocardial substrate metabolism by altering circulating substrate levels augmented the heterogeneity (Plate 35-1) and, further, revealed a paradoxical response of the myocardial ^{11}C-palmitate kinetics to glucose loading.[58,59] The preferential fatty acid oxidation in the fasted state, when circulating free fatty acid levels are high and insulin levels are low, is reflected on the clearance curve by the large relative size of the rapid clearance curve component and the steepness of its slope (Plate 35-1 and Fig. 35-6). Oral glucose loading followed by an increase in circulating glucose levels, by increased insulin secretion, and a decline in circulating free fatty acid levels results in a shift in myocardial substrate selection toward glucose, so for the same amount of cardiac work less free fatty acid is oxidized.[58] The clearance curve morphology reflects this situation by a decline in the relative size of the rapid clearance curve component with a less steep slope. Yet in about half of the patients studied, glucose loading resulted in a "paradoxical response." The relative size of the rapid clearance curve component and the steepness of its slope increased rather than decreased (Fig. 35-6). Furthermore, as demonstrated in a subsequent investigation,[59] glucose loading enhanced the heterogeneity of regional clearance rates. The number of paradoxically responding regions appeared to correlate to the degree of impairment in global left ventricular function.

The observations made thus far with PET in patients with idiopathic dilated cardiomyopathy seem puzzling and internally inconsistent. The "normal rates" of blood flow and increased rates of oxidative metabolism are a surprise in view of the markedly elevated wall stress and tension development as major determinants of myocardial oxygen consumption. On the other hand, it is possible that this increase in demand is offset by a lower contractile state as another important determinant of myocardial oxygen demand. The heterogeneous ^{11}C-palmitate uptake and clearance rates further seem inconsistent with the observed homogeneity and blood flow in oxidative metabolism. Yet it is possible that the myopathic process selectively targets the initial metabolic steps of fatty acid metabolism, including their initial sequestration and subsequent β-oxidation. Thus "sick" myocytes may primarily rely on glucose as its preferred substrate.

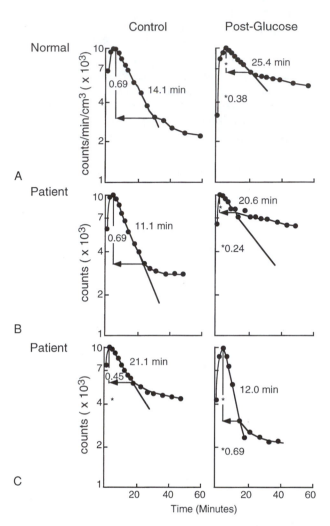

Fig. 35-6. Myocardial time–activity curves derived from serially acquired PET images in the fasted state (left) and following glucose utilization. Note the biexponential clearance pattern in the normal volunteer (**A**). The relative size of the rapid clearance curve component is 69 percent, and the clearance half-time is 14.1 minutes. Glucose loading induces a marked change in the clearance curve morphology. The relative size of the rapid clearance curve component declines to 38 percent; the clearance half-time increases to 25.4 minutes. (**B & C**) The time–activity curves were obtained for patients with ischemic cardiomyopathy. Note the normal response pattern to glucose loading in the patients shown in **B**. In contrast, the patient in **C** exhibits a paradoxical response. In the fasting state, the relative size of the rapid clearance curve component is mildly reduced yet markedly increases after glucose loading. Furthermore, the steepness of the slope markedly increases as indicated by the shorter clearance half-times. (From Schelbert et al.,[58] with permission.)

MECHANICAL EFFICIENCY IN NONISCHEMIC CARDIOMYOPATHY

One study in eight patients with nonischemic cardiomyopathy and an average left ventricular ejection fraction of only 22 ± 5 percent correlated indices of external cardiac work with the tissue clearance rate of ^{11}C-acetate from the left ventricular myocardium (defined as k_{mono}) as a measure of myocardial oxygen consumption.[57] External work was estimated by echocardiography from the product of the stroke volume index, peak systolic pressure, and heart rate or from hemodynamic parameters as the product of stroke volume and the difference between mean arterial blood pressure and capillary wedge pressure normalized to the body surface area. The ratio of these stroke work indices to oxidative metabolism as determined with ^{11}C-acetate represented a measure of mechanical efficiency. This index markedly increased (by 35 percent for the echocardiographically derived and 68 percent for the hemodynamically derived external work index) during nitroprusside infusion associated with an increase in ejection fraction, cardiac output, and stroke work. These findings suggest the possibility of estimating noninvasively the mechanical efficiency of the left ventricular myocardium. Such estimates may prove useful for monitoring pharmacologic interventions in terms of a more efficient use of oxygen and other substrates and energy conversion.

Ischemic Cardiomyopathy

Different from idiopathic dilated cardiomyopathy, blood flow and metabolism studies with PET can have direct diagnostic and therapeutic implications in patients with ischemic cardiomyopathy. As discussed above, confluent, discrete reductions in blood flow corresponding to distinct coronary vascular territories are characteristic for ischemic cardiomyopathy. The question is whether the impairment in regional contractile function associated with such flow reductions can be reversed or improved through interventional restoration of blood flow. A concordant reduction in regional glucose utilization as evident on myocardial ^{18}F-2-fluoro-2-deoxyglucose uptake images predicts with a rather high degree of accuracy that segmental function does not improve following revascularization. Conversely, the persistence of exogenous glucose utilization, as expressed in the form of a blood flow–metabolism mismatch heralds the presence of viable myocardium and thus predicts with 80 to 90 percent accuracy postrevascularization improvement in segmental systolic wall motion.[60–65]

Table 35-6. Effect of Revascularization and Left Ventricular Ejection Fraction

Author	No. of pts.	Extensive Mismatch Region				Small or No Mismatch Region			
		No.[a]	Pre-LVEF	Post-LVEF	P	No.	Pre-LVEF	Post-LVEF	P
Tillisch et al.[60]	17	11	30 ± 11	45 ± 14	< 0.05	6	30 ± 11	31 ± 12	NS
Marwick et al.[65]	24	9	37 ± 11	40 ± 9	NS	15	38 ± 13	38 ± 13	NS
Carrel et al.[62]	21	21	34 ± 14	52 ± 11	< 0.01	—	—	—	—
Lucignani et al.[63]	14	13	38 ± 5	48 ± 4	< 0.001	—	—	—	—
Depré et al.[68]	23	[b]	43 ± 18	52 ± 15	< 0.001	[b]	35 ± 9	23 ± 8	NS

[a] Number of patients with and without mismatches.
[b] Values not given.

More pertinent to chronic coronary artery disease patients with poor left ventricular function, poor long-term survival, severely limited physical activity, and a high preoperative mortality are questions of whether blood flow metabolism imaging with PET can identify patients with the poorest survival and can aid in selecting patients who are likely to benefit most from surgical revascularization in terms of congestive heart failure symptoms, global left ventricular function, and long-term survival. If the answer is yes, blood flow metabolism findings on PET would decisively alter the risk-benefit ratio of surgical revascularization and thus significantly affect the therapeutic decision making process.

There is in fact considerable evidence that PET offers predictive information on the postrevascularization outcome of global left ventricular function. As summarized in Table 35-6, the presence of blood flow–metabolism mismatches or persistent though altered glucose metabolic activity involving at least 15–25 percent of the left ventricular myocardium results in postrevascularization improvement of the left ventricular ejection fraction. On the other hand, such improvement is unlikely to occur if there are only small mismatches (less than 5 percent of the left ventricular myocardium) or if blood flow–metabolism matches only are present.[60,62,63,66–68] It is important to note that such improvement may occur slowly and over periods of at least several months,[69] as exemplified in a case report.[70] In this patient with an ejection fraction of 16 percent, early after revascularization there was a modest improvement. Subsequent serial measurements revealed a progressive increase to 47 percent at 12 months after revascularization. "Redifferentiation" of abnormal (dedifferentiated) cells frequently associated with blood flow–metabolism mismatches may require time for reconstruction or reexpression of myofibers and of the contractile machinery.[68,71,72] It may account for the slow yet progressive improvement in left ventricular performance.

One of the above questions addressed the identification of patients with high future morbidity and mortality and whether revascularization of such patients would avert catastrophic events such as an acute myocardial infarction or death. Several follow-up studies have demonstrated higher morbidity and, in two studies, higher mortality of patients exhibiting blood flow–metabolism mismatches.[73–76] One investigation provided information on the outcome of 129 patients with coronary artery disease over a 17 ± 9 month period after myocardial blood flow and glucose uptake imaging on PET.[76] Nearly half of the patients underwent revascularization. Nonfatal ischemic events were most frequent in patients with blood flow–metabolism mismatches on pharmacologic treatment. Based on the Cox proportional hazard model, mismatches and failure to revascularize were independent predictors of such ischemic events as unstable angina or an acute nonfatal myocardial infarction. Thirteen patients died during the follow-up period. Multivariate analysis implicated the left ventricular ejection fraction and age as independent predictors of cardiac deaths. It is important to note that in this study the patients exhibited a wide range of left ventricular ejection fractions. In patients who died, the ejection fraction averaged 22 ± 13 percent compared to 39 ± 14 percent in patients without a nonfatal ischemic event.

In a more recent study of 93 patients followed over an average 13.6 months, not the left ventricular ejection fraction but the presence of a blood flow–meta-

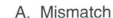

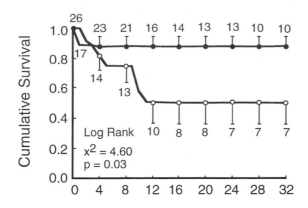 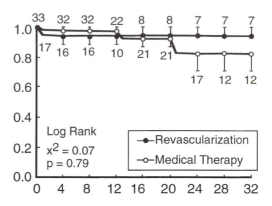

Months of Follow-up

Fig. 35-7. Survival of patients with markedly depressed left ventricular ejection fractions according to the blood flow metabolism patterns and revascularization and medical treatment. **(A)** Note the rather poor 2-month survival of patients with blood–flow metabolism mismatches on medical treatment, in contrast to the significantly better survival of patients with blood–flow metabolism mismatches submitted to surgical revascularization. **(B)** More patients without mismatches survived following revascularization than did those on medical therapy, but the difference was statistically insignificant. The survival data suggest that blood flow metabolism mismatches identify high risk patients who, at the same time, appear to benefit most in terms of survival from surgical revascularization. (From Di Carli et al.,[75] with permission.)

bolism mismatch and the lack of surgical revascularization proved to be predictors of cardiac death.[75] In these patients with end-stage coronary artery disease, the left ventricular fraction was more uniformly decreased, averaging 26 ± 6 percent. The cumulative survival for patient subgroups according to the absence or presence of blood flow–metabolism mismatches and according to treatment (pharmacologic versus revascularization). Again, based on a Cox model analysis, the extent of a blood flow–metabolism mismatch had a negative effect on survival ($P < 0.02$), whereas revascularization positively affected survival ($P < 0.04$). Fig. 35-7 depicts the cumulative survival for each subgroup.

In addition to increasing long-term survival, the quest for amelioration or even relief of congestive heart failure-related symptoms represents another goal of surgical revascularization in patients with ischemic cardiomyopathy. Preliminary data reported in the above described clinical investigations suggested that such improvement can indeed be predicted from the blood flow metabolism patterns on PET. For instance, 71 percent of the patients with extensive blood flow–metabolism mismatches revealed on follow-up an improvement from NYHA class III or IV to class I or II at 13 months after surgi-

cal revascularization. This particular question, however, has been explored in more detail in another clinical investigation.[77] That study compared the extent of prerevascularization blood flow–metabolism mismatches (Plate 35-2) to the long-term improvement in physical activity. It applied a specific activity scale that expressed physical activity in metabolic units.[78] Patients were admitted to a structured interview prior to and after as long as 32 months following coronary artery bypass grafting. As depicted in Fig. 35-8, there was a direct, statistically significant correlation between the extent of the blood flow–metabolism mismatch and the postrevascularization change in physical activity. This improvement in the specific activity scale was most prominent in patients with a blood flow–metabolism mismatch that affected at least 20 percent or more of the left ventricular myocardium.

CONCLUSIONS

Each of the three tomographic imaging techniques can contribute uniquely to the diagnosis of heart failure, elucidation of its underlying etiology, characterization of its severity, and the decision making pro-

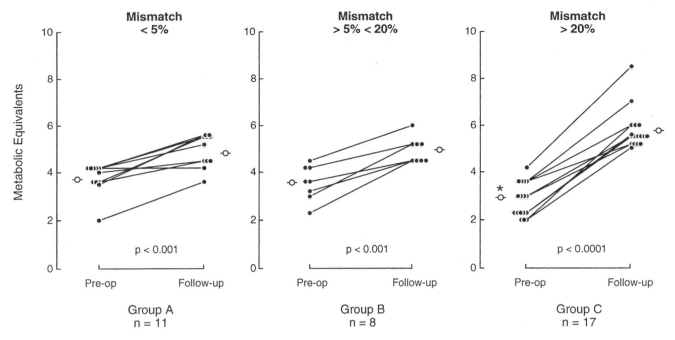

Fig. 35-8. Improvement in the specific activity scale (expressed in metabolic equivalents) following revascularization. The patients are grouped into those with no or only small mismatches (**A**) those with small mismatches (**B**) and those with mismatches involving more than 20 percent of the left ventricular myocardium (**C**). Note that the patient group with the largest blood flow metabolism mismatches exhibited the greatest improvement in metabolic equivalents and thus benefited most from surgical revascularization in terms of relief of congestive heart failure symptoms. (From Di Carli et al.,[77] with permission.)

cess regarding the most appropriate therapeutic course of action; and they help monitor responses to treatment. At present, cine MRI and ultrafast CT primarily focus on delineating the structure and mechanical function of the heart. As such, they are most useful for gauging the severity of heart failure and the responses of mechanical function to pharmacologic and revascularization interventions. The potential of MR for characterizing metabolic abnormalities, though promising, remains currently largely unexplored and thus underutilized. On the other hand, it is this particular aspect of the failing heart that can and already has been most extensively explored with PET. In fact, patterns of blood flow and metabolism contain considerable prognostic information on patients with ischemic cardiomyopathy considered for surgical revascularization. Abnormal patterns of substrate metabolism in idiopathic dilated cardiomyopathy as delineated with PET or of high energy phosphate concentrations and their changes in response to manipulation of circulating substrate levels may in the future lead the way to novel pharmacologic interventions. Lastly, merging the metabolic information obtained by PET with the anatomic and functional information obtained by MRI or CT may result in even more detailed, accurate characterization of the failing ventricle and en-

hance the accuracy of predicting long-term therapeutic outcomes.

ACKNOWLEDGMENTS

The author thanks Diane Martin for preparing the illustrations and gratefully acknowledges Eileen Rosenfeld's skillful assistance in preparing this manuscript. This work was supported in part by the Director of the Office of Energy Research, Office of Health and Environmental Research, Washington, DC; by research grants HL 29845 and HL 33177, National Institutes of Health, Bethesda, MD; and by an Investigative Group Award by the Greater Los Angeles Affiliate of the American Heart Association, Los Angeles, CA.

REFERENCES

1. Mogelvang J, Thomsen C, Mehlsen J et al: Evaluation of left ventricular volumes measured by magnetic resonance imaging. Eur Heart J 1986;7:1016–1021
2. Mogelvang J, Stubgaard M, Thomsen C, Henriksen O: Evaluation of right ventricular volumes measured by magnetic resonance imaging. Eur Heart J 1988;9: 529–533

3. Van Rossum A, Visser F, Sprenger M et al: Evaluation of magnetic resonance imaging for determination of left ventricular ejection fraction and comparison with angiography. Am J Cardiol 1988;62:628–633

4. Sechtem U, Pflugfelder P, Gould R, Cassidy M, Higgins C: Measurement of right and left ventricular volumes in healthy individuals with cine MR imaging. Radiology 1987;163:697–702

5. Sakuma H, Fujita N, Foo T et al: Evaluation of left ventricular volume and mass with breath-hold cine MR imaging. Radiology 1993;188:377–380

6. Semelka R, Tomei E, Wagner S et al: Normal left ventricular dimensions and function. Interstudy reproducibility of measurements with cine MR imaging. Radiology 1990;174:763–768

7. Buser P, Auffermann W, Holt W et al: Noninvasive evaluation of global left ventricular function with use of cine nuclear magnetic resonance. J Am Coll Cardiol 1989;13:1294–1300

8. Suzuki J, Caputo G, Masui T et al: Assessment of right ventricular diastolic and systolic function in patients with dilated cardiomyopathy using cine magnetic resonance imaging. Am Heart J 1991;122:1035–1040

9. Fujita N, Haretiala J, O'Sullivan M et al: Assessment of left ventricular diastolic function in dilated cardiomyopathy with cine magnetic resonance imaging. Effect of an angiotensin converting enzyme inhibitor, benazepril. Am Heart J 1993;125:171–178

10. Katz J, Milliken M, Stray-Gundersen J et al: Estimation of human myocardial mass with MR imaging. Radiology 1988;169:495–498

11. Sechtem U, Sommerhoff B, Markiewicz W et al: Regional left ventricular wall thickening by magnetic resonance imaging. Evaluation in normal persons and patients with global and regional dysfunction. Am J Cardiol 1987;59:145–151

12. Auffermann W, Chew W, Wolfe C et al: Normal and diffusely abnormal myocardium in humans. Functional and metabolic characterization with P-31 MR spectroscopy and cine MR imaging. Radiology 1991;179:253–259

13. Sechtem U, Pflugfelder P, Cassidy M et al: Mitral or aortic regurgitation. Quantification of regurgitant volumes with cine MR imaging. Radiology 1988;167:425–430

14. Pflugfelder P, Sechtem U, White R et al: Noninvasive evaluation of mitral regurgitation by analysis of left atrial signal loss in cine magnetic resonance. Am Heart J 1989;117:1113–1119

15. Fujita N, Chazouilleres A, Hartiala J et al: quantification of mitral regurgitation by velocity-encoded cine nuclear magnetic resonance imaging. J Am Coll Cardiol 1994;23:951–958

16. Saeed M, Wendland M, Sakuma H et al: Coronary artery stenosis. Detection with contrast-enhanced MR imaging in dogs. Radiology 1995;196:79–84

17. Manning W, Li W, Edelman R: A preliminary report comparing magnetic resonance coronary angiography with conventional angiography. N Engl J Med 1993;328:828–832

18. Whitman G, Chance B, Bode H et al: Diagnosis and therapeutic evaluation of a pediatric case of cardiomyopathy using phosphorus-31 nuclear magnetic resonance spectroscopy. J Am Coll Cardiol 1985;5:745–749

19. Doherty N, Seelos K, Suzuki J et al: Application of cine nuclear magnetic resonance imaging for sequential evaluation of response to angiotensin-converting enzyme inhibitor therapy in dilated cardiomyopathy. J Am Coll Cardiol 1992;19:1294–1302

20. Roig E, Georgiou D, Chomka E et al: Reproducibility of left ventricular myocardial volume and mass measurements by ultrafast computed tomography. J Am Coll Cardiol 1991;18:990–996

21. Cutrone J, Georgiou D, Khan S et al: Right ventricular mass measurement by electron beam computed tomography. Validation with autopsy data. Invest Radiol 1995;30:64–68

22. Rumberger J, Reed J: Quantitative dynamics of left ventricular emptying and filling as a function of heart size and stroke volume in pure aortic regurgitation and in normal subjects. Am J Cardiol 1992;70:1045–1050

23. Bleiweis M, Mao S, Brundage B: Total biventricular volume and total left ventricular volume by ultrafast computed tomography. Prediction of left ventricular mass. Am Heart J 1994;127:667–673

24. Pietras R, Wolfkiel C, Veselik K et al: Validation of ultrafast computed tomographic left ventricular volume measurement. Invest Radiol 1991;26:28–34

25. Hajduczok Z, Weiss R, Stanford W, Marcus M: Determination of right ventricular mass in humans and dogs with ultrafast cardiac computed tomography. Circulation 1990;82:202–212

26. Feiring A, Rumberger J: Ultrafast computed tomography analysis of regional radius-to-wall thickness ratios in normal and volume-overloaded human left ventricle. Circulation 1992;85:1423–1432

27. Hirose K, Reed J, Rumberger J: Serial changes in regional right ventricular free wall and left ventricular septal wall lengths during the first 4 to 5 years after index anterior wall myocardial infarction. J Am Coll Cardiol 1995;26:394–400

28. Hirose K, Reed J, Rumberger J: Serial changes in left and right ventricular systolic and diastolic dynamics during the first year after an index left ventricular Q wave myocardial infarction. J Am Coll Cardiol 1995;25:1097–1104

29. Chareonthaitawee P, Christian T, Hirose K, Gibbons R, Rumberger J: Relation of initial infarct size to extent of left ventricular remodeling in the year after acute myocardial infarction. J Am Coll Cardiol 1995;25:567–573

30. Rumberger J, Bell M: Measurement of myocardial perfusion and cardiac output using intravenous injection methods by ultrafast (cine) computed tomography. Invest Radiol, suppl. 1992;2:40–46

31. Louie E, Lin S, Reynertson S et al: Pressure and volume loading of the right ventricle have opposite effects on left ventricular ejection fraction. Circulation 1995;92:819–824

32. Wisenberg G, Schelbert HR, Hoffman EJ et al: In vivo quantitation of regional myocardial blood flow by positron emission computed tomography. Circulation 1981;63:1248–1258

33. Yamashita K, Tamaki N, Yonekura Y et al: Regional wall thickening of left ventricle evaluated by gated positron emission tomography in relation to myocardial perfusion and glucose metabolism. J Nucl Med 1991;32:679–685

34. Kuhle W, Porenta G, Huang S-C et al: Quantification of regional myocardial blood flow using ^{13}N-ammonia

and reoriented dynamic positron emission tomographic imaging. Circulation 1992;86:1004–1017

35. Muzik O, Beanlands RSB, Hutchins GD et al: Validation of nitrogen-13-ammonia tracer kinetic model for quantification of myocardial blood flow using PET. J Nucl Med 1993;34:83–91

36. Krivokapich J, Huang SC, Hoffman EJ et al: Noninvasive detection of functionally significant coronary artery stenoses with exercise and PET. J Nucl Med 1988;29:837–838

37. Buxton DB, Nienaber CA, Luxen A et al: Noninvasive quantitation of regional myocardial oxygen consumption in vivo with [1-^{11}C] acetate and dynamic positron emission tomography. Circulation 1989;79:134–142

38. Armbrecht JJ, Buxton DB, Brunken RC, Phelps ME, Schelbert HR: Regional myocardial oxygen consumption determined noninvasively in humans with [1-^{11}C] acetate and dynamic positron tomography. Circulation 1989;80:863–872

39. Schön HR, Schelbert HR, Najafi A et al: C-11 labeled palmitic acid for the noninvasive evaluation of regional myocardial fatty acid metabolism with positron computed tomography. I. Kinetics of C-11 palmitic acid in normal myocardium. Am Heart J 1982;103:532–547

40. Schelbert HR, Henze E, Schön HR et al: palmitic acid for the noninvasive evaluation of regional myocardial fatty acid metabolism with positron computed tomography. IV. In vivo demonstration of impaired fatty acid oxidation in acute myocardial ischemia. Am Heart J 1983;106:736–750

41. Rosamond TL, Abendschein DR, Sobel BE, Bergmann SR, Fox KAA: Metabolic fate of radiolabeled palmitate in ischemic canine myocardium. Implications for positron emission tomography. J Nucl Med 1987;28:1322–1329

42. Ratib O, Phelps ME, Huang SC et al: Positron tomography with deoxyglucose for estimating local myocardial glucose metabolism. J Nucl Med 1982;23:577–586

43. Phelps ME, Hoffman EJ, Selin CE et al: Investigation of [^{18}F] 2-fluoro-2-deoxyglucose for the measure of myocardial glucose metabolism. J Nucl Med 1978;19:1311–1319

44. Gambhir SS, Schwaiger M, Huang SC, et al: Simple noninvasive quantification method for measuring myocardial glucose utilization in humans employing positron emission tomography and fluorine-18 deoxyglucose. J Nucl Med 1989;30:359–366

45. Hoffman EJ, Phelps ME, Wisenberg G, Schelbert HR, Kuhl DE: Electrocardiographic gating in positron emission computed tomography. J Comput Assist Tomogr 1979;3:731–739

46. Hoffman EJ, Huang SC, Phelps ME: Quantitation in positron emission computed tomography. J Comput Assist Tomogr 1979;3:299–308

47. Iida H, Rhodes C, de Silva R et al: Myocardial tissue fraction. Correction for partial volume effects and measure of tissue viability. J Nucl Med 1991;32:2169–2175

48. Yamamoto Y, De Silva R, Rhodes C et al: A new strategy for the assessment of viable myocardium and regional myocardial blood flow using ^{15}O-water and dynamic positron emission tomography. Circulation 1992;86:167–178

49. Schelbert H: Principles of Positron Emission Tomography. pp. 1140–1168. In Marcus ML, Skorton DJ, Wolf GL (eds): Cardiac Imaging. WB Saunders, Philadelphia, 1991

50. Eisenberg JD, Sobel BE, Geltman ED: Differentiation of ischemic from nonischemic cardiomyopathy with positron emission tomography. Am J Cardiol 1987;59:1410–1414

51. Vaghaiwalla Mody F, Brunken R, Warner-Stevenson L et al: Differentiating cardiomyopathy of coronary artery disease from nonischemic dilated cardiomyopathy utilizing positron tomography. J Am Coll Cardiol 1991;17:373–383

52. Czernin J, Müller P, Chan S et al: Influence of age and hemodynamics on myocardial blood flow and flow reserve. Circulation 1993;88:62–69

53. Krivokapich J, Smith GT, Huang SC et al: N-13 ammonia myocardial imaging at rest and with exercise in normal volunteers. Quantification of absolute myocardial perfusion with dynamic positron emission tomography. Circulation 1989;80:1328–1337

54. Fung C, Czernin J, Müller P et al: Noninvasive demonstration of normal myocardial perfusion reserve in patients with dilated idiopathic cardiopathy. J Am Coll Cardiol 1992;19:120A

55. Neglia D, Parodi O, Gallopin M et al: Myocardial blood flow response to pacing tachycardia and to dipyridamole infusion in patients with dilated cardiomyopathy without overt heart failure. Circulation 1995;92:796–804

56. Chan S, Warner-Stevenson L, Brunken R, Krivokapich J, Phelps ME: Myocardial oxygen consumption in patients with idiopathic dilated cardiomyopathy. J Nucl Med 1990;31:773

57. Beanlands R, Armstrong W, Hicks R et al: The effects of afterload reduction on myocardial carbon 11-labeled acetate kinetics and noninvasively estimated mechanical efficiency in patients with dilated cardiomyopathy. J Nucl Cardiol 1994;1:3–16

58. Schelbert HR, Henze E, Sochor H et al: Effects of substrate availability on myocardial C-11 palmitate kinetics by positron emission tomography in normal subjects and patients with ventricular dysfunction. Am Heart J 1986;111:1055–1064

59. Sochor H, Schelbert H, Schwaiger M, Henze E, Phelps M: Studies of fatty acid metabolism with positron emission tomography in patients with cardiomyopathy. Eur J Nucl Med 1986;12:S66–S69

60. Tillisch J, Brunken R, Marshall R et al: Reversibility of cardiac wall motion abnormalities predicted by positron tomography. N Engl J Med 1986;314:884–888

61. Tamaki N, Yonekura Y, Yamashita K et al: Positron emission tomography using fluorine-18 deoxyglucose in evaluation of coronary artery bypass grafting. Am J Cardiol 1989;64:860–865

62. Carrel T, Jenni R, Haubold-Reuter S et al: Improvement of severely reduced left ventricular function after surgical revascularization in patients with preoperative myocardial infarction. Eur J Cardiothorac Surg 1992;6:479–484

63. Lucignani G, Paolini G, Landoni C et al: Presurgical identification of hibernating myocardium by combined use of technetium-99m hexakis 2-methoxyisobutylisonitrile single photon emission tomography and fluorine-18 fluoro-2-deoxy-D-glucose positron emission tomography in patients with coronary artery disease. Eur J Nucl Med 1992;19:874–881

64. Tamaki N, Ohtani H, Yamashita K et al: Metabolic

activity in the areas of new fill-in after thallium-201 reinjection. Comparison with positron emission tomography using fluorine-18-deoxyglucose. J Nucl Med 1991;32:673–678

65. Marwick T, MacIntyre W, Lafont A, Nemec J, Salcedo E: Metabolic responses of hibernating and infarcted myocardium to revascularization. A follow-up study of regional perfusion, function, and metabolism. Circulation 1992;85:1347–1353

66. Marwick T, Nemec J, Lafont A, Salcedo E, MacIntyre W: Prediction by postexercise fluoro-18 deoxyglucose positron emission tomography of improvement in exercise capacity after revascularization. Am J Cardiol 1992;69:854–859

67. Besozzi MC, Brown MD, Hubner KF et al: Retrospective post therapy evaluation of cardiac function in 208 coronary artery disease patients evaluated by positron emission tomography. J Nucl Med 1992;33:885

68. Depré C, Vanoverschelde J-LJ, Melin J et al: Structural and metabolic correlates of the reversibility of chronic left ventricular ischemic dysfunction in humans. Am J Physiol 1995;268:H1265–H1275

69. Vanoverschelde J, Melin J, Depré C et al: Time-course of functional recovery of hibernating myocardium after coronary revascularization. Circulation, suppl. I 1994;90:378

70. Luu M, Stevenson L, Brunken R et al: Delayed recovery of revascularized myocardium after referral for cardiac transplantation. Am Heart J 1990;119:668–670

71. Vanoverschelde J-L, Wijns W, Depré C et al: Mechanisms of chronic regional postischemic dysfunction in humans. New insights from the study of noninfarcted collateral-dependent myocardium. Circulation 1993;87:1513–1523

72. Maes A, Flameng W, Nuyts J et al: Histological alterations in chronically hypoperfused myocardium. Correlation with PET findings. Circulation 1994;90:735–745

73. Eitzman D, Al-Aouar Z, Kanter H et al: Clinical outcome of patients with advanced coronary artery disease after viability studies with positron emission tomography. J Am Coll Cardiol 1992;20:559–565

74. Tamaki N, Kawamoto M, Takahashi N et al: Prognostic value of an increase in fluorine-18 deoxyglucose uptake in patients with myocardial infarction. Comparison with stress thallium imaging. J Am Coll Cardiol 1993;22:1621–1627

75. Di Carli M, Davidson M, Little R et al: Value of metabolic imaging with positron emission tomography for evaluating prognosis in patients with coronary artery disease and left ventricular dysfunction. Am J Cardiol 1994;73:527–533

76. Lee K, Marwick T, Cook S et al: Prognosis of patients with left ventricular dysfunction, with and without viable myocardium after myocardial infarction. Circulation 1994;90:2687–2694

77. Di Carli M, Farbod A, Schelbert H et al: Quantitative relation between myocardial viability and improvement in heart failure symptoms after revascularization in patients with ischemic cardiomyopathy. Circulation 1995;92:3436–3444

78. Goldman L, Hashimoto B, Ef C, Loscalzo A: Comparative reproducibility and validity of systems for assessing cardiovascular functional class. Advantages of a new specific activity scale. Circulation 1981;64:1227–1234

36 Acute Ischemic Heart Failure: Pathophysiology and Management

Kanu Chatterjee
Stuart J. Hutchison
Tony M. Chou

The definition of acute heart failure has not been firmly established. However, in clinical practice it is recognized when symptoms of heart failure develop rapidly within hours and days (but not necessarily abruptly after the acute insult) in patients without prior evidence of cardiac decompensation. Exacerbation of symptoms in patients with established chronic heart failure is not usually regarded as acute heart failure. Myocardial, pericardial, and valvular dysfunction can produce acute heart failure; however, the pathophysiologic mechanisms and the hemodynamic abnormalities are different and distinct (in these various conditions). In clinical practice myocardial dysfunction following acute myocardial infarction is the most frequent cause of acute heart failure. Left ventricular volume overload resulting from acute mitral or aortic regurgitation is another important cause of acute left heart failure. Acute predominant right ventricular infarction and massive or submassive pulmonary embolism can produce predominant severe right heart failure. Cardiac tamponade with pericardial effusion can also produce a low output state and hypotension rather acutely (discussed in the Chapter on Pericardial Disease). This chapter will focus on the most common cause of acute heart failure, myocardial infarction and ischemia.

ACUTE HEART FAILURE

Heart Failure in Acute Myocardial Infarction: Pathophysiology

The severity of pump failure complicating acute myocardial infarction is variable. It can be mild with only clinical evidence of pulmonary congestion, or it can be severe with florid pulmonary edema, hypotension, low cardiac output, and clinical features of cardiogenic shock. The prognosis of pump failure complicating myocardial infarction is directly related to its severity. Before the introduction of reperfusion therapy the incidence of mild heart failure in acute myocardial infarction varied between 20 and 40 percent, with the hospital mortality varying between 10 and 17 percent.[1] During the era of reperfusion therapy the incidence of heart failure had declined. Before widespread use of thrombolytic therapy for reperfusion, the incidence of cardiogenic shock remained fairly constant: approximately 8 percent for several years.[2] The mortality among patients with cardiogenic shock also remained fairly constant, between 70 and 80 percent, despite widespread use of vasodilators, vasopressors, and intraaortic balloon pump counterpulsation. In the GISSI trial the incidence of severe pulmonary edema and cardiogenic shock was 2–4 percent.[3] The mortality of patients with cardiogenic shock, with intravenous streptokinase therapy, remained at 70 percent.

Acute pump failure following myocardial infarction results from impaired regional and global systolic function and regional and global diastolic dysfunction. Mechanical complications such as mitral regurgitation due to papillary muscle infarction, left-to-right shunt due to interventricular septal rupture, and cardiac tamponade from free wall rupture can produce severe acute heart failure. Atrial and ventricular tachyarrhythmias, bradyarrhythmias including heart block, abnormalities of electrolytes, acid-base dysequilibrium, and abnormalities of pulmonary gas exchange may contribute to pump failure during acute myocardial infarction. Concomitant with systolic and diastolic dysfunction following acute myocardial injury, compensatory mechanisms are activated and overt clinical heart failure may result owing to inadequate compensatory changes to maintain pump function.

Changes in Contractile Function

Total cessation or marked reduction in coronary blood flow due to the formation of occlusive thrombi at the site of fissured or ruptured atheromatous plaque produces rapid impairment of the contractile function of the myocardium at risk.[4–6] The degree of impairment of contractile function may range from hypokinesis (reduced myocardial shortening) to akinesis (lack of myocardial shortening) to dyskinesis (systolic lengthening of the myocardium). The degree and duration of impairment of contractile function of the myocardium at risk is related not only to the degree of reduction of anterograde flow but also to the presence or absence of collateral flow. In the absence of residual flow myocardial necrosis rapidly ensues, and the wavefront of necrosis extends from the subendocardium to the epicardium.[7] Without reestablishment of adequate flow the necrosis of myocardium at risk is usually completed within 3–6 hours. Concurrent with the onset of ischemia and necrosis, the contractile function of affected myocardium rapidly deteriorates.

Acute myocardial ischemia produces characteristic alterations in regional ventricular function in the acutely ischemic segments, the nonischemic areas directly adjacent to the ischemic region, and the remote nonischemic areas.[8] Within a few seconds of total interruption of blood flow, systolic shortening of the ischemic myocardium decreases, and the ischemic region performs little or no effective work. With continued ischemia, systolic shortening is replaced by late systolic and then holosystolic lengthening or bulging. Marked bulging occurs primarily during isovolumic systole, and the ischemic segments demonstrate akinesis during the ejection phase. Paradoxical shortening of the ischemic myocardium occurs during isovolumic relaxation and early diastole. The systolic bulging indicates that work is being performed on, rather than by, the ischemic region. Lengthening during systole and shortening during isovolumic relaxation of the acutely ischemic myocardial segments suggests that these paradoxical changes in wall motion of the is-

chemic region occur passively. However, the acutely ischemic myocardium may retain some initial residual contractile function, as it has been demonstrated that acute inotropic stimulation may decrease the paradoxical systolic bulging of the ischemic region. Necrotic myocardium, however, does not have any residual contractile function. Asynchronous force generation by the mildly ischemic and more severely ischemic myocardial segments also can produce paradoxical systolic bulging. The late shortening of the ischemic myocardium that occurs after systole may also represent the presence of residual contractile function and delayed relaxation. With experimental acute ischemia, the extent of postsystolic shortening is predictive of the magnitude of recovery of function following reperfusion.

Myocardial segments directly adjacent to the acute ischemic region may also demonstrate abnormalities of systolic function. Functional impairments occur in the overlying nonischemic subepicardium or in the lateral nonischemic border even though coronary blood flow in these areas may remain normal. The functional impairments of this nonischemic and normally perfused myocardium adjacent to the acutely myocardial segments may be due to mechanical tethering to the abnormally contracting ischemic region. Increased regional wall stress, consequent on acute ischemia, may also contribute to impaired systolic function of this adjacent nonischemic myocardial segments. Nonischemic myocardial segments remote from the acutely ischemic or infarcting myocardium also demonstrate altered systolic function. Augmented shortening or hyperfunction of these nonischemic areas has been demonstrated in both experimental studies and patients with acute myocardial infarction. The hyperfunctioning of the remote nonischemic areas probably results from the increased use of the Frank-Starling mechanism secondary to an ischemia-induced increase in left ventricular diastolic pressure and a regional intraventricular unloading effect. Increased sympathetic stimulation may also be contributory; however, hyperkinesis of the nonischemic regions has been documented in the presence of β-blockade and in experimental studies with isolated hearts that lack reflex neurohumoral responses.

Systolic hyperfunction of remote nonischemic myocardial segments contributes to maintain overall left ventricular pump function in patients with acute myocardial infarction. A significant portion of the increase in shortening of the nonischemic segments is expended in paradoxically stretching the ischemic region during isovolumic systole. It reduces the amount of effective shortening by nonischemic areas available for overall left ventricular ejection. Thus the acutely ischemic nonfunctioning dyskinetic myocardial segments impose a mechanical disadvantage on the nonischemic areas, and this mechanical disadvantage is directly related to the amount of paradoxical systolic bulging in the ischemic region. The pathophysiologic mechanism of severe left ventricular systolic dysfunction resulting from acute aneurysm formation in patients with myocardial infarction is related to these abnormalities and the interactions of systolic function of the ischemic and nonischemic myocardial segments.

Hyperkinesis of the remote nonischemic areas, however, does not occur uniformly in all patients with acute myocardial infarction. With significant coronary artery stenosis in the nonischemic areas, hypokinesis instead of hyperkinesis may be observed. Interruption of collateral blood flow to the distal remote nonischemic segments from acute coronary artery occlusion to the ischemic zone may also impair systolic function of the nonischemic segments. Patients with acute myocardial infarction and hyperkinesis of the nonischemic areas are more likely to have single vessel than multivessel coronary artery disease. In contrast, asynergy at remote nonischemic segments is more likely to indicate three-vessel coronary artery disease, which is associated with a higher mortality rate. Patients with augmented systolic function of the nonischemic zone also tend to have higher left ventricular ejection fractions and lower in-hospital mortality. Thus changes in the systolic function of the remote nonischemic areas in patients with acute myocardial infarction have important prognostic significance.

The cellular and biochemical bases for depressed contractile function of the acutely ischemic myocardium are likely to be multifactorial.[9] A rapid decrease in the tissue content of creatinine phosphate in the ischemic zone along with a fall in the ATP levels and increased tissue lactic acid values and a decrease in intracellular pH contribute to the impairment of contractile function of the ischemic myocardium. A rapid increase in inorganic phosphate concentration and a decrease in the phosphocreatinine/inorganic phosphate ratio may be substantially mitigated by a concomitant reduction in myofilament sensitivity to calcium which leads to decreased contractility and energy requirements may decrease contractile function. An ischemia-induced fall in myocardial tension is accompanied by a rapid decrease in action potential duration, which may decrease calcium release by the sarcoplasmic reticulum. Circulating catecholamine levels increase during the early phase of acute myocardial infarction, particularly in patients with clinical heart failure and impaired left ventricular systolic function. Increased catecholamines can produce a number of detrimental effects, including induction of arrhythmias, increased myocardial oxygen consumption, and oxygen wasting due to mitochrondrial uncoupling. Elevated circulating free fatty acid levels resulting from metabolic effects of catecholamines increase myocardial oxygen consumption.

Oxygen-derived free radicals generated during acute myocardial ischemia, may contribute to myocardial damage and myocardial dysfunction. Oxygen-derived free radicals produced particularly during reperfusion may cause structural damage of the myocardium by various mechanisms, including dysfunction of the membrane phospholipids and mitochondria. Vascular endothelium is also damaged with increased vascular permeability. Endothelium-derived relaxing factors are inactivated by oxygen-derived free radicals. This vascular endothelial dysfunction may produce secondary ischemia to the myocardium and impair its contractile function.

Prolonged ischemia without reperfusion produces irreversible myocardial damage and irrecoverable myocardial function. The biochemical and cellular abnormalities of irreversible damage include marked glycogen depletion, diffuse mitochondrial swelling, altered matrix of the mitochondria, deranged plasmalemma of the sarcolemma, severe depletion of ATP content, and an inability to resynthesize creatinine phosphate. An inability to maintain ionic gradients across the cell membrane and to control cell volume also characterizes irreversible myocardial damage. Moreover, calcium overload has been implicated as a potential mechanism for irreversible myocardial injury during prolonged ischemia. Accumulation of intracellular calcium and mitochondrial calcium overloading decrease ATP production, contributing to irreversible cell damage.

The extent of myocardial ischemic injury is the major determinant of the changes in the global left ventricular volumes and ejection fraction. When the extent of myocardial injury reaches a threshold level, the left ventricular ejection fraction declines, despite activation of intrinsic and extrinsic compensatory mechanism.[10] When the extent of myocardial injury involves 10 percent or more of the left ventricular perimeter, the ejection fraction declines with little or no change in left ventricular stroke volume. This implies that the decrease in ejection fraction is associated with an increase in left ventricular end-diastolic volume. Overt clinical heart failure occurs when 25–40 percent of the left ventricular perimeter is involved with ischemic injury. With the involvement of 30–40 percent or more of left ventricular myocardium, clinical features of cardiogenic shock with marked impairment of ventricular systolic function is observed. With severe impairment of left ventricular systolic function, not only is there an increase in left ventricular end-systolic and end-diastolic volume, there is also a decrease in stroke volume that may be associated with decreased cardiac output and hypotension.

Diastolic Dysfunction

Regional and global diastolic dysfunction[1,8,10] is common with acute myocardial infarction. Paradoxical shortening of the ischemic segments occurs during isovolumic relaxation, and the early diastolic phase is probably due to elastic recoil of the passably stretched ischemic myocardial segments or to persistent late systolic active shortening. The nonischemic myocardial segments lengthen during the isovolumic relaxation phase and may be due to tethering of ischemic and nonischemic areas. This asynchronous wall motion during isovolumic relaxation is associated with a decreased rate of left ventricular pressure fall as reflected by a decrease in peak negative dP/dt and an increase in the time constant of left ventricular pressure fall, which may reflect changes in the intrinsic relaxation properties of the ischemic myocardium and altered loading conditions. The abnormalities of wall motion during isovolumic relaxation phase may impair left ventricular early diastolic filling. Prolonged relaxation is associated with a higher left ventricular diastolic pressure, which retards diastolic filling and decreases diastolic filling time. The concurrent reduction of systolic emptying results in a higher end-systolic volume, which increases inflow impedance and contributes to abnormal ventricular filling. The changes in global left ventricular compliance and myocardial stiffness are variable with acute myocardial infarction. The changes in left ventricular compliance following myocardial infarction are related to time after the onset of infarction, changes in right ventricular volume and function, ventricular interaction, changes in pericardial pressure, and the presence or absence of systemic vasoconstriction. Substantial left ventricular dilatation can occur within a few hours of the onset of acute infarction, particularly in patients with large anterior infarcts. There may be a disproportionate increase in left ventricular diastolic pressure, suggesting decreased compliance, which contributes to the development of pulmonary edema. However, even in patients with large myocardial infarctions a slower increase in left ventricular volume during the subacute or chronic postinfarction phases may not be associated with a concomitant increase in pulmonary capillary wedge pressure. A progressive increase in left ventricular end-diastolic volume from the time of hospital discharge to 1 year has been documented without a substantial increase in left ventricular diastolic pressure in patients with anterior wall myocardial infarction. Thus during the subacute and early chronic phases of myocardial infarction the global left ventricular compliance may not change; and in some patients the pressure–volume relation may shift rightward. During the acute phase of myocardial infarction, however, the global left ventricular compliance is generally reduced, probably reflecting alterations in the viscoelastic properties of ischemic and necrotic tissue due to cellular and interstitial edema.

Abnormal regional and global diastolic function during acute infarction is associated with abnormal filling of the left ventricle, which is usually reflected in an elevated left ventricular filling pressure. Although elevations in left ventricular diastolic pressure may be associated with improved ventricular function due to increased use of the Frank-Starling mechanism by the nonischemic myocardium, elevations in left ventricular diastolic pressure may cause pulmonary venous congestion and pulmonary edema. In patients with acute myocardial infarction, there appears to be an optimal level of left ventricular filling pressure that maximizes stroke volume with minimal adverse hemodynamic complications. This so-called optimal filling pressure corresponds to mean pulmonary capillary wedge pressures in the range of 15–20 mmHg. The maximal use of the Frank-Starling mechanism by the nonischemic myocardium in this optimal filling range provides a maximal increase in stroke volume. A rise in left ventricular filling pressure beyond this optimal range, however, is associated with pulmonary venous congestion. Furthermore, excessive elevations in left ventricular diastolic pressure and volume increase the diastolic wall stress and myocardial oxygen demand. Subendocardial ischemia in the nonischemic zones may also occur because of an increase in subendocardial wall stress and concomitant reduction in transmyocardial perfusion pressure gradient.

Ventricular remodeling after acute myocardial infarction contributes to the abnormalities of both systolic and diastolic function.[11] Ventricular remodeling consists of chamber enlargement, myocyte hypertrophy and thinning, and architectural changes of the matrix. Infarct expansion, which may begin within 24 hours after acute myocardial infarction, is acute dilatation and thinning of the infarct zone. Infarct expansion occurs more frequently in patients with anterior wall infarction, transmural infarcts, and infarcts above a critical size when the infarction involves 10 percent or more of the left ventricular mass. Myocyte thinning and cell slippage with structural derangement are thought to be the predominant mechanism for infarct expansion. Although no further myocardial necrosis occurs, infarct expansion increases ventricular volume and wall stress as well as myocardial oxygen consumption. Remodeling changes may be generalized and may involve nonischemic regions. These remodeling changes, involving ischemic and nonischemic regions, may produce progressive ventricular dilatation and reduction of systolic and diastolic function. Activation of neurohormonal systems with vasoconstrictive antinatriuretic and mitogenic effects is also thought to be an important mechanism for ventricular remodeling.

Infarct expansion during the acute phase of myocardial infarction may lead to several complications, including congestive heart failure, formation of mural thrombus, and cardiac rupture. Infarct expansion has been associated with increased mortality in patients with acute myocardial infarction.

Systolic and diastolic dysfunction during acute myocardial infarction is potentially reversible with reperfusion of the ischemic myocardium (Fig. 36-1). With experimental myocardial infarction it has been demonstrated that if the ischemic myocardium is reperfused within 5 minutes systolic function promptly returns to normal, whereas diastolic dysfunction may require 30–45 minutes to resolve. If reperfusion does not occur within 15 minutes of ischemia, abnormalities of function may persist more than 3 hours before returning to normal. When reperfusion occurs after several hours of ischemia, functional recovery may be incomplete and markedly delayed. This pro-

longed impairment in myocardial function, despite reestablishment of adequate coronary blood flow and myocardial perfusion, has been termed "stunned myocardium."[12,13] Clinical studies have also demonstrated that prompt and adequate reperfusion may be associated with rapid recovery of systolic and diastolic myocardial function. Delayed reperfusion, however, may be associated with persistent and permanent myocardial dysfunction with minimal or no functional recovery. The severity and duration of dysfunction of the ischemic reperfused myocardium are related to the severity and duration of myocardial ischemia. The mechanism of stunned myocardium remains unclear and controversial.[9] With experimental myocardial infarction, persistent ultrastructural cellular injury has been observed even after reperfusion of the ischemic myocardium. These ultrastructural changes include the presence of abnormal intermyofibrillar and intermyofilament edema, glycogen depletion, and generalized mitochondrial and sarcolemmal damage. Ultrastructural changes of cellular injury may recover with time after reperfusion. With experimental myocardial infarction it has been demonstrated that there is rapid restoration of the creatinine pool, whereas nucleotide pools remain depleted in functional postischemic reperfused myocardium. These findings suggest that limitation of the mitochondrial energy production is not the mechanism of stunning of the myocardium, and that delayed resynthesis of adenine nucleotides may be contributory. Although a convincing relation between cell death and severe depletion of adenine nucleotides has been reported, the relation between re-

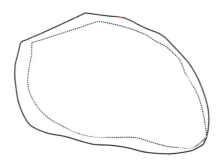

LVEDP - 23 mmHg
EF   - 0.34
SWI - 26 g-m/M^2

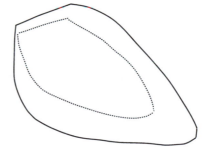

LVEDP - 12 mmHg
EF   - 0.71
SWI - 71 g-m/M^2

Fig. 36-1. Superimposed left ventricular end-diastolic (solid line) and end-systolic frames (dotted line) from contrast ventriculograms of a patient before and after revascularization by coronary artery bypass surgery. Note the recovery of global and regional left ventricular systolic function of the ischemic reperfused myocardium. Improvement in hemodynamics also occured after reperfusion. LVEDP, left ventricular end-diastolic pressure; EF, ejection fraction; SWI, stroke work index.

pletion of adenine nucleotide pools and the return of cardiac function has not been firmly established.

There are several clinical implications of stunned myocardium. After reperfusion therapy the recovery of function may not occur immediately, and it is important to maintain supportive therapy in patients with severe pump failure following myocardial infarction. The stunned myocardial segments are responsive to inotropic stimulation. Therefore with inotropic stimulation not only can one recognize the presence of stunned myocardium, it can also be used to support myocardial function following reperfusion therapy. The other clinical implication of stunned myocardium is the timing of assessment of changes in left ventricular function after reperfusion therapy. Early assessment, within a few hours or a few days after reperfusion, may not provide the information about the final recovery of left ventricular function.

Clinical and Hemodynamic Subsets of Heart Failure Complicating Myocardial Infarction

Systolic and diastolic dysfunction resulting from acute myocardial ischemic injury are associated with hemodynamic abnormalities that can be used to categorize patients with pump failure into clinically

meaningful subsets; these categories in turn provide guidelines for appropriate therapeutic strategies.[14–16] The two major hemodynamic abnormalities, low cardiac output and increased pulmonary capillary wedge pressure, correlate with clinical manifestations of hypoperfusion and pulmonary congestion. Thus clinical manifestations of the hemodynamic abnormalities can also be used to categorize patients with acute myocardial infarction (Table 36-1).

The patients with no clinical evidence of hypoperfusion or pulmonary congestion have relatively normal hemodynamics, with a cardiac index higher than 2.2 L/m^2 and pulmonary capillary wedge pressure less than 18 mmHg. These patients are categorized to clinical and hemodynamic subset 1. In patients in clinical or hemodynamic subset 2, clinical evidence of pulmonary congestion is present with no evidence of hypoperfusion. In these patients the pulmonary capillary wedge pressure is elevated (more than 18 mmHg), but the cardiac index is normal (2.2 L/m^2 or higher). In patients in subset 3, evidence of hypoperfusion is present in the absence of congestive symptoms, and the hemodynamic abnormalities are characterized by a pulmonary capillary wedge pressure less than 18 mmHg and cardiac output decreased to less than 2.2 L/m^2. In patients in subset 4, symptoms of hypoperfusion and pulmonary congestion are pres-

Table 36-1. Clinical and Hemodynamic Subsets in Acute Myocardial Infarction

Classification System	Clinical Features	Hemodynamic Features	Approx. Proportion of Patients (%)	Hospital Mortality (%)
Killip class				
1	No signs of congestive heart failure		40–50	6
2	S3 gallop, bibasilar rales		30–40	17
3	Acute pulmonary edema		10–15	38
4	Cardiogenic shock		5–10	81
Cedars-Sinai clinical subsets				
1	No pulmonary congestion or tissue hypoperfusion		25	1
2	Pulmonary congestion only		25	11
3	Tissue hypoperfusion only		15	18
4	Pulmonary congestion and tissue hypoperfusion		35	60
Cedars-Sinai hemodynamic subsets				
1		PCW ≤ 18; CI > 2.2	25	3
2		PCW > 18; CI > 2.2	25	9
3		PCW ≤ 18; CI ≤ 2.2	15	23
4		PCW > 18; CI ≤ 2.2	35	51

Abbreviations: PCW, pulmonary capillary wedge pressure (mmHg); CI, cardiac index (L·min^{-1}·sq m^{-1}).

ent along with severe hemodynamic abnormalities characterized by a low cardiac index (less than 2.2 L/m^2) and elevated pulmonary capillary wedge pressure exceeding 18 mmHg.

Categorization of patients with acute infarction into clinical or hemodynamic subsets allows assessment of immediate prognosis. The hospital mortality of patients in clinical or hemodynamic subset 1 is approximately 1–3 percent, whereas in subset 2 the mortality increases to 9–11 percent. In patients in subset 3, the hospital mortality is considerably higher (18–23 percent), and the mortality is highest in subset 4 (50–60 percent). The patients in subset 4 can be further categorized into those with clinical features of cardiogenic shock and those without. In patients with clinical features of cardiogenic shock, the hemodynamics indicate severe depression of cardiac function, usually with a left ventricular stroke work index of 20 g m^{-1} · sq m^{-1} or less and a pulmonary capillary wedge pressure greater than 25 mmHg. The cardiac index in these patients is usually less than 1.5 L/m^2. The hospital mortality among patients with the hemodynamic abnormalities of cardiogenic shock usually exceeds 80 percent despite aggressive supportive therapy.

Recognition of various clinical and hemodynamic subsets also allows appropriate therapeutic interventions. For example, patients in subset 1 do not require any specific therapy except adequate reperfusion of ischemic myocardium. Patients in subset 2 may require diuretics or nitroglycerin to relieve congestive symptoms. In patients in subset 3 the primary objective of therapy is to improve cardiac output and ameliorate hypoperfusion. Patients in subset 4, however, require aggressive support therapy to maintain adequate pump function and reperfusion therapy.

MANAGEMENT OF ACUTE HEART FAILURE COMPLICATING MYOCARDIAL INFARCTION

The management approach to patients with acute myocardial infarction can be outlined based on clinical presentation and specific complications. Patients with uncomplicated acute myocardial infarction (subset 1) with ST segment elevation in the presenting ECG should be considered for early reperfusion therapy. The method of choice of reperfusion therapy remains debatable and depends on various factors including the availability of various thrombolytic agents, the availability of the cardiac catheterization laboratory, and the team of intervention cardiolo-

gists experienced in nonpharmacologic reperfusion technique.

Available data indicate that the use of the front-loaded tissue-type plasminogen activator (t-PA) regimen is more likely to recanalize the infarct-related artery rapidly and establish adequate blood flow to the ischemic myocardium than is intravenous streptokinase.[17] With front-loaded t-PA followed by intravenous heparin therapy the reduction in mortality among patients with acute myocardial infarction appears to be greater than that with intravenous streptokinase. When intravenous thrombolytic therapy is contraindicated or its usefulness for establishing adequate blood flow to the ischemic myocardium remains in doubt or when the diagnosis of acute myocardial infarction based on clinical presentation or ECG changes remains uncertain, primary angioplasty of the infarct-related coronary artery should be considered to establish adequate blood flow to the ischemic myocardium.[18] Many institutions now preferentially use primary angioplasty rather than intravenous thrombolytic therapy particularly in hemodynamically unstable patients, although its effectiveness in reducing mortality compared to thrombolytic therapy has not been firmly established.

Irrespective of what method of reperfusion therapy is chosen, all patients with documented or suspected acute myocardial infarction should be considered for reperfusion therapy, which has the greatest potential to decrease the extent of myocardial injury, the development of heart failure, and mortality. In addition to reperfusion therapy, all patients with acute myocardial infarction should be treated with aspirin and heparin if the patient has received t-PA as the thrombolytic agent. Intravenous heparin infusion is also indicated in patients with acute anterior wall myocardial infarction to decrease the incidence of thromboembolic complications. Intravenous β-blocker (metoprolol) therapy is also indicated, particularly in patients who did not receive reperfusion therapy. It should be emphasized that in patients who receive intravenous thrombolytic therapy such as t-PA the administration of intravenous metoprolol can be associated with a decreased incidence of reinfarction and postinfarction ischemia. Routine use of intravenous nitroglycerin in patients with acute myocardial infarction has not been associated with any substantial reduction in mortality.[19] Thus nitroglycerin is used to relieve ischemic pain and to decrease pulmonary venous pressure in patients with pulmonary venous congestion. Routine use of intravenous magnesium has also not been found beneficial in patients with acute myocardial infarction.[19] Thus magnesium therapy is restricted in selected patients with ventricular arrhythmias, particularly those who develop polymorphous ventricular tachycardia. Angiotensin-converting enzyme (ACE) inhibitors decrease hospital mortality and improve the long-term prognosis.[19,20]

Pulmonary Congestion Without Hypoperfusion (Subset 2)

Mild pulmonary congestion is common in patients with acute myocardial infarction and is clinically evidenced by the presence of bilateral pulmonary rales with mild or no dyspnea. The hemodynamic abnormality in such patients is usually a modest increase in pulmonary capillary wedge pressure (18–25 mmHg) resulting from increased left ventricular diastolic pressure associated with decreased compliance. In addition to mild dyspnea and pulmonary rales, an S3 gallop is appreciated in some patients. Chest radiography usually reveals evidence of mild to moderate pulmonary venous congestion. Hemodynamic monitoring is not required for the diagnosis or for initial therapy of these patients.

The treatment is directed to maintain adequate arterial oxygenation with supplemental oxygen and to relieve pulmonary venous congestion by decreasing pulmonary venous pressure with diuretic, or nitroglycerin, or both. Initially, a single dose of intravenous furosemide 20–40 mg should be administered. Furosemide decreases the pulmonary capillary wedge and right arterial pressures without causing any significant change in heart rate, cardiac output, or mean atrial pressure in patients with acute myocardial infarction with clinical heart failure.[21] The pulmonary capillary wedge and right atrial pressures are reduced with furosemide before any substantial increase in urinary output is seen and appear to correlate to the concurrent increase in peripheral venous capacitance. Also, in response to nitroglycerin the pulmonary capillary wedge pressure falls, and cardiac output usually does not decrease in patients with overt left ventricular failure. However, when there is an excessive decrease in pulmonary capillary wedge pressure or when the initial pulmonary capillary wedge pressure is low, cardiac output may decrease with a further decrease in pulmonary capillary wedge pressure, resulting in hypotension and reflex tachycardia.[22] Intravenous nitroglycerin not only causes venodilatation but can produce significant arterial dilatation. Nitroglycerin increases compliance of large arteries and may cause a significant reduction in central aortic pressure, which might not be reflected during monitoring of the peripheral arterial pressure. Nitroglycerin also improves ventriculo-aortic coupling, which may be contributory to improved left ventricular performance.

It should be appreciated, however, that in approximately 10 percent of patients with acute myocardial infarction nitroglycerin and nitrates can produce a paradoxical response characterized by bradycardia and hypotension.[22] Soon after the administration of intravenous or nonparenteral nitroglycerin or nitrates, sinus bradycardia or junctional escape rhythm along with hypotension may develop. The precise mechanism for this paradoxical response remains unclear, but it is likely due to activation of the Bezold-Jarisch reflex resulting from stimulation of cardiac mechanoreceptors producing cardioinhibitory and vasodepressor responses. These paradoxical responses can be prevented by administration of atropine or by atrial pacing.

Sodium nitroprusside is another vasodilator that can be used to decrease pulmonary capillary wedge pressure. Sodium nitroprusside has a balanced effect on venous capacitance and arterial resistance vessels. In patients with left ventricular failure, in response to sodium nitroprusside there is a substantial decrease in pulmonary capillary wedge pressure along with an increase in cardiac output.[22] In patients with normal pulmonary capillary wedge pressure, however, or when there is an excessive decrease in pulmonary capillary wedge pressure, hypotension along with decreased cardiac output and reflex tachycardia may occur. Intravenous sodium nitroprusside can produce variable effects on myocardial ischemia.[22] In some studies a deleterious effect on coronary hemodynamics and worsening myocardial ischemia have been observed. In other studies, however, a beneficial response has been reported, particularly in patients with evidence of heart failure. The changes in mortality and clinical outcome in patients with acute myocardial infarction treated with sodium nitroprusside have also been variable. In some studies a reduction in mortality and a favorable clinical outcome has been observed, whereas in others increased mortality has been observed particularly in patients without clinical heart failure.[22]

For treatment of pulmonary venous congestion in patients without evidence of low cardiac output, intravenous nitroglycerin is preferable to sodium nitroprusside. However, if there is evidence of low cardiac output as well as increased systemic vascular resistance, sodium nitroprusside may provide an advantage over nitroglycerin in increasing cardiac output.

Acute Pulmonary Edema Without Shock

Patients with acute pulmonary edema but no shock also belong to the clinical and hemodynamic subset 2. The clinical profile and hemodynamic abnormalities, however, are different from those in patients with mild pulmonary congestion. Acute respiratory distress with tachypnea, tachycardia, and sometimes peripheral cyanosis along with extensive bilateral pulmonary rales with or without bronchospasm are recognized in almost all patients. Radiologic evidence for frank bilateral pulmonary edema is invariably present. Moderate to severe hypoxemia (decrease in arterial PO_2) and retention of carbon dioxide (increased $PaCO_2$) are also common. Immediate determination of the hemodynamic status is rarely feasible until the patient is stabilized. When determined, hemodynamic measurements usually reveal a pulmonary capillary wedge pressure exceeding 25 mmHg with normal or slightly decreased cardiac output. Sinus tachycardia, marked elevation of systemic vascular resistance, and elevated blood pressures are frequently observed. In addition to marked impairment of both diastolic and systolic left ventricular function, transient severe mitral regurgitation appears to be the underlying mechanism of such severe hemodynamic abnormalities in these patients. Acute pulmonary edema complicating myocardial infarction is associated with a mortality rate of 30–50 percent, and so prompt intervention to reverse the hemodynamic abnormalities is necessary.

Immediate therapy consists of administration of supplemental oxygen (60–100 percent) by face mask, intravenous morphine, and sublingual nitroglycerin or nitroglycerin spray. Intravenous diuretics such as furosemide are administered concurrently. Arterial blood gases should be determined and endotracheal intubation considered early if arterial PO_2 of at least 60 mmHg cannot be maintained by face mask ventilation. Intravenous nitroglycerin should be started at 5–10 μg/min and the dose increased by 5–10 μg/min every 10 minutes to lower arterial systolic pressure to not less than 100 mmHg. If the patient remains hypertensive, intravenous sodium nitroprusside may be added at 5–10 μg/min with a slow increase of the infusion rate by 5–10 μg/min every 10–15 minutes, depending on the response.

An echocardiographic and Doppler evaluation should be considered in all patients to assess the severity of left ventricular dysfunction and the presence and severity of mitral regurgitation. All patients should be considered for immediate reperfusion therapy. In many institutions, primary angioplasty is considered to be the most effective method for establishing adequate blood flow to the ischemic myocardium. If facilities for immediate cardiac catheterization and angioplasty are not available, intravenous thrombolytic agents should be used unless contraindicated. Hemodynamic monitoring to guide aggressive supportive therapy is fre-

Table 36-2. Management of Patients with Pulmonary Congestion Without Hypoperfusion (Subset 2)

Patients with mild pulmonary congestion
- Supplemental oxygen by nasal cannula or face mask
- Sublingual nitroglycerin (0.4 mg) and chewable aspirin (160 mg)
- Intravenous furosemide (20–40 mg)
- Intravenous nitroglycerin (5–10 μg/min initial dose, increasing by 5–10 μg/min every 5–10 minutes until 200 μg/min dose is reached or there is 10% decrease in mean BP in normotensives and 30% decrease in mean BP in hypertensives
- Chewable aspirin (160 mg)
- Intravenous thrombolytic therapy
- Avoid hemodynamic monitoring in the absence of clinical deterioration

Acute pulmonary edema without hypotension or hypertension
- Supplemental oxygen (60–100%) by face mask, intubation and mechanical ventilation (early than late), if arterial PO_2 < 60 mmHg, increasing PCO_2 or decreasing arterial pH
- Sublingual nitroglycerin 0.4 mg followed by IV nitroglycerin (as above)
- Intravenous furosemide (40 mg)—may be repeated depending on response
- Chewable aspirin (160 mg)
- Consider catheterization and primary angioplasty if facilities are available
- Intravenous thrombolytic therapy when catheterization is not feasible
- Doppler echocardiography to evaluate the presence and severity of mitral regurgitation; sodium nitroprusside in the presence of significant mitral regurgitation
- Hemodynamic monitoring for maintenance vasodilatory therapy

Abbreviations: BP, blood pressure; IV, intravenous.

quently required in these patients, even after thrombolysis or angioplasty. Patients with persistent pulmonary edema, despite adequate supportive therapy, should be considered for cardiac catheterization, and in all patients the presence of significant mitral regurgitation should be evaluated. The management approach to patients with pulmonary congestion without hypoperfusion is summarized in the Table 36-2.

Hypoperfusion Without Pulmonary Congestion (Subset 3)

When there is clinical evidence of hypoperfusion, such as decreased urine output, mental obtundation, and cool periphery, and hypotension is present without signs and symptoms of pulmonary venous congestion, hypovolumic shock or predominant right ventricular infarction should be considered. True hypovolumic shock is an uncommon complication of acute myocardial infarction and should be confirmed by determining the hemodynamic status. With hypovolumic shock the right atrial pressure is low, pulmonary capillary wedge pressure is less than 18 mmHg, and cardiac index is less than $2.2 \, L \cdot min^{-1} \cdot sq \, m^{-1}$. The precise mechanisms of hypovolumic shock in acute myocardial infarction are unclear. Aggressive diuretic therapy, excessive use of vasodilators, and in some instances diaphoresis and vomiting may contribute to the hypovolumic state. The treatment of hypovolumic shock consists of rapid administration of intravenous fluids, 50–100 ml every 15–20 minutes under close clinical and hemodynamic observation until the pulmonary capillary wedge pressure is elevated to 14–18 mmHg. This range of pulmonary capillary wedge pressure has been recognized as the optimal left ventricular filling pressure in patients with acute myocardial infarction.[23] After maintaining adequate filling pressure with volume replacement therapy, the use of intravenous inotropic drugs, particularly dobutamine, may be required if hypotension persists with an inadequate increase in cardiac output. In such patients significant impairment of left ventricular pump function should be suspected, and additional supportive therapy with continued volume replacement should be given. Management of right ventricular infarction is discussed in subsequent sections.

Cardiogenic Shock (Subset 4)

Cardiogenic shock is the most serious complication of acute myocardial infarction and carries a poor prognosis. Cardiogenic shock is diagnosed when there is sustained hypotension with a systolic blood pressure of less than 90 mmHg with evidence of decreased tissue perfusion. Impaired tissue perfusion is manifested clinically by diminished urine output (< 20 ml/h), mental obtundation, and confusion resulting from impaired cerebral perfusion. Cold, clammy skin and diaphoresis, which are clinical manifestations of an activated sympathoadrenergic system, are frequently observed in patients with cardiogenic shock. The clinical syndrome of hypotension and hypoperfusion results from severe cardiac hypofunction. Severe hypofunction may be caused by extensive acute myocardial necrosis, acute myocardial infarction of less severity with prior loss of myocardial function resulting from old myocardial infarction, and less commonly by large areas of ischemic

nonfunctioning but viable myocardium along with only modest areas of myocardial infarction. Autopsy studies indicate that in patients with cardiogenic shock there is usually involvement of at least 35–40 percent of the total left ventricular mass.[1,10]

The incidence of cardiogenic shock in acute myocardial infarction is on average 7.5 percent and does not appear to have changed significantly in recent years.[2] The overall mortality associated with cardiogenic shock without prompt, adequate reperfusion of the ischemic myocardium also has remained unchanged (approximately 78 percent).[2] Cardiogenic shock tends to occur more frequently in older patients, patients with anterior myocardial infarctions, and patients with prior Q-wave myocardial infarction. In addition, they are more likely to have a preinfarction history of angina and congestive heart failure. Some studies have shown a higher prevalence of diabetes mellitus in patients with cardiogenic shock.[24,25]

Cardiogenic shock complicating myocardial infarction can occur in various clinical settings: (1) within a few hours or at the onset of acute myocardial infarction; (2) with the development of mechanical complications, such as severe mitral regurgitation due to papillary muscle infarct or rupture or left-to-right shunt due to ventricular septal rupture; (3) late shock due to stuttering myocardial necrosis with progressively worsening left ventricular function.

The prognosis of patients who develop shock syndrome within a few hours or at the onset of myocardial infarction is poor. During the Multicenter Investigation of the Limitation of Infarct Size (MILIS) study, 2.5 percent of patients with myocardial infarction were found to be in cardiogenic shock during the initial evaluation, and shock developed in another 3 percent of patients during hospitalization.[26] The in-hospital mortality of patients with cardiogenic shock complicating myocardial infarction is 70–100 percent.[24] Up to 50 percent of patients expire within 10 hours of the onset of cardiogenic shock, suggesting that the shock syndrome is a rapidly lethal condition.[27] Supportive therapy with vasopressor and inotropic agents has not caused any improvement in prognosis. Intraaortic balloon counterpulsation, although a helpful nonpharmacologic intervention for stabilizing patients, may not improve the prognosis of patients with cardiogenic shock. Many uncontrolled studies have suggested that the overall mortality is 87–100 percent among patients with cardiogenic shock despite treatment with intraaortic balloon counterpulsation.[1] However, one small randomized study suggested that patients assigned to intra aortic balloon counterpulsation therapy had improved in-hospital and 1-year survivals, regardless of whether coronary revascularization was attempted.[28] However, without adequate reperfusion therapy, a substantial benefit in survival is unlikely despite aggressive supportive therapy, including the use of intraaortic balloon counterpulsation.

Intravenous thrombolytic therapy does not appear to decrease mortality among patients with cardiogenic shock. In the GISSI study,[3] for patients with Killip class IV there was a 30-day mortality rate of 69.9 percent with intravenous streptokinase compared to 70.1 percent with placebo. In the international trial in which more than 20,000 patients with acute myocardial infarction were randomized to streptokinase and tissue plasminogen activator (t-PA) the in-hospital mortality in patients treated with streptokinase was 64.9 percent, and with t-PA it was 78.1 percent.[29] In the ISIS-2 trial, in patients with acute myocardial infarction and systolic blood pressure of less than 100 mmHg there was a lower mortality rate after treatment with streptokinase compared to that with placebo.[30] However, many patients enrolled in this study did not meet the conventional criteria for cardiogenic shock. In the GUSTO trial a survival advantage with streptokinase over t-PA was reported for patients with cardiogenic shock.[17] These patients, however, still had a significant mortality rate regardless of the thrombolytic regimen used (55–78 percent). The reason for the lack of survival benefit with intravenous thrombolytic therapy in patients with cardiogenic shock is not clear but may be related to the decreased perfusion pressure and low cardiac output associated with inadequate concentration of the thrombolytic agent in the infarct-related artery.

A number of uncontrolled studies have reported that primary angioplasty may decrease mortality of patients with cardiogenic shock complicating acute myocardial infarction (Table 36-3). The patency rates of the infarct-related artery appears to be high: 60–100 percent (average 75 percent).[31–54] The success rate for primary angioplasty in the setting of cardiogenic shock is significantly lower (approximately 73 percent) than the success rate among compensated patients undergoing primary angioplasty. Of the patients in whom primary angioplasty is successful, in-hospital survival rates were on average 75 percent, which compares favorably with the 22 percent survival rate of those who had failed angioplasty. These uncontrolled studies indicate that primary angioplasty may be of benefit in reducing the mortality of patients with cardiogenic shock, presumably due to the increased likelihood of establishing adequate flow to the ischemic myocardium. It should be emphasized, however, that there have been no randomized controlled studies examining the efficacy of primary angioplasty in cardiogenic shock complicating acute myocardial infarction. Nevertheless, the presently available data suggest that reperfusion therapy by primary angioplasty should be considered in patients with cardiogenic shock if feasible.

It is emphasized that despite adequate reperfusion of the ischemic myocardium, the mechanical function of salvaged ischemic myocardium may not recover immediately because of stunning. Supportive treatment is almost always necessary despite reperfusion therapy in patients with cardiogenic shock.

Pharmacologic Supportive Treatment

The combination of vasopressor, inotropic, and vasodilator agents is frequently required to stabilize patients with severe pump failure and cardiogenic shock.[1] In patients with severe hypotension, initially a vasopressor agent such as phenylephrine, norepinephrine, or dopamine (vasopressor doses) is used to maintain adequate arterial pressure. Concurrently, intraaortic balloon counterpulsation therapy should be instituted, and reperfusion therapy is initiated. The systemic hemodynamic status is determined as soon as it is feasible and the pharmacologic supportive therapy adjusted according to the hemodynamic profile and the hemodynamic responses to therapy. Reperfused viable ischemic "stunned" myocardium responds to inotropic stimulation, and low doses of dobutamine ($2–10 \ \mu g \cdot kg^{-1} \cdot min^{-1}$) may increase stroke volume and cardiac output. With large doses of dobutamine, however, contractile function of ischemic myocardium may deteriorate owing to an induced imbalance between myocardial oxygen supply and demand. Furthermore, larger doses of dobutamine may induce tachycardia and hypotension. If the increase in cardiac output with dobutamine is inadequate, intravenous phosphodiesterase inhibitors such as amrinone, milrinone, or enoximone can be added. A combination of dobutamine and a phosphodiesterase inhibitor produces a greater increase in cardiac output and a greater reduction in pulmonary capillary wedge pressure than when either agent is used alone. However, such combination therapy also has a greater potential to induce hypotension and tachycardia. If cardiac output remains low and if systemic vascular resistance and pulmonary capillary wedge pressures are elevated, sodium nitroprusside can be added. Concomitant use of nitroglycerin and diuretics should be considered if the pulmonary capillary wedge, right atrial, and pulmonary artery pressures remain elevated. The stepwise therapeutic

Table 36-3. Coronary Angioplasty for Cardiogenic Shock

Study	No. of Patients	Year	Reperfusion Rate	Mortality		
				Total	+ Reperfusion	− Reperfusion
O'Neill et al. [33]	27	1985	24/27 (88)	8/27 (30)	6/24 (25)	2/3 (67)
Brown et al. [36]	28	1985	17/28 (61)	16/28 (58)	7/17 (42)	9/11 (82)
Shani et al. [34]	9	1986	6/9 (67)	3/9 (33)	NA	NA
Heuser et al. [35]	10	1986	6/10 (60)	4/10 (40)	1/6 (17)	3/4 (75)
Disler et al. [42]	7	1987	5/7 (71)	4/7 (57)	2/5 (40)	2/2 (100)
Laramee et al. [37]	39	1988	33/39 (86)	16/39 (41)	NA	NA
Lee et al. [38]	24	1988	13/24 (54)	12/24 (50)	3/13 (23)	9/11 (82)
Stack et al. [39]	43	1988	NA	25/43 (58)	NA	NA
Ellis et al. [43]	61	1989	42/61 (69)	20/61 (32)	6/42 (14)	13/19 (68)
Gacioch and Topol [41]	25	1989	18/25 (72)	11/25 (44)	4/18 (22)	7/7 (100)
Verna et al. [44]	7	1989	7/7 (100)	1/7 (14)	1/7 (14)	0/0
Meyer et al. [46]	25	1990	22/25 (88)	12/25 (47)	9/22 (41)	3/3 (100)
Hibbard et al. [47,50]	45	1992	28/45 (62)	20/45 (44)	8/28 (29)	12/17 (71)
Moosvi et al. [48,51]	38	1990	29/38 (76)	18/38 (47)	11/29 (38)	7/9 (78)
Eltchaninoff et al. [49]	33	1991	25/33 (76)	12/33 (36)	6/25 (24)	6/8 (75)
Lee et al. [40]	69	1991	49/69 (71)	31/69 (45)	15/49 (31)	16/20 (80)
Brodie et al. [52]	22	1991	15/22 (68)	11/22 (50)	NA	NA
Bengston et al. [32]	46	1992	39/46 (85)	20/46 (43)	NA	NA
Seydoux et al. [53]	21	1992	18/21 (86)	9/21 (43)	6/18 (33)	0/3 (0)
O'Keefe et al. [54]	79	1993	65/79 (82)	35/79 (44)	24/65 (37)	11/14 (79)
Total	658		461/615 (75)	288/658 (44)	109/368 (30)	100/131 (76)

Abbreviations: NA, not available; +, with; −, without.
Data represent patient numbers (percentages in parentheses).
(Adapted from Bates and Topol,[31] with permission.)

approach based on hemodynamics is outlined in Figure 36-2.

Decreased aortic impedance associated with systolic unloading has the potential to increase forward stroke volume along with a decrease in left ventricular end-systolic and end-diastolic volumes and left ventricular diastolic and pulmonary capillary wedge pressures. Systemic hemodynamic improvement is not uniformly seen; and in the absence of cardiac reserve, hemodynamic improvement with intra-aortic balloon counterpulsation may be minimal.[1]

Intraaortic balloon counterpulsation therapy may decrease the risk of acute reocclusion of the infarct-related artery after angioplasty and reduce the adverse cardiac event rate, including death, stroke, reinfarction, the need for emergent surgical revascularization, and recurrent ischemia. Increased survival has been reported with the use of intraaortic balloon counterpulsation in conjunction with reperfusion therapy.[24]

In hospitals without a cardiac catheterization laboratory, intraaortic balloon counterpulsation may be useful for stabilizing patients with cardiogenic shock and for their transfer to institutions where facilities for revascularization are available. In a nonran-domized retrospective study, use of intraaortic balloon counterpulsation and transfer of patients to such centers and appropriate revascularization was associated with a survival rate of 69 percent compared to a 7 percent survival rate among patients treated conservatively.[24]

The use of intraaortic balloon counterpulsation may maintain arterial diastolic pressure and improve coronary hemodynamics, allowing the use of vasodilators and inotropic agents without the risk of reducing coronary perfusion pressure. Although clinical data are scanty and the results of randomized trials are not available, use of intraaortic balloon counterpulsation has emerged as important supportive therapy for management of patients with cardiogenic shock. The device can be safely instituted, including in patients who receive thrombolytic therapy.

The use of intraaortic balloon counterpulsation is not without complications. Complication rates up to 30 percent have been reported, and they tend to occur more frequently in elderly patients, women, and those with peripheral vascular disease. Vascular complications such as ischemic lower extremities, damage to the femoral artery, and local bleeding are most frequent; but other complications such

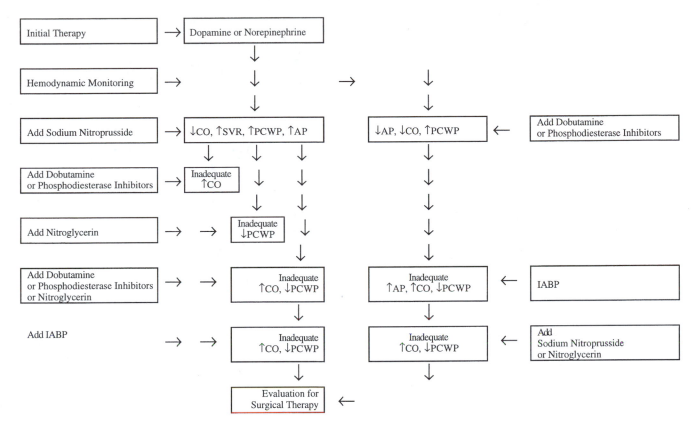

Fig. 36-2. Supportive therapeutic approach for hypotension and cardiogenic shock complicating acute myocardial infarction.

as bowel infarction, hemolysis, thrombocytopenia, gas leak, aortic dissection, retroperitoneal bleeding, injury to abdominal viscera, and cholesterol embolism may also occur. Furthermore, elderly patients, patients with multiple previous infarcts, those with massive irreversible myocardial necrosis, and those with late and slow onset of cardiogenic shock are least likely to benefit from intraaortic balloon counterpulsation therapy. Nevertheless, this technique remains an important nonpharmacologic supportive treatment for the management of cardiogenic shock.

Mechanical Defects Complicating Acute Myocardial Infarction

Postinfarction myocardial ruptures, including septal, papillary muscle, or free wall ruptures are life-threatening mechanical complications that are potentially correctable when rapidly recognized; and some lives can be salvaged.[55-58] These mechanical defects can produce severe hemodynamic abnormalities and clinical features of cardiogenic shock despite often occurring in the setting of having a relatively

smaller myocardial infarction and less extensive coronary artery disease.[59,60]

Rupture of a free wall is a sudden, usually fatal complication of acute myocardial infarction. It is the most common form of ventricular myocardial rupture, being 8–10 times more common than papillary muscle rupture.[61] The overall incidence with acute myocardial infarction is approximately 3 percent, and it occurs in 10–20 percent of patients who die from complications of acute infarction.[61-63] Immediate recognition and intervention salvage occasional patients with acute rupture; patients with subacute rupture have a better prognosis when diagnosed early and surgically corrected.[64,65]

Rupture occurs most frequently in the free wall of the left ventricle (80–90 percent) and less commonly in the right ventricle.[63,66,67] Rarely, rupture occurs at multiple sites, including the atria, and may be associated with concurrent papillary muscle or interventricular septal rupture.[68,69] Infarct expansion, uncontrolled hypertension, absence of collaterals, and thrombolytic therapy have been thought to predispose to free wall rupture.[70] The path after rupture through the free wall may be direct; but it is often serpiginous and more commonly occurs at an eccentric position rather than through the center of the necrotic area, near the junction between the normally contracting noninfarcted myocardium and dyskinetic infarcted myocardium, suggesting that local shear forces contribute to the disruption of tissue.[71]

Approximately 90 percent of free wall ruptures occur during the first week of the onset of myocardial infarction, but approximately 25–35 percent of all ruptures occur within the first 24 hours of the diagnosis of acute myocardial infarction.[61,63] Most frequently, rupture occurs abruptly and unexpectedly in a patient with an otherwise uncomplicated myocardial infarction. Chest pain atypical for myocardial ischemia or for pericarditis, repetitive emesis, and unexplained restlessness and agitation sometimes precede the abrupt collapse and cardiac arrest.[62,63,72]

The clinical risk factors include female gender, first myocardial infarction, persistent hypertension, the use of glucosteroids or nonsteroidal antiinflammatory drugs and early ambulation.[60,72,73] The impact of thrombolytic therapy on the risk of the free wall rupture has not been established. Small clinical studies have suggested that free wall rupture may occur more frequently after thrombolytic therapy, but prospective studies have failed to confirm such findings.[74–78]

Diagnosis of free wall rupture in clinical practice is difficult, and a strong clinical suspicion is required based on the presence of vague symptoms, the risk factors, and some ECG changes. A deviation from the expected evolutionary changes in the ST-T segment during the first 72 hours after acute myocardial infarction, atypical T wave changes, and persistent, progressive, or recurrent ST elevations are frequently seen in patients with impending and established free wall ruptures.[62,79] Sinus bradycardia and atrioventricular (AV) junctional rhythm may precede tamponade, which also may produce electromechanical dissociation. Echocardiography is the technique of choice for the diagnosis of rupture complicating myocardial infarction.[80] Hemodynamic monitoring is not necessary but when available shows equalization of the diastolic pressure. Immediate pericardiocentesis may be diagnostic and may transiently improve hemodynamics.[81–84] In some patients inotropic agents and volume loading transiently improve hemodynamics.[81] Emergency thoracotomy with repair of the rupture is the only definitive treatment and may salvage some patients with subacute rupture.[64] If sudden acute rupture occurs, resulting in abrupt severe tamponade, salvage is rare.

Mitral Regurgitation with Acute Myocardial Infarction

The severity, pathogenesis, and prognosis of acute ischemic mitral regurgitation is variable. The prevalence of mitral regurgitation has been assessed by various diagnostic techniques, and the incidence varies according to the investigative techniques utilized in the studies. The prevalence of mitral regurgitation in acute infarction diagnosed by auscultation has been reported to range between 17 and 55 percent.[81,83] With echocardiography performed within 48 hours to 3 months after infarction, the incidence of mitral regurgitation in ischemic heart disease has been reported to range between 20 and 56 percent.[85–87] With the advent of reperfusion therapy for acute myocardial infarction and the use of primary or rescue angioplasty as modalities for reperfusion, opportunities have been available to assess the incidence and severity of mitral regurgitation by angiographic studies within a few hours of the onset of symptoms.[88] The incidence of mitral regurgitation of any severity detected by contrast ventriculography performed within 6 hours of the onset of symptoms is approximately 19 percent, but the incidence of early severe mitral regurgitation is only about 4 percent.

The pathogenesis of mitral regurgitation in acute ischemic syndrome is also variable. Mild mitral regurgitation is common in patients with acute myocardial infarction and can be detected in up to 50 percent of patients. It usually results from mild papillary dysfunction or dysfunction of the ventricular muscle where the papillary muscle is anchored.[89] Asynchronous left ventricular contraction and relaxation, particularly involving the posterolateral wall of the left ventricle, may also produce mild mitral regurgitation. Mild ischemia of the papillary muscle or the left ventricular wall supporting the papillary muscle may impair adequate tension development and shortening, which can be associated with inadequate coaptation of the mitral leaflets, producing relatively mild mitral regurgitation. The mitral regurgitation in these circumstances can be late systolic or pansystolic. Mitral regurgitation due to mild papillary muscle dysfunction is frequently transient and does not produce any hemodynamic compromise. Clinically, a late systolic or a pansystolic murmur is recognized without other findings of severe left ventricular volume overload or secondary pulmonary hypertension. Transthoracic echocardiography and Doppler examination reveals mild mitral regurgitation.

In patients with acute ischemic syndrome, severe mitral regurgitation can occur within a few hours of the onset of symptoms.[88] Early severe mitral regurgitation in patients with acute infarction appears to be more common in females and the elderly. Associated cerebrovascular disease, diabetes, prior myocardial infarction, and prior coronary artery bypass surgery appear to be other risk factors for this complication of acute myocardial infarction. In approximately 68 percent of patients, severe triple- or double-vessel coronary artery disease are present. Posterolateral myocardial infarction is the most frequent site of infarction associated with early severe mitral regurgitation. The pathogenesis of early severe mitral regurgitation in patients with acute ischemic syndromes is not clear. With experimental myocardial infarction in animals, ischemia or limited infarction of the papillary muscle does not produce severe mitral regurgitation.[1] Involvement of the ventricular wall supporting the papillary muscle by ischemic injury, in addition to damage to the papillary muscle, is necessary to produce severe mitral regurgitation.[59] Papillary muscle ischemia or infarction also produces lengthening and elongation of the papillary muscle involved. With the onset of isovolumic systole there is inadequate development of tension in the papillary muscle and adjacent ventricular wall, which allows instantaneous onset of mitral regurgitation due to inadequate coaptation of the leaflets of the mitral valve. Malcoaptation of the mitral leaflets continues during the ejection phase owing to inadequate shortening of the papillary muscle, which allows pansystolic mitral regurgitation. Asymmetric left ventricular and mitral annular enlargement and abnormal ventricular torsion along its long axis have also been thought to be important contributing factors in the pathogenesis of early severe mitral regurgitation with acute myocardial infarction. These pathogenic mechanisms of severe mitral regurgitation demonstrated in experimental animals with acute myocardial infarction have been confirmed by angiographic and echocardiographic studies in patients with acute ischemic syndrome.[88,90,91] Transthoracic, transesophageal, echocardiographic, and Doppler studies demonstrate regional wall motion abnormality and papillary muscle dysfunction. Incoordinate ventricular contraction and relaxation, asymmetric ventricular enlargement, and abnormalities of annular function can also be demonstrated by echocardiographic study.

Mitral regurgitation in patients with acute ischemic syndromes tends to occur more frequently owing to dysfunction of the posteromedial papillary muscle and adjacent left ventricular wall than to the anterolateral papillary muscle.[92] The blood supply of the papillary muscles is derived from the branches of epicardial coronary arteries that transverse the wall of the ventricle and run the length of the papillary muscle (end-arteries). The subendocardial position of the papillary muscles and the vascular anatomy predispose to papillary muscle ischemia.[93] The posteromedial papillary muscle receives blood supply usually from a single epicardial coronary artery (i.e., the posterior descending) and makes it most vulnerable to ischemia. The anterolateral papillary muscle has a dual blood supply from the both the anterior descending and the left circumflex coronary arteries.[94,95] Posterolateral or inferior myocardial infarction results from occlusion of the posterior descending coronary artery or of the circumflex coronary artery, which also supplies posteromedial papillary muscle. This vascular anatomy explains the increased frequency of severe mitral regurgitation in the acute ischemic syndrome in patients with inferoposterior or posterolateral myocardial infarction.

Early severe mitral regurgitation can induce severe hemodynamic abnormalities, including hypotension, low cardiac output, and a marked increase in pulmonary venous pressure and secondary pulmonary hypertension. With significant mitral regurgitation, left atrial pressure increases disproportionately, not only because of a sudden increase in left atrial volume load but also owing to a lack of increase in left atrial size in response to volume overload. A marked increase in left atrial pressure causes a passive increase in pulmonary capillary wedge pressure and postcapillary pulmonary hypertension. Right heart failure ensues owing to a sudden increase in right ventricular ejection impedance. Because of an increase in left ventricular diastolic volume resulting from mitral regurgitation, the left ventricle moves along the steeper portion of its pressure–volume curve, causing a disproportionate increase in end-diastolic pressure. With a concomitant increase in left ventricular end-systolic wall stress (end-systolic pressure) the left ventricular forward stroke volume declines. Forward stroke volume also decreases proportionate to the severity of mitral regurgitation. When a small or limited infarction is associated with severe mitral regurgitation, the left ventricular global ejection fraction may be maintained owing to regurgitation-mediated decreased left ventricular ejection empedance. However, in patients with a large infarction or prior myocardial infarction, the left ventricular ejection fraction is usually significantly lower than normal because the magnitude of depression of global contractile function is not compensated by decreased ejection impedance resulting from mitral regurgitation. Clinical presentations of early severe mitral regurgitation are usually a sudden onset of severe pulmonary venous congestion and acute pulmonary edema. Signs and symptoms of severe pulmonary venous congestion are observed in approximately 46 percent of these patients.[88] It is of interest that in approximately 54 percent of patients with early severe mitral regurgitation signs and symptoms of pulmonary venous congestion are absent initially. A mitral regurgitation murmur is detected by auscultation in approximately 56 percent of these patients but is absent in approximately 44 percent.[88] Echocardiographic evaluations, however, are highly sensitive and reliable for the detection of mitral regurgitation. Thus echocardiographic and Doppler studies are recommended in all patients with suspected early mitral regurgitation.

Papillary muscle rupture is infrequent (1 percent of postinfarction patients), and the clinical course is fulminant, accounting for 1–5 percent of postinfarction deaths,[96] with half of the mortality within the first 24 hours after diagnosis.[97] Partial rupture causes severe mitral insufficiency, and complete rupture leads to torential mitral insufficiency.[98]

Rupture of the posteromedial papillary muscle occurs 6–12 times more frequently than rupture of the anterolateral papillary muscle; and it is seen more frequently with inferoposterior myocardial infarction.[94–97] In approximately half of the patients there is underlying single-vessel coronary disease,[59] and in 50 percent of patients with papillary muscle rupture the infarction size is comparatively small (area less than 6 cm^2).[59,96]

Papillary muscle rupture usually occurs between days 2 and 7, but 20 percent of ruptures occur within the first 24 hours of infarction.[59,93] The clinical presentation is characterized by a sudden onset of severe pulmonary edema with or without hypotension. Abrupt onset of cardiogenic shock may also indicate papillary muscle rupture. A loud holosystolic apical murmur is usually present and may have a crescendo-decrescendo quality. If the mitral regurgitation is severe, the murmur may be soft or absent because of equalization of atrial and ventricular pressures and impaired left ventricular function.[59,98,99] A palpable trill is uncommon and is appreciated in only 20–30 percent of patients. The first heart sound is softer in intensity owing to postcapillary pulmonary hypertension. A prominent left ventricular S3 gallop indicates elevated left ventricular end-diastolic pressure. Right ventricular failure is evident from the elevated jugular venous pressure, left parasternal lift, and a right ventricular S3 gallop.

The ECG usually shows evidence of recent inferior or posterior infarction, but the ECG changes are sometimes nonspecific and Q waves may be absent. Severe pulmonary edema is invariably present on chest radiography. Assessment of the severity of regurgitation (regurgitation index) is possible with radionuclide ventriculography, but in clinical practice this technique is seldom used for diagnosis. Echocardiography and Doppler studies are the investigations of choice and should be performed in all patients suspected of developing mitral regurgitation.

Transthoracic echocardiography (sensitivity 45–50 percent) is less sensitive than transesophageal echocardiography (sensitivity 100 percent) for visualizing the disrupted mitral valve,[90,100–102] but it is highly sensitive for detecting (by color Doppler studies) the resultant mitral insufficiency (100 percent).[100,103] Echocardiography also demonstrates the underlying regional wall motion abnormality at the site of infarction and excludes ventricular septal rupture or free-wall rupture. A partial papillary muscle rupture can also be diagnosed by two-dimensional echocardiography.[90,91]

An early giant V wave is detected in the pulmonary capillary wedge pressure tracing when hemodynamics are determined. However, tall peaked V waves may also be present with a ventricular septal defect due to increased left atrial venous return in the presence of a normal compliance of the left atrium. A reflected V wave in the pulmonary artery pressure tracing, however, is diagnostic of subacute or acute severe mitral regurgitation. Reflux of oxygenated blood from the left atrium may occur in patients with acute severe mitral regurgitation; and sampling of blood in the distal pulmonary artery branches, suggesting a left-to-right shunt, may reveal higher saturation. Thus the diagnosis may be confused with ventricular septal rupture. Therefore in the presence of suspected severe mitral insufficiency, blood should be sampled at the main pulmonary artery level.

As in many patients with postinfarction papillary muscle rupture, the infarctions are relatively small and residual ventricular function may be preserved; mitral regurgitation is potentially correctable by surgery. Therapy is therefore directed to early surgery after stabilizing the patients, if possible.

When the blood pressure is adequate, vasodilator drugs such as nitroprusside or hydralazine can be used to reduce regurgitant volume by decreasing systemic impedance to left ventricular ejection and by decreasing the mitral valve regurgitant orifice area, thereby increasing resistance at the mitral valve.[104–106] Nitroprusside and hydralazine reduce the pulmonary capillary wedge pressure regurgitant volume and V wave magnitude, and they increase cardiac output. Intravenous nitroglycerin reduces the capillary wedge pressure and regurgitant volume, but it has a less salutary effect on forward stroke volume and cardiac output.

Vasodilator agents cannot be used initially in patients with severe hypotension. In such patients intraaortic balloon counterpulsation should be instituted promptly to augment diastolic arterial pressure, reduce left ventricular impedance and regurgitant volume, and increase forward stroke volume and cardiac output.[107] Subsequently, vasodilator agents or inotropes (or both) can be added to further improve hemodynamics. Many patients can be stabilized with aggressive pharmacotherapy and intraaortic balloon counterpulsation.

As perioperative reinfarction influences the prognosis adversely,[108] if the hemodynamic state permits, cardiac catheterization should be performed to delineate the coronary anatomy with a view to coronary artery bypass surgery at the time of mitral valve repair or replacement. Occasionally, in patients with early severe mitral insufficiency without papillary muscle rupture, coronary angioplasty of the infarct-related vessel has been shown to improve mitral insufficiency and the hemodynamic status.[109,110] Presumably, papillary muscle ischemia rather than infarction is the cause of mitral regurgitation in these patients, and correction of ischemia allows improvement of papillary muscle function and a decrease in mitral regurgitation. In most patients, however, coronary artery bypass surgery with or without mitral valve surgery is required for early severe mitral regurgitation.[88]

Mitral valve replacement or reparative surgery should be performed before other organ failure develops. The surgical mortality is approximately 30–40 percent. The survival of patients with shock who do not have surgery is negligible, and so early surgery is indicated in these patients. Without surgery, mortality is 50 percent in 24 hours and 94 percent within 8 weeks.[97] With early surgery, a salvage rate of 60–70 percent of patients may be expected.[111,112]

Ventricular Septal Rupture

Ventricular septal rupture occurs in 0.5–2.0 percent of patients with acute myocardial infarction and accounts for 1–5 percent of all deaths resulting from myocardial infarction.[93,113] The incidence of ventricular septal rupture is similar for anterior and inferior myocardial infarction.[94,114] Most ventricular septal ruptures occur between the third and seventh day after acute myocardial infarction, although some ruptures can occur as early as the first day or as late as 2 weeks.[93,115]

Most frequently, ventricular septal rupture occurs after a first myocardial infarction, and it is usually located in the low interventricular septum.[69,116] Multiple sites of rupture are observed in 40 percent of patients.[117] Complex ruptures, which are usually serpiginous rather than direct through the infarcted myocardium, may occur in association with ruptures of other structures such as papillary muscles.[69,118] Lack of septal collateral flow, regional distortion, infarct expansion, and local shear stress appear to be the important factors for the development of ventricular septal rupture.[70,116] Thrombolytic therapy does not appear to increase the incidence of ventricular septal rupture, and its relation to the genesis of postinfarction septal rupture is controversial.[119] Single-vessel disease is found in 30–50 percent of patients, and the infarct may be relatively small.[116,120]

Ventricular septal rupture produces a left-to-right shunt that increases the volume load on the right and left ventricle and increases the left ventricular diastolic pressure, left atrial pressure, and pulmonary artery pressure. There is a substantial increase in right atrial and right ventricular diastolic pressures. The systemic cardiac output is substantially decreased, and the magnitude of reduction is related to the magnitude of the left-to-right shunt. The larger the left-to-right shunt, the greater is the reduction in systemic output. The magnitude of the left-to-right shunt depends on the relative resistance at the site of the interventricular septal defect and the pulmonary and systemic vascular resistance. If the defect is large there is little resistance at the site of the defect, and therefore the magnitude of the left-to-right shunt is primarily determined by the relative resistance in the pulmonary vascular bed and the systemic vascular bed. In patients with ventricular septal rupture following myocardial infarction the defect is usually large, and therefore the pulmonary vascular and systemic vascular resistances determine primarily the magnitude of the left-to-right shunt. Right ventricular function is also a determinant for the prognosis of patients with ventricular septal rupture. Impaired left ventricular function associated with disproportionately elevated left ventricular diastolic pressure and elevated right atrial pressure is associated with poor prognosis. Left ventricular dysfunction is also associated with high operative mortality for repair of ventricular septal rupture.

The clinical presentation is characterized by the appearance of a new pansystolic murmur and worsening congestive heart failure. Approximately 50 percent of patients have a palpable trill along the lower left sternal border.[121] There is both right and left-sided S3 gallop and an increase in intensity of the pulmonic component of the second heart sound due to associated pulmonary hypertension. Pulmonary edema is less abrupt and the clinical tempo less dramatic than in patients with papillary muscle rupture. The clinical spectrum ranges from mild to moderate pulmonary edema to cardiogenic shock.[122] The ECG shows variable and nonspecific abnormalities, except for evidence of myocardial infarction.[122]

Two-dimensional echocardiography is the investigation of choice for diagnosis of the septal defect. It also reveals regional wall motion abnormalities and changes in right and left ventricular function. Doppler studies demonstrate transseptal flow across the defect.[100,103,123] Venous injection of agitated saline may demonstrate negative contrast in the right ventricle. Transthoracic or transesophageal echocardiography also provide assessment of left and right ventricular function, which influences the perioperative prognosis.[124]

Hemodynamic monitoring is not required for the diagnosis of ventricular septal rupture, but it is useful for assessing the response to therapy. Right heart catheterization reveals an increase in the right atrial, right ventricular diastolic, and pulmonary artery pressures. Pulmonary capillary wedge pressure is also elevated. Oximetry demonstrates an oxygen step-up detectable at the right ventricular level as well as at the pulmonary artery level (Fig. 36-3). A recirculation peak is seen on the thermodilution cardiac output curve.

With conservative therapy, the mortality of postinfarction ventricular septal rupture is approximately 24 percent during the first 24 hours, 46 percent at 1 week, and up to 82 percent at 2 months.[93] Early surgical repair is preferable, and the operative mortality is approximately 27 percent in patients without cardiogenic shock,[93,94] although it, can be as high as 50 percent for patients in cardiogenic shock.[116,125] Over-

all survival is 50–70 percent. The operative mortality is higher in patients with inferoposterior septal defects. Technical difficulties and the need for concurrent mitral valve repair or replacement and tricuspid valve repair may account for the poorer prognosis in these patients. The operative mortality is higher in older patients and in those with a markedly impaired left ventricular ejection fraction. Nevertheless, the survivors of surgery usually have a better long-term prognosis and functional class. Low mortality rate has been observed during long-term follow-up, and approximately 50 percent of patients survive for 10 years after successful corrective surgery.[126]

Like patients with papillary muscle infarction, the operative mortality is reduced if the patients can be stabilized prior to surgery. The most effective supportive therapy is use of intraaortic balloon counterpulsation, which reduces the magnitude of the left-to-right shunt and increases forward stroke volume. The vasodilators that have the potential to decrease both pulmonary and systemic vascular resistance, such as nitroprusside, may be ineffective and indeed can increase the magnitude of the left-to-right shunt. If the magnitude of reduction in pulmonary vascular resistance is proportionately greater than that of systemic vascular resistance, the left-to-right shunt increases. The vasodilators that have relatively less effect on the pulmonary vascular bed but more effect on the systemic vascular bed may be more effective in reducing the magnitude of the left-to-right shunt. In this regard, hydralazine appears to be better than sodium nitroprusside or nitroglycerin. After institution of intraaortic balloon counterpulsation, addition

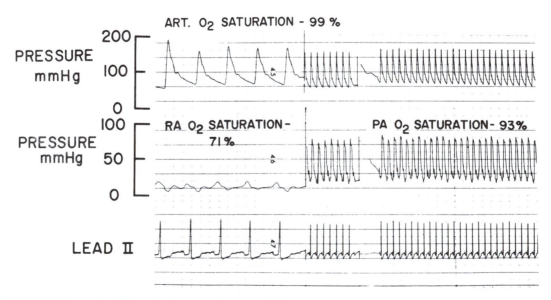

Fig. 36-3. Diagnosis of ventricular septal rupture by oximetry. There is a step-up in oxygen saturation in the pulmonary artery blood sample compared to that in the right atrial blood sample.

Table 36-4. Management Strategies for Cardiogenic Shock

Cardiogenic shock within a few hours of onset of infarction
    Coronary angiography and primary angioplasty of infarct-related artery or revascularization surgery
    Vasopressor to maintain arterial pressure
    Intraaortic balloon counterpulsation
    Supportive pharmacotherapy according to hemodynamics
    Left ventricular assist device as a bridge to cardiac transplant in refractory patients
Papillary muscle rupture and severe mitral regurgitation
    Supportive therapy with intravenous nitroprusside or intravenous hydralazine
    Intraaortic balloon counterpulsation: first in hypotensive patients, then add vasodilators
    Addition of inotropic agents for further hemodynamic improvement
    Cardiac catheterization and corrective surgery as early as possible
Ventricular septal rupture
    Intraaortic balloon counterpulsation
    Add vasodilators, preferably hydralazine
    Add inotropic agent for further hemodynamic improvement
    Corrective surgery as early as possible with or without prior catheterization

---

of hydralazine may reduce the magnitude of the left-to-right shunt and increase forward cardiac output. Addition of dobutamine also may increase forward cardiac output. The management approach of patients with cardiogenic shock with or without mechanical defects is summarized in Table 36-4.

RIGHT VENTRICULAR INFARCTION

Pathoanatomy

Right ventricular infarction is an important etiology of acute right heart failure. Isolated right ventricular myocardial infarction, in the absence of left ventricular myocardial infarction, is rare, with the incidence only 3–1 percent in autopsy studies.[127] Associated right ventricular myocardial infarction is a common (up to 40 percent) complication of left ventricular inferoposterior infarction.[128] The severity of right ventricular myocardial infarction is traditionally graded into four anatomic types.[127] With type 1, less than 50 percent of the inferior wall of the right ventricle is involved in addition to the inferior wall of the left ventricle and the posteroinferior part of the interventricular septum. With type II, more than 50 percent of the right ventricular inferior wall is involved. With type III, in addition to the inferior wall of the right ventricle less than 50 percent of the anterior wall of the right ventricle is involved. With type IV there is extensive necrosis of the free wall of the right ventricle in addition to its inferior wall. The hemodynamic abnormalities such as low output state are likely to occur with types III and IV right ventricular myocardial infarction. Types III and IV right ventricular myocardial infarction are almost always due to total occlusion of the right coronary artery proximal to the right ventricular branches, often in association with significant stenosis of the left anterior descending artery.

Diagnosis

The clinical diagnosis[128–130] of right ventricular myocardial infarction requires awareness of the association of right ventricular myocardial infarction in patients with inferoposterior wall myocardial infarction. Right ventricular myocardial infarction may be clinically silent. Combinations of hypotension, elevated jugular venous pressure, and clear lung fields occur usually in patients with severe right ventricular myocardial infarction.[1] However, if findings of right heart failure are detected in the absence of overt left ventricular failure, such as pulmonary edema and left ventricular S3 gallop, right ventricular myocardial infarction should be suspected. An obvious Kussmaul's sign—defined as lack of decrease or an increase in the jugular venous pressure during the inspiratory phase of respiration—appears to be highly specific for the diagnosis of right ventricular myocardial infarction,[1] but Kussmaul's sign is not appreciated in many patients. Significant pulsus paradoxus is also a relatively uncommon finding in patients with right ventricular myocardial infarction. These findings, however, reflect the hemodynamic abnormalities of effusive-constrictive pericarditis and suggest that abnormal ventricular filling characteristics, as are seen with pericardial tamponade or constrictive pericarditis, may occur. Tricuspid regurgitation in the absence of clinical evidence for significant pulmonary arterial hypertension also suggests significant right ventricular failure.

The ECG reveals an ST segment elevation of more than 1 mm in lead V_1 and V_4R in the presence of inferior wall myocardial infarction.[129] When the magnitude of ST elevation in lead V_4R is at least 0.5 mm, a sensitivity of 83 percent and a specificity of 77 percent have been reported. ST segment elevations may extend from V_3R to V_7R in some patients with extensive right ventricular myocardial necrosis. With marked right ventricular dilatation and its anterior displacement, ST segment elevations can be observed in the anterior precordial leads extending from leads V_1 to V_5 or V_6. With right ventricular myocardial infarction associated with inferior wall infarction, the magnitude of the Q wave in lead III is usually greater than the magnitude of the Q wave in lead AVF. When the magnitude of ST segment depression in leads V_1 and V_2 is less than 50 percent of the magnitude of ST segment elevation in leads II, III, and AVF, right ventricular dysfunction is frequently observed.

Myocardial scintigraphy with technetium 99m pyrophosphate reveals uptake of the radionuclide in the area of the right ventricle in approximately 40 percent of patients with acute inferior wall myocardial infarction.[128] Radionuclide ventriculography and echocardiography are employed to assess right and left ventricular function. With right ventricular myocardial infarction, the right ventricular ejection fraction is usually less than 40 percent, and there is regional dyskinesis or akinesis.[1] Dilatation of the right ventricle with impaired systolic function and dyskinesis or akinesis of the right ventricular wall segments strongly suggest right ventricular myocardial infarction. Echocardiography reveals a wall motion abnormality of the inferior wall of the left ventricle. Echocardiography is necessary in the differential diagnosis of cardiac tamponade and right ventricular myocardial infarction, as the altered hemodynamics seen with right ventricular myocardial infarction may be similar to those seen with tamponade.[1,131]

The hemodynamic abnormalities associated with right ventricular myocardial infarction are variable and are related to the extent of right ventricular necrosis and severity of associated left ventricular dysfunction. Hemodynamic tests reveal a disproportionate elevation of right atrial pressure compared to the rise in pulmonary capillary wedge pressure, and the right atrial/pulmonary capillary wedge pressure ratio is 0.86 or more. If the right atrial pressure is 10 mmHg or more and the right atrial/wedge pressure ratio exceeds 0.86, the sensitivity and specificity of these hemodynamic abnormalities for the diagnosis of right ventricular myocardial infarction are 82 percent and 97 percent, respectively.[1] It has been

suggested that the volume expansion can unmask the hemodynamics of right ventricular myocardial infarction. With marked right ventricular dilatation, the hemodynamic abnormalities may be similar to those of effusive-constrictive pericarditis. Equalization of right and left ventricular end-diastolic pressures and a "dip and plateau" type of right ventricular diastolic pressure pulse may be observed (Fig. 36-4). An increase in intrapericardial pressure and the constraining effect of the pericardium appear to comprise the mechanism of these hemodynamic abnormalities.[132]

Low Output State

PATHOPHYSIOLOGY

Bradyarrhythmias that may be complicated by a low output state are frequently seen with right ventricular infarction. The incidence of complete AV block may be as high as 20 percent and may produce hypotension and the low output state.[133] The loss of timed atrial contribution in ventricular filling appears to be the predominant mechanism of decreased stroke volume. The increase in heart rate by ventricular pacing alone may induce a further reduction in stroke volume. Thus in patients who develop AV block, AV sequential pacing is desirable to maintain adequate ventricular filling and to increase cardiac output.[134]

Only about 10 percent of patients with right ventricular infarction develop cardiogenic shock or severe low output state. The mechanism of decreased cardiac output in right ventricular myocardial infarction is decreased left ventricular preload. In dogs with induced isolated right ventricular myocardial infarction, the left ventricular transmural pressure (left ventricular diastolic pressure minus intrapericardial pressure) declines when the right ventricular transmural pressure increases.[132,135] Similarly, the left ventricular diastolic volume decreases when right ventricular dimensions increase. A number of interacting mechanisms contribute to decreased left ventricular preload.[133] A decrease in right ventricular stroke volume resulting from right ventricular failure is the major determinant for decreased left ventricular preload. After isolated right ventricular infarction in dogs, the decreased right ventricular stroke work index is associated with increased right ventricular transmural pressure and volume, suggesting a significant depression of right ventricular pump function.[132,135] In isolated right ventricular myocardial infarction in

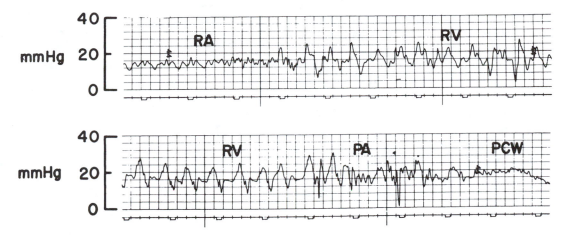

Fig. 36-4. Hemodynamic abnormalities during severe right ventricular infarction showing disproportionate elevation of right atrial (RA) pressure compared to that of pulmonary capillary wedge pressure (PCW) pressure and equalization of RA and PCW pressures. Right ventricular (RV) pressure waveform shows square root sign constraining effect of pericardium.

dogs, volume expansion with intravenous fluid can be associated with a substantial increase in right ventricular stroke volume along with an increase in right ventricular transmural pressure and diastolic volume.[135] The improved right ventricular Starling function results in an increase in left ventricular preload, as evidenced by increased left ventricular transmural pressure and left ventricular diastolic volume. It should be emphasized, however, that if the right ventricular diastolic pressure is already significantly elevated, intravenous fluid does not increase the right ventricular preload owing to the constraining effect of the pericardium. In addition to impaired contractile function of the right ventricle, the increase in right ventricular afterload and its resistance to ejection contributes to impaired right ventricular pump function. With right ventricular dilatation, its wall stress increases, which is one of the major components of afterload. In the presence of intact pericardium and with right ventricular dilatation there is an increase in intrapericardial pressure associated with a passive increase in left ventricular end-diastolic pressure. Thus there is also an increase in left atrial and pulmonary venous pressure. An increase in pulmonary venous pressure is associated with an obligatory increase in pulmonary artery pressure, which offers a greater resistance to right ventricular ejection. Pulmonary hypertension therefore is another contributing factor to impaired right ventricular pump function and the reduction in its stroke output.

Left and right ventricular filling may also be compromised owing to increased intrapericardial pressure. In experimental isolated right ventricular infarction, the intrapericardial pressure increases and there is an equalization of right and left ventricular diastolic pressures. When the pericardium is removed, along with a decrease in pericardial pressure the equalization of the diastolic pressures is no longer present.[132] These findings suggest that relatively nonelastic pericardium exerts a constraining effect on ventricular filling and contributes to the low left ventricular preload. The orientation and function of the intraventricular septum is also an important determinant of changes in left ventricular compliance and preload.[136] The intraventricular septum shifts toward the left ventricle during diastole, which further decreases left ventricular preload. Right atrial ischemia is associated with ineffective right atrial contraction, which in turn decreases right ventricular filling. In the presence of tricuspid regurgitation, right ventricular forward stroke volume decreases in proportion to the severity of tricuspid regurgitation.

THERAPEUTIC APPROACH

The therapeutic approach to correct low cardiac output is directed at increasing the left ventricular preload. With experimental right ventricular infarction in dogs, after removal of the pericardium the left ventricular stroke volume increases.[132] However, pericardial decompression as a therapeutic approach to improve systemic output in patients with acute right ventricular myocardial infarction has not been confirmed in clinical studies. The other physiologic mechanisms that can potentially augment right ventricular stroke volume and therefore increase left ventricular preload are (1) increased right ventricular Frank-Starling function; (2) decreased right ventricular afterload; and (3) increased right ventricular contractile function.

Early reperfusion therapy to recanalize the infarct-related artery should always be considered for the relief of right ventricular ischemia, as it enhances contractile function. In patients with cardiogenic shock, primary angioplasty of the infarct-related artery is preferable to intravenous thrombolytic therapy. Without establishing adequate flow, recovery of right ventricular systolic function does not occur sufficiently to reverse the shock state.

The improvement in right ventricular pump function by the Frank-Starling mechanism during volume expansion depends on the initial right and left ventricular filling pressures and the severity of the right ventricular systolic dysfunction. When marked right ventricular dilatation is present and its transmural pressure is already significantly elevated (right atrial pressure exceeding 10–15 mmHg) a further increase in right ventricular volume and its filling pressure during volume loading is not accompanied by any significant increase in its stroke volume, as the right ventricle operates on the relatively flat portion of its function curve.[135] Furthermore, during volume expansion the right or left ventricular volume may not increase despite a substantial increase in left ventricular diastolic pressures, suggesting a further reduction in left ventricular compliance. Thus in patients with already elevated right atrial and pulmonary capillary wedge pressure, intravenous fluid therapy is not indicated and may be harmful.

Several vasodilators have been used in an attempt to reduce pulmonary artery pressure to decrease resistance to right ventricular ejection. Sodium nitroprusside occasionally increases systemic output, but it also may cause hypotension. The magnitude of improvement in cardiac output and right ventricular ejection fraction with nitroprusside is also much less compared to that with inotropic agents such as dobutamine.

Positive inotropic agents such as dobutamine and dopamine have been found to effectively improve the right ventricular ejection fraction and increase systemic output. However, dopamine can also increase pulmonary artery pressure and hence the right ventricular ejection resistance, which may curtail the magnitude of increase in cardiac output. It must be emphasized that β-adrenergic agonists are likely to increase myocardial oxygen consumption, and so the

Table 36-5. Therapy of Right Ventricular Myocardial Infarction

Asymptomatic: observe. Avoid diuretics and venodilators, which may induce hypotension and low cardiac output.

Symptomatic, low cardiac output.
  Normotensive or hypotensive with pulmonary capillary wedge (PCWP) or right atrial (RAP) pressure < 15 mmHg: intravenous fluids to increase PCWP and/or RAP to 15–18 mmHg. If cardiac output does not increase or remains inadequate, add a positive inotropic agent (preferably dobutamine).
  Hypertensive with PCWP or RAP > 15 mmHg: add a vasodilator. If cardiac output remains inadequate, add a positive inotropic agent (preferably dobutamine).
  Hypotensive with PCWP and/or RAP > 15 mmHg: add a positive inotropic agent (preferably dopamine).

Atrioventricular sequential pacing in the presence of atrioventricular block and subsequent therapy as for symptomatic, low cardiac output.

Right ventricular assist or pulmonary artery counterpulsation in selected refractory patients.

potential exists for enhancing myocardial ischemia. Also, excessive tachycardia may result, which may compromise right and left ventricular filling. Intravenous phosphodiesterase inhibitors, such as amrinone and milrinone, have been used to improve right ventricular systolic function and decrease pulmonary artery pressure. It has been shown that with phosphodiesterase inhibitors the right ventricular ejection fraction can increase along with an increase in right ventricular stroke volume. There is a suggestion that left ventricular diastolic function may improve with phosphodiesterase inhibitors. It should be emphasized, however, that phosphodiesterase inhibitors can also produce systemic vasodilatation and decrease systemic vascular resistance. In some patients a combination of dobutamine and phosphodiesterase inhibitors is necessary to maximize the increase in cardiac output. It is apparent that in patients with low output state and hypotension hemodynamic monitoring is preferable for assessing the response to therapy. The guidelines for management of low output state in patients with right ventricular myocardial infarction are summarized in Table 36-5.

REFERENCES

1. Chatterjee K: Complications of acute myocardial infarction. Curr Probl Cardiol 1993;18:1–79
2. Goldberg RJ, Gore JM, Alpert JS et al: Cardiogenic

shock resulting from acute myocardial infarction. A fourteen year community wide perspective. N Engl J Med 1991;325:1117–1122

3. Gruppo Italiano per 10 Studio della Streptochinasi della'Infarto Miocardico (GISSI): Effectiveness of intravenous streptokinase thrombolytic treatment in acute myocardial infarction. Lancet 1986;1:397–402

4. Falk E, Shah PK, Fuster V: Coronary plaque disruption. Circulation 1995;92:657–671

5. Davies MJ, Thomas AC: Plaque fissuring. The cause of acute myocardial infarction, sudden ischemic death, and crescendo angina. Br Heart J 1985;53:363–373

6. DeWood MA, Spores J, Notske R et al: Prevalence of total coronary occlusion during the early hours of transmural myocardial infarction. N Engl J Med 1981;303:897–902

7. Reimer KA, Jennings RB: The "wave front phenomenon" of myocardial ischemic cell death. II. Transmural progression of necrosis within the framework of ischemic bed size (myocardium at risk) and collateral flow. Lab Invest 1979;40:633–644

8. Lew W, LeWinter MM: Acute myocardial infarction. Pathophysiology. pp. 7.112–7.133. In Chatterjee K, Parmley WW (eds): Cardiology. Vol. 2. Lippincott-Raven, Philadelphia, 1991

9. Taegtmeyer H: Biochemistry of acute myocardial infarction. pp. 29–52. In Francis GS, Alpert JS (eds): Coronary Care. 2nd Ed. Little, Brown, Boston, 1995

10. Shah PK, Francis GS: Pump failure, shock and cardiac rupture in acute myocardial infarction. pp. 289–324. In: Francis GS, Alpert JS (eds): Coronary Care. 2nd Ed. Little, Brown, Boston, 1995

11. Pfeffer MA, Braunwald E: Ventricular remodeling after myocardial infarction. Experimental observations and clinical implications. Circulation 1990;81:1161–1172

12. Braunwald E, Kloner RA: The stunned myocardium. Prolonged postischemic ventricular dysfunction. Circulation 1982;66:1146

13. Williamson BD, Lim MJ, Buda AJ: Transient left ventricular filling abnormalities (diastolic stunning) after acute myocardial infarction. Am J Cardiol 1990;66:897–903

14. Forrester JS, Diamond G, Chatterjee K et al: Medical therapy of acute myocardial infarction by application of hemodynamic subsets (Part 1). N Engl J Med 1976;295:1356–1362

15. Forrester JS, Diamond G, Chatterjee K et al: Medical therapy of acute myocardial infarction by application of hemodynamic subsets (Part 2). N Engl J Med 1976;295:1404–1413

16. Killip T, Kimball JT: Treatment of myocaridal infarction in a coronary care unit. A two year experience with 250 patients. Am J Cardiol 1967;20:457–464

17. GUSTO Investigators: An international randomized trial comparing four thrombolytic strategies for acute myocardial infarction. N Engl J Med 1993;329:673–682

18. Grines CL, Browne KF, Marco J et al: A comparison of immediate angioplasty with thrombolytic therapy for acute myocardial infarction. The primary angio-

plasty in myocardial infarction study group. N Engl J Med 1993;328:673–679

19. ISIS Collaborative Group. ISIS-4 (Fourth International Study of Infarct Survival): A randomized trial comparing oral captopril versus placebo, oral mononitrate versus placebo, and intravenous magnesium sulphate versus control among 58,043 patients with suspected acute myocardial infarction. Lancet 1995;345:669–685

20. GISSI-3 (Gruppo Italiano per lo Studio Della Sopravvivenza Nell' Infarto Miocardico): GISSI-3. Effects of lisinopril and transdermal glyceryl trinitrate singly and together on 6-week mortality and ventricular function after acute myocardial infarction. Lancet 1994;343:1115–1122

21. Dikshit K, Vyden JK, Forrester JS et al: Renal and extrarenal hemodynamic effects of furosemide in congestive heart failure after acute myocardialinfarction. N Engl J Med 1973;288:1087–1090

22. Chatterjee K, Parmley WW: The role of vasodilator therapy in heart failure. Prog Cardiovasc Dis 1977;19:301–325

23. Crexells C, Chatterjee K, Forrester JS et al: Optimal level of left heart filling pressures in acute myocardial infarction. N Engl J Med 1973;289:1263–1266

24. Chou TM, Amidon TM, Ports TA, Wolfe CL: Cardiogenic shock. Thrombolysis or angioplasty. J Intens Care Med 1995;11:37–48

25. Califf RM, Bengtson JR: Cardiogenic shock. N Engl J Med 1994;330:1724–1730

26. Hands ME, Rutherford JD, Muller JE et al: The in-hospital development of cardiogenic shock after myocardial infarction. Incidence, predictors of occurrence, outcome and prognostic factors. The MILIS study group. J Am Coll Cardiol 1989;14:40–48

27. Scheidt S, Ascherian R, Killip T: Shock after acute myocardial infarction. A clinical and hemodynamic profile. Am J Cardiol 1970;26:556–564

28. Waksman R, Weiss AT, Gotsman MS, Hasin Y: Intra-aortic balloon counterpulsation improves survival in cardiogenic shock complicating acute myocardial infarction. Eur Heart J 1993;14:71–74

29. International Study Group: In-hospital mortality and clinical course of 20,891 patients with suspected acute myocardialinfarction randomized between alterplase and streptokinase with or without heparin. Lancet 1990;336:71–75

30. Second International Study of Infarct Survival Collaborative Group (ISIS-2): Randomized trial of intravenous streptokinase, oral aspirin, both or neither among 17,187 cases of suspected acute myocardial infarction: ISIS-2. Lancet 1988;2:349–360

31. Bates ER, Topol EJ: Limitations of thrombolytic therapy for acute myocardial infarction complicated by congestive heart failure and cardiogenic shock. J Am Coll Cardiol 1991;81:1077–1084

32. Bengston JR, Kaplan AJ, Pieper KS et al: Prognosis in cardiogenic shock after acute myocardial infarction in the interventional era. J Am Coll Cardiol 1992;20:1482–1489

33. O'Neill WW, Erbel R, Laufer N et al: Coronary angioplasty therapy of cardiogenic shock complicating

acute myocardialinfarction [abstract]. Circulation, suppl. III 1985;72:309

34. Shani J, Rivera M, Geengart A et al: Percutaneous transluminal coronary angioplasty in cardiogenic shock [abstract]. J Am Coll Cardiol 1986;7:219A

35. Heuser RR, Goss JE, Ramo BW et al: Coronary angioplasty in the treatment of cardiogenic shock. The therapy of choice [abstract]. J Am Coll Cardiol 1986; 7:219A

36. Brown TM, Ianne LA, Gorden DF et al: Percunaneous myocardial reperfusion reduces mortality in acute myocardial infarction complicated by cardiogenic shock [abstract]. Circulation, suppl. III 1985: 309

37. Laramee LA, Rutherford BD, Ligon RW et al: Coronary angioplasty for cardiogenic shock following myocardial infarction [abstract]. Circulation, suppl. II 1988;78:634

38. Lee L, Bates ER, Pitt B et al: Percutaneous transluminal coronary angioplasty improves myocardial infarction complicated by cardiogenic shock. Circulation 1988;78:1345–1351

39. Stack RS, Califf RM, Hinohara T et al: Survival and cardiac event rates in the first year after emergency coronary angioplasty for acute myocardial infarction. J Am Coll Cardiol 1988;11:1141–1149

40. Lee L, Erbel R, Brown TM et al: Multicenter registry of term survival. J Am Coll Cardiol 1991;17: 599–603

41. Gacioch GM, Topol EJ: Frontiers in cardiogenic shock management. Integration of angioplasty and new support devices [abstract]. Circulation, suppl. II 1989;80:624

42. Disler L, Haitas B, Benjamin J et al: Cardiogenic shock in evolving myocardial infarction. Treatment by angioplasty and streptokinase. Heart Lung 1987; 16:649–652

43. Ellis SG, O'Neill WW, Bates ER et al: Implications for patient triage from survival and left ventricular functional recovery analyses in 500 patients treated with coronary angioplasty for acute myocardial infarction. J Am Coll Cardiol 1989;13:1251–1259

44. Verna E, Repetto S, Boscarini M et al: Emergency coronary angioplasty in patients with severe left ventricular dysfunction or cardiogenic shock after acute myocardial infarction. Eur Heart J 1989;10: 958–966

45. O'Keefe JJ, Rutherford BD, McConahay DR et al: Early and late results of coronary angioplasty without antecedent thrombolytic therapy for acute myocardial infarction. Am J Cardiol 1989;64:1221–1230

46. Meyer P, Blanc P, Baudouy M, Morand P: Treatment of primary cardiogenic shock by coronary transluminal angioplasty during the acute phase of myocardial infarction. Arch Mal Coeur Vaiss 1990; 83:329–334

47. Hibbard MD, Holmes DRJ, Gersh BJ, Reeder GS: Coronary angioplasty for acute myocardial infarction complicated by cardiogenic shock [abstract]. Circulation, suppl. III 1990;82:308

48. Moosvi AR, Villanueva L, Gheorghiade M et al: Early revascularization improves survival in cardiogenic shock [abstract]. Circulation, suppl. III 1990; 82:308

49. Eltchaninoff H, Simpfendorfer C, Whitlow PL: Coronary angioplasty improves both early and 1 year survival in acute myocardial infarction complicated by cardiogenic shock [abstract]. J Am Coll Cardiol 1991; 17:167A

50. Hibbard MD, Holmes DRJ, Bailey KR et al: Percutaneous transluminal coronary angioplasty in patients with cardiogenic shock. J Am Coll Cardiol 1992;19: 639–646

51. Moosvi AR, Khaja F, Villanueva L et al: Early revascularization improves survival in cardiogenic shock complicating acute myocardial infarction. J Am Coll Cardiol 1992;19:907–914

52. Brodie BR, Weintraub RA, Stuckey TD et al: Outcomes of direct coronary angioplasty for acute myocardial infarction in candidates and non-candidates for thrombolytic therapy. Am J Cardiol 1991;67: 7–12

53. Seydoux C, Goy JJ, Beuret P et al: Effectiveness of percutaneous transluminal coronary angioplastyin cardiogenic shock during acute myocardial infarction. Am J Cardiol 1992;69:968–969

54. O'Keefe JJ, Bailey WL, Rutherford BD, Hartzler GO: Primary angioplasty for acute myocardial infarction in 1,000 consecutive patients. Results in an unselected population and high-risk subgroups. Am J Cardiol 1993;72:107G–115G

55. Blanche C, Khan SS, Chaux A, Matloff JM: Postinfarction ventricular septal defect in the elderly. Analysis and results. Ann Thorac Surg 1994;57: 1244–1247

56. Daggett WM: Postinfarction ventricular septal defect repair. Retrospective thoughts and historical perspectives. Ann Thorac Surg 1990;50:1006–1009

57. Cooley DA: Repair of postinfarction ventricular septal defect. J Card Surg 1994;9:427–429

58. Ivert T, Almdahl SM, Lunde P, Lindblom D: Postinfarction left ventricular pseudonaneurysm—echocardiographic diagnosis and surgical repair. Cardiovasc Surg 1994;2:463–466

59. Nishimura RA, Schaff HV, Shub C et al: Papillary muscle rupture complicating acute myocardial infarction. Analysis of 17 patients. Am J Cardiol 1983; 51:373–377

60. Mann JM, Roberts WC: Rupture of the left ventricular free wall during acute myocardial infarction. Analysis of 138 necropsy patients and comparison with 50 necropsy patients with acute myocardial infarction without rupture. Am J Cardiol 1988;62: 847–859

61. Bates RJ, Beutler S, Resnekov L, Anagnostopoulos CE: Cardiac rupture—challenge in diagnosis and management. Am J Cardiol 1977;40:429–437

62. Oliva PB, Hammil SC, Edwards WD: Cardiac rupture, a clinically predictable complication of acute myocardialinfarction. Report of 70 cases with clinicopathologic correlations. J Am Coll Cardiol 1993;22: 720–726

63. Salem BI, Lagos JA, Haikal M, Gowda S: The potential impact of the thrombolytic era on cardiac rupture complicating acute myocardial infarction. Angiology 1994;45:931–936

64. Windsor HM, Chang VP, Shanahan MX: Postinfarction cardiac rupture. J Thorac Cardiovasc Surg 1982; 84:755–761

65. Cengel A, Metin M, Yener A, Dortlemez O, Dortlemez H: Subacute rupture of the free left ventricular wall following acute myocardial infarction. Successful surgery in a case. Jpn Heart J 1990;31: 745–748

66. Mann JM, Roberts WC: Rupture of the left ventricular free wall during acute myocardialinfarction. Analysis of 138 necropsy patients and comparison with 50 necropsy patients with acute myocardial infarction without rupture. Am J Cardiol 1988;62: 847–859

67. Bansal RC, Pai RG, Hauck AJ, Isaeff DM: Biventricular apical rupture and formation of pseudoaneurysm. Unique flow patterns by Doppler and color flow imaging. Am Heart J 1992;124:497–500

68. Maeta H, Imawaki S, Shiraishi Y, Shinohara T, Shimizu A: Repair of both papillary and free wall rupture following acute myocardial infarction. J Cardiovasc Surg (Torino) 1991;32:828–832

69. Edwards BS, Edwards WD, Edwards JE: Ventricular septal rupture complicating acute myocardial infarction. Identification of simple and complex types in 53 autopsied hearts. Am J Cardiol 1984; 54:1201–1205

70. Jugdutt BI, Michorowski BL: Role of infarct expansion in rupture of the ventricular septum after acute myocardial infarction. A two-dimensional echocardiographic study. Clin Cardiol 1987;10:641–652

71. Lewis AJ, Burchell HB, Titus JL: Clinical and pathologic features of postinfarction cardiac rupture. Am J Cardiol 1960;23:45–53

72. Rasmussen S, Leth A, Kjoller E, Pedersen A: Cardiac rupture in acute myocardial infarction. A review of 72 consecutive cases. Acta Med Scand 1979; 205:11–16

73. Bionck G, Morgensen PL, Nyquist O et al: Studies of myocardial rupture with tamponade in acute myocardial infarction. I. Clinical features. Chest 1972;61: 4–6

74. Makamura F, Minamino T, Higashino Y et al: Cardiac free wall rupture in acute myocardial infarction. Ameliorative effect of coronary reperfusion. Clin Cardiol 1992;15:244–250

75. Ohman EM, Topol EJ, Callif RM et al: An analysis of the cause of early mortality after administration of thrombolytic therapy. The Thrombolysis Angioplasty in Myocardial Infarction Study Group. Coron Artery Dis 1993;4:957–964

76. Massel DR: How sound is the evidence that thrombolysis increases the risk of cardiac rupture? Br Heart J 1993;69:284–287

77. Califf RM, Fortin DF, Tenaglia AN, Íane DC: Clinical risks of thrombolytic therapy. Am J Cardiol 1992;69: 12A–20A

78. Honan MB, Harrell FE, Reimer KA et al: Cardiac rupture and timing of thrombolytic therapy. A meta-analysis [abstract]. Circulation, suppl II 1988;78: 502A

79. London RE, London SB: The electrocardiographic sign of acute hemopericardium. Circulation 1962;25: 780

80. Desoutter P, Halphen C, Haiat R: Two-dimensional echographic visualization of free ventricular wall rupture in acute anterior myocardial infarction. Am Heart J 1984;108:1360–1361

81. Maisel AS, Gilpin EA, Klein L et al: The murmur of papillary muscle dysfunction in acute myocardial infarction. Clinical features and prognostic implications. Am Heart J 1988;112:705–711

82. Coma CI, Lopez SJ, Gonzalez GA, Jadraque LM: Hemodynamic effect of dextran, dobutamine, and pericardiocentesis in cardiac tamponade secondary to subacute heart rupture. Am Heart J 1987;114: 78–84

83. Heikkila J: Mitral incompetence complicating acute myocardial infarction. Br Heart J 1967;29:220–223

84. Cohn LH: Surgical management of acute and chronic cardiac mechanical complications due to myocardial infarction. Am Heart J 1981;102:1049–1060

85. Brazilai B, Gessler C Jr, Perez JE et al: Significance of Doppler-detected mitral regurgitation in acute myocardial infarction. Am J Cardiol 1988;61: 220–223

86. DeServi S, Vaccari L, Assandri J et al: Clinical significance of mitral regurgitation in patients with recent myocardial infarction. Eur Heart J, suppl. F 1988;9: 5–9

87. Loperfido F, Biasucci LM, Pennestri F et al: Pulsed Doppler echocardiographic analysis of mitral regurgitation after myocardial infarction. Am J Cardiol 1986;58:692–697

88. Teheng JE, Jackman JD Jr, Nelson CL et al: Outcome of patients sustaining acute ischemic mitral regurgitation during myocardial infarction. Ann Intern Med 1992;117:18–24

89. David TE: Techniques and results of mitral valve repair for ischemic mitral regurgitation. J Card Surg, suppl. 1994;9:274–277

90. Chirillo F, Totis O, Cavarzerani A et al: Transesophageal echocardiographic findings in partial and complete papillary muscle rupture complicating acute myocardial infarction. Cardiology 1992;81:54–58

91. Hanlon JT, Conrad AK, Combs DT, McLellan BA, Doolan K: Echocardiographic recognition of partial papillary muscle rupture. J Am Soc Echocardiogr 1993;6:101–103

92. Estes EJ, Dalton FM, Entman ML, Dixon HD, Hackel DB: The anatomy and blood supply of the papillary muscles of the left ventricle. Am Heart J 1966;71: 356–362

93. Sharma SK, Seckler J, Israel DH et al: Clinical cardiographic and anatomic findings in acute severe ischimic mitral regurgitation. Am J Cardiol 1992;70: 277–280

94. Friedman HF, Kuhn LA, Katz, AM: Clinical and electrocardiographic features of cardiac rupture following acute myocardial infarction. Am J Med 1971; 50:709–720

95. Vlodaver Z, Edwwards JE: Rupture of ventricular septum or papillary muscle complicating myocardial infarction. Circulation 1977;55:815–822

96. Wei JY, Hutrchins GM, Bulkley BH: Papillary muscle rupture in fatal acute myocardial infarction. A potentially treatable form of cardiogenic shock. Ann Intern Med 1979;90:149–52

97. Sanders RJ, Neubuerger KT, Ravin A: Rupture of papillary muscles. Occurrence of rupture of the posterior muscle in posterior myocardial infarction. Dis Chest 1957;31:316–323

98. Barbour DJ, Roberts WC: Rupture of a left ventricular papillary muscle during acute myocardial infarc-

tion. Analysis of 22 necropsy patients. J Am Coll Cardiol 1986;8:558–565

99. Forrester JS, Diamond G, Freedman S et al: Silent mitral insufficiency in acute myocardial infarction. Circulation 1971;44:877–883

100. Kishon Y, Iqbal A, Oh JK et al: Evolution of echocardiographic modalities in detection of postmyocardial infarction ventricular septal defect and papillary muscle rupture. Study of 62 patients. Am Heart J 1993;126:667–675

101. Zotz RJ, Dohmen G, Genth S, Erbel R, Meyer J: Diagnosis of papillary muscle rupture after acute myocardial infarction by transthoracic and transesophageal echocardiography. Clin Cardiol 1993;16:665–670

102. Sakai K, Nakamura K, Hosoda S: Transesophageal echocardiographic findings of papillary muscle rupture. Am J Cardiol 1991;68:561–563

103. Smyllie JH, Sutherland GR, Geuskens R et al: Doppler color flow mapping in the diagnosis of ventricular septal rupture and acute mitral regurgitation after myocardial infarction. J Am Coll Cardiol 1990;15:1449–1455

104. Yoran C, Yellin EL, Becker RM et al: Mechanism of reduction of mitral regurgitation with vasodilator therapy. Am J Cardiol 1979;43:773–777

105. Greenberg BH, Massie BM, Brundage BH et al: Beneficial effects of hydralazine in severe mitral regurgitation. Circulation 1978;58:273–279

106. Chatterjee K, Parmley WW, Swan HJ et al: Beneficial effects of vasodilator agents in severe mitral regurgitation due to dysfunction of subvalvar apparatus. Circulation 1973;48:684–690

107. Gold HK, Leinbach RC, Sanders CA et al: Intra-aortic balloon pumping for ventricular septal defect or mitral regurgitation complicating acute myocardial infarction. Circulation 1973;47:1191–1196

108. Dellborg M, Held P, Swedberg K, Vedin A: Rupture of the myocardium. Occurrence and risk factors. Br Heart J 1985;54:11–16

109. Le FC, Metzger JP, Lachurie ML et al: Treatment of severe mitral regurgitation caused by ischemic papillary muscle dysfunction. Indications for coronary angioplasty. Am Heart J 1992;123:860–865

110. Heuser RR, Maddoux GL, Goss JE et al: Coronary angioplasty for acute mitral regurgitation due to myocardial infarction. A non-surgical treatment preserving mitral valve integrity. Ann Intern Med 1987;107:852–855

111. Replogle RL, Campbell CD: Surgery for mitral regurgitation associated with ischemic heart disease. Results and strategies. Circulation, suppl. I 1989;79:122–125

112. Kay JH, Zubiate P, Mendez MA et al: Surgical treatment of mitral insufficiency secondary to coronary artery disease. J Thorac Cardiovasc Surg 1980;79:12–18

113. Hutchins GM: Rupture of the interventricular septum complicating myocardial infarction. Pathological analysis of 10 patients with clinically diagnosed perforations. Am Heart J 1979;97:165–173

114. Roberts WC, Ronan JAJ, Harvey WP: Rupture of the left ventricular free wall (LVFW) or ventricular septum (VS) secondary to acute myocardial infarction (AMI). An occurrence virtually limited to the first transmural AMI in hypertensive individuals [abstract]. Am J Cardiol 1975;35:166

115. Sanders RJ, Kern WH, Blount SG: Perforation of the interventricular septum complicating myocardial infarction. Am Heart J 1956;51:736–748

116. Radford MJ, Johnson RA, Daggett WJ et al: Ventricular septal rupture. A review of clinical and physiologic features and an analysis of survival. Circulation 1981;64:545–553

117. Hill JD, Lary D, Kerth WJ, Gerbode F: Acquired ventricular septal defects. Evolution of an operation, surgical technique, and results. J Thorac Cardiovasc Surg 1975;70:440–450

118. Mann JM, Roberts WC: Acquired ventricular septal defect during acute myocardial infarction. Analysis of 38 unoperated necropsy patients and comparison with 50 unoperated necropsy patients without rupture. Am J Cardiol 1988;62:8–19

119. Kleiman NS, Terrin M, Jueller H et al: Mechanisms of early death despite thrombolytic therapy. Experience from the Thrombolysis in Myocardial Infarction Phase II (TIMI II) study. J Am Coll Cardiol 1992;19:1129–1135

120. Killen DA, Reed WA, Wathanacharoen S, McCallister BD, Bell HH: Postinfarctional rupture of the interventricular septum. J Cardiovasc Surg (Torino) 1981;22:113–126

121. Perloff JK, Talano JV, Ronan JAJ: Non-invasive techniques in acute myocardial infarction. Prog Cardiosc Dis 1971;13:437–464

122. Khan MM, Patterson GC, O'Kane HO, Adgey AA: Management of ventricular septal rupture in acute myocardial infarction. Br Heart J 1980;44:570–576

123. Stevenson JG, Kawabori I, Dooley T, Guntheroth WG: Diagnosis of ventricular septal defect by pulsed Doppler echocardiography. Sensitivity, specificity and limitations. Circulation 1978;58:322–326

124. Moore CA, Nygaard TW, Kaiser DL, Cooper AA, Gibson RS: Postinfarction ventricular septal rupture. The importance of location of infarction and right ventricular function in determining survival. Circulation 1986;74:45–55

125. Feneley MP, Chang VP, O'Rourke MF: Myocardial rupture after acute myocardial infarction. Ten year review. Br Heart J 1983;49:550–556

126. Davies RH, Dawkins KD, Skillington PD et al: Late functional results after surgical closure of acquired ventricular septal defect. J Thorac Cardiovasc Surg 1993;106:592–598

127. Isner J, Roberts WC: Right ventricular infarction complicating left ventricular infarction secondary to coronary heart diseases. Am J Cardiol 1978;42:885–894

128. Sharpe DN, Botvinick EH, Shames DM et al: The non-invasive diagnosis of right ventricular infarction. Circulation 1978;57:483–490

129. Lopez-Sendon J, Coma-Cannella I, Aleasena S et al: Electrocardiographic findings in acute right ventricular infarction. Sensitivity and specificity of electrocardiographic alterations in right precordial leads V_4R, V_3r, V_1, V_2 and V_3. J Am Coll Cardiol 1985;6:1273–1279

130. Baigre RS, Hag A, Morgan CD: The spectrum of right ventricular involvement in inferior wall myocardial infarction. A clinical, hemodynamic and non-invasive study. J Am Coll Cardiol 1983;1:1396–1404

131. Lorell B, Leinbach RC, Pohost GM et al: Right ventricular infarction. Clinical diagnosis and differentiation from cardiac tamponade and pericardial constriction. Am J Cardiol 1979;43:465–471

132. Goldstein JA, Vlahakes GJ, Verrier ED et al: The role of right ventricular systolic dysfunction and elevated intrapericardial pressure in the genesis of low output in experimental right ventricular infarction. Circulation 1982;65:513–522

133. Chatterjee K: Right ventricular infarction. Pathogenesis of low output. pp. 317–328. In Vincent JL (ed): Update in Intensive Care on Emergency Medicine. Vol. 5. Springer-Verlag, New York, 1988

134. Topol EJ, Goldschlager N, Ports TA et al: Hemodynamic benefit of atrial pacing in right ventricular myocardial infarction. Ann Intern Med 1982;96: 594–597

135. Goldstein JA, Vlahakes GJ, Verrier ED et al: Volume loading improves low cardiac output in experimental right ventricular infarction. J Am Coll Cardiol 1983; 2:270–278

136. Mikell FL, Asinger RW, Hodges M: Functional consequences of interventricular septal involvement in right ventricular infarction. Echocardiographic, clinical, and hemodynamic observations. Am Heart J 1983;105:393–401

37 Chronic Heart Failure: Diagnosis and Management

Barry M. Massie
Mohamad H. Yamani

In a book entirely devoted to the subject of heart failure, one might question the need for an "overview" such as this one. Indeed, it is for the very reason that the specific approaches to diagnosing and treating the patient with heart failure have been covered in such great detail in multiple chapters that the editors thought a more general and coherent overview was required. Little unique information is covered in this chapter. Rather, its goal is to provide the clinician with a guide to the management of this complex syndrome. The reader is encouraged to refer to the appropriate chapters for a more detailed discussion of specific topics with more comprehensive citations of the relevant literature. It should be noted that this overview is limited to chronic heart failure in adult patients, and it focuses primarily on heart failure secondary to left ventricular systolic dysfunction.

GUIDELINES FOR THE MANAGEMENT OF HEART FAILURE

Heart failure the only common cardiovascular condition in the developed regions of the world that is associated with a rising incidence, prevalence, and number of deaths.[1] Many of these statistics are driven by the aging of the population,[2] as heart failure is predominantly a condition of the elderly; but the upward trends persist even after correction for age. The care of patients with heart failure places a tremendous burden on health care resources. For instance,

in 1993 the last figure for which statistics are available, congestive heart failure (CHF) was listed as the primary diagnosis in 875,000 hospital discharges in the United States with the resulting 6.5 million days of care at an estimated cost exceeding $8 billion.[3] CHF was also responsible for more than 11 million physician visits and is, with the exception of hypertension, the leading cardiovascular cause for office visits.[4] Although this litany of statistics is gloomy enough in its own right, it is particularly surprising and disappointing in view of the major advances that have occurred in the pathophysiologic understanding of heart failure and its treatment. Despite a series of trials demonstrating the feasibility of preventing heart failure and improving the survival of patients affected by this condition,[5-8] the morbidity and mortality rates for these patients continues to rise. One plausible explanation for this paradox is that physicians have been slow to incorporate these new advances into their clinical practices.[9] This discordance has been the rationale for developing guidelines for the management of heart failure, four of which have been published by governmental and professional organizations over the last several years.[10-13] This chapter refers extensively to these guidelines, updating them where appropriate. The strength of these guidelines is that they are based on extensive review of the literature and provide clear, evidence-based recommendations; but the universality of such recommendations is limited by the complexity and heterogeneity of this syndrome and the need for the clinician to individualize management decisions. Furthermore, the rapid progress of re-

551

search and evolution of treatment approaches may render even recent recommendations obsolete or incorrect. No doubt this chapter will suffer from the same limitations.

PREVENTION OF HEART FAILURE

Before discussing the management of heart failure, it is particularly appropriate to discuss the prevention of this condition, because ultimately this is where the emphasis must be placed.[1] As with most cardiovascular conditions, preventive measures are important at each phase of the natural history of heart failure. As indicated in Table 37-1, these measures can be subdivided into primary prevention when applied to patients with intact left ventricular function, secondary prevention when applied to patients with left ventricular damage and dysfunction but without overt heart failure, and tertiary prevention when the goal is to prevent progression or mortality in patients who already suffer from clinical heart failure. With regard to primary prevention, the objective is to modify risk factors for subsequent

---

Table 37-1. Strategies to Prevent Heart Failure and Its Progression

Primary prevention[a]
    Treat hypertension (especially systolic hypertension)
    Treat hyperlipidemia
Secondary prevention[b]
    ACE inhibitor
    β-Blocker
    Secondary prevention post-MI
        Aspirin
        β-Blocker
        Antihyperlipidemic therapy
        Anticoagulation
        Coronary revascularization in appropriate patients
Tertiary prevention[c]
    ACE inhibitor
    β-Blocker
    Digoxin
    Secondary prevention post-MI (see Secondary prevention, above)
    Intensive home monitoring and intervention

Abbreviations: ACE, angiotensin-converting enzyme; MI, myocardial infarction.
[a] Prior to onset of left ventricular dysfunction or cardiac disease.
[b] After onset of left ventricular dysfunction or coronary artery disease but without congestive heart failure.
[c] After onset of heart failure, to delay progression and prevent events.

---

heart failure. Rigorous treatment of hypertension and, perhaps most particularly, predominantly systolic hypertension in elderly patients can have a profound effect on reducing the number of new cases of heart failure.[14,15] In the Systolic Hypertension in the Elderly Program, new cases of heart failure were reduced by 54 percent using this intervention. On a statistical basis, it is likely that aggressive antihypertensive therapy in elderly patients may be the most powerful preventive measure available. Aggressive antihyperlipidemic therapy shows the same promise. In the 4S trial conducted in patients with manifest atherosclerotic disease, new cases of congestive heart failure were reduced by 30 percent with aggressive lowering of low density lipoprotein (LDL) cholesterol.[16] In patients with underlying coronary artery disease, it is also likely that aspirin and warfarin, by preventing recurrent coronary events, can also prevent heart failure. Other obvious approaches to primary prevention include properly timed surgery for valve lesions and prudent consumption of alcohol.

Secondary preventive approaches have received the greatest attention because of the findings with angiotensin-converting enzyme (ACE) inhibitors in patients with asymptomatic left ventricular dysfunction or post-myocardial infarction.[5,6,17,18] Growing evidence supports the ability of β-blockers to prevent the progression of asymptomatic left ventricular dysfunction to overt heart failure in patients with underlying coronary artery disease and those with nonischemic cardiomyopathy[19,20] (see Ch. 47). Revascularization is also clearly beneficial in selected patients with left ventricular dysfunction and significant coronary artery disease (see Ch. 51). Finally, each of the approaches advocated for primary prevention can still play an important role in secondary prevention.

Tertiary prevention is probably a misnomer but is used to describe treatments that alter the natural history of patients with clinical heart failure. The ACE inhibitors are the most established medications with this benefit,[8] but strong evidence suggest that β-blockers can accomplish the same goal[19,20] (see Ch. 47). Again, the role of coronary revascularization in appropriate patients and the importance of antihypertensive, lipid-lowering, and antithrombotic therapy should not be minimized.

DIAGNOSIS AND EVALUATION OF HEART FAILURE

Definition

Although heart failure is common and most physicians believe they "know it when they see it," it is in fact difficult to define. Most clinically useful definitions are empiric rather than mechanistic. The following definition was used in the Agency for Health Care Policy and Research (AHCPR) guidelines.[10]

> Heart failure is a clinical syndrome or condition characterized by (1) signs and symptoms of intravascular and interstitial volume overload, including shortness of breath, rales, and edema, and/or (2) manifestations of inadequate tissue perfusion, such as fatigue or poor exercise tolerance. These signs and symptoms result when the heart is unable to generate a cardiac output sufficient to meet the body's demands.

Many subclassifications are subsumed into this definition. Heart failure has been divided into "high output" when the cardiac output is elevated but still is not sufficient to meet requirements (e.g., thyrotoxicosis, severe anemia, beriberi) or "low output" when cardiac dysfunction is responsible. The term "left-sided" heart failure is used to describe patients whose primary symptoms are related to pulmonary congestion and low cardiac output, whereas patients whose primary manifestations are edema, ascites, and elevated jugular venous pressures are characterized as having "right-sided" heart failure. This latter distinction may be misleading, as the most frequent cause of "right-sided" heart failure is left ventricular dysfunction with pulmonary hypertension, and patients are often inappropriately treated because they lack obvious evidence of left ventricular failure. Terms such as "forward" and "backward" heart failure, connoting the presence of low output manifestations and fluid retention, respectively, have generally passed from use.

Despite the myriad terms used to describe heart failure, several subclassifications are important because they affect diagnostic and therapeutic approaches. The first relates to the etiology of cardiac dysfunction. Heart failure may be due to ischemic heart disease, left ventricular muscle disease (nonischemic cardiomyopathy), valvular abnormalities, intracardiac shunts (or more complex congenital deformities), or extracardiac conditions (including pericardial disease). Many of these etiologies are amenable to specific therapies that may ameliorate or reverse heart failure, and they should be sought and excluded. On the other hand, specific therapy is not available for most cardiomyopathies and heart failure due to coronary artery disease in the absence of ongoing ischemia. A second important distinction is between heart failure due to left ventricular systolic dysfunction, usually characterized by a dilated left ventricle and reduced left ventricular ejection fraction (<35–40 percent) and left ventricular dia-

stolic dysfunction, which is often recognized by a process of exclusion. These conditions require different diagnostic and therapeutic approaches.

Recognition of Heart Failure

In its classic presentation with exertional dyspnea, orthopnea, and paroxysmal dyspnea and the physical findings of pulmonary rales, third heart sound, elevated jugular venous pressure, and peripheral edema, chronic heart failure is easy to recognize. However, it is critical to appreciate that only a few patients present with all or even most of these findings. In one report 20 percent of patients with reduced ejection fractions met no clinical criteria for heart failure.[21] Another found that only a few of those with ejection fractions of 30 percent or less had exertional dyspnea,[22] although the latter symptom appears to be the most sensitive. Table 37-2 shows the sensitivity and specificity of the "classic" historical and physical examination findings in one series of heart failure patients.[23] It should be noted that symptoms such as orthopnea and paroxysmal dyspnea are uncommon. Indeed, particularly in the elderly patient, heart failure may present atypically, with complaints of fatigue, altered mental status or confusion, or even nausea, abdominal pain, or loss of appetite due to hepatic congestion or bowel edema. Conversely, the symptoms of heart failure may be nonspecific. Dyspnea, fatigue, and edema are not uncommon in older patients and sedentary individuals. They may reflect deconditioning, venous insufficiency, pulmonary abnormalities, or medication effects. Perhaps as many as half of the patients ultimately diagnosed as having heart failure have previously received treatment for respiratory disease (especially bronchodilators) or gastrointestinal problems or have been thought to have venous insufficiency.

The physical examination also has significant limitations, as shown in Table 37-2. Indeed, many patients with moderate or even severe heart failure have no physical findings. A third heart sound has been reported as being relatively sensitive in some studies[21] but not in others,[23] and its detection is variable.[24,25] Similarly, elevated jugular venous pressures, especially as elicited by the hepatojugular reflux maneuver, have been found to be a sensitive sign by some[26] but not by others.[23] Pulmonary rales are frequently absent with chronic heart failure, even with markedly elevated pulmonary capillary wedge pressures.[27,28]

Thus heart failure should be considered in any patient with complaints of exertional shortness of

Table 37-2. Sensitivity, Specificity, and Predictive Value of Symptoms and Physical Findings for Diagnosing Heart Failure

Symptom or Sign	Sensitivity (%)	Specificity (%)	Predictive Accuracy[a] (%)
Exertional dyspnea	66	52	23
Orthopnea	21	81	2
Paroxysmal nocturnal dyspnea	33	76	26
History of edema	23	80	22
Resting heart rate >100 bpm	7	99	6
Rales	13	91	21
Third heart sound	31	95	61
Jugular venous distension	10	97	2
Edema (on examination)	10	93	3

[a] Percent of patients with heart failure in whom each sign was correctly identified.
(Adapted from Harlan et al.,[23] with permission.)

breath or edema and in elderly persons presenting with nonspecific, nonlocalized symptoms. Suspicion should be heightened in individuals with known or suspected coronary artery disease, chronic hypertension, diabetes, or alcohol abuse. A negative physical examination should not exclude the diagnosis.

The most frequent procedure used to confirm or exclude the diagnosis of heart failure is the chest radiograph.[9] Unfortunately, it too is relatively unhelpful. Although evaluation of the pulmonary vasculature provides considerable insight into left atrial and pulmonary artery pressures during acute heart failure, the adaptive ability of the lungs to mobilize fluid leaked from capillaries in patients with chronically elevated pulmonary venous pressures makes these signs insensitive in chronic heart failure.[28,29] The most sensitive radiographic sign is cardiomegaly, but considerable left ventricular enlargement may not be apparent on radiographs. As discussed below, an echocardiogram is the preferred test when the diagnosis of heart failure is being considered.

Diagnostic Testing

The goals of additional diagnostic testing in patients found or suspected to have heart failure are several: (1) to confirm the diagnosis of a primary cardiac pathology; (2) to identify abnormalities amenable to specific interventions or treatments; and (3) to determine the underlying pathophysiology (e.g., systolic versus diastolic dysfunction). The several published guidelines are in close agreement in their recommendations for diagnostic testing (Table 37-3). Routine blood tests are suggested to (1) detect severe anemia (a potential cause of dyspnea or high output heart failure); (2) assess renal function and electrolytes

(renal failure may mimic heart failure, and renal function is important to monitor during treatment; hyponatremia is a marker of heart failure severity, and hypokalemia or hyperkalemia require treatment or may limit ACE inhibitor therapy); and (3) measure liver function tests (cirrhosis may mimic heart failure; hepatic dysfunction may be caused by heart failure; hemochromatosis often affects the liver). A urinalysis is recommended to detect proteinuria and glycosuria. Thyroid function testing is recommended in patients with atrial fibrillation or unexplained sinus tachycardia and in selected elderly patients, as thyrotoxicosis and myxedema are two of the most readily treatable causes of heart failure. Serum iron and ferritin levels can identify patients with hemochromatosis, another disorder, albeit rare, that is amenable to therapy.

Although the limitations of the chest radiograph have been discussed, it is still recommended that accompanying pulmonary disease be excluded and a baseline provided if the patient's status changes, although an echocardiogram provides more useful data on cardiac size and valvular abnormalities. An electrocardiogram can confirm the rhythm, identify many old myocardial infarctions, and determine if conduction abnormalities, which may be indicative of infiltrative disorders, are present.

An echocardiogram is recommended in essentially all patients with heart failure. This single procedure addresses, at least in part, all three goals of the diagnostic evaluation. It provides important qualitative and quantitative assessment of the size and function of both ventricles and the degree of hypertrophy. Using Doppler techniques, the degree of pulmonary hypertension can be estimated. This test, if technically adequate, identifies any significant valvular abnormality, pericardial effusion, and most congenital

Table 37-3. Guideline Recommendations for Evaluation of Heart Failure Patients

Procedure	AHCPR[10]	AHA/ACC[11]	Canadian[12]	European[13]
Routine laboratory tests	CBC, Cr, lytes, LFTs, albumin, UA	CBC, BUN, Cr, lytes, Mg, Ca, PO$_4$, glucose, albumin, UA	CBC, BUN, Cr, lytes, LFTs, uric acid	CBC, BUN, Cr, lytes, LFTs, UA
Additional laboratory tests	T$_4$, TSH (afib, elderly)	TSH (afib, selected patients), ferritin (selected patients)	TSH (selected patients), ferritin (selected patients)	TSH
Other standard tests	Radiography, ECG	Radiography, ECG	Radiography, ECG	Radiography, ECG
LV function measurement	All patients (echo preferred)	All patients (echo)	All patients (echo or nuclear)	Not stated
Doppler echo	All patients	All patients	All patients	All patients
Nuclear EF	Alternative to echo		Recommended	Alternative to echo
Stress testing with imaging	Selected patients with prior MI	Selected patients with prior MI or unexplained HF	When revascularization is being considered	Indications no stated
Coronary angiography	Select patients with angina or severe ischemia	Selected pts with angina or severe ischemia or unexplained HF	Patients with angina	Selected patients with ischemia
Ambulatory ECG	Discouraged unless Sx	Discouraged unless Sx	Discouraged unless Sx	Useful
Endomyocardial biopsy	Discouraged	Selected patients	Discouraged except anthracycline toxicity	Limited utility
Measurement of exercise capacity	Selected patients	Selected patients	Not recommended	Not recommended
Follow-up	Clinical assessment	Serial testing discouraged	Not discussed	Not discussed

Abbreviations: Cr, creatinine; lytes, electrolytes; LFTs, liver function tests; UA, urinalysis; afib, atrial fibrillation; HF, heart failure; Sx, symptoms; MI, myocardial infarction; EF, ejection fraction; LV, left ventricular; CBC, complete blood count; T$_4$, thyroxine; TSH, thyroid-stimulating hormone; echo, echocardiography; BUN, blood urea nitrogen.

defects. The finding of a left ventricular aneurysm or segmental dysfunction associated with wall thinning is suggestive of underlying coronary artery disease, but the echocardiogram has often been misleading in distinguishing ischemic from nonischemic cardiomyopathies. Although not a definitive test, it can also suggest infiltrative disease and thyrotoxicosis. In the presence of preserved left ventricular systolic function, diastolic abnormalities are suggested, particularly if severe left ventricular hypertrophy is found and altered left ventricular diastolic filling patterns are observed (although the latter finding is nonspecific).[30–32]

Radionuclide angiography provides an alternative method for examining left ventricular function but yields far less overall information than the echocardiogram; it is not recommended for most patients. Nuclear tests to evaluate ischemia are discussed below. Ambulatory electrocardiograms are not recommended unless the patient has symptoms of a possible arrhythmia, such as syncope or near syncope. Ventricular arrhythmias are common but in general should not be sought, as treatment is not recommended unless symptoms are present. In some patients with atrial fibrillation, ambulatory monitoring may demonstrate an uncontrolled ventricular response that can exacerbate or even cause heart failure, although exercise testing may be a better way to assess heart rate responses. Pulmonary function testing is often undertaken but adds little for the patient with impaired left ventricular function without audible bronchospasm. Testing to quantify exercise capacity may be helpful in patients whose symptoms are difficult to assess by history or who appear to have substantial discrepancies between their symptoms and the apparent severity of heart failure. Concomitant measurements of respiratory gas exchange and oxygen utilization may be of some value but are primarily helpful for assessing suitability for transplantation.

Because left ventricular function and heart failure can be assessed noninvasively, cardiac catheterization is indicated primarily to assess valvular lesions or to evaluate coronary artery disease (see below). Right heart catheterization and hemodynamic monitoring should be reserved for unstable patients or as part of a transplant evaluation. Endomyocardial biopsy has largely fallen from favor as a routine part of the assessment of heart failure patients. In the past, biopsies were employed to detect active myocarditis, but immunosuppressive therapy administered based on histologic evidence of myocarditis has not proved beneficial.[33] Therefore unless more specific markers of response to therapy are identified, the role of endomyocardial biopsy is limited to detecting specific, but rare, treatable infiltrative diseases such as sarcoidosis and eosinophilic myocarditis.

Assessment for Revascularization

Coronary artery disease is the most common cause of heart failure.[2] Unfortunately, the role of coronary revascularization in these patients has not been clarified in clinical trials. Much of the literature on this subject is not directly relevant (e.g., deals with revascularization for patients with angina and mildly reduced ejection fractions rather than overt heart failure) and often borders on being anecdotal.[34] Nonetheless, it is apparent that selected patients benefit from revascularization with an improvement in left ventricular function, symptoms, and prognosis; the difficulty lies in identifying the appropriate candidates. This subject is extensively reviewed and referenced in an article[34] and in Chapter 22 (see also Ch. 51).

Based on the reasonable assumptions that the best candidates for revascularization are those with the greatest amount of viable but jeopardized myocardium and the most severe demonstrable ischemia, the AHCPR and AHA/ACC guidelines recommend a stratified approach to diagnostic testing.[10,11] First, it should be recognized that because of advanced age and severe co-morbidity, most patients with heart failure are not candidates for coronary revascularization. However, among the patients who are potential candidates and are amenable to such an intervention, those with symptomatic angina probably have the most to gain in terms of symptom amelioration and, most likely, prognosis. For these patients coronary angiography may be the most cost-effective approach to evaluation, although stress testing followed by angiography is an appropriate alternative pathway. Patients with known coronary disease, as evidenced by a prior myocardial infarction or a history of angina, may also have substantial ischemia; but in most cases some form of stress test is the appropriate initial approach. Patients with no current or previous angina or myocardial infarction, particularly in the absence of diabetes or multiple risk factors, are the least likely to have significant coronary disease. It is not clear whether additional testing is warranted in these individuals.

There is also considerable controversy on the optimal strategy for noninvasive testing. There are two goals of testing: (1) identifying myocardium that is contracting but is potentially ischemic with exercise or stress (e.g., jeopardized myocardium); and (2) detecting dysfunctional myocardium that is viable and may recover contractile function following revascularization (e.g., hibernating myocardium). Myocardial perfusion scintigraphy and stress echocardiography have their advocates, although there is greater experience with the former approach. Positron emission tomography (PET), which allows independent assessment of blood flow and metabolism, is the gold standard, but excellent results have been obtained with thallium scintigraphy using rest-redistribution protocols to examine viability.[35] (see Ch. 53).

The approach to revascularization in patients identified as having significant myocardial ischemia or dysfunction due to myocardial hibernation is yet another area of controversy. Clearly, coronary bypass surgery carries a higher initial risk but also has been demonstrated to improve prognosis in patients with left ventricular dysfunction[34] (see Ch. 53). Indeed, the goal in such patients should be "complete" revascularization, which is usually not accomplished with angioplasty. On the other hand, patients at high risk for surgery or poor target vessels may receive some benefit, particularly with regard to ischemic symptoms, from angioplasty of selected vessels.

GENERAL MEASURES: COUNSELING, DIET, AND ACTIVITY RECOMMENDATIONS

As with any chronic disease that severely affects the quality and quantity of life, optimal management of heart failure requires good communication between health care providers and the patient and patient's family. Important issues for discussion include patient education, medication compliance, life style modifications and adaptations, dietary and activity recommendations, and the need for advance directives.[10] These issues have been reviewed elsewhere[36] and are covered in Chapter 41.

MEDICATIONS FOR HEART FAILURE DUE TO SYSTOLIC DYSFUNCTION

The number of medications that have been evaluated for chronic heart failure has increased in recent years. This chapter reviews only those currently available for chronic therapy, which are divided into four classes: diuretics, positive inotropic agents, peripheral vasodilators, and neurohormonal antagonists. In addition, several clinically oriented reviews of the pharmacologic therapy of CHF have been published.[37–39] The reader is referred to Chapter 55 on investigational therapies and those on each class of medications for more complete discussion of mechanisms and results.

Diuretics

Salt and water retention resulting from activation of neurohormonal systems comprise a hallmark of chronic heart failure. Although it is often apparent on physical examination, it may be subclinical or, in mild cases, absent. Even when there is no evidence of fluid retention, normal intravascular volumes may be associated with markedly elevated ventricular filling pressures, particularly during activity. Thus diuretics produce rapid hemodynamic and clinical improvement in most symptomatic patients, although they have not been subjected to rigorous trials with clinical endpoints. However, aggressive diuresis is associated with further activation of the renin-angiotensin-aldosterone system and the sympathetic nervous system, as well as with electrolyte imbalances, so it is preferable to combine these agents with ACE inhibitors in most cases. Some patients with mild symptoms obtain adequate symptom relief from ACE inhibitors alone, but they are the exception rather than the rule. In contrast, asymptomatic patients with left ventricular dysfunction usually do not require diuretic therapy.

The pharmacology and clinical use of diuretics have been reviewed[40] and are covered in detail in Chapter 42. Thiazide diuretics may be sufficient in patients with mild symptoms and are preferable in hypertensive individuals, as they provide more prolonged blood pressure control.[37] Loop diuretics are required in most patients with moderate to severe symptoms. Because an intraluminal threshold must be exceeded to obtain the desired effect, greater diuresis is best achieved by increasing the amount of each dose. Divided doses are appropriate to prolong the period of diuresis. When it is difficult to obtain an adequate diuresis or if the total daily dose becomes high (above 320 mg of furosemide), a useful strategy is to combine diuretics with different sites of action. Metolazone, because it is effective even in patients with substantial reductions in glomerular filtration rate, is often used in this setting[41]; and the combination of metolazone and a loop diuretic is the most effective approach to stabilizing refractory patients.[42] However, caution must be exercised to avoid severe electrolyte disturbances, and intermittent metolazone administration is preferred. The addition of low doses of spironolactone (12.5–50.0 mg a day) may also be helpful, even in patients receiving ACE inhibitors, although careful monitoring of K^+ is essential.

Because of the impressive results of the ACE inhibitor trial and the desire to avoid hypotension and renal dysfunction while administering these agents, many physicians are underutilizing diuretics. A noteworthy diuretic withdrawal trial demonstrated that a large number of heart failure patients require diuretic treatment, and that substitution of an ACE inhibitor is not usually sufficient.[43]

Positive Inotropic Drugs

Although there are many pharmacologic approaches to increasing myocardial contractility, most remain investigational or require parenteral administration[39] (see Ch. 55). Only the digitalis glycosides are discussed here, and the reader is referred to Chapters 43 and 46 for additional information on these and other inotropic agents.

The use of digitalis has engendered enormous controversy for more than 200 years, but well designed trials have now clarified its role. In patients with well characterized left ventricular systolic dysfunction and symptomatic heart failure, digoxin withdrawal has been consistently associated with clinical deterioration.[44–47] Deterioration was noted irrespective of whether patients were receiving background therapy with diuretics alone or diuretics plus ACE inhibitors. Although the withdrawal design may be biased in favor of the drug and cannot establish safety, the Digitalis Investigators Group (DIG) has resolved these issues.[48] In that study with nearly 8000 randomized patients with New York Heart Association (NYHA) class I–III CHF, digoxin treatment had neither a beneficial nor an adverse effect on all-cause mortality. There was a significant decrease in deaths due to CHF but a counterbalancing trend toward an increase in deaths ascribed to arrhythmias and acute myocardial infarction. The DIG trial, like previous studies, found that digoxin therapy was associated with a 28 percent reduction in patients hospitalized for CHF (from 32.5 percent to 25.1 percent). This benefit tended to be greater in patients with lower ejection fractions, nonischemic cardiomyopathy, more severe symptoms, and larger cardiothoracic (CT) ratios on radiography.

These data firmly establish a role for digoxin therapy in patients who have symptomatic CHF with reduced systolic function, and in those with atrial fibrillation and other forms of supraventricular tachycardia. Debate will continue concerning its use in patients with dilated cardiomyopathy and few symptoms and when it should be initiated in relation to other medications. In the latter regard, data support the use of digoxin in conjunction with diuretics alone or in combination with ACE inhibitors. Older studies, albeit anecdotal, convincingly show benefits of digoxin as the sole therapy.[49]

As this chapter is being prepared, two other positive inotropic agents are available on a noninvestigational basis for chronic oral therapy outside the United States: ibopamine in several countries in Europe and Latin America and vesnarinone in Japan. The efficacy of ibopamine was never convincingly demonstrated in placebo-controlled trials, and it has been found to increase mortality among patients with severe heart failure.[50]

Published results with vesnarinone suggested that this novel agent with multiple mechanisms of action had considerable promise in the management of CHF.[51] However, the recently completed VEST trial, which enrolled more than 3500 patients with NYHA class III and IV CHF not only failed to confirm these earlier results, but found that vesnarinone in the previously studied 60 mg dose *increased* all-cause mortality by 26 percent. This trial also provided no indication of improved quality of life to counterbalance this risk. These results suggest that chronic oral positive inotropic therapy with agents other than digoxin has little role in the management of CHF.

Intravenous positive inotropic therapy with dobutamine, and much less frequently with the phosphodiesterase inhibitor milrinone, is also used intermittently or chronically in end-stage patients. Controlled data with this approach are limited, but anecdotally it appears effective in mitigating symptoms and preventing hospitalizations, although it is likely that this treatment increases arrhythmias and mortality.[52–54] This approach is best reserved for bridging to transplantation or for patients who cannot be discharged from the hospital on conventional or nonparenteral investigational drugs (see Ch. 52).

Direct-Acting Vasodilators

It has been nearly three decades since the rationale for vasodilator therapy evolved from the recognition that cardiac performance could be modulated by altering its loading conditions and that vasoconstriction is a frequent accompaniment of chronic heart failure. During that period a wide variety of vasoactive medications have been investigated, and most have been found to produce acute, and in some cases sustained, hemodynamic improvement (see Ch. 44). However, among the nonparenteral direct-acting vasodilators, only hydralazine and several nitrate preparations have been shown to positively affect clinical endpoints. Indeed, the list of vasodilators that have not been effective or have had adverse effects is long and includes prazosin and other α-blockers, minoxidil, flosequinan, epoprostenol, and several calcium channel blockers.

The best evidence for a beneficial effect of direct-acting vasodilators comes from the V-HeFT studies,[55,56] which showed that chronic therapy with hydralazine 300 mg a day and isosorbide 160 mg a day increased exercise tolerance and prolonged survival. Symptom and exercise improvement were at least as great as with enalapril, but the latter agent was associated with a lower mortality rate. Because of the latter finding and the better side effect profile of ACE inhibitors, direct-acting vasodilators are used primarily in patients who are not candidates for ACE inhibitors or who do not tolerate them. Nitrates and hydralazine are also reasonable agents to add for patients who remain symptom-limited on optimal therapy with diuretics, ACE inhibitors, and digoxin, although controlled data are not available to support this approach.[57] Because mitral regurgitation is frequent in severe CHF and is afterload-dependent, hydralazine may be particularly useful when regurgitation is substantial.[58] Nitrate tolerance limits the efficacy of these agents, but its impact can be limited by ensuring a nitrate-free period of at least 10 hours.

The greatest interest has surrounded the use of calcium channel blockers to treat CHF, as these agents are both potent vasodilators and effective for other cardiovascular conditions. This subject is reviewed in detail in Chapter 48, but an overview of the results suggests that by and large these agents produce adverse effects in patients with symptomatic heart failure or severe left ventricular dysfunction.[59-61] An exception may be amlodipine, which improved exercise in one small study[62] and had a neutral effect on mortality in a large morbidity and mortality trial with the acronym PRAISE.[63] This trial enrolled 1153 patients with severe NYHA class III and IV CHF and ejection fractions of less than 30 percent. Overall, there was no difference in mortality between the amlodipine and placebo-treated patients, establishing for the first time the safety of a calcium channel blocker in patients with CHF. An interesting finding was that the patients clinically classified as having nonischemic cardiomyopathy had 45 percent lower mortality on amlodipine. Because this unique finding remains unexplained, corroboration from the ongoing PRAISE II trial in nonischemic cardiomyopathy is required before this drug can be recommended for the treatment of heart failure, but these results make it possible to recommend amlodipine for the treatment of angina and hypertension in patients with reduced ejection fractions or symptomatic heart failure.

Neurohormonal Antagonists

The major advance in the treatment of CHF over the past two decades has been the discovery of ACE inhibitors and their role in this syndrome. Although the use of these agents followed logically from the recognition that plasma renin activity and other components of the renin-angiotensin-aldosterone system are elevated in CHF, it is now clear that ACE inhibitors are effective even in patients with normal circulating levels of these hormones[64] (see Ch. 45). This discordance is likely explained by the importance of the tissue renin-angiotensin system, the inhibition of kinin metabolism by ACE inhibitors and resulting increase in prostaglandin levels and stimulation of endothelium-derived relaxing factor release, and the indirect sympathoinhibition mediated by reduced angiotensin II levels. It is also clear that the benefits of ACE inhibition go beyond their hemodynamic effects, which are modest compared to those of direct vasodilators and positive inotropic drugs.

The clinical benefits of ACE inhibitors on prognosis and symptoms have been demonstrated in a series of positive trials in patients with severe CHF,[7] mild to moderate symptoms (the original Captopril Multicenter Study, SOLVD, and V-HeFT-II),[8,56,65] and chronic or post-myocardial infarction asymptomatic left ventricular systolic dysfunction (SOLVD, SAVE, AIRE, and others).[5,6,16,18] These results indicate that ACE inhibitors should be administered to all patients with documented low ejection fractions, regardless of whether symptomatic CHF is present.

The few absolute contraindications to using ACE inhibitors in CHF are hypersensitivity or life-threatening angioedema (even if not precipitated by an ACE inhibitor) and hyperkalemia (uncorrected K^+ of more than 5.5 mmol/L). Moderate hyperkalemia or renal insufficiency with serum creatinine concentrations up to 3.0 mg/dl should not preclude ACE inhibitor therapy but does indicate the need for careful monitoring. ACE inhibitors can be initiated without difficulty in most patients, although the occasional excessive decline in blood pressure or occurrence of renal dysfunction or hypokalemia mandate starting at low dosages and careful monitoring. Patients at higher risk for these adverse effects are those with low pretreatment blood pressure (systolic pressure less than 100 mmHg), intravascular volume depletion, hyponatremia (serum Na^+ less than 135 mmol/L), baseline K^+ more than 5.0 mmol/L, and diabetes. In such patients, an initial captopril dose of 6.25 mg may be administered, and the blood pressure should be observed 1 to 2 hours after the dose. In other patients the initial doses can be higher (captopril 12.5 mg tid or enalapril 2.5 mg bid). Telephone follow-up to determine whether symptoms of hypotension have occurred is advisable, and renal function and K^+ should be assessed within a week. The doses should be gradually titrated to captopril 50 mg tid or enalapril 10 mg bid as tolerated, even if the patient has improved at lower dosages. Although ACE inhibitor usage is increasing, even among primary care physicians,[9] most physicians prescribe doses well below those shown to be effective in the trials listed above.

It is unclear whether the angiotensin II blockers are similarly effective, and adequate placebo-controlled trials with these agents have not been performed. Because many of the potential effects of ACE inhibitors are not mediated by reduced levels of angiotensin II, it should not be assumed that specific antagonists have the same benefits (see Chs. 45 and 55). Therefore angiotensin II blockers are not recommended for CHF, except as an alternative to other vasodilators in patients who are intolerant to ACE inhibitors (usually due to angioedema, severe rashes, or intolerable cough). There is no evidence that they produce less renal dysfunction.

The renin-angiotensin system is not the only neurohormonal system activated in CHF. In particular, there is increased sympathetic activity, which may play an important role in the progression of the cardiac dysfunction. The use of β-blockers in CHF, although counterintuitive, is not new (see Ch. 47). However, only recently have trials provided evidence of clinical benefit. Experience with three highly different agents[20,66,67] has now shown that chronic therapy consistently improves left ventricular function, as assessed by the ejection fraction, and prevents progression and hospitalizations. There are favorable trends toward mortality reduction in the CIBIS trials and with carvedilol, but the number of events are small and the carvedilol experience is only short term.

Clearly this is a promising new avenue for the treatment of CHF, but several issues remain unresolved. There is a suggestion in several studies that β-blockade may be more effective in patients with nonischemic cardiomyopathy,[66,67] but it has not been a consistent finding.[20] It is uncertain when during the course of CHF that β-blockade should be initiated. There is evidence that these drugs may be particularly effective in preventing progressive symptoms and left ventricular remodeling during early heart failure[19] (unpublished data) but also favorable results in moderate to severe heart failure.[20,66,67] Patients with decompensated heart failure or volume overload, however, are not candidates, as early deterioration is frequent. It is also uncertain whether all β-blockers produce comparable effects. Positive results have been reported with metoprolol and bisoprolol (both β_1 selective agents), carvedilol (a nonselective β-blocker with α-blocking activity), and bucindolol (a nonselective agent with vasodilating activity). Whether one agent is superior remains to be determined. Finally, given the impressive results with β-blockers, it is reasonable to query whether ACE inhibitors provide additional benefit. This question is important, as in the absence of an answer CHF patients are likely to be routinely treated with three or four drugs, and side effects or hypotension may limit the use of one or more of them.

As the use of β-blocker usage for heart failure widens from a limited number of investigators to inexperienced practitioners, several points must be emphasized. First, only stable patients should be started on these agents; it is not the therapy to add to the regimen of a refractory, hemodynamically compromised patient. Second, the initial dosages should be small—the equivalent of 2.5 mg metoprolol once or twice a day or one-twentieth the smallest pill available in the United States. Third, 10 percent or more of the patients deteriorate early, but many of these patients can be gradually titrated to target doses. In patients with severe symptoms and elevated filling pressures, a useful strategy is to increase the diuretic dosage at the time of initiating β-blockers.

SUGGESTED APPROACH TO THE PHARMACOLOGIC THERAPY OF CHF SECONDARY TO SYSTOLIC DYSFUNCTION

Figure 37-1 outlines a recommended approach to the pharmacologic treatment of CHF and left ventricular dysfunction, based on published guidelines and the authors' practices.[10,11,12,38] The severity of symptoms, shown along the base of the diagram, is the primary determinant of drug usage. Medications for which there is strong evidence of efficacy in the indicated group of patients are shown in solid-bordered bars, whereas promising but as yet unproved agents are shown in the dash-bordered bars.

In patients who are identified as having left ventricular systolic dysfunction (ejection fractions of less than 35–40 percent) without symptoms, the only proved therapy is an ACE inhibitor, which should be initiated in all such individuals. Data from the postmyocardial infarction β-blocker trials and studies with carvedilol suggest that this class of agent may have an important role in such patients as well[19] (unpublished data, Australia–New Zealand Carvedilol Study). Trials are required to determine whether one or the other or a combination of the two is the optimal approach. At this point it might be prudent to use

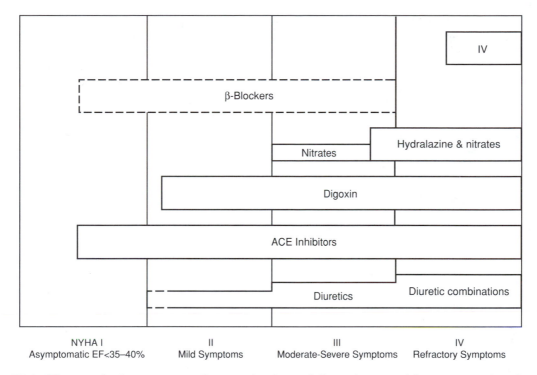

Fig. 37-1. Pharmacologic treatment of congestive heart failure. Agents with an uncertain role: A-II blockers, amlodipine, vesnarinone.

the combination in post-infarction patients: an ACE inhibitor for nonischemic patients with ejection fractions less than 30 percent (where these drugs have been more effective)[5,6] and a β-blocker, with or without an ACE inhibitor, for nonischemic cardiomyopathies with higher ejection fractions.

In symptomatic patients, initial therapy usually consists of a combination of diuretics and ACE inhibitors, started together or in sequence. A few patients with mild symptoms and no evidence of fluid retention may be managed with ACE inhibitors alone. Digoxin should be added if the patient remains symptomatic on these two drugs, although many clinicians utilize digoxin in all symptomatic patients now that its safety has been established. Patients who continue to be symptomatic on all three drugs (often referred to as standard triple therapy) may respond to increasing doses of diuretics or to the addition of a direct-acting vasodilator, such as a nitrate. With increasing symptoms (NYHA class III), more aggressive use of diuretics and vasodilators, including hydralazine particularly in patients with substantial mitral regurgitation, is appropriate. Advanced class III and class IV patients often require combination diuretic regimens, with loop diuretics supplemented by metolazone or spironolactone (or both). Patients

refractory to all of these approaches may benefit from intermittent or chronic intravenous inotropic therapy with dobutamine.

As indicated in Figure 37-1, the role of β-blockers remains unsettled, but data are adequate to support the use of these agents in patients with mild to moderate symptoms with the objective of preventing progression. Their role in severely symptomatic patients is uncertain, at least prior to full stabilization.

Several other promising agents with as yet undefined roles are listed at the bottom of Figure 37-1. The angiotensin II blockers are logical alternatives to ACE inhibitors in intolerant individuals, but they should be considered a second choice. In pilot studies the combination of ACE inhibitors and angiotensin II blockers has been tolerated and anecdotally helpful in occasional individuals. Amlodipine is promising for patients with nonischemic cardiomyopathy and might be considered an alternative to hydralazine and nitrates as a fourth line of therapy in these patients, but the data for β-blockers is more robust.

Cardiac transplantation has an important, albeit quantitatively limited, role in the management of patients with refractory heart failure. The selection of candidates and appropriate timing of transplantation are important issues but are beyond the scope of this manuscript. The reader is referred to Chapters 52 and 53 in which these topics are discussed in detail.

MANAGEMENT OF THE PATIENT WITH HEART FAILURE AND PRESERVED SYSTOLIC FUNCTION

The proportion of patients carrying the diagnosis of heart failure who are found to have preserved left ventricular systolic function (ejection fractions of more than 45 percent) is estimated to be 20–40 percent, and this percentage rises among the elderly[30–32,68] (see Chs. 25 and 39). However, before the clinical picture is attributed to heart failure, other causes should be excluded, including anemia, thyroid abnormalities, and pulmonary disease. Valvular abnormalities must also be ruled out. Intermittent ischemia often induces episodic symptoms and signs of heart failure without accompanying chest pain, particularly when underlying left ventricular hypertrophy or diabetes is present. Stress testing may be helpful when planning therapy for these patients, even if revascularization is not being considered. If all these explanations are excluded, amyloidosis should also be considered, albeit specific therapy is not available. However, after complete evaluation, most patients are not found to have a specific etiology but, rather, to have multiple contributory causes, including hypertension, left ventricular hypertrophy, diabetes, and coronary disease; and the symptoms are ascribed to diastolic dysfunction. The clinical presentation of heart failure due to diastolic dysfunction overlaps considerably with that of systolic dysfunction, although the former patients usually do not have severe symptoms and often have episodic heart failure. On examination they are less likely to have third heart sounds and usually do not have severe cardiomegaly.

Unfortunately, but not surprisingly in view of its multifactorial nature, heart failure due to diastolic dysfunction is often difficult to treat, even though it tends to carry a more benign prognosis.[68,69] There is no specific therapy for diastolic heart failure, although calcium channel blockers have been advocated.[70] In the absence of specific therapy, there are three primary goals of treatment: to reduce symptoms, to control hypertension and reverse consequent left ventricular hypertrophy, and to prevent myocardial ischemia.

Diuretics provide the most symptom relief if fluid retention is a feature. Thiazide diuretics are also the most effective therapy for isolated or predominantly systolic hypertension[14,71] and during chronic diuretic therapy tends to produce the greatest regression of left ventricular hypertrophy,[72,73] which is an important mechanism of diastolic dysfunction. Hypertension is not only the main stimulus to left ventricular hypertrophy in these patients; it also is a frequent precipitant of ischemia and therefore should be aggressively controlled. β-Blockers and ACE inhibitors complement diuretics well, and calcium blockers are another effective alternative. Central sympatholytics may also mitigate episodic hypertensive episodes. Nitrates have been found useful for preventing ischemia,[11] but they may cause dizziness and postural symptoms. β-Blockers and calcium channel blockers can also be used to treat ischemia. Because tachycardia is often poorly tolerated in these patients, the former agents should be used when the basal or exercise heart rate is excessive.

ANCILLARY THERAPY IN HEART FAILURE PATIENTS

Congestive heart failure usually does not present as an isolated problem, and a number of accompanying conditions complicate its management. Some of the more common and important issues are discussed below.

Treatment of Hypertension

Hypertension places an additional load on the failing heart, so aggressive treatment of hypertension is warranted. Indeed, patients with CHF often feel and do better when their pressures are at the low end of normal. Unless the patient becomes symptomatic from hypotension or develops renal dysfunction or angina due to renal or coronary hypoperfusion, systolic blood pressures of 90 mmHg or even lower should be accepted, although target pressures of 110–120 mmHg are reasonable. Drugs that lower blood pressure, such as diuretics, ACE inhibitors, and vasodilators, form the cornerstone of therapy for CHF. Therefore only rarely are additional antihypertensive drugs required. Central sympatholytics are effective; but given the most recent data on β-blockers (initiated at low doses) and amlodipine, they are the more preferable choices.

Treatment of Angina

When angina persists in patients with heart failure, revascularization is the favored approach in suitable candidates. Nitrates should be the initial therapeutic approach. Until recently other antianginal drugs were considered relatively contraindicated, but it is now apparent that the cautious use β-blockers and amlodipine are additional options.

Treatment of Arrhythmias

Both supraventricular and ventricular arrhythmias are common in patients with heart failure and often become difficult management problems[74] (see Ch. 49). In patients who develop atrial fibrillation, it is desirable but not always possible to restore and maintain sinus rhythm.[75] Poor rate control may exacerbate left ventricular dysfunction, and a coordinated atrial contraction may improve stroke volume. Unfortunately, the only medication likely to be helpful in this setting is amiodarone. Digoxin, directly or indirectly by improving the heart failure, appears to maintain sinus rhythm. There were significantly fewer hospitalizations for supraventricular tachycardia with digoxin in the DIG trial.[48]

Because sudden, presumably arrhythmic, deaths account for 40–50 percent of deaths in heart failure patients and because ventricular arrhythmias are an indicator of worse prognosis, the finding of symptomatic and even asymptomatic ventricular ectopy is often considered ominous.[74] Patients with symptoms suggestive of an arrhythmia, such as syncope or near-syncope, require careful evaluation. Those with demonstrated sustained or symptomatic ventricular tachycardia on monitoring or during electrophysiologic testing should be treated with amiodarone or undergo implantable defibrillator placement.[76,77]

Patients with asymptomatic ventricular ectopy, including moderately long burst of ventricular tachycardia, present a dilemma.[74] Although these findings may indicate a poor prognosis, there is no evidence that treatment improves this prognosis. Indeed, with the exception of amiodarone, most anti-arrhythmic agents are likely to increase mortality. Nor is there convincing evidence that electrophysiologic testing or other procedures such as signal-averaged electrocardiograms or heart rate variability can identify asymptomatic patients who are likely to benefit from drug or device therapy. Two trials have evaluated amiodarone in such individuals but unfortunately reached opposite conclusions. The Argentinean GESICA study found that amiodarone 300 mg daily prolonged survival and prevented both sudden and non-sudden death in a group of patients with severe CHF primarily due to nonischemic cardiomyopathy.[78] In contrast, a Veterans Administration cooperative study using a 400 mg daily dosage in patients with predominantly NYHA class II CHF due in most cases to coronary artery disease found no benefit, despite a significant rise in ejection fraction and successful suppression of asymptomatic ventricular arrhythmias.[79] The most likely explanation for these discordant findings is that the benefits of amiodarone may be conveyed by its β-blocking activity and be limited to nonischemic cardiomyopathy.[80] In any case, pharmacologic therapy for asymptomatic ventricular arrhythmias is not encouraged.

Anticoagulation

Although heart failure increases the risk of thromboembolism, there are no controlled clinical trials to govern recommendations for anticoagulation in the heart failure population. What few data are available have been summarized[81] and are reviewed in Chapter 50. Patients with atrial fibrillation are at particularly high risk and should receive warfarin anticoagulation. Anticoagulation is also recommended for patients with a history of thromboembolism and those with mobile intracardiac thrombi. However, the rate of arterial thromboembolism in patients who are in sinus rhythm is low, 2.0–2.4 percent in large studies. When this low rate is balanced against the increased risk of bleeding in these patients due to fluctuating liver function and their overall poor prognosis, anticoagulation does not seem warranted.

The use of aspirin in heart failure patients is also controversial. Most of these patients have underlying coronary artery disease, for which aspirin is often administered but for which evidence of efficacy for long-term therapy is limited. What makes this problematic is that there is a suggestion that aspirin may interfere with the benefit of ACE inhibitor therapy (see Ch. 50). At this time, aspirin is discouraged in patients with nonischemic heart failure and may not be appropriate in patients with ischemic heart disease who are remote from a myocardial infarction or unstable ischemic syndrome.

Important Drug Interactions

From the foregoing, it is apparent that CHF is a condition that requires polypharmacy. Because of its effects on renal and hepatic function, drug metabolism is likely to be abnormal. Thus care must be taken to avoid drug interactions and excessive dosing. The most obvious drug interactions are those that involve digoxin (quinidine and amiodarone) and warfarin (amiodarone). A more frequent problem is the interaction of ACE inhibitors with aspirin and other nonsteroidal antiinflammatory agents (see Ch. 50). The latter interfere with the benefits of ACE inhibitors but, more importantly, may act together to reduce renal blood flow.[82]

FOLLOW-UP OF PATIENTS WITH HEART FAILURE

Each of the guidelines recommend that patients be followed primarily by clinical assessments, including a quantitative assessment of the patient's activity tolerance and symptoms and careful physical examination. Serial testing procedures are discouraged because they are poorly reproducible and are insensitive to either deterioration or improvement. Exceptions to this recommendation include assessments for transplantation and the evaluation of findings such as new heart murmurs or abrupt changes in clinical course.

CONCLUSION

Congestive heart failure is a common disorder that is responsible for a large number of hospitalizations and physician visits. There have been important advances in the diagnosis and treatment of heart failure, but many have not been adequately incorporated into practice.[9] Guidelines have attempted to rectify this deficiency by providing clear recommendations in areas where data are available to support them. This chapter summarized the primary recommendations of several guidelines and has incorporated the results of many recent trials. Given the scope of the material covered, many important areas have received only cursory coverage. As a result, the reader is encouraged to follow the references to the many chapters in this book that provide comprehensive discussions on each of these topics.

REFERENCES

1. Massie BM, Shah NB: The heart failure epidemic. Magnitude of the problem and potential mitigating approaches. Curr Opin Cardiol 1996;11:221–6
2. Kannel WB, Ho K, Thom T: Changing epidemiological features of cardiac failure. Br Heart J, suppl. 2 1994; 72:3–9
3. National Center for Health Statistics: 1993 Summary. National Hospital Discharge Survey. Vital and Health Statistics. Series 13, No. 121. pp. 1–63. NCHS, Hyattsville, MD, 1995
4. National Center for Health Statistics: National Ambulatory Medical Care Survey, 1989 Summary. Vital and Health Statistics, Series 13, No. 110. DHHS publication. 92–1774. NCHS, Hyattsville, MD, 1992
5. SOLVD Investigators: Effect of enalapril on mortality and the development of heart failure in asymptomatic patients with reduced left ventricular ejection fractions. N Engl J Med 1992;327:685–691
6. Pfeffer MA, Braunwald E, Moyé LA et al: Effect of captopril on mortality and morbidity in patients with left ventricular dysfunction after myocardial infarction. N Engl J Med 1992;327:669–677
7. CONSENSUS Trial study group. Effects of enalapril on mortality in severe congestive heart failure. Results of the Cooperative North Scandinavian Enalapril Survival Study (CONSENSUS). N Engl J Med 1987;316: 1429–1435
8. SOLVD Investigators: Effect of enalapril on survival in patients with reduced left ventricular ejection fractions and congestive heart failure. N Engl J Med 1991; 325:293–302
9. Edep ME, Shah NB, Tateo I, Massie BM: Differences in practice patterns in managing heart failure between cardiologists, family practioners, and internists [abstract]. J Am Coll Cardiol 1996;27:367A
10. Konstam MA, Dracup K, Baker DW et al: Heart Failure. Evaluation and Care of Patients with Left-Ventricular Systolic Dysfunction. Agency for Health Care Policy and Research Publication 94–0612, Rockville, MD, June 1994
11. American College of Cardiology/American Heart Association Committee on Evaluation and Management of Heart Failure: Guidelines for the evaluation and management of heart failure. J Am Coll Cardiol 1995;26: 1376–1398
12. Johnstone DE, Abdulla A, Arnold JM et al: Diagnosis and management of heart failure. Canadian Cardiovascular Society Consensus Conference. Can J Cardiol 1994;10:613–631
13. Task Force on Heart Failure of the European Society of Cardiology: Guidelines for the diagnosis of heart failure. Eur Heart J 1995;16:741–751
14. SHEP Cooperative Research Group: Prevention of stroke by antihypertensive treatment in older persons with isolated systolic hypertension. Final results of the Systolic Hypertension in the Elderly Program (SHEP). JAMA 1991;265:3255–3264
15. Dahlöf B, Lindholm LH, Hannson L et al: Morbidity and mortality in the Swedish Trial in Old Patients with Hypertension (STOP Hypertension). Lancet 1991;338:1281–1285
16. Kjekshus J, Pedersen T: Lowering of cholesterol with simvastatin may prevent development of heart failure in patients with coronary heart disease [abstract]. J Am Coll Cardiol 1995;25:282A
17. Acute Infarction Ramipril Efficacy (AIRE) Study Investigators: Effects of ramipril on mortality and morbidity of survivors of acute myocardial infarction with clinical evidence of heart failure. Lancet 1993;342: 821–828
18. Ambrosioni E, Borghi C, Magnani B: The effect of the angiotensin-converting-enzyme inhibitor zofenopril on mortality and morbidity after anterior myocardial infarction. N Engl J Med 1995;332:80–85
19. Colucci WS, Packer M, Bristow MR et al: Carvedilol inhibits clinical progression in patients with mild heart failure. Circulation, suppl. I 1995;92:395
20. Packer M, Bristow MR, Cohn JN et al: The effect of

carvedilol on morbidity and mortality in patients with chronic heart failure. N Engl J Med 1996;334:1349–55

21. Marantz PR, Tobin JN, Wassertheil-Smoller S et al: The relationship between left-ventricular systolic function and congestive heart failure diagnosed by clinical criteria. Circulation 1988;77:607–612

22. Mattleman SJ, Hakki A, Iskandrian AS et al: Reliability of bedside evaluation in determining left ventricular function: correlation with left ventricular ejection fraction determined by radionuclide ventriculography. J Am Coll Cardiol 1983;1:417–420

23. Harlan WR, Oberman A, Grimm R et al: Chronic congestive heart failure in coronary artery disease. Clinical criteria. Ann Intern Med 1977;86:133–138

24. Ishmail AA, Wing S, Ferguson J et al: Interobserver agreement by auscultation in the presence of a third heart sound in patients with congestive heart failure. Chest 1987;91:870–873

25. Gadsbøll N, Høilund-Carlsen PF, Nielsen GG et al: Symptoms and signs of heart failure in patients with myocardial infarction. Reproducibility and relationship to chest x-ray, radionuclide ventriculography, and right heart catheterization. Eur Heart J 1989;10:1017–1028

26. Butman SM, Ewy GA, Standen JR, Kern KB, Hahn E: Bedside cardiovascular examination in patients with severe chronic heart failure. Importance of rest or inducible jugular venous distension. J Am Coll Cardiol 1993;22:968–974

27. Stevenson LW, Perloff JK: The limited reliability of physical signs for estimating hemodynamics in chronic heart failure. JAMA 1989;261:884–888

28. Chakko CS, Woska D, Martinez H et al: Clinical, radiographic, and hemodynamic correlations in chronic congestive heart failure. Conflicting results may lead to inappropriate care. Am J Med 1991;90:353–359

29. Dash H, Lipton MJ, Chatterjee K, Parmley WW: Estimation of pulmonary artery wedge pressure from chest radiograph in patients with chronic congestive cardiomyopathy and ischaemic cardiomyopathy. Br Heart J 1980;44:322–329

30. Grossman W: Diastolic dysfunction in congestive heart failure. N Engl J Med 1991;325:1557–1564

31. Goldsmith SR, Dick C: Differentiating systolic from diastolic heart failure. Pathophysiologic and therapeutic considerations. Am J Med 1993;95:645–655

32. Bonow RO, Udelson JE: Left ventricular diastolic dysfunction as a cause of congestive heart failure. Mechanisms and management. Ann Intern Med 1992;117:502–510

33. Mason JW, O'Connell JB, Herskowitz A et al: A clinical trial of immunosuppressive therapy for myocarditis. N Engl J Med 1995;333:269–275

34. Baker DW, Jones R, Hodges J et al: Management of heart failure. III. The role of revascularization in the treatment of patients with moderate or severe left ventricular systolic dysfunction. JAMA 1994;272:1528–1534

35. Bonow RO, Dilsizian V, Cuocolo A, Bacharach SL: Identification of viable myocardium in patients with chronic coronary artery disease and left ventricular dysfunction. Comparison of thallium scintigraphy with reinjection and PET imaging with ^{18}F-fluorodeoxyglucose. Circulation 1991;83:26–37

36. Dracup K, Baker DW, Dunbar SB et al: Management of heart failure. II. Counseling, education, and lifestyle modifications. JAMA 1994;272:1442–1446

37. Baker DW, Konstam MA, Bottorff M, Pitt B: Management of heart failure. I. Pharmacologic treatment. JAMA 1994;272:1361–1366

38. Massie BM: A personal perspective on the treatment of heart failure in 1994. Curr Opin Cardiol 1994;9:255–263

39. Massie BM, Shah NB: Future approaches to pharmacologic therapy for congestive heart failure. Curr Opin Cardiol 1995;10:229–237

40. Cody RJ, Kubo SH, Pickworth KK: Diuretic treatment for the sodium retention of congestive heart failure. Arch Intern Med 1994;154:1905–1914

41. Ellison DH: The physiologic basis of diuretic synergism. Its role in treating diuretic resistance. Ann Intern Med 1991;114:886–894

42. Kiyingi A, Mield MJ, Pawsey CC et al: Metolazone and the treatment of severe refractory congestive heart failure. Lancet 1990;335:29–31

43. Grinstead WC, Francis MJ, Marks GF et al: Discontinuation of chronic diuretic therapy in stable congestive heart failure secondary to coronary artery disease or to idiopathic dilated cardiomyopathy. Am J Cardiol 1994;73:881–886

44. DiBianco R, Shabetai R, Kastuk W et al: A comparison of oral milrinone, digoxin, and their combination in the treatment of patients with chronic heart failure. N Engl J Med 1989;320:677–683

45. Captopril-Digoxin Multicenter Research Group: Comparative effects of therapy with captopril and digoxin in patients with mild to moderate heart failure. JAMA 1988;259:539–544

46. Packer M, Gheorghiade M, Young JB et al: Withdrawal of digoxin from patients with chronic heart failure treated with angiotensin-converting-enzyme inhibitors. N Engl J Med 1993;329:1–7

47. Uretsky BF, Young JB, Shahidi FE et al: Randomized study assessing the effect of digoxin withdrawal in patients with mild to moderate chronic congestive heart failure. Results of the PROVED trial. J Am Coll Cardiol 1993;22:955–962

48. Results of the Digitalis Investigators Group Trial. Presented at Scientific Session of the American College of Cardiology, Orlando, March 1996

49. Christian HA: Digitalis therapy. Satisfactory effects in cardiac cases with regular pulse-rate. Am J Med Sci 1919;157:593–602

50. Results of the PRIME-II trial. Presented at Scientific Session of the American College of Cardiology, Orlando, March 1996

51. Feldman AM, Bristow MR, Parmley WW et al: Effects of vesnarinone on morbidity and mortality in patients with heart failure. N Engl J Med 1993;149–155

52. Liang CS, Sherman L, Doherty J et al: Sustained improvement of cardiac function in patients with congestive heart failure after short-term infusion of dobutamine. Circulation 1984;69:113–119

53. Miller LW: Outpatient dobutamine for refractory congestive heart failure. Advantages, techniques, and results. J Heart Lung Transplant 1991;10:482–487

54. Dies F, Knell MJ, Whitlow P et al: Intermittent dobutamine in ambulatory outpatients with chronic cardiac failure [abstract]. Circulation, suppl. II 1986;74:38

55. Cohn JN, Archibald DG, Ziesche S et al: Effect of vasodilator therapy on mortality in chronic congestive

heart failure. Results of a Veterans Administration cooperative study. N Engl J Med 1986;314:1547–1552

56. Cohn JN, Johnson G, Ziesche S et al: A comparison of enalapril with hydralazine-isosorbide dinitrate in the treatment of chronic congestive heart failure. N Engl J Med 1991;325:303–310

57. Massie BM, Packer M, Hanlon JT, Combs DT: Combined captopril and hydralazine therapy for refractory heart failure. A feasible and efficacious regimen. J Am Coll Cardiol 1983;2:338–345

58. Haeusslein EA, Greenberg BH, Massie BM: The influence of mitral regurgitation on the hemodynamic response to vasodilators in chronic congestive heart failure. Chest 1991;100:1312–1315

59. Packer M: Pathophysiologic mechanisms underlying the adverse effects of calcium channel-blocking drugs in patients with chronic heart failure. Circulation, suppl. IV 1989;80:59–67

60. Elkayam U, Amin J, Mehra A et al: A prospective, randomized, double-blind, crossover study to compare the efficacy and safety of chronic nifedipine therapy with that of isosorbide dinitrate and their combination in the treatment of chronic congestive heart failure. Circulation 1990;82:1954–1961

61. Goldstein RE, Boccuzzi SJ, Cruess D, Nattel S: Diltiazem increase late-onset congestive heart failure in post-infarction patients with early reduction in ejection fraction. Circulation 1991;83:52–60

62. Packer M, Nicod P, Khandheria BR et al: Randomized, multicenter, double-blind, placebo-controlled evaluation of amlodipine in patients with mild-to-moderate heart failure [abstract]. J Am Coll Cardiol 1991;17:274A

63. Packer M, O'Connor CM, Ghali JK et al: Effect of amlodipine on morbidity and mortality in severe chronic heart failure. N Engl J Med (in press)

64. Massie BM, Amidon T: Angiotensin converting enzyme inhibitor therapy for congestive heart failure. Rationale, results, and current recommendations. pp. 380–399. In Hosenpud JD, Greenberg BH (eds): Congestive Heart Failure. Springer-Verlag, New York, 1993

65. Captopril Multicenter Research Group: A placebo controlled trial of captopril in refractory chronic congestive heart failure. J Am Coll Cardiol 1983;2:755–763

66. Waagstein F, Bristow MR, Swedberg K et al: Beneficial effects of metoprolol in idiopathic dilated cardiomyopathy. Lancet 1993;342:1441–1446

67. CIBIS Investigators and Committees: A randomized trial of β-blockade in heart failure. The Cardiac Insufficiency Bisoprolol Study (CIBIS). Circulation 1994;90:1765–1773

68. Vasan RS, Benjamin EJ, Levy D: Prevalence, clinical features and prognosis of diastolic heart failure. An epidemiologic perspective. J Am Coll Cardiol 1995;26:1565–1574

69. Cohn JN, Johnson GR, Shabetai R et al: Ejection fraction, peak exercise oxygen consumption, cardiothora-cic ratio, ventricular arrhythmias, and plasma norepinephrine as determinants of prognosis in heart failure. The V-HeFT VA Cooperative Studies Group. Circulation, suppl. VI 1993;87:5–16

70. Setaro JF, Zaret BL, Schulman DS, Black HR, Soufer R: Usefulness of verapamil for congestive heart failure associated with abnormal left ventricular diastolic filling and normal left ventricular systolic performance. Am J Cardiol 1990;66:981–986

71. MRC Working Party: Medical Research Council trial of treatment of hypertension in older adults. Principal results. BMJ 1992;304:405–412

72. Liebson PR, Grandits GA, Dianzumba S et al: Comparison of five antihypertensive monotherapies and placebo for change in left ventricular mass in patients receiving nutritional-hygienic therapy in the Treatment of Mild Hypertension Study (TOMHS). Circulation 1995;91:698–706

73. Gottdiener JS, Reda DJ, Massie BM et al: Effect of single-drug therapy on reduction of left ventricular mass in mild to moderate hypertension. Comparison of 6 antihypertensive agents with placebo. Circulation (in press)

74. Stevenson WG: Mechanisms and management of arrhythmias in heart failure. Curr Opin Cardiol 1995;10:274–281

75. Chun SH, Sager PT, Stevenson WG et al: Long-term efficacy of amiodarone for the maintenance of normal sinus rhythm in patients with refractory atrial fibrillation or flutter. Am J Cardiol 1995;76:47–50

76. Stevenson WG, Stevenson LW, Middlekauff HR, Saxon LA: Sudden death prevention in patients with advanced ventricular dysfunction. Circulation 1993;88:2953–2961

77. Saxon LA, Wiener I, DeLurgio DB et al: Implantable defibrillators for high-risk patients with heart failure who are awaiting cardiac transplantation. Am Heart J 1995;130:501–506

78. Doval HC, Nul DR, Grancelli HO et al: Randomised trial of low-dose amiodarone in severe congestive heart failure. Grupo de Estudio de la Sobrevida en la Insuficiencia Cardiaca en Argentina (GESICA). Lancet 1994;344:493–498

79. Singh SN, Fletcher RD, Fisher SG et al: Amiodarone in patients with congestive heart failure and asymptomatic ventricular arrhythmia. Survival Trial of Antiarrhythmic Therapy in Congestive Heart Failure. N Engl J Med 1995;333:77–82

80. Massie BM, Fisher SG, Radford M et al: Effect of amiodarone on clinical status and left ventricular function in patients with congestive heart failure. Circulation 1996;93:2318–34

81. Baker DW, Wright RF: Management of heart failure. IV. Anticoagulation for patients with heart failure due to left ventricular systolic dysfunction. JAMA 1994;272:1614–1618

82. Packer M: Interaction of prostaglandins and angiotensin II in the modulation of renal function in congestive heart failure. Circulation, suppl. I 1988;77:64–73

38 Pediatric Heart Failure: Pathophysiology, Clinical Presentation and Treatment

Andrew N. Redington

The clinical syndrome of heart failure is difficult to define precisely in adults, and it is even more so in pediatric practice. Cellular metabolic disease, structural myocardial disease, congenital malformations of the heart and great arteries with consequent pressure and volume overload, cyanosis, myocardial ischemia, arrhythmia, and the effects of surgery can occur alone or coexist. Furthermore, each may have different implications for the developing myocardium when compared to its adult counterpart. Indeed, it is only with the knowledge of the developmental aspects of the myocardium and pulmonary and systemic beds that the etiology, clinical presentation, and therapy can be understood.

MYOCARDIAL DEVELOPMENT

The physiologic changes in the circulation at birth are the greatest to which the body could be exposed. Transition from the fetal circulation to the normal postnatal circulation is associated with abrupt changes in the loading conditions of the heart. At the first breath, the right ventricular afterload falls precipitously and continues to fall over the first few postnatal weeks. Conversely, the low resistance placental bed is removed from the systemic circulation, and left ventricular afterload increases severalfold. Not surprisingly, then, the left ventricular mass increases, and the right ventricular mass decreases relative to body weight during the first few weeks of postnatal life.[1] It is now fairly well established that the increase in left ventricular mass is related not only to an increase in cell size but also to cell hyper-

plasia.[2] Just how long the myocardium has the capacity for cell division remains uncertain, however. Myocyte growth does occur, with, the cross-sectional area of each myocyte increasing while the myocyte lengthens.[3]

The energetics of the myocyte are also rapidly changing. After birth there is a massive increase in mitochondrial volume, coincident with a change to oxidative metabolism; unlike in the fetal heart, the primary substrate for energy transfer changes to long-chain fatty acid. Intracellular calcium handling also undergoes a rapid maturational change after birth. The volume fraction of the sarcoplasmic reticulum increases[4]; and although not demonstrated in humans, there is an increase in calcium-sensitive ATPase activity after birth.[5] These changes go along with the clinical finding of an apparently greater sensitivity to exogenously provided ionized calcium in small neonates, particularly after open heart surgery.

There are also changes in contractile protein isoform expression. It is interesting that the right and left ventricles show little difference in isoform expression from fetal to adult life. Nonetheless, both ventricles show age-related changes in myosin light chains.[6] In the human fetal ventricle there is a light chain indistinguishable from that of the adult atrium.[6] It disappears, however, such that the normal adult ventricular myosin isoforms are expressed within a few weeks of birth. Going along with the changes in response to exogenous ionized calcium, there is a greater amount of phosphorylated tropomyosin in the fetal heart than in the adult heart. The mechanical implications of this change are uncertain but may be related to the increased myocardial lengthening rate required in the reduced filling time available in the relatively tachycardic fetal heart.

The mechanical properties of the myocardium also evolve during fetal and early ex utero life. Although there is a greater resting tension for any degree of stretch (i.e., ventricular compliance is lower), paradoxically ventricular filling is far more dependent on atrial systole in the fetus than in newborns.[7,8] Loss of the mechanical augmentation of atrial systole (during tachyarrhythmias, for example) can therefore lead to a profound change in cardiac output. Furthermore, the ability of the neonatal myocardium to develop tension is lower than that seen in the adult myocardium at equivalent resting length. Whether it is a direct reflection of cellular myocardial activity or an effect of a proportionately greater extramyocardial cellular volume has been speculated, the latter being more likely but difficult to prove.

The response of the myocardium to loading conditions also varies with age. Its response to inotropic stimulation is variable and may be related to changes in the arginine–nitric oxide pathway that occur during the first few days of life. Furthermore, the newborn heart has a relatively higher diastolic volume and, as mentioned earlier, poorer chamber compliance. Thus increased volume load or dilatation response to increased afterload (such as occurs with coarctation of the aorta) leads to a more profound increase in left atrial pressure than might otherwise be expected.

Finally, the cardiac output is exquisitely dependent on acute changes in heart rate.[9] Although chronic changes in heart rate can be well tolerated (as in the case of congenital complete heart block), acute cardiovascular collapse can occur at both slow and fast rates, and this sensitivity is inversely related to postnatal age. Thus supraventricular tachycardia with a heart rate of 250–300 beats per minute almost uniformly leads to heart failure if sustained in the neonate, whereas the same heart rate may be well tolerated in the same child at age 3 months.

EXTRACARDIAC ADAPTATION

Pulmonary Vascular Bed

The airless lungs of the fetus have a significantly greater resistance to flow than the systemic vascular bed. Inflation of the lungs at birth leads to an abrupt fall in resistance and an increase in pulmonary blood flow. This increased pulmonary blood flow leads to an increase in the left atrial pressure, which in turn leads to closure of the flap of the foramen ovale. Clo-

sure of the arterial duct is usually a spontaneous event occurring within the first few minutes to the first few days of life; hence the series-parallel circulation of the fetus becomes a solely series circulation. There then follows a variable decline in the pulmonary vascular resistance over the first few days or weeks of life. This natural reduction is obviated by many disease states. Birth asphyxia, structural heart disease, independent lung disease, and so on impose secondary effects on the pulmonary vascular bed. In the presence of a large ventricular septal defect, for example, the pulmonary vascular resistance may not reach its nadir until several weeks after birth. Thus the evolution of heart failure may have the pulmonary vascular resistance as its major determinant. Anomalous left coronary artery arising from the pulmonary artery is a perfect example. Although perfused with deoxygenated blood, symptoms do not arise until the pulmonary vascular resistance falls to a level that does not sustain coronary perfusion. Patients are rarely symptomatic therefore within the first 2–3 weeks of life.

Oxygen Delivery

The relatively low oxygen tension and obligatory mixing that occurs in the fetus leads to a relatively high hematocrit and a rightward shift of the oxyhemoglobin dissociation curve via the 2,3-diphosphoglycerate mechanism.[10,11] There is a normal fall in the hematocrit and hemoglobin concentration during the first few weeks of life, reaching a nadir at approximately 3 months of age. Coincident with this phase is a gradual change from the fetal hemoglobin pattern to an adult one. This normal maturational change is, to some extent, attenuated in cyanotic congenital heart disease but tends not to be the case in the infant with normoxic heart disease. Thus at the same time the left-to-right shunt is increasing in some of these patients the oxygen-carrying capacity and oxygen extraction ratio are decreasing. This "physiologic anemia" further compounds the hemodynamic effects of such conditions; unphysiologic anemia is therefore particularly important to avoid.

Duct-Dependent Circulation

The specific diseases that lead to a duct-dependent circulation are discussed in detail later in the chapter. Nonetheless, it is pertinent at this stage, when considering developmental aspects of heart failure, to outline this group of problems.

The persistence of an arterial duct in itself can lead

to heart failure. There are certain conditions in congenital heart disease whereby *closure* of the arterial duct leads to rapid onset and often severe or fatal heart failure.

The normal mechanism of closure of the arterial duct probably reflects a balance between the arginine–nitric oxide pathway and changes in prostaglandin synthesis. It is now well known that administration of indomethacin to the mother during pregnancy can lead to constriction of the arterial duct in the normal fetus. After birth this mechanism (blockade of prostaglandin synthesis) is used as a therapeutic tool to rid the often premature baby of an unwanted open arterial duct. As in most vascular structures, the nitric oxide pathway also plays a role. Inhibition of nitric oxide synthesis in the neonatal lamb leads to ductal constriction, independent of the prostaglandin pathway.[12] It is administration of exogenous prostaglandins, not nitric oxide donors, that are used therapeutically to maintain ductal patency.[13] Prostaglandins E_2 and E_1 have been used routinely and are approximately 10 times more effective than PGI_2 for example. Indeed, the use of prostaglandin to maintain ductal patency has probably been the most significant advance in the treatment of congenital heart disease since the early 1970s. With fetal diagnosis of congenital anomalies becoming ever more common, the prophylactic use of prostaglandins to avoid the adverse effects of normal duct closure in some cardiac lesions is becoming more widespread. Nonetheless, a significant number of patients present with a variety of symptoms upon closure of the arterial duct.

Patients with total or partial reduction of antegrade blood flow directly from the heart to the pulmonary artery (e.g., pulmonary atresia, severe tetralogy of Fallot) have so-called duct-dependent pulmonary circulation. In these patients the normal programmed closure of the arterial duct leads to decreased pulmonary blood flow and presentation with severe cyanosis; "heart failure," which is rare, occurs as a secondary phenomenon. More important, in terms of the current discussion, are those patients with a duct-dependent systemic circulation. By and large, these patients have hypoplasia of the left-sided structures (e.g., mitral atresia, aortic atresia, coarctation, or interruption of the aorta—see below). In these patients, normal systemic blood flow is supported by the right ventricle. Blood ejected from the right ventricle either passes to the lungs or through the arterial duct to the body. The pulmonary/systemic blood flow ratio largely depends on the pulmonary/systemic vascular resistance ratio which can be used to advantage for management of such patients (see below). Clearly, however, closure of the

arterial duct leads to a marked reduction in tissue perfusion. If there is an adequate-size left ventricle and potentially adequate left ventricular output (as in the case of simple coarctation), it is the lower body that is primarily starved of oxygen delivery. In such cases as hypoplastic left heart syndrome the entire body is hypoperfused. The physiologic consequences of this potential difference are minimal, however, because closure of the arterial duct under any of these circumstances can lead to severe acidemia, a feedback loop of worsening myocardial performance, and ultimately death. Thus even with simple coarctation, an arterial pH of 6.8 with a base deficit in excess of 20 is not unusual. This condition clearly has widespread, general effects despite potentially adequate upper body blood flow. Prostaglandin infusion, with consequent reopening of the arterial duct, can lead to prompt, satisfying improvement in these patients. Tissue perfusion and acidemia improve, myocardial performance recovers, and an advantageous feedback loop is established. The ability to stabilize a patient and correct the physiologic or metabolic abnormalities prior to surgical relief of the obstructive lesion has transformed the results of such surgery.

MECHANICAL/PHYSIOLOGIC SUBSTRATES FOR HEART FAILURE IN INFANTS AND CHILDREN

Left Heart Obstructive Lesions

Closure of the arterial duct in patients with left-sided obstructive lesions leads to one of the severest forms of heart failure seen in children. Table 38-1 lists some of the most important causes. Although most of these conditions present with identical symptoms, their implications may be different. Mitral atresia with the hypoplastic left heart syndrome is still considered by some to be an inoperable condition,

Table 38-1. Left-sided Obstructive Lesions Leading to Neonatal Heart Failure

Cor triatriatum
Supravalvular mitral stenosis
Valvular mitral stenosis
Mitral atresia/absent left atrioventricular connection
Subaortic stenosis (rare)
Critical valvular aortic stenosis
Supravalvular aortic stenosis (rare)
Coarctation or interruption of the aortic arch

whereas simple coarctation of the aorta can be surgically repaired with a low risk of morbidity and mortality.

Myocardial Dysfunction

Although secondary myocardial dysfunction can occur in almost any form, and may indeed be part of the definition of heart failure in neonates and infants, there is a long list of what might be considered primary myocardial problems that present during the neonatal period and childhood. Two major groups are considered: inherited cardiomyopathies and secondary myocardial diseases.

INHERITED CARDIOMYOPATHIES

"Hypertrophic" inherited cardiomyopathies are the commonest form. Some of these disorders are truly related to increased myocardial cellular numbers or mass, whereas others are related to the deposition of abnormal amounts of metabolic products, so-called storage disorders (Table 38-2). It is beyond the remit of this chapter to discuss each in detail. Suffice it to say that many of the inherited cardiomyopathies, particularly the storage disorders, are difficult to treat and tend to lead to progressive cardiac and extracardiac problems. The abnormal deposition of mucopolysaccharides, for example (Hurlers syndrome being the commonest), leads to progressive myocardial hypertrophy in some, valvular lesions with stenosis and regurgitation in others, and even sudden death due to obstructive deposition in coronary arteries in later years.[14] The hypertrophic cardiomyopathy associated with Noonan syndrome is also variable. Heart failure during the neonatal period with the need for transplantation has been described, whereas in others it may follow a benign course. Although superficially similar to familial hypertrophic obstructive cardiomyopathy, the long-term implications for sudden death seem to be different, being

much lower in the Noonan-related hypertrophic cardiomyopathy. In general, treatment of these abnormalities is expectant, as there are relatively few indications for specific treatment.

SECONDARY MYOCARDIAL DYSFUNCTION

Secondary myocardial dysfunction is far more common than the primary dysfunction described above. To some extent, there is an element of myocardial dysfunction with all forms of childhood heart failure. In this section we concentrate on the abnormalities related to decreased contractility, as the major determinant of symptoms (Table 38-3).

Birth Asphyxia

Birth asphyxia is probably the commonest cause of myocardial dysfunction.[15,16] It remains subclinical in many, but in others it can be an important clinical sequela of prolonged birth asphyxia. The causes of birth asphyxia are protean, but the effects on the myocardium are usually specific. Decreased myocardial contractility, particularly in the watershed area of the posterior wall of the left ventricle close to the mitral valve, is characteristic. The consequent rise in left atrial pressure leads to tachypnea and sometimes frank heart failure with pulmonary edema. When it is severe, myocardial infarction can occur with recovery being uncertain.[17,18] For most cases the problem resolves completely over the course of a few days, and only supportive treatment is usually required. Whether recovery is via metabolic adaptation or by myocardial cell division and replacement is unknown and is a question common to the sometimes remarkable recovery in myocardial performance seen with other conditions (see below).

Myocarditis

Neonatal myocarditis probably results from a transmitted viral infection during pregnancy. It can present with profound myocardial dysfunction, often requiring prolonged intensive care with ventilatory

---

Table 38-2. Some Inherited "Hypertrophic" Cardiomyopathies

Truly hypertrophic: familial hypertrophic obstructive cardiomyopathy, Noonan syndrome

Storage disorders: glycogen storage diseases, mucopolysaccharidoses, lipid storage diseases, respiratory chain abnormalities (inherited mitochondrial metabolic disorders)

Miscellaneous: endocardial fibroelastosis, hypothyroidism, hyperinsulinism

---

Table 38-3. Some Causes of Secondary Myocardial Dysfunction

Birth asphyxia
Duct-dependent systemic circulation (see text)
Myocarditis
Anomalous origin of the left coronary artery from the pulmonary artery
Miscellaneous coronary anomalies
Chronic tachyarrhythmia

and inotropic support. Its presentation in older children tends to be similar to the pattern described in adults. A preceding viral illness is common, but such is the frequency of these illnesses in children this is hardly surprising. A specific viral antigen or antibody response is infrequently isolated. Specific treatment is as uncertain for children as it is in adults. Immunosuppression with steroids and other agents has had mixed success. An innovation is the use of pooled immunoglobulins. In one nonrandomized study there appeared to be a temporal relation between improved myocardial performance and administration of this agent.[19] Subsequent anecdotal experience suggests that this therapy may have a role but is still experimental.

Anomalous Left Coronary Artery from the Pulmonary Artery

An interesting condition and of particular interest to adult cardiologists, anomalous left coronary artery arising from the pulmonary artery reflects possibly the purest form of myocardial hibernation seen in humans. This relatively simple structural anomaly can lead to major myocardial dysfunction; it is not due to the myocardium being bathed with deoxygenated blood (from the pulmonary artery) but to the decreased perfusion pressure that evolves during the first few weeks of life as the pulmonary vascular resistance and pulmonary artery pressure fall. Sudden death can occur, but the more usual presentation is progressive symptoms of heart failure.

Echocardiography reveals a grossly dysfunctional, usually incoordinate left ventricle. A left ventricular shortening fraction of less than 5 percent is not unusual. Associated papillary muscle dysfunction with mitral valve incompetence is a common associated feature. The most interesting phenomenon is the rapid response of the myocardium to reperfusion. Urgent surgery is indicated, which usually consists of reimplantation of the anomalous coronary artery into the aorta. If the immediate perioperative period is survived, dramatic recovery of left ventricular performance may occur within just a few days. A normal left ventricular shortening fraction can be achieved within 2–3 weeks of surgery. We and others have shown complete resolution of major wall motion abnormalities over the longer term.[201] Although poorly studied, it is compelling to think that such prompt and complete recovery reflects the metabolic hibernation of myocardium with subsequent restitution as the most likely mechanism.

Tachyarrhythmias

Chronic tachyarrhythmias can lead to decreased myocardial contractility. In some it is clearly the result of a feedback loop associated with deteriorating tissue perfusion, which is most commonly the case with neonatal supraventricular tachycardia, for example. These children, often with a heart rate of 300–350 bpm, develop a clinical spiral of increasing heart failure with decreasing tissue perfusion and consequent acidemia, followed by reduced myocardial performance. In others a more chronic and invidious effect on myocardial performance is seen. Chronic atrial flutter, ectopic atrial tachycardia, or long R-P tachycardia may be tolerated for many months or years. Ultimately, however, left ventricular contractile dysfunction occurs, the exact mechanism of which is uncertain. What is clear, however, is that restitution of normal sinus rhythm may lead to restoration of myocardial contractile function and is always worth persuing.

LESIONS ASSOCIATED WITH LEFT-TO-RIGHT SHUNT

There are many anatomic causes of a large left-to-right shunt in children with congenital heart disease (Table 38-4).

Atrial Septal Defect

Although the atrial septal defect is the exemplar of isolated left-to-right shunt, its long-term effects are so different from the rest of this group of disorders it is considered separately. The degree of left-to-right shunting across an atrial septal defect is related not only to its size but the downstream physiology. Relatively subtle differences in left and right ventricular inflow resistance can lead to major changes in the degree of left-to-right shunting.[21] Thus in the presence of abnormal left ventricular function or anatomic lesions affecting the left side of the heart, the left-to-right shunt tends to be large. An isolated atrial septal defect (be it a secundum, sinus venosus, or primum defect) is usually well tolerated. Even though the magnitude of the left-to-right shunt may be similar to that of a ventricular septal defect re-

Table 38-4. Causes of a Left-to-Right Shunt in Children

Atrial septal defect
Ventricular septal defect
Aortopulmonary window
Arterial duct
Aortopulmonary collateral arteries

quiring urgent surgery, symptoms are usually limited. "Heart failure," as such, rarely occurs before the fourth to fifth decade of life and is usually a consequence of progressive and marked right ventricular dilatation. Whether surgical closure influences the development of the long-term deleterious effects of an atrial septal defect remains controversial, particularly the case for surgical closure when performed during adult life.[22] Conceptually, however, it seems likely that early surgery, before the onset of right ventricular dilatation and arrhythmia, will prove to be durable in the long term, but it remains to be seen.

High Perfusion Pressure Left-to-Right Shunt

The remainder of the group listed in Table 38-4 are unified not only by a left-to-right shunt but increased perfusion pressure of the pulmonary vascular bed. This combination has two consequences: early onset of symptoms and the possibility of developing early pulmonary vascular disease. Their implications and management are therefore different from that of atrial septal defect. Symptoms are rare within the first few days or weeks of life, a consequence of the naturally elevated pulmonary vascular resistance seen at birth. The elevated resistance limits the shunting that can occur across these anatomic lesions, and the delayed fall in resistance associated with these lesions prolongs the clinical course. Ultimately, however, most of the patients, particularly when the communication between the left and the right side of the heart is large, develop symptoms of heart failure. The symptoms are progressive, mirroring the fall in pulmonary vascular resistance.

The exact cause of the heart failure, be it systolic or diastolic, has been poorly elucidated. In a study of left ventricular pressure dimension analysis, patients with ventricular septal defect and heart failure (characterized by tachypnea, growth failure, and hepatomegaly) were found to have reduced contractility, as measured by the slope of the end-systolic pressure dimension relation, compared with those without features of congestive heart failure,[23] despite treatment with furosemide and digoxin. This information is important as it has previously been suggested that systolic function may be within normal limits in these patients, and treatment with agents to increase contractility (e.g., digoxin) were thought to be inappropriate. The role of such therapy is discussed later.

Spontaneous closure of the arterial duct and smaller ventricular septal defects can occur, but most patients with a nonlimiting defect require sur-gery, which not only relieves symptoms but obviates the possibility of the development of irreversible pulmonary vascular disease. Paradoxically, the development of pulmonary vascular disease reduces the symptoms, and failure to recognize this situation as a potential cause of improvement can lead to disaster. Medical therapy for high pressure/high flow heart failure in these infants is reserved for those in whom surgery is not necessary or during the period leading up to surgical correction; it is considered later in the chapter.

VALVULAR LESIONS

Although rheumatic disease is now rarely seen in the West, the spectrum of stenotic and regurgitant cardiac valves is encountered in the congenitally malformed heart. The presentation and assessment of these lesions are not dissimilar to that for the corresponding adult lesions.

RIGHT VENTRICLE AS SYSTEMIC VENTRICLE

Several lesions, both pre and postoperative, lead to the scenario of the right ventricle as the systemic ventricle. In its classic form, congenitally corrected transposition with no associated anomalies results in the right ventricle acting exclusively as the systemic ventricle. Mustard or Senning repair (both atrial redirection procedures) of transposition of the great arteries is now rarely performed, although there is a large cohort of these patients who were repaired 10–25 years ago who are now entering their adult lives with the morphologically right ventricle acting as their systemic pumping chamber. These patients give us a better insight into this problem than those with more complex forms of heart disease, in whom perhaps the right ventricle is the only pumping chamber in the ventricular mass. For the sake of brevity, patients with this more complex morphology are excluded from the subsequent discussion.

The long-term concerns regarding the durability of the right ventricle to perform as the systemic ventricle in the circulation led to introduction of the arterial switch operation for transposition of the great arteries. These concerns, based on some of the long-term data available in patients with congenitally corrected transposition, may be misplaced. Congenitally corrected transposition can be diagnosed at postmortem examination as an incidental finding after death due to old age. Right ventricular failure can occur, but it is usually associated with tricuspid valve failure. The morphologically tricuspid valve may be abnormal in congenitally corrected transposition (e.g., Ebstein's anomaly of the tricuspid valve), and it is this abnormality, rather than primary myocardial dysfunction, that often results in symptoms.

Under the circumstances of the Mustard or Senning procedure, the morphologically tricuspid valve is rarely abnormal. Primary right ventricular myocardial failure is relatively rare during the first two to three decades after the procedure. Right ventricular volume at both end-systole and end-diastole tends to be increased; and the ejection fraction, both at rest and on exercise, is reduced in these patients.[24,25] Furthermore, the response of the right ventricle, in terms of its work–function curve, suggests a larger increment in end-diastolic pressure per unit increase in myocardial workload. Most of these patients remain asymptomatic for many years. Although maximal exercise ability is impaired in most detailed studies of exercise performance, submaximal exercise and the physiologic response to it is usually normal. Furthermore, longitudinal deterioration is difficult to demonstrate. There appears to be no relation between the length of follow-up after operation and the degree of right ventricular dysfunction. In one unique study, there was no change in exercise performance or the right ventricular ejection fraction in a cohort of older patients followed over an average of 5 years.[26] A small number of patients develop primary myocardial failure of the right ventricle after such repairs, however. There are some data to suggest that preoperative events may be just as important as the postoperative loading conditions under such circumstances. Evidence of myocardial damage prior to reparative surgery comes from the demonstration of preoperative myocardial isoenzyme release[27] and postoperative right ventricular wall motion abnormalities being present prior to surgery.[28]

Successful surgery for congenital heart lesions has only been available since the mid-1960s. The longer-term evolution of such problems requires documentation, particularly as additional acquired heart disease may develop. This area is a specialty within itself and is not discussed further here.

CLINICAL SYNDROME OF HEART FAILURE IN CHILDREN

There is no single feature that defines cardiac failure in children. Rather, it is a constellation of symptoms. Such is the diversity of underlying pathophysiology, it should not be assumed that heart failure represents decreased myocardial contractility. Indeed, for most, myocardial contractility may be normal or increased despite symptoms and signs of "heart failure."

Physical Signs

FAILURE TO THRIVE

The failure of normal somatic growth during infancy and early childhood has many causes. It is a frequent feature in the presence of important congenital heart disease. It almost certainly reflects the additional energy expenditure consequent to the other symptoms of heart failure and the failing circulation as a whole, but it is clearly exacerbated if the symptoms of heart failure lead to decreased caloric intake.

TACHYPNEA

Tachypnea is the most usual presenting feature of heart failure in children. Whether due to downstream obstructive disease (venous hypertension) or increased pulmonary blood flow (as with a left-to-right shunt), alveolar edema and decreased lung compliance are seen almost universally. In the neonate and young infant the generation of tidal volume is achieved less by chest wall movement and more by diaphragmatic excursion because of the more perpendicular orientation of the ribs with respect to the spine in the small child. Thus increased diaphragmatic activity is associated with indrawing of the intercostal muscles, sternal recession, and Harrison's sulci (indrawing of the lower part of the lateral rib cage). In older children, especially those with chronic symptoms, perceived shortness of breath is rare at rest. Recognized shortness of breath on exercise is more unusual and may become apparent only during the fourth or fifth year of life, when school activities expose it.

PERIPHERAL PULSES

The peripheral pulses may be normal. In the presence of significant left-sided lesions or any other problem that reduces cardiac output, the peripheral pulses are weaker; more importantly and particularly in younger children, a core-to-peripheral temperature gap is exposed, even at rest. High output cardiac failure is seen in patients with aortopulmonary connections (e.g., arterial duct, aortopulmonary window) and more rarely with aortic valve regurgitation. The bounding, or collapsing, peripheral pulse is a sensitive, specific sign in these patients.

VENOUS PRESSURE

The assessment of jugular venous pressure in small children is difficult, so a clinical surrogate is required. Pediatric cardiologists thus use hepatic congestion as a marker for an elevated systemic venous pressure. The pattern of enlargement can be used in a similar way to the pattern of change in jugular venous pressure. Pulsatility with atrial systole suggests decreased right ventricular compliance, or tricuspid stenosis. Systolic expansion goes along with important tricuspid regurgitation, as seen in Ebstein's anomaly, for example. Although conceptually one might imagine otherwise, it is also temporarily durable. The hepatic size changes over the course of a few minutes and promptly reflects changes in right atrial pressure. In older children the jugular venous pressure can be analyzed directly, in the usual way.

CARDIAC ENLARGEMENT

Some degree of cardiac enlargement is usual with childhood heart failure, but is a fairly nonspecific sign. A right ventricular impulse is more specific and is seen whenever there is important associated right ventricular dilatation or hypertrophy.

HEART SOUNDS

The pediatric cardiologists' near obsession with the pulmonary component of the second heart sound is justified. Its presence and intensity as well as its relation to the aortic component of the second heart sound, are important, relatively specific markers of disease. Indeed, much of clinical decision making regarding the need for closure of a ventricular septal defect, for example, is based on the intensity of the pulmonary component to the second heart sound accentuation, reflecting elevated pulmonary arterial diastolic pressure. No one piece of information is taken in isolation; and if in doubt, cardiac catheterization is indicated. Nonetheless, for most cases it is a reliable clinical sign.

The presence of a gallop rhythm can be difficult to interpret. In the presence of a heart rate above 150 bpm (which is not unusual in an ill child for any reason), it may be difficult to distinguish the physiologic third heart sound of the normal heart from a summation or fourth heart sound of the abnormal one.

MURMURS

The diagnosis and assessment of heart failure rarely rests on the presence or absence of a heart murmur. The underlying cause may of course be diagnosable from typical physical signs, including a heart murmur. This subject is not discussed further.

PERIPHERAL EDEMA

Peripheral edema is a remarkably uncommon feature of heart failure in children. It is occasionally seen in association with pleural effusions and ascites when there is severe right ventricular diastolic dysfunction or in more complex cases such as in children after a Fontan operation (atrio- or veno-pulmonary connection). Indeed, the presence of peripheral edema suggests a problem other than that of the heart when seen in children (e.g., nephrotic syndrome), such is its rarity in association with congenital heart lesions.

INVESTIGATION OF HEART FAILURE IN CHILDREN

Chest Radiography

Occasionally the chest radiograph is pathognomonic of the underlying structural lesion (e.g., supracardiac total anomalous pulmonary venous congestion) causing heart failure. More usually, nonspecific cardiac enlargement with pulmonary vascular changes is seen. It is possible to distinguish between pulmonary venous and pulmonary arteriolar enlargement but may be difficult particularly as they are so frequently seen together.

Electrocardiography

It is beyond the scope of this chapter to describe all the maturational changes in the electrocardiogram (ECG) that occur during the first weeks, months, and years of life. Suffice it to say that changes in the normal maturational pattern occur with significant congenital anomalies. Unexpected chamber dominance for age may be an important clue to the underlying problem. More specific features are also seen. Ischemia with ST segment depression or even elevation is frequently seen with the myocardial dysfunction associated with asphyxia. Similarly ST segment changes, and even transient Q waves are seen with the reversible ischemia of anomalous left coronary artery arising from the pulmonary artery (see above). Finally, the underlying arrhythmic cause of heart failure, be it acute or chronic, may be apparent on the 12-lead ECG.

Cross-Sectional Echocardiography with Doppler Studies

The practice of pediatric cardiology has been transformed by cross-sectional echocardiographic screening for structural lesions. It is also widely used to assess myocardial performance. Today most of the lesions described in Tables 38-1 to 38-4 can be diagnosed using echocardiographic imaging alone. Diagnostic cardiac catheterization for structural lesions is rare. The size and physiologic implications of these structural lesions can also be readily assessed. Thus with a combination of imaging and Doppler evaluation it is usually possible to assess the potential impact of a ventricular septal defect and the possible later need for surgery, even in the newborn without symptoms. Evaluation of progression of lesions is also almost exclusively performed by a combination of cross-sectional echocardiography and Doppler studies. The size of the defects, valve physiology, and the magnitude of shunting is now a part of the day-to-day routine evaluation of most defects, as it is for acquired heart disease in adults.

The direct assessment of myocardial performance and how it is affected by structural abnormalities has received less attention. Some of the methods developed for noninvasive evaluation of myocardial performance in adults can be translated to assessment of the smaller heart with congenital heart disease, but some cannot.

Systolic Myocardial Performance

Left ventricular ejection fraction remains the commonest index of myocardial performance measured using echocardiography. Its interpretation is more difficult in children because of associated abnormalities. Being a highly load-dependent index, left atrioventricular valve regurgitation, shunting through ventricular septal defects, and the presence of extracardiac abnormalities must all be taken into account.

To overcome this problem, less load-dependent derivatives have been developed.[29] The velocity of circumferential fiber shortening helps to distinguish some of the effects of a variable heart rate, but perhaps the most widely applied clinical and experimental method for assessing ventricular systolic performance in children relates the rate-corrected velocity of circumferential fiber shortening to left ventricular end-systolic wall stress. Although it requires measurement of peak systolic blood pressure, a calibrated carotid or axillary arterial pulse tracing, and simultaneous left ventricular M-mode recording, these indices have been applied to the assessment of

systolic function in a wide range of congenital lesions, both before and after operation.[30,31] One can argue the validity of many of the assumptions that are implicit in such an analysis, particularly when there is a congenitally malformed heart. As important, however, are the interpretation and relevance of such data. Sequential data are rarely available, and the long-term implications of a value recorded outside the 95 percent confidence limits is difficult to determine. Whether such measurements can be used to assess the value of surgical strategies or other therapeutic intervention remains to be seen.

Diastolic Function

Diastolic function is as difficult to assess as systolic performance of the heart affected by structural congenital abnormalities. One might argue that its relevance to symptomatology and subsequent therapeutic measures is greater. Ventricular filling in the fetus is most dependent on atrial systolic function. With increasing gestation and ex utero age this dependence becomes less. Nonetheless, loss of atrial systole and shortening of diastolic filling time can have catastrophic implications for myocardial performance as a whole. This explanation is the probable one for the cardiovascular collapse associated with supraventricular tachycardia, for example, where both effects are seen. Restrictive left ventricular physiology (again by obviating the atrial augmentation to cardiac output) is also poorly tolerated in young children. At this point it is worth remembering that, perhaps dissimilar to adult heart failure, the right ventricle (even when in subpulmonary position) may be equally important as a cause of heart failure in children. Extreme right ventricular systolic dysfunction is rare, but right ventricular diastolic dysfunction is common. The right ventricle may be too small (as in the case of pulmonary stenosis or atresia) or have abnormal diastolic physiology.[32] The manifestations of restrictive right ventricular physiology, for example, may be different from that seen when there is biventricular restriction. Thus unlike reports generated from adult populations,[33] the Doppler inflow characteristics of the restrictive right ventricle may superficially appear to be normal. Antegrade diastolic pulmonary arterial flow (which is possible to generate because of the low pulmonary vascular resistance seen when there is isolated right ventricular restrictive disease) may be the best marker of such physiology. Such abnormalities are only just being explored but have already been shown to be the single most important cause of low cardiac output and of right heart failure immediately after repair of tetralogy of Fallot.[34] The difficulties encountered assessing the right ventricle when it is acting as the systemic ventricle have already been alluded to. The issues are widespread but include the validity of use of measurements previously established for the left ventricle, the correct comparative group, and the relation of indices of ventricular performance to global performance (e.g., assessed by exercise function studies).

Exercise Function Studies

Because of age limitations, exercise function studies to assess global circulatory performance are restricted to children over the age of 7–8 years. Nonetheless, some important patterns emerge, particularly during the postoperative evaluation. After cardiopulmonary bypass, some degree of chronotropic incompetence (if defined by a lower than expected peak heart rate at maximal workload) is almost uniformly seen. The exact nature of this phenomenon is poorly understood, however, as chronotropic evolution during exercise is often normal during submaximal exercise. The same problem arises when one assesses maximal oxygen consumption. Maximal oxygen consumption after almost any form of congenital heart repair is generally reduced. The reasons for this reduction are multiple and have been related to ventricular systolic and diastolic dysfunction, residual hemodynamic abnormalities, and so on. Nonetheless, many of these patients are asymptomatic in day-to-day life. Again, the submaximal evolution of oxygen consumption can remain normal over a wide range. Indeed, with some conditions supranormal oxygen consumption and cardiac output are seen at submaximal workloads even after complete repair of the congenital heart defect. It is likely therefore that metabolic mechanisms that have evolved prior to surgery may take many years to resolve afterward.

All of these features must be taken into account when assessing global circulatory performance in children. The additional effects of age, somatic growth, puberty, and other neurohumeral changes are further confounding factors. Single point analysis, comparing an individual at a fixed point in time against expected normal ranges is therefore discouraged. The value of exercise testing is more relevant to the sequential analysis of an individual's performance.

TREATMENT

As for any other heart disease, if heart failure is related to an anatomic problem, relief of the anatomic problem is the primary treatment. This point is particularly important in children with congenital heart disease. Nonetheless, there are situations where medical therapy is required both before and after surgical intervention. To some extent, the treatment of dilated cardiomyopathy in a child follows the broad principles established for dilated cardiomyopathy in the adult; these aspects are not explored in detail here. More important is the physiologic consequences of treatment for children with specific congenital heart disease. In general, the amount of data available on which to base decision making is sparse, and the exact roles of the various agents available are unconfirmed by large randomized studies. Nonetheless, many classes of drugs are used to treat heart failure in children.

Developmental Considerations

ABSORPTION

The absorption of enterally administered drugs may vary considerably over the first few weeks and months of life. At birth the gastric pH is near neutral, but it falls to normal within a few hours of life. Other gastric secretions evolve more slowly. Absolute hydrogen ion secretion and pepsin and intrinsic factor levels increase during the first 3 months of life, and pancreatic exocrine activity reaches adult levels by the end of the first year. Peristalsis is also variable in neonates but reaches adult rates by the second half of the first year.

With heart failure, gastric emptying and peristalsis may be reduced, and vomiting and possetting are more likely. All of these factors may influence the absorption and distribution of orally administered drugs.

DRUG DISTRIBUTION

Infants and children have a greater body weight/fat ratio than adults. The water concentration of neonatal adipose tissue, for example, is approximately twice that of adults. The volume of distribution of water-soluble drugs is therefore greater in children. Protein binding by drugs is affected by the presence of fetal albumin, total serum albumin, globulin, and protein concentrations, and their binding sites and affinity. All of these factors change in the presence of malnutrition and the natural evolution of protein levels. For example, normal adult albumin and total protein-binding capacity increases to reach adult levels by about the first birthday.

DRUG METABOLISM AND ELIMINATION

Phase one reactions—oxidation, reduction, hydrolysis, and hydroxylation—mature rapidly within the first few weeks of life. Phase two reactions, in the liver—glucuronidation, sulfation, and acetylation—may remain relatively immature until about age 5 years. Thus the hepatic modification of many drugs may be different from that of adults. The maturation of renal function, similarly, does not follow a uniform pattern. Tubular reabsorption is probably normal from birth, but the glomerular filtration rate gradually rises during the first few months of life. Finally, renal blood flow seems to have a narrower limits for autoregulation, particularly during the first few days of life, and so small changes in cardiac output can lead to large changes in renal function.

Diuretics

The most common combination of diuretic therapy for this age group is a loop diuretic plus a potassium-sparing diuretic, as for adult heart disease. The mode of action in children is similar and the range of complications the same. Unlike adults, children are more prone to overdiuresis with consequent hypovolemia and renal hypoperfusion. Infants are at most risk because they are least able to adjust their fluid intake and most prone to fluid-losing states, such as diarrhea and vomiting. Hyponatremia is a particular problem in children, particularly young children, in whom low-sodium milk preparations may provide inadequate supplementation under such circumstances.

Aminophylline is used in some intensive care units as a diuretic. It enhances renal perfusion by renovascular adenosine receptor blockade, which may be particularly effective when administered with a loop diuretic such as furosemide. This synergistic effect of the two drugs probably acts by influencing autoregulatory mechanisms, which unhelpfully reduce renal blood flow when there is a borderline cardiac output, particularly in small children. The use of aminophylline is clearly limited by its potential effects on heart rate automaticity. Aminophylline and theophylline levels must be monitored if an infusion is given.

Digoxin

Digoxin increases the availability of calcium for myocardial contraction by inhibiting the sarcolemmal sodium-potassium ATPase (Na^+/K^+-ATPASE). It remains widely used in pediatric practice for primary myocardial disorders and heart failure associated with shunts, despite an almost complete lack of data to support any long-lasting hemodynamic effects. Changes in load-dependent, and load-independent indices of ventricular performance have been shown in infants and neonates with large left-to-right shunts, but little clinical benefit can be proved with digoxin.[35] With primary myocardial failure the rationale for its use is more conceptually understandable but equally poorly demonstrated in children.

The potential for digoxin toxicity also must be taken into account. Absorption is variable from the gastrointestinal tract, approximately 50–75 percent being absorbed from an oral dose. There is a wide individual variation, and drug levels must be measured whenever it used in children. Although infants appear to tolerate larger doses and higher levels of digoxin than adults, there are no data to support a specific dose regimen to achieve higher levels.

It seems remarkable that such a widely used drug has so few experimental or clinical data to support its use an inotrope or otherwise. It remains a highly effective drug for the management of supraventricular tachyarrhythmias, however; and this application is, for some units, its only currently established therapeutic role.

Vasodilators

Vasodilators are now frequently used to treat heart failure. Intravenous vasodilators (nitrodilators and phosphodiesterase inhibitors) are most commonly used on the intensive care unit in the acutely ill child with primary myocardial failure or after heart surgery.

The use of nitrodilators before surgery was widespread a decade ago. Because of effects on the pulmonary vascular bed, however, some drugs are detrimental, reducing systemic blood flow by increasing the left-to-right shunt.[36] They have largely been replaced by the newer phosphodiesterase inhibitors. Amrinone and milrinone are often used in North America whereas enoximone, an imidazole derivative, is more commonly employed in Europe. All of these drugs undergo extensive hepatic metabolism, enoximone being metabolized to an active sulfoxide, which then undergoes renal elimination. This process must be taken into account when deciding on dosage.

Angiotensin-Converting Enzyme Inhibitors

The chronic administration of vasodilators has largely centered around the use of angiotensin-converting enzyme (ACE) inhibitors. Unlike digoxin, many publications show the benefit of ACE inhibitors for treatment of low output and high output heart failure in the presence of a left-to-right shunt.[37,38] In a small subgroup, ACE inhibitors can be detrimental, however. In these patients a differential effect on pulmonary and systemic vascular resistance is seen, whereby the pulmonary vascular resistance falls more than its systemic counterpart.[39] This reaction leads to an increased left-to-right shunt and decreased systemic perfusion, as with other vasodilators (see below). For most patients, however, the reverse is true, there being a relative reduction in systemic vascular resistance with improved systemic perfusion and a reduced left-to-right shunt.[40] There are few data for children with chronic primary myocardial failure or decreased ventricular performance secondary to previous surgical interventions. Nonetheless, in one study of its use in these patients, enalapril was particularly effective.[41]

Systemic hypotension can occur, particularly when there has been chronic diuretic therapy and hyponatremia. Overall, the dose of captopril is much higher than that traditionally given to adults; 3–4 mg/kg per day may be well tolerated, but particular care must be taken to monitor the use of these agents in children with renal artery stenosis or borderline renal function.[42]

CONCLUSIONS

The etiology of heart failure in children has a wide anatomic and physiologic substrate. Unlike in adult practice, ischemic cardiomyopathy is rare and high output failure common. There are clearly marked individual variations as well as major superimposed effects of developmental changes. There is also a remarkable lack of data available regarding the effectiveness of medical therapy. Nonetheless, because of the impact of surgical and nonsurgical techniques on reducing or closing shunts, the implications for heart failure in children are much less sinister than chronic heart failure in adults. There remains a small proportion of patients with primary or secondary myocardial dysfunction, however. The specific information available for the role of treatment and even assessment of myocardial failure in these children is limited.

REFERENCES

1. Anversa P, Olivetti G, Loud AV: Morphometric study of early postnatal development in the left and right ventricular myocardium of the rat. I. Hypertrophy, hyperplasia and binucleation of myocytes. Circ Res 1980; 46:495–502

2. Korecky B, Rakusan K: Normal and hypertrophic growth of the rat heart. Changes in cell dimensions and number. Am J Physiol 1978;234:H123–H128

3. Legatto MJ: Cellular mechanisms of normal growth in the mammalian heart. II. A quantitative comparison between the right and left ventricular myocytes in the dog from birth to five months of age. Circ Res 1979; 44:263–279

4. Page E, Buecker JL: Development of dyadic junctional complexes between sarcoplasmic reticulum and plasmalemma in rabbit left ventricular myocardial cells. Morphometric analysis. Circ Res 1981;48:519–522

5. Nayler WG, Fassold E: Calcium accumulation and ATPase activity of cardiac sarcoplasmic reticulum before and after birth. Cardiovasc Res 1977;11:231–237

6. Price KM, Littler WA, Cummins P: Human atrial and ventricular myosin light-chain subunits in the adult and during development. Biochem J 1980;191: 571–580

7. Davies P, Dewar J, Tynan M, Ward R: Post-natal development changes in the length-tension relationship of cat papillary muscles. J Physiol (Lond) 1975;253: 95–102

8. Friedman WF: The intrinsic physiologic properties of the developing heart. Prog Cardiovasc Dis 1972;15: 87–111

9. Anderson PAW, Glick KL, Killam AP, Mainwaring RD: The effect of heart rate on in utero left ventricular output in the fetal sheep. J Physiol (Lond) 1986;372: 557–573

10. Versmold HT, Linderkamp O, Dohlemann C et al: Oxygen transport in congenital heart disease. Influence of fetal haemoglobin, red cell pH and 2,3-diphosphoglycerate. Pediatr Res 1976;10:566–570

11. Berman W Jr, Woods SC, Yabek SM et al: Systemic oxygen transport in patients with congenital heart disease. Circulation 1987;75:360–368

12. Abrams SE, Walsh KP, Diamond M, Clarkson MJ, Coker SJ: Nitric oxide is a potential arterial duct dilator in neonatal lambs [abstract]. Br Heart J, suppl. 1994;71:P63

13. Heymann MA: Pharmacologic use of prostaglandin E_1 in infants with congenital heart disease. Am Heart J 1981;101:837–843

14. Gatzoulis MA, Vellodi A, Redington AN: Cardiac involvement in mucopolysaccharidoses. Effects of allogenic bone marrow transplant. Arch Dis Child 1995;73: 259–260

15. Rowe RD, Hoffman T: Transient myocardial ischemia of the newborn infant. A form of severe cardiorespiratory distress in full-term infants. J Pediatr 1981;97: 243–250

16. Burnard ED, James LS: Failure of the heart after undue asphyxia at birth. Pediatrics 1961;28:545–565

17. Finley JP, Howman-Giles RB, Gilday DL, Bloom KR, Rowe RD: Transient myocardial ischemia of the newborn infant demonstrated by thallium myocardial imaging. J Pediatr 1979;94:263–270

18. Donnelly WH, Bucciarelli RL, Nelson RM: Ischemic papillary muscle necrosis in stressed newborn infants. J Pediatr 1980;96:295–200

19. Drucker NA, Colan SD, Lewis AB et al: Gamma-globulin treatment of acute myocarditis in the paediatric population. Circulation 1994;89:252–257

20. Carvalho JS, Redington AN, Oldershaw PJ et al: Analysis of left ventricular wall motion before and after reimplantation of anomalous left coronary artery in infancy. Br Heart J 1991;65:218–222

21. Manning PB, Mayer JE, Snaders SP et al: Unique features and prognosis of primum ASD presenting in the first year of life. Circulation 1994;90:30–35

22. Konstantinides S, Glebel A, Olschewski M et al: Comparison of surgical and medical therapy for atrial septal defect in adults. N Engl J Med 1995;333:469–473

23. Stewart JM, Hintze TH, Woolf PK et al: Nature of heart failure in patients with ventricular septal defect. Am J Physiol 1995;269:(Heart Circ Physiol 38): H1473–H1480

24. Graham TP, Atwood GF, Boucek RJ, Boerth RC, Bender HW: Abnormalities of right ventricular function following Mustard's operation for transposition of the great arteries. Circulation 1975;52:678–684

25. Arciniegas E, Farooki ZQ, Hakimi M, Perry BL, Gree E: Results of the Mustard operation for dextro-transposition of the great arteries. J Thorac Cardiovasc Surg 1981;81:580–585

26. Wong KY, Venables AW, Kelly MJ, Kalff V: Longitudinal study of ventricular function after the Mustard operation for transposition of the great arteries. A long-term follow-up. Br Heart J 1988;60:316–323

27. Boucek TP: Myocardial injury in infants with congenital heart disease. Evaluation by creatinine kinase MB isoenzyme analysis. Am J Cardiol 1982;50:129–134

28. Redington AN, Rigby ML, Oldershaw PJ, Gibson DG, Shinebourne EA: Right ventricular function 10 years after the Mustard procedure. Analysis of size, shape and wall motion. Br Heart J 1989;62:455–461

29. Colan SD, Barrow KM, Newmann A: Left ventricular end-systolic wall stress-velocity of fiber shortening relation. A load independent index of myocardial contractility. J Am Coll Cardiol 1984;4:715–724

30. Colan SD, Borow KM, Neumann A: Use of the calibrated carotid pulse tracing for calculation of left ventricular pressure and wall stress throughout ejection. Am Heart J 1985;109:1306–1310

31. Colan SD, Barrow KM, MacPherson D et al: Use of the indirect axillary pulse tracing for noninvasive determination of ejection time, upstroke time, and left ventricular wall stress throughout ejection in infants and young children. Am J Cardiol 1984;53:1154–1158

32. Redington AN, Penny D, Rigby ML, Hayes A: Antegrade diastolic pulmonary arterial flow as a marker of right ventricular restriction after complete repair of pulmonary atresia with intact septum and critical pulmonary valve stenosis. Cardiol Young 1992;2: 382–387

33. Appleton CP, Hatle LK, Popp RL: Demonstration of restrictive ventricular physiology by Doppler echocardiography. J Am Coll Cardiol 1988;4:757–768

34. Cullen S, Shore D, Redington AN: Characterization of restrictive right ventricular physiology after repair of tetralogy of Fallot. Implications for the early postoperative course. Circulation 1995;91:782–789

35. Redington AN, Carvalho JS, Shinebourne EA: Does digoxin have a place in the treatment of congenital heart disease? Cardiovasc Drugs Ther 1989;3:21–24

36. Beekman RH, Rocchini AP, Rosenthal A: Haemodynamic effects of hydralazine in infants with a large ventricular septal defect. Circulation 1982;65: 523–528

37. Friedman WF, George BL: Treatment of congestive heart failure by altering loading conditions of the heart. J Pediatr 1985;106:697–706

38. Artman M, Graham TP: Guidelines for vasodilator therapy of congestive heart failure in infants and children. Am Heart J 1987;113:994–1005

39. Boucek MM, Chang RL: Effects of captopril on the distribution of left ventricular output with ventricular septal defect. Pediatr Res;24:499–503

40. Frenneaux M, Stewart RAH, Newman CMH, Hallidie-Smith KA: Enalapril for severe heart failure in infancy. Arch Dis Child 1989;64:219–223

41. Seguchi M, Nakazawa M, Momma K: Effect of enalapril on infants and children with congestive heart failure. Cardiol Young 1992;2:14–19

42. Leversha AM, Wilson NJ, Clarkson PM et al: Efficacy and dosage of enalapril in congenital and acquired heart disease. Arch Dis Child 1994;70:35–39

39 Heart Failure in Elderly Patients: Focus on Diastolic Dysfunction

Lip-Bun Tan
Stephen G. Ball

This chapter covers two conceptually different but clinically overlapping subjects: heart failure in elderly patients and heart failure due to diastolic dysfunction. This juxtaposition is neither arbitrary nor inappropriate. Heart failure is disproportionately a condition of older individuals (Fig. 39-1), with a prevalence in the United States of 1 percent at 25–54 years, 4.5 percent at 65–74 years, and 10 percent above age 75.[1] More than 80 percent of heart failure patients are 65 years or older, and they account for a disproportionate number of the heart failure deaths and hospitalizations.[1,2] With the widespread availability of noninvasive tests of left ventricular function, it has become clear that many patients with the syndrome of congestive heart failure do not have impaired contractile performance but, rather, presumptively have symptoms based on diastolic dysfunction.[3–5] Importantly, this latter pathophysiology is disproportionately present in older patients.

The two requisite elements for developing any treatment strategy are an understanding of the nature of the problem and the availability of treatment options. Available data covering these two elements in relation to the management of heart failure in the elderly population and diastolic heart failure are beginning to emerge but are still rather limited. In particular, there is a paucity of clear evidence from large-scale trials evaluating the efficacy of any treatment strategy in these two interrelated subgroups of the heart failure population. Furthermore, although an arbitrary definition of "elderly" may seem straightforward, the relation between "elderly" and "biologic age," which is more relevant to clinical practice, is not. The lack of a satisfactory definition of "diastolic heart failure" compounds the difficulties of discussing these topics.

Large-scale trials allow comparisons of various treatment strategies, and by far the simplest and most certain outcome to measure is mortality. However, in the very elderly population, mortality reduction may be seen more as delaying death than prolonging life. Many elderly patients with severe heart failure are less concerned with quantity of life than with quality of life and gaining symptomatic benefit. Studies on mortality reduction alone may therefore be less relevant. However, assessments of the quality of life provide "soft" endpoints, rather than the "hard" endpoint of death. Objective measures such as exercise time as surrogates of "benefit" are fraught with difficulties because many older patients are unable to perform exercise tests for a multitude of reasons unrelated to their cardiac condition. Such factors partly account for the scanty data available to us from clinical trials to determine treatment for elderly patients.

Appropriately controlled evaluations of therapy for diastolic heart failure are also scarce, and large-scale trials are nonexistent. Current methods for evaluating diastolic function are technically difficult to perform and more problematic to interpret. Moreover, in a large proportion of cases of left ventricular dysfunction, diastolic dysfunction is closely linked to systolic dysfunction.[4–7] Patients with pure diastolic dysfunction are not readily identified and entered

581

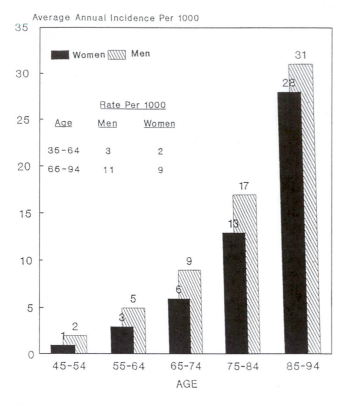

Average Annual Incidence Per 1000

■ Women ▨ Men

Rate Per 1000

Age	Men	Women
35–64	3	2
66–94	11	9

AGE

Fig. 39-1. Increased incidence of heart failure with age during a 30-year follow-up study in Framingham. (From Kannel and Belanger,[1] with permission.)

into studies. Often these patients suffer from multiple illnesses, such as diabetes, hypertension, peripheral vascular disease, angina pectoris, pulmonary insufficiency, and dementia, which may be more limiting and more lethal than the cardiac condition. Their cardiac prognosis is better than for those with systolic dysfunction,[3] which would dictate the need for both larger numbers and longer-term follow-up for comparable mortality trials. To date, no drug has been found that improves lusitropism without affecting the inotropic state of the myocardium.

PATHOPHYSIOLOGY OF THE AGING CARDIOVASCULAR SYSTEM

Even in normal individuals aging produces profound effects on the cardiovascular system.[8–10] The effects are exacerbated by accompanying diseases, such as hypertension, atherosclerosis, and diabetes, and are probably mitigated somewhat by regular exercise and moderate sodium intake.[11,12] Some of the most noticeable alterations occur in the peripheral vasculature, particular in the large elastic arteries, as evi-

denced by the rise in systolic blood pressure with age. The anatomic and histologic correlates of these changes include vascular hypertrophy, with increased intimal thickness, increased collagen content with altered characteristics, and elastin fragmentation. This process results in reduced vascular distensibility and compliance, enhancing the pulsatile load faced by the left ventricle during systole.

On an anatomic basis, the most consistent cardiac change with aging is progressive left ventricular hypertrophy, resulting from increasing wall thickness without an alteration in cavity dimensions,[10] which may reflect in part the vascular changes but is probably not fully explained by them. On a histologic and molecular basis, the myocardial changes are more substantial.[8,9,13] There is a modest degree of myocyte enlargement and increased collagen deposition. In animal models there are alterations in contractile protein expression and calcium handling. Another feature of the aging heart is the cumulative attrition of cardiomyocytes, resulting in an estimated loss of about 35 percent of the total myocytes previously present during early adulthood.[14,15] There are suggestions in experimental animals that cardiomyocytes can regenerate in certain circumstances,[15,16] but it is believed that the incidence is too low to be of any clinical consequence. Other changes in the heart include thickening and calcification of the aortic and mitral valves and subvalvular structures, which may lead to clinically significant aortic stenosis and less frequently mitral regurgitation.[8,17] Aortic root dilatation may lead to significant aortic regurgitation. Each of these changes can be exacerbated by chronic hypertension.

These changes in the cardiovascular system with aging are associated with several physiologic alterations that have important clinical ramifications during conditions of stress and disease. Although contractile performance is generally maintained at rest, it displays impaired responsivity to exercise adrenergic stimulation.[8,9,18,19] In contrast to systolic function, diastolic function and left ventricular filling decline with age.[12,20,21] These factors, together with impaired chronotropic responses with aging and changes in skeletal muscle,[8,9] are responsible for the progressive decline in exercise capacity in older individuals. Myocyte loss and impaired functional reserve also partly explain why elderly patients have a worse prognosis and are more vulnerable to cardiogenic shock after myocardial infarction,[22] why they have a poorer prognosis once they develop congestive heart failure,[22] and why they are more vulnerable to developing cardiogenic shock.

GENERAL STRATEGY FOR TREATING THE ELDERLY PATIENT

The overall objectives of treating heart failure include the relief of symptoms, thereby improving the quality of life (a major determinant of which is functional capacity), and the extension of survival. In elderly patients the former objectives are often considered more important than the last objective. It is usually, then, the quality of life and not longevity that is of paramount importance. Often the major goal in medicine for the elderly individual is to enable him or her to continue an independent and satisfactory life. In the absence of evidence indicating that any of currently available drugs, such as angiotensin-converting enzyme (ACE) inhibitors, or other treatment modalities are able to improve prognosis for those with purely diastolic heart failure, the treatment priority for this condition is essentially symptomatic benefit.

The cornerstone of therapy is identification of the primary and secondary defects that produce the syndrome of heart failure (Table 39-1). Identifying the primary defect is important because in geriatric medicine a large part of clinical management is palliative therapy. For instance, an elderly patient may present with severe congestion secondary to heart failure. A common tendency is to treat the secondary defects by using diuretics and vasodilators (preferably ACE inhibitors) with insufficient thought given to the primary defect, allowing an uncommon cause, such as pericardial constriction, to remain undiag-

nosed. Had this primary defect been identified and corrected, the secondary defects of fluid retention and vasoconstriction would resolve. A rational treatment strategy is based on a precise diagnosis (which may be more difficult to ascertain in the frail and elderly) and a good understanding of the pathophysiologic processes involved. The tendency to minimize diagnostic testing is misplaced, as these patients are often the most difficult to evaluate clinically and are more intolerant of inappropriate interventions.

Secondary defects, such as fluid retention and excessive vasoconstriction, are compensatory and adaptive mechanisms invoked to maintain as normal a cardiac output and blood pressure as possible in response to primary cardiac dysfunction; they are mediated by neuroendocrine activation. Together with the primary defects, they produce the symptoms and signs of heart failure. The tertiary defects are the detrimental effects produced as a result of therapeutic attempts (or failure) to treat the condition.

Treatment of Primary Defects

With congestive heart failure the primary defect must lie in the heart. The only definitive treatment for heart failure consists of removing the primary defect. Although it is usually not possible, a diligent search for reversible causes is important. Several of these causes warrant particular consideration in the older population. Two forms of valvar disease may appear without a history. The most common is cal-

---

Table 39-1. Defects Associated with Heart Failure and Their Management

Defect	Management
Primary	
Pump dysfunction	Establish cause and interventional remedy as indicated (see text)
Myocardial depression	Positive inotropic support, mechanical assist (in acute phases)
Secondary (via neurohumoral activation)	
Fluid retention and congestion	Fluid and salt restriction, diuretics, venodilators
Vasoconstriction	ACE inhibition, nitrates, hydralazine, losartan
Organ hypoperfusion	Inotropes or volume replacement if appropriate
Flow redistribution	ACE inhibition, low-dose dopamine, inotropes
Arrhythmia	Correct tertiary defects, treat myocardial ischemia, antiarrhythmic therapy
Tertiary (secondary to therapeutic attempts)	
Electrolyte imbalance	Monitor biochemistry, correct imbalance, potassium-sparing diuretics, ACE inhibition
Arrhythmia	Avoid proarrhythmic agents
Organ hypoperfusion	Decrease diuretics and vasodilators
Maldistribution of flow	Avoid α-adrenergic inhibitors
Progressive myocardial injury	ACE inhibition, avoid inotropes
Skeletal muscle deconditioning	Avoid bed rest, exercise rehabilitation

cific aortic stenosis, which may present with unexplained dyspnea or overt heart failure. Less frequent is mitral regurgitation of subvalvar origin due to ruptured chordae tendineae in patients with myxomatous mitral valves or degenerative disease. Echocardiography can exclude these diagnoses. Thyroid dysfunction can also present with signs and symptoms of heart failure. Acute heart failure with rapid atrial fibrillation is most common, although subclinical hyperthyroidism, even with maintained sinus rhythm, and hypothyroidism can also cause heart failure. Therefore thyroid function testing should be undertaken.

Other specific interventions of particular relevance in elderly patients include the discontinuation of cardiodepressant drugs, control of arrhythmia, insertion of pacemakers for complete heart block and severe chronotropic incompetence, revascularization for recurrent acute heart failure due to myocardial ischemia, aspiration of pericardial fluid, or stripping of pericardium in the presence of constrictive pericarditis. The most common defect causing heart failure is cardiac myocyte loss, as a consequence of myocardial infarction, myocarditis, cardiomyopathy, or senescence. There is as yet no definitive therapy for this type of defect. At present, therapy should be directed at preventing further loss of cardiomyocytes in order to stem the progression of ventricular dysfunction.

An important question about management is whether surgical intervention can help the patient. Investigations can determine if a surgical option is possible. The decision to proceed to surgery is dependent on establishing that the symptoms and objective functional impairment truly result from a surgically correctible defect. In elderly patients concomitant disease may be a major influencing factor. Immediate operative risks must also be weighed against potential improvements in symptoms and prognosis. The likelihood that a patient will return to the same, if not an improved, mental status and functional independence is an important consideration when undertaking major surgery. In general, however, although mortality and morbidity rates for heart surgery are higher in old patients,[23–26] they are acceptable in appropriately selected patients (6–10 percent among patients requiring isolated coronary bypass or valve replacement operations). Most patients have improved functional status postoperatively.[27]

The success of the treatment, be it surgical or medical, should also be evaluated objectively by how well cardiac function has been improved after the therapy. Improvements in cardiac function would be indicated by improvements in cardiac reserve, exercise capacity, and symptoms. However, exercise tolerance and symptoms are subjective endpoints and indirect indicators of cardiac function. They may not truly reflect changes in cardiac function after treatment. An objective indicator of cardiac function is cardiac reserve,[28,29] and evidence of such an improvement should be sought if feasible. Cardiac pumping reserve in normal subjects and cardiac patients with various disorders before and after intervention is represented in Figure 39-2. When the cardiac reserve is insufficient even to maintain an adequate power output at rest (cardiogenic shock), death ensues.[30]

Treatment of Secondary Defects

Symptoms of congestion arise owing to the secondary defects of heart failure. In the event of failure of the heart as a pump or a normal heart facing excessive hemodynamic burden (e.g., hypertension or arteriovenous shunting), the heart relies on the cardiovascular compensatory mechanisms to maintain adequate circulation. From the therapeutic point of view, it is more important to normalize cardiac load by instituting treatment, such as antihypertensive therapy and removal of the stimulus to high-output states (e.g., treating anemia and thyrotoxicosis), than to deal with the compensatory mechanisms and decompensation. Elderly patients are likely to carry the burden of disproportionately high systolic pressures associated with aging large arteries. Anemia, whether dietary or disease-related, should not be overlooked.

The compensatory mechanisms activated during heart failure are similar to those seen with hemorrhagic shock. Unlike in hypovolemic shock, however, fluid retention and vasoconstriction worsen heart failure. Decompensation occurs during heart failure when some of these compensatory mechanisms become inadequate or excessive. The strategy of therapy should be directed at optimizing the beneficial compensatory mechanisms without the accompanying detrimental effects.

Fluid and salt retention occur as an attempt to invoke the Starling effect through ventricular distension and is a compensatory mechanism but may result in troublesome congestion. Too much fluid and salt retention results in tissue edema, which impedes tissue perfusion and reduces vasodilatory capacity. Gut and hepatic congestion impair absorption and metabolism, contributing to cardiac cachexia, and importantly rendering oral medication less effective. The ensuing hypoalbuminemia further worsens the edema. Pulmonary edema causes ill-tolerated symp-

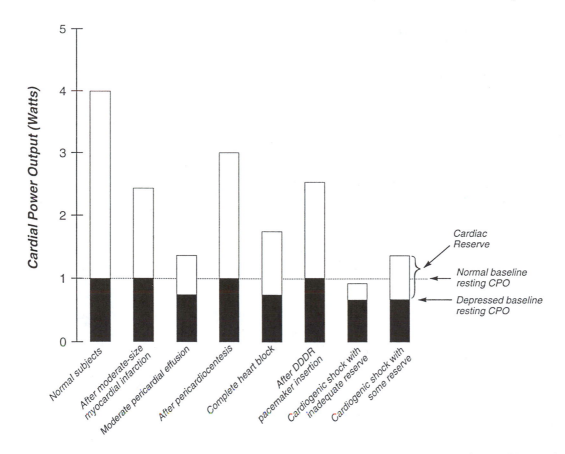

Fig. 39-2. Cardiac function in normal and diseased states. Cardiac performance is depicted by cardiac power output at the baseline resting state (height of the dark portion of each bar). The increment from this point to the peak (the height of the blank portion of each bar) represents the cardiac pumping reserve. *Dashed horizontal line* represents the baseline resting cardiac power output of an average-sized adult normal human subject.

toms (orthopnea, effort dyspnea), impairs gaseous exchange and mechanics of ventilation, and increases the work of ventilatory muscles, which in turn imposes unnecessary extra demand on cardiac performance. Excessive cardiac dilatation causes functional atrioventricular valve regurgitation, reducing ventricular pumping efficiency. Diuretics and venodilators are effective drugs for this condition.[30]

Neuroendocrine responses to cardiac hypofunction aim to increase the cardiac pumping rate and force, as well as vasoconstriction, in an attempt to maintain normal blood pressure and to divert the limited blood flow to the vital organs; but the resulting vasoconstriction may further impair cardiac function by excessive loading, and the released hormones are potentially arrhythmogenic and cardiotoxic.[32–34] Excessive vasoconstriction imposes higher afterload on the heart due to activation of the sympathetic, renin-angiotensin, and vasopressin systems. There is also a suggestion of increased endothelin levels. The vasoconstriction is exacerbated by diuretic therapy because of the resultant stimulation of the renin-angio-

tensin system and release of vasopressin. Excessive vasoconstriction of the renal arterioles eventually leads to reduction in the renal blood flow and glomerular filtration rates. The resulting azotemia and oliguria compound the management of heart failure. Chronic overstimulation of the sympathetic system causes myocardial norepinephrine depletion and β-adrenoceptor down-regulation, resulting in sympathetic hyporesponsiveness, especially in older individuals,[18] and diminished myocardial chronotropic and inotropic reserves. ACE inhibition is the appropriate treatment, but agents that improve cardiac performance, such as digoxin, may secondarily reduce the neurohumoral activation. The stretching of atrial and ventricular walls releases atrial and brain natriuretic peptides, which counterbalance, albeit insufficiently, the fluid and salt retention and vasoconstriction of catecholamines, angiotensin, and aldosterone.

Myocardial hypertrophy (which serves to reduce ventricular wall stress and augment function) is another compensatory mechanism; but when it is excessive, as in hypertrophic cardiomyopathy or hypertensive heart disease, it causes diastolic dysfunction and renders the subendocardial region more prone to ischemia. Hypertensive left ventricular hypertrophy regresses with effective long-term therapy, particularly that of the systolic pressure. Although short-term trials have suggested an advantage of ACE inhibitors,[35] diuretics may provide better results because of their ability to produce sustained systolic control.[36,37] It is important to note that some myocardial hypertrophy secondary to myocyte loss may be a beneficial compensatory mechanism and should not be suppressed.[38]

Management of Tertiary Defects

It is inevitable that interventions that alter physiologic homeostatic controls lead to complications. Some of these tertiary defects can be detrimental. The commonest is probably electrolyte imbalance. The powerful loop diuretics lead to loss of potassium and magnesium, either of which can contribute to and precipitate tachyarrhythmias. Diuretic therapy for heart failure can also paradoxically lead to significant hyponatremia ("paradoxical" because natriuresis is one of the desired effects). Hyponatremia during heart failure is particularly difficult to treat and is associated with a poor prognosis.[39] Diuretics can also induce intravascular hyponatremia which may lead to worsening hypoperfusion of organs and postural hypotension. Diuretics must be used carefully to avoid these complications.[40,41]

Each type of vasodilator has preferential effects on different vascular beds. Such selective or, perhaps better termed, indiscriminate vasodilation often counters the natural redistribution of blood flow, which aims to preserve flow to vital organs in low-output states. For instance, the redistribution of blood flow, especially during exercise, is largely effected by sympathetic vasoconstriction. The use of α-adrenergic blockers counteracts this action, and it is not surprising to find that prazosin does not improve exercise tolerance or the prognosis for heart failure patients.[42,43] Vasodilators that shunt blood into the splanchnic or cutaneous vasculature similarly do not improve exercise capacity. ACE inhibitors may worsen the renal function of patients who are dependent on angiotensin-induced renal efferent arteriole vasoconstriction to maintain glomerular filtration rates. Certain positive inotropic agents (e.g., catecholamines) are known to be cardiotoxic, causing arrhythmias and cardiac myocyte necrosis.[44,45] These iatrogenic tertiary defects should be minimized by judicious use of therapeutic agents.

SPECIFIC FEATURES OF TREATING HEART FAILURE IN ELDERLY PATIENTS

Pharmacologic and Pathophysiologic Considerations

Drug treatment at either extreme of the age spectrum requires special attention. The elderly patient population has a greater tendency than the young patient to concomitant problems, both medical and social, and a greater propensity for adverse drug reactions. Several pharmacokinetic and pharmacodynamic factors contribute to this state. Malabsorption problems are not uncommon in elderly patients; but when compounded by congestive cardiac failure, enteral drug absorption (e.g., of diuretics) may be significantly compromised such that a parenteral route of administration must be considered. Because of increased body fat and decreased lean body mass and serum albumin, there is a tendency for maldistribution of cardiac drugs. Decreased renal function and liver metabolism lead to decreased elimination, resulting in accumulation of drugs. Lower doses must be used in such cases. Renal handling of electrolytes is also impaired with aging. Introduction of diuretic and ACE inhibition therapy in these patients should always be closely monitored.

Changes in the cardiovascular system also render the elderly patient more prone to side effects of drugs. Because of decreased cardiac reserve, these patients are more susceptible to the negative inotropic effects of drugs, which may precipitate heart failure. One of the diagnostic steps when dealing with older patients first presenting with heart failure is to determine if the heart failure is drug-induced. Such drugs as β-adrenergic inhibitors, calcium antagonists, or antiarrhythmic agents prescribed for other reasons may have to be withdrawn or replaced.

The pacemaker and conduction tissues in geriatric hearts are often abnormal, rendering these patients more vulnerable to heart block sinus node dysfunction. Drugs with negative chronotropic or negative dromotropic effects must be used with great caution.[46,47] Another hallmark of presbycardia is reduced ventricular compliance. Any agent that compromises the diastolic filling duration, such as is seen in conjunction with reflex tachycardia with vasodilating drugs, may worsen congestion and reduce cardiac output and blood pressure. Myocardial hypertrophy in older patients may also render the subendocardial regions more vulnerable to ischemia.

In the elderly patient, baroreceptor and autonomic malfunction and loss of arterial compliance compound the likelihood of hypotension and organ underperfusion when diuretics or antihypertensive medications are prescribed. In combination with atherosclerosis, which is common in elderly patients, these effects can result in ischemia of the "watershed" regions of the central nervous system, resulting in brain stem ischemia or transient ischemic attacks. Patients taking these drugs should therefore be closely monitored regarding their hydration status and postural hypotension.

Social factors and impairment of hearing, sight, and cognitive functions may add to the difficulties of treatment.

Principles of Prescribing Cardiovascular Drugs

It is a useful adage to adopt when prescribing for any patient (but in particular for older individuals) that drug treatment for non-life-threatening conditions should be started at low doses and increased stepwise according to need while avoiding side effects. However, with life-threatening conditions, such as serious arrhythmias or severe acute left ventricular failure in moribund patients, appropriate doses of effective drugs are administered. Once the patient is stable, the doses can then be reduced in stages to the minimum effective maintainance dose to minimize unwanted side effects.

In general, closer monitoring of responses and side effects is required when treating elderly heart failure patients than in younger patients for the pathophysiologic and pharmacologic reasons described above. Elderly patients are also more likely to be receiving other drugs. Careful review and coordination of medications is important. The chances of serious drug interactions are greater with polypharmacy. Possible drug interactions should be assiduously checked whenever introducing a new drug. A particular issue in heart failure patients is the frequent concomitant use of ACE inhibitors and nonsteroidal antiinflammatory drugs (NSAIDs). The NSAIDs may reduce the efficacy of ACE inhibitors, but more importantly the combination may impair or irreversibly damage renal function when renal perfusion is tenuous.[48]

Compliance is a major issue when prescribing for all patients but particularly in some elderly individuals because of the multiplicity of drugs they may receive and their declining mental functioning. Simple regimens are more likely to produce better compliance. Cost may be a factor, as many elderly patients are responsible for some or all of their medication expenses. Abrupt diuresis may be a particular problem because of impaired bladder control or obstruction, and thought should be given to the best regimen for the life style of the individual.

Finally, the population of elderly heart failure patients is heterogeneous. Interindividual variability is greater than that in younger populations. It must therefore be reemphasized that particularly close monitoring of compliance, efficacy, and side effects of treatment is required when treating this group of patients.

Practical Therapeutic Strategy

Treatment of acute and chronic heart failure and the use of various pharmacologic and nonpharmacologic therapies is considered in other chapters. In this section we highlight features specifically relevant to treating elderly patients.

EVALUATION FOR SURGICAL INTERVENTION

Having stressed the importance of diagnosing the primary defects of heart failure, especially the surgically treatable defects, factors other than purely medical ones often must be taken into account when determining whether an elderly patient should be put forward for cardiac surgery. Chronologic age and multiple pathologies are known risk factors for surgery complications, but advances have steadily reduced the risks of operation.[23–25] If successful, surgery can often produce an outcome superior to that achieved with the best medical therapy.[27] Thus weighing the potential risks and benefits of surgery is a severe test of the skill of the clinician. In this regard there is increasing disapproval of those who practice ageism. Obviously, the final decision on whether to undertake the operation rests with the patient, but this decision is heavily influenced by what information and opinions are conveyed by the clinician. As far as possible, objective information based on physiologic measurements (on cardiovascular and other systems) and other scientific data including local outcome data for procedures is provided in preference to subjective, biased opinions.

INTERVENTIONAL THERAPY

Patients with surgically correctable primary defects should be considered for operation at the appropriate time. Such interventions include the following.

1. Valve replacement can be done with low mortality in most patients with aortic stenosis, but the outcome is worse when surgery of a second valve or coronary surgery is required.[24,25]
2. Valvoplasty should be considered, especially for mitral stenosis. Aortic valvoplasty for calcific aor-

tic stenosis has not provided long-term relief and should be reserved for situations in which the only objective is temporary palliation.

3. Pericardiocentesis or fashioning a pericardial window should always be undertaken for pericardial effusion.
4. Pericardial stripping for pericardial constriction can be performed, although the risks are relatively high.
5. Repair of shunts, especially for postmyocardial infarction ventricular septal defects, may be done.
6. Permanent pacemaker insertion, which is cost-effective, can be undertaken for symptomatic complete heart block, although its indication for purely congestive cardiac failure is still being debated and investigated.
7. Coronary bypass surgery or angioplasty in the absence of angina may improve heart failure symptoms and quality of life of patients who have significant segments of left ventricular wall with demonstrable reversible akinesia or hypokinesia due to ischemic or hibernating myocardium.

NONPHARMACOLOGIC THERAPY

The general measures include asking the patients to stop smoking, stop or reduce ethanol intake, and institute fluid and salt restriction, rehabilitation, and counseling.[49] Excessive ethanol intake not only exacerbates alcoholic cardiomyopathy, it increases the propensity for atrial fibrillation, negative inotropism, and, in cases of beer or lager, excessive fluid intake. Fluid restriction may allow lower doses of diuretics to be used and, when combined with checks of daily weights, would forestall impending congestive decompensation and the need for frequent hospitalization.

Bed rest is particularly treacherous in elderly individuals.[50] Edematous patients are more prone to develop bedsores. Prolonged bed rest enhances the development of venous thrombosis and pulmonary embolism. Bed rest causes deconditioning, resulting in reduced exercise tolerance and aerobic capacity, muscular atrophy, and muscle weakness. Enforced bed rest should no longer form a routine part of the management of patients in congestive heart failure, except for those with acute myocarditis and those whose edema is unresponsive to a modern diuretic and vasodilator regimen. In contrast, activity should be encouraged in a prudent manner.[49,50] Although no data are as yet available on whether exercise training prolongs life, there is clear evidence that it improves exercise capacity and other measures associated with improved prognosis.[51,52]

MEDICAL THERAPY

Depending on the specific problems at hand, the general medical therapy that can be instituted are listed in Table 39-2. Specific pharmacologic treatments are shown in Table 39-1. For chronic heart failure, a recommended treatment strategy is shown in Table 39-3.

Diuretics are still the mainstay pharmacologic treatment of acute and chronic heart failure.[31] In patients with fluid retention, no other drug therapy can alleviate symptoms and improve exercise tolerance to the same extent as diuretics.[53] However, because of the metabolic disturbances and neurohormonal activation commonly induced by diuretics,[40,41] ACE inhibitors should generally be co-administered. Thiazide diuretics are used only for the mildest forms of heart failure and with concomitant hypertension. Loop diuretics are more powerful than thiazide and may be less liable to cause metabolic disturbances at low doses. The commonly used loop diuretics are furosemide and bumetanide, although the slower and longer action of torsemide is better tolerated by some elderly patients.

Due to the diminished renal function with aging, diuretic therapy should be more closely monitored

Table 39-2. General Medical Treatment for Heart Failure Patients

Problem	Management
Hypoxia	O_2 + airway pressure (artificial ventilation)
Anemia	Investigation, hematinics, transfusion
Nausea	Antiemetics
Anxiety	Counseling, anxiolytics
Depression	Counseling, antidepressants
Dietary deficiencies	Protein and vitamin supplements
Hypoalbuminemia	Protein supplements, albumin transfusion
Thromboembolism	Prophylactic aspirin, anticoagulation
Respiratory infection	Avoid smoking, influenza vaccination

Table 39-3. Medical Treatment Strategy for Chronic Heart Failure in Elderly Patients

Degree of Failure	Treatment
Mild	Thiazide or loop and K⁺-sparing diuretics, ACE inhibitor
Moderate	Loop and K⁺-sparing diuretics, ACE inhibitor/other vasodilators, digoxin
Severe	As above, intravenous (IV) loop diuretics with or without metolazone, IV low-dose dopamine, IV positive inotropes, intermittent IV dobutamine, (hemofiltration, ultrafiltration)

than in young patients. In practice, there is no real substitute for checking serum electrolytes, urea, and creatinine regularly during diuretic therapy. Oral potassium supplementation is not effective and does not replenish the loss of magnesium. Therefore it is better to combine loop diuretic treatment with an ACE inhibitor and possibly a potassium-sparing diuretic. Hyponatremia should be avoided because, unlike marked deficits in potassium or magnesium, which can be easily dealt with by judicious infusion of these electrolytes, significant hyponatremia is much more difficult to correct and probably equally arrhythmogenic.

Patients already on oral diuretics sometimes decompensate and become congested, which may be compounded by gut edema compromising drug absorption. Such patients are best admitted to hospital for a period of treatment with intravenous diuretics. High dose infusion of furosemide (up to 500 mg IV per day) or bumetanide (up to 15 mg IV per day) is sometimes needed. Combination with a thiazide diuretic (especially metolazone) can result in marked diuresis in patients with intractable congestion. However, such therapy can be potent, inducing alarming electrolyte imbalance (especially hyponatremia).

Another way to deal with intractable congestion is the concurrent use of low dose dopamine. To avoid giving too much fluid, the dopamine is necessarily infused at fairly high concentration; and it should be given via a central line to avoid painful thrombophlebitis. Congestion unresponsive to this drug may require addition of positive inotropic agents. Finally, it should be emphasized that heart failure patients are dependent on renal function for their well-being. Preservation of their renal function is of paramount

importance, without which medical therapy is well nigh impossible because dialysis or filtration are generally not well tolerated by heart failure patients, especially elderly ones.

Vasodilators are firmly established for treatment of heart failure. The rationale is to unload the heart. Both preload and afterload reduction contribute to reducing the ventricular wall stress and improving forward flow. However, excessive preload reduction may impair stroke volume, especially in patients without substantial left ventricular dilatation and in those with prominent diastolic dysfunction. Excessive afterload reduction may compromise coronary perfusion, thereby exacerbating myocardial ischemia and, especially in elderly patients, symptomatic hypotension. Indiscriminate vasodilation of the splanchnic and cutaneous beds may result in less flow available to the skeletal muscles during exercise.

It is accepted that ACE inhibitors, which have vasodilation as part of their mechanism of action, are standard treatment for chronic heart failure because of their beneficial effects on prognosis and progressive left ventricular dysfunction.[54] Although their effects on exercise tolerance have been more variable,[55] they consistently prevent hospitalizations and clinical episodes of worsening heart failure.

When administering ACE inhibitors to elderly patients, there are two specific adverse effects to avoid. Excessive hypotension should be avoided by carefully introducing the drug under close supervision for those particularly at risk. These patients can usually be identified by their low pretreatment blood pressures (systolic pressure ≤ 100 mmHg, prior symptoms of dizziness, abnormal renal function, or hyponatremia). Patients should not be too dehydrated at the time of introduction; those on high doses of diuretics, especially with demonstrable postural fall in pressure, are at particular risk. The most problematic adverse effect of ACE inhibition is impairment of renal function, which tends to be a particular issue in the elderly patient. Activation of the renin-angiotensin system in the kidney is a natural attempt to increase glomerular filtration by constriction of the efferent arterioles, thereby increasing filtration pressure. In some patients ACE inhibition induces a reduction in filtration rate and overall renal function. Individuals at greatest risk for worsening renal function are those with baseline abnormalities, borderline arterial pressure, and diabetes. The latter group also has a predisposition to hyperkalemia. It is therefore important to monitor the creatinine and potassium levels soon after introduction of the ACE inhibitor and after upward dose adjustment (several days to 1 week, depending on the baseline blood pressure and renal function). Baseline renal dysfunction is not a contraindication for ACE inhibitor therapy; but if levels continue to increase, particularly after downward adjustment of diuretics when feasible, the ACE inhibitor must be withdrawn or used at a lower dose.

The combination of ACE inhibitor and NSAIDs should be avoided if possible and monitored closely if utilized, as NSAID therapy also impairs renal compensation to reduced blood flow by inhibiting prostaglandin synthesis.[48] For instance, acute gouty attacks should be treated with colchicine or corticosteroids in high risk heart failure patients on an ACE inhibitor, and acetaminophen is preferred for pain relief, rather than NSAIDs. In patients with significant unilateral renal artery stenosis, ACE inhibition may result in chemical autonephrectomy that is undetectable by serum urea and creatinine estimations if the other kidney is normal enough to take over the function. If the stenosis is bilateral, the consequence may be renal deterioration resulting in the need for dialysis or filtration.

In patients unable to use ACE inhibitors, nitrates offer an alternative. Long-acting nitrate preparations able to provide sustained benefit, with a drug-free period of at least 6 hours during the day, is recommended (e.g., sustained-release isosorbide mononitrate 30–80 mg per day). Combination with hydralazine may be justified according to trial data and the claims that hydralazine may lessen nitrate tolerance. Nitrates may be added to ACE inhibitors in patients who remain symptomatic or in those with concomitant angina.

Inotropic agents are used under the premise that if the heart is failing strengthening the myocardial contraction may be beneficial. However, the experience with several inotropic agents has been unfavorable, with both phosphodiesterase inhibitors and β-adrenoreceptor agonists increasing mortality during chronic therapy.[44] Although these adverse results may be unique to these agents,[56,57] it is possible that excessive stimulation accelerates myocardial damage or precipitates lethal arrhythmias.[44,58] Therefore positive inotropic therapy should be used judiciously.

Digitalis preparations are the oldest drugs still in use as modern cardiovascular therapy and are still the only oral positive inotropic agents available worldwide for chronic oral therapy. After many years of controversy, a series of well controlled studies in appropriately selected patients with established systolic dysfunction established that digoxin withdrawal is associated with clinical deterioration and worsening symptoms and exercise tolerance.[59–61]

The preliminary findings from the Digitalis Investigators Group trial (see Chapter 43 for more complete discussion) have shown conclusively that digoxin has a neutral effect on survival, indicating that it is not a dangerous drug when used appropriately. Nonetheless, without evidence that this agent has a beneficial effect on survival, its role is primarily in patients with atrial fibrillation and those who remain symptomatic despite therapy with diuretics and ACE inhibitor or vasodilators.[62]

Because of its narrow therapeutic window, monitoring serum digoxin levels may be required especially in older patients, who often have impaired or fluctuating renal function and variable pharmacokinetics. Because digoxin is usually given in low dosages to avoid toxicity, its positive inotropic effect is less at rest than during exercise,[63] and as such it has an important property: inotropic stimulation when it is needed (i.e., during exertion). This property may be an advantage and may explain why digoxin has not had the adverse effects of more powerful inotropic drugs.

Intermittent prolonged dobutamine infusion may produce symptomatic and functional benefits that persists for days to weeks after cessation of the infusion; and it may be used in patients with severe heart failure when other medical therapy fails. The beneficial effects are thought to be related to pharmacologic conditioning effects not dissimilar to those obtained after exercise training. Such therapy must, however, be instituted under close supervision due to the arrhythmogenic potential of the drug.[65]

β-Adrenoreceptor blockers and other experimental agents continue to be investigated for heart failure. These medications are discussed in depth elsewhere (see Ch. 47). Particular caution and appropriate experience are required before using these medications in elderly patients.

Treatment of Acute Heart Failure

Acute heart failure occurs more frequently in elderly patients. The usual causes are cardiogenic shock following acute myocardial infarction, acute ischemic left ventricular dysfunction presenting as "flash" pulmonary edema, and acute valvar insufficiency. Each of these entities is dealt with elsewhere in this book, but a few points relevant to the elderly patient deserve emphasis.

It has been estimated that cardiogenic shock occurs when the infarction results in a loss of 40 percent or more of the myocardium.[66] By the time the advanced age of 90 years is reached, an estimated loss of 35 percent of the myocardium would have occurred through natural attrition.[14] It is not surprising that the incidence of cardiogenic shock after acute myocardial infarction is higher in elderly patients irrespective of previous myocardial infarction.

Despite the worse prognosis of elderly patients when they develop acute heart failure, some of the usual therapeutic approaches may not be feasible. Most of these conditions require surgical intervention, which may not be appropriate in elderly patients with concomitant illnesses or excessive debilitation. The medical therapy is similar in old and young patients, consisting mainly of diuretics, intravenous inotropes or vasodilators (or both), and antiischemic therapy when indicated. If these maneuvers achieve stability, the issue of revascularization or valve surgery can be reevaluated.

SPECIFIC FEATURES OF TREATING DIASTOLIC HEART FAILURE

The incidence and prevalence of diastolic heart failure that requires treatment is unknown. It has been stated that up to 40 percent of patients with heart failure have primarily diastolic dysfunction, although a figure of 20 percent is cited more frequently.[3–5] The derivation of these figures is uncertain, and well designed prospective studies are not available. In general, the diagnosis of heart failure due to diastolic dysfunction is one of exclusion.[67–69] First, noncardiac etiologies for the presenting symptoms and signs, such as pulmonary disease and edema of other causes, must be eliminated. Second, systolic dysfunction must be excluded by appropriate noninvasive or invasive techniques. In particular, mitral insufficiency, which can produce apparently normal ejection fraction measurements despite significantly impaired contractility, must be considered. Third, other cardiac causes of heart failure that may be associated with preserved systolic function, such as aortic stenosis and most importantly intermittent ischemia, must be excluded.

Unfortunately, there is no good test to measure diastolic function and hence "rule in" diastolic heart failure. One of the most widely cited studies showing the importance of diastolic dysfunction illustrates the problem.[70] Among 58 patients with a clinical diagnosis of congestive heart failure and normal systolic left ventricular function (radionuclide left ventricular ejection fraction > 45 percent), about 40 percent were found to have impaired diastolic function with a peak filling rate of less than 2.5 end-diastolic volume(s). This retrospective study may have

been biased by the type of patients referred for testing. Furthermore, this result may be an overestimate because the normal range for the peak filling rate was determined from 14 normal healthy volunteers (age range 31–55 years) who were significantly younger than the patients studied (mean age 68 ± 12 years). The normal range of 4.04 ± 0.77 end-diastolic volume (EDV)/s obtained in this study was substantially higher than the value of 3.1 ± 0.6 EDV/s in those less than 50 years of age and 2.6 ± 0.6 in those 50 years or older.[71]

Pari passu with natural attrition of cardiomyocytes as part of the aging process[14] is the increased myocardial collagen content with senescence.[15] Using Doppler indices age has been shown to be a predominant determinant of left ventricular diastolic function[69,72]—so much so that it is impossible to distinguish age-related changes from clinically important diastolic dysfunction in the individuals. The age association with left ventricular diastolic dysfunction persists even during exercise.[73] Care should therefore be exercised when interpreting the results of noninvasive investigations to avoid a false-positive diagnosis of diastolic heart failure.

Few data are available regarding the prognosis of isolated diastolic heart failure. In the V-HeFT study, a small subgroup of patients with heart failure but a normal left ventricular ejection fraction (> 45 percent) had significantly lower mortality than those with a reduced ejection fraction despite the fact that the two subgroups had similar exercise intolerance.[74] There was no direct assessment of diastolic dysfunction in this study to establish whether the subgroup with a "normal" ejection fraction indeed had diastolic failure. In the AIRE study, in which patients were admitted with clinical evidence of heart failure even if transient after a myocardial infarction,[75] the ejection fraction was measured in a representative subgroup of 553 patients. About half of these patients had ejection fractions above 40 percent and a lower mortality rate than those with lower ejection fractions. Again there were no direct measurements of diastolic function, but little benefit appeared to accrue to these patients from ACE inhibitor treatment.

There are virtually no data from clinical trials in patients with diastolic dysfunction, and clinicians are confronted with confusing and conflicting information. For instance, β-adrenergic inhibitors have been considered to be beneficial in the treatment of diastolic dysfunction, but students of physiology know that adrenergic stimulation enhances myocardial relaxation by reducing myofilament sensitivity to calcium, accelerating the sequestration of calcium into sarcoplasmic reticulum and increasing the rate of cross-bridge turnover.[6,68] When treating "pure" diastolic dysfunction, reduction of preload was claimed to be "not indicated" because it "may exacerbate the existing impairment in ventricular filling,"[8] and yet clinicians have found that diuretics are indispensable in patients with fluid retention due to diastolic dysfunction.[76] Similarly, calcium blockers are sometimes considered beneficial, but physicians are cautioned about using vasodilators because they may induce excessive hypotension in an underfilled left ventricle.

Practical Therapeutic Strategy

INTERVENTIONAL THERAPY

As with the treatment of any patient manifesting clinical features of heart failure, the most important step of management is to determine the primary defect(s) giving rise to heart failure. It is therefore essential to establish the diagnosis. Therapeutic attempts should therefore be based on dealing with the causes of diastolic dysfunction, whereas the symptoms can be ameliorated by dealing with the secondary defects of heart failure and avoiding the tertiary defects (see above).

Once the cause of the diastolic dysfunction has been established, treatment is directed at preventing or correcting the etiologic agents or processes. In practice, the commonest causes of diastolic heart failure are hypertensive and ischemic heart disease, restrictive and hypertrophic cardiomyopathies, and pericardial diseases. For hypertensive diastolic heart failure with preserved left ventricular systolic function, the primary aim is to lower the blood pressure, preferably over the entire 24 hours of each day, including during exertion or stress. Once this goal has been achieved, drugs may be selected secondarily to target specific goals, such as regression of ventricular hypertrophy,[35] cardioprotection,[34] and prevention or regression of myocardial fibrosis.[77]

With ischemic heart failure the processes leading to diastolic dysfunction are complex and include failure of relaxation due to ischemia, ischemic contracture, asynchronous relaxation, hibernating or stunned myocardium, and aneurysm formation. The definitive treatment is revascularization, and this step may have to be considered for patients who are not troubled by angina. When revascularization is not feasible or not available, medical treatment should consist first of antiischemic agents. Positive inotropic and other agents that cause reflex tachycardia should be avoided.

Clearly pericardial surgery is indicated for con-

striction and recurrent effusion. Cardiac tumors require resection. Examples of treatment of restrictive cardiomyopathy include chelation therapy for hemochromatosis and steroid therapy for sarcoid heart disease. Endocardial fibroelastosis requires treatment of the hypereosinophilic syndrome with steroid and cytotoxic drugs and if necessary plasma exchange and leukophoresis to prevent progression, as well as surgical removal of the endocardial fibrous layer. Surgical resection may also be required for hypertrophic cardiomyopathy when the hypertrophied myocardium causes too much impedance to flow in and out of the ventricle. Alternatively, selective embolization of penetrating coronary arteries supplying the hypertrophied segments may be beneficial.

NONPHARMACOLOGIC THERAPY

Endurance exercise training has been shown to improve diastolic filling in elderly subjects who have reduced diastolic function[78] and in patients with dilated cardiomyopathy.[79] The improvement in peak oxygen consumption correlated with improvements in diastolic filling characteristics.

Atrioventricular sequential pacing can also improve diastolic function by preserving atrial contraction and optimizing the atrioventricular delay. The alteration in the ventricular excitation pattern can also be helpful in hypertrophic cardiomyopathy patients.

PHARMACOTHERAPY

In terms of ventricular dynamics, the principles of therapy can be classified according to the following objectives.

1. Increase ventricular diastolic compliance by improving biochemical properties governing cardiomyocyte relaxation,[80,81] which may be best accomplished by β-adrenoreceptor stimulation or phosphodiesterase inhibition (although no such agents are available for chronic oral therapy) or by regression of myocardial hypertrophy and interstitial fibrosis (e.g., using ACE inhibitors[77] or other antihypertensive therapy).
2. Lower the operating point along the left ventricular pressure–volume relation by reducing total blood volume with diuretics and by venodilatation, taking the precaution of not excessively reducing the ventricular preload.
3. Maintain atrial systolic contribution to ventricular filling by maintaining sinus rhythm and an appropriate AV interval, controlling the arrhythmia, and artificial AV sequential pacing.

4. Preserve or prolong the diastolic filling period using negative chronotropic agents such as β-adrenoreceptor blockers and verapamil (which induce negative inotropic effects) or digoxin and oral amiodarone (which are devoid of negative inotropism).

5. Allow the ventricle to empty more completely so more can go into the ventricle during subsequent diastole. It is accomplished by reducing afterload, removing outflow obstruction, and using negative inotropic agents (e.g., β-adrenoreceptor blockers, verapamil) for hypertrophic obstructive cardiomyopathy, or aortic valve replacement for aortic regurgitation.

6. Shorten the ventricular systolic phase using vasodilatory adrenergic stimulatory agents, phosphodiesterase inhibitors, nitric oxide-contributing agents (e.g., nitrates, nitroprusside), or thyroxine.

7. Possibly remove pericardial constraint by pericardiectomy.

The selection of treatment option(s) should be guided by the pathophysiologic findings from investigations. Owing to the difficulty of interpreting the results from investigations, clinical treatment of diastolic dysfunction and heart failure has been largely empiric. Hence it must be guided by the outcome of therapeutic attempts.

Monitoring Efficacy of Treatment

It has been stated that "the rationale for treating patients with diastolic failure is to improve exercise tolerance by diminishing or suppressing upward shifts in the diastolic pressure–volume relation."[6] At the end of an excellent review on clinical methods of evaluating diastolic performance, Little and Downes concluded that "it is unlikely that a single easily interpreted index of LV diastolic performance will ever be developed."[82] A major challenge facing clinicians and researchers attempting to treat this condition is how to assess the efficacy of potential treatment modalities.

It is difficult and not desirable to identify the treatment effects on lusitropic properties in isolation from inotropic, chronotropic, and dromotropic effects and from effects on ventricular preload and afterload. The main problems are that: (1) clinical methods of measuring diastolic function may be too inaccurate to detect small changes; (2) most therapies also affect systolic function, so improvement may be due to changes in systolic function; or (3) the lack of overall improvement may have been due to the positive lusitropic effects being negated by the deleterious inotro-

pic or chronotropic effects. For many patients, careful symptom assessment is the best guide to managing therapy. If unreliable, it may be supplemented by quantitative measurements of exercise capacity. From the foregoing discussion, it should be apparent that the definition, assessment, and treatment of diastolic dysfunction remain a challenge to cardiac research.

REFERENCES

1. Kannel WB, Belanger AJ: Epidemiology of heart failure. Am Heart J 1991;121:951–957
2. Gillum RF: Epidemiology of heart failure in the United States. Am Heart J 1993;1042–1047
3. Vasan RS, Benjamin EJ, Levy D: Prevalence, clinical features and prognosis of diastolic heart failure. An epidemiologic perspective. J Am Coll Cardiol 1995;26:1565–1574
4. Grossman W: Diastolic dysfunction in congestive heart failure. N Engl J Med 1991;325:1557–1564
5. Bonow RO, Udelson JE: Left ventricular diastolic dysfunction as a cause of congestive heart failure. Mechanisms and management. Ann Intern Med 1992;117:502–510
6. Brutsaert DL, Sys SU, Gillebert TC: Diastolic failure. Pathophysiology and therapeutic implications. J Am Coll Cardiol 1993;22:318–325
7. Tan LB, Cubkcu A: What factors determine exercise capacity in left ventricular dysfunction? Eur Heart J 1996;17:168–170
8. Wei JY: Age and the cardiovascular system. N Engl J Med 1992;327:1735–1739
9. Lakatta EG: Cardiovascular regulatory mechanisms in advanced age. Physiol Rev 1993;7:413–467
10. Gerstinblith G, Frederiksen J, Yin FC et al: Echocardiographic assessment of a normal adult population. Circulation 1977;56:273–278
11. Avolio AP, Fa-Quan D, We-Quiang L et al: Effects of aging on arterial distensibility in populations with high and low prevalence of hypertension. Comparison between urban and rural communities. Circulation 1985;71:202–210
12. Fleg JL, Shapiro Ep, O'Connor F et al: Left ventricular diastolic filling in older male athletes. JAMA 1995;273:1371–1375
13. Lakatta EG: Myocardial adaptations in advanced age. Basic Res Cardiol, suppl. 2 1993;88:125–33
14. Olivetti G, Melissari M, Capasso JM, Anversa P: Cardiomyopathy of the aging human heart. Myocyte loss and reactive cellular hypertrophy. Circ Res 1991;68:1560–1568
15. Anversa P, Palackal T, Sonnenblick E et al: Myocyte cell loss and myocyte cellular hyperplasia in the hypertrophied aging rat heart. Circ Res 1990;67:871–885
16. Anversa P, Fitzpatrick D, Argani S, Capasso JM: Myocyte mitotic division in the aging mammalian rat heart. Circ Res 1991;69:1159–1164
17. Kitzman DW, Scholz DG, Hagen PT, Ilstrup DM, Edwards WD: Age-related changes in normal human hearts during the first 10 decades of life. Part II (Maturity). A quantitative anatomic study of 765 specimens

from subjects 20–99 years old. Mayo Clin Proc 1988; 63:137–46

18. White M, Roden R, Minobe W et al: Age-related changes in β-adrenergic neuroeffector systems in the human heart. Circulation 1994;90:1225–1238

19. Fleg JL, O'Connor F, Gerstenblith G et al: Impact of age on the cardiovascular response to dynamic upright exercise in healthy men and women. J Appl Physiol 1995;78:890–900

20. Schulman SP, Lakatta EG, Fleg JL et al: Age-related decline in left ventricular filling at rest and exercise. Am J Physiol 1992;263:H1932–H1938

21. Kitzman DW, Higginbotham MB, Cobb FR et al: Exercise intolerance in patients with heart failure and preserved left ventricular systolic function. Failure of the Frank-Starling mechanism. J Am Coll Cardiol 1991; 17:1065–1072

22. Rich MW, Bosner MS, Chung MK, Shen J, McKenzie JP: Is age an independent predictor of early and late mortality in patients with acute myocardial infarction. Am J Med 1992;92:7–13

23. Peterson ED, Cowper PA, Jollis JG et al: Outcomes of coronary artery bypass graft surgery in 24,461 patients aged 80 years or older. Circulation, suppl. II 1995;92:85–91

24. Katz NM, Hannan RL, Hopkins RA, Wallace RB: Cardiac operations in patients aged 70 years and over. Mortality, length of stay, and hospital charge. Ann Thorac Surg 1995;60:96–100

25. Elayda MA, Hall RJ, Reul RM et al: Aortic valve replacement in patients 80 years and older. Operative risks and long-term results. Circulation, suppl. II 1993;88:11–16

26. Mills SA: Risk factors for cerebral injury and cardiac surgery. Ann Thorac Surg 1995;59:1296–1299

27. Jaeger AA, Hlatky MA, Paul SM, Gortner SR: Functional capacity after cardiac surgery in elderly patients. J Am Coll Cardiol 1994;24:104–108

28. Tan LB: Clinical and research implications of new concepts in the assessment of cardiac pumping performance in heart failure. Cardiovasc Res 1987;21:615–622

29. Tan LB: Evaluation of cardiac dysfunction, cardiac reserve and inotropic response. Postgrad Med J, suppl. 1 1991;67:10–20

30. Tan LB, Littler WA: Measurement of cardiac reserve in cardiogenic shock. Implications for prognosis and management. Br Heart J 1990;64:121–128

31. Cody RJ, Kubo SH, Pickworth KK: Diuretic treatment for the sodium retention of congestive heart failure. Arch Intern Med 1994;154:1905–1914

32. Packer M: Pathophysiology of chronic heart failure. Lancet 1992;340:88–92

33. Packer M: The neurohormonal hypothesis. A theory to explain the mechanism of disease progression in heart failure. J Am Coll Cardiol 1992;20:248–254

34. Tan LB, Jalil JE, Pick R, Janicki JS, Weber KT: Cardiac myocyte necrosis induced by angiotensin II. Circ Res 1991;69:1185–1195

35. Dahlof B, Pennert K, Hansson L: Reversal of left ventricular hypertrophy in hypertensive patients. A meta-analysis of 109 treatment studies. Am J Hypertens 1992;5:95–110

36. Liebson PR, Grandits GA, Dianzumba S et al: Comparison of five antihypertensive monotherapies and placebo for change in left ventricular mass in patients receiving nutritional-hygienic therapy in the Treatment of Mild Hypertension Study (TOMHS). Circulation 1995;9:698–706

37. Massie BM: Effect of diuretic therapy on hypertensive left ventricular hypertrophy. Eur Heart J, suppl. G 1992;13:53–60

38. Tan LB, Hall AS: Cardiac remodelling. Br Heart J 1994;72:315–316

39. Lee WH, Packer M: Prognostic importance of serum sodium concentration and its modification by converting-enzyme inhibition in patients with severe heart failure. Circulation 1986;73:257–267

40. Bayliss J, Norell M, Canepa-Anson R, Sutton G, Poole-Wilson PA: Untreated heart failure. Clinical and neuroendocrine effects of introducing diuretics. Br Heart J 1987;57:17–22

41. Kubo SH, Clark M, Laragh JH, Borer JS, Cody RJ: Identification of normal neurohormonal activity in mild congestive heart failure and stimulating effect of upright posture and diuretics. Am J Cardiol 1987;60:1322–1328

42. Cohn JN, Archibald DG, Phil M et al: Effect of vasodilator therapy on mortality in chronic congestive heart failure. Results of a Veterans Administration Cooperative Study. N Engl J Med 1986;314:1547–1552

43. Markham RV, Corbett JR, Gilmore A, Pettinger WA, Frish BG: Efficacy of prazosin in the management of chronic congestive heart failure. A six-month randomized, double-blind, placebo-controlled study. Am J Cardiol 1983;51:1346–1352

44. Packer M: The development of positive inotropic agents for chronic heart failure. How have we gone astray? J Am Coll Cardiol, suppl. A 1993;22:119–126

45. Benjamin IJ, Jalil TE, Tan TB et al: Isoproterenol-induced myocardial fibrosis in relation to myocyte necrosis. Circ Res 1989;65:667–670

46. Cowan JC, Baig MW, Tan LB: Disorders of the heart. In: Davies DM (ed) Textbook of Adverse Drug Reactions. 4th Ed. pp. 99–171. Oxford University Press, Oxford, 1991

47. Stolarek I, Scott PJ, Caird FI: Physiological changes due to age. Implications for cardiovascular drug therapy. Drugs Aging 1991;1:467–476

48. Sturrock ND, Struthers AD: Non-steroidal anti-inflammatory drugs and angiotensin converting enzyme inhibitors. A commonly prescribed combination with variable effects on renal function. Br J Clin Pharmacol 1993;354:343–348

49. Dracup K, Baker DW, Dunbar SB et al: Management of heart failure. II. Counseling, education, and lifestyle modifications. JAMA 1994;272:1442–1446

50. Editorial: On bedresting in heart failure. Lancet 1990; 336:975–976

51. Coats AJ: Exercise rehabilitation in chronic heart failure. J Am Coll Cardiol, (suppl. A) 1993;22:172–177

52. McKelvie RS, Teo KK, McCartney N et al: Effects of exercise training in patients with congestive heart failure. A critical review. J Am Coll Cardiol 1995;25:789–796

53. Grinstead WC, Francis MJ, Marks GF et al: Discontinuation of chronic diuretic therapy in stable congestive heart failure secondary to coronary artery disease or to idiopathic dilated cardiomyopathy. Am J Cardiol 1994;73:881–886

54. Garg R, Yusuf S: Overview of randomized trials of angiotensin-converting enzyme inhibitors on mortality

and morbidity in patients with heart failure. Collaborative Group on ACE Inhibitor Trials. JAMA 1995; 273:1450–1456

55. Swedberg K, Gundersen T: The role of exercise testing in heart failure. J Cardiovasc Pharmacol, suppl. 9 1993;22:13–17

56. Feldman AM: Classification of positive inotropic agents. J Am Coll Cardiol 1993;22:1223–1227

57. Remme WJ: Inodilator therapy for heart failure. Early, late, or not at all? Circulation, suppl. IV 1993; 87:97–107

58. Katz AM: The cardiomyopathy of overload. An unnatural growth response in the hypertrophied heart. Ann Intern Med 1994;121:363–371

59. DiBianco R, Shabetai R, Kastuk W et al: A comparison of oral milrinone, digoxin, and their combination in the treatment of patients with chronic heart failure. N Engl J Med 1989;320:677–683

60. Packer M, Gheorghiade M, Young JB et al: Withdrawal of digoxin from patients with chronic heart failure treated with angiotensin-converting-enzyme inhibitors. Results of the RADIANCE study. N Engl J Med 1993;329:1–7

61. Uretsky BF, Young JB, Shahidi FE et al: Randomized study assessing the effect of digoxin withdrawal in patients with mild to moderate chronic congestive heart failure. Results of the PROVED trial. J Am Coll Cardiol 1993;22:955–962

62. Yusuf S, Garg R, Held P, Gorlin R: Need for a large randomized trial to evaluate the effects of digitalis on morbidity and mortality in congestive heart failure. Am J Cardiol, suppl. G 1992;69:64–70

63. Tan LB, Murray RG, Tweddel AC, Hutton I: Cardiotonic effect of digitalis in sinus rhythm during exercise. pp. 455–460. In: Erdmann E, Greeff K, Skou JC (eds) Cardiac Glycosides 1785–1985. Springer-Verlag, New York, 1986

64. Tan LB: The search for an ideal positive inotropic agent. Eur J Clin Pharmacol 1986;30:509–512

65. Miller LW, Mirkle EJ, Hermann V: Outpatient dobutamine for end-stage congestive heart failure. Crit Care Med 1990;18:530–533

66. Page DL, Caulfield JB, Kastor JA, DeSantis RW, Sanders CA: Myocardial changes associated with cardiogenic shock. N Engl J Med 1971;285:133–137

67. Gaasch WH: Diagnosis and treatment of heart failure based on left ventricular systolic or diastolic dysfunction. JAMA 1994;271:1276–1280

68. Lenihan DJ, Gerson MC, Hoit BD, Walsh RA: Mechanisms, diagnosis, and treatment of diastolic heart failure. Am Heart J 1995;130:153–166

69. Vasan RS, Benjamin EJ, Levy D: Congestive heart failure with normal left ventricular systolic function. Clinical approaches to the diagnosis and treatment of diastolic heart failure. Arch Intern Med 1996;156: 146–157

70. Soufer R, Wohlgelernter D, Vita NA et al: Intact systolic left ventricular function in clinical congestive heart failure. Am J Cardiol 1985;55:1032–1036

71. Iskandrian AS, Hakki A: Age-related changes in left ventricular diastolic performance. Am Heart J 1986; 112:75–78

72. Benjamin EJ, Levy D, Anderson KM et al: Determinants of Doppler indexes of left ventricular diastolic function in normal subjects (the Framingham Heart Study). Am J Cardiol 1992;70:508–515

73. Swinne CJ, Shapiro EP, Lima SD, Fleg JL: Age-associated changes in left ventricular diastolic performance during isometric exercise in normal subjects. Am J Cardiol 1992;691:823–826

74. Cohn JN, Johnson G: Heart failure with normal ejection fraction. The V-HeFT study. Circulation, suppl. III 1990;81:48–53

75. AIRE Study Investigators: Effect of ramipril on mortality and morbidity of survivors of acute myocardial infarction with clinical evidence of heart failure. Lancet 1993;342:821–828

76. ACC/AHA Task Force Report: Guidelines for the evaluation and management of heart failure. J Am Coll Cardiol 1995;26:1376–1398

77. Brilla CG, Janicki JS, Weber KT: Cardioreparative effects of lisinopril in rats with genetic hypertension and left ventricular hypertrophy. Circulation 1991;83: 1771–1779

78. Levy WC, Cerqueira MD, Abrass IB, Schwartz RS, Stratton JR: Endurance exercise training augments diastolic filling at rest and during exercise in healthy young and older men. Circulation 1993;88:116–126

79. Belardinelli R, Georgiou D, Cianci G et al: Exercise training improves left ventricular diastolic filling in patients with dilated cardiomyopathy. Clinical and prognostic implications. Circulation 1995;91: 2775–2784

80. Katz AM: Interplay between inotropic and lusitropic effects of cyclic adenosine monophosphate on the myocardial cell. Circulation, suppl. I 1990;82:7–11

81. Perreault CL, Williams CP, Morgan JP: Cytoplasmic calcium modulation and systolic versus diastolic dysfunction in myocardial hypertrophy and failure. Circulation suppl. VII 1993;87:31–37

82. Little WC, Downes TR: Clinical evaluation of left ventricular diastolic performance. Prog Cardiovasc Dis 1990;32:273–290

40 Large Trials and Meta-analyses

Robert S. McKelvie
Salim Yusuf

Chronic congestive heart failure (CHF) is a syndrome that is the end result of a number of types of cardiac damage and resulting compensatory mechanisms. Patients usually have multiple symptoms and experience high rates of hospitalization, morbidity, and mortality, leading to limitation of daily activities and a poor quality of life. Therefore treatment of these patients not only focuses on symptomatic relief but includes strategies that decrease morbidity and mortality.[1] Detailed studies on a small number of patients are useful for examining physiologic mechanisms related to a particular therapy, and these data can then be used to justify the design of large trials that can reliably assess the effects on mortality and morbidity. However, even if a beneficial effect on a surrogate outcome such as exercise tolerance has been demonstrated, it cannot necessarily guarantee that mortality and morbidity will be reduced. This apparent inconsistency has been seen with a number of studies where improvements in exercise tolerance, ejection fraction, or ventricular arrhythmias did not lead to benefits on clinically relevant outcomes.[2–5]

The observation that improvements in surrogate endpoints do not always correlate with clinical benefit should not be surprising because a number of complex and interrelated factors may contribute to the clinical condition of a CHF patient, making the clinical course highly variable and unpredictable. In such situations there is no substitute for directly examining the effects of an intervention on mortality and morbidity. Approaches to reliably ascertain the clinical effect of therapy requires minimizing all sources of "error" ("noise" or, more formally, variance) during the evaluation.[1] These "errors" can generally be classified into those due to systematic biases or to random errors.[6] Randomized, double-blind, controlled trials are used to avoid various systematic biases. This design avoids biases in patient allocation and endpoint ascertainment as well as minimizing imbalances at entry in known and unknown risk factors between those on the active treatment and those on standard treatment. Random errors are chiefly due to the play of chance and are most effectively minimized by increasing the number of patients in a study. By having a large enough sample size, an appropriate number of events are expected to occur so plausible differences can be detected.

Large clinical trials could be conducted efficiently by simplifying all aspects of the protocol if the chief aim is to assess the effects of therapy on mortality or morbidity in CHF patients. This is because the outcome measures (e.g., mortality, hospitalizations) can be unbiasedly and relatively accurately documented with simple procedures for data collection and can therefore be applied efficiently to large numbers of patients. Studying large numbers of patients also provides more reliable information of the impact of a therapy on less common but clinically important adverse effects (e.g., neutropenia). Large clinical trials are also required because most treatments are likely to have only a moderate impact on major outcomes. The expectation of moderate benefits is not surprising given the great heterogeneity of the etiology and pathophysiology of CHF, the unpredictability of survival among apparently similar patients, and the various mechanisms (e.g., arrhythmias, pump failure, myocardial infarction) that can lead to death. The use of a particular therapy would generally be expected to influence only a few of the various mechanisms that lead to clinical deterioration or death, thereby making it unlikely that any therapy would have more than a moderate effect on the course of CHF. Therefore as has been found with many treatments for other common cardiovascular diseases, the expected risk reduction would be no greater than 20–25 percent.[7,8] However, given the high prevalence of CHF and the high rates of mortality and morbidity, even a 15–20 percent risk reduction in mortality or major morbidity is of great clinical importance.

The results of randomized controlled trials of various therapies for CHF patients are discussed in this chapter. We discuss vasodilators, angiotensin-converting enzyme inhibitors (ACE-Is), β-blockers, inotropic agents, antiarrhythmic drugs, and calcium channel blockers. Newer therapeutic approaches such as angiotensin II receptor antagonists and exercise training are also briefly discussed. We recognize that these and other trials are discussed in greater detail in other chapters. Our goal is to place these trials into a broader perspective.

DIRECT-ACTING VASODILATORS

The initial rationale for the use of direct-acting vasodilators in CHF patients was to decrease the left ventricular afterload or preload by decreasing peripheral vascular resistance or increasing venous capacitance, thereby decreasing the load imposed on the failing ventricle. This hypothesis was extensively tested in the Vasodilator in Heart Failure (V-HeFT) I trial.[9] In this study 642 patients who were taking digoxin and diuretic were randomized to receive placebo, prazosin, or the combination of hydralazine plus isosorbide dinitrate. There was no beneficial effect on any outcome with prazosin. Compared to placebo the hydralazine–isosorbide dinitrate combination resulted in a significant increase in ejection fraction at 8 weeks and 1 year. A trend toward fewer deaths ($P < 0.093$ using the prespecified method of analysis) was observed for the combination therapy group. V-HeFT-I demonstrated that not all vasodilators have the same effect on CHF and suggested that the combination of hydralazine and nitrates may be beneficial. In the subsequent V-HeFT-II study, the hydralazine-isosorbide dinitrate combination was compared to the ACE inhibitor enalapril.[10] The latter regimen was associated with a significantly better 2-year survival, but exercise tolerance was better with the direct-acting vasodilator regimen.

Because V-HeFT-I involved two vasodilators, it is uncertain whether the observed favorable trend represents the effect of one of these agents or the combination. Experience with agents that have isolated or predominant arterial vasodilating actions, such as minoxidil, prostacyclin, flosequinan, and calcium channel blockers (see below), has not been favorable.[11,12] In contrast, small controlled studies have suggested that nitrates alleviate symptoms and improve exercise tolerance, although these effects may be limited by tolerance, and larger trials during the immediate postinfarction period also indicated a beneficial effect of nitrates.[13,14] Thus it is tempting to ascribe the V-HeFT-I results to the nitrate component. However, both ISIS-4 and GISSI-3 showed only a small beneficial effect of nitrates on short-term survival in large groups of unselected postinfarction patients,[15,16] although whether such an effect might be present during long-term therapy or in patients selected for heart failure or left ventricular dysfunction is uncertain. At this time, therefore, the role of direct-acting vasodilators, particularly in patients already receiving ACE-Is, remains unsettled.

ANGIOTENSIN-CONVERTING ENZYME INHIBITORS

More than 10,000 patients with varying severity of left ventricular dysfunction have been randomized into trials that have assessed the benefits of ACE-Is. These trials have assessed the impact of ACE-Is on mortality, hospitalization for CHF, exercise tolerance, ventricular function, and quality of life.[17] Another goal in some of these trials was to determine whether the early institution of therapy could reduce the rate of progression of patients from asymptomatic to symptomatic left ventricular dysfunction.[18]

Effects on Mortality

The Cooperative North Scandinavian Enalapril Survival Study (CONSENSUS) trial was the first to examine the effects of ACE-I inhibitor on mortality in CHF patients.[19] Patients who remained in New York Heart Association (NYHA) functional class IV despite 2 weeks of maximum therapy with diuretics, digoxin, and non-ACE-I vasodilators were randomized to either enalapril or a placebo group for an average of 6 months. The enalapril group had a significant ($P = 0.003$) reduction in mortality, as well as improvements in NYHA functional class, and reductions in heart size and the need for diuretics. In the Studies of Left Ventricular Function (SOLVD) treatment trial symptomatic patients mainly in NYHA class II and III were randomized to either placebo or enalapril for an average of 41 months.[20] There was a 16 percent ($P = 0.0036$) reduction in total mortality risk and a 22 percent ($P = 0.0045$) reduction in risk due to progressive heart failure deaths.

The use of long-term ACE-I therapy has also been studied in patients with left ventricular dysfunction or heart failure following myocardial infarction. In the Survival and Ventricular Enlargement (SAVE) trial patients at 3–16 days after myocardial infarction with an ejection fraction less than 40 percent but without overt heart failure or symptoms of myocardial ischemia were randomized to receive either captopril or placebo for an average of 42 months.[21] There was a reduction of all-cause mortality of 19 percent ($P = 0.19$) and of cardiovascular mortality of 21 percent ($P = 0.014$) in the group taking captopril. In the SAVE trial the significant reduction in cardiovascular mortality was consistent in those on and not on antifailure therapy (diuretics or digoxin) at baseline, suggesting that background antifailure therapy does not significantly modify the effect of the ACE-I. The Acute Infarction Ramipril Efficacy (AIRE) trial[22] randomized patients who had clinical evidence of heart failure on days 3–10 after the index myocardial infarction to either ramipril or placebo for an average of 15 months. There was a 27 percent ($P = 0.002$) reduction in total mortality in the ramipril group. The collective data from several small randomized trials in CHF of a variety of ACE-Is also demonstrate similar results on reduction in mortality.[17]

The effects of ACE-I inhibitor therapy in patients with asymptomatic left ventricular dysfunction (ejection fraction less than 35 percent) have been examined in the SOLVD prevention trial.[18] Patients were randomized to receive either enalapril or placebo for an average treatment period of 37 months. There was an 8 percent ($P = 0.30$) reduction in total mortality and a 12 percent ($P = 0.12$) reduction in cardiovascular mortality found for the enalapril group. This trial demonstrated prevention of hospitalization for CHF and prevention of CHF (see later). During the study more patients assigned to the placebo than to the enalapril group received digoxin, diuretics, or ACE-Is that were not part of the study regimen. This practice may have accounted for the lack of significant difference in the mortality endpoint between the two groups, as the reduction in mortality with enalapril was chiefly due to a lower incidence of heart failure.

In the trials that included patients with overt heart failure[19,20,22] there was an immediate reduction in mortality with the institution of ACE-I therapy, with the benefits sustained up to 4 years. In patients with asymptomatic left ventricular dysfunction[18,21] benefits were not observed for at least 12–18 months; thereafter mortality was reduced during the rest of the long-term treatment in the trial. The latter indicates that there may be a period during which left ventricular remodeling has to be prevented during asymptomatic left ventricular dysfunction in order to limit the development of heart failure, which ultimately translates into reduced mortality.

The data from the V-HeFT-II trial indicate that ACE-Is are superior to hydralazine–isosorbide. They also suggest that there may be little relation between the ability of a drug to improve the ejection fraction and exercise tolerance compared with its effects on mortality or morbidity. In this trial 804 patients were randomized to receive either hydralazine–isosorbide dinitrate or the ACE-I enalapril.[23] There was a trend to fewer deaths (153 versus 132; $P = 0.08$) in the group taking enalapril, but the improvements in ejection fraction and exercise tolerance were significantly greater in the group taking the combination vasodilator therapy.

Effects on Development of Heart Failure and Hospitalization Rate

The ACE-Is have been demonstrated to reduce morbidity and the development of heart failure in asymptomatic and symptomatic patients with left ventricular dysfunction. In the SOLVD prevention trial[18] there was a 37 percent reduction in the development of CHF, a 43 percent reduction in the development of CHF and need for CHF therapy, a 36 percent reduction in the first hospitalization, and a 44 percent reduction in multiple hospitalizations for CHF. Also the incidence of death or development of CHF was significantly decreased (by 29 percent), and death or hospitalization for CHF was significantly decreased (by 20 percent). The SOLVD treatment trial demonstrated that in patients with established heart failure ACE-I therapy significantly decreased the risk of one or more hospitalizations.[20] This study also demonstrated a 26 percent ($P < 0.0001$) reduction in the combined endpoint of deaths or hospitalizations for CHF in patients taking the enalapril. The results from the SAVE trial are consistent with those found in the SOLVD trials.[21] A 37 percent risk reduction ($P < 0.001$) for the development of CHF and a 22 percent ($P = 0.019$) risk reduction for the development of CHF requiring a hospital admission were found in SAVE. The results from the AIRE trial have also demonstrated a 19 percent ($P = 0.008$) risk reduction for the first validated event in any individual patient of death, reinfarction, stroke, or the development of severe or resistant heart failure.[22]

Several additional trials have examined the effect of ACE-Is in larger but less selected groups of acute postinfarction patients.[15,16,24] In contrast to SAVE, the effects on survival were smaller. This difference can be attributed to the much shorter period of treatment and follow-up (4–6 weeks) or to the inclusion of patients with preserved left ventricular function. The favorable effect of a 6-week course of ACE-I therapy on the combined endpoint of death and severe CHF after 6 weeks and mortality at 1 year in the SMILE study, which entered patients only with presumably large anterior infarctions,[25] suggests that the size of the infarction and the severity of subsequent left ventricular dysfunction are important determinants of benefit in this setting.

Effects on Ischemic Events

In CHF patients it has been demonstrated that the occurrence of a new myocardial infarction increases the risk of subsequent death by up to eightfold, and that one-third of all deaths are preceded by a major ischemic event.[26] Similar data have been reported by Rutherford et al.[27] from the SAVE trial. These data emphasize that reductions in ischemic events should be an integral part of the management of patients with left ventricular dysfunction.

The SOLVD trials demonstrated that 25 percent of patients in the placebo group developed myocardial infarction or were hospitalized for unstable angina during the 3.5 years of follow-up.[26] Treatment with enalapril reduced the incidence of myocardial infarction by 23 percent ($P = 0.001$) and hospitalizations for unstable angina by 22 percent ($P = 0.0001$). There were reductions in both fatal and nonfatal myocardial infarctions, although the effects of reducing nonfatal infarction were twice as great as those seen with reducing fatal myocardial infarction. In contrast, whereas the reduction in hospital admissions for worsening heart failure with enalapril was observed shortly after randomization, the effects on ischemic events were not apparent for at least 6 months and peaked at 36 months. This delay in ischemic events resembles the pattern observed in trials of cholesterol lowering[28,29] and suggests that the mechanism of benefit is not due to acute hemodynamic changes. Instead the benefits are likely due to structural changes in the vessel wall.[30]

The SAVE trial[21] demonstrated a 25 percent reduction ($P = 0.015$) of the risk of recurrent myocardial infarction in patients in the captopril group. In SAVE there was also a significant reduction in the need for revascularization procedures, although there was no impact on unstable angina. There were few myocardial infarctions diagnosed in the AIRE trial,[22] and this trial did not demonstrate an impact on myocardial infarction rates. The observation that ramipril had less effect on ischemic events than has

been previously found may relate to the relatively short follow-up (only 15 months), the high noncompliance rate to treatment allocation by 1 year, and the limited number of myocardial infarctions. Combining the results from the SOLVD, SAVE, and AIRE trials there is still a significant reduction in myocardial infarction rates with ACE-I by about 20 percent.[30] Collectively, therefore, these data indicate that in patients with low ejection fractions ACE-Is prevent major ischemic events such as myocardial infarction, unstable angina, and the need for revascularization procedures (Table 40-1).

Subgroup Effects

Subgroup analyses of the SOLVD and SAVE trials indicate that treatment was beneficial in a large number of subgroups identified, including both genders, left ventricular dysfunction of different etiologies, and different background therapies. However, it appears that the reductions in mortality and hospitalizations for heart failure were greater for patients with more severe degrees of left ventricular dysfunction. It also appears that by comparing the results in the CONSENSUS I, AIRE, the SOLVD treatment trial, and the SOLVD prevention trial the benefits in terms of absolute and relative risk reductions, especially on mortality, were greater in those with more marked symptoms. A meta-analysis of all available ACE-I trials in patients with left ventricular dysfunction and heart failure has been performed, with the results demonstrating benefit for patients in these subgroups. The benefits were greater among patients with more severe left ventricular dysfunction (Tables 40-2A and 40-2B).[17]

Conclusions

The results of the trials of ACE-I therapy clearly demonstrate their benefits in CHF patients. There is a significant reduction in mortality and morbidity (progression of heart failure or hospitalization) due to heart failure. Table 40-3 demonstrates the number of events prevented or delayed by treating 1000 patients with an ACE-I for 3 years. As can be seen, ACE-Is have a significant impact on the development of heart failure, hospitalizations, ischemic events, and death in the group with no heart failure but an ejection fraction of 0.35 or lower and the group with heart failure with an ejection fraction of 0.35 or lower. Therefore these data suggest that the use of ACE-Is could be cost-effective and even lead to a substantial reduction in health care costs for patients with overt heart failure.

Table 40-1. Effect of Enalapril on the Development of Myocardial Infarction, Hospitalization for Worsening Angina, and Cardiac and Total Mortality in the SOLVD Combined Trials

Outcome	No. of Events (%) Placebo	No. of Events (%) Enalapril	Risk reduction (95% CI)	Z-score	P-value
Myocardial infarction					
Fatal	157 (4.6)	139 (4.1)	14 (−8,32)	1.32	0.19
Nonfatal	230 (6.8)	169 (5.0)	29 (13,4)	3.39	0.001
Either	362 (10.6)	288 (8.5)	23 (11,3)	3.38	0.001
Hospitalization for angina[a]	595 (17.5)	499 (14.7)	20 (9,29)	3.61	0.001
MI or hospitalization for angina	859 (25.3)	707 (20.8)	22 (14,2)	4.89	0.0001
Cardiac deaths, nonfatal MI	918 (27.0)	758 (22.3)	21 (13,2)	4.72	0.0001
Cardiac deaths, nonfatal MI, or hospitalization for angina	1350 (39.7)	1117 (32.9)	22 (16,2)	6.20	0.0001
All deaths, nonfatal MI, or hospitalization for angina	1422 (41.8)	1205 (35.5)	20 (14,2)	5.82	0.0001

Abbreviations: MI, myocardial infarction; Z, score: Z test for difference between two proportions; CI: confidence level. Numbers in parentheses are percents.

[a] The data above regarding hospitalization for angina includes both the primary or secondary discharge diagnosis. The numbers of patients hospitalized with a primary diagnosis of worsening angina are: Prevention trial (329 placebo versus 296 enalapril, Z = 1.61) Treatment trial (204 placebo versus 166 enalapril, Z = 2.55) and combined trials (533 placebo versus 462 enalapril, Z = 2.84).

Table 40-2A. Total Mortality by Various Subgroups Based on Sex, Age, NYHA Class, Etiology, and Ejection Fraction[a]

Subgroup (No. of Trials)	Allocation: No. of Events/No. Randomization (%) ACE Inhibitors	Allocation: No. of Events/No. Randomization (%) Controls	Odds Ratio (95% CI)
Sex (n = 80)			
Male	485/2937 (16.5)	558/2462 (22.7)	0.76 (0.65–0.88)
Female	117/871 (13.4)	144/716 (20.1)	0.79 (0.59–1.06)
Age (years) (n = 27)			
≤60	240/1614 (14.9)	294/1407 (20.9)	0.72 (0.59–0.89)
>60	355/1936 (18.3)	395/1574 (25.1)	0.81 (0.67–0.97)
NYHA class[b] (n = 28)			
I	39/193 (20.2)	45/181 (24.9)	0.75 (0.46–1.23)
II	265/1930 (13.7)	296/1622 (18.2)	0.83 (0.68–1.01)
III	227/1376 (16.5)	262/1103 (23.8)	0.76 (0.60–0.96)
IV	71/253 (28.1)	96/213 (45.1)	0.55 (0.36–0.84)
Etiology (n = 24)			
Ischemic heart disease	415/1997 (20.8)	488/1757 (27.8)	0.77 (0.65–0.91)
Nonischemic heart disease[c]	173/1132 (15.3)	187/1006 (18.6)	0.80 (0.62–1.04)
EF (n = 16)			
≤ 0.25	287/1129 (25.4)	351/1039 (33.8)	0.69 (0.57–0.85)
> 0.25	209/1335 (15.7)	208/1138 (18.3)	0.98 (0.78–1.23)
All patients (n = 32)	611/3870 (15.8)	709/3235 (21.9)	0.77 (0.67–0.88)

[a] Data on sex were missing on two patients and not available from two trials. Data on age were missing on eight patients and not available from four trials. Data on NYHA class were missing on seven patients and not available from three trials. Data on etiology were missing on 18 patients and not available from eight trials. Data on ejection fraction (EF) were missing on 340 patients and not available from 16 trials. Data on EF were not available because EF was not an entry criteria in 14 trials.

[b] In one of the trials of rampiril, eight patients were classified as NYHA class II–III and thus included in NYHA class III for analysis, and six patients were classified as NYHA class III–IV and thus included in NYHA class IV.

[c] Includes ischemic heart disease not confirmed.

(From Garg et al.,[17] with permission.)

Table 40-2B. Total Mortality or Hospitalization for Congestive Heart Failure by Various Subgroups Based on Sex, Age, NYHA Class, Etiology, and Ejection Fraction[a]

Subgroup (No. of Trials)	Allocation: No. Events/No. Randomization (%)		Odds Ratio (95% CI)
	ACE Inhibitors	Controls	
Sex (n = 30)			
Male	673/2937 (22.9)	818/2462 (33.2)	0.63 (0.55–0.73)
Female	176/871 (20.2)	211/716 (29.5)	0.78 (0.59–1.04)
Age, (years) (n = 27)			
≤60	358/1614 (22.2)	438/1407 (31.1)	0.71 (0.59–0.86)
>60	483/1936 (24.9)	581/1574 (36.9)	0.79 (0.66–0.95)
NYHA class[b] (n = 28)			
I	53/193 (27.5)	63/181 (34.8)	0.69 (0.44–1.09)
II	376/1930 (19.5)	461/1622 (28.4)	0.68 (0.57–0.81)
III	304/1376 (22.1)	377/1103 (34.2)	0.58 (0.46–0.73)
IV	117/253 (46.2)	129/213 (59.2)	0.69 (0.43–1.10)
Etiology (n = 24)			
Ischemic heart disease	566/1997 (28.3)	704/1757 (40.1)	0.63 (0.54–0.74)
Nonischemic heart disease[c]	263/1132 (23.2)	292/1006 (29.0)	0.72 (0.57–0.91)
EF (n = 16)			
≤ 0.25	381/1129 (33.7)	499/1039 (48.0)	0.53 (0.43–0.65)
> 0.25	315/1335 (23.6)	337/1138 (29.6)	0.85 (0.69–1.04)
All patients (n = 32)	854/3810 (22.4)	1036/3178 (32.6)	0.65 (0.57–0.74)

[a] Data on sex were missing on two patients and not available from two trials. Data on age were missing on eight patients and not available from four trials. Data on NYHA class were missing on seven patients and not available from three trials. Data on etiology were missing on 18 patients and not available from eight trials. Data on ejection fraction (EF) were missing on 340 patients and not available from 16 trials. Data on EF were not available because EF was not an entry criteria in 14 trials.

[b] In one of the trials of rampiril, eight patients were classified as NYHA class II–III and thus included in NYHA class III for analysis, and six patients were classified as NYHA class III–IV and thus included in NYHA class IV.

[c] Includes ischemic heart disease not confirmed.

(From Garg et al.,[17] with permission.)

Table 40-3. Implications of Routine Use of ACE Inhibitors in Patients with Low Ejection Fractions (Based on the SOLVD Trial Results)

Parameter	Events Prevented or Delayed by Treating 1000 Patients with an ACE-I for 3 Years	
	EF ≤ 0.35 + CHF	EF ≤ 0.35 + No CHF
Development of CHF	NA	90
Hospitalization for CHF	200	65
Myocardial infarction or unstable angina	40	35
Deaths	50	15

Abbreviations: CHF, congestive heart failure; EF, ejection fraction; NA, not applicable; ACE-I, angiotensin-converting enzyme inhibitor.

The data from these large trials provide a rational basis for the use of ACE-Is in patients with asymptomatic or symptomatic left ventricular dysfunction. Currently, the recommended approach is to treat these patients as early as possible with an ACE-I.

POSITIVE INOTROPIC AGENTS

There are a number of ways to classify positive inotropic drugs. One generally accepted classification is outlined in Table 40-4, which incorporates the major clinical and laboratory considerations in relation to these agents.[31] Aside from digitalis, most of these agents have been developed since the mid-1970s and are used for short-term management of CHF.[32–36]

Nondigitalis Therapy for Heart Failure

A number of agents with positive inotropic activity but with chemical structures and mechanisms of action different from those of digitalis or catechola-

Table 40-4. General Classification of Positive Inotropic Agents and Overview of Their Current Status for Intervention

Positive Inotropic Drug Groups	Clinical Application as Positive Inotropic Therapy	
	Acute/Short Term	Long Term
Digitalis	+	+
Catecholamines and related compounds		
β-Adrenergic agonists	+	−
α-Adrenergic agonists	−	−
Dopaminergic agents	+ (Dopamine)	Unlikely
Phosphodiesterase inhibitors	+	Unlikely
Others		
Direct adenylate cyclase agonists	?	?
Calcium sensitizers	?	?
H₂-receptor agonists	?	?
Endogenous substances (glucagon; thyroid hormone)	?	?

mines have been investigated.[37,38] The phosphodiesterase inhibitors (PDE-I) comprise an alternative group of drugs that have been demonstrated to have positive inotropic and vasodilator activity.[39–42] Their main mechanism of action is through inhibition of phosphodiesterase producing increased cyclic adenosine monophosphate (cAMP). The use of an agent to increase cAMP was considered rational for CHF patients, as the production of cAMP is deficient in failing human hearts, especially those in the terminal stages.[43,44]

Amrinone was the first of the (PDE-I) group to undergo extensive clinical evaluation. Intravenous administration of amrinone in the short-term was found to produce marked hemodynamic improvement.[45–48] More long-term clinical studies demonstrated that amrinone was active when given orally as a positive inotrope and vasodilator.[49–51] However, these studies were not large-scale randomized double-blind placebo-controlled trials, and little was known about the long-term efficacy and safety of amrinone.

DiBianco et al.[52] gave oral amrinone to 173 CHF patients who were predominantly NYHA class II to III. They found that 52 of these patients had an adequate exercise test response (increased exercise time by more than 2 minutes) and were free of limiting side effects while taking amrinone. These 52 responders to amrinone were then randomized in a double-blind fashion to continue to receive the active medication (31 patients) or were withdrawn and placed on placebo (21 patients). After a 12-week follow-up there was no significant difference observed for indices of left ventricular size and function, systolic time intervals, or maximal exercise time between those on amrinone and those on placebo. Episodes of worsened CHF severe enough to require termination of the double-blind treatment were as frequent in patients taking placebo as those on amrinone. However, side effects (including elevation of serum liver enzymes, reduced platelet counts, and gastrointestinal and central nervous complaints) were more common in the patients taking amrinone.

Another study examined the effects of amrinone using a prospective double-blind randomized controlled trial in 99 NYHA functional class II–IV CHF patients.[53] After 12 weeks of therapy there was no significant difference found between the two groups or compared to baseline with regard to symptoms, NYHA functional class, left ventricular ejection fraction, cardiothoracic ratio, frequency and severity of ventricular ectopy, or mortality. Adverse reactions were significantly more frequent with amrinone, occurring in 83 percent of patients and necessitating withdrawal in 34 percent. Therefore these findings were consistent with those found in the study by DiBianco et al.[52]

After these two reports no further studies of amrinone were performed partly because of the findings and partly because the Sterling Winthrop Research Institute had developed a promising analog of amrinone called milrinone. Milrinone, in studies of heart failure, has been found to increase the cardiac index and exercise tolerance and reduce ventricular filling pressure and systemic vascular resistance.[42,54–62] Furthermore, milrinone was shown to improve diastolic ventricular function[56] and to complement captopril.[63]

DiBianco et al.[64] compared the effects of oral placebo, milrinone, digoxin, and their combination on the exercise capacity and clinical course of patients in sinus rhythm with symptomatic mild to moderate heart failure. There were 230 patients randomized to one of the four groups, and they were followed up 12 weeks after randomization. Milrinone and digoxin each increased exercise time compared to placebo, but there was no difference between the active medications; nor was the combination of digoxin and milrinone better than the active drugs individually. Left ventricular ejection fraction was significantly improved by digoxin but not by milrinone. There was an increase in ventricular arrhythmias in patients receiving milrinone. Therefore in this study, although milrinone increased exercise capacity and decreased symptoms of heart failure it did not offer any advantage over digoxin therapy. Furthermore, milrinone aggravated ventricular arrhythmias.

The results of a meta-analysis of 21 small randomized trials of PDE-I and β-adrenergic agonists (β-AAs) suggested that excess mortality (PDE-I odds ratio 1.58, 95 percent CI 1.04–2.41; β-AA odds ratio 2.07, CI 1.23–3.49) was associated with the use of these agents.[65] These results must be interpreted cautiously because of the potential multiple actions of these agents, short duration of the trials, uncertainty regarding unpublished data, and the lack of use of ACE-Is. The results emphasized the importance of performing a large, long-term randomized controlled trial to assess mortality prior to these agents being incorporated into clinical practice.

A larger randomized double-blind placebo-controlled trial has since been reported that was designed to assess the effects of milrinone on mortality and morbidity in CHF patients.[66] In this trial 1088 NYHA functional class III or IV CHF patients were randomized to receive either oral milrinone or placebo, and the median follow-up was 6.1 months. Milrinone therapy resulted in a 28 percent increase in all-cause mortality ($P = 0.038$) and a 34 percent increase in cardiovascular mortality ($P = 0.016$). This effect was greatest in patients in NYHA functional class IV, who had a 53 percent increase in mortality ($P = 0.006$). There was no beneficial effect on survival found for any subgroup. Patients treated with milrinone had more hospitalizations (44 percent versus 39 percent; $P = 0.041$), were withdrawn from double-blind therapy more frequently (12.7 percent versus 8.7 percent; $P = 0.041$), and had serious cardiovascular reactions, including hypotension ($P = 0.006$) and syncope ($P = 0.002$), more often than patients given placebo. The results from this trial demonstrated definitively that there was no benefit to milrinone therapy in CHF patients.

Enoximone is another PDE-I that has been evaluated in CHF patients.[67] In this study 102 patients in NYHA functional class II or III were randomized to receive either enoximone or placebo in a double-blind randomized placebo-controlled trial. There were no significant differences in symptom score or exercise capacity between enoximone and placebo after 4 months of therapy. The dropout rate was greater ($P < 0.02$) with enoximone (46 percent) than with placebo (25 percent). There were five deaths in the enoximone group and none in the placebo group ($P < 0.05$) after 4 months of treatment. This study

demonstrated that enoximone produced no clinical benefit compared to placebo; and although it was not designed as a mortality trial, the high mortality rate raises concerns about the detrimental effect of enoximone.

Pimobendan exerts a positive inotrope effect that is mediated by a combination of sensitizing myocardial contractile proteins to intracellular calcium, a PDE-I effect, and a vasodilator action.[68–73] One study[74] examined the efficacy and safety of pimobendan in 198 ambulatory CHF patients with NYHA class III or IV symptoms. The patients were all taking digoxin and diuretics, and 80 percent were taking an ACE-I and 14 percent were taking a non-ACE-I vasodilator. Patients were randomized to receive daily either placebo or 2.5, 5.0, or 10 mg of pimobendan. After 12 weeks of follow-up, compared to placebo, the 5.0 mg of pimobendan significantly increased exercise duration 121.6 ± 19.1 seconds ($P < 0.001$), whereas the 10 mg dose increased exercise duration by only 81.1 ± 19.5 seconds ($P = 0.05$). Compared to placebo the 5.0 mg dose produced a significant improvement in the quality of life measure (Minnesota Living with Heart Failure Questionnaire), by 8.5 ± 2.3 units ($P < 0.01$). There was a total of 23 all-cause hospitalizations in the placebo group, which was significantly higher than the 33 in the three groups treated with pimobendan ($P < 0.01$). There were no significant differences between the placebo and pimobendan groups with respect to changes in ejection fraction, plasma norepinephrine levels, proarrhythmic effect, or number of patients with a significant adjustment in background therapy. Furthermore, there was no difference in mortality between the placebo and pimobendan groups. Obviously, larger trials with longer follow-up of this medication are required to confirm these effects and assess the effect on mortality and morbidity. Also studies are needed on patients with milder forms of CHF and those with end-stage heart failure with symptoms at rest. At present, further development of this drug has been terminated.

Vesnarinone is a PDE-I that may be an exception to the other previously studied drugs in this group, such as amrinone and milrinone. In contrast to agents that act exclusively by increasing the levels of cAMP, vesnarinone slows the heart rate, prolongs the action potential, and suppresses the delayed outward potassium current.[75,76] In one study CHF patients in NYHA functional classes II–IV were randomized to 120 or 60 mg of vesnarinone per day compared to placebo.[77] After 253 patients had been enrolled, randomization to the 120 mg vesnarinone group had to be stopped because of a significant increase in early mortality in this group (16 deaths in the vesnarinone 120 mg per day group versus 6 patients in the control group). Thereafter patients were randomly assigned to either 60 mg of vesnarinone per day (239 patients) or placebo (238 patients). At the end of the 6-month follow-up the group taking 60 mg vesnarinone had fewer patient deaths or worsening heart failure than those in the placebo group (26 versus 50 patients; $P = 0.003$), a 50 percent (95 percent confidence interval = 20–69 percent) risk reduction. Similarly, there were fewer deaths among the vesnarinone-treated patients (13 versus 33 patients; $P = 0.002$). Patients taking vesnarinone had a greater improvement in quality of life than those in the placebo group, but this effect was entirely accounted for by the imputation method, which scored death as the "worst" quality of life score. The main side effect was reversible neutropenia, which occurred in 2.5 percent of the patients taking vesnarinone. Therefore this study demonstrated that vesnarinone has a narrow therapeutic range with the higher dose (120 mg per day) resulting in greater mortality compared to placebo. The lower dose (60 mg per day), however, appears to reduce mortality and morbidity as well as improve quality of life scores. Unfortunately, despite these promising results, the much larger Vesnarinone Evaluation of Survival Trial (VEST) which recently ended found an adverse effect of vesnarinone survival. These findings are discussed in Chapter 46.

There is only limited information about other non-digitalis positive inotropic agents. Xamoterol is a β_1 selective partial agonist. In one placebo-controlled study in patients with mild to moderate heart failure comparing xamoterol and digoxin there was an improvement in exercise duration and improved breathlessness and tiredness, whereas no similar benefits were observed with digoxin.[78] Another study in patients ($n = 516$) with more severe CHF (NYHA functional class III–IV) demonstrated increased mortality (9.1 percent versus 3.7 percent; $P = 0.02$) within the first 100 days of randomization.[79] Oral ibopamine was designed specifically to deliver a dopamine congener to the circulation.[31] A number of studies suggest that long-term ibopamine administration is capable of improving symptoms and perhaps exercise capacity in CHF patients.[80–84] However, as discussed in Chapter 46, a larger trial found little of these benefits and a high mortality rate in patients with severe CHF treated with ibopamine.

Digitalis Therapy for Heart Failure

Digitalis has been the mainstay of heart failure therapy for more than two centuries. However, the use of digoxin in patients with heart failure remains controversial, reflected by the inconsistency of the use of digoxin across the world. A survey from participants in the SOLVD Registry found that digoxin use ranged from 80 percent in patients with four signs of CHF and a left ventricular ejection fraction of less than 20 percent to approximately 20 percent in patients with only one sign of CHF and an ejection fraction of 36–45 percent. Overall, approximately 50 percent of patients with left ventricular dysfunction with or without symptoms of heart failure from the United States were taking digoxin compared with only 24 percent from Belgium and 41 percent from Canada.

At least 15 randomized controlled trials of digitalis in CHF patients have been identified.[64,78,85–97] The first two trials enrolled patients without clear evidence of CHF,[85,86] and the third included patients with atrial fibrillation.[87] Several small trials evaluated CHF patients using a crossover design with treatment periods of 2–3 months each.[88–92,94] Almost all patients were withdrawn from previous chronic use of digitalis and randomized to receive placebo or digoxin.

Lee et al.[88] found a significant improvement in heart failure score (based on clinical and radiographic changes) in the digoxin-treated patients, although similar patients deteriorated clinically during the control and active treatment phases. Retrospective analysis suggested that a third heart sound, an enlarged heart, and a low ejection fraction correlated with benefit among responders. No improvement in ejection fraction was found with digoxin. Fleg et al.[89] reported no difference in exercise capacity, physical findings, or symptoms between the digoxin and placebo arms in a study of 40 patients. Taggart et al.[90] found no clear evidence of a benefit with digoxin in 22 patients (worsening CHF developed in four patients given placebo versus two given digoxin). After screening 380 patients, Guyatt et al.[91] included 30 patients in their study and reported results obtained in the 20 who completed the treatment. Patients benefited with respect to symptoms, clinical assessment of CHF, exercise capacity (6-minute walking distance), and ejection fraction during the treatment period compared with the placebo phase. The large proportion of patients excluded or with missing endpoint data makes interpretation of the results difficult.

In a double-blind crossover study, Pugh et al.[92] studied 44 patients and observed that 11 (25 percent) deteriorated clinically while taking placebo compared with only 5 (11 percent) who deteriorated taking digoxin. Most patients who deteriorated could be stabilized by increasing the dose of diuretics. Only two patients required reintroduction of digoxin. Benefit from digoxin could not be predicted based on a third heart sound, hemodynamic criteria, echocardiographic measures, or heart size.

Four larger trials compared digoxin with placebo or a second active drug. Only the results comparing the digoxin group to the placebo group are discussed here. In the captopril–digoxin trial[93] 1986 patients were randomized to receive digoxin or placebo. All patients had an ejection fraction of less than 40 percent, and 85 percent of patients had NHYA class I or II CHF. After 6 months there was a favorable nonsignificant improvement in exercise time in the digoxin group compared with the placebo group, and the ejection fraction increased by 4 percent in the digoxin group versus 1 percent in the placebo group ($P < 0.05$). Of the total, 8 patients given digoxin and 19 given placebo had to be hospitalized due to CHF. There were seven deaths in the digoxin group and six in the placebo group. In the xamoterol–digoxin trial,[78] 204 patients were randomized to receive digoxin or placebo; 80 percent were in NYHA class I or II. A fixed daily dose of 0.25 mg digoxin was administered. In patients who completed the 3-month double-blind phase, there was no difference in exercise duration between treatment groups. There was no difference in symptoms between groups, although decreases in peripheral edema and rales were found among digoxin-treated patients. No deaths occurred in the digoxin group compared with one in the placebo group. In the milrinone–digoxin trial,[64] 111 patients were randomized to receive digoxin or placebo. After 3 months the ejection fraction increased by 1.7 percent in the digoxin group and decreased by 2.0 percent in the placebo group ($P < 0.01$). Exercise tolerance in patients receiving digoxin increased by 14 percent compared with those given placebo ($P < 0.05$). Three patients in the digoxin group and four in the placebo group died during treatment. None of the above trials reported a preferential benefit in any particular subgroup. In another multicenter trial,[97] 133 patients with a documented myocardial infarction resulting in regional wall motion abnormalities and mild CHF were randomized to digoxin or placebo for 1 year. Digoxin resulted in improvement in quality of life and NYHA class compared with the placebo group ($P < 0.05$). No differences in exercise tolerance were observed.

The results of two parallel trials of digoxin withdrawal versus placebo have been reported.[95,96] In a study of 88 heart failure patients in sinus rhythm who were not on ACE-Is, Uretsky et al.[95] reported that patients withdrawn from digoxin showed deterioration of ejection fraction and exercise capacity on the treadmill, although digoxin withdrawal had no effect on NYHA class or the 6-minute walk test. In a larger trial of 178 patients with a low ejection frac-

tion and on ACE-Is, Packer et al.[96] reported a significant favorable effect of digoxin on ejection fraction, exercise capacity on the treadmill, the 6-minute walk test, and the frequency of worsening CHF compared with the placebo group.

The effect of digoxin on survival among patients following myocardial infarction or with heart failure has been analyzed by several investigators using existing databases.[98–104] In several studies it was suggested that digoxin might increase the risk of sudden death or mortality among subgroups of patients with frequent ventricular ectopy.[98,99] In some of these studies[103,104] digoxin use was associated with a significantly higher risk of death than among those not using digoxin, after adjustment for differences in risk factors. However, other studies suggested that the higher mortality seen among digoxin-treated patients was largely due to a higher incidence of adverse risk factors. In these studies after statistical adjustments, the apparently higher mortality associated with digoxin use was not statistically significant. A critical review of these studies indicates that the effect of digoxin on survival cannot be assessed reliably by retrospective analyses of databases but, rather, requires large, randomized, controlled trials.[105]

Although there have been numerous randomized trials conducted to evaluate the effect of digoxin, these trials have had several limitations. First, all of the trials except one have been withdrawal trials; therefore it is not possible to evaluate the impact of initiation of digoxin compared with placebo. Second, none of these trials was of sufficient size or duration to provide reliable information on mortality. Third, patients with a relatively preserved ejection fraction have not been included in most of these trials, and therefore extrapolation of the available data from trials that enrolled only patients with low ejection fraction are limited. Fourth, patients received concomitant ACE-I therapy in only one of these trials. Given these limitations, the need to evaluate the effect of digoxin on morbidity and mortality in a broad spectrum of patients with heart failure and concurrent ACE-I therapy was apparent. This has been accomplished in the Digitalis Investigators Group (DIG) trial, whose preliminary results are discussed in Chapter 43.

β BLOCKER THERAPY

The first report demonstrating that the use of β-blocker therapy in idiopathic dilated cardiomyopathy and resting tachycardia improved the clinical condition of patients was published in 1975.[106] Since then a number of studies have demonstrated the effect of β-blocker therapy in patients with heart failure.[107–117] These studies showed beneficial effects on cardiac function, symptoms, and exercise performance, but none was designed to assess the effects of β-blocker therapy on mortality and morbidity.

In the Metoprolol in Dilated Cardiomyopathy (MDC) trial,[118] 383 patients with idiopathic dilated cardiomyopathy and NYHA functional class II or III heart failure were randomized to either metoprolol or placebo and followed up after 12 months of therapy. Approximately 80 percent of the patients in both groups were taking digoxin and ACE-Is. There were 34 percent fewer primary endpoints (95 percent confidence interval -6 to 62 percent; $P = 0.058$) in the metoprolol than the placebo group (2 metoprolol and 19 placebo patients deteriorated to the point of needing transplantation, with 23 and 19, respectively, dying). The increases in ejection fraction and exercise tolerance along with the decrease in pulmonary capillary wedge pressure were significantly greater in the metoprolol group than in the placebo group between baseline and 12 months. This study showed that β-blocker therapy decreases clinical deterioration while alleviating symptoms and improving cardiac function. Unfortunately, the study was not adequately powered to determine if β-blocker therapy has a beneficial effect on mortality, so another larger trial is needed to determine if there is a beneficial effect on this outcome measure.

The Cardiac Insufficiency Bisoprolol Study (CIBIS) was designed to examine the effect of bisoprolol, compared to placebo, on survival. The mean follow-up was 1.9 years, and the patients received background diuretic and vasodilator (90 percent of cases received ACE-I) therapy.[119] A total of 641 patients (approximately 50 percent with ischemic heart disease) were randomized to either placebo (321 patients) or bisoprolol (320 patients). Only 50 percent of the study patients reached the target dose of 5 mg bisoprolol daily. There was no significant difference observed in mortality between the two groups (67 patients died on placebo, 53 died on bisoprolol; $P = 0.22$; relative risk 0.80, 95 percent confidence interval 0.56–1.15). Bisoprolol significantly improved the functional status of the patients; fewer patients in the bisoprolol group required hospitalization for cardiac decompensation (90 on placebo versus 61 on bisoprolol; $P < 0.01$), and more patients improved by at least one NYHA class (48 on placebo versus 68 on bisoprolol; $P = 0.04$). Subgroup analysis demonstrated that in patients without a history of ischemic heart disease the mortality rate was significantly less in those taking bisoprolol (42 of 187, or 22.5 percent, of patients died on placebo; 18 of 151, or 12

percent, of patients died on bisoprolol; $P = 0.01$). There is no clear explanation for this suggested differential effect of β-blockade related to etiology. The lower than expected mortality rate in the placebo group and the fact that 50 percent of the patients did not achieve the target bisoprolol dose are possible reasons a significant effect on mortality may not have been observed. The more recent results with carvedilol, which provide additional evidence of a benefit with β-blockade in CHF, are discussed in Chapter 47. Other trials are required to assess whether β-blockers have a long-term beneficial effect on mortality. Also future trials should stratify patients according to etiology, especially according to history of myocardial infarction.

No large trials have been designed to specifically examine the effect of β-blocker therapy in patients with heart failure due to ischemic heart disease. There are, however, five trials that reported separately the effects of β-blocker therapy in postmyocardial infarction patients with or without CHF.[120–124] The pooled mortality data from these studies show that there is an approximately 20–30 percent reduction in mortality in the patients taking β-blockers.[125] The results must be interpreted cautiously because of the large number of trials not reporting subset data on heart failure. In the Norwegian timolol trial[121] mortality data were stratified according to heart size as determined on chest radiographs prior to randomization. There were three classifications described (Fig. 40-1): normal, borderline (men 500–550 ml/m^2) or definitely enlarged (men more than 550 ml/m^2; women more than 500 ml/m^2). Mortality was reduced with β-blockers by approximately 40 percent in each group; but because of the higher absolute risk associated with cardiac enlargement, the number of lives saved per 100 patients treated (Fig. 40-1) was greatest in the group with cardiac enlargement.[125] Analysis of the data derived from the BHAT trial[124,126] also demonstrates that the greatest number of lives saved is in the group with heart failure.[125] The results from both BHAT[124] and the Norwegian timolol trial[121] indicate that sudden deaths were reduced more than nonsudden deaths.[125] It should be emphasized that the patients in the postmyocardial infarction trials had mild to moderate heart failure; therefore the effects of β-blocker therapy in patients with more severe left ventricular dysfunction have not been determined. The results of the overview by Held[125] support the use of β-blocker therapy in patients with heart failure and ischemic heart disease, but the results should be interpreted cautiously for a number of reasons. In many trials mortality outcome data for CHF patients are not reported, and it is not clear whether this is due to failure of data collection or the analysis.

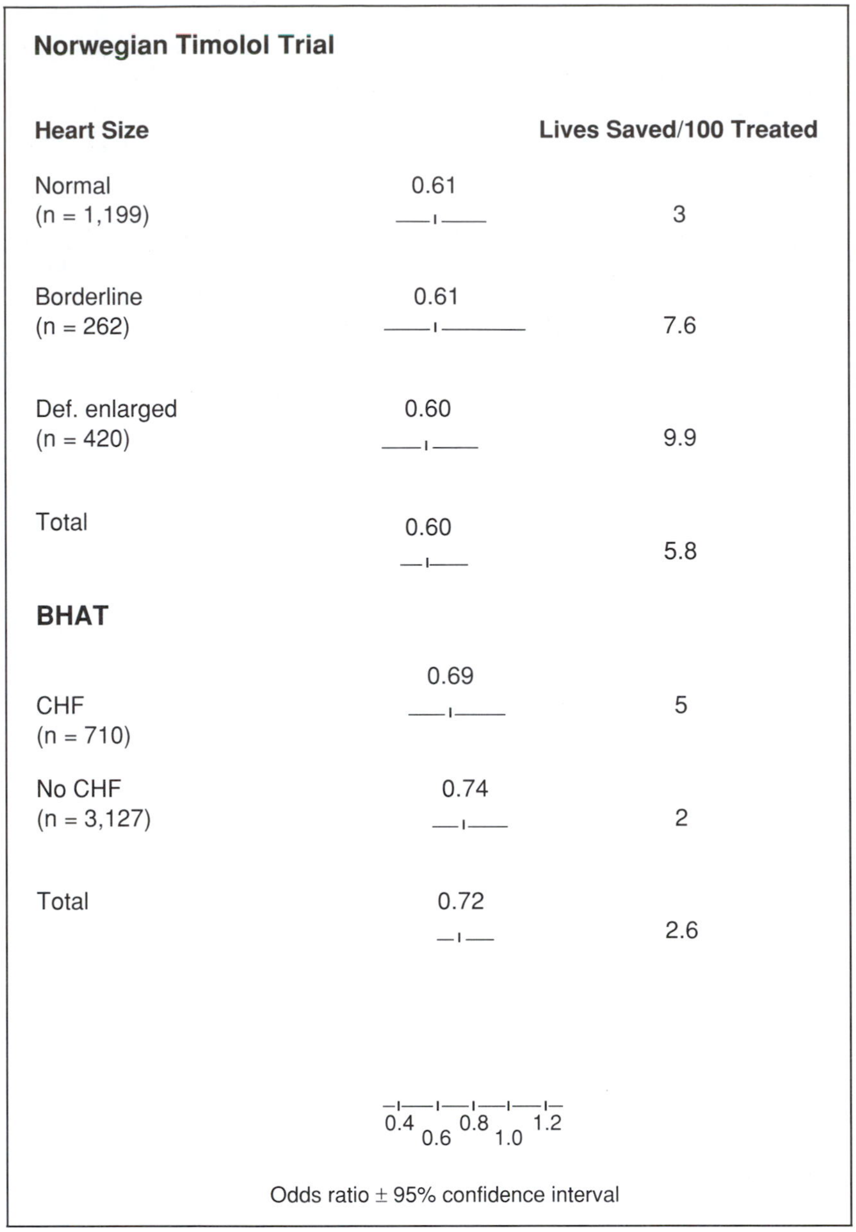

Norwegian Timolol Trial

Heart Size		Lives Saved/100 Treated
Normal (n = 1,199)	0.61 —ı—	3
Borderline (n = 262)	0.61 —ı—	7.6
Def. enlarged (n = 420)	0.60 —ı—	9.9
Total	0.60 —ı—	5.8

BHAT

CHF (n = 710)	0.69 —ı—	5
No CHF (n = 3,127)	0.74 —ı—	2
Total	0.72 —ı—	2.6

```
—ı—ı—ı—ı—ı—
0.4   0.8   1.2
   0.6   1.0
```

Odds ratio ± 95% confidence interval

Fig. 40-1. Odds of death and number of lives saved divided by baseline heart size and by history of heart failure in two large trials (Norwegian timolol trial[121] and BHAT[124]). Odds ratio ± 95% confidence interval. (From Held,[125] with permission.)

Furthermore, the possibility exists that less promising results related to β-blocker therapy were not reported, which would bias the results in favor of active therapy. The definition of heart failure was not consistent among the various trials, making it difficult to know if the same types of patient were being compared among trials. A more appropriate interpretation of the results of this overview is that a prospective randomized controlled trial of β-blocker compared to placebo is required to assess the effects in CHF patients from the full range of NYHA functional classes.

Avezum et al.[127] reported a systematic overview of 16 trials that examined the effect of β-blockade on mortality, hospitalization for CHF, transplantation, and symptoms in patients with heart failure. Their results suggested (Table 40-5) a modest reduction of mortality (10–20 percent), a large reduction in hospitalization rate for CHF (40–50 percent), and reduction of the need for transplantation (about 70 percent). Patients taking β-blockers were also found to have a significant improvement in NYHA functional classification (odds ratio 0.56 ± 0.57; $P = 0.01$). A major limitation to this overview was the lack of com-

Table 40-5. β-Blockers for Heart Failure: Systematic Overview

Endpoint	No. of Trials	Treatment Events/Total	Control Events/Total	Odds Ratio (95% CI)	P
Mortality	8	89/702	97/630	0.87 (0.55–1.18)	0.28
Hospitalization	4	114/548	185/551	0.51 (0.25–0.78)	0.0007
Transplantation	5	5/658	17/578	0.30 (−0.55 to 1.15)	0.11

(From Avezum et al.,[127] with permission.)

plete data on all endpoints. The results of this study further emphasize the need to perform a prospective randomized controlled trial with several thousand patients to assess whether the apparent benefits suggested by overview studies are real or inflated owing to selection biases.

CALCIUM CHANNEL BLOCKERS

There is a theoretic rationale for using calcium channel blockers in patients with heart failure. These drugs have a strong arteriolar vasodilator effect and an antiischemic effect; they improve left ventricular relaxation and prevent calcium entry into myocardial cells.[128] Therefore it is not surprising that this group of drugs has been tried in CHF patients.

The fact that nifedipine has a powerful vasodilator effect has encouraged its use in the treatment of CHF patients, but the results with this drug have been disappointing. In a study by Agostoni et al.,[129] nifedipine (20 mg three times daily) was compared to captopril (50 mg three times daily) with an 8-week follow-up in 18 patients with dilated cardiomyopathy who were optimally treated with digitalis and diuretic drugs. The captopril but not the nifedipine treatment improved exercise tolerance and symptoms. In fact, some patients on nifedipine had deterioration of symptoms. Elkayam et al.[130] compared the effect of 8 weeks of isosorbide dinitrate (40 mg four times daily), nifedipine (20 mg four times daily), and their combination in patients with mild to moderate heart failure. This study demonstrated a significantly higher incidence of heart failure worsening, necessitating enhanced diuretic therapy, hospitalization, or both in patients treated with nifedipine alone or in combination with isosorbide dinitrate. These and other studies[128,131] suggest that nifedipine should not be used in CHF patients.

Diltiazem has also been examined in heart failure patients. The Multicenter Diltiazem Postinfarction Trial evaluated the effect of diltiazem (240 mg daily) on mortality and reinfarction in 1237 patients 3–15 days after the onset of myocardial infarction and compared it with the effect of placebo in 1232 similar patients.[132] In 490 patients with evidence of pulmonary congestion on the chest radiograph, diltiazem was associated with an increased number of cardiac events. Furthermore, Goldstein et al.[133] demonstrated that the likelihood of developing chronic heart failure with diltiazem was inversely related to the degree of left ventricular dysfunction. Therefore the use of diltiazem therapy should be avoided in patients with left ventricular dysfunction.

Experience with verapamil has been limited because of the known negative inotropic effect of the drug and the warning by the manufacturer concerning the risk of developing heart failure. The Danish study on the effect of verapamil death or reinfarction in survivors of myocardial infarction included patients with heart failure.[134] This placebo-controlled trial examined the effects of verapamil, 120 mg three times daily started 7–15 days after the infarction in 1775 patients who were followed for a mean of 16 months. Patients who could not have their heart failure symptoms controlled on 160 mg or less of (Lasix) furosemide daily were excluded from the study. Verapamil did not have a beneficial effect in patients with heart failure.

Data suggest that at least some calcium channel blockers can be used safely in patients with heart failure, although they do not provide clear evidence of benefit. A preliminary report of a placebo-controlled study of amlodipine (a peripherally selective dihydropyridine that produces little if any reflex tachycardia) in 118 patients with NYHA class II or III CHF taking diuretics, digoxin, and in most cases ACE-Is revealed a small but statistically significant improvement in exercise tolerance and symptoms.[135]

Although this finding requires confirmation, it provided the background for the Prospective Randomized Amlodipine Survival Evaluation trial (PRAISE) in which 1153 patients with advanced NYHA class III and IV CHF and an ejection fraction of 30 percent or less on baseline therapy with diuretics, digoxin, and ACE inhibitors were randomized to amlodipine 10 mg per day or placebo. For the entire study group, there was no statistically significant effect on the primary endpoint of death and life-threatening cardiovascular events (38.9 percent in the amlodipine group, 42.3 percent in the placebo group; $P = 0.30$). A surprising and noteworthy finding was a 31 percent reduction in this endpoint and a 45 percent decrease in mortality in the group thought to have primary cardiomyopathy. Additional studies are planned to confirm this observation. V-HeFT-III evaluated felodipine in a smaller population of milder heart failure patients. This study found no significant adverse or beneficial effect of the calcium channel blocker, although the trial was underpowered to detect an effect of even moderate size. Taken together, these trials indicate that at least some calcium channel blockers can be administered safely to patients with heart failure and severe left ventricular dysfunction for indications such as angina and hypertension, but they do not support the usage of these agents specifically for the indication of heart failure.

OTHER THERAPEUTIC INTERVENTIONS IN HEART FAILURE PATIENTS

Congestive heart failure is a complex process and probably represents the end result of a number of pathophysiologic processes. As a result it might be expected that a number of therapeutic agents are required to treat the syndrome successfully. Although other therapeutic modalities are being assessed for the treatment of heart failure, not enough data have accumulated to allow confident conclusions regarding the efficacy of these therapies.

Angiotensin II receptor antagonists comprise a relatively new class of pharmacologic blockers of the renin-angiotensin system (RAS).[136–138] In normal and diseased human hearts (idiopathic and ischemic cardiomyopathy), the major conversion of angiotensin I to angiotensin II by the local RAS involves specific serine proteases termed the angiotensin I convertases,[139] and ACE-Is play only a minor role in the conversion of angiotensin I to angiotensin II.[140] Although ACE inhibition has been found to acutely decrease circulating angiotensin II, chronic treatment causes a build-up of circulating angiotensin II to normal levels.[140,141] These findings have led to consideration of the use of angiotensin II (A-II) receptor antagonists in patients with CHF. Experimental hemodynamic studies in ischemic heart failure have shown that losartan (an A-II antagonist) and captopril cause similar acute hemodynamic, hormonal, and renal effects without changing the left ventricular weight/body weight ratio, mean aortic pressures,

or heart rates when compared with placebo.[142,143] A study comparing the effects of enalapril with losartan in 106 patients with symptomatic CHF and a mean ejection fraction of 25 percent has been reported.[144] Exercise capacity and clinical status were similar after treatment with losartan or enalapril for 12 weeks. The results of these studies suggest that an A-II antagonist may be as effective in the treatment of heart failure as ACE-Is. Much more work is needed with the A-II antagonists to further assess the effects of this agent on symptoms and mortality in CHF patients.

Natural history data suggest that one-half of all heart failure patients die suddenly, presumably from a lethal ventricular arrhythmia. In general, antiarrhythmic agents have not been shown to modify this outcome and are not routinely recommended.[145] The GESICA trial has indicated that amiodarone holds some promise for reducing mortality due to heart failure.[146] These results were not confirmed in the Veteran's Affairs Cooperative Study of amiodarone in NYHA functional class III and IV CHF patients.[147] Clearly more studies are needed to assess the role of antiarrhythmic therapy in heart failure patients.

Many studies have demonstrated that there is no significant relation between ejection fraction and exercise capacity in CHF patients.[148–152] Also pharmacologic therapies that acutely improve central hemodynamics do not produce a concomitant improvement in functional capacity.[153,154] This has encouraged some investigators to assess the effects of exercise training in patients with heart failure.[155] A number of studies have assessed the effects of exercise training in this patient group, but only a few, representing fewer than 100 CHF patients, have used a randomized controlled design.[155] These studies have demonstrated that exercise training results in improved exercise capacity and reduced neurohormone levels.[155,156] There is still a need to evaluate the effects of exercise training on long-term functional capacity, patient compliance, and mortality outcome. At the present time there is an ongoing randomized controlled trial (EXERT) designed to determine the effects of 12 months of exercise training on the 6-minute walk test performance, peak oxygen uptake during incremental exercise testing, muscle strength, quality of life, and cardiac function.[155] This trial is being performed in Hamilton and Edmonton, Canada, with reporting of data planned for 1997.

CONCLUSION

Although many studies have examined the effects of various therapeutic strategies in CHF patients, there is still much work to do in order to improve the way these patients are treated. Only ACE-Is have been shown to significantly reduce mortality and morbidity in CHF patients. Even with ACE-I therapy the mortality rate for these patients remains unacceptably high, which supports the importance of finding other ways to treat these patients. A report in preliminary form in 1996, showed a neutral effect on mortality and some evidenced benefit of this drug. β-Blocker trials are required in patients with idiopathic congestive cardiomyopathy and those with ischemic cardiomyopathy to determine the effects of this group of drugs on mortality and morbidity. Additional studies are needed to determine the role of antiarrhythmic and exercise therapy. The use of calcium channel blockers in CHF patients should be limited, as there are no data to suggest that they are of any benefit for this group of patients. The only exception may be the calcium channel blocker amlodipine, but more studies are required to better define the role of this agent for the treatment of CHF patients. Future studies also need to determine the effects of combination therapy (e.g., ACE-Is and A-II antagonists) on clinical symptoms, morbidity, and mortality in CHF patients.

REFERENCES

1. Yusuf S, Garg R: Design, results and interpretation of randomized, controlled trials in congestive heart failure and left ventricular dysfunction. Circulation, suppl. VII 1993;87:115
2. Uretsky BF, Jessop M, Konstam MA et al: Multicenter trial of oral enoximone in patients with moderate to moderately severe congestive heart failure. Lack of benefit compared with placebo. Enoximone Multicenter Trial Group. Circulation 1990;82:774
3. Xamoterol Group. Xamoterol in severe heart failure. Lancet 1990;336:1
4. Packer M, Carver JR, Rodeheffer RJ et al: Effect of oral milrinone in mortality in severe chronic congestive heart failure. N Engl J Med 1991;325:1468
5. Cardiac Arrhythmia Suppression Trial (CAST) Investigators: Preliminary report. Effect of encainide and flecainide on mortality in a randomized trial of arrhythmia suppression after myocardial infarction. N Engl J Med 1989;321:406
6. Yusuf S, Collins R, Peto R: Why do we need some large, simple randomized trials? Stat Med 1984;3:409
7. Yusuf S, Wittes J, Friedman L: Overview of results of randomized clinical trials in heart disease. I. Treatments following myocardial infarction. JAMA 1988;260:2088
8. Yusuf S, Wittes J, Friedman L: Overview of results of randomized clinical trials in heart disease. II. Unstable angina, heart failure, primary prevention with aspirin and risk factor modification. JAMA 1988;260:2259
9. Cohn JN, Archibald DG, Ziesche S et al: Effect of vasodilator therapy on mortality in chronic congestive heart failure. Results of a Veterans Administration cooperative study. N Engl J Med 1986;314:1547
10. Cohn JN, Johnson G, Ziesche S et al: A comparison of enalapril with hydralazine-isosorbide dinitrate in the treatment of chronic congestive heart failure. N Engl J Med 1991;325:303
11. Franciosa JA, Jordan RA, Wilen MM, Leddy CL: Minoxidil in patients with chronic heart failure. Contrasting hemodynamic and clinical effects in a controlled trial. Circulation 1984;70:63
12. Packer M: Physiological mechanisms underlying the adverse effects of calcium channel-blocking drugs in patients with chronic heart failure. Circulation, suppl. IV 1989;80:59
13. Franciosa JA, Cohn JN: Effect of isosorbide dinitrate in response to submaximal and maximal exercise in patients with congestive heart failure. Am J Cardiol 1979;43:1009
14. Yusef S, Sleight P, Held P, McMahon S: Routine medical management of myocardial infarction. Lessons from overviews of recent randomized controlled trials. Circulation, suppl. II 1990;82:117
15. Gruppo Italiano per Io Studio della Soprawivenza Nell'Infarto Miocardico: GISSI-3. Effects of lisinopril and transdermal glyceryl trinitrate singly and together on 6-week mortality and ventricular function after acute myocardial infarction. Lancet 1994;343:1115
16. ISIS-4 Collaborative Group: ISIS-4. A randomised factorial trial assessing early oral captopril, oral mononitrate, and intravenous magnesium sulphate in 58,050 patients with suspected myocardial infarction. Lancet 1995;345:669
17. Garg R, Yusuf S: Overview of randomized trials of angiotensin-converting enzyme on mortality and morbidity in patients with heart failure. JAMA 1995;273:1450
18. SOLVD Investigators: Effect of enalapril on mortality and the development of heart failure in asymptomatic patients with reduced left ventricular ejection fractions. N Engl J Med 1992;327:685
19. CONSENSUS Trial Study Group: Effects of enalapril on mortality in severe congestive heart failure. N Engl J Med 1987;316:1429
20. SOLVD Investigators: Effect of enalapril on survival in patients with reduced left ventricular ejection fractions and congestive heart failure. N Engl J Med 1991;325:293
21. Pfeffer MA, Braunwald E, Moyé LA et al: Effect of captopril on mortality and morbidity in patients with left ventricular dysfunction after myocardial infarction. Results of the Survival and Ventricular Enlargement Trial. N Engl J Med 1992;327:669
22. Acute Infarction Ramipril Efficacy (AIRE) Study Investigators: Effect of ramipril on mortality and morbidity of survivors of acute myocardial infarction with clinical evidence of heart failure. Lancet 1993;342:821
23. Cohn JN, Johnson G, Ziesche S et al: A comparison of enalapril with hydralazine-isosorbide dinitrate in the treatment of chronic congestive heart failure. N Engl J Med 1991;325:303
24. Chinese Cardiac Study Group: Oral captopril versus placebo among 13,634 patients with suspected acute myocardial infarction. Interim report from the Chinese Cardiac Study. Lancet 1995;345:686

25. Ambrosioni E, Borghi C, Magnani B: The effect of the angiotensin-converting enzyme inhibitor zofenopril on mortality and morbidity after anterior myocardial infarction. The Survival of Myocardial Infarction Long-Term Evaluation (SMILE). N Engl J Med 1995; 332:80

26. Yusuf S, Pepine CJ, Garces C et al: Effect of enalapril on myocardial infarction and unstable angina in patients with low ejection fractions. Lancet 1992;340: 1173

27. Rutherford JD, Pfeffer MA, Moyé LA et al: Effects of captopril on ischemic events after myocardial infarction. Circulation 1994;90:1731

28. Frick MH, Elo O, Haapa K et al: Helsinki Heart Study. Primary prevention trial with gemfibrozil in middle-aged men with dyslipidemia. N Engl J Med 1987;317:1237

29. Scandinavian Simvastatin Survival Study Group: Randomised trial of cholesterol lowering in 4444 patients with coronary heart disease; the Scandinavian Simvastatin Survival Study (4S). Lancet 1994;344: 1383

30. Lonn EM, Yusuf S, Jha P et al: Emerging role of angiotensin-converting enzyme inhibitors in cardiac and vascular protection. Circulation 1994;90:2056

31. Leier CV: Current status of non-digitalis positive inotropic drugs. Am J Cardiol 1992;69:120G

32. Tuttle RR, Mills J: Dobutamine. Development of a new catecholamine to selectively increase cardiac contractility. Circ Res 1975;36:185

33. Beregovich J, Bianchi C, D'Angelo R et al: Hemodynamic effects of a new inotropic agent (dobutamine) in chronic cardiac failure. Br Heart J 1975;37:629

34. Akhtar N, Mikulic E, Cohn JN, Chaudhury MH: Hemodynamic effects of dobutamine in patients with severe heart failure. Am J Cardiol 1975;36:202

35. Leier CV, Webel J, Bush CA: The cardiovascular effects of the continuous infusion of dobutamine in patients with severe heart failure. Circulation 1977;56: 468

36. Unverferth DV, Magorien RD, Altschuld R et al: The hemodynamic and metabolic advantages gained by a three-day infusion of dobutamine in patients with congestive cardiomyopathy. Am Heart J 1983;106:29

37. Farah A, Alousi AA: New cardiotonic agents. A search for a digitalis substitute. Life Sci 1978;22:1139

38. Packer M: Vasodilator and inotropic drugs for chronic heart failure. Distinguishing hype from hope. J Am Coll Cardiol 1988;12:1299

39. Wilmshurst PT, Thompson DS, Jenkins BS et al: Hemodynamic effects intravenous amrinone in patients with impaired left ventricular function. Br Heart J 1983;49:77

40. Konstam MA, Cohen ST, Weiland DS et al: Relative contribution of inotropic and vasodilator effects to amrinone-induced hemodynamic improvement in congestive heart failure. Am J Cardiol 1986;57:242

41. Baim DS, McDowell AV, Cherniles J et al: Evaluation of a new bipyridine inotropic agent—milrinone—in patients with severe congestive heart failure. N Engl J Med 1983;309:748

42. Jaski BE, Fifer MA, Wright RF et al: Positive inotropic and vasodilator actions of milrinone in patients with severe congestive heart failure. J Clin Invest 1985;75:643

43. Feldman MD, Copelas L, Gwanthmey JK et al: Deficient production of cyclic AMP. Pharmacologic evidence of an important cause of contractile dysfunction in patients with end-stage heart failure. Circulation 1987;75:331

44. Wilmshurst PT, Walker JM, Fry CH et al: Inotropic and vasodilator effects of amrinone on isolated human tissue. Cardiovasc Res 1984;18:302

45. Benotti JR, Grossman W, Braunwald E et al: Hemodynamic assessment of amrinone. A new inotropic agent. N Engl J Med 1978;299:1373

46. LeJemtel TH, Keung E, Sonnenblick EH et al: Amrinone. A new non-glycoside, non-adrenergic cardiotonic agent effective in the treatment of intractable myocardial failure in man. Circulation 1979;59:1098

47. Siskind SJ, Sonnenblick EH, Forman R et al: Acute substantial benefit of inotropic therapy with amrinone on exercise hemodynamics and metabolism in severe congestive heart failure. Circulation 1981;64: 966

48. Klein NA, Siskind SJ, Frishman WH et al: Hemodynamic comparison of intravenous amrinone and dobutamine in patients with chronic congestive heart failure. Am J Cardiol 1981;48:170

49. LeJemtel TH, Keung E, Ribner HS et al: Sustained beneficial effects of oral amrinone on cardiac and renal function in patients with severe congestive heart failure. Am J Cardiol 1980;45:123

50. Wynne J, Malacoff RF, Benott JR et al: Oral amrinone in refractory congestive heart failure. Am J Cardiol 1980;45:1245

51. Weber KT, Andrews V, Janicki JS et al: Amrinone and exercise performance in patients with chronic heart failure. Am J Cardiol 1981;48:164

52. DiBianco R, Shabetai R, Silverman BD et al: Oral amrinone for the treatment of chronic congestive heart failure. Results of a multicenter randomized double-blind and placebo-controlled withdrawal study. J Am Coll Cardiol 1984;4:855

53. Massie B, Bourassa M, DiBianco R et al: Long-term oral administration of amrinone for congestive heart failure. Lack of efficacy in a multicenter controlled trial. Circulation 1985;71:963

54. Borow KM, Come PC, Neumann A et al: Physiologic assessment of the inotropic, vasodilator and afterload reducing effects of milrinone in subjects without cardiac disease. Am J Cardiol 1985;55:1204

55. Ludmer PL, Wright RF, Arnold JM et al: Separation of the direct myocardial and vasodilator actions of milrinone administered by an intracoronary infusion technique. Circulation 1986;73:130

56. Monrad ES, McKay RG, Baim DS et al: Improvement in indexes of diastolic performance in patients with congestive heart failure treated with milrinone. Circulation 1984;70:1030

57. Cody RJ, Muller FB, Kubo SH et al: Identification of the direct vasodilator effect of milrinone with an isolated limb preparation in patients with chronic congestive heart failure. Circulation 1986;73:124

58. Sinoway LS, Maskin CS, Chadwick B et al: Long-term therapy with a new cardiotonic agent, WIN 47203. Drug-dependent improvement in cardiac performance and progression of the underlying disease. J Am Coll Cardiol 1983;2:327

59. Simonton CA, Chatterjee K, Cody RJ et al: Milrinone in congestive heart failure. Acute and chronic hemo-

dynamic and clinical evaluation. J Am Coll Cardiol 1985;6:453

60. Timmis AD, Smyth P, Jewett DE: Milrinone in heart failure. Effects on exercise hemodynamics during short term treatment. Br Heart J 1985;54:42

61. White HD, Ribeiro JP, Hartley LH, Colucci WS: Immediate effects of milrinone on metabolic and sympathetic responses to exercise in severe congestive heart failure. Am J Cardiol 1985;56:93

62. Likoff MJ, Weber KT, Andrews V et al: Milrinone in the treatment of chronic cardiac failure. A controlled trial. Am Heart J 1985;110:1035

63. LeJemtel TH, Maskin CS, Mancini D et al: Systemic and regional hemodynamic effects of captopril and milrinone administered alone and concomitantly in patients with heart failure. Circulation 1985;72:364

64. DiBianco R, Shabetai R, Kostuk W et al: A comparison of oral milrinone, digoxin, and their combination in the treatment of patients with chronic heart failure. N Engl J Med 1989;320:677

65. Yusuf S, Teo KK: Inotropic agents increase mortality in patients with congestive heart failure. Circulation, Suppl. III 1990;82:673

66. Packer M, Carver JR, Rodeheffer RJ et al: Effect of oral milrinone on mortality in severe chronic heart failure. N Engl J Med 1991;325:1468

67. Uretsky BF, Jessup M, Konstam MA et al: Multicenter trial of oral enoximone in patients with moderate to moderately severe congestive heart failure. Lack of benefit compared with placebo. Circulation 1990; 82:774

68. Verdouw PD, Hartog JM, Duncker DJ et al: Cardiovascular profile of pimobendan, a benzimadazole-pyridazinone derivative with vasodilating and inotropic properties. Eur J Pharmacol 1986;126:21

69. Pouleur H, Hanet C, Shroder E et al: Effects of pimobendan (UDCG 115 BS) on left ventricular inotropic state in conscious dogs and in patients with heart failure. J Cardiovasc Pharmacol, suppl. 2 1989;14:S18

70. Permanette B, Sebening H, Hartmann F, Klein G: Acute effects of intravenous UDCG 115 BS (pimobendan) on the cardiovascular system and left ventricular pump function. J Cardiovasc Pharmacol, suppl. 2 1989;14:S36

71. Ruegg JC: Effects of new inotropic agents on calcium sensitivity of contractile proteins. Circulation, suppl. III 1986;73:I78

72. Fujino K, Sperelakis N, Solaro RJ: Sensitization of dog and guinea pig heart myofilaments to calcium activation and the inotropic effect of pimobendan. Comparison with milrinone. Circ Res 1988;63:911

73. Solaro RJ, Fujino K, Sperelakis N: The positive inotropic effect of pimobendan involves stereospecific increases in the calcium sensitivity of cardiac myofilaments. J Cardiovasc Pharmacol, suppl. 2 1989;14:S7

74. Kubo SH, Gollub S, Bourge R et al: Beneficial effects of pimobendan on exercise tolerance and quality of life in patients with heart failure. Results of a multicentre trial. Circulation 1992;85:942

75. Iijima T, Taira N: Membrane current changes responsible for the positive inotropic effect of OPC-8212, a new inotropic agent, in single ventricular cells of guinea pig heart. J Pharmacol Exp Ther 1987; 240:659

76. Rapundalo ST, Lathrop DA, Harrison SA et al: Cyclic AMP-dependent and cyclic AMP-independent actions of a novel cardiotonic agent, OPC-8212. Naunyn Schmiedebergs Arch Pharmacol 1988;338:692

77. Feldman AM, Bristow MR, Parmley WW et al: Effects of vesnarinone on morbidity and mortality in patients with heart failure. N Engl J Med 1993;329:149

78. German and Austrian Xamoterol Study Group: Double-blind placebo controlled comparison of digoxin and xamoterol in chronic heart failure. Lancet 1988; 1:489

79. Xamoterol in Severe Heart Failure Study Group: Xamoterol in severe heart failure. Lancet 1990;336:1

80. Rajfer SI, Rossen JD, Douglas FL et al: Effects of long term therapy with oral ibopamine on resting and exercise capacity in patients with heart failure. Relationship to the generation of N-methyldopamine and to plasma norepinephrine levels. Circulation 1986; 73:740

81. Condorelli M, Mattioli G, Caponneto S et al: The long term efficacy of ibopamine in treating patients with severe heart failure. A multicenter investigation. J Cardiovasc Pharmacol, suppl. 8 1989;14:83

82. Rolandi E, Savino F, Cantoni V et al: Long term therapy of chronic congestive heart failure with ibopamine. A multicenter trial. J Cardiovasc Pharmacol, suppl. 8 1989;14:93

83. Van Heldhuisen DJ, Man in't Veld AJ, Dunselman PHJM et al: Double-blind, placebo-controlled study of ibopamine and digoxin in patients with mild to moderate heart failure. Results of The Dutch Ibopamine Multicenter Trial (DIMT). J Am Coll Cardiol 1993;22:1564

84. Van Heldhuisen DJ, Brouwer J, Man in't Veld AJ et al: Progression of mild untreated heart failure during six months follow-up and clinical and neurohumoral effects of ibopamine and digoxin as monotherapy. Am J Cardiol 1995;75:796

85. Starr J, Luchi RJ: Blind study on the action of digitoxin on elderly women. Am Heart J 1969;78:740

86. Kirsten E, Rodstein M, Iuster Z: Digoxin in the aged. Geriatrics 1973;1:95

87. Dobbs SM, Kenyon WI, Dobbs RJ: Maintenance digoxin after an episode of heart failure. Placebo-controlled trial in outpatients. BMJ 1977;1:749

88. Lee C, Johnson RA, Bingham JB: Heart failure in outpatients. N Engl J Med 1982;306:699

89. Fleg JL, Gottlieb SH, Lakatta EG: Is digoxin really important in treatment of compensated heart failure? Am J Med 1982;73:244

90. Taggart AJ, Johnston GD, McDevitt DG: Digoxin withdrawal after cardiac failure in patients with sinus rhythm. J Cardiovasc Pharmacol 1983;5:229

91. Guyatt GH, Sullivan MJ, Fallen EL et al: A controlled trial of digoxin in congestive heart failure. Am J Cardiol 1988;61:371

92. Pugh SE, White NJ, Aronson JK et al: Clinical, hemodynamic and pharmacologic effects of withdrawal and reintroduction of digoxin in patients with heart failure in sinus rhythm after long term treatment. Br Heart J 1989;61:529

93. Captopril-Digoxin Multicenter Research Group: Comparative effects of therapy with captopril and digoxin in patients with mild to moderate heart failure. JAMA 1988;259:539

94. Fleg JL, Rothfeld B, Gottlieb SH, Wright J: Effect of maintenance digoxin therapy on aerobic performance and exercise left ventricular function in mild to mod-

erate heart failure due to coronary artery disease. A randomized, placebo, controlled crossover trial. J Am Coll Cardiol 1991;17:743

95. Uretsky BF, Young JB, Shahidi FE et al: Randomized study assessing the effect of digoxin withdrawal in patients with mild to moderate chronic congestive heart failure. Results of the PROVED Trial. J Am Coll Cardiol 1993;22:955

96. Packer M, Gheorghiade M, Young JB et al: Withdrawal of digoxin from patients with chronic heart failure treated with angiotensin converting-enzyme inhibitors. N Engl J Med 1993;329:1

97. Drexler H, Schumacher M, Siegrist J et al: Effect of captopril and digoxin on quality of life and clinical symptoms in patients with coronary artery disease and mild heart failure. J Am Coll Cardiol 1992;19:260A

98. Moss AJ, Davis HT, Conrad DL et al: Digitalis-associated cardiac mortality after myocardial infarction. Circulation 1981;64:1150

99. Bigger AJ, Fleiss JL, Rolnitzky LA et al: Effect of digitalis treatment on survival after acute myocardial infarction. Am J Cardiol 1985;55:623

100. Ryan TJ, Bailey KR, McCabe CH et al: The effects of digitalis on survival in high-risk patients with coronary artery disease. Circulation 1983;67:735

101. Byington R, Goldstein S: Association of digitalis therapy with mortality in survivors of acute myocardial infarction. Observations in the Beta-Blocker Heart Attack Trial. J Am Coll Cardiol 1985;6:976

102. Muller JE, Turi ZG, Stone PH et al: Digoxin therapy and mortality after myocardial infarction. Experience in the MILIS Study. N Engl J Med 1986;314:265

103. Mancini DM, Benotti JR, Elkayam U et al: Antiarrhythmic drug use and high serum levels of digoxin are independent adverse prognostic factors in patients with chronic heart failure [abstract]. Circulation suppl. II 1991;84:243

104. Sweeney MO, Moss AJ, Eberly S, Andrews M: Factors associated with sudden cardiac death in survivors of acute myocardial infarction [abstract]. Circulation, suppl. II 1991;84:20

105. Yusuf S, Wittes J, Bailey K, Furberg C: Digitalis—a new controversy regarding an old drug. The pitfalls of inappropriate methods. Circulation 1986;73:14

106. Waagstein F, Hjalmarson Å, Varnauskas E, Wallentin I: Effect of chronic beta-adrenergic receptor blockade in congestive cardiomyopathy. Br Heart J 1975;37:1022

107. Swedberg K, Hjalmarson Å, Waagstein F, Wallentin I: Beneficial effects of long-term β-blockade in congestive cardiomyopathy. Br Heart J 1980;44:117

108. Swedberg K, Hjalmarson Å, Waagstein F, Wallentin I: Adverse effects of β-blockade withdrawal in patients with congestive cardiomyopathy. Br Heart J 1980;44:134

109. Swedberg K, Hjalmarson Å, Waagstein F, Wallentin I: Prolongation of survival in congestive cardiomyopathy by β-receptor blockade. Lancet 1979;1:1374

110. Waagstein F, Hjalmarson Å, Swedberg K, Wallentin I: β-Blockers in dilated cardiomyopathies. They work. Eur Heart J, suppl. A 1983;4:173

111. Engelmeier RS, O'Connell JB, Walsh R et al: Improvement in symptoms and exercise tolerance by metoprolol in patients with dilated cardiomyopathy. A double-blind, randomized, placebo-controlled trial. Circulation 1985;72:536

112. Heilbrunn SM, Shah P, Bristow MR et al: Increased β-receptor density an improved hemodynamic response to catecholamine stimulation during long-term metoprolol therapy in heart failure from dilated cardiomyopathy. Circulation 1989;79:483

113. Sano H, Kawabata N, Yonezawa K et al: Metoprolol was more effective than captopril for dilated cardiomyopathy in Japanese patients. Circulation, suppl. II 1989;80:118

114. Waagstein F, Caidahl K, Wallentin I et al: β-blockade in congestive cardiomyopathy. Effects of short- and long-term metoprolol treatment followed by withdrawal and readmission of metoprolol. Circulation 1989;80:551

115. Nemanich JW, Veith RC, Abrass IB, Stratton JR: Effects of metoprolol on rest and exercise cardiac function and plasma catecholamines in chronic congestive heart failure secondary to ischemic or idiopathic cardiomyopathy. Am J Cardiol 1990;66:843

116. Andersson B, Hedner T, Lundqvist-Blomström C, Waagstein F: Exercise hemodynamics and myocardial metabolism during chronic β-blockade in severe heart failure. J Am Coll Cardiol 1991;18:555

117. Woodley SL, Gilbert EM, Anderson JL et al: β-blockade with bucindolol in heart failure caused by ischemic versus idiopathic dilated cardiomyopathy. Circulation 1991;84:2426

118. Waagstein F, Bristow MR, Swedberg K et al: Beneficial effects of metoprolol in idiopathic dilated cardiomyopathy. Lancet 1993;342:1441

119. CIBIS Investigators and Committees: A randomized trial of β-blockade in heart failure. The Cardiac Insufficiency Bisoprolol Study (CIBIS). Circulation 1994;90:1765

120. Baber NS, Evans DW, Howitt G et al: Multicenter post-infarction trial of propranolol in 49 hospitals in the United Kingdom, Italy and Yugoslavia. Br Heart J 1980;44:96

121. Norwegian Multicenter Study Group: Timolol-induced reduction in mortality and reinfarction in patients surviving acute myocardial infarction. N Engl J Med 1981;304:801

122. Australian and Swedish Pindolol Study Group: The effect of pindolol on the two year mortality after complicated myocardial infarction. Eur Heart J 1983;4:367

123. European Infarction Study Group: European Infarction Study (EIS). A secondary prevention study with slow-release oxprenolol after myocardial infarction. Morbidity and mortality. Eur Heart J 1984;5:189

124. Chadda K, Goldstein S, Byinton R, Curb JD: Effect of propranolol after acute myocardial infarction in patients with congestive heart failure. Circulation 1986;73:503

125. Held P: Effects of beta blockers on ventricular dysfunction after myocardial infarction. Tolerability and survival effects. Am J Cardiol 1993;71:39C

126. Beta-Blocker Heart Attack Research Group: A randomized trial of propranolol in patients with acute myocardial infarction. I. mortality results. JAMA 1982;247:1707

127. Avezum A, Tsuyuki RT, Yusuf S: Beta blockers for heart failure. A systematic overview. Eur Heart J (in press, 1996)

128. Elkayam U, Shotan A, Mehra A, Ostrzega E: Calcium channel blockers in heart failure. J Am Coll Cardiol, suppl. A 1993;22:139A

129. Agostoni PG, DeCesare N, Doria E et al: Afterload reduction. A comparison of captopril and nifedipine in dilated cardiomyopathy. Br Heart J 1986;55:391

130. Elkayam U, Amin J, Mehra A et al: A prospective, randomized, double-blind, crossover study to compare the efficacy and safety of chronic nifedipine therapy with that of isosorbide dinitrate and their combination in the treatment of chronic congestive heart failure. Circulation 1990;82:1954

131. Parameshwar J, Poole-Wilson A: The role of calcium antagonists in the treatment of chronic heart failure. Eur Heart J, suppl. A 1993;14:38

132. Multicenter Diltiazem Postinfarction Trial Research Group: The effect of diltiazem on mortality and reinfarction after myocardial infarction. N Engl J Med 1988;319:385

133. Goldstein RE, Boccuzzi SJ, Cruess D, Nattel S: Diltiazem increases late-onset congestive heart failure in post infarction patients with early reduction in ejection fraction. Circulation 1991;83:52

134. Danish Study Group on Verapamil in Myocardial Infarction: Secondary prevention with verapamil after myocardial infarction. Am J Cardiol 1990;66:331

135. Packer M, Nicod P, Khandheria BR et al: Randomized, multicenter, double-blind, placebo-controlled evaluation of amlodipine in patients with mild-to-moderate heart failure. J Am Coll Cardiol 1991;17:274A

136. Tsunoda K, Abe K, Hagino T et al: Hypotensive effect of losartan, a nonpeptide angiotensin II receptor antagonist, in essential hypertension. Am J Hypertens 1993;1:28

137. Weber MA: Clinical experience with the angiotensin II receptor antagonist losartan. A preliminary report. Am J Hypertens 1992;5:247

138. Kang PM, Landau AJ, Eberhardt RT, Frishman WH: Angiotensin II receptor antagonists. A new approach to blockade of the renin-angiotensin system. Am Heart J 1994;127:1388

139. Urata H, Healy B, Stewart RW et al: Angiotensin II-forming pathways in normal and failing human hearts. Circ Res 1990;66:883

140. Bumpus FM: Angiotensin I and II. Some early observations made at the Cleveland Clinic Foundation and recent discoveries relative to angiotensin II formation in human heart. Hypertension, suppl. III 1991;18:122

141. Lindpaintner K, Jin M, Wilhelm MJ et al: Intracardiac generation of angiotensin and its physiologic role. Circulation, suppl. I 1988;77:18

142. Raya TE, Fonken SJ, Lee RW et al: Hemodynamic effects of direct angiotensin II blockade compared to converting enzyme inhibition in rat model of heart failure. Am J Hypertens 1991;4:334S

143. Fitzpatrick MA, Rademaker MT, Charles CJ et al: Angiotensin II receptor antagonism in bovine heart failure. Acute hemodynamic, hormonal, and renal effects. Am J Physiol 1992;263:H250

144. Lang RM, Yellin L, McKelvie RS et al: Comparative effects of Losartan and enalapril on exercise capacity and clinical status of patients with heart failure [abstract]. Circulation, suppl. I 1994;90:602

145. Teo KK, Yusuf S, Furberg CD: Effects of prophylactic antiarrhythmic drug therapy in acute myocardial infarction. JAMA 1993;270:1589

146. Doval HC, Nul DR, Grancelli HO et al: Randomized trial of low-dose amiodarone in severe congestive heart failure. Lancet 1994;344:493

147. Singh SN, Fletcher RD, Gross-Fisher S et al: Amiodarone in patients with congestive heart failure and asymptomatic ventricular arrhythmias. Survival trial of antiarrhythmic therapy in congestive heart failure. N Engl J Med 1995;333:77

148. Higginbotham MB, Morris KG, Conn EH et al: Determinants of variable exercise performance among patients with severe left ventricular dysfunction. Am J Cardiol 1983;51:52

149. Franciosa JA, Park JA, Levine B: Lack of correlation between exercise capacity and indices of resting left ventricular performance in heart failure. Am J Cardiol 1981;47:33

150. Szlachcic J, Massie BM, Kramer BL et al: Correlates and prognostic implications of exercise capacity in chronic congestive heart failure. Am J Cardiol 1985;55:1037

151. Port S, McEwan P, Cobb FR: Influence of resting ventricular function on left ventricular response to exercise in patients with coronary artery disease. Circulation 1981;63:856

152. Liang C-S, Stewart DK, LeJemtel TH et al: Characteristics of peak aerobic capacity in symptomatic and asymptomatic subjects with left ventricular dysfunction. Am J Cardiol 1992;69:1207

153. Maskin CS, Forman R, Sonneblick EH et al: Failure of dobutamine to increase exercise capacity despite hemodynamic improvement in severe congestive heart failure. Am J Cardiol 1983;51:177

154. Drexler H, Banhardt U, Meinertz T et al: Contrasting peripheral short-term and long-term effects of converting enzyme inhibition in patients with congestive heart failure. A double-blind, placebo-controlled trial. Circulation 1989;79:491

155. McKelvie RS, Teo KK, McCartney N et al: Effects of exercise training in patients with congestive heart failure. A critical review. J Am Coll Cardiol 1995;25:789

156. Coats JS, Adamopoulos S, Radaelli A et al: Controlled trial of physical training in chronic heart failure. Exercise performance, hemodynamics, ventilation and autonomic function. Circulation 1992;85:2119

41 Nonpharmacologic Interventions

Martin J. Sullivan
Mary H. Hawthorne

Although the incidence of coronary artery disease, stroke, and myocardial infarction is decreasing and better pharmacologic agents are available to treat hypertension, the prevalence of chronic heart failure (CHF) is increasing even after adjustment for an aging population.[1] Studies[2,3] suggest that 1–2 percent of the adult population in the United States (2 million to 3 million people) have CHF. Pharmacologic therapy has resulted in dramatic reductions in mortality and morbidity rates associated with heart failure and may even reduce the occurrence of new-onset CHF in patients with asymptomatic left ventricular (LV) systolic dysfunction.[4] However, the development of new pharmacologic agents has been limited; and even with maximal medical therapy, mortality remains high in patients with functional class III or IV symptoms. Most are seriously disabled, requiring intensive follow-up and often repeated hospitalizations. Prolonging life with this disorder may increase disease prevalence and the number of patients requiring long-term follow-up for symptomatic CHF. Therefore an important goal in this field is the development of nonpharmacologic interventions that can improve quality of life and alleviate symptoms in these patients.

This chapter reviews four types of interventions: (1) exercise training and rehabilitation; (2) psychological and biobehavioral interventions; (3) nutrition; and (4) patient education and self-care strategies. Each of these areas is an essential co-intervention to pharmacologic therapy for treatment of patients with heart failure.

EXERCISE TRAINING AND REHABILITATION

Although pharmacologic therapy is the cornerstone of treatment for this disorder, a growing number of studies demonstrate that exercise training in patients with LV systolic dysfunction and CHF can improve exercise performance and reduce exertional symptoms without adversely affecting LV geometry or contractility.[5–14] In addition to demonstrating diminished symptoms and aerobic capacity, studies have also shown that sympathetic activation is reduced after exercise conditioning in patients with CHF, raising the possibility that long-term exercise may stabilize the course of progressive systolic dysfunction in patients with this disorder. Long-term aerobic exercise is an active therapy that involves patients in their own care and gives them a chance to affect their own outcome. Quality of life has been shown to significantly improve after cardiac rehabilitation in patients with CHF, related to improved exercise tolerance.[15] These results indicate that long-term aerobic exercise may represent an important adjunctive treatment strategy for patients with severe systolic dysfunction and may alleviate symptoms and improve exercise tolerance is comparable to that obtained from pharmacologic therapy.[16]

Physiology of Exercise Training

Exercise training in normal subjects leads to a number of important physiologic adaptations that may be beneficial in patients with cardiac diseases. In

617

normal subjects exercise training leads to an improvement in both submaximal[17] and maximal[18-20] exercise performance, favorably affects blood lipid levels,[21] and may act to delay the development of coronary artery disease.[22] Improved exercise tolerance in normal subjects is mediated through central hemodynamic changes and peripheral adaptations. Although stroke volume increases during exercise, LV systolic function is generally not improved by exercise in normal subjects. During submaximal exercise after training the heart rate is decreased, cardiac output is unchanged, and blood lactate levels are reduced. These results are associated with increased aerobic enzyme content, glycogen content, and capillary density in skeletal muscle[23] and decreased circulating catecholamine levels during submaximal exercise.[24] Studies have demonstrated that exercise training in patients with coronary artery disease leads to an increase in peak oxygen consumption, a training bradycardia, and an increase in peak arteriovenous oxygen difference.[25-28] Although exercise stroke volume may improve in selected patients after 12 months of intense exercise training,[8,29] most studies have not demonstrated an improvement in stroke volume, LV ejection fraction, or intracardiac filling pressures after training.[25-28] Thus peripheral adaptations that lead to more efficient oxygen extraction, including an increase in peak muscle blood flow[28] and increased aerobic enzyme content in skeletal muscle,[30] play an important role in the response to training in patients with coronary artery disease and preserved systolic LV function. The work rate at which angina and myocardial ischemia occurs is increased after exercise training. Although some studies have demonstrated an increase in the rate–pressure product at the onset of LV ischemia during exercise after exercise training, most have shown no change in this index of myocardial oxygen consumption after training. It has been difficult to demonstrate that the amount of myocardium that becomes ischemic during exercise is reduced with training.[29-32] Studies by Froelicher et al.[31] and Sebechts et al.[32] demonstrated some improvement in ischemia by thallium scintigraphy in patients with angina after exercise training, although their results were not conclusive. In addition to improving exercise capacity, a number of studies have demonstrated that exercise training improves depression and anxiety in patients who are status after myocardial infarction.[33,34] This finding may have important consequences, as these psychosocial factors are associated with a worse prognosis for this disorder.

Exercise Physiology in Patients with Severe Systolic LV Dysfunction

Although increased intrapulmonary pressures may be important for producing dyspnea during acute heart failure, several lines of evidence indicate that

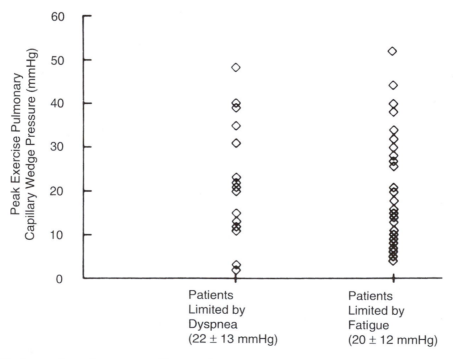

Fig. 41-1. Peak exercise pulmonary capillary wedge pressure in patients limited by dyspnea versus those limited by fatigue. (Data from Sullivan et al.[39])

these are not the primary factors limiting exercise in stable ambulatory patients with chronic heart failure. Massie et al.[35] demonstrated no relation between peak exercise pulmonary capillary wedge pressure and peak VO_2 in patients with chronic heart failure. When examining ventilatory control in this disorder,[36] we have demonstrated that during short-term maximal exercise in patients with CHF, 70 percent of patients are limited by leg fatigue; and increased pulmonary dead space and ventilation during exercise are related to decreased cardiac output and not to increased pulmonary wedge pressures. As illustrated in Figure 41-1 pulmonary wedge pressures are not higher in patients limited by dyspnea than in those limited by fatigue, suggesting that exertional dyspnea is not primarily due to pulmonary venous congestion in this disorder.

Studies of patients with severe systolic LV dysfunction suggest that exercise intolerance is due primarily to the early onset of anaerobic metabolism in skeletal muscle.[37-40] Two factors have been identified that may contribute to this response in patients: reduced muscle perfusion during exercise[35,39] and alterations in skeletal muscle histology and biochemistry, which include decreased aerobic enzyme content, decreased type I fiber content, reduced mitochondrial volume density, and decreased capillarization.[40-43] Previous studies using magnetic resonance spectroscopy (^{31}P-MRS) have demonstrated that early anaerobic metabolism occurs independently of reduced blood flow[37,44] and is not due solely to skeletal muscle atrophy.[45,46] Studies in our laboratory have demonstrated that lactate appearance at a given submaximal work rate in patients with severe LV systolic dysfunction and CHF is not closely related to muscle blood flow but is inversely related to aerobic enzyme content in skeletal muscle ($r = -0.74; p = 0.02$).[40] These data suggest that intrinsic alterations in skeletal muscle histology and biochemistry play an important role in determining exercise tolerance in patients with this disorder. The concept that the skeletal muscle metabolic response to exercise plays the primary role in determining exercise tolerance here provides a physiologic rationale for utilizing exercise training as a potential means to improve exertional symptoms in patients with CHF.

Exercise Training for Patients with Severe LV Dysfunction

It has long been held that exercise was contraindicated in patients with CHF. In the past, bed rest was useful for producing a diuresis in some CHF patients with fluid overload. However, with the advent of loop diuretics and vasodilators, uncontrolled edema is a problem in only a few patients with LV systolic dysfunction; thus most patients are ambulatory. Although a small number of patients with severe systolic LV dysfunction have been included in earlier training studies,[6-8] it has only been since the mid-1980s that research has been directed specifically at examining the training response in this group of patients. Studies from our institution by Conn et al.[9] demonstrated an increase in peak exercise capacity in patients with LV ejection fractions of 13–25 percent after 4–37 months of exercise conditioning. These changes were accompanied by an increase in peak exercise oxygen pulse with no exercise-related complications. Studies by Kellermann et al.[47] and Hoffmann et al.[48] have also demonstrated an increase in peak exercise performance after training in patients with LV dysfunction but noted no change in LV ejection fraction, no alterations in wall motion abnormalities, and no exercise-related morbidity.

Studies in our laboratory[11,12] examined the effects of 4–6 months of exercise conditioning in patients with class I–III CHF due to systolic LV dysfunction (LV ejection fraction 24 ± 10 percent). Before and after training, patients underwent maximal graded bicycle exercise with hemodynamics measurements. Patients exercised for 4 hours per week and improve their functional class from 2.4 ± 0.6 to 1.3 ± 0.7 ($P < 0.01$). Peak VO_2 (Fig. 41-2A) increased from 16.8 ± 3.7 ml·kg^{-1}·min^{-1} to 20.6 ± 4.7 ml·kg$^-$·min^{-1} (both $P < 0.01$) after training. Cardiac output was unchanged during submaximal exercise (Fig. 41-2B) and tended to increase at maximal exercise from 8.9 ± 2.9 to 9.9 ± 3.2 L/min ($P = 0.13$). Heart rate (Fig. 41-2C) was reduced at rest and during submaximal exercise but did not change at maximal exercise. Systemic arteriovenous oxygen (AV-O_2) difference (Fig. 41-2D) was increased at rest, unchanged during submaximal exercise, and increased at peak exercise from 13.1 ± 1.4 to 14.6 ± 2.3 ml/dl ($P < 0.05$). Arterial, right atrial, pulmonary capillary wedge, and pulmonary artery pressures at rest and during exercise were unchanged after training. Stroke volume was unchanged at rest but tended to increase during exercise, although these changes did not reach statistical significance (P 0.12). Resting and exercise LV ejection fraction, LV end-systolic volume, and LV end-diastolic volume were not significantly altered by training, and there were no changes in rest or exercise wall motion abnormalities.

Leg blood flow, leg oxygen delivery, leg vascular resistance, and leg AV-O_2 difference did not change at rest or during submaximal exercise after training. Blood flow to the single leg increased at peak exercise from 2.5 ± 0.7 to 3.0 ± 0.8 L/min ($P < 0.01$), as

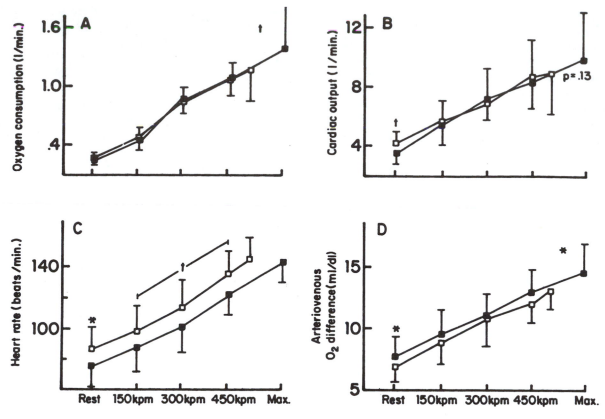

Fig. 41-2. Resting and exercise oxygen consumption, cardiac output, heart rate, and systemic arteriovenous oxygen difference in patients before (open squares) and after (closed squares) training. *$P < 0.05$; †$P < 0.01$ by Wilcoxon signed rank test. (From Sullivan et al.,[11] with permission.)

did leg oxygen delivery. Arterial and femoral venous lactate concentrations were markedly reduced during submaximal exercise but were unchanged at rest or maximal exercise after training. Similarly, training decreased the femoral arteriovenous lactate difference and leg lactate production during submaximal exercise. The VO_2 at which the ventilatory anaerobic threshold occurred, assessed by blinded inspection of breath-by-breath data using the ventilatory equivalents method, increased from 10.1 ± 1.2 to 12.1 ± 2.6 ml·kg^{-1}·min^{-1} ($P < 0.01$) (Fig. 41-3), accompanied by an increase in exercise time at a fixed submaximal work rate from 938 ± 410 seconds to 1429 ± 691 seconds. There was no relation between the change in peak VO_2 after exercise training and any hemodynamic variable measured during the baseline exercise study. Specifically, the rest and peak exercise LV ejection fraction, stroke volume, cardiac output, VO_2, systemic AV-O_2 difference, leg AV-O_2 difference, and femoral vein oxygen saturation were unrelated to the response to training.

Although our study was uncontrolled, the results indicate that exercise training may improve both submaximal and maximal exercise capacity in pa-

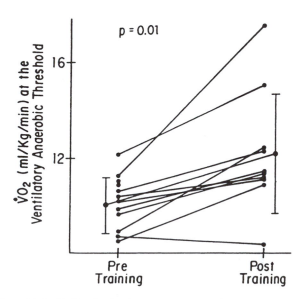

Fig. 41-3. Individual changes in ventilatory anaerobic threshold with exercise training for 12 patients with chronic heart failure. (From Sullivan et al.,[12] with permission.)

tients with mild to moderate heart failure and systolic LV dysfunction. Improved peak cardiac output contributed to improved peak VO_2 in some patients, although peripheral adaptations, including increased skeletal muscle vascular conductance and oxygen extraction and decreased skeletal muscle lactate production, were primarily responsible for the training effect in our patients. Previous studies have identified markedly reduced aerobic enzyme content in skeletal muscle in patients with this disorder;[40-44] it is possible that exercise training may act in part by reversing these biochemical alterations and increasing aerobic enzyme activity in skeletal muscle.[30] Possibly one of the most important findings of this study was that submaximal exercise endurance was markedly improved in our patients. It was accompanied by improved dyspnea and fatigue during activities of daily living, such as grocery shopping and walking up hills.

A study by Minotti et al.[38] examined forearm metabolism by ^{31}P-MRS before and after one-arm training in five patients with CHF. The slope of the increase in the inorganic phosphate/phosphocreatine ratio during exercise was lower after training, indicating a delay in anaerobic metabolism. It was accompanied by no changes in forearm muscle mass or

blood flow, suggesting that biochemical alterations in skeletal muscle led to improved exercise performance. An important study by Coats et al.[13] also examined exercise training in patients with chronic heart failure (LV ejection fraction 16 ± 8 percent) employing a crossover design with the investigators blinded to training status. Patients demonstrated a significant improvement in peak VO_2 and a decrease in heart rate during submaximal exercise after training. In addition, these authors demonstrated a decline in peak VO_2 to baseline values after a period of detraining, indicating that improved peak VO_2 was not due solely to familiarization with the exercise protocol. Symptom scores, assessed by a modified Likert questionnaire, were also improved in patients after training.

An important finding in this study was that sympathetic nervous system activation was reduced after training. Figure 41-4 illustrates a decrease in sympathetic nervous system activation as indicated by power spectral analysis in an individual patient after training. The increase in low frequency variability after training indicates an increase in parasympathetic activation, and the decrease in low frequency amplitude represents a decrease in sympathetic activation. Because reduced parasympa-

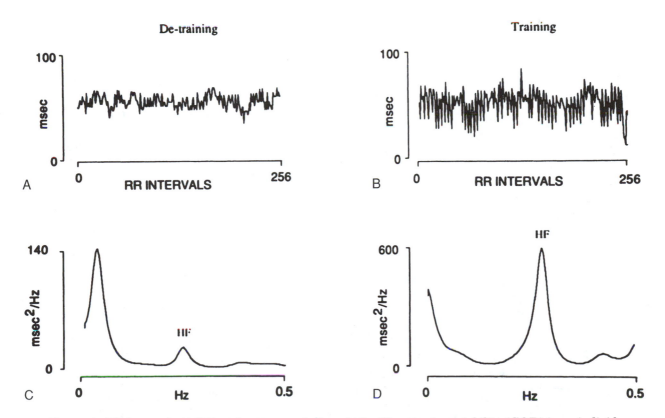

Fig. 41-4. RR intervals **(A&B)** and power spectral analysis of heart rate variability **(C&D)** in an individual patient after detraining **(A&C)** and in training **(B&D)**. The increase in HF (high frequency) component indicates increased parasympathetic control after training. (From Coats et al.,[13] with permission.)

thetic activation and reduced heart rate variability have been linked to an increased incidence of sudden death, these findings raise the possibility that exercise training may reduce the potential for arrhythmias with this disorder. The finding that neuroendocrine activation is reduced in patients with CHF suggests that long-term exercise may decrease afterload and thereby delay progressive LV dysfunction in patients with this disorder. This point is important because all therapies that have proved to be beneficial during long-term follow-up in CHF have been shown to decrease sympathetic nervous system activation.

Rehabilitation for Patients with Angina and CHF

Arvan[49] examined the exercise training response in 85 patients with coronary artery disease subdividing subjects into four groups based on a high or low LV ejection fraction (LVEF) (more than or less than 0.40) and the presence or absence of a positive exercise treadmill test for ischemia. Patient groups with an LVEF more than 0.40 with or without ischemia and those with an LVEF less than 0.40 without ischemia all demonstrated a training effect as indicated by an increase in peak VO_2 and a decrease in submaximal exercise heart rate. Patients with severe LV systolic dysfunction and ischemia did not demonstrate a training effect, although 5 of 11 had angina on the posttraining exercise test, which may have limited the utility of peak VO_2 measurements. These results suggest that high risk patients with a reduced LVEF and significant ongoing ischemia may not benefit from exercise training. Although our anecdotal experience indicates that many of these patients have improved exercise tolerance after training, patients with ischemia and severe LV dysfuncion should probably undergo angiography and, if possible, myocardial revascularization prior to exercise training. Previous studies have indicated that this group may accrue the largest absolute mortality reduction from surgical intervention (or possibly angioplasty)[50,51]

What is the best course of action for patients with severe LV systolic dysfunction, CHF, and ongoing LV ischemia in whom surgery or angioplasty is not an option? Although studies are not available in this group, it is possible that an intensive multidisciplinary approach to reduce risk factors, alter diet, improve psychosocial functioning, and increase exercise performance may benefit these patients. This assumption is based on angiographic trials[52-58] that have demonstrated delayed progression or regression of coronary artery atherosclerotic lesions in pa-

tients who have undergone intensive risk factor modification interventions. A number of these studies also demonstrated a reduction in angina[52,55,56] and cardiac events[54,56,58] in treated patients. Analysis of outcomes of the first seven angiographic regression studies demonstrates a 50–60 percent reduction in cardiac events in treated patients in these trials.

The Heidelberg Trial[57] and the Lifestyle Heart Trial[55] have examined cardiac rehabilitation-based interventions on coronary anatomy and ischemia in patients with coronary artery disease. In both trials, treated patients exercised aerobically and followed a low fat diet (10–20 percent of calories from fat). In the Lifestyle Heart Trial[55] patients also were involved in weekly support groups aimed at reducing hostility and isolation as well as stretching and meditation practices aimed at achieving the relaxation response. Both of these trials demonstrated that at least 30 percent of treated patients achieved definite angiographic regression. Although the change in percent diameter stenosis with treatment was small in these studies, it is important to note that these small changes were associated with a reduction in angina frequency[55] and in stress-induced ischemia assessed by quantitative thallium scanning[57] or positron emission tomography (PET) scanning.[55] These trials set the stage for a new era in cardiac rehabilitation for patients with coronary artery disease and offer hope for patients with CHF and angina in whom surgery or angioplasty is not possible. At the Duke Center for Living we have incorporated this multidisciplinary intensive approach into both long-term rehabilitation and short-term cardiac retreat programs. The Healing the Heart program at Duke combines exercise, nutritional counseling to reduce fat intake to less than 20 percent of calories, patient support groups, aerobic exercise, and stress reduction. We believe that psychosocial interventions may not only improve quality of life and may reduce adverse events but also allow patients to make a stronger commitment to making life style changes. Although definitive studies examining multifactorial risk factor interventions in patients with LV systolic dysfunction, CHF, and angina are not available, it is possible that a combination of moderate aerobic exercise, low fat diet, lipid management, and stress reduction therapy can produce beneficial results. Future studies are needed to assess outcomes in this high risk population after multifactorial cardiac rehabilitation interventions.

Summary and Recommendations

Based on studies and the experience at our institution[6,9,11,12] and others,[7,8,10,13-15,47,49] it appears that medically stable patients with moderate heart failure and severe systolic LV dysfunction benefit from participation in long-term aerobic exercise conditioning programs. Patients with persistent rales and uncontrolled edema on maximal medical therapy with digoxin, diuretics, and vasodilators have not been included in most previous studies and generally do not participate in exercise programs at the Duke Center for Living. However, a preliminary report by Myers et al.[15] has demonstrated that patients with functional class III or IV CHF can achieve important benefits from a progressive walking program, including improved peak VO_2, anaerobic threshold, quality of life as well as a decrease in symptoms. The results of this study suggest that even selected patients with severe CHF benefit from moderate exercise conditioning. Some patients with CHF experience a temporary increase in fluid accumulation 2–6 weeks after starting exercise, which may represent an increase in circulating plasma volume due to exercise. This change should be managed by increasing diuretics and careful patient follow-up; it does not preclude continued exercise. If the patient continues to have worsening CHF symptoms, the exercise training should be stopped or exercise intensity reduced until symptoms are alleviated. Exercise intensity can commence at 40–70 percent of peak VO_2 in patients without ischemia with the training range increased to 60–80 percent of peak VO_2 over 6–12 weeks. In patients with CHF and ongoing LV ischemia, coronary angiography and revascularization is recommended prior to cardiac rehabilitation. If revascularization is not possible, intensive multifactorial rehabilitation efforts, including exercise, low fat diet, lipid management, and stress reduction, are likely the optimal strategy. The goals in this group are to reduce LV ischemia and symptomatic angina and improve exercise tolerance and quality of life.

One meta-analysis in patients with coronary artery disease suggested a benefit of exercise training on long-term morbidity and mortality.[59] However, most of these patients have preserved LV systolic function, and these results may not apply to patients with severe systolic dysfunction. Although patients with LV systolic dysfunction, especially in the setting of ischemia, have a higher risk for exercise-related complications, it appears that this risk is relatively small when compared to the high incidence of non-exercise-related sudden death reported in clinical series for these patients. Analogous to the coronary artery bypass grafting experience, it is possible that patients with severe LV systolic dysfunction can achieve a benefit in terms of morbidity or mortality from exercise training precisely because they are at highest risk. However, studies examining the long-term effects of exercise training on morbidity and

mortality in patients with LV dysfunction are currently unavailable and are needed in this area. In light of other studies, it appears that patients with severe LV dysfunction and stable class I–III heart failure controlled on medical therapy achieve a clinically important improvement in exercise performance and symptoms through exercise conditioning comparable to that achieved by vasodilator therapy. Cardiac rehabilitation offers improved exercise tolerance and quality of life and represents a valuable therapeutic adjunct to the pharmacologic management of patients with CHF.

PSYCHOLOGICAL AND BIOBEHAVIORAL INTERVENTIONS

Our understanding of the role of emotional and psychological issues in patients with CHF and of biobehavioral interventions in their management is limited. However, a body of research is accumulating that provides evidence that psychosocial factors, including depression, anxiety, and social isolation, play an important role in the clinical course of patients with CHF and are significant predictors of mortality in these patients.[60–63] Work has been reported from our laboratory that documents significant relations among mood disturbance, functional status, and quality of life in a sample of patients with CHF.[61] Twenty-nine patients with class II–IV heart failure were enrolled in a project at Duke University Medical Center to evaluate the feasibility of outpatient support of patients and their families by nurse-practitioners. Subjects were followed for a period of 6 months. Major variables measured at four data points (baseline and 1, 3, and 6 months) included functional status (measured by the Heart Failure Functional Status Inventory: HFFSI),[63] emotional status using the Profile of Mood States (POMS),[64] overall quality of life using Ferrans' and Powers" Quality of life Index-Cardiac III (QLI-III),[65] and Mishel's Uncertainty in Illness Index (MUIS).[66]

In our study the HFFSI scores were directly related to all major psychological and quality of life variables. These results indicate that quality of life in patients with heart failure is related not only to VO_2 but to mood state as well. As such, emotional factors are important variables in functional outcomes and quality of life and raise the possibility that psychology-based interventions may improve quality of life in this patient group. The findings of our study are consistent with the findings of Dracup and associates, who documented the relation of emotions to functional capacity in a group of patients awaiting cardiac transplantation.[63] In a more recent study of

46 patients evaluated for cardiac transplantation, Burnett and associates found that patients with high anxiety and limited ego defenses had higher mortality rates than patients with low anxiety scores and greater ego strength.[67]

Research findings that document the relation of emotions to functional outcomes in patients with heart failure are important given what has also been documented about emotions and adverse events with other types of cardiac illness. Previous studies have documented that mortality rates for patients with coronary heart disease are significantly higher in patients diagnosed with affective disorders such as depression; in fact, affective disorders are related to an increased risk for myocardial infarction, dysrhythmias, sudden cardiac death, and more rapid disease progression.[68–70] In a landmark study, Frasure-Smith and associates documented a higher mortality rate among patients with depression following myocardial infarction.[71] Among 222 patients followed for 6 months after hospital discharge, the diagnosis of major depression was a significant predictor of mortality; depressed patients had a sixfold risk for death compared with that of controls. Work done by Williams and associates at our institution has also been groundbreaking in understanding the link between stress, hostility, social isolation, and coronary heart disease (CAD); these factors have been found to be important risk factors for adverse outcomes in patients with CAD.[72]

A number of physiologic mechanisms may explain the link between psychosocial factors with events in patients with coronary artery disease and CHF, including increased neurohumoral activation, altered immunologic reactivity, increased blood lipids, coronary vasoconstriction, and altered heart rate variability (HRV).[73] Decreased HRV has been shown to be an important risk factor for mortality among patients who are postmyocardial infarction and those with CHF.[74–76] Such understanding raises the possibility that interventions designed to alter psychological factors could result in significant improvement in quality of life as well as clinical outcomes and mortality for patients with significant LV dysfunction. A study by Moser et al.[77] supports this concept; these authors examined central hemodynamics via right heart catheterization before and after mental relaxation in patients with CHF. This group demonstrated that patients with advanced heart failure could use biofeedback to exert voluntary control over regional vascular tone. In this study, mental relaxation reduced systemic vascular resistance, improved cardiac output, and increased skin temperature.[77] An important study by Kostis et al.[78] furthered this concept by examining a multimodal nonpharmacologic intervention in the treatment of patients with CHF. Twenty patients were randomly assigned to one of three treatment arms: (1) combined nonpharmacologic intervention consisting of graduated exercise training, dietary modification, and cognitive-behavioral therapy designed for stress management and coping with depressive affect, anger, or anxiety; (2) digoxin titrated to achieve a blood level between 0.8 and 2.0 mg/ml; and (3) double-blind placebo. Kostis and associates found significant improvement in functional status and psychological variables for patients participating in the intervention arm.[78] Outcome measures indicated that after 12 weeks of the study the patients receiving multimodal therapy demonstrated significantly improved functional capacity, reduced body weight, and improved affective state. In contrast, digoxin improved the ejection fraction without a corresponding improvement in exercise tolerance or psychological measures. It is interesting to note that depression tended to worsen in placebo-treated patients in this trial. These results suggest that multidisciplinary interventions may lead to important functional improvements in patients with this disorder.

Biobehavioral Strategies

The goal of biobehavioral techniques such as relaxation and stress reduction strategies is to enable individuals to consciously achieve physiologic self-regulation of the autonomic nervous system, bringing involuntary responses (heart rate, blood pressure, respirations, and muscle tension) under voluntary control.[79] Among the most effective of the various methods is relaxation. Regardless of the relaxation technique selected, *physiologic self-regulation* involves daily use of the following three steps.[80]

1. Assessing oneself for physiologic cues to stress
2. Learning biobehavioral skills to evoke inner peace, calmness, and relaxation
3. Assessing body cues or responses to biobehavioral techniques

Relaxation techniques are taught to patients within the context of their importance for reducing overall stress as a life style change rather than perfecting an exercise that is performed twice a day.

Hyman and associates[81] conducted a meta-analysis of 48 studies that examined the effects of 10 types of relaxation training on various clinical problems (e.g., hypertension, pain, and headache). This analysis demonstrated moderate to high effects for the studies that examined the effects of relaxation training in patients with hypertension. This analysis also

Table 41-1. Relaxation Strategies
Autogenic training: repetition of autosuggestive phrases to oneself to induce mental and physical relaxation.
Benson's relaxation response: requires a four-step process: (1) quiet environment; (2) use of a mental device such as a word or phrase to be repeated; (3) adopting a passive attitude through focused attention; (4) using a comfortable position to induce relaxation.
Biofeedback: provides feedback about autonomic responses (blood pressure heart rate, galvanic skin response, muscle tension) through instrumentation, which may assist patients in recognizing and controlling these responses to promote relaxation.
Jacobsen's progressive relaxation: contracting and relaxing various muscle groups in a progressive fashion until total body relaxation is achieved.
Other effective techniques: hypnosis, imagery, Lamaze, meditation, music therapy, rhythmic breathing, transcendental meditation (TM), yoga, zen.
(Data from Newton and Froelicher[129] and Hyman et al.[81])

indicated that of the techniques examined Progressive Muscle Relaxation (PMR)[81] and meditation were the most effective for producing a sustained reduction in blood pressure over time. The authors posit that these methods may be most effective because of their simplicity and ease of use compared with the more complicated methods such as Benson's Relaxation Response or biofeedback. The most commonly utilized relaxation techniques are listed in Table 41-1.

In summary, available information suggests that significant patient benefits can be achieved from interventions designed to treat the emotional responses to illness and the accompanying sympathetic activation, which may increase the patient's risk for adverse cardiac events. To accomplish such treatment goals, the first step we recommend at our facility is a comprehensive psychosocial evaluation. Among factors evaluated are: anger, hostility, depression, and available sources of emotional and social support. Identified needs can be addressed in several ways; the attending physician can provide direct care and counseling, or the patient can undergo individual psychotherapeutic evaluation and intervention from other available staff.

SELF-CARE STRATEGIES AND PATIENT EDUCATION

The treatment of patients with heart failure is often difficult, not only because of the nature and severity of the associated symptoms but also because of the complex treatment protocols that place substantial demands on the patient and family in terms of knowledge, cooperation, and active participation.[82–84] As a consequence, recurrent episodes of heart failure requiring hospitalization for treatment characterize the illness trajectory for many of these patients. Heart failure patients, particularly those over age 65, have the highest hospital readmission rate (40–57 percent) of all reported patient groups.[85–87] Furthermore, data suggest that a significant portion of patient crises could be avoided through interventions to improve compliance with prescribed management protocols and recognition of the early warning signs of clinical problems.

Four primary conditions are necessary for the success of self-care.

1. The patient must have the cognitive ability, desire, and requisite knowledge base to interpret the meaning and salience of symptoms.
2. A family member or "significant other" is needed to provide tangible and emotional support in caregiving.
3. Close professional follow-up is needed by a physician and nurse team during the transition period from hospital to home and during subsequent periods of instability.
4. Treatment plans must include primary prevention and treatment of co-morbid problems, such as diabetes.

A careful assessment of the patient and family member's ability to provide self-care is needed as soon as possible when formulating the patient's treatment plan. Patient education is begun early in the hospital setting with the realization that learning may be compromised while patients are in this setting. Thus effective patient education is contingent on adequate follow-up care and close monitoring of the patient during the first few weeks after the patient's hospital discharge. It can be achieved through nursing home visits, phone calls, or weekly clinic visits until the patient's condition is stable.[83,88]

There has been limited research to identify the specific learning needs of patients with heart failure. Hagenhoff and associates[89] surveyed the most important learning needs in a sample of heart failure patients. The needs were ranked according to importance using a five-point Likert scale and the results compared with responses from a sample of hospital nurses. The most important identified learning needs were (1) medications, (2) anatomy and physiology (3) cardiac risk factors, (4) guidelines about what to do in an emergency (including CPR training), and (5) diet.

Table 41-2. Content for
Patient Education

Normal anatomy and physiology of the heart and circulation
Definition of heart failure
Reasons for signs and symptoms of worsening failure
Concepts of cardiac risk factor reduction
Pulse taking
Activity conservation and progression
When to phone the physician
Emergency plans
Dietary restrictions (sodium, fluids, calories, lipids)
Weight management
Medications (actions, side effects, interactions)
Management of co-morbid conditions
Health promotion and primary prevention
Psychological aspects of illness
Importance of compliance
Community resources
Follow-up care

(From Doyle.[130])

The Agency for Health Care Policy and Research (AHCPR)[60] guidelines for the evaluation and care of patients with LV systolic dysfunction underscore the importance of patient and family counseling. In addition to self-care strategies related to activity, diet, and treatment, patients must be informed about the exact nature of their illness, including the symptoms of worsening failure and what to do if they occur. According to the guidelines, patients are encouraged to complete advance directives regarding their health care preferences. An overview of the content that should be included in patient education for heart failure patients is included in Table 41-2. Table 41-3 contains a listing of self-care strategies that can be used to organize a discharge plan for this patient population.

DIET AND NUTRITION IN CHF PATIENTS

Sodium Restrictions

Restriction of dietary sodium has been considered to be an essential component in the treatment of heart failure and remains a recommended treatment modality, even with the availability of effective diuretic therapy.[82,90–96] Volpe and associates,[97] in the only recent available controlled trial concerning dietary sodium restrictions in patients with heart failure, reported the results of administering a high salt diet (250 mEq/day for 6 days) on hemodynamics, salt-regulating hormones, and renal excretory response in a sample of patients with mild heart failure (NYHA class I or II, ejection fraction less than 50 percent). Twelve untreated patients with idiopathic or ischemic cardiomyopathy (medication therapy withheld for a 3-week washout period before the study and for its duration) were compared with 12 normal subjects. In normal subjects the high sodium diet was associated with a significant increase in LV end-diastolic volume, ejection fraction, and stroke volume and with a reduction in total peripheral vascular resistance (all $P < 0.001$). Measures of atrial natriuretic factor (ANF) levels increased ($P < 0.05$), whereas plasma renin activity and aldosterone levels fell. In the heart failure group the end-diastolic volume increased significantly, but with no rise in ejection fraction or stroke volume or change in peripheral resistance. Plasma ANF levels also failed to increase in response to salt loading. Aldosterone and renin supression were similar in both groups. CHF patients were found to have significantly higher cumulative sodium balances than their normal counterparts ($P < 0.05$). This study, although it provides scientific support for the practice of dietary sodium restrictions, does not extend our understanding regarding the degree sodium needs to be restricted in heart failure patients.

Current recommendations for dietary sodium restrictions as an important adjunct to diuretic therapy are detailed in Table 41-4. These guidelines are consistent with AHCPR[60] recommendations. In our clinical practice, severe sodium restrictions (less than 2 g/day) are instituted only in patients with significant congestive symptoms who are refractory to

---

Table 41-3. Self-Care Activities

---

1. Daily weight-taking on waking, before breakfast, in the same clothes, using the same scale.
2. Report a weight gain over 3 pounds in 1 week (without a change in diet).
3. Maintain a low salt diet; include low sodium foods in diet and avoid those high in sodium.
4. Take all medications as prescribed; know the names, dosages, side effects, and actions of each medication.
5. Report any side effects or problems with medications.
6. Know the symptoms of heart failure; promptly report shortness of breath, increased fatigue, swelling of ankles or abdomen, an increased need to use the bathroom more frequently, or frequent colds.
7. Participate in regular exercise and stress reduction techniques as prescribed.
8. Plan daily activities in advance in order to conserve energy.

(From Bushnell.[84])

Table 41-4. Stepped Approach to Sodium Restriction and Diuretic Therapy

NYHA Class	Sodium Restrictions	Diuretic Therapy
II	Eliminate added salt from table and avoid heavily salted foods	Thiazide or low dose loop diuretic
III	Eliminate salt from cooking and the table (1.2–1.8 g Na$^+$/day)	Loop diuretic with progressive dosing
IV	Reduce sodium intake to <1 g/day by adding low Na$^+$ foods	Loop + K$^+$-sparing diuretic

(Data from Smith.[98])

increased diuretics and medication adjustments. Sodium restrictions in the frail elderly or the malnourished patient also have the potential to compound the effects of diminished appetite or compromised absorption due to gastrointestinal edema. Aggressive diuresis and sodium restrictions can also result in dehydration, which can interfere with a patient's capacity for exercise.

Dietary sodium restrictions are in need of controlled evaluation because there is evidence that such restrictions may result in adverse events in certain patient subgroups. For instance, several studies have found that in normotensive individuals total cholesterol and low-density lipoprotein (LDL) cholesterol change inversely with the salt intake.[99,100] There is also substantial evidence of variable responses to sodium associated with both gender and ethnicity.[100,101] Fluid intake restriction must be considered for patients with refractory symptoms or those with severe or symptomatic hyponatremia. Many clinicians use this measure sparingly because of the accompanying thirst sensation in many of these patients, which significantly reduces quality of life.

Alcohol Intake

In the absence of data evaluating the effects of the ingestion of alcohol in patients with heart failure, conventional wisdom dictates that alcohol, a known myocardial depressant, should be restricted. There are substantial data indicating that alcohol should be completely avoided by the patient with an alcohol-induced cardiomyopathy, as abstinence can result in significant improvement in clinical status[102] and because continued consumption is associated with a 3-year mortality of 80 percent.[103] Sometimes, however, it is not clear whether the etiology of heart failure is alcohol. Therefore in all patients with idiopathic cardiomyopathy in whom alcohol may be a contributing factor to heart failure, it is our practice to eliminate alcohol use. The long-term effects of alcohol on the course of other types of heart failure patients is unknown. A conservative approach is recommended in the AHCPR clinical practice guideline: Alcohol intake is discouraged, with patients who continue to drink advised to limit intake to no more than one drink a day.[60]

Nutrition

Our evolving understanding of the pathophysiology of heart failure indicates that the importance of an adequate diet and the potential benefits of dietary supplementation in the treatment of heart failure have been greatly underestimated. There are three reasons for specific nutritional interventions (calorie/nutrient intake) in patients with CHF: (1) malnutrition; (2) obesity; (3) coronary artery disease, angina, and hyperlipidemia. Malnutrition is not limited to those patients with the obvious cachexia and muscle wasting associated with terminal heart failure. One study reported that as many as 30–50 percent of hospitalized heart failure patients were undernourished.[104] This point is important for the clinician to recognize in light of what we are learning about the importance of adequate nutrition to myocardial performance; there is substantial evidence that with malnutrition these patients experience protein-energy metabolism, a catabolic state where lean muscle mass, including myocardial muscle mass, is significantly reduced.[105,106] Contractile energy reserves are also significantly reduced,[107–109] and potentially toxic metabolites may be produced.

Patients with CHF are at risk for malnutrition because of increased demands for energy occurring along with diminishing resources. These factors are summarized as follows:

1. *Decreased intake:* Heart failure patients are older, experience higher rates of poverty and depression, and are at risk for diminished appetite due to the multiple medications they take.
2. *Increased nutritional losses due to malabsorption.*[104]
3. *Increased nutritional requirements:* Resting metabolic rates have been found to be 18 percent

higher when compared with normal age-matched adults.[110]

Malnutrition among heart failure patients is also associated with immunocompromise, poor wound healing, and significantly more mortality and morbidity in the hospitalized heart failure patient.[104,105,111] Guidelines for nutritional assessment in heart failure patients are outlined in Table 41-5.

It is well accepted that control of body weight is important in the management of heart failure, as with added weight there is a concomitant increase in circulating volume and myocardial workload.[118] Obesity, in and of itself, is known to be an independent predictor of mortality and increases the risk for the development of heart failure in both men and women.[103,118,119] For patients who need to achieve weight loss, caloric restriction is recommended. Women should generally be restricted to 900–1200 calories and men to 1200–1500. The goal is to achieve a weight loss of 1–2 lb per week[15]; weight loss can be enhanced by the addition of exercise, which may obviate the need for significant caloric restriction. It has also been documented that even modest weight loss (8–10 lb) in patients with morbid obesity and related cardiomyopathy can result in a significant decrease in ventricular wall mass.[120] As outlined previously, patients with CHF due to coronary artery disease who have ongoing ischemia might benefit from a low fat diet (less than 20–25 percent of calories from fat). Care must be taken to provide adequate protein and calorie intake in these cases.

Nutritional Supplementation (Micronutrients and Antioxidants)

Some evidence raises the possibility that the inclusion of specific micronutrients can replenish myocardial energy stores, stabilize cellular metabolism, or counteract toxic substances such as cytokines. Attention has been directed toward the effects of one such agent, coenzyme Q_{10} (CoQ_{10}), on left ventricular function in dilated cardiomyopathy.[121-125] CoQ_{10} is a vitamin-like essential substance that has a key role in oxidative phosphorylation and synthesis of ATP. Other functions performed by this substance are membrane stabilization and as a naturally occurring antioxidant.[125] Research concerning this substance evolved in conjunction with evaluation of patients with cardiomyopathy who were found to have deficiencies in this substance in endomyocardial biopsy samples; the level of deficiency was associated with the amount of LV dysfunction.

The effectiveness of CoQ_{10} has been evaluated in

Table 41-5. Essential Elements of Nutritional Assessment in Patients with CHF

Assess laboratory values
    Serum albumin
    Transferrin
    T lymphocyte count
    Skin testing[112,113]

Calculate RWR: relative body weight = actual weight/IBW (%)
    Use age-specific weight-for-height tables (e.g., Metropolitan Life Insurance tables); recent guidelines indicate that lean body mass decreases with age, thus weights for older individuals should increase over time up to 10–20 pounds.[114,115]

Evaluate patient for risk for malnutrition and/or obesity based on RW[116]
    At risk = RW < 80% or loss of 10–20% body weight for age
    Obesity = RW > 120%
    Morbid obesity = RW > 200%

Identify physiologic risk factors for malnutrition[117]
    Diminished taste and smell
    Inadequate dentition
    Dementia
    Acute illness
    Malabsorption
    Increased metabolic rate

Identify social factors contributing to risk for malnutrition
    Social isolation
    Alcoholism
    Low income
    Depression
    Learning or reading disability

Estimate daily sodium, potassium and fluid intake:

Evaluate adequacy of diet via 24-hour diet recall or diary: estimate adequacy of caloric intake and nutritional balance
    Caloric requirements should include stress factor for illness or increased resting metabolic rate (1500–1800 cal/day)
    Diet composition < 30% fat, 15% carbohydrate, 55% carbohydrate[115]

Alternate method for weight evaluation[114]
    Body mass index (BMI) = weight kg/(height in meters)^2 or = weight lb (height in inches)^2 (BMI has the highest correlation with measurements of body fat composition)
        Obesity = BMI > 27.5 kg/m^2
        Morbid obesity = BMI > 40 kg/m^2

Abbreviations: RWR, relative weight reduction; IBW, ideal body weight; RW, relative weight.

a series of uncontrolled and placebo-controlled, double-blind experiments. A large Italian multicenter uncontrolled study reported by Baggio and associates[123] used CoQ$_{10}$ as an adjunctive treatment for a sample of patients with class II and III failure. Preliminary results of the study indicate that after 3 months of test treatment among 1113 patients clinical improvements were noted in more than 50 percent of patients reporting each of the following signs and symptoms: cyanosis, edema, rales, liver enlargement, jugular reflux, dyspnea, palpitations, sweating, arrhythmias, insomnia, vertigo, and nocturia. Although it is difficult to draw conclusions from this uncontrolled trial, of note is the low occurrence of adverse effects and ease of administration reported by this large group of participants.

Controlled research has demonstrated that CoQ$_{10}$ can improve exercise tolerance in patients with stable angina pectoris.[121] Several controlled trials have demonstrated that patients with LV dysfunction may improve in subjective functional assessment (e.g., fatigue and dyspnea) accompanied by increased ejection fraction and fractional shortening and decreased cardiac size. Such improvements are hypothesized to be the result of improvements in the energy supply to the myocardium with correction of metabolic deficits in the myocardium, specifically the impairment of energy-dependent calcium ion transport across the sarcoplasmic reticulum, where there is interference with the excitation-contraction-relaxation coupling sequence.

Much interest has also been generated in the use of vitamins A, C, and E for antioxidant therapy.[126,127] Vitamin E has been demonstrated to be successful for its use in the treatment of familial hypercholesterolemia. Research indicates that the usefulness of this agent can be extended to attenuating adverse effects of toxic metabolites in myocytes. In a study of rats administration of vitamin E in the form of probucol significantly reduced the adverse myocardial effects of adriamycin, resulting in improved LV function and lowered mortality.[128] This success is attributed to the reduction of a significant antioxidant deficit associated with the effects of adriamycin on myocyte metabolism.

CONCLUSIONS AND RECOMMENDATIONS

Although relatively few studies have examined nonpharmacologic therapy in CHF patients, data suggest that these treatment strategies may have significant clinical benefits. Based on recent studies[6,9,14,15,17–19] and the experience at our institution,[5,11,12] it

---

Table 41-6. General Guidelines for Exercise Training for Patients with CHF

Step I: Screen patient for relative contraindications
 Symptomatic ventricular tachycardia (VT)
 Active myocarditis
 Pseudoaneurysm

Step II: Exercise testing to set training range and evaluate safety of exercise. Training may be contraindicated in patients with
 Exertional hypotension
 Severe ischemia at low levels of exercise (should have revascularization if possible, prior to exercise)
 Sustained exercise-induced VT

Step III: Begin patient's choice of low level exercise as tolerated three or four times a week
 Walking
 Exercise bicycle
 Low level weight lifting with 15 repetitions

Step IV: Accelerate program as tolerated with goal set at 45 minutes at 75% VO$_2$; more strenuous forms of exercise such as jogging and water aerobics can be added as tolerance improves.

Note: It is not uncommon for patients who have been exercising for approximately 6 weeks to need an increase in diuretic dosage. Care must be taken that this does not discourage the patient from continuing exercise training.

---

appears that medically stable patients with moderate heart failure and severe systolic LV dysfunction may benefit from participation in long-term aerobic exercise conditioning programs (as outlined in Table 41-6). Some patients with CHF experience a temporary increase in fluid accumulation 2–6 weeks after starting exercise, which may represent an increase in circulating plasma volume due to exercise. It should be managed by increasing diuretics and careful patient follow-up; it does not preclude continued exercise. If the patient continues to have worsening CHF symptoms, exercise training should be stopped or exercise intensity reduced until symptoms improve. Exercise intensity can commence at 40–70 percent of peak VO$_2$ in patients without ischemia with the training range increased to 60–80 percent of peak VO$_2$ over 6–12 weeks. In patients with CHF and ongoing myocardial ischemia, coronary angiography and revascularization is recommended prior to cardiac rehabilitation. If revascularization is not possible, intensive multifactorial rehabilitation efforts, including exercise, low fat diet, lipid management, and stress reduction, would likely be the optimal strategy. The goals in this group are to reduce ischemia and symptomatic angina and improve exercise tolerance and quality of life.

Improved patient education and nursing follow-up

offers the possibility of reducing morbidity. Biobehavioral interventions may also improve quality of life and offer the potential to improve outcomes. Although definitive studies examining multimodal interventions in patients with LV systolic dysfunction, CHF, and angina are not available, it is possible that a combination of strategies, including moderate aerobic exercise, diet management, and stress reduction therapy, may produce beneficial results. Future studies are needed to assess the effects of multifactorial cardiac rehabilitation interventions on clinical outcomes and quality of life in this high risk population.

ACKNOWLEDGMENTS

This study was supported by grant HL-17670 from the National Heart, Lung, and Blood Institute, Bethesda, MD, and by General Medical Research Funds from the Veterans Administration Medical Center, Durham, NC. M.J.S. was supported by an established investigatorship from the American Heart Association.

REFERENCES

1. Ghali JK, Cooper R, Ford E: Trends in hospitalization rates for heart failure in the United States, 1973–1986. Arch Intern Med 1990;150:769
2. Kannel WB, Belanger AJ: Epidemiological of heart failure. Am Heart J 1991;121:951
3. Schocken DD, Arrieta MI, Leaverton PE, Ross EA: Prevalence and mortality rate of congestive heart failure in the United States. J Am Coll Cardiol 1992; 20:301
4. Pfeffer MA, Braunwald E, Moye LA et al: Effect of captopril on mortality and morbidity in patients with left ventricular dysfunction after myocardial infarction. Results of the survival and ventricular enlargement trial. N Engl J Med 1992;10:669
5. Letac B, Cribier A, Desplanches JF: A study of left ventricular function in coronary patients before and after physical training. Circulation 1977;56:375
6. Cobb FR, Williams RS, McEwan P et al: Effects of exercise training on ventricular function in patients with recent myocardial infarction. Circulation 1982; 66:100
7. Lee AP, Ice R, Blessey R et al: Long-term effects of physical training on coronary patients with impaired ventricular function. Circulation 1979;60:1519
8. Hagberg JM, Ehsani AA, Holloszy JO: Effect of 12 months of intense exercise training on strike volume in patients with coronary artery disease. Circulation 1983;67:1194
9. Conn EH, Williams RS, Wallace AG: Exercise responses before and after physical conditioning in patients with severely depressed left ventricular function. Am J Cardiol 1982;49:296
10. Coats AJS, Adamopoulos S, Meyer TE et al: Effects of physical training in chronic heart failure. Lancet 1990;335:631
11. Sullivan MJ, Higginbotham MB, Cobb FR: Exercise training in patients with severe left ventricular dysfunction. Hemodynamic and metabolic effects. Circulation 1988;78:506
12. Sullivan MJ, Higginbotham MB, Cobb FR: Exercise training in patients with chronic heart failure delays ventilatory anaerobic threshold and improves submaximal exercise performance. Circulation 1989;79: 324
13. Coats AJS, Adamopoulos S, Radaelli A et al: Controlled trial of physical training in chronic heart failure. Exercise performance, hemodynamics, ventilation, and autonomic function. Circulation 1992;85: 2119
14. Giannuzzi P, Temporelli PL, Gattone M et al: Eami-exercise training in anterior myocardial infarction. An ongoing multicenter randomized trial. Chest 1992;101:3155
15. Myers MG, Baigrie RS, Kavanagh T et al: Benefits of physical training in patients with heart failure [abstract]. Circulation, suppl. I 1992;86:400
16. Minotti JR, Massie BM: Exercise training in heart failure patients. Does reversing the peripheral abnormalities protect the heart? Circulation 1992;85:2323
17. Henriksson J: Training induced adaptation of skeletal muscle and metabolism during submaximal exercise. J Physiol (Lond) 1977;270:661
18. Seals DR, Hagberg JM, Hurley BF et al: Endurance training in older men and women. Cardiovascular responses to exercise. J Appl Physiol 1984;57:1024
19. Blomqvist CG, Saltin B: Cardiovascular adaptations to physical training. Annu Rev Physiol 1983;45:169
20. Scheuer J, Tipton CM: Cardiovascular adaptations to physical training. Annu Rev Physiol 1977;39:221
21. Wood PD, Haskell WL, Blair SM: Increased exercise level and plasma lipoproteins. Metabolism 1983;32: 31
22. Peters PK, Cady LD, Bischoff DB: Physical fitness and subsequent myocardial infarction in healthy workers. JAMA 1983;249:3052
23. Saltin B, Gollnick PD: Skeletal muscle adaptability. Significance for metabolism and performance. In Peachey LD (ed): The Handbook of Physiology. The Skeletal Muscle System. American Physiological Society, Bethesda 1982
24. Peronnet F, Cleroux J, Perrault H et al: Plasma norepinephrine response to exercise before and after training in humans. J Appl Physiol 1981;51:812
25. Clausen JP: Circulatory adjustments to dynamic exercise and effect of physical training in normal subjects and patients with coronary artery disease. Prog Cardiovasc Dis 1976;18:459
26. Varnauskas E, Bergman H, Houk P, Bjorntorp P: Hemodynamic effects of physical training in coronary patients. Lancet 1966;2:8
27. Detry JM, Rousseau M, Vandenbroucke G et al: Increased arteriovenous oxygen difference after physical training in coronary heart disease. Circulation 1971;44:109
28. Clausen JP, Trap-Jensen J: Effects of training on the distribution of cardiac output in patients with coronary artery disease. Circulation 1970;42:611
29. Hagberg JM: Physiologic adaptations to prolonged

high-intensity exercise training in patients with coronary artery disease. Am Coll Sports Med 1991;23:661

30. Ferguson RJ, Taylor AW, Cote P et al: Skeletal muscle and cardiac changes with training in patients with angina pectoris. Am J Physiol, suppl. H 1982;243:830

31. Froelicher V, Jensen D, Genter F et al: A randomized trial of exercise training in patients with coronary artery disease. JAMA 1984;252:1291

32. Sebrechts CP, Klein JL, Ahnve S: Myocardial perfusion changes following 1 year of exercise training assessed by thallium-201 circumferential count profiles. Am Heart J 1986;112:1217

33. Health and Public Policy Committee, American College of Physicians. Cardiac rehabilitation services. Ann Intern Med 1988;109:671

34. Taylor CB, Houston-Miller N, Ahn DK et al: The effects of exercise training programs on psychosocial improvement in uncomplicated postmyocardial infarction patients. J Psychosom Res 1986;30:581

35. Massie BM: Exercise tolerance in congestive heart failure. Role of cardiac function, peripheral blood flow, and muscle metabolism and effect of treatment. Am J Med, suppl. 3A 1988;84:75

36. Sullivan MJ, Higginbotham MB, Cobb FR: Increased exercise ventilation in chronic heart failure. Intact ventilatory control despite hemodynamic and pulmonary abnormalities. Circulation 1988;77:552

37. Massie BM, Conway M, Rajagopalan B et al: Skeletal muscle metabolism during exercise under ischemic conditions. Evidence for abnormalities unrelated to blood flow. Circulation 1988;78:320

38. Minotti JR, Johnson EC, Hudson TL: Skeletal muscle response to exercise training in congestive heart failure. J Clin Invest 1990;86:751

39. Sullivan MJ, Knight JD, Higginbotham MB et al: Relation between central and peripheral hemodynamics during exercise in patients with chronic heart failure. Muscle blood flow is reduced with maintenance of arterial perfusion pressure. Circulation 1989;80:769

40. Sullivan MJ, Green HJ, Cobb FR: Altered skeletal muscle metabolic response to exercise in chronic heart failure. Relationship to hemodynamics and skeletal muscle aerobic enzyme activity. Circulation 1991;84:1597

41. Mancini DM, Coyle E, Coggan A et al: Contribution of intrinsic skeletal muscle changes to ^{31}P NMR skeletal muscle metabolic abnormalities in patients with chronic heart failure. Circulation 1989;80:1338

42. Drexler H, Riede U, Münzel T: Alterations of skeletal muscle in chronic heart failure. Circulation 1992;85:1751

43. Sullivan MJ, Green HJ, Cobb FR: Skeletal muscle biochemistry and histology in ambulatory patients with long-term chronic heart failure. Circulation 1990;81:518

44. Wilson JR, Fink L, Maris J et al: Evaluation of energy metabolism in skeletal muscle of patients with heart failure with gated phosphorus-31 nuclear magnetic resonance. Circulation 1985;71:57

45. Mancini DM, Walter G, Reichek N et al: Contribution of skeletal muscle atrophy to exercise intolerance and altered muscle metabolism in heart failure. Circulation 1992;85:1364

46. Sullivan MJ, Charles HC, Negro-Villar R: Early skeletal muscle anaerobic metabolism occurs independent of muscle atrophy in heart failure. Circulation, suppl. II 1988;84:7

47. Kellermann JJ, Ben-Ari E, Fisman E et al: Physical training in patients with ventricular impairment. Adv Cardiol 1986;34:131

48. Hoffmann A, Duba J, Lengyel M, Majer K: The effect of training on physical working capacity of MI patients with LV dysfunction. Eur Heart J, suppl. G 1987;8:43

49. Arvan S: Exercise performance of the high risk acute myocardial infarction patient after cardiac rehabilitation. Am J Cardiol 1988;62:197

50. Alderman EL, Fisher LD, Litwin P: Results of coronary artery surgery in patients with poor left ventricular function (CASS). Circulation 1983;68:785

51. Vigilante GJ, Weintraub WS, Klein LW et al: Improved survival with coronary bypass surgery in patients with three-vessel coronary disease and abnormal left ventricular function. Matched case-control study in patient with potentially operable disease. Am J Med 1987;82:697

52. Brown G, Albers JJ, Fisher LD: Regression of coronary artery disease as a result of intensive lipid-lowering therapy in men with high levels of apolipoprotein B. N Engl J Med 1990;323:289

53. Kane JP, Malloy MJ, Ports TA: Regression of coronary atherosclerosis during treatment of familial hypercholesterolemia with combined drug regimens. JAMA 1990;264:3007

54. Buchwald H, Varco RL, Matts JP: Effect of partial ileal bypass surgery on mortality and morbidity from coronary heart disease in patients with hypercholesterolemia. Report of the Program on the Surgical Control of the Hyperlipidemias (POSCH). N Engl J Med 1990;323:946

55. Ornish D, Brown SE, Scherwitz LW: Can lifestyle changes reverse coronary heart disease? The Lifestyle Heart Trial. Lancet 1990;336:129

56. Watts GF, Lewis B, Brunt JNH: Effects on coronary artery disease of lipid-lowering diet, or diet plus cholestyramine, in the St. Thomas' Atherosclerosis Regression Study (STARS). Lancet 1992;339:563

57. Schuler G, Hambrecht R, Schlierf G et al: Regular exercise and low-fat diet. Effects on progression of coronary artery disease. Circulation 1992;86:1

58. Vogel RA: Comparative clinical consequences of aggressive lipid management, coronary angioplasty and bypass surgery in coronary artery disease. Am J Cardiol 1992;69:1229

59. O'Connor GT, Buring JE, Yusuf S: An overview of randomized trials of rehabilitation with exercise after myocardial infarction. Circulation 1989;80:234

60. Agency for Health Care Policy and Research: Heart Failure: Evaluation and Care of Patients with Left-Ventricular Systolic Dysfunction. US Department of Health and Human Services, Washington, DC, 1994

61. Hawthorne MH, Hixon ME: Functional status, mood disturbance and quality of life in heart failure. p. 309. In Funk SG, Tornquist EM, Champagne MT, Weise R (eds): Key Aspects of Caring for the Acutely Ill. Springer, New York, 1995

62. Adams KF, Califf RA, Harrell FE et al: Clinical characteristics not hemodynamics predict outcome in end-stage heart failure—The FIRST trial experience [abstract]. J Heart Failure 1995;2:34

63. Dracup KC, Walsden JA, Stevenson LW et al: Quality of life in patients with advanced heart failure. J Heart Lung Transplant 1992;11:273

64. McNair D, Lorr M, Droppelman L: Profile of Mood

States. EdiTS/Educational and Industrial Testing Service, San Diego, 1992

65. Ferrans CE, Powers MJ: Psychometric assessment of Quality of Life Index. Res Nurs Health 1992;15:29

66. Mishel MH: The Mishel Uncertainty in Illness Manual: School of Nursing, University of North Carolina, Chapel Hill, 1990

67. Burnett CK, Suetta CA, Dunlap SH et al: Psychological predictors of survival in patients evaluated in cardiac transplantation [abstract]. J Heart Failure 1995; 2:618

68. Meyerberg RJ, Castellanos A: Cardiac arrest and sudden cardiac death. p. 742. In Braunwald E (ed): A Textbook of Cardiovascular Medicine. 3rd Ed. WB Saunders, Philadelphia, 1988

69. Ruberman W, Weinblatt E, Goldberg JD et al: Psychological influences on mortality after myocardial infarction. N Engl J Med 1984;311:552

70. Shuster JL, Stern TA, Tesar GE: Psychological problems and their management. p. 483. In Wenger NK, Hellerstein HK (eds): Rehabilitation of the Coronary Patient. Churchill Livingstone, New York, 1992

71. Frasure-Smith N, Lesperance F, Talajic M: Depression following myocardial infarction. JAMA 1993; 270:1819

72. Williams RB, Barefoot JC, Califf RM et al: Prognostic importance of social and economic resources among medically treated patients with angiographically documented coronary artery disease. JAMA 1992;267: 520

73. Littman AB: Review of psychosomatic aspects of cardiovascular disease. Psychother Psychosom 1993;60: 148

74. Van Ravenswaajj-Arts CMA, Kollee LAA, Hopman JCW et al: Heart rate variability. Ann Intern Med 1993;118:436

75. Saul JP, Arai Y, Berger RD et al: Assessment of autonomic regulation in chronic congestive heart failure by heart rate spectral analysis. Am J Cardiol 1988; 61:1292

76. Bigger JT Jr, Fleiss JL, Steinman RC et al: Frequency of domain measures of heart period variability and mortality after myocardial infarction. Circulation 1992;85:164

77. Moser DK, Dracup K, Woo MA et al: Voluntary control of vascular tone using skin temperature biofeedback in patients with advanced heart failure [abstract]. Circulation, suppl. I 1992;86:104

78. Kostis JB, Rosen RC, Cosgrove N et al: Nonpharmacologic therapy improves functional and emotional status in congestive heart failure. Chest 1994;106: 996

79. Guzzetta CE, Dossey BM: Cardiovascular Nursing. Mosby, St. Louis, 1992

80. Achterberg J, Dossey B, Kolkmeier L: Rituals of Healing. Bantam, New York, 1992

81. Hyman RB, Feldman HR, Harris RB et al: The effects of relaxation training on clinical symptoms. A meta-analysis. Nurs Res 1989;38:216–220

82. Bousquet GL: Congestive heart failure. J Card Nurs 1990;4:35

83. Quaal SJ: The person with heart failure and cardiogenic shock. In Guzzetta CE, Dossey EM (eds): Cardiovascular Nursing: Holistic Practice. Mosby, St. Louis, 1992

84. Bushnell FK: Self-care teaching for congestive heart failure patients. Gerontol Nurs 1992;18:27

85. Berkman S. Dumas S, Gastfriend J et al: Predicting hospital readmission of elderly cardiac patients. Health Social Work 1987;12:21

86. Gooding J, Jette AM: Hospital readmissions among the elderly. J Am Geriatr Soc 1985;33:595

87. Vinson JM, Rich MW, Sperry JC et al: Early readmission of elderly patients with congestive heart failure. J Am Geriatr Soc 1990;38:1290

88. Frasure-Smith N, Prince R: Long-term follow-up of the ischemic heart disease life stress monitoring program. Psychosom Med 1989;51:485

89. Hagenhoff BD, Feutz C, Conn VS et al: Patient education needs as reported by congestive heart failure patients and their nurses. J Adv Nurs 1994;19:685

90. Dracup K, Baker DW, Dunbar SB et al: Management of heart failure. II. Counseling, education, and lifestyle modifications. JAMA 1994;272:1442

91. Snively WD, Beshear DR, Roberts KT: Sodium restricted diet. Review and current status. Nurs Forum 1974;13:59

92. Dahl L: Salt and hypertension. Am J Clin Nutr 1972; 25:231

93. Hopkins BE, Rogers R: Sodium restrictions in heart failure. Med J Aust 1972;1:370

94. Dyckner T, Wester P-O: Salt and water balance in congestive heart failure. Acta Med Scand, suppl. 1986;707:27

95. Smith TW, Braunwald E, Kelly RA: The management of heart failure. p. 485. In Braunwald E (ed): Heart Disease: A Textbook of Cardiovascular Medicine. 3rd Ed. WB Saunders, Philadelphia, 1988

96. Gottlieb SH: Heart failure. p. 737. In Barker LR, Burton JR, Zieve PD (eds): Principles of Ambulatory Medicine. Williams & Wilkins, Baltimore, 1991

97. Volpe M, Tritto C, DeLuca N et al: Abnormalities of sodium handling and of cardiovascular adaptation during high salt diet in patients with mild heart failure. Circulation 1993;88:1620

98. Smith TW: Heart failure. p. 187. In Wyngaarden JB, Smith LH, Bennett JC (eds): Cecil Textbook of Medicine. 19th Ed. WB Saunders, Philadelphia, 1992

99. Fliser D, Norwack R, Allendorf-Otswald N et al: Serum lipid changes on low salt diet. Am J Hypertens 1993;6:320

100. Ames RP: Hyperlipidemia in hypertension. Causes and prevention. Am Heart J 1991;122:1219

101. Flack JM, Ensrud KE, Mascioli S et al: Racial and ethnic modifiers of the salt-blood pressure response. Hypertension 1991;17:1–115

102. Molgaard H, Kristensen BO, Baandrup U: Importance of abstention in alcoholic heart disease. Int J Cardiol 1990;26:373

103. Wynne J, Braunwald E: The cardiomyopathies and myocarditides. p. 1410. In Braunwald E (ed): Heart Disease: A Textbook of Cardiovascular Medicine. 3rd Ed. WB Saunders, Philadelphia, 1988

104. Freeman LM, Roubenoff R: The nutrition implications of cardiac cachexia. Nutr Rev 1994;52:340

105. Ansari A: Syndromes of cardiac cachexia and the cachectic heart. Prog Cardiovasc Dis 1987;30:45

106. Morrison WL, Edwards RHT: Cardiac cachexia. BMJ 1991;302:301

107. Tian R, Reis M, Bak R et al: Does reduced energy

supply contribute to heart failure [abstract]? Circulation, suppl. I 1994;90:112

108. Katz AM: The cardiomyopathy of overload. An unnatural growth response in the hypertrophied heart. Ann Intern Med 1994;121:363

109. Swan HJC: Left ventricular dysfunction in ischemic heart disease. Fundamental importance of the fibrous matrix. Cardiovasc Drugs Ther 1994;8:305

110. Scheffers J, Vaitkevicius VG, Fisher ML et al: Elevated resting metabolic rate in congestive heart failure [abstract]. Circulation, suppl. I 1994;90:602

111. Paccagnella A, Calo MA, Caenaro G et al: Cardiac cachexia and postoperative nutrition management. J Parent Ent Nutr 1994;18:409

112. Heizer WD: Weight loss. p. 15. In Dombrand L, Hoole AS, Pickard CG (eds): Manual of Clinical Problems in Adult Ambulatory Care. Little, Brown, Boston, 1992

113. Grant JP, Custer PB, Thurlow J: Current techniques of nutritional assessment. Surg Clin North Am 1981; 61:437

114. Blackman MR: Obesity. p. 1028. In Barker LR, Burton JR, Zieve PD (eds): Principles of Ambulatory Medicine. Williams & Williams, Baltimore, 1991

115. Baron RB: Obesity. p. 8. In Dombrant L, Hoole AS, Pickard CG (eds): Manual of Clinical Problems in Adult Ambulatory Care. Little, Brown, Boston, 1992

116. NIH Consensus Development Panel on the Implications of Obesity: Ann Intern Med 1985;103:1073

117. Robbins LJ: Evaluation of weight loss in the elderly. Geriatrics 1989;44:31

118. Gotto AM, Farmer JA: Risk factors for coronary heart disease. p. 1153. In Braunwald E (ed): Heart Disease: A Textbook of Cardiovascular Medicine. 3rd Ed. WB Saunders, Philadelphia, 1988

119. Pi-Sunyer F: Obesity. p. 1162. In Wyngaarden JB, Smith LH, Bennett JC (eds): Cecil Textbook of Medicine. WB Saunders, Philadelphia, 1992

120. MacMahon SW, Wilcken DEL, Macdonald GJ: The effect of weight reduction on left ventricular mass. A randomized controlled trial in young, overweight, hypertensive patients. N Engl J Med 1986;314:334

121. Kamikawa T, Kobayashi A, Yamashita T et al: Effects of coenzyme Q_{10} on exercise tolerance in chronic stable angina pectoris. Am J Cardiol 1985;56:247

122. Morisco C, Trimarco B, Cordorelli M: Effect of coenzyme Q_{10} therapy in patients with congestive heart failure. A long-term multicenter randomized study. Clin Investigator, suppl. 8 1993;71:S134

123. Baggio E, Gandini R, Plancher AC et al: Italian multicenter study on the safety and efficacy of coenzyme Q_{10} as adjunctive therapy in heart failure. Clin Investigator, suppl. 1993;71:S145

124. Pogessi L, Galanti G, Comeglio M et al: Curr Ther Res 1991;49:878

125. Mortensen SA: Perspectives on therapy of cardiovascular diseases with coenzyme Q_{10} (ubiquinone). Clin Investigator, suppl. 8 1993;71:S116

126. Rivlin RS: Disorders of vitamin metabolism. Deficiencies, metabolic abnormalities, and excesses. p. 1170. In Wyngaarden JB, Smith LH, Bennett JC (eds): Cecil Textbook of Medicine. 3rd Ed. WB Saunders, Philadelphia, 1992

127. Manson JE, Walter CW, Meir JS et al: Vitamins C, E and carotene and incidence of coronary heart disease in women [abstract]. Circulation, suppl I. 1994; 90:128

128. Siveski-Illiskovic N, Kaul N, Singal PK: Probucol promotes endogenous antioxidants and provides protection against adriamycin-induced cardiomyopathy in rats. Circulation 1994;89:2829

129. Newton KM, Froelicher ESS: Education of the patient and family. In-hospital phase. pp. 715–738. In Underhill SL, Woods SL, Froelicher ESS, Halpenny CJ (eds): Cardiac Nursing. Lippincott-Raven, Philadelphia, 1989

130. Doyle B: Nursing challenge. The patient with end-stage heart failure. pp. 311–355. In Kern LS (ed): Cardiac Critical Care. Aspen, Rockville, MD, 1988

42 Diuretic Therapy

Robert J. Cody

We hope that the results reported in this paper will lead to a more general and accurate use of suitable diuretics in the treatment of edema, and possibly to the discovery of further helpful therapeutic agents.

Binger and Keith[1]

The mechanisms by which the transition from asymptomatic left ventricular dysfunction to symptomatic congestive heart failure occurs remain obscure, as patients with similar degrees of left ventricular dysfunction exhibit a wide range of symptoms. A feature of this symptomatic transition is the onset of sodium retention. Most simply stated, sodium retention results from the inability of the body to excrete sodium at a rate commensurate with dietary sodium intake. This process also occurs with heart failure as a result of the functional impairment that takes place in response to decreased renal blood flow (Fig. 42-1). Over time, the net retention of sodium, with resultant edema, produces rales, peripheral edema, hepatomegaly with ascites, and increased blood volume, with increased cardiac filling pressures. These findings are in fact the hallmark of congestive heart failure. Pragmatic utilization has been the basis for diuretic utilization, although formal studies and clinical trial outcomes are lacking. Use of angiotensin-converting enzyme (ACE) inhibitors for early stages of heart failure suggests that diuretic use may be delayed until later stages of the disease, but this judgment is based largely on conjecture. This chapter summarizes the rationale and current use of diuretics for the treatment of the edema and sodium retention of congestive heart failure.

FACTORS CONTRIBUTING TO SODIUM RETENTION AND EDEMA IN HEART FAILURE

Chronic congestive heart failure is characterized by decreased left ventricular systolic function and, in most cases, abnormal diastolic function. The resultant decrease of cardiac output and increased ventricular end-diastolic pressure set the stage for sodium retention. Decreased cardiac output and increased systemic resistance produce decreased renal blood flow, and the magnitude of renal blood flow reduction is correlated with decreased cardiac output.[2] Diminished renal blood flow is a stimulus for activation of neurohormonal vasoconstriction pathways, particularly the renin system,[3–5] which produces vasoconstriction and aldosterone secretion. Total body water, extracellular fluid, and plasma volume are increased compared to controls.[5] With heart failure, there may be a range of blood volume expansion, reflected in renin system suppression and increased cardiac filling pressures (Fig. 42-2). These hemodynamic responses become the basis for sodium retention.

Under most conditions, sodium excretion is primarily determined by the glomerular filtration rate. The reduction of glomerular filtration rate in congestive heart failure is highly correlated with hemodynamic parameters, where the greatest reduction of cardiac output and renal blood flow are associated with the greatest reduction of glomerular filtration rate.[2,6,7] Renal blood flow and function tend to decrease with age in normal subjects, and an age effect can be superimposed on the overall reduction in

635

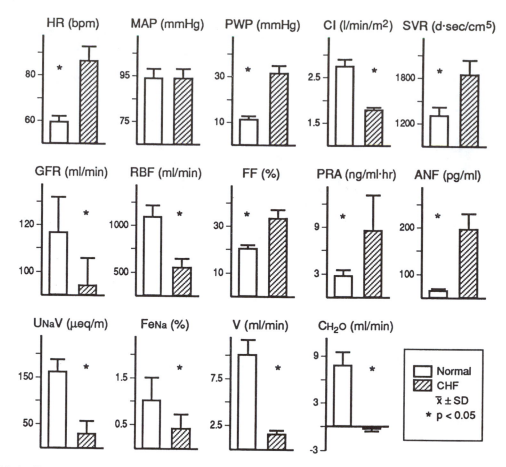

Fig. 42-1. Comparison of systemic hemodynamics, renal hemodynamics, renal excretory function, and neurohormonal levels in normal subjects and patients with moderate to severe congestive heart failure. (Data from Cody et al.,[9])

renal blood flow and function due to the heart failure process.[2,6,7] The resultant diminished delivery of sodium to the distal nephron at the level of the macula densa becomes a potent stimulus for renin release.[8] Aldosterone, the second factor governing sodium excretion, further increases sodium retention at the distal nephron at the expense of potassium excretion. Although current therapy of heart failure may improve cardiac output and renal blood flow, no current oral therapy has uniformly improved the glomerular filtration rate.

In addition to activation of the renin system, other neurohormonal factors that promote retention of sodium and water include vasopressin, norepinephrine, and the vasoconstrictor prostaglandins.[3,4] The effect of vasopressin is primarily the promotion of free water retention, rather than sodium retention; and it typically contributes to hyponatremia.

In carefully controlled metabolic studies, patients were divided into groups that achieved either neutral sodium balance or sodium retention in response to 100 mEq sodium intake.[9] In the patients who retained sodium, there was a relative increase of blood urea nitrogen, plasma renin activity, and urinary aldosterone excretion. Patients in neutral balance exhibited relatively normal renal and neurohormonal function.

ROLE OF DIETARY SODIUM

It is important to emphasize that the clinical effectiveness of diuretics depends on adherence to a restricted sodium diet.[10] Experimental animal data have demonstrated that chronic sodium restriction increases sodium uptake from the tubular lumen at the level of the distal nephron.[11,12] It is not possible to eliminate dietary sodium entirely; therefore a more useful goal is limitation of sodium intake. A dietary history is necessary to identify hidden sources of sodium intake. Patients should be instructed to limit their daily intake of sodium to approximately 2500 mg, although this amount can be further reduced depending on the severity of the edema.

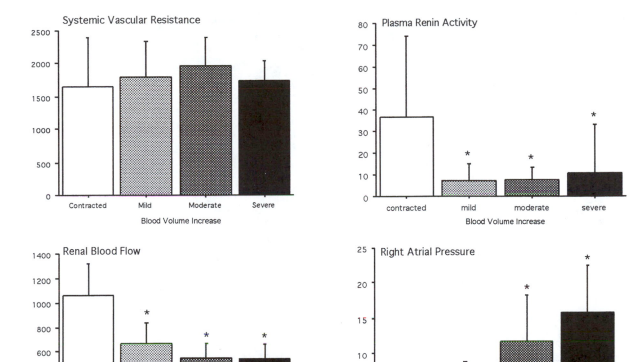

Fig. 42-2. Blood volume, measured by ^{125}I-albumin, is given on the x axis as a percent of normal blood volume. Four groups of heart failure patients on digoxin and diuretics, but no ACE inhibitors, are identified: contracted (n = 4; −12 ± 6 percent < normal), mild increase (n = 8; 14 ± 3 percent > normal), moderate increase (n = 7; 25 ± 3 percent > normal), and severe increase (n = 8; 40 ± 10 percent > normal). Systemic vascular resistance (dyne/s × cm⁵) was not different for the groups. With progressive increase of blood volume, plasma renin activity (ng/ml × h) was suppressed. The expansion of blood volume is associated with progressive reduction of renal blood flow (ml/min). The increase of blood volume is also associated with a progressive increase of right atrial pressure (mmHg). Thus despite diuretic therapy, there may be a range of blood volume expansion, which influences both renin release and cardiac filling pressures.

ENDPOINTS FOR EVALUATION OF DIURETICS

The sites of action of diuretics are shown in Figure 42-3, and the overall effects of diuretics[13,14] and their relevance to heart failure[14] have been summarized elsewhere. Traditionally, diuretic agents have been developed for the treatment of hypertension or relief of edema (heart failure, cirrhosis, nephrotic syndrome, chronic renal failure), rather than treatment of heart failure per se.[15] Consequently, efficacy endpoints have been weight loss and increased urine output. In future evaluations of diuretic compounds, it may be necessary to assess endpoints that reflect efficacy for specific disease states, such as congestive heart failure (Table 42-1). There is no laboratory test or other objective marker by which one can quantify the presence or absence of edema. For this reason the Sodium Retention Score was developed[16] (Table 42-2) to tract the extent of edema, particularly in clinical trials.

PHARMACOKINETICS OF DIURETIC THERAPY

Loop Diuretics

The term loop diuretic has evolved to encompass pharmacologic compounds that exert their primary action on the thick ascending loop of Henle. To reach the intraluminal site of action, these organic acids

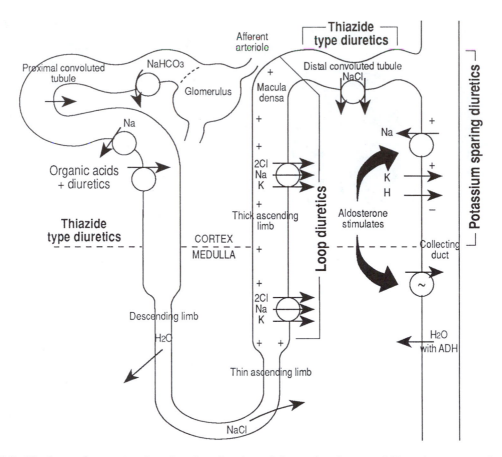

Fig. 42-3. Nephron, demonstrating the site of action of the major classes of diuretic compounds. (From Cody et al.,[14] with permission.)

Table 42-1. Current Versus Suggested Endpoints for Evaluation of a Diuretic Drug in Congestive Heart Failure

Current endpoints
    Weight reduction
    Increased urinary output
    Symptomatic improvement
Suggested future endpoints
    Improved quality of life score (subjective improvement)
    Improved sodium retention score (clearance of physical findings of edema)
    Sodium excretion and diuresis[a]
    Improved exercise capacity
        Maximal (modified Naughton protocol)
        Submaximal (6-minute walk)
    Assessment of the extent of neurohormonal activation and electrolyte supplementation
    Documented hemodynamic and vascular effect
    Mortality

[a] Correlated with pharmacokinetics.

must first be secreted into the proximal tubule via the organic acid pathway (Fig. 42-3). Once in the lumen, active reabsorption of chloride is inhibited in both the medullary and cortical portions of the loop of Henle. Decreased sodium reabsorption also occurs, as the chloride ion is co-transported with sodium and potassium.

The three loop diuretics traditionally used in the United States to treat the edema of heart failure are ethacrynic acid, furosemide, and bumetanide. Use of ethacrynic acid has diminished, and torsemide is a currently approved diuretic with some pharmacologic advantages. After oral administration, furosemide has 40 percent bioavailability, bumetanide 80 percent, and torsemide more than 90 percent. All three agents are extensively bound to plasma proteins and are rapidly secreted by the organic acid pathway of the proximal tubule.[14] Diminished diuresis and a prolonged renal elimination of the drug may be expected during heart failure, when renal dysfunction is evident. Torsemide, however, has two active metabolites, which probably accounts for its longer elimination half-life of 3 hours. Residual loop diuretic concentration is eliminated by nonrenal

Table 42-2. Proposed Sodium Retention Score	
Score	Criteria
Rales	
0	None present
1	Lower one-third of lungs
2	Lower two-thirds lungs
3	Throughout lungs
Peripheral pitting edema	
0	None present
1	Trace edema
2	Edema at the ankle level
3	Edema present above the ankle
4	Anasarca
Weight change	
−1	Decreased weight
0	No change in weight
1	Increased weight
Hepatomegaly	
0	Absent
1	Present
Third sound gallop	
0	Absent
1	Present
Increased jugular venous pressure	
0	Absent
1	Present

Range of possible scores: −1 to 11.

mechanisms including hepatic degradation and excretion. Because of the differences in bioavailability and potency, equivalent doses of bumetanide, furosemide, and torsemide are 1, 40, and 20 mg, respectively.

Thiazides

Thiazide diuretics are derivatives of the benzothiadiazine structure. Like loop diuretics, they are organic acids and are highly protein-bound. Because they cannot be filtered, they gain access to the tubular lumen via the organic acid secretory pathway of the proximal tubule. Traditionally, intraluminal thiazides have been thought to inhibit the active transport of chloride and passive movement of sodium in the cortical portion of the ascending loop of Henle. Approximately 10 percent of the filtered sodium is left to be reabsorbed at this and more distal sites in the nephron. Metolazone is a thiazide diuretic that historically was thought to function similar to carbonic anhydrase inhibitors in the proximal tubule.

Therefore it was commonly added to a loop diuretic for synergistic effect in patients resistant to monotherapy. Subsequent data indicate that the additive response observed with metolazone, used in combination with a loop diuretic, is due to its sodium blockade at the distal portion of the nephron.[17,18]

Differences among pharmacokinetic characteristics of thiazide-type agents are minimal. Of those highlighted in Table 42-3, peak values range from 2 to 6 hours. Chlorothiazide and hydrochlorothiazide have the shortest duration of action, 6 to 12 hours, and may be administered twice a day if needed. Similar to the loop diuretics, endogenous organic acid metabolic end products may accumulate in renal failure and compete with diuretics for access into the lumen. Thiazides do not provide a broad dose–response range. Because of these combined problems, thiazides are not generally used in patients with glomerular filtration rates less than 30 ml/min. Indapamide is the only thiazide that undergoes substantial hepatic metabolism, with only 7 percent found unchanged in the urine. Chlorothiazide is the only thiazide available in a soluble form, which permits intravenous administration. This point is of enormous clinical value when the drug is administered in combination with a loop diuretic for the intravenous treatment of acute decompensation, for refractory sodium retention, or when oral intake is not possible. Absorption of oral chlorothiazide or metolazone may be impaired by delayed gastric absorption.

Potassium-Sparing Diuretics

Although potassium-sparing diuretics uniformly act at the distal nephron and collecting duct, their effect is achieved by different mechanisms. One mechanism is mediated by aldosterone and antagonized by spironolactone, a competitive receptor antagonist. The effects of triamterene and amiloride are independent of mineralocorticoids, and they act by direct inhibition of sodium transport. Differing from spironolactone, these two drugs must first reach their site of action by means of glomerular filtration and the organic base secretory pathway of the proximal tubule. Overall, these agents decrease sodium reabsorption and potassium excretion, and they may potentiate hyperkalemia.

The pharmacokinetic properties of the potassium-sparing diuretics help explain their differences in onset and duration of action; these properties have been summarized elsewhere.[14,19] Gastrointestinal absorption is 90 percent with spironolactone, 30 percent with amiloride if administered with food, and even lesser absorption with triamterene due to in-

Table 42-3. Diuretic Pharmacokinetics

Drug	Route	Onset	Peak	Duration	Dosage[a]
Loop diuretics					
Furosemide	IV	5 min	30 min	2 hours	20–120 mg
	PO	30 min	1–2 hours	6–8 hours	20–160 mg qd or bid
Bumetanide	IV	5 min	30–45 min	2 hours	0.5–1.0 mg
	PO	0.5–1.0 hour	1–2 hours	4–6 hours	0.5–2.0 mg qd
Torsemide	IV	5 min	15–30 min	12–16 hours	20–100 mg
	PO	30 min	1 hour	12–16 hours	20–100 mg qd
Thiazides					
Chlorothiazide	IV	15 min	30 min	2 hours	250–500 mg q12h
	PO	1–2 hours	4 hours	6–12 hours	250–500 mg bid
Chlorthalidone	PO	2 hours	2–6 hours	24–72 hours	50–100 mg qd
Hydrochlorothiazide	PO	2 hours	4–6 hours	6–12 hours	25–50 mg qd
Indapamide	PO	1–2 hours	2 hours	36 hours	2.5–5.0 mg qd
Metolazone	PO	1 hour	2 hours	12–24 hours	5–10 mg qd
Potassium-sparing agents					
Spironolactone	PO	3 days[b]	1–2 hours	2–3 days	25–200 mg/day
Triamterene	PO	2–4 days	2–4 hours	7–9 hours	100 mg bid
Amiloride	PO	2 hours	3–4 hours	24 hours	5–10 mg qd

[a] Clinically accepted dosages and intervals in heart failure that are not strictly determined by pharmacokinetics.
[b] Although plasma levels are detected in 2 hours, the maximum diuretic effect is seen within 3 days.

traproduct variability. Onset of diuretic action occurs rapidly, 2–4 hours with amiloride and triamterene. This effect may persist 24 hours despite early peak plasma concentrations and an elimination half-life of 6–9 hours. After a single oral dose of spironolactone, peak serum concentrations of the parent drug are seen within 1–2 hours, and the active metabolites peak in 2–4 hours. A more gradual onset of diuresis is exhibited, with the maximum effect occurring in 3 days. When spironolactone therapy is discontinued, diuresis may continue for 2–3 days secondary to the longer half-life of the metabolites. Triamterene and amiloride are both excreted unchanged in the urine. In contrast, spironolactone undergoes extensive hepatic metabolism.

ALTERED PHARMACOKINETICS AND PHARMACODYNAMICS

Each diuretic has altered pharmacokinetics and pharmacodynamics in heart failure; furosemide is highlighted to demonstrate the changes that occur during the heart failure process. Unique to the concept of diuretic therapy is the fact that the urinary diuretic concentration does not reflect merely drug elimination. The renal tubular urine concentration is the amount of the drug delivered to its primary site of action at the luminal side of tubular cells. Consequently, the route of administration and blood concentration are important only to the extent that they influence the delivery of effective concentrations of diuretic to the primary site of action within the tubular lumen.

The response to diuretics can be altered in two general ways. First, a pharmacokinetic effect can occur, whereby the concentration of diuretic that reaches the tubular lumen is reduced, such as decreased gastrointestinal absorption. The pharmacokinetics of the intravenous formulations of the loop diuretics are virtually unaltered during heart failure, unless the glomerular filtration rate is less than 30 ml/min. Typically, this level is reached only with moderate to severe chronic renal insufficiency and only the most severe cases of congestive heart failure.[2,6]

The pharmacokinetics of oral furosemide are altered by the heart failure process in that absorption may be prolonged, thereby delaying the time to appearance and peak concentration of furosemide within the urine. Thus after oral administration the absorption of furosemide and bumetanide is prolonged, 0.5–1.0 hour longer than that observed in healthy subjects; it is less altered with torsemide.[20–23] With prolonged absorption, the time to peak concentrations within the urine is prolonged twofold, and elimination rates are one-half those of normal subjects. These pharmacokinetic effects explain why intravenous furosemide is significantly more effective than oral furosemide in the decompensated patient and why torsemide efficacy and bioavailability for the intravenous and oral formulations is virtually identical.

Second, a pharmacodynamic effect can occur, whereby the target organ response to a given drug concentration is diminished. In this case, natriuresis and diuresis are diminished relative to the normal response. The pharmacodynamic responses to both intravenous and oral furosemide are altered with heart failure. Compared to normal subjects, the rate of sodium excretion in heart failure patients is reduced at any given renal tubular furosemide concentration. The "ceiling dose," defined as the dose above which further incremental sodium excretion is minimal, in patients with heart failure is twice that of normal subjects. Thus, if the ceiling dose in normals is 80 mg, the ceiling dose in heart failure patients is 160 mg.[20,24,25]

A pharmacodynamic effect also occurs with chronic, long-term use of these agents. In this situation an adequate concentration of drug is achieved at the site of action, but the natriuretic and diuretic responses are diminished. With long-term loop diuretic therapy, hypertrophy of the distal tubule occurs, fostering enhanced distal tubular sodium reabsorption which counterbalances inhibition of reabsorption of the thick ascending limb of the loop of Henle achieved by the diuretic (Fig. 42-4).[11,12,26] All

of the loop diuretics demonstrate a shift in the dose–response curve.[21,25,27–29] Diuresis may ensue with alterations in the disease process (i.e., increasing cardiac output with afterload reduction or instituting combination diuretic therapy), discussed below.

RESPONSES TO INITIATION OF DIURETIC THERAPY

The hemodynamic response to diuretic therapy has been characterized primarily in the setting of pulmonary edema. The acute hemodynamic response consists of a vasodilator effect[30] and reduction of cardiac filling pressures.[30–32] During acute decompensated heart failure, changes in cardiac output vary from an increase or no change to significant reduction; and changes in hemodynamics can proceed or lag, affecting the initiation of diuresis. Studies have reported vasoconstriction[33] or initial vasodilation followed by vasoconstriction[34] with acute or short-term follow-up. A review of the cited literature therefore reveals

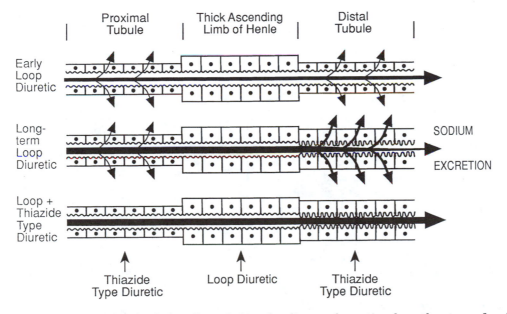

Fig. 42-4. Adaptation of distal tubule cells and altered sodium reabsorption from the stage of early loop diuretic therapy to long-term loop diuretic therapy. In the latter, there is hypertrophy of the distal tubular cells. (**Top**) Early loop diuretic therapy is associated with proximal and distal nephron sodium reabsorption, but the blockade of sodium reabsorption in the thick ascending limb of Henle results in overall net sodium excretion. (**Middle**) With long-term high-dose loop diuretic therapy, modest proximal sodium reabsorption occurs, followed by blockade of sodium reabsorption at the thick ascending limb. Distal nephron tubular cell hypertrophy occurs, and marked reabsorption of sodium at this point offsets the favorable effect of the loop diuretic, resulting in attenuated sodium excretion. (**Bottom**) Addition of a thiazide-type diuretic to a chronic loop diuretic blocks proximal and distal nephron sodium reabsorption. The latter prevents the accentuated sodium reabsorption seen in the middle panel, with an overall additive or even synergistic effect with the loop diuretic, so sodium excretion is markedly enhanced. (From Cody et al.,[14] with permission.)

a divergent range of hemodynamic responses to diuretics, although most acute studies demonstrate reduced cardiac filling pressures.[30-32]

Loop diuretics have been shown to decrease renal vasculature resistance and to increase total and cortical renal blood flow as previously summarized.[14] However, this reaction may be related to the severity of the heart failure, as a group of patients with moderate chronic congestive heart failure, after 3–4 weeks of oral furosemide, did not significantly alter renal blood flow.[35]

It is difficult to isolate a single neurohormonal factor as being primarily responsible for the overall hemodynamic and regional hemodynamic response to diuretics. In general, sodium depletion and diuretic therapy tend to increase renin and aldosterone.[9,33-36] Sympathetic nervous system activity also increases in response to diuretics.[9,35,36]

PRACTICAL CONSIDERATIONS

Intravenous Diuretics for Acute Decompensation of Heart Failure

Intravenous diuretic therapy may be used acutely in several clinical situations. With pulmonary edema the obvious benefit of acute intravenous diuretic therapy is the rapid clearance of pulmonary congestion, mediated by natriuresis and diuresis, reduced intravascular volume, and vasodilation. As subacute decompensation is a prelude to pulmonary edema, the goals of intravenous diuretic therapy are similar to these for treatment of pulmonary edema. Acute intravenous diuretic therapy may also be used to supplement chronic oral therapy for sodium retention to augment diuresis in the outpatient setting. The primary goal of intravenous diuretic therapy is the elimination of edema; concerns regarding adverse activation of neurohormonal activity and electrolyte depletion are of lesser importance, although potassium and magnesium intake should be supplemented. For acute reversal of sodium retention and fluid overload, therapy with a loop diuretic is indicated. It should be given intravenously, to a ceiling dose that is twice the normal dose (e.g., furosemide 80 mg, bumetanide 2 mg, torsemide 40 mg), and increased as necessary, combined with other agents. A thiazide-type diuretic in combination with a loop diuretic is often highly effective. However, an oral thiazide-type diuretic, particularly metolazone, may require several days to achieve its maximal favorable response owing to delayed absorption. The ability to utilize intravenous chlorothiazide (Diuril) is often overlooked.[14,19] Unlike hydrochlorothiazide, chlorothiazide can be given intravenously in a dose of 250–500 mg, which is equivalent to an oral hydrochlorothiazide dosage of 25–50 mg; when combined with a loop diuretic, it produces greater diuresis than the loop diuretic alone. This subject is discussed further in the section dealing with resistance to diuretics.

Oral Diuretics for Chronic Management of Heart Failure

Traditionally, there has been a consensus in clinical practice that diuretics are the therapy of choice for symptomatic heart failure, and that they represent the mainstay of therapy in most patients. A survey among hospital- and office-based internists and office-based cardiologists revealed that 53 percent of physicians employed diuretics as initial therapy for heart failure in patients with normal sinus rhythm; an additional 30 percent used a combination of diuretics and digitalis as initial therapy.[37] The severity of sodium retention provides a guide to appropriate diuretic therapy (Table 42-4). When left ventricular dysfunction is asymptomatic and there is no clinical evidence of sodium retention, diuretics may not be required. It is generally advisable, however, that all heart failure patients should be instructed in moderate dietary salt intake (approximately 2–3 g of sodium per day).

Table 42-4. Recommended Use of Diuretics for Congestive Heart Failure

Asymptomatic left ventricular dysfunction
    Establish moderate sodium intake
    Angiotensin-converting enzyme (ACE) inhibitor

Mild sodium retention
    Thiazide-type diuretic or low dose loop diuretic
    Continue moderate sodium intake
    Combine with an ACE inhibitor

Moderate sodium retention
    Loop diuretic, adjusting for renal function if necessary
    Continue moderate sodium intake
    Combine with an ACE inhibitor

Severe sodium retention
    Large dose loop diuretic combined with a thiazide-type diuretic
    Continue moderate sodium intake
    ACE inhibitor, unless contraindicated
    Consider addition of a potassium-sparing diuretic

Treatment measures for refractory sodium retention
    Intermittent intravenous loop diuretic
    Short-term infusion of a loop diuretic
    Intensified combination oral diuretic therapy
    Intravenous positive inotropic therapy
    Ultrafiltration or dialysis

In view of the outcome of numerous clinical trials,[38,39] there is a mandate for earlier use of ACE inhibitors. By blocking the renin system (decreased angiotensin II and aldosterone), the development of sodium retention may be delayed. However, ACE inhibitors should not be considered "diuretics." In fact, their efficacy may be attenuated as sodium retention develops.[9] The clinical response to ACE inhibitors may be inadequate when given as single therapy,[40,41] and the co-administration of diuretics is required. For relief of edema and congestive symptoms, diuretic therapy is more effective than an ACE inhibitor when given as single therapy.[42]

Dietary sodium intake should be restricted throughout all stages of heart failure. Patients with mild sodium retention and relatively normal renal function can be treated with sodium restriction and a thiazide-type diuretic. As sodium retention progresses to a more moderate range, a loop diuretic is indicated, with adjustment for renal function if necessary. Use of a thiazide-type diuretic in combination with a loop diuretic is often effective. A potassium-sparing diuretic may be added to reduce oral potassium supplements and to enhance diuresis. While the combination of an ACE inhibitor with a potassium-sparing diuretic could produce hyperkalemia, this problem typically does not occur in the severe heart failure patient who also requires oral potassium supplementation to prevent hypokalemia[43] and when the serum creatinine is less than 2.5 mg/dl. However, this point has not been tested in a large clinical trial. The efficacy and safety of this approach is being tested in the Randomized Aldactone Efficacy Study (RALES) trial, where placebo or one of several doses of spironolactone will be added to the combination of furosemide and an ACE inhibitor in a double-blind, randomized design.

The difficulty with any diuretic treatment algorithm is that the endpoint for reversal of sodium retention is poorly defined. Alternate approaches to the assessment of diuretic therapy of heart failure are therefore required.[15,16]

Management of Diuretic Resistance

Patients should be considered to have "diuretic resistance" when they demonstrate progressive edema despite escalating oral or intravenous diuretic therapy. The factors that contribute to diuretic resistance have been summarized elsewhere.[14,19,25,26] Renal insufficiency can reduce tubular secretion of the diuretic as well as the filtered load of sodium. Therefore patients with decreased renal function due to heart failure[2] or superimposed age[2,8] frequently have reduced responses to diuretics. In addition, studies have demonstrated that indomethacin and other nonsteroidal antiinflammatory agents reduce the maximal response to furosemide.[44] Mesenteric congestion may limit the absorption and bioavailability of orally administered medications.

Finally, patients with refractory volume overload frequently do not comply with their extensive medication regimens exactly as prescribed. This situation may be due to intentional deletion, misunderstanding, or self-modification. Ineffective limitation of dietary sodium intake produces a greater physiologic resistance to a given diuretic dose.

Several therapeutic interventions can be used to augment diuretic responses in patients with refractory edema. Escalating the dosage of intravenous loop diuretics is the most common approach, and the dosage should be rapidly doubled until the desired effect is produced. An ultrahigh dose of loop diuretic may be effective,[45,46] although the overall response to ultrahigh doses is often unimpressive. Alternatively, and perhaps more physiologic (Fig. 42-4), is the combination of a thiazide and a loop-type diuretic in view of the structural hypertrophy of the distal nephron described earlier. Although precise dose limits are difficult to define, when a patient achieves a requirement, for instance, of 240 mg of furosemide daily, addition of an intravenous (chlorothiazide) or oral thiazide-type diuretic is more effective than further increases of the loop diuretic. The combination of loop/thiazide diuretic is more effective than ultrahigh doses of a loop diuretic alone or switching from one loop diuretic to another.

Patients with heart failure should weigh themselves on a regular basis. When there is a more than 3- to 5-pound weight gain over the course of 1 week, the patient can temporarily add a short-term (3–5 days) oral thiazide-type diuretic for enhanced sodium excretion. This strategy allows the dose of loop diuretic to be kept constant, avoiding prescription changes or errors that can occur with frequent changes in loop diuretic doses. Furthermore, by using supplemental thiazide-type diuretics only on an intermittent basis, one tends to reduce the cumulative long-term diuretic exposure. One of the most dangerous combinations is high dose loop diuretic plus persistent high dose metolazone. This regimen can produce excessive electrolyte depletion and renal dysfunction. Another approach is based on the concept that continuous infusion of a loop diuretic is more effective than intermittent bolus administration in terms of net sodium excretion.[47,48] Careful metabolic studies have demonstrated greater net sodium excretion using this approach, compared to intermittent bolus administration, despite comparable amounts of bumetanide appearing in the urine. Although such data have not primarily been collected in the chronic congestive heart failure population, it would be reasonable to assume comparable efficacy.

As a more aggressive approach, dialysis, hemofiltration, and ultrafiltration have been successfully utilized for the management of sodium retention during heart failure.[49,50] However, the latter approaches are generally not required in the absence of coexistent renal failure (glomerular filtration rate less than 30 ml/min) and when combined intravenous loop and thiazide regimens can be utilized.

ADVERSE EFFECTS

The adverse effects of diuretic drugs in heart failure patients have been summarized elsewhere.[14,19] Most of these are the result of altered renal tubular electrolyte transport and therefore may be related to the intensity and duration of therapy. Electrolyte disorders are the most common adverse effects of all diuretics. Chronic diuretic use may produce hypokalemia, hyponatremia, hypocalcemia, hypomagnesemia, hyperuricemia, and metabolic alkalosis. The reported incidence for these electrolyte and metabolic disorders is anywhere from 14 to 60 percent.[19]

The most common problem is hypokalemia, mediated by direct transport into the tubular lumen and hypersecretion of aldosterone, which blocks distal reabsorption. Most heart failure patients require concomitant use of potassium supplements to correct hypokalemia. Hypokalemia and hypomagnesemia may be associated with myalgias, leg cramps, and an increase in ventricular arrhythmias. As high grade ventricular arrhythmias and sudden death are frequently observed with heart failure,[51,52] the adverse effect of diuretics on electrolyte balance is of particular concern. However, the direct relation of electrolyte imbalance and the occurrence of ventricular arrhythmias has not been adequately assessed in a prospective manner. Hyponatremia is a common occurrence in the setting of chronic heart failure, especially when large doses of diuretics are utilized.[53] There is no specific therapy for this problem at the current time, although vasopressin antagonists are under development. Hyponatremia may correct with chronic ACE inhibitor therapy.[54] Limitation of free water intake should be utilized when serum sodium decreases to less than 125 mg/dl. In addition to activation of the renin system, diuretic usage can increase vasopressin, producing a reduction of free water clearance, which together with uncontrolled sodium intake results in hyponatremia.

Additional adverse effects may be seen with loop diuretics.[14,19] Hyperuricemia occurs in 18–40 percent of patients and may precipitate an acute episode of gout, but it typically occurs in patients with a history of gout. Gastrointestinal disturbances are more frequent with ethacrynic acid than with furosemide or bumetanide but occur in fewer than 10 percent of patients. Ototoxicity has also been reported to appear with the use of ethacrynic acid more than furosemide, but in fewer than 5 percent of patients. Concurrent administration of other ototoxic drugs (e.g., aminoglycosides) may potentiate this problem. Glucose intolerance may occur with loop diuretics but to a lesser extent than is seen with thiazide diuretics. In patients with heart failure diuretics may activate neurohormonal pathways,[3,4,33–36] but long-term activation of neurohormones by diuretics has not been demonstrated. Furthermore, the association between diuretic-induced neurohormonal stimulation and increased mortality has not been conclusively demonstrated.

Some adverse effects are specific for certain drug classes. For instance, hyperkalemia with potassium-sparing agents occurs in 2–10 percent of patients.[19] However, few controlled studies have evaluated the efficacy of adding potassium-sparing diuretics in this setting. Particular concern exists for the use of spironolactone, combined with a loop diuretic and ACE inhibitor, in regard to excess retention of potassium, although it is not the practical experience among physicians who treat heart failure. This question is now under formal evaluation by the RALES investigators. The first dose-range study has been reported,[55] with encouraging safety and efficacy results, and a survival trial with severe heart failure is under way.

ELECTROLYTE SUPPLEMENTATION

Electrolyte abnormalities and supplementation have been previously summarized.[19] Most commonly, diuretic-induced hypokalemia is associated with metabolic alkalosis and a coexisting chloride deficit. Therefore chloride is the preferred salt of potassium, rather than gluconate or bicarbonate, for supplementation in this setting.[19] Administration of potassium by the intravenous route is recommended to correct moderate to severe potassium deficits, with or without the occurrence of cardiac arrhythmias. This route is also useful when oral replacement is not feasible or not tolerated owing to a decrease in gastrointestinal motility. Oral, slow-release potassium chloride preparations utilize various wax matrix and microencapsulated products for chronic management of diuretic-induced hypokalemia. Patient preference and cost should be considered during product selection. Generally, patients require 40–120 mEq/day to maintain potassium homeostasis. Chronic diuretic therapy also leads to hypomagnesemia. Potassium and magnesium become interrelated, since magnesium is a cofactor in the appropriate function of the Na^+/K^+-ATPase pump. Therefore hypokalemia may persist until the magnesium deficiency is corrected. Although normal serum magnesium concentrations range from 1.6 to 2.0 mEq/L, only 1 percent of magnesium is found extracellularly, so serum and urinary concentrations do not accurately reflect the total body content.

Monitoring Safety and Efficacy

Because the primary indication for diuretic therapy is the relief of symptoms and signs of sodium retention, it is common practice to monitor the clinical response to diuretics by following the patient's weight and symptoms pending newer approaches to endpoint evaluation.[15] Clinically, when there is a satisfactory reduction in dyspnea, orthopnea, and peripheral edema, it is possible to reduce the dose of diuretics to maintenance levels. Many patients on intensive diuretic regimens are treated to achieve a "dry" weight endpoint, beyond which continued therapy may result in greater degrees of renal insufficiency, neurohormonal activation, or orthostatic hypotension. Unfortunately, this endpoint is not readily identified. Patients who are also taking vasodilators may be particularly susceptible to orthostasis. It has been observed for both hypertension and congestive heart failure that the magnitude of blood pressure reduction (and vasodilation) in response to ACE inhibitors is greater in the presence of sodium depletion and diuretic therapy. Although the combination of a diuretic with an ACE inhibitor provides a favorable clinical result, excessive diuresis can produce marked hypotension.[56] From the standpoint of safety, diuretics should be withheld or the dosage decreased when excessive hypotension occurs or is anticipated, prior to the onset of ACE inhibitor therapy.

FUTURE THERAPIES FOR SODIUM RETENTION AND EDEMA

Despite the long-standing desire for a more effective means to treat the edema of congestive heart failure,[1] there has not been a novel approach to the management of sodium retention in decades. Abnormalities of aldosterone, arginine vasopressin, and natriuretic peptides have been identified; and their impact on edema is rather obvious. However, the absence of practical templates for the development of specific antiedema therapy for the management of heart failure persists.

Natriuretic Peptides

Initial human studies with atrial natriuretic peptide (ANP), the first available natriuretic peptide, were conducted during the 1980s.[57] The response to ANP has been previously summarized.[58,59] In normal subjects, ANP was associated with diuretic and natriuretic effects. The renin-angiotensin system was suppressed, and a vasodilator effect was evident. Intraarterial administration of ANP confirmed a dose-dependent direct vasodilator effect.[60]

The response during severe heart failure did not uniformly match that of normal subjects. A vasodilator response was demonstrated,[57,60,61] but suppression of the renin system was less striking. More importantly, although a "significant" increase of sodium and water excretion was observed,[61] the magnitude of sodium or water excretion was not commensurate with clinically effective diuresis.[57] Evidence suggests that the renal response to ANP was attenuated with more severe heart failure. "Brain" natriuretic peptide (BNP) is so called because of its initial localization in central nervous system sources. BNP can be considered an alternate approach to enhancing sodium and water excretion in humans and induction of vasodilation. In preliminary studies there is a reduction of pulmonary wedge pressure, an increase of stroke volume, and a reduction of systemic vascular resistance—all markers of a systemic vasodilator effect and the kind of response desired during heart failure patients.[62,63]

Urodilatin is the ANP sequence [ANF (95–126)] with a cis–cis bridge similar to that of human ANP [ANF (98–126)] and other natriuretic peptides. It is produced by the kidney and is isolated from the urine, thereby functionally positioned to have importance in the management of sodium and water balance. During human heart failure infusion of urodilatin produces a small, but significant, increase of urine flow and sodium excretion associated with vasodilation.[64] Although these changes are statistically significant, the clinical impact of urodilation remains to be demonstrated, and diuresis is not of the range seen with a diuretic compound.

Chronic augmentation of endogenous natriuretic peptides may represent a more logical approach to edema management. ANP degradation by neutral

Table 42-5. Pharmacologic Approaches to Enhanced Natriuretic Peptide Activity

Increase of plasma natriuretic peptides
  ANP [ANF (99–126)]
  Urodilatin [ANF (95–126)]
  BNP

Inhibition of neutral endopeptidase degradation of endogenous ANP
  Pfizer
    Candoxatril (orally active)
    Candoxatrilat (intravenous)
  Bristol-Myers Squibb
    SQ 28603
  Miles
    Sinorphan/Bay y 7432 (orally active)
  Schering
    SCH 34826

Additional approaches
  Combined NEP/ACE inhibitors

endopeptidase (NEP) can be prevented with specific NEP inhibitors, thereby increasing the circulating level of endogenous ANP. Early studies with two NEP inhibitors—intravenous candoxatrilat and the oral form candoxatril—were well tolerated in animal models and enhanced the diuretic, natriuretic, and hypotension effects of ANP.[65–67] These NEP inhibitors display classic competitive inhibitor effects. Candoxatrilat, the active form of the prodrug candoxatril, is given orally and changed to the active compound candoxatrilat by hepatic hydrolysis. With both experimental and human heart failure, diuresis, vasodilation, and suppression of the renin system have been observed and thus have potential application to attenuate the progression of heart failure decompensation. These compounds require greater evaluation at early stages of heart failure. At later stages of heart failure, with established edema and renal dysfunction, neurohormonal and hemodynamic abnormalities offset the benefit of ANP augmentation. Approaches to augmentation of endogenous ANP are summarized in Table 42-5.

Arginine Vasopressin Antagonists

Neurohormonal abnormalities during heart failure have been targets for pharmacologic inhibition since the early 1980s. Among these abnormalities, an increase of circulating arginine vasopressin (AVP) has been identified, and abnormalities of both the V1 and V2 AVP receptor have been characterized. Reduction of free water clearance and hypotension are two manifestations of abnormal V2 AVP activity. A specific antagonist of either the V2 or combined V1/V2 recep-

tor is logical, and its development is under way. Preliminary data with the AVP antagonist OPC-31260 indicate an increase of free water clearance and hemodynamic improvement.[68]

REFERENCES

1. Binger MW, Keith NM: Effect of diuretics in different types of edema. JAMA 1933;101:2009
2. Cody RJ, Ljungman S, Covit AB et al: Regulation of glomerular filtration rate in chronic congestive heart failure patients. Kidney Int 1988;34:361
3. Cody RJ: Neurohormonal influences in the pathogenesis of congestive heart failure. p. 73. In Weber K (ed): Heart Failure. WB Saunders, Philadelphia, 1989
4. Francis GS, Goldsmith SR, Levine TB, Cohn JN: The neurohormonal axis in congestive heart failure. Ann Intern Med 1984;101:370–377
5. Anand IS, Ferrari R, Kalra GS et al: Edema of cardiac origin studies of body water and sodium, renal function, hemodynamic indices, and plasma hormones in untreated congestive cardiac failure. Circulation 1989;80:299–305
6. Cody RJ, Torre S, Clark M, Pondolfino K: Age-related hemodynamic, renal, and hormonal differences in patients with congestive heart failure. Arch Intern Med 1989;149:1023–1028
7. Cody RJ: Assessment of neurohormonal parameters in congestive heart failure. Determination of sodium and water regulation. p. 25. In Morganroth J, Moore EN (eds): Congestive Heart Failure. Martinus Nijhoff, Boston, 1987
8. Skott O, Briggs JP: Direct demonstration of macula densa mediated renin secretion. Science 1987;237:1618–1620
9. Cody RJ, Covit AB, Schaer GL et al: Sodium and water balance in chronic congestive heart failure. J Clin Invest 1986;77:1441–1452
10. Wilcox CS, Mitch WE, Kelly RA et al: Response to furosemide. I. Effect of salt intake and renal compensation. J Lab Clin Med 1983;102:450–458
11. Ellison D, Velazquez H, Wright FS: Adaptation of the distal convoluted tubule of the rat. Structural and functional effects of dietary salt intake and chronic diuretic infusion. J Clin Invest 1989;83:113–126
12. Stanton B, Kaissling B: Adaptation of distal tubule and collecting duct to increased sodium delivery. II. Na$^+$ and K$^+$ transport. Am J Physiol 1988;255:F1269–F1275
13. Wilcox CS: Diuretics. p. 2133. In Brenner BM, Rector FC Jr (eds): The Kidney. Saunders, Philadelphia, 1991
14. Cody RJ, Kubo SH, Pickworth KK: Diuretic utilization for the sodium retention of congestive heart failure. Arch Intern Med 1994;154:1905–1914
15. Cody RJ: Clinical trials of diuretic therapy in congestive heart failure. Research needs and clinical considerations. J Am Coll Cardiol, suppl. 1993;21:165A
16. Cody RJ: The need for a sodium retention score in clinical trials of heart failure. Clin Pharmacol Ther 1993;54:7
17. Brater DC, Pressley RH, Anderson SA: Mechanism of the synergistic combination of metolazone and bumetanide. J Pharmacol Exp Ther 1985;233:70

18. Oster JR, Epstein M, Smoller S: Combined therapy with thiazide-type and loop diuretic agents for resistant sodium retention. Ann Intern Med 1983;99:405

19. Cody RJ, Pickworth KK: Approaches to diuretic therapy and electrolyte imbalance in congestive heart failure. p. 37. In Deedwania PC (ed): Update in Congestive Heart Failure. WB Saunders, Philadelphia, 1994

20. Brater DC, Seiwell R, Anderson S: Absorption and disposition of furosemide in congestive heart failure. Kidney Int 1982;22:171

21. Brater DC, Day B, Burdette A, Anderson S: Bumetanide and furosemide in heart failure. Kidney Int 1984; 26:183

22. Friedel HA, Buckley MMT: Torsemide: a review of its pharmacological properties and therapeutic potential. Drugs 1991;41:81

23. Brater DC, Leinfelder J, Anderson SA: Clinical pharmacology of torsemide, a new loop diuretic. Clin Pharmacol Ther 1987;42:187

24. Brater DC: Clinical pharmacology of loop diuretics. Drugs, suppl. 1991;3:14

25. Brater DC: Resistance to loop diuretics. Why it happens and what to do about it. Drugs 1985;30:427

26. Ellison DH: The physiologic basis of diuretic synergism. Its role in treating diuretic resistance. Ann Intern Med 1991;114:886

27. Vargo D, Kramer WG, Black PK et al: The pharmacokinetics of torsemide in patients with congestive heart failure. Clin Pharmacol Ther 1994;56:9

28. Brater DC, Chennavasin P, Seiwell R: Furosemide in patients with heart failure. Shift in dose-response curves. Clin Pharmacol Ther 1980;28:182

29. Ward A, Heel RC: Bumetanide. A review of its pharmacodynamic and pharmacokinetic properties and therapeutic use. Drugs 1984;28:426–464

30. Lal S, Murtagw JG, Pollock AM et al: Acute hemodynamic effects of furosemide in patients with normal and raised left atrial pressures. Br Heart J 1969;31: 711–717

31. Magrini F, Niarchos AP: Hemodynamic effects of massive peripheral edema. Am Heart J 1983;105:90–94

32. Stampfer M, Epstein SE, Beiser DG et al: Hemodynamic effects of diuresis at rest and during intense upright exercise in patients with impaired cardiac function. Circulation 1968;37:900–911

33. Francis GS, Siegel RM, Goldsmith SR et al: Acute vasoconstrictor response to intravenous furosemide in patients with chronic congestive heart failure. Ann Intern Med 1985;103:1–6

34. Ikram H, Chan W, Espiner EA, Nicholls MG: Hemodynamic and hormone responses to acute and chronic furosemide therapy in congestive heart failure. Clin Sci 1980;59:443–449

35. Kubo SH, Clark M, Laragh JH et al: Identification of normal neurohormonal activity in mild congestive heart failure and stimulating effect of upright posture and diuretics. Am J Cardiol 1987;60:1322–1328

36. Bayliss J, Norell M, Canepa-Anson R et al: Untreated heart failure. Clinical and neuroendocrine effects of introducing diuresis. Br Heart J 1987;57:17–22

37. Hlatky MA, Fleg JL, Hinton PC et al: Physician practice in the management of congestive heart failure. J Am Coll Cardiol 1986;8:966–970

38. Cody RJ: Comparing ACE inhibitor trial results in patients with acute myocardial infarction. Arch Intern Med 1994;154:2029

39. Cody RJ: ACE inhibitors. Mechanisms, pharmacodynamics, and clinical trials in heart failure. Cardiol Rev 1994;3:145

40. Odemuyiwa O, Gilmartin J, Kenny D, Hall RJC: Captopril and the diuretic requirements in moderate and severe chronic heart failure. Eur Heart J 1989;10:586

41. Anand IS, Kalra GS, Ferrari R et al: Enalapril as initial and sole treatment in severe chronic heart failure with sodium retention. Int J Cardiol 1990;28:341

42. Richardson A, Bayliss J, Scriven AJ et al: Double-blind comparison of captopril alone against furosemide plus amiloride in mild heart failure. Lancet 1987;2:709

43. Ikram H, Webster MWI, Nicholls MG et al: Combined spironolactone and converting-enzyme inhibitor therapy for refractory heart failure. Aust NZ J Med 1986; 16:61

44. Channavasin P, Seiwell R, Brater DC: Pharmacokinetic-dynamic analysis of the indomethacin-furosemide interaction in man. J Pharmacol Exp Ther 1980; 215:77

45. Brater DC: Resistance to diuretics. Emphasis on a pharmacological perspective. Drugs 1981;22:477

46. Gerlag PG, Meijel J: High-dose furosemide in the treatment of refractory congestive heart failure. Arch Intern Med 1988;148:286

47. Copeland JG, Campbell DW, Plachetka JR et al: Diuresis with continuous infusion of furosemide after cardiac surgery. Am J Surg 1983;46:796

48. Rudy DW, Voelker JR, Greene PK et al: Loop diuretics for chronic renal insufficiency. A continuous infusion is more efficacious than bolus therapy. Ann Intern Med 1991;115:360

49. Agostoni PG, Marenzi GD, Pepi M et al: Isolated ultrafiltration in moderate congestive heart failure. J Am Coll Cardiol 1993;21:424

50. Rubin J, Ball R: Continuous ambulatory peritoneal dialysis as treatment of severe congestive heart failure in the face of chronic renal failure. Report of eight cases. Arch Intern Med 1986;146:1533

51. Holmes J, Kubo SH, Cody RJ, Kligfield P: Arrhythmias in ischemic and nonischemic dilated cardiomyopathy. Prediction of mortality by ambulatory electrocardiography. Am J Cardiol 1985;55:146

52. Gradman A, Deedwania P, Cody R et al: Predictors of total mortality and sudden death in mild to moderate heart failure. J Am Coll Cardiol 1989;14:564

53. Schaer GL, Covit AB, Laragh JH, Cody RJ: Association of hyponatremia with increased renin activity in chronic congestive heart failure. Impact of diuretic therapy. Am J Cardiol 1983;51:1635

54. Packer M, Medina N, Yushak H: Correction of dilutional hyponatremia in severe chronic heart failure by converting enzyme inhibition. Ann Intern Med 1984; 100:782

55. Pitt B: The Randomized Aldactone Evaluation Study (RALES). Parallel dose finding study. J Am Coll Cardiol 1995;25:45A

56. Cody RJ, Franklin KW, Laragh JH: Postural hypotension during tilt with chronic captopril therapy of severe congestive heart failure. Am Heart J 1982;103: 480

57. Cody RJ, Atlas SA, Laragh JH et al: Atrial natriuretic factor in normal subjects and heart failure patients. Plasma levels and renal, hormonal and hemodynamic response to peptide infusion. J Clin Invest 1986;78: 1362

58. Cody RJ, Atlas SA, Laragh JH: Physiological and pharmacological studies of atrial natriuretic factor, a natriuretic and vasoactive peptide. J Clin Pharmacol 1987;27:927

59. Atlas SA, Cody RJ, Laragh JH: Atrial natriuretic peptide in heart failure. p. 19. In Braunwald E (ed): Heart Disease. Saunders, Philadelphia, 1992

60. Kubo SH, Atlas SA, Laragh JH, Cody RJ: Maintenance of forearm vasodilator action of atrial natriuretic factor in congestive heart failure secondary to ischemic or idiopathic dilated cardiomyopathy. Am J Cardiol 1992;69:1306

61. Fifer MA, Molina CR, Quiroz A et al: Hemodynamic and renal effects of atrial natriuretic peptide in congestive heart failure. Am J Cardiol 1990;65:211

62. Marcus LS, Hart D, Packer M et al: Hemodynamic effects of synthetic human brain natriuretic peptide infusion in patients with severe congestive heart failure. A placebo controlled, crossover trial. J Am Coll Cardiol 1995;25:235A

63. Abraham WT, Lowes BD, Ferguson DA et al: Systemic hemodynamic and renal excretory effects of a continuous 4-hour infusion of human brain natriuretic peptide in patients with heart failure. J Am Coll Cardiol 1995; 25:236A

64. Elsner D, Muders F, Muntze A et al: Efficacy of prolonged infusion of urodilatin [ANP-(95-126)] in patients with congestive heart failure. Am Heart J 1995; 129:766

65. Margulies K, Cavero P, Seymour A et al: Neutral endopeptidase inhibition (NEP-I) enhances natriuresis via renal tubular mechanisms. Kidney Int 1990;38:67

66. Elsner D, Munzel A, Kromer EP, Riegger GAJ: Effectiveness of endopeptidase inhibition (candoxatril) in congestive heart failure. Am J Cardiol 1992;70:494

67. Munzel T, Kurz S, Holtz J et al: Neurohormonal inhibition and hemodynamic unloading during prolonged inhibition of ANF degradation in patients with severe chronic heart failure. Circulation 1992;86:1089

68. Naitoh M, Suzuki H, Murakami M et al: Effects of oral AVP receptor antagonists OPC-21268 and OPC-31260 on congestive heart failure in conscious dogs. Am J Physiol 1994;267:H2245

43 Cardiac Glycosides

David M. Kaye
Ralph A. Kelly
Thomas W. Smith

Although clinical experience with cardiac glycosides spans more than two centuries, important issues regarding their mechanism(s) of action and appropriate role in the management of heart failure remain controversial. In his classic monograph, William Withering described in detail aspects of therapeutic properties and toxicity of the common foxglove plant *Digitalis purpurea*.[1] Subsequently during the nineteenth century it was thought that digitalis only offered beneficial actions in patients with dropsy in whom the pulse was rapid or irregular. This notion has been the subject of lengthy debate and has been resolved only partially by several prospective controlled trials that document the safety and efficacy of the digitalis glycosides in patients with moderate to severe heart failure, as discussed below.

The term cardiac glycoside or digitalis glycoside refers to a large family of more than 300 steroids or steroid glycosides that exert characteristic positively inotropic and electrophysiologic actions on the myocardium. Of interest, the leaves of *Digitalis purpurea* (foxglove) contain a number of digitalis glycosides, including digitoxin. Digoxin is a semisynthetic derivative made from the leaves of *Digitalis lanata*. Ouabain, in contrast, is obtained from the seeds of *Strophanthus gratus*. These steroid glycosides share a steroid nucleus (Fig. 43-1), with an α, β-unsaturated lactone ring attached to carbon-17. In the absence of the sugar residues, the portion of the molecule that includes the steroid and unsaturated lactone ring is termed a genin, or aglycone. Although these compounds share similar pharmacologic actions with their parent compounds, they are in general less potent and their action is of short duration. The molecular basis for the inhibitory actions of these drugs on Na^+/K^+-ATPase remains uncertain. Originally, biologic activity was thought to require the presence of the unsaturated lactone ring, the C-14 β-hydroxyl group, and a *cis* stereochemical conformation of the steroid nucleus at the junctions of the A-B and C-D rings. The importance of the lactone ring and the *cis*-A-B and C-D ring junctions has been challenged by the observations of Thomas et al.[2] Data show that certain derivatives of prednisone, prednisolone, and progesterone can exert biologic actions similar to those of the cardiac glycosides. More detailed descriptions of the sources, chemistry, and structure–activity relations of the cardiac glycosides may be found in standard texts.[3,4]

CARDIAC GLYCOSIDES: INHIBITORS OF Na^+/K^+-ATPase

The early work of Wiggers and Stimson[5] conclusively showed that digitalis glycosides exerted a positive inotropic effect in the intact heart, augmenting the positive dP/dt under isovolumic conditions in the set-

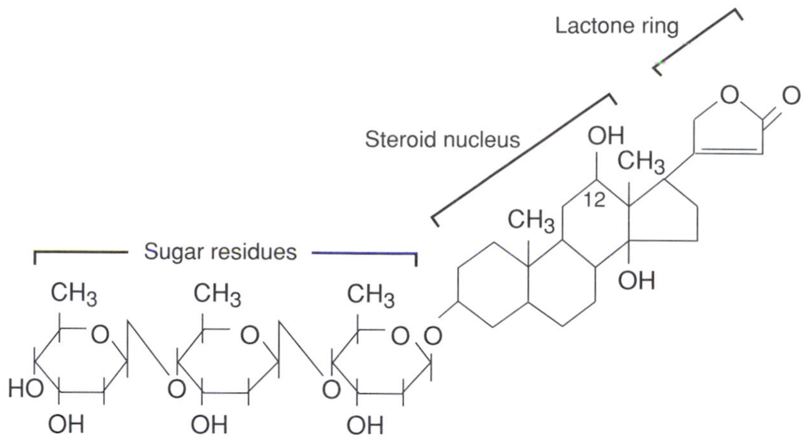

Fig. 43-1. Molecular structure of digoxin.

ting of constant heart rate and afterload. However, the mechanism by which this response occurred remained unclear for another 30 years until the plasma membrane Na$^+$/K$^+$-ATPase was discovered in the crab peripheral nerve,[6] and it became apparent that digitalis glycosides inhibit the active transport of monovalent cations across the cell membrane. Furthermore, it was evident that there was a direct relation between myocardial contractility and intracellular sodium activity.[7]

Sarcolemmal Na$^+$/K$^+$-ATPase, the enzymatic representation of the plasma membrane sodium pump, is an integral membrane protein that is responsible for translocating sodium and potassium ions across the cell membrane using energy provided by hydrolysis of the terminal high-energy ATP phosphate.[8] All cardioactive steroids share the property of being potent, highly specific inhibitors of this intrinsic membrane transport protein. Of note, primary amino acid sequence data indicate a remarkable degree of homology among these ion-translocating "P-type" ATPases, suggesting that they represent a family of evolutionary ancient enzymes. This class of ATPases, which includes the sarcoplasmic reticulum and plasma membrane Ca^{2+}-ATPases and the H$^+$/K$^+$-ATPase of the stomach and colon, share a similar catalytic cycle that involves formation of a phosphorylated aspartyl intermediate.[9,10]

The Na$^+$/K$^+$-ATPase is a heterodimer composed of two α-subunits and two β-subunits. Each subunit exists in multiple isoforms, but the α-subunit contains the binding site for digitalis glycosides.[11,12] The α-subunit has 10 transmembrane domains and a molecular mass of approximately 113 KDa.[10] All known functional aspects of Na$^+$/K$^+$-ATPase enzyme activity (binding sites for Na$^+$, K$^+$, Mg^{2+}, ATP, and as cardiac

glycosides) are known to be associated with the α-subunit. Site-directed mutagenesis studies of this subunit have indicated that the amino acid composition of the membrane-spanning domain H$_1$, the extracellular domain between H$_1$ and H$_2$, and the extracellular loop between H$_7$ and H$_8$ transmembrane domains are closely associated with binding of ouabain.[10] The β-subunit is a glycoprotein with a molecular mass of approximately 55 kDa, the function of which remains uncertain. An interaction site between the α- and β-subunits has been described on the extracellular loop between the H$_7$ and H$_8$ transmembrane domains of the α-subunit.[13]

A clearer understanding has emerged of the overall physicochemical basis by which enzymatic activity results in the exchange of three intracellular sodium ions for two extracellular potassium ions, as depicted in Figure 43-2. It is believed that the binding of three Na$^+$ ions to the cytosolic aspect of the enzyme allows phosphorylation to proceed, causing a conformational change to occur. This change expose Na$^+$ ions to the extracellular surface, where they are released; and potassium may bind in their place (it is unclear as to whether these sites are the same). The binding of extracellular K$^+$ promotes dephosphorylation, with subsequent translocation of the cation to the cytoplasm. During the phase in which Na$^+$/K$^+$-ATPase binds to K$^+$ the cardiac glycoside binding domain is relatively less accessible, providing one explanation for why increased extracellular K$^+$ reverses some of the toxic effects of these drugs.[14]

The factors responsible for regulating the expression of the relevant genes that encode the α- and β-subunits are largely unknown, although a role for thyroid hormone has been extensively studied.[15,16] In addition, available data suggest that increased

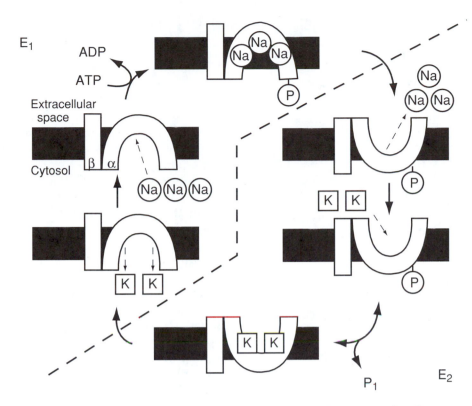

Fig. 43-2. Simplified Albers-Post model of Na$^+$ and K$^+$ translocation across the plasma membrane by Na$^+$/K$^+$-ATPase, showing the two major conformational states of the enzyme with their respective phosphorylation profile (From Lingrel,[140] with permission.)

expression of Na$^+$/K$^+$-ATPase can be induced by aldosterone in cultured cardiomyocytes.[17] Up-regulation of Na$^+$/K$^+$-ATPase by digitalis has been demonstrated in a number of cell types including HeLa cells, chick heart cells, skeletal myotubes, and guinea pig myocardium.[18–21] Similar findings have been reported in human erythrocytes obtained from patients receiving chronic digoxin therapy,[22] although Schmidt and colleagues did not observe any up-regulation of Na$^+$/K$^+$-ATPase in specimens of the left ventricle obtained at necropsy from patients treated with digoxin.[23] Allen et al.[24] examined the influence of heart failure on Na$^+$/K$^+$-ATPase mRNA abundance and protein content in the left ventricle (obtained at the time of transplantation) and compared it to that in nonfailing donor hearts not allocated for transplantation. They demonstrated no significant differences in either mRNA abundance or protein content as detected by ^{3}H-ouabain binding, although there was a trend for the latter to be reduced in the heart failure samples. These findings should be interpreted with caution however, owing to the small sample size and the use of digoxin in all of the heart failure patients studied.

BASIC MECHANISMS OF DIGITALIS ACTION DURING HEART FAILURE

Although congestive heart failure generally develops as the consequence of diminished contractile performance, profound alterations in autonomic activity and cardiovascular reflex function are additional features. In this regard, emerging information indicates that the cardiac glycosides may exert beneficial actions on these disturbances.

Positive Inotropic Effect

The positive inotropic effect of the cardiac glycosides has been known for more than 70 years, characterized by an increase in stroke work or tension generation at a given preload in both normal and failing myocardium. It is now widely believed that these actions are brought about by an increase in the availability of intracellular Ca^{2+},[25–28] which occurs as a consequence of the inhibitory action of the cardiac

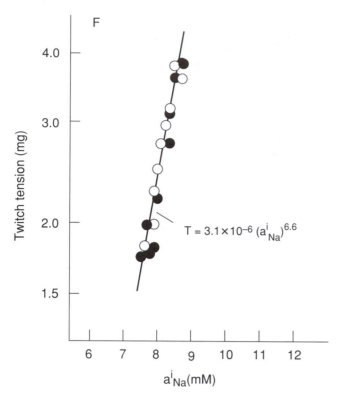

Fig. 43-3. Note the steep relation between increasing intracellular Na$^+$ and developed tension. (From Im and Lee,[31] with permission.)

glycosides on Na$^+$ and K$^+$ transport at the plasma membrane and a rise in intracellular Na$^+$.

Through the development of sensitive methods for determining intracellular Na$^+$ and Ca^{2+} concentrations ([Na$^+$]$_i$ and [Ca^{2+}]$_i$, respectively), compelling evidence has linked the positive inotropic actions of the cardiac glycosides to an increase in [Na$^+$]$_i$.[29,30] Indeed, there is a steep relation between [Na$^+$]zi and tension development (Fig. 43-3).[31] Exposure to subtoxic concentrations of cardiac glycosides, which results in a doubling of twitch tension development, increases the [Na$^+$]$_i$ concentration by approximately 2 mM at most, explaining why earlier workers were unable to document a role for sodium in the action of cardiac glycosides using less sensitive techniques. The concept of the dependence on increased [Na$^+$]$_i$ as a mechanism for the positive inotropic response has been further supported by experiments in which [Na$^+$]$_i$ has been perturbed by other means, such as tetrodotoxin, which reduces [Na$^+$]$_i$, and the treppe phenomenon, during which an increase in stimulus frequency results in increased [Na$^+$]$_i$ accompanied by increased contractility.[32,33] Within this framework, the sarcolemmal Na$^+$/Ca^{2+} exchanger assumes a major role (Fig. 43-4). By inhibiting the active extrusion of intracellular Na$^+$ ions in exchange for extra-

cellular K$^+$ ions, cardiac glycosides slow the outward movement of intracellular Ca^{2+} ions in exchange for extracellular Na$^+$ ions during the polarized state of the cell and may increase the transsarcolemmal entry of extracellular Ca^{2+} in exchange for intracellular Na$^+$ via the Na$^+$/Ca^{2+} exchanger during depolarization, leading to Ca^{2+} accumulation. Measurements of intracellular calcium transients using sensitive fluorescent indicators and ion sensitive microelectrodes, however, indicate a minimal effect of cardiac glycosides on diastolic [Ca^{2+}]$_i$.[27] The reason for this finding is the rapid sequestration of intracellular Ca^{2+} by the sarcoplasmic reticulum, which is largely inaccessible to microelectrodes and most fluorescent indicators. The increased [Ca^{2+}]$_i$ only becomes apparent during systole with the release of Ca^{2+} stored in the sarcoplasmic reticulum. At rapid heart rates Na$^+$ influx via the fast Na$^+$ channel may be sufficiently great to approach the maximum inotropically effective [Na$^+$]$_i$, thereby diminishing the positive inotropic effect of cardiac glycosides at high contraction frequencies. Despite its reliance on the Na$^+$/Ca^{2+} exchanger for its actions, it is unclear whether digitalis alters the expression of this important protein. Studer et al.[35] demonstrated increased Na$^+$/Ca^{2+} exchanger mRNA and protein in patients with failing hearts, many of whom were receiving digoxin, but no casual relation was established.

In addition to augmenting peak systolic Ca^{2+} through Na$^+$/Ca^{2+} exchange, digitalis under some circumstances increase Ca^{2+} influx through sarcolemmal voltage-sensitive Ca^{2+} channels.[26] The exact mechanism and relative contribution of an increase in the calcium current (I$_{Ca}$) to [Ca^{2+}]$_i$ is unclear. It is possible that the increased I$_{CA}$ is a positive feedback response to increased intracellular Ca^{2+}, possibly related to increased phosphorylation of L-type Ca^{2+} channels. Other direct or indirect mechanisms have been proposed to contribute, in part, to the positive inotropic actions of cardiac glycosides, including (1) evidence for an enhancing effect on sarcoplasmic reticulum (SR) calcium release through an interaction of digoxin with the SR Ca^{2+} release channel[36] and (2) a role for the Na$^+$/H$^+$ exchanger, whereby the increase in [Ca^{2+}]$_i$ occurring as a consequence of Na$^+$/K$^+$-ATPase inhibition leads to intracellular proton accumulation and a subsequent further rise in [Na$^+$]$_i$ mediated via Na$^+$/H$^+$ exchange.[37]

Actions on the Autonomic Nervous System

As described elsewhere (see Ch. 14), a characteristic feature of heart failure is activation of the sympathetic nervous system in conjunction with a reduc-

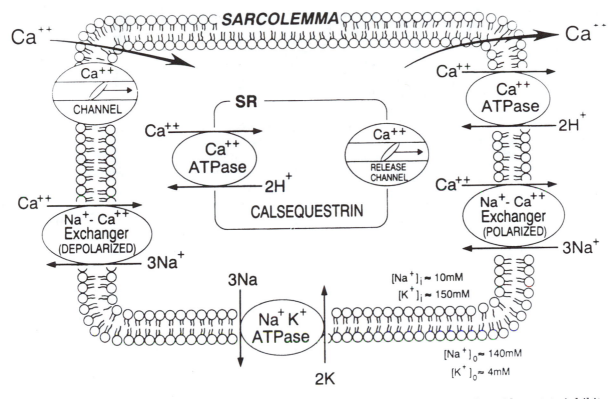

Fig. 43-4. Effect of Na⁺ pump inhibition on cellular Ca^{2+} homeostasis. Cardiac glycosides act to inhibit the Na⁺/K⁺-ATPase leading to net accumulation of intracellular Na⁺, which tends to limit Ca^{2+} extrusion by the Na⁺/Ca^{2+} exchanger. As a consequence the net intracellular Ca^{2+} accumulation occurs, which is rapidly sequestered by the sarcoplasmic reticulum (SR). This additional Ca^{2+} is available for release during cellular depolarization, augmenting contractile performance. The left-hand side of the diagram is intended to indicate events taking place during cellular depolarization and on the right during the state of polarization. It should be noted that the Na⁺/Ca^{2+} exchanger is sensitive to membrane voltage (given that it is electrogenic) and therefore tends to operate in a "reverse" mode during cell depolarization. Net Ca^{2+} extrusion is dependent on the Na⁺ gradient, which in turn can be altered by Na⁺/K⁺-ATPase inhibition (From Smith et al.,[34] with permission.)

tion in the gain (or sensitivity) of reflex responses to perturbations in the arterial blood pressure and ventricular filling pressures. Of relevance to the present discussion, abundant data suggest that the digitalis glycosides can alter various aspects of autonomic function.

A number of early investigators noted that, depending on the particular experimental conditions, digitalis could elicit vasoconstriction in a number of vascular beds, including the coronary arteries[38] and forearm.[39,40] These effects were typically noted in experimental animals or humans with normal heart function. The mechanism underlying these effects appears to be complex, in large part mediated by augmented sympathetic nervous outflow (*vide infra*) and to a lesser extent due to a transient direct inhibition of vascular smooth muscle Na⁺/K⁺-ATPase, with consequent increased intracellular Ca^{2+} and thus de-

veloped tension.[41,42] More recently it has been suggested that digitalis may increase the activity of type III, cGMP-inhibited cAMP phosphodiesterase in vascular smooth muscle, it having been shown that cardiac glycosides diminish the vasodilatory actions of amrinone and milrinone in isolated rat aortic rings and in the forearm vasculature of patients with heart failure.[43,44]

In addition to a direct vascular effect, a wealth of data support the notion that digitalis exerts a number of its actions via neurally mediated mechanisms. Vatner et al.[38] showed that ouabain caused coronary vasoconstriction in conscious dogs but that this action could not be demonstrated during general anesthesia. Further work has shown that this phenomenon appears to be explained by increased sympathetic outflow from the brain,[45-48] typically being seen with potentially toxic or rapidly administered doses. The genesis of this sympathoexcitatory effect in normal animals is not completely understood but appears be mediated by or near the area postrema.[49,50] Other actions of digitalis on the sympathetic nervous system have also been described including the release of norepinephrine from postganglionic nerve terminal varicosities through a Ca^{2+}-dependent exocytotic process[51] and inhibitory effects on catecholamine reuptake.[52]

In addition to sympathetic nervous stimulation, digitalis exerts effects on efferent parasympathetic nerves. These actions include increased nerve firing mediated through central mechanisms and facilitation of the action of acetylcholine at muscarinic cholinergic receptors.[45]

Extensive literature supports the concept that digitalis glycosides can augment baroreceptor discharge sensitivity under normal circumstances[46,53,54] and in experimental[55] and clinical heart failure (as discussed below). The mechanism by which this alteration in baroreceptor discharge sensitivity occurs is unclear, although a direct effect on the Na^+/K^+-ATPase of baroreceptor cells in the carotid sinus has been suggested by Wang et al. based on studies involving direct perfusion of the isolated carotid sinus with ouabain.[55] Of interest, digitalis glycosides have also been shown to potentiate chemoreceptor discharge activity in animals and humans.[56,57]

Effects of Chronic Digoxin Therapy on the Autonomic Nervous System

In contrast to the relatively large number of acute studies of the effects of digitalis glycosides on autonomic function in heart failure, the chronic effects of digoxin therapy on reflex function or sympathetic tone have not been well characterized. Alicandri et al.[58] presented the first long-term data on this issue, demonstrating that digoxin (and captopril) reduced plasma norepinephrine levels. In a study of patients with moderate to severe heart failure, Kaye et al.[59] demonstrated similar levels of integrated sympathetic nervous activity by comparing the whole-body spillover rate for norepinephrine in individuals treated with or without digoxin. There was, however, a nonsignificant trend toward higher cardiac sympathetic activity in subjects not receiving digoxin compared to those treated with digoxin. Krum et al. showed in 26 patients that chronic (4–8 weeks) digoxin treatment was associated with a reduction in plasma norepinephrine and an increase in heart rate variability, although there were no control (nondigoxin-treated) individuals available for comparison in this study.[60]

Electrophysiologic Effects

A comprehensive review of the electrophysiologic actions of digitalis is beyond the scope of the present discussion and may be found elsewhere.[25,61] The electrophysiologic actions of digitalis at therapeutic concentrations probably reflect a combination of direct actions on specialized cells comprising the conducting system within the heart and the result of actions on the autonomic nervous system. At clinically relevant concentrations digoxin reduces sinoatrial node firing, an effect mediated largely by an increase in vagal tone. The vagotonic action of digoxin also increases the maximum diastolic potential in atrial tissue. Similarly, the important antiarrhythmic actions of digitalis at the atrioventricular (AV) node are also largely dependent on alterations in autonomic tone. Nontoxic doses of digitalis administered to humans cause a slowing of AV node conduction and increased refractoriness. These actions are abolished by atropine[62] and by cardiac denervation in the setting of human cardiac transplantation. Interestingly, the parasympathomimetic actions of digitalis have also been shown to increase heart rate variability when analyzed in both time and frequency domains.[63]

The toxic arrhythmogenic actions of the cardiac glycosides also reflect the combined result of direct cellular effects and indirect autonomic effects. During exposure to high concentrations of the cardiac glycosides, isolated myocardial preparations demonstrate "after-depolarizations," a result of cellular Ca^{2+} overload with consequent spontaneous release of Ca^{2+} from the sarcoplamsic reticulum.[64] At toxic levels, sympathoexcitation also appears to contribute to the range of arrhythmias that may be observed.[50]

THERAPEUTIC ACTIONS OF DIGITALIS GLYCOSIDES DURING HUMAN HEART FAILURE

Although digitalis preparations have been used to treat symptoms of congestive heart failure for at least 200 years, debate continues regarding the risk benefit ratio for patients in sinus rhythm. Surprisingly this issue has been systematically addressed only since the mid-1970s.

Acute Hemodynamic Effects

Since the late 1940s numerous studies have indicated that acute administration of digitalis is associated with beneficial effects on a number of hemodynamic parameters, including cardiac index, left ventricular filling pressure, and systemic vascular resistance in patients with heart failure.[39,65,66] Administration of cardiac glycosides in normal individuals results in either no change or a slight decline in cardiac output. This result is not surprising, as cardiac output is determined not only by myocardial contractility but by the prevailing loading conditions of the heart and by the heart rate. Thus although digitalis glycosides do increase contractility in nonfailing cardiac tissue, adjustments in autonomic reflexes (and possibly other direct effects of digoxin) usually prevent a detectable increase in cardiac output.[67]

With the advent of more sophisticated methods for hemodynamic investigation, additional beneficial effects of acute digitalis administration have been documented in patients with heart failure. Ribner and colleagues[68] demonstrated a significant increase in cardiac output and significant falls in pulmonary capillary wedge pressure, right atrial pressure, and heart rate 6 hours after the intravenous administration of 1 mg of digoxin. These measurements were also performed during exercise, where again statistically significant beneficial effects on the same parameters were evident. Other investigators have also documented favorable hemodynamic effects of acute intravenous digoxin during human heart failure. Gheorghiade et al.[69] demonstrated favorable effects of digoxin on cardiac index, stroke work, and pulmonary capillary wedge pressure in patients with severe heart failure who were initially treated with diuretics and vasodilators but remained in overt heart failure. Of note in this study and others,[70] variability in hemodynamic response to acute digitalis administration is attributable in large part to the degree of hemodynamic abnormality present prior to digoxin administration. In general, data from these studies indicate that the administration of digoxin to patients with heart failure is most likely to result in a beneficial response where overt hemodynamic decompensation exists, in contrast to the patient with ventricular dysfunction and a well compensated hemodynamic profile.

In addition to the influence of the baseline hemodynamic status in determining the digoxin response, the cause and pathophysiology of heart failure in the individual patient are important. Although concerns have been raised regarding the administration of digoxin to individuals with acute or recent myocardial infarction (as discussed below), there are no data examining the influence of heart failure etiology (e.g., ischemic versus idiopathic) on the hemodynamic effects of digoxin administration for any given level of ventricular dysfunction. With regard to the influence of pathophysiology, a special distinction should be drawn between systolic and diastolic ventricular dysfunction in the context of digitalis use. Although the foregoing discussion clearly supports a beneficial effect of acute digitalis therapy in systolic dysfunction, there is little evidence that digitalis provides benefit to patients with heart failure due principally to "diastolic dysfunction" or to patients with restrictive/constrictive physiology. Conceptually, the rise in intracellular Ca^{2+} that is central to the effects of digitalis could conceivably worsen abnormal myocardial relaxation during diastole. Furthermore, in patients with hypertrophic cardiomyopathy, particularly those with outflow tract obstruction, it is possible that digitalis could worsen the subaortic outflow gradient. Although in general slowing of the ventricular rate is beneficial when treating patients with symptomatic diastolic dysfunction and atrial arrhythmias, drugs other than the cardiac glycosides are usually preferable.

In a related context, the acute or chronic therapeutic value of digitalis in the hypertrophied or dilated nonfailing heart remains uncertain. With the development of hypertrophy, and before the onset of overt failure, the work capacity of the myocardium tends to be reduced at any given left ventricular end-diastolic pressure. By exerting a positive inotropic effect, digitalis augments the myocardial work capacity and may thus reduce end-diastolic volume and end-diastolic pressure.[67] Under these circumstances, these drugs may not necessarily increase cardiac output at rest but could increase the inotropic reserve.

There have been several reports investigating the hemodynamic effects of digoxin in conjunction with other vasoactive compounds in subjects with heart failure. These studies have been reviewed in detail by Tisdale and Gheorghiade[71] and Tauke et al.[72] A number of workers have demonstrated synergistic hemodynamic effects when evaluating combination therapy with digoxin and vasodilators, including captopril,[73,74] sodium nitroprusside,[75] hydralazine,[76] and nifedipine.[77] In limited studies the combination of digoxin with dobutamine has not been shown to result in a hemodynamic profile superior to either agent alone.[78]

Acute Effects on the Autonomic Nervous System

In light of data demonstrating that digoxin may alter several aspects of autonomic function during experimental heart failure, attention has been directed at defining these actions in humans with heart failure. This line of investigation has been given added impetus by a number studies that clearly associate disturbances of autonomic function (particularly sympathetic nervous system activity) and survival after heart failure.[79-81]

Among the alterations in autonomic activity observed with heart failure, disturbed baroreceptor function and sympathoexcitation are two targets at which digitalis has been proposed to act. To address the first issue, Ferguson[82] examined baroreflex-mediated changes in forearm vascular resistance at various levels of lower body negative pressure before and after administration of a rapid-acting intravenous digitalis preparation. After treatment with the cardiac glycoside there was a restoration toward the profile expected under conditions of normal baroreflex function. In a related study, Ferguson and colleagues also showed that digitalis administration augmented the increase in muscle sympathetic nerve firing during various degrees of cardiopulmonary baroreceptor unloading in patients with heart failure[83] (Fig. 43-5). In this study, administration of an-

other positively inotropic agent (dobutamine) did not appear to modify reflex function, suggesting a specific action of digitalis. In conjuction with these effects on reflex function, sympathoinhibition was also seen, perhaps as a result of improved baroreflex sensitivity. Goldsmith et al.[84] also examined the effects of acute digitalis administration on reflex and sympathetic nervous function using norepinephrine kinetics and tilt-testing. In this study, however, there were no apparent effects on sympathetic nervous activity or the reflex response to head-down tilt.

A number of other acute studies of digitalis administration have suggested beneficial effects of cardiac glycosides on neurohormonal parameters in patients with heart failure. Studies by Ribner and colleagues[68] and Covit et al.[85] demonstrated significant reductions in plasma norepinephrine, renin activity, and aldosterone after the acute administration of intravenous digoxin to patients with New York Heart Association (NYHA) class III to IV heart failure. Interestingly, a blunting of the acute sympathoexcita-

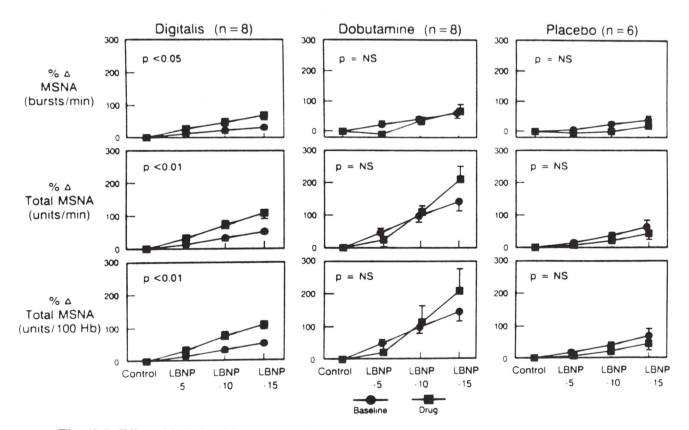

Fig. 43-5. Effect of digitalis, dobutamine, and placebo on muscle sympathetic nerve activity (MSNA) in response to varying degrees of lower body negative pressure (LBNP), which unloads cardiopulmonary baroreceptors. Data are expressed as percentage change in firing rate (top panels), total integrated MSNA (middle panels), or integrated MSNA corrected for heart rate (bottom panels). (From Ferguson et al.,[83] with permission.)

tory effects of exercise (as manifested by increased plasma norepinephrine and renin activity) was also documented after acute digoxin administration in heart failure patients.[68]

Chronic Digoxin Therapy for Heart Failure

A critical appraisal of digitalis' role in the treatment of heart failure was not systematically addressed until the late 1960s. A number of these early studies, however, are difficult to interpret because of the limited descriptive data regarding the diagnosis and severity of heart failure. An early trial with adequate design was reported in 1977 by Dobbs et al.,[86] who conducted a study of chronic digoxin therapy using a double-blind placebo-controlled single-crossover format in 46 patients with heart failure of varying etiology. Thirty-four percent ($M = 16$) of the patients receiving placebo deteriorated, eight of whom improved upon reinstitution of digoxin. Interpretation of this study is complicated by the fact that nearly one-third of the subjects were in atrial fibrillation, and their clinical outcomes were not distinguished from those in sinus rhythm.

During the early 1980s Fleg et al.[87] performed a double-blind, placebo-controlled, crossover study of chronic digoxin therapy in 30 NYHA class II–III patients (i.e., mild to moderate heart failure) over 3 months. In this study there were no significant differences apparent between placebo- and digoxin-treated subjects using a number of clinical endpoints, including orthopnea, paroxysmal nocturnal dyspnea, and exercise tolerance. Discontinuation of digoxin therapy did, however, result in significant deterioration of left ventricular function, as assessed echocardiographically. Using a similar format, Taggart et al.[88] were also able to show beneficial effects of digoxin on left ventricular function in patients with mild heart failure.

Lee and colleagues[89] conducted a double-blind, placebo-controlled crossover trial of 25 patients with heart failure. In contrast to the previous two studies, significant positive effects of digoxin were seen in relation to a clinical heart failure score that consisted of an assessment of dyspnea, the presence or absence of rales, heart rate, signs of right-sided congestion, and chest radiographic abnormalities. Furthermore, it was apparent that subjects with evidence of more advanced heart failure due to systolic dysfunction were more likely to benefit, as discussed above in the context of the acute hemodynamic effects of digoxin administration. Aside from the inclusion of patients with more severe heart failure, an additional possi-

ble reason for the difference in results between this trial and that of Fleg et al. was the use of higher daily digoxin doses with monitoring of serum digoxin concentrations.

Four additional trials were reported in 1988. Guyatt et al.[90] studied 20 patients with moderate to severe heart failure using a variety of endpoints, including a heart failure score, exercise capacity, and echocardiographic indices of contractile function. None of the patients deteriorated while receiving digoxin, but seven worsened during the placebo phase. Of interest, those subjects who deteriorated during the placebo period had evidence of more severe heart failure. A small, albeit significant improvement in exercise capacity and ejection fraction were also seen with digoxin therapy. Another small scale study by Haerer and colleagues, conducted over 3 weeks, showed a beneficial effect of digoxin on left-sided filling pressures and cardiac output.[91]

The Captopril-Digoxin Multicenter Research Group trial[92] was the first randomized, placebo-controlled prospective trial to have sufficient power to begin to address the appropriate role for digoxin in the drug treatment of heart failure. It evaluated the effects of captopril, digoxin, or placebo therapy in 300 patients maintained on diuretic therapy. Most of these patients had only mild heart failure, and the study design excluded patients who became unstable during digoxin withdrawal in preparation for randomization, thus potentially reducing the number of patients who might benefit most from digitalis therapy. Subjects randomized to digoxin therapy showed a significant increase in left ventricular function, unlike their counterparts receiving captopril. Furthermore, either digoxin or captopril similarly reduced the need for increased diuretic therapy or hospitalization compared to patients receiving placebo. In contrast, unlike captopril, digoxin did not significantly improve exercise tolerance in this study, in contrast to the PROVED and RADIANCE trials (see below).

In 1985 the German and Austrian Xamoterol Study Group also presented their findings in patients with mild heart failure randomized to xamoterol, digoxin, or placebo.[93] Digoxin improved clinical indices of heart failure but not exercise capacity. Many factors confound the complete interpretation of this study, including the mild degree of heart failure (106 of the 433 subjects were NYHA class I) and the presence of active angina in more than 50 percent of the patients.

Another multicenter trial by DiBianco et al. examined the relative benefits of milrinone or digoxin compared to placebo in 230 patients with moderate to severe heart failure.[94] After 3 months, digoxin significantly improved left ventricular function and exercise capacity compared to placebo. In addition, digoxin was significantly less likely to exhibit proarrhythmic effects in comparison to milrinone.

Although the foregoing data generally support the notion that digoxin is beneficial in patients with heart failure in sinus rhythm, this issue has been more satisfactorily addressed by the PROVED and RADIANCE trials. The PROVED trial[95] examined the effects of randomized double-blind withdrawal of digoxin treatment in patients initially stabilized on combination digoxin and diuretic therapy. This study included 88 patients with NYHA class II to III heart failure and an average left ventricular ejection fraction (LVEF) of 29 ± 2 percent, all patients having an LVEF of 35 percent or less. After digoxin withdrawal, placebo-treated subjects displayed an increased incidence of treatment failure (increased diuretic requirement, need for hospital treatment), reduced exercise capacity (treadmill time), reduced left ventricular function, and increased body weight in comparison to the digoxin-treated group.

As a consequence of the compelling evidence supporting a beneficial role for angiotensin-converting enzyme (ACE) inhibitor therapy for heart failure, a number of trials involving digoxin have been structured to address the role of combination therapy. In addition to favorable acute hemodynamic effects, Gheorghiade and colleagues[73] demonstrated that the combination of digoxin and captopril increased exercise capacity significantly, in contrast to either agent alone. The largest and most comprehensively designed trial is the RADIANCE trial.[96] In many aspects the design of this trial was similar to the PROVED trial. In the RADIANCE study 178 patients with heart failure of severity comparable to that of individuals in the PROVED study were randomized to digoxin withdrawal or continuation after a run-in phase during which therapy consisted of digoxin, a diuretic, and an ACE inhibitor (captopril or enalapril). In comparison to patients who continued digoxin therapy, the subjects switched to placebo showed a significantly greater probability of worsening heart failure (Fig. 43-6), reduced exercise tolerance, worsening quality of life indices and poorer left ventricular function.

Taken together, the PROVED and RADIANCE trials support the use of digoxin therapy in patients with chronic heart failure who are in sinus rhythm. Of particular importance, RADIANCE supports the use of digoxin in the era of ACE inhibitor therapy. However, it is important to emphasize that these trials suffer from several limitations inherent in the withdrawal design.[72,97] First, all participants had been maintained on digoxin, thus introducing a se-

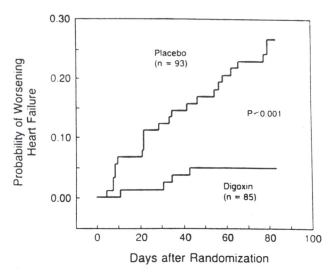

Fig. 43-6. Kaplan-Meier plot of data from the RADIANCE trial indicating a significantly greater likelihood of patients receiving placebo (after randomized withdrawal of digoxin) to experience worsening heart failure, even with continuing diuretic and ACE inhibitor treatment. (From Packer et al.,[96] with permission.)

lection bias for patients who were better responders. Second, and more relevant to the issue of the effect of digoxin on mortality and the potential of a hazard associated with digoxin therapy, all those who entered had evidenced that they could tolerate digoxin for at least 3 months without experiencing lethal or symptomatic arrhythmias. Third, it appears likely that chronic therapy with some inotropic agents, such as milrinone and flosequinan, accelerates the deterioration of cardiac function in a way which becomes apparent only when these drugs are withdrawn.[98,99]

Results of the Digitalis Investigators Group Trial

To address the unresolved key issues of the effect of chronic digoxin therapy on mortality and the long-term clinical course of patients with congestive heart failure, a multicenter U.S. National Heart, Lung, and Blood Institute (NHLBI) sponsored trial, the Digoxin Investigators Group (DIG) study was undertaken.[97,100,101] It was a prospective, randomized, double-blind, placebo-controlled trial of digoxin in patients with mild to moderate heart failure. Although the results have been presented in preliminary form,[102] the final results of this trial have not yet been published. Altogether 7788 patients in sinus rhythm with left ventricular ejection fractions of 45 percent or more (although a subset of 1000 patients with symptomatic heart failure was also included) on diuretics and ACE inhibitors were randomized and followed on blinded therapy for a mean of 37 months (28–58 months). Because previous studies have suggested that benefits of digoxin were greater in patients with more severe symptoms and left ventricular dysfunction, it is noteworthy that this population had relatively mild heart failure (69 percent had NYHA class I or II symptoms, and the mean left ventricular ejection fraction was 32 percent). Importantly, most patients had not previously been receiving digoxin.

The prespecified primary endpoint was all-cause mortality, and there was absolutely no difference in this endpoint between the treatment groups (odds ratio 1.0). There was also no difference in cardiovascular deaths, which constituted 85 percent of the total. However, there was a significant 14 percent reduction in deaths due to worsening heart failure, which was essentially balanced by an increase in deaths ascribed to arrhythmia and acute myocardial infarction. The designated secondary endpoint was cardiovascular hospitalizations. The numbers listed in Table 43-2 are the number of patients who were hospitalized at least once during the course of the study, although many of these patients had multiple hospitalizations. Hospitalizations for any cardiovascular reason and those for worsening heart failure were significantly reduced by 10 percent and 28 percent, respectively. Overall, digoxin was generally well tolerated, and serious toxicity was uncommon, with 75 hospitalizations for suspected digoxin toxicity in the active therapy group and 35 in the placebo group.

Additional analyses from this study will provide a wealth of information for the clinician. Several trends were apparent from the preliminary results. When subgroup analyses were performed on the combined endpoint of heart failure-related mortality and hospitalizations, there was greater benefit at the lower range of ejection fractions and in the patients with a nonischemic etiology than in those with an ischemic etiology for heart failure. There were also trends toward more benefit in patients with class III or IV than in those with I or II symptoms and those with larger cardiothoracic ratios on chest radiographs.

Thus the DIG trial has confirmed that digoxin prevents clinical worsening of heart failure, as judged by hospitalizations; and digoxin accomplishes it without evidence of either a decreased or an increased risk of death. These results suggest that digoxin is an appropriate therapy for patients with symptomatic heart failure when used in conjunction with ACE inhibitors and diuretics.

PHARMACOLOGY OF DIGITALIS GLYCOSIDES

Digoxin is by far the most commonly prescribed cardiac glycoside preparation. Digitoxin is also available for clinical use. Reviews of the pharmacokinetics and metabolism of these and other cardiac glycosides can also be found elsewhere.[103,104]

The pharmacokinetics and pharmacodynamics of digoxin have been well characterized, allowing it to be used safely in a broad range of clinical circumstances. Irrespective of the route of administration (oral or intravenous), digoxin is excreted in an exponential fashion with an elimination half-life of 36–48 hours in patients with normal renal function. As a result this constitutes a daily loss of approximately one-third of body stores. Given the fact that digoxin is secreted or reabsorbed to only a limited extent at the tubular level (see below) the glomerular filtration rate (or creatinine clearance) is a key consideration when determining individual patient dosing schedules. Various nomograms have been constructed for estimating the relation between renal function and daily digoxin elimination. A reasonable approximation of the daily percentage loss is given by the formula:

$$\% \text{ Daily loss} = 14 + \frac{\text{creatinine clearance (ml/min)}}{5}$$

The constant in this equation (14 percent) is intended to account for nonrenal excretion of digoxin, and it should be noted that this factor may vary considerably. In patients with prerenal azotemia, digoxin clearance may correlated more closely with urea clearance, implying that the drug may undergo some degree of tubular reabsorption.[105] Conversely, some degree of renal tubular secretion of digoxin has been proposed,[106] and it may be the explanation of altered digoxin clearance in the context of acute vasodilator therapy in patients with heart failure.[107] Although most of the digoxin eliminated by the kidney is unchanged, some may appear as the inactive metabolite dihydrodigoxin, which arises by bacterial (*Eubacterium lentum*) transformation by the enteric flora.[108] Significant bacterial metabolism occurs in up to 10 percent of patients, thereby increasing the digoxin clearance rate. It should also be noted that digoxin exhibits a high degree of tissue binding, resulting in a large volume of distribution, averaging 4–7 L/kg, and therefore is not effectively cleared by dialysis. Infants and neonates appear to handle digoxin in a fashion similar to adults, although renal tubular secretion may be more important.[109] Of further importance to pediatric and obstetric practice, digoxin does cross the placenta, and the digoxin concentration in umbilical venous blood approaches that seen in maternal blood. Digoxin is one of the few cardiovascular drugs for which there is a large literature on its use in the treatment of fetal arrhythmias, and it appears to be safe and effective. Children typically tolerate (and require) higher serum levels of digoxin than adolescents and adults for controlling the ventricular rate of supraventricular arrhythmias and for heart failure.

Gastrointestinal absorption of digoxin occurs passively, increasing in rate and proportion with decreasing molecular polarity (digoxin being of intermediate polarity). In patients with normal gastrointestinal function the oral bioavailability of most currently available tablet preparations is approximately 65–75 percent. The highest bioavailability is currently available in an encapsulated gel preparation, which is reported to exhibit 90–100 percent absorption.[110] Considerable interindividual variation in digoxin absorption exists. Patients with malabsorption syndromes may absorb the drug poorly and erratically, although subjects with pancreatic insufficiency and steatorrhea appear to absorb the drug normally.

Apart from pharmacokinetic issues arising from gastrointestinal absorption and renal function, various drug interactions have the potential to significantly alter serum concentrations of digoxin. Some of these interactions are listed in Table 43-1.

Dosing Schedules

While individual patient profiles dictate particular dosing schedules, broad guidelines can be derived based on the pharmacokinetic principles already outlined. In general, there is usually no need to treat patients with an acute loading dose of digoxin, except in the setting of supraventricular arrhythmias where other drugs have been ineffective or are contraindicated. Because of the close proximity of therapeutic and toxic concentrations of digoxin, rapid loading protocols must be approached with caution and close

Table 43-1. Drug Interactions with Digoxin

Drug	Mechanism of Interaction	Mean Magnitude of Interaction (%)
Cholestyramine	Adsorption of digoxin	↓ 25
Kaolin pectin	Adsorption of digoxin	?
Bran	Adsorption of digoxin	↓ 20
Antacids	?	↓ 25
Neomycin	?	↓ 28
Sulfasalazine	?	↓ 18
PAS	?	↓ 22
Bepridil	?	↑ 34
Phenytoin	?	↓ 30
Propafenone	?	↑ 100
Erythromycin	↑ Bioavailability due to ↓ metabolism by gut flora	↑ 43–116
Tetracycline		
Quinidine	?↓ Bioavailability, ↓ volume of distribution, ↓ renal and nonrenal clearance	↑ 100
Amiodarone	↓ Renal and nonrenal clearance	↑ 70–100
Verapamil	↓ Renal and nonrenal clearance	↑ 70–100
Diltiazem	?↓ Renal and nonrenal clearance	Zero to small ↑
Nicardipine	?	↑ 15
Tiapamil	?	↑ 60
Spironolactone	↓ Renal and nonrenal clearance	↑ 30
Triamterene	↓ Nonrenal clearance	↑ 20
Indomethacin (preterm infants)	?↓ Renal clearance	↑ 50

Mean magnitude of interaction refers to the degree of alteration in bioavailability or serum concentration.
(Modified from Smith et al.,[34] with permission.)

monitoring. For patients with normal renal function, a daily dosing regimen of 0.25 or 0.50 mg of digoxin results in a steady-state total body digoxin content of 0.67 or 1.35 mg, respectively, within approximately 1 week (i.e., five half-lives). If a loading dose is to be given, the oral administration of 0.9 mg or 1.8 mg of digoxin in divided doses over 24 hours results in plasma levels that approach those seen at steady state with either 0.25 mg or 0.50 mg daily, given normal renal function. In adults, an intravenous loading protocol comprising a total of 0.50 to 0.75 mg/45 kg (100 lb) body weight in divided doses over 24 hours is unlikely to result in toxicity, again given normal renal function. Dosing schedules for pediatric applications may be found elsewhere.[34] Various nomograms have been developed for determining maintenance dose requirements of digoxin based on lean body mass and renal function, but they provide no substitute for frequent and careful observation of the patient.

In the absence of a supraventricular arrhythmia where control of the ventricular rate provides some index of dosing efficacy, it is often difficult to accurately judge the state of digitalization. Current data suggest that up to approximately 80 percent of the maximum inotropic effect of digoxin is obtained when the serum concentration is in the range of 1.0–1.5 ng/ml at 24 hours after the dose.[111,112] In general, other "markers" of the state of digitalization, such as electrocardiographic ST-T wave changes, are of relatively little use, having limited sensitivity and specificity.

HEART FAILURE AND DIGITALIS TOXICITY

When assessing the potential benefits of any therapeutic strategy, appropriate consideration must also be given to factors that may contribute to individual variation in sensitivity to digitalis and most importantly to potential adverse effects (Table 43-2). In the context of digoxin treatment for heart failure, those individuals likely to benefit most from its use are often those at greatest risk for adverse effects. Of paramount importance are disturbances of electrolyte homeostasis, which are often seen with severe heart failure per se or as a consequence of diuretic or ACE inhibitor therapy.

Alterations in the serum potassium concentration are particularly important. Aside from its own electrophysiologic effects, hypokalemia increases Na^+/K^+-ATPase sensitivity to digoxin, at least in part by virtue of the role of potassium in promoting dephosphorylation of Na^+/K^+-ATPase, a state associ-

Table 43-2. Factors Influencing Individual Sensitivity to Digitalis
Type and severity of heart disease
Serum electrolyte disturbances
Hypokalemia or hyperkalemia
Hypomagnesemia
Hypercalcemia
Hyponatremia
Acid-base disturbances
Concomitant drug administration
Anesthetics
Catecholamines and sympathomimetics
Antiarrhythmic drugs
Thyroid disturbance
Altered renal function
Autonomic nervous activity
Respiratory disease

ated with reduced digoxin affinity. Secondarily, hypokalemia (< 2.5 mEq) favors intracellular Na^+ accumulation. Furthermore, chronic hypokalemia has been reported to reduce Na^+/K^+-ATPase protein (as reflected by ^{3}H-ouabain binding) in rat skeletal muscle[113] but not in the myocardium, which could thereby reduce the volume of distribution of the drug resulting in higher plasma concentrations for a given dose and level of renal function. In contrast, hyperkalemia reduces myocardial sensitivity to cardiac glycosides by virtue of the mechanisms described above. However, hyperkalemia itself favors cell depolarization, particularly in AV nodal conducting tissue, thereby exacerbating digitalis-induced AV block. Thus disturbances of potassium on either side of the physiologic range may contribute to digitalis-mediated prolongation of conduction. As a result, particular caution should be observed when concurrently administering digitalis with diuretics, ACE inhibitors, β-blockers, and nonsteroidal antiinflammatory drugs, and in individuals with impaired renal function.

Disturbances of other electrolytes may also influence myocardial sensitivity to cardiac glycosides. Hypomagnesemia may also favor increased digitalis sensitivity, perhaps by virtue of its role in Na^+/K^+-ATPase cycling. Again, concomitant diuretic therapy is of clinical importance in this respect. However, the correlation between serum Mg^{2+} and intracellular Mg^{2+} is weak, leaving the optimal range for serum Mg^{2+} in digoxin-treated heart failure patients unclear. Hypercalcemia may increase ventricular automaticity, possibly in a synergistic fashion with digitalis.

Aside from issues related to electrolyte control, other coexistent disease may alter individual sensitivity to digitalis glycosides. Hypothyroidism is associated with a significantly increased elimination half-life, whereas the converse is true of hyperthyroidism. Patients with chronic obstructive pulmonary disease may be at increased risk of proarrhythmic phenomena as a consequence of their propensity to disturbances of acid-base control and hypoxemia.

Although clear evidence supports the use of digoxin during heart failure, mention should be made of specific forms of myocardial disease in which this use remains controversial or may be associated with increased risk of toxicity. Of prime importance is the use of digoxin for acute myocardial infarction associated with heart failure. To date, there is no evidence of an increased incidence of arrhythmia in patients treated with digitalis glycosides during the acute phase of their infarct.[114,115] However, other data have suggested that mortality might be higher in digoxin-treated individuals with heart failure and ventricular arrhythmia following myocardial infarction.[116,117] Other studies, however, do not support these data.[118–120] In view of this uncertainty, a reasonable approach may be to use digoxin only in the setting of heart failure and acute or recent myocardial infarction where other alternatives are inappropriate or inadequate for the management of supraventricular arrhythmias. Apart from myocardial infarction, the use of digoxin in patients with active myocardial ischemia also deserves consideration. In one study[121] digoxin treatment improved myocardial perfusion in patients with coronary artery disease and left ventricular dysfunction, whereas in other instances worsening of angina may be observed. Digoxin toxicity may also be more common in cardiac amyloidosis, possibly due to the enhanced affinity of amyloid protein for digoxin.[122]

The specific electrophysiologic and electrocardiographic manifestations associated with digitalis toxicity are well known and have been described in detail elsewhere,[34,61] as have the extracardiac phenomena. The most important factor when managing digoxin toxicity is maintenance of a high level of suspicion, particularly in individuals with a propensity toward the development of toxicity. In all cases, optimization of the serum potassium is important, in conjunction with temporary cessation of the drug. Bradyarrhythmias, whether sinus bradycardia or as a consequence of sinoatrial or AV nodal conduction delay, may respond to atropine or require temporary pacing depending on the presence of hemodynamic compromise.

Digoxin-induced tachyarrhythmias may demand more urgent attention, particularly ventricular tachycardia. Phenytoin and lidocaine are effective in this setting, whereas other agents (particularly class 1a) may be difficult to use safely, especially in the presence of concomitant conduction disturbances. Ultra-short-acting β-blockers, such as esmolol, may also be helpful. Although electrical cardioversion is safe in the absence of digoxin toxicity, it may be hazardous in the setting of digitalis-induced arrhythmias.

For the individual with actually or potentially life-threatening digoxin toxicity, the use of digoxin-specific polyclonal antibody Fab fragments provides a means of rapidly reversing the effects of digoxin or digitoxin with few adverse effects.[123–125]

ENDOGENOUS CARDIAC GLYCOSIDE–LIKE SUBSTANCES

The demonstration of a high degree of conservation of the molecular identity and sensitivity to digitalis glycosides of Na^+/K^+-ATPase across many species has led to the concept that the cardiac glycoside-binding site may act as a receptor for some endogenous factor.[126] A complete review of this topic is beyond the scope of this chapter and may be found elsewhere.[126–128] Although most attention has been directed at ligands that may potentially interact with the glycoside-binding site, it should also be noted that other endogenous compounds can modify Na^+/K^+-ATPase protein content and activity, including catecholamines, insulin, thyroid hormone, and mineralocorticoids, generally by directly altering the intracellular sodium concentration.

Consonant with the idea that cardiac glycoside-like compounds could influence the regulation of sodium (and potassium) homeostasis, much of the work related to the identification of potential candidate compounds and their physiologic actions has been performed in relation to hypertension. A number of workers have suggested the presence of a compound in ultrafiltrates of plasma from hypertensive humans or experimental animals that augments the response to various vasoconstrictors.[129,130] Others have demonstrated the presence of a factor in the plasma of hypertensive individuals that reduces $^{22}Na^+$ efflux from leukocytes and inhibits Na^+/K^+-ATPase.[131,132] Speculation has also arisen as the presence of endogenous glycosides within the central nervous system in the context of blood pressure regulation and the control of sympathetic nervous activity.[133,134] Attention has also been given to the presence of such factors in the plasma of uremic individuals based on observations of depressed sodium pump activity[135] and reports of false-positive digoxin radioimmunoassays.[136,137] Considerable debate continues to surround the existence of a putative endogenous digitalis-like factor, and controversy surrounds its potential chemical nature. Proposed candidates include a number of low-molecular-weight peptides, a variety of steroid derivatives, and even ouabain itself (see Kelly and Smith[127] for an extensive review, also[138,139]).

Despite ongoing interest, there is as yet no proof that a true endogenous ligand for the digitalis-binding site on Na$^+$/K$^+$-ATPase exists; nor is there convincing evidence that an as yet uncharacterized endogenous Na$^+$/K$^+$-ATPase inhibitor plays any role in blood pressure regulation or sodium homeostasis. A more immediate clinical issue relates to the potential for misinterpretating digoxin radioimmunoassays, resulting in falsely elevated plasma digoxin estimations. False-positive or falsely elevated immunoassay results are most often encountered in patients with end-stage renal failure, pregnant women, neonates, and possibly acromegalic individuals. These technical difficulties are often related to the use of digoxin assay systems in which an antibody of inadequate affinity and specificity is used in the radioimmunoassay.

REFERENCES

1. Withering W: An account of the foxglove and some of its medical uses, with practical remarks on dropsy, and other diseases. p. 231. In: Classics of Cardiology. Dover Publications, Baltimore, MD, 1941
2. Thomas R, Gray P, Andrews J: Digitalis: its mode of action, receptor, and structure-activity relationships. In: Advances in Drug Research. Academic Press, San Diego, 1989
3. Guntert TW, Linde HHA: Chemistry and structure-activity relationships of cardioactive steroids. p. 13. In: Handbook of Experimental Pharmacology: Cardiac Glycosides. Springer-Verlag, Berlin, 1981
4. Marshall PG: Steroids. Cardiotonic glycosides and aglycones. In: Rodd's Chemistry of Carbon Compounds. Elsevier, Amsterdam, 1970
5. Wiggers CJ, Stimson B: Studies on the cardiodynamic actions of drugs. III. The mechanism of cardiac stimulation by digitalis and g-strophanthin. J Pharmacol Exp Ther 30:251, 1927
6. Skou JC: The influence of some cations on an adenosine triphosphatase from peripheral nerves. Biochim Biophys Acta 23:394, 1957
7. Luttgau HC, Niedergeke R: The antagonism between Ca and Na ions on the frog's heart. J Physiol (Lond) 142:486, 1958
8. Skou JC: The Na,K-pump. Methods Enzymol 156:1, 1988
9. Pedersen PL, Carafoli E: Ion motive ATPases. Trends Biol Sci 12:146, 1987
10. Lingrel JB, Kuntzweiler T: Na$^+$,K$^+$-ATPase. J Biol Chem 269:19659, 1994
11. Shull GE, Greeb J, Lingrel JB: Molecular cloning of three distinct forms of the Na$^+$,K$^+$-ATPase α-subunit from rat brain. Biochemistry 25:8125, 1986
12. Urayama T, Sweadner KJ: Ouabain sensitivity of the alpha 3 isozyme of rat Na$^+$,K$^+$ATPase. Biochem Biophys Res Commun 156:796, 1988
13. Lemas MV, Hamrick M, Takeyasu K, Fambrough DM: 26 Amino acids of an extracellular domain of the Na,K ATPase alpha-subunit are sufficient for assembly with the Na,K ATPase beta-subunit. J Biol Chem 269:8255, 1994
14. Wallick ET, Schwartz A: Interaction of cardiac glycosides with Na$^+$,K$^+$-ATPase. Methods Enzymol 156:201, 1988
15. Horowitz B, Hensley CB, Quintero M et al: Differential regulation of Na$^+$,K$^+$ ATPase α_1, α_2 and β subunit mRNA and protein levels by thyroid hormone. J Biol Chem 265:14308, 1990
16. Orlowski J, Lingrel JB: Thyroid and glucocorticoid hormone regulate the expression of multiple Na,K-ATPase genes in cultured neonatal rat cardiac myocytes. J Biol Chem 265:3462, 1990
17. Ikeda U, Hyman R, Smith TW, Medford RM: Aldosterone-mediated regulation of Na$^+$,K$^+$ ATPase gene expression in adult and neonatal rat cardiocytes. J Biol Chem 266:12058, 1991
18. Bluschke V, Bonn R, Greefe K: Increase in the (Na$^+$-K$^+$)-ATPase activity in heart muscle after chronic treatment with digitoxin or potassium deficient diet. Eur J Pharmacol 37:189, 1976
19. Brodie C, Sampson SR: Effects of chronic oubain treatment on [^{3}H]ouabain binding sites and electrogenic component of membrane potential in cultured rat myotubes. Brain Res 247:121, 1985
20. Kim D, Marsh JD, Barry WH, Smith TW: Effects of growth in low potassium medium or ouabain on membrane Na,K-ATPase, cation transport, and contractility in cultured chick heart cells. Circ Res 55:39, 1984
21. Rayson BM: Rates of synthesis and degradation of Na$^+$-K$^+$ ATPase during chronic ouabain treatment. Am J Physiol 356:C75, 1989
22. Erdmann E, Werdan K, Krawietz W: Influence of digitalis and diuretics on ouabain binding sites on human erythrocytes. Klin Wochenschr 62:87, 1984
23. Schmidt TA, Holm-Nielsen P, Kjeldsen K: No upregulation of digitalis glycoside receptor (Na,K-ATPase) concentration in human left ventricle samples obtained at necropsy after long term digitalisation. Cardiovasc Res 25:684, 1991
24. Allen PD, Schmidt TA, Marsh JD, Kjeldsen K: Na,K-ATPase expression in normal and failing human left ventricle. Basic Res Cardiol 87:87, 1992
25. Eisner DA, Smith TW: The Na-K pump and its effectors in cardiac muscle. p. 863. In Fozzard HA, Haber E, Katz AM, Morgan HE (eds): The Heart and Cardiovascular System. Lippincott-Raven, Philadelphia, 1992
26. Marban E, Tsien RW: Enhancement of cardiac calcium current during digitalis inotropy. Positive feedback regulation by intracellular calcium. J Physiol (Lond) 329:589, 1982

27. Wier WG, Hess P: Excitation-contraction coupling in cardiac Purkinje fibres. Effects of cardiotonic steroids on the intracellular [Ca^{2+}] transient, membrane potential and contraction. J Gen Physiol 83:395, 1984

28. Morgan JP, Blinks JR: Intracellular Ca^{2+} transients in the cat papillary muscle. Can J Physiol Pharmacol 60:524, 1982

29. Deitmer JW, Ellis D: The intracellular sodium activity of cardiac Purkinje fibres during inhibition and re-activation of the Na-K pump. J Physiol (Lond) 284:241, 1978

30. Eisner DA, Lederer WJ: Does sodium pump inhibition produce the positive inotropic effects of strophanthidin in mammalian cardiac muscle. J Physiol (Lond) 296:75, 1979

31. Im WB, Lee CO: Quantitative relation of twitch and tonic tensions to intracellular Na$^+$ activity in cardiac Purkinje fibres. Am J Physiol 247:C478, 1984

32. Eisner DA, Lederer WJ, Sheu SS: The role of intracellular sodium activity in the action of anti-arrhythmic action of local anesthetics in sheep Purkinje fibres. J Physiol (Lond) 340:163, 1983

33. Lederer WJ, Sheu SS: Heart rate dependent changes in intracellular sodium activity and twitch tension in sheep cardiac Purkinje fibres. J Physiol (Lond) 345:44, 1983

34. Smith TW, Braunwald E, Kelly RA: The management of heart failure. p. 464. In Braunwald E (ed): Heart Disease. A Textbook of Cardiovascular Medicine. WB Saunders, Philadelphia, 1992

35. Studer R, Reinecke H, Bilger J et al: Gene expression of the cardiac Na$^+$-Ca^{2+} exchanger in end-stage human heart failure. Circ Res 75:443, 1994

36. McGarry SJ, Williams AJ: Digoxin activates sarcoplasmic reticulum Ca^{2+} release channels. A possible role in cardiac inotropy. Br J Pharmacol 108:1043, 1993

37. Kim D, Cragoe EJ Jr, Smith TW: Relations among sodium pump inhibition, Na-Ca and Na-H exchange activation, and Ca-H interaction in cultured chick heart cells. Circ Res 60:185, 1987

38. Vatner SF, Higgins CB, Franklin D et al: Effects of a digitalis glycoside on coronary and systemic dynamics in conscious dogs. Circ Res 28:470, 1971

39. Mason DT, Braunwald E, Karash RB, Bullock FA: Sudies on digitalis. X. Effects of ouabain on forearm vascular resistance and venous tone in normal subjects and in patients with heart failure. J Clin Invest 43:532, 1964

40. Ross JJ, Waldhausen JA, Braunwald E: Studies on digitalis. I. Direct effects on peripheral vascular resistance. J Clin Invest 39:930, 1960

41. Lang S, Blaustein MP: The role of the sodium pump in the control of vascular tone in the rat. Circ Res 46:463, 1980

42. Blatt CM, Marsh JD, Smith TW: Extracardiac effects of digitalis. p. 209. In: Digitalis Glycosides. Grune & Stratton, Orlando, 1985

43. Harris AL, Silver PJ, Lemp BM, Evans DB: The vasorelaxant effect of milrinone and other vasodilators are attenuated by ouabain. Eur J Pharmacol 145:133, 1989

44. Jondeau G, Klapholz M, Katz SD et al: Control of arteriolar resistance in heart failure. Partial attenuation of specific phosphodiesterase inhibitor-mediated vasodilation by digitalis glycosides. Circulation 85:54, 1992

45. McLain PL: Effects of cardiac glycosides on spontaneous efferent activity in vagus and sympathetic nerves of cats. Int J Neuropharmacol 8:379, 1969

46. McLain PL: Effects of ouabain on spontaneous afferent activity in the aortic and carotid sinus nerves of cats. Neuropharmacology 9:399, 1970

47. Lathers CM: Effects of timolol on autonomic neural discharge associated with ouabain induced arrhythmia. Eur J Pharmacol 64:95, 1982

48. Gillis RA: Cardiac sympathetic nerve activity. Changes induced by ouabain and propranolol. Science 166:508, 1969

49. Somberg JC, Kuhlman JE, Smith TW: Localization of the neurally mediated coronary vasoconstrictor effect of digoxin. Circ Res 49:226, 1981

50. Somberg JC, Smith TW: Localization of the neurally-mediated arrhythmogenic effects of digitalis. Science 204:321, 1979

51. Kranzhofer R, Haass M, Kurz T et al: Effect of digitalis glycosides on norepinephrine release in the heart. Dual mechanisms of action. Circ Res 68:1628, 1991

52. Sharma VK, Pottick LA, Banerjee SP: Ouabain stimulation of noradrenaline transport in guinea pig heart. Nature 386:817, 1980

53. Quest JA, Gillis RA: Effect of digitalis on carotid sinus baroreceptor activity. Circ Res 35:247, 1974

54. Zucker IH, Peterson TV, Gilmore JP: Ouabain increases left atrial stretch receptor discharge in the dog. J Pharmacol Exp Ther 212:320, 1980

55. Wang W, Chen JS, Zucker IH: Carotid sinus baroreceptor sensitivity in experimental heart failure. Circulation 81:1959, 1991

56. Schmitt G, Guth V, Muller-Limmroth W: Uber die Wirkung von Digitalis und Strophanthin auf die Aktionpotentiale der Chemorezeptoren in Glomus caroticum der Katze. Z Biol 110:316, 1958

57. Schobel HP, Ferguson DW, Clary MP, Somers VK: Differential effects of digitalis on chemoreflex responses in humans. Hypertension 23:302, 1994

58. Alicandri C, Fariello R, Boni E et al: Captopril versus digoxin in mild to moderate chronic heart failure. A crossover study. J Cardiovasc Pharmacol 9:S61, 1987

59. Kaye DM, Lambert GW, Lefkovits J et al: Neurochemical evidence of cardiac sympathetic activation and increased central nervous system norepinephrine turnover in severe congestive heart failure. J Am Coll Cardiol 23:570, 1994

60. Krum H, Bigger JT, Goldsmith RL, Packer M: Effect of long term digoxin therapy on autonomic function in patients with chronic heart failure. J Am Coll Cardiol 25:289, 1995

61. Friedman P: Therapeutic and toxic electrophysiologic effects of cardiac glycosides. p. 29. In: Digitalis Glycosides. Grune & Stratton, Orlando, 1985

62. Carlton RA, Miller PH, Grettinger JS: Effects of ouabain, atropine, and ouabain and atropine on A-V nodal conduction in man. Circ Res 20:283, 1967

63. Kaufman ES, Bosner MS, Bigger JT et al: Effects of digoxin and enalapril on heart period variability and response to head-up tilt in normal subjects. Am J Cardiol 72:95, 1993

64. Ferrier GR: Digitalis arrhythmias. Role of oscillatory afterpotentials. Prog Cardiovasc Dis 19:459, 1997

65. McMichael J, Sharpey-Schafer EP: The action of intravenous digoxin in man. Q J Med 52:123, 1944

66. Lagerlof H, Werko L: Studies on the circulation in man. The effect of cedilanid (lanatoside C) on cardiac output and blood pressure in the pulmonary circulation in patients with compensated and decompensated heart disease. Acta Cardiol 4:1, 1944

67. Braunwald E: Effects of digitalis on the normal and the failing heart. J Am Coll Cardiol 5:51A, 1985

68. Ribner B, Plucinski DA, Hsieh AM et al: Acute effects of digoxin on total systemic vascular resistance in congestive heart failure due to dilated cardiomyopathy. A hemodynamic-hormonal study. Am J Cardiol 56:896, 1985

69. Gheorghiade M, St Clair J, St Clair C, Beller GA: Hemodynamic effects of intravenous digoxin in patients with severe heart failure initially treated with diuretics and vasodilators. J Am Coll Cardiol 9:849, 1987

70. Cohn K, Selzer A, Kersh ES et al: Variability of hemodynamic response to acute digitalization in chronic cardiac failure due to cardiomyopathy and coronary artery disease. Am J Cardiol 31:461, 1975

71. Tisdale JE, Gheorghiade M: Acute hemodynamic effects of digoxin alone or in combination with other vasoactive agents in patients with heart failure. Am J Cardiol 69:34G, 1992

72. Tauke J, Goldstein S, Gheorghiade M: Digoxin for chronic heart failure. A review of the randomized controlled trials with special attention to the PROVED and RADIANCE trials. Prog Cardiovasc Dis 37:49, 1994

73. Gheorghiade M, Hall V, Lakier J, Goldstein S: Comparative hemodynamic and neurohumoral effects of intravenous captopril and digoxin and their combinations in patients with severe heart failure. J Am Coll Cardiol 13:134, 1989

74. Cantelli I, Vitolo A, Lombardi G et al: Combined hemodynamic effects of digoxin and captopril in patients with congestive heart failure. Curr Ther Res 36:323, 1984

75. Raabe DS: Combined therapy with digoxin and nitroprusside in heart failure complicating acute myocardial infarction. Am J Cardiol 43:990, 1979

76. Ribner HS, Zucker MJ, Staisor C et al: Vasodilators as a first-line therapy for congestive heart failure. A comparative hemodynamic study of hydralazine, digoxin and their combination. Am Heart J 114:91, 1987

77. Cantelli I, Pavesi PC, Rarchi C et al: Acute hemodynamic effects of combined therapy with digoxin and nifedipine in patients with chronic heart failure. Am Heart J 106:308, 1983

78. Bonelli J, Jancuska M: Comparison of digoxin and dobutamine in patients with severe dilatative cardiomyopathy. Int J Clin Pharmacol Ther Toxicol 27:120, 1989

79. Cohn J, Levine T, Olivari M et al: Plasma norepinephrine as a guide to prognosis in patients with chronic congestive heart failure. N Engl J Med 311:819, 1984

80. Swedberg K, Eneroth P, Kjekshus J et al: Hormones regulating cardiovascular function in patients with severe congestive heart failure and their relation to mortality. Circulation 82:1730, 1990

81. Kaye DM, Lefkovits J, Jennings G et al: Cardiac norepinephrine spillover as a prognostic marker in severe heart failure. Circulation, suppl. I88:I107, 1993

82. Ferguson DW: Baroreflex-mediated circulatory control in human heart failure. Heart Failure 6:3, 1990

83. Ferguson DW, Berg WJ, Saunders JS et al: Sympathoinhibitory responses to digitalis glycosides in heart failure patients. Circulation 80:65, 1989

84. Goldsmith SR, Simon AB, Miller E: Effect of digitalis on norepinephrine kinetics in congestive heart failure. J Am Coll Cardiol 20:858, 1992

85. Covit AB, Schaer GI, Sealy JE et al: Suppression of the renin-angiotensin system by intravenous digoxin in chronic congestive heart failure. Am J Med 75:445, 1983

86. Dobbs SN, Kenyon WI, Dobbs RJ: Maintenance digoxin after an episode of heart failure. Placebo controlled trial in outpatients. BMJ 1:749, 1977

87. Fleg L, Gottlieb SH, Lakatta EG: Is digoxin really important in compensated heart failure? Am J Med 73:244, 1982

88. Taggart AJ, Johnston GD, McDevitt DG: Digoxin withdrawal after cardiac failure in patients with sinus rhythm. J Cardiovasc Pharmacol 5:229, 1983

89. Lee DCS, Johnson RA, Bingham JB et al: Heart failure in outpatients. A randomized trial of digoxin versus placebo. N Engl J Med 306:699, 1982

90. Guyatt GH, Sullivan MJJ, Fallen EL et al: A controlled trial of digoxin in congestive heart failure. Am J Cardiol 61:371, 1988

91. Haerer W, Bauer U, Hetzel M, Fehske J: Long-term effects of digoxin and diuretics in congestive heart failure. Results of a placebo-controlled randomized double-blind study. Circulation, suppl. II 78:53, 1988

92. Captopril Digoxin Multicenter Research Group: Comparative effects of therapy with captopril and digoxin in patients with mild to moderate heart failure. JAMA 259:539, 1988

93. German and Austrian Xamoterol Study Group: Double-blind placebo-controlled comparison of digoxin and xamoterol in chronic heart failure. Lancet 1:489, 1988

94. DiBianco R, Shabetai R, Kostuk W et al: A comparison of oral milrinone, digoxin, and their combination in the treatment of patients with chronic heart failure. N Engl J Med 320:677, 1989

95. Uretsky BF, Young JB, Shahidis et al: Randomized study assessing the effect of digoxin withdrawal in patients with mild to moderate chronic congestive heart failure. Results of the PROVED trial. J Am Coll Cardiol 22:955, 1993

96. Packer M, Gheorghiade M, Young J et al: Withdrawal of digoxin from patients treated with angiotensin converting enzyme inhibitors. N Engl J Med 329:1, 1993

97. Smith TW: Digoxin in heart failure. N Engl J Med 329:51, 1993

98. Cheesebro JH, Browne KF, Fenster PE, Garland WT, Konstam MA: The hemodynamic effects of chronic oral milrinone therapy. A multicenter controlled trial. J Am Coll Cardiol 11:144A, 1988

99. Packer M, Rouleau J, Swedberg K et al: Effect of flosequinan on survival in chronic heart failure. Preliminary results of the PROFILE study. Circulation, suppl. I 88:301, 1993

100. Kelly RA, Smith TW: Digoxin in heart failure. Implications of recent trials. J Am Coll Cardiol, suppl. A 22:107A, 1993

101. Yusuf S, Garg R, Held P et al: Need for a large trial to evaluate the effects of digitalis on morbidity and mortality in congestive heart failure. Am J Cardiol 69:64G, 1992

102. Results of the Digoxin Investigators Group (DIG) trial. Presented at the 45th Scientific Sessions of the American College of Cardiology, March 26, 1996, Orlando, FL

103. Smith TW: Digitalis Glycosides. Grune & Stratton, Orlando, 1985

104. Greef K, Wirth KE: Pharmocokinetics of Strophanthus glycosides. p. 57. In Greef K (ed): Handbook of Experimental Pharmacology, Springer-Verlag, Berlin, 1981

105. Halkin H, Sheiner LB, Peck CC et al: Determinants of the renal clearance of digoxin. Clin Pharmacol Ther 17:385, 1975

106. Steiness E: Renal tubular secretion of digoxin. Circulation 50:103, 1974

107. Cogan JJ, Humphreys MH, Carlson CJ et al: Acute vasodilator therapy increases renal clearance of digoxin in patients with congestive heart failure. Circulation 64:973, 1981

108. Lindenbaum J, Rund DG, Butler VP: Inactivation of digoxin by the gut flora. Reversal by antibiotic therapy. N Engl J Med 305:789, 1981

109. Rogers MC, Willerson JT, Smith TW: Serum digoxin in the human fetus, neonate, and infant. N Engl J Med 287:1010, 1972

110. Johnson BF, Lindenbaum J, Budnitz E et al: Variability of steady-state digoxin kinetics during administration of tablets or capsules. Clin Pharmacol Ther 39:306, 1986

111. Lewis RP: Clinical use of serum digoxin concentrations. Am J Cardiol 69:97G, 1992

112. Kolibash AJ, Lewis RP, Bourne DW et al: Extension of the serum digoxin concentration-response relationship to patient management. J Clin Pharmacol 29:300, 1989

113. Klausen T, Kjeldsen K, Norgaard A: Effects of denervation on sodium, potassium and [H^3] binding in muscle of normal and potassium depleted rats. J Physiol (Lond) 345:123, 1983

114. Lown B, Klein MD, Barr I et al: Sensitivity to digitalis drugs in acute myocardial infarction. Am J Cardiol 30:388, 1972

115. Reichansky I, Conradson TB, Holmberg S et al: The effect of intravenous digoxin on the occurrence of ventricular tachyarrhythmias in acute myocardial infarction in man. Am Heart J 91:705, 1976

116. Moss AJ, Davis HT, Conard DL et al: Digitalis-associated cardiac mortality after myocardial infarction. Circulation 64:1150, 1981

117. Bigger JT, Fleiss JL, Rolnitzky LM et al: Effect of digitalis on survival after acute myocardial infarction. Am J Cardiol 55:623, 1985

118. Ryan TJ, Bailey KR, McCabe CH et al: The effects of digitalis on survival in high-risk patients with coronary artery disease. Circulation 67:735, 1983

119. Madsen EB, Gilpin E, Henning H et al: Prognostic importance of digitalis after acute myocardial infarction. J Am Coll Cardiol 3:681, 1984

120. Muller JE, Turi ZG, Stone PH et al: Digoxin therapy and mortality after myocardial infarction. Experience in the MILIS study. N Engl J Med 314:265, 1986

121. Vogel R, Kirch D, LeFree M et al: Effects of digitalis on resting and isometric exercise myocardial perfusion in patients with coronary artery disease and left ventricular dysfunction. Circulation 56:355, 1977

122. Rubinow A, Skinner M, Cohen AS: Digoxin sensitivity in amyloid cardiomyopathy. Circulation 63:1285, 1981

123. Antman EM, Wenger TL, Butler VP Jr et al: Treatment of 150 cases of life-threatening digitalis intoxication with digoxin-specific Fab antibody fragements. Final report of a multicenter study. Circulation 81:1744, 1990

124. Woolf AD, Wenger T, Smith TW, Lovejoy FH: The use of digoxin-specific Fab fragments for severe digitalis intoxication in children. N Engl J Med 326:1739, 1992

125. Kelly RA, Smith TW: Recognition and management of digitalis toxicity. Am J Cardiol 69:108G, 1992

126. Kelly RA, Smith TW: The search for the endogenous digitalis. An alternative hypothesis. Am J Physiol 256:C937, 1989

127. Kelly RA, Smith TW: Endogenous cardiac glycosides. Adv Pharmacol 25:263, 1994

128. De Wardener HE, Clarkson EM: Concept of a natriuretic hormone. Physiol Rev 65:658, 1985

129. Huang CT, Cardons N, Michelakis AM: Existence of a new vasoactive factor in experimental hypertension. Am J Physiol 238:E25, 1978

130. Plunkett WC, Hutchins PM, Gruber KA, Buckalew VM: Evidence for a vascular sensitizing factor in the plasma of saline-loaded dogs. Hypertension 4:581, 1982

131. Hamlyn JM, Ringel R, Schaeffer J et al: A circulating inhibitor of ($Na^+ K^+$) ATPase associated with essential hypertension. Nature 300:650, 1982

132. Kelly RA, O'Hara DS, Goldszer RC et al: Endogenous digitalis-like inhibitors from human plasma. p. 649 In: The Sodium Pump. Company of Biologists, Cambridge, 1985

133. Halperin J, Schaeffer R, Galvey L, Malone S: Ouabain-like activity in human cerebrospinal fluid. Proc Natl Acad Sci USA 80:6101, 1983

134. Halperin JA, Martin AM, Malave S: Increased digitalis-like activity in human cerebrospinal fluid after expansion of the extracellular volume. Life Sci 37:561, 1985

135. Smith EKM, Welt LG: The red blood cells as a model for the study of uremic toxins. Arch Intern Med 126:827, 1970

136. Kelly RA, O'Hara DS, Canessa ML, Mitch WE, Smith TW: Characterisation of digitalis-like factors in human plasma. Interactions with NaK-ATPase and crossreactivity with cardiac glycoside-specific antibodies. J Biol Chem 260:11396, 1985

137. Lackner TE, Lau BW, Parvin C, Valdes R: Endogenous digoxin-like immunoreactivity in elderly patients with normal serum creatinine concentrations. Clin Pharmacol 7:449, 1988

138. Gottlieb SS, Rogowski AC, Weinberg M et al: Elevated concentrations of endogenous ouabain in patients with congestive heart failure. Circulation 86:420, 1992

139. Kelly RA, Smith TW: Is ouabain the endogenous digitalis? Circulation 86:694, 1992

140. Lingrel JB, Van Huyse J, O'Brien W et al: Structure function studies of the Na, K/ATPase. Kidney 44:S32, 1994

44 Vasodilator Therapy

Carl V. Leier

This chapter contains information relevant to the use of direct-acting vasodilators during heart failure. Emphasis is placed on the prototypical agents nitrates and hydralazine. Other vasodilating agents, such as calcium channel blockers and sympatholytic drugs, and agents with indirect or secondary vasodilating properties (e.g., angiotensin-converting enzyme inhibitors, digitalis) are discussed elsewhere in this book.

development and success of the angiotensin-converting enzyme (ACE) inhibitors. Hence for heart failure management today, direct-acting vasodilators are best viewed as agents capable of supporting or supplementing other interventions and therapies. Whether direct-acting vasodilation will earn a more prominent role in heart failure therapeutics awaits the development and study of new, tolerable, safe, more effective agents.

INTRODUCTION

In 1956 Burch reported that elevated venous pressure and symptoms of heart failure could be reduced with the sympatholytic agent hexamethonium.[1] About a decade later, Gould et al.[2] published their findings on the favorable hemodynamic and clinical effects of phentolamine, an α-adrenergic blocker, on congestive heart failure. Studies on direct-acting vasodilators for heart failure proliferated during the 1970s and 1980s.

Direct-acting vasodilators have never entered a golden era of heart failure management. The role of vasodilator therapy (e.g., nitroprusside, intravenous nitroglycerin) in acute heart failure was abbreviated by other agents (e.g., dobutamine), mechanical assists (e.g., intraaortic balloon counterpulsation), and aggressive interventional approaches (e.g., angioplasty, cardiac surgery). With chronic heart failure, the growing popularity of long-term hydralazine–nitrate combination therapy during the 1980s after the V-HeFT I trial[3] showed favorable results with this combination on survival, was largely upstaged by the

RATIONALE FOR VASODILATION IN CONGESTIVE HEART FAILURE

Congestive heart failure (CHF) is, in part, characterized by excessively elevated afterload and preload (Fig. 44-1A). Afterload, generally defined for the intact heart as systolic ventricular wall stress, increases during CHF secondary to a rise in aortic impedance, systemic (and pulmonic) vascular resistance, and ventricular chamber size (Laplace effect). Unfortunately, the increase in afterload evokes further deterioration of ventricular function. Preload is the state of diastolic (presystolic) cardiomyocyte stretch; and, as described by the Frank-Starling relation, an increase in myocyte stretch augments the systolic performance (rate and extent) of the subsequent contraction. Although a rise in preload may enhance systolic performance to a certain degree in patients with ventricular dysfunction, this mechanism provides inadequate cardiac compensation for most CHF patients, and thus the ventricle and heart continue to fail during systole despite increasing ventricular filling pressure, diastolic volume, and pre-

A. Effects of elevated afterload and preload on ventricular dysfunction

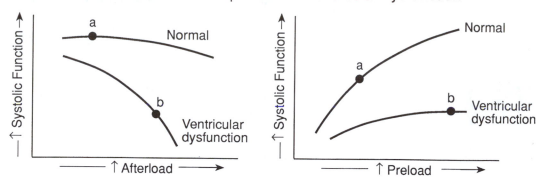

B. Response of the failing ventricle to afterload and preload reducing therapy

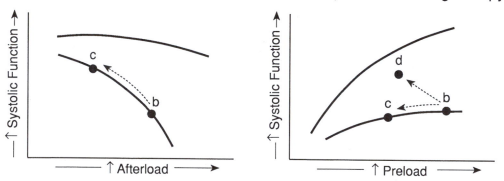

Fig. 44-1. Conceptual relations between ventricular systolic function and the loading conditions, afterload and preload. **(A)** Development of ventricular dysfunction and heart failure causes a downward shift in the afterload–ventricular systolic function curve (*left*) and the preload–ventricular systolic function curve (*right*: Frank-Starling relation). (*Left*) The usual increase in afterload with heart failure causes further deterioration of ventricular systolic function; shift of point *a* in normals to point *b* in patients with ventricular systolic failure and elevated afterload. (*Right*) The downward shift in the preload-ventricular function curve and normal point *a* by ventricular dysfunction (and rise in afterload) is usually accompanied in heart failure by movement to the right, point *b*, via fluid retention and venoconstriction. The movement to point *b* is viewed as an attempt to improve ventricular function by "going up the Frank-Starling curve." For patients with substantial ventricular dysfunction and decompensated heart failure, movement to point *b* results in excessive fluid retention, edema, and "congestion," usually with minimal improvement of ventricular function (flat segment of the depressed curve). **(B)** Ventricular systolic responses to afterload reduction (*left*) and preload reduction (*right*). (*Left*) "Unloading" the failing ventricle of excessive systolic wall stress usually elicits improvement of systolic function (moving *b* to point *c*). (*Right*) Unloading the failing ventricle of excessive preload with preload-reducing agents (e.g., venodilators, diuretics) moves point *b* to *c* and reduces ventricular filling pressures, wall stress, edema, and "congestion." Combined afterload-preload reduction also augments systolic function (point *d*).

load. Fluid retention by the kidneys, venoconstriction and central shifts in blood volume, and the inability of the failing ventricle to eject its contents account for the elevation in ventricular filling pressure, volume, and preload in CHF. The Frank-Starling curve in the presence of severe ventricular dysfunction (and accompanying elevated afterload) is depressed to the point where further increases in ventricular filling pressure, volume, and preload achieve little change in systolic performance; in fact,

any additional fluid retention at this stage simply increases ventricular/venous/capillary pressures to cause pulmonary and peripheral edema and "congestion." The various mechanisms (e.g., activation of the sympathetic nervous system and renin-angiotensin-aldosterone axis) responsible for elevated afterload and preload in CHF and a more detailed discussion of the concepts of afterload and preload in CHF are presented elsewhere in this book.

Vasodilation can improve the abnormal central hemodynamics of CHF by reducing, or "unloading," the excessive afterload and preload afflicting the failing heart (Fig. 44-1B). Direct-acting vasodilators are a means of delivering vasodilatation or afterload and preload reduction to the congested, vasoconstricted heart failure patient. From a historical perspective, the direct-acting vasodilators nitroprusside, organic nitrates, and hydralazine are the agents most responsible for bringing the concepts of afterload and preload reduction into the therapeutics of human heart failure.[4,5] By decreasing an elevated afterload in CHF, the heart responds to vasodilator therapy with an increase in stroke volume and cardiac output and a decrease in systolic wall stress and myocardial oxygen consumption. By reducing elevated ventricular filling pressures and excessive preload, vasodilator therapy (particularly agents with venodilating properties), diuretics, or both reduce venous-capillary pressures, edema, and "congestion."

Table 44-1. Potential Uses and Benefits of Vasodilator Therapy for Heart Failure

Afterload reduction }
Preload reduction } acute or long-term, left and right heart.

Reduction of valvular regurgitation.

As alternative therapy for intolerance to angiotensin-converting enzyme (ACE) inhibitors.

Treatment for concomitant angina pectoris or other symptoms and signs of ischemic heart disease (e.g., nitrates, calcium channel blockers).

Generally promotes a favorable balance of myocardial oxygen supply and demand.

Supplemental agents to other antihypertensive therapy in the control of concomitant systemic hypertension.

As a means of withdrawing patients with severe congestive heart failure (CHF) from infusions of cardiovascular support drugs (e.g., dobutamine, dopamine); notable agent for this purpose is hydralazine.

Reduction or reversal of ventricular hypertrophy, chamber size, and remodeling.

May improve ventricular diastolic function (e.g., nitrates, calcium channel blockers).

Favorable effect on atrial size, function, and rhythms.

Preferential augmentation of regional blood flow (e.g., hydralazine to enhance renal blood flow).

May reduce hospitalization for some CHF patients.

Favorable effect on survival (hydralazine–nitrate combination).

Table 44-2. Potential Disadvantages of Direct-Acting Vasodilators for Heart Failure

Compared to angiotensin-converting enzyme inhibitors, current vasodilating agents used in CHF therapy:
Appear to be less effective in reducing symptoms
Generally evoke more adverse effects (i.e., less well tolerated)
Have less survival benefit

The rise in cardiac output (via afterload reduction) and peripheral vasodilation elicited by direct-acting vasodilators may increase nonnutritive blood flow to peripheral sites and organs greater than any increase in nutritive or effective flow.

Pharmacodynamic tolerance occurs during repeated dosing of certain vasodilating agents (e.g., nitrates).

Direct-acting vasodilating agents can activate or exacerbate neurohormonal systems (e.g., sympathetic nervous system, renin-angiotensin-aldosterone axis).

Certain vasodilators have other pharmacologic properties (e.g., positive inotropy, phosphodiesterase inhibition), which is detrimental in some CHF patients.

The major clinical issues and concerns, potential benefits, and possible disadvantages pertaining to the general use of vasodilators during heart failure are listed in Tables 44-1 and 44-2. These points are self-explanatory, and most are addressed later in the chapter; a few deserve emphasis. The principal clinical applications for the direct-acting vasodilators include (1) substitute therapy for moderate to severe CHF when ACE inhibitors are not tolerated; (2) supplemental therapy when CHF is complicated by uncontrolled hypertension, angina, or CHF symptoms while treated with digitalis, diuretics, and ACE inhibitors; and (3) primary therapy for certain conditions, such as urgent-emergent hypertension, valvular regurgitation, acute cardiogenic pulmonary edema, and dobutamine-dependent CHF. The vasodilator combination hydralazine and isosorbide dinitrate is currently the only therapy other than ACE inhibitors and selected β-blockers to improve survival of CHF patients[3]; however, the vasodilator combination is generally not particularly well tolerated, and its survival benefit is less in magnitude.[6] By reducing afterload, ventricular wall stress, ventricular filling pressures, and occasionally heart rate and coronary resistance, vasodilators generally have a favorable effect on the myocardial oxygen supply–demand balance.

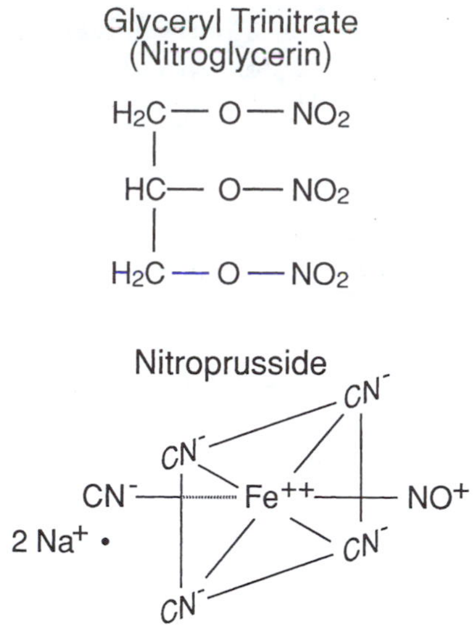

Glyceryl Trinitrate
(Nitroglycerin)

$$H_2C - O - NO_2$$

$$HC - O - NO_2$$

$$H_2C - O - NO_2$$

Nitroprusside

Fig. 44-2. Molecular structures of nitroglycerin and nitroprusside, the agents most commonly used for acute vasodilator therapy.

ACUTE, SHORT-TERM VASODILATOR THERAPY

The most commonly employed agents for acute vasodilator therapy of heart failure are sublingual and intravenous nitroglycerin and intravenous nitroprusside (Fig. 44-2).

Nitroglycerin (Glyceryl Trinitrate)

Through intermediary nitrosothiols, nitroglycerin acts on guanylate cyclase of smooth muscle cells to generate cyclic guanosine monophosphate (cGMP).[7,8] cGMP elicits relaxation of the smooth muscle cells with consequent vasodilation of arterial and venous vasculature. Some of the vasodilation may also be mediated by nitrate-induced prostacyclin and prostaglandin (PG) E production by endothelium.[7,9-11] Nitroglycerin is rapidly cleared (plasma half-life of 1–3 minutes) by vascular extraction, hydrolysis in blood, and hepatic glutathione nitrate reductase.[12-15] Because nitroglycerin undergoes brisk metabolism and clearance, blood levels are directly related to the route and rate of administration.

CLINICAL CARDIOVASCULAR PHARMACOLOGY

Nitrate therapy via sublingual tablet, lingual-buccal spray, or intravenous infusion lowers ventricular filling pressures, diastolic wall stress, and preload

within 3–5 minutes after administration (Fig. 44-3).[12,16-26] Systemic venodilation with a peripheral shift of intracardiac and central venous blood volume is viewed as the predominant preload-reducing mechanism of nitrates. Other properties of nitrates during heart failure likely contribute to its preload-reducing effects and account for additional hemodynamic benefits; by reducing intramyocardial venous pressure and congestion (via lowering right atrial and coronary sinus pressure), augmenting myocardial perfusion and energetics, and perhaps favorably affecting intracellular metabolism (e.g., calcium movement), nitrates may improve ventricular diastolic function and thus further reduce elevated ventricular filling pressures.

Sublingual, lingual-buccal, and intravenous nitrate administration at standard doses also reduces systemic vascular resistance, aortic impedance, and ventricular afterload (Fig. 44-3). During heart failure, this effect results in enhanced ventricular systolic performance and emptying, increased stroke volume and cardiac output, smaller ventricular volumes, and if present a decrease in valvular (aortic or mitral) regurgitation (with further reduction in ventricular filling pressure and volume).[12,16-23,27-29]

The effects of acute nitrate therapy on coronary blood flow and myocardial energetics have not been adequately addressed in human CHF, but it is likely that acute nitrate therapy favorably affects myocardial perfusion and oxygenation and the overall oxygen supply/demand ratio.[17,30-32] By reducing ventricular wall stress and volume, nitrates are capable of decreasing myocardial oxygen consumption; and by reducing the vascular resistance of coronary arteries and lengthening diastolic time, these agents enhance myocardial perfusion. The hemodynamic and clinical improvement noted after acute nitrate therapy in patients with acute heart failure is likely to result, in part, from the favorable energetic profile (myocardium) of nitrates in this clinical setting.

In human CHF, intravenous nitroglycerin decreases limb vascular resistance with augmentation of limb blood flow.[17] Interestingly, renal and hepatosplanchnic vasculature behaves differently. Hepatosplanchnic vascular resistance and blood flow are unaltered, whereas renal vascular resistance may increase modestly or remain unchanged during nitrate infusion in CHF.[17]

CLINICAL INDICATIONS AND APPLICATION

General Indications

Although not heavily supported by large, controlled clinical trials, acute nitrate therapy appears to render clinical or hemodynamic improvement in a num-

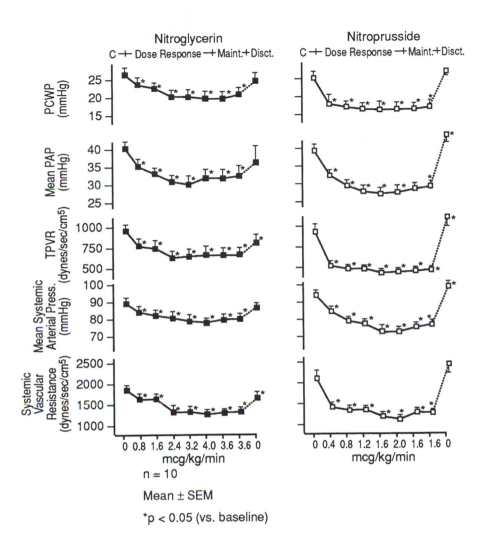

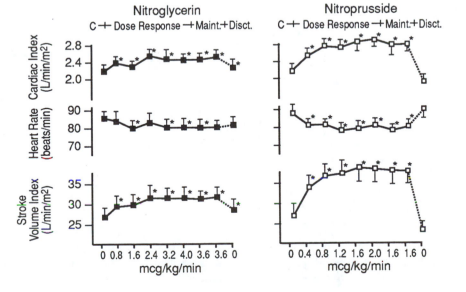

Fig. 44-3. Central hemodynamic responses to infusions of nitroglycerin and nitroprusside in patients with severe congestive heart failure. C, baseline control, PAP, pulmonary artery pressure; PCWP, pulmonary capillary wedge pressure; TPVR, total pulmonary vascular resistance. (Adapted from Leier et al.,[17] with permission.)

ber of heart failure situations and conditions.[17-26] Sublingual (tablet), lingual-buccal (spray), or intravenous nitroglycerin effectively reduces elevated ventricular filling pressures and the congestive symptoms and dyspnea of acute heart failure, cardiogenic pulmonary edema, and severely decompensated chronic CHF. The effects of acute nitrate therapy appear to be most dramatic when these conditions are caused or complicated by occlusive coronary artery disease or ischemic myocardium. I commonly administer sublingual nitroglycerin (one to three tablets over 10–15 minutes) as the initial therapy after diagnosing acute cardiogenic pulmonary edema, such that symptomatic improvement can occur during the institution of other management activities (e.g., attaining venous access, administering a diuretic, obtaining an electrocardiogram). Select chronic CHF patients can be instructed to effectively self-medicate their occasional episode of acute decompensation with nitroglycerin tablets or spray; this form of intervention can often avert another visit to the emergency room (and subsequent hospitalization) and replaces the visit with telephone or outpatient clinic management or, at least, makes the trip and visit to the emergency room a more comfortable one. Lastly, intravenous nitroglycerin can be added to other cardioactive support therapy (e.g., dobutamine or dopamine) if additional preload-afterload reduction or myocardial antiischemic effects are needed over the short term (generally less than 48 hours).

Administration

Nitroglycerin tablets are administered sublingually in 0.3–0.6 mg doses every 3–10 minutes (up to 3 or 4 doses) as needed to reduce the moderate to severe resting dyspnea of acute heart failure. Lingual-buccal spray can be employed in a similar fashion. The onset of action ranges from 3 to 6 minutes, and the effects can persist 15–30 minutes.

Intravenously administered nitroglycerin is usually started at a low dose (e.g., 0.2 $\mu g \cdot kg^{-1} \cdot min^{-1}$) and increased as needed to attain the desired hemodynamic or clinical endpoints. Hemodynamic responses are seen by 3–5 minutes and plateau at 10–15 minutes during a continuous infusion. If administered over a number of hours, the infusion rate may have to be increased to overcome the development of pharmacodynamic tolerance.

Potential Undesirable Effects

Compared to most other cardiovascular support drugs, nitrates are relatively safe to use. Symptoms related to arterial vasodilation (e.g., flushing, head-ache, systemic hypotension) are the most prominent and, if problematic, can be reduced or eliminated by simply decreasing the dose. In contrast to nitroprusside, a fall in systemic arterial oxygen saturation during the infusion and rebound hemodynamic deterioration after withdrawal are uncommon for nitrates.[17] Although infrequent, mild methemoglobinemia can develop during prolonged, high dose infusions of nitroglycerin.[33-35]

Some CHF patients experience no hemodynamic changes after standard acute nitrate dosing (pharmacodynamic resistance).[36] Although the mechanism(s) for this drug resistance is not well delineated, it is most commonly associated with high right atrial pressures and marked peripheral edema. Diuretic therapy can reverse the pharmacodynamic resistance to acute nitrate therapy.

Pharmacodynamic tolerance (loss of drug response during continued administration) is a relatively constant feature of continuous (i.e., uninterrupted) nitrate therapy and can occur as early as 4–8 hours after initiating a nitroglycerin infusion.[17,37,38] Reasonable approaches to this clinical problem for acute nitrate therapy include treating any fluid volume retention (diuretics), keeping the infusion short term (less than 72 hours), and advancing the infusion rates as needed over the short-term treatment period. Tolerance is usually not encountered during sublingual or lingual-buccal administration.

Nitroprusside

The structure of sodium nitroprusside is presented in Figure 44-2. Nitroprusside delivers its smooth muscle relaxation effects through the generation of nitric oxide and nitrosothiols, which stimulate guanylate cyclase to increase intracellular cGMP.[7,8] Its powerful vasodilating properties are apparent as early as 60–90 seconds after administration and dissipate for the most part within 20–30 minutes following discontinuation.[17,39,40] Sodium nitroprusside is converted to cyanide in blood, vascular tissue, and the liver.[40] The circulating cyanide is promptly metabolized by the liver to thiocyanate and prussic acid, averting cyanide toxicity in most nitroprusside-treated patients. Prussic acid has a particular affinity for methemoglobin. Because of its long half-life (3–4 days via renal clearance), thiocyanate can accumulate and occasionally evoke thiocyanate toxicity, particularly in patients with renal dysfunction or during a prolonged nitroprusside infusion at a high dose.

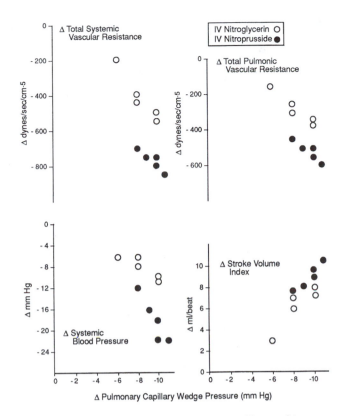

Fig. 44-4. Comparative hemodynamic effects of intravenously administered nitroglycerin and nitroprusside in severe heart failure. For any reduction in left ventricular filling pressure (estimated by pulmonary capillary wedge pressure), nitroprusside elicits a greater drop in systemic and pulmonic vascular resistances. (Adapted from Haas and Leier,[41] with permission.)

CLINICAL CARDIOVASCULAR PHARMACOLOGY

The central hemodynamic effects, mediated by nitroprusside's rather powerful preload- and afterload-reducing properties, are illustrated in Figure 44-3. As noted in Figures 44-3 and 44-4, nitroprusside has a far more aggressive arterial/arteriolar-dilating profile than that of intravenously administered nitroglycerin.[17,41]

Several mechanisms contribute to the nitroprusside-induced fall in ventricular filling pressure and preload during heart failure. Foremost is its ability, via vasodilation, to shift the expanded central blood volume to the periphery. The decreased afterload promotes ventricular systolic emptying and decreases valvular regurgitation with consequent reduction in ventricular diastolic pressure and volume. In patients with severe CHF, nitroprusside may enhance renal blood flow and elicit a mild diuresis and drop in intravascular volume.[42] The decrease in cardiac volume, particularly as confined to the limited

pericardial space, accounts for most of the fall in ventricular filling pressures; and nitroprusside may favorably affect overall ventricular diastolic function.[43,44]

Afterload reduction accounts for most of the improvement in ventricular systolic performance to nitroprusside in patients with severe CHF (Fig. 44-1). As such, with proper dosing, clinically significant systemic hypotension is averted through the augmentation of stroke volume, cardiac output, and perhaps baroreceptor function.[17,19,39,45,46] The nitroprusside-induced fall in ventricular afterload is secondary to its vigorous systemic arteriolar dilating properties, but its ability to improve other components of aortic impedance (e.g., decreased aortic wave reflectance and increased aortic compliance) and reduce ventricular volumes likely contribute as well.[47-49]

With human CHF, standard dosing of nitroprusside decreases limb vascular resistance with a consequent rise in limb blood flow.[17] Renal vascular resistance decreases as well, but the response in renal blood flow depends considerably on concomitant changes in systemic blood pressure; a modest to no reduction in systemic (renal) arterial pressure is usually accompanied by increased flow, whereas a greater fall in pressure evokes little to no augmentation of renal flow.[17,42,50] Hepatosplanchnic vascular resistance and blood flow are not altered significantly with standard doses of nitroprusside for human CHF.[17]

Nitroprusside can alter myocardial energetics and perfusion in a number of ways. With human CHF, proper dosing of nitroprusside reduces myocardial oxygen consumption, its indirect measurement parameters (e.g., double or triple product, systolic stress–time integral), and its determinants by reducing systolic (and diastolic) wall stress.[17,39,43-49,51-55] However, in the presence of inadequate ventricular filling pressures, refractory marked ventricular dysfunction, or excessive dosing, nitroprusside can adversely affect myocardial perfusion and energetics by reducing coronary perfusion pressure, increasing the heart rate (which increases oxygen consumption and decreases diastolic coronary perfusion time), and reflexly exacerbating sympathetic nervous system tone and renin-angiotensin release. Unless heart rate is altered, nitroprusside has little overall effect on diastolic coronary perfusion time.[56] In contrast to nitroglycerin, nitroprusside has the potential to adversely affect regions of myocardial ischemia through a "coronary steal" mechanism; its powerful arteriolar dilating properties may divert blood from ischemic or marginal regions to nonthreatened, already well perfused areas. Early studies suggest that this consideration is indeed relevant to human conditions caused or complicated by myocardial ischemia.[57,58] Elevated methemoglobin levels generated by prolonged high infusion rates or renal dysfunction could adversely affect myocardial oxygenation as well.[40]

GENERAL INDICATIONS AND APPLICATION

Indications

Nitroprusside is one of the most powerful, easily managed vasodilators available for use in humans. However, because of its rather aggressive vasodilating effects and compared to nitroglycerin its high side effect profile and potentially greater propensity to adversely affect myocardial perfusion and energetics, nitroprusside is reserved for patients whose hemodynamic status is severely and acutely compromised; typically, it is these conditions for which acute nitrate therapy provides inadequate afterload-preload reduction. Conditions for which nitroprusside offers the optimal short-term afterload-preload reduction until more definitive intervention (e.g., valvular surgery) is instituted are (1) acute myocardial infarction and severe heart failure complicated by uncontrolled accelerated or malignant hypertension, marked mitral valvular regurgitation (e.g., ischemic or ruptured papillary muscle), ruptured interventricular septum, or a large infarction with decompensated hemodynamics not responsive to acute nitrate therapy; and (2) acute volume- or pressure-overload heart failure secondary to a variety of conditions, many catastrophic (e.g., acute aortic or mitral valvular regurgitation, uncontrolled hypertensive heart failure). Nitroprusside is often employed to augment, via afterload-preload reduction, the cardiovascular and hemodynamic properties of other modalities (e.g., dobutamine or dopamine infusions).[59-61] Once again, nitroprusside is best viewed currently as short-term, powerful vasodilator support until a mechanical assist (e.g., intraaortic balloon counterpulsation) and definitive intervention (e.g., emergent coronary bypass or valvular surgery) are instituted.

Nitroprusside may have a role, albeit limited, in the management of chronic CHF. Stevenson et al.[62] employed this agent to hemodynamically and clinically stabilize patients with advanced severe CHF and determine their optimal level of response to vasodilation, which was then targeted with orally administered vasodilators. Nitroprusside has also been employed to assess the reversibility of elevated pulmonary vascular resistance and pulmonary hypertension for evaluation of a patient's candidacy for heart transplantation.

Administration

Nitroprusside is usually started at 0.1–0.3 $\mu g \cdot kg^{-1} \cdot min^{-1}$ and advanced as needed to safely achieve the usual clinical and hemodynamic endpoints (decreased systemic and pulmonic vascular resistances, decreased ventricular filling pressures, increased systemic perfusion, and decreased symptoms) without provoking significant hypotension or reflex tachycardia.

Precautions and Potential Undesirable Effects

Hypotension is the most common adverse effect of nitroprusside administration and is generally secondary to excessive dosing, inadequate ventricular filling pressure, or insufficient ventricular systolic function and reserve. The hypotension, if severe or prolonged, can evoke hypoperfusion and dysfunction of an organ system (e.g., prerenal azotemia).[63] Nitroprusside can exacerbate myocardial ischemia via a fall in coronary perfusion pressure, reflex tachycardia, "coronary steal" (see above), occasional mild arterial desaturation, and a rise in methemoglobinemia. In general, hypotension, organ hypoperfusion, and myocardial ischemia are uncommon with proper patient and dose selection.

Abrupt discontinuation of nitroprusside can elicit "rebound" hemodynamic and clinical deterioration.[64] Measures employed to avert this threatening situation include more gradual withdrawal, conversion to intravenous nitroglycerin, or the addition of certain agents with vasodilating properties (e.g., ACE inhibitors, sympatholytic agents).

Thiocyanate and cyanide toxicities (including death) are rare during standard short-term dosing ($\leq 3 \ \mu g \cdot kg^{-1} \cdot min^{-1}$ for less than 72 hours).[40,65,66] Renal dysfunction and prolonged, high dose infusions increase the likelihood of these complications. An occasional patient experiences some systemic arterial desaturation during nitroprusside secondary to exacerbation of a pulmonic ventilation–perfusion mismatch.[67-69] Although rather uncommon, nitroprusside has been associated with a fall in platelet number and function.[70]

LONG-TERM VASODILATOR THERAPY

Except for certain clinical situations (e.g., CHF complicated by valvular regurgitation, intolerance to ACE inhibitors), vasodilator drugs are not generally regarded as first-line therapy for long-term management of CHF. At the present time, the vasodilators most commonly selected for chronic use in CHF patients are nitrates and hydralazine.

Nitrate Preparations

The oral and transdermal nitrate preparations are more appropriately directed at long-term management of CHF.[71–82] In contrast to the intravenous and sublingual preparations, the oral and transdermal nitrates evoke only mild afterload reduction unless relatively high doses are employed. Therefore their role in long-term CHF therapy is to supplement other preload reduction therapy or to ameliorate a patient's complicating problems (e.g., angina).

The basic pharmacology of nitroglycerin was presented earlier in the chapter; its molecular structure shown in Figure 44-2. Isosorbide dinitrate and mononitrate are shown in Figure 44-5. Isosorbide dinitrate is readily absorbed by the gastrointestinal tract but is subject to first-pass metabolism by the liver with an overall bioavailability of 20–25 percent. The terminal (second compartment) half-life of the oral preparation is about 4 hours. Isosorbide dinitrate is metabolized by the liver to isosorbide 2- or 5-mononitrate, both with vasodilating properties and half-lives of 2–3 and 4–6 hours respectively. The largest portion of the biologic activity of isosorbide dinitrate is thought to be mediated by its 5-mononitrate metabolite. Isosorbide 5-mononitrate is now available as an oral preparation. It is well absorbed (nearly 100 percent), not affected by hepatic first-pass extraction, and minimally (less than 10 percent) protein-bound. It is metabolized by denitration in serum to inactive isosorbide and mononitrate glucuronide.

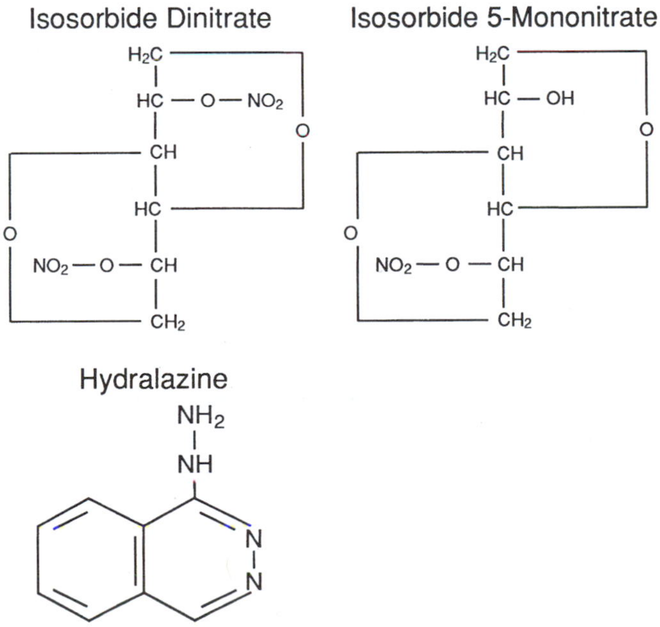

CLINICAL CARDIOVASCULAR PHARMACOLOGY

Standard doses of transdermal nitroglycerin and orally administered nitrates (e.g., isosorbide dinitrate or mononitrate) decrease mean atrial and ventricular filling pressures, with more modest effects on vascular resistances and ventricular afterload. This response is likely mediated through venodilation, but improvement of ventricular diastolic function is a contributory factor for some CHF patients.[71–76,78–82] Higher doses (e.g., isosorbide dinitrate at $\geq$ 40 mg PO) can elicit enough of a reduction in vascular resistance and afterload to generate a clinically significant rise in stroke volume and cardiac output.[80] For "more balanced" long-term preload and afterload reduction, the nitrate preparations are combined with other vasodilators (e.g., hydralazine).[3,83,84]

Nitrates have a favorable pharmacologic profile relative to myocardial perfusion and energetics. By reducing ventricular wall stress, nitrates lower myocardial oxygen demand; and by decreasing ventricular filling pressure more than aortic diastolic pressure, nitrates can increase coronary perfusion pressure. Although nitrates also have favorable coronary vasodilating properties, their net effect on coronary blood flow is modulated by the myocardial oxygen demand.[72]

Long-term administration of combination isosorbide dinitrate–hydralazine improves survival of patients with chronic CHF.[3] In fact, the first demonstration of any therapy reducing mortality in chronic CHF was rendered through the isosorbide dinitrate–hydralazine combination (V-HeFT I trial).[3] Whether this survival benefit is mediated through the nitrate or hydralazine has not yet been determined; the favorable effects of nitrates on myocardial energetics, and perhaps ventricular remodeling[85] and dysrhythmias,[86] make this drug group a reasonable contender.

CLINICAL INDICATIONS AND APPLICATIONS

Clinical Indications

Although nitrates have not been approved for CHF by the U.S. Food and Drug Administration (FDA), available data suggest that nitrates may be useful in a number of CHF scenarios. CHF complicated or

Fig. 44-5. Molecular structures of the vasodilators most commonly employed for chronic management of CHF. Nitroglycerin is shown in Figure 44-2.

exacerbated by episodic myocardial ischemia, angina, or angina-equivalent symptoms may respond favorably to nitrate therapy. The clinical and laboratory manifestations of diastolic dysfunction, particularly if caused by myocardial ischemia, may improve during nitrate therapy.[21,27,76] For CHF patients who cannot tolerate ACE inhibitors, long-term nitrate–hydralazine combination therapy should be considered part of the therapeutic plan to improve survival.[3] Long-term nitrate therapy may also be considered during the postinfarction period to reduce detrimental ventricular remodeling and the development of CHF in postinfarct patients who cannot tolerate ACE inhibitors,[85] although this specific application requires further study and documentation in humans.

Administration

The usual doses for CHF range from 0.5 to 2.0 inches of 2 percent nitroglycerin ointment, 20–60 mg of isosorbide dinitrate, and 10–30 mg of isosorbide 5-mononitrate. Pharmacodynamic tolerance, the bane of chronic nitrate therapy, has necessitated modifications in the dosing schedule. Continued effectiveness requires interrupted or delayed dosing; for example, nitroglycerin ointment is most effective as a morning dose with another dose 8 hours later followed by a 16 hour dosing gap (4–8 hours of which is drug-free). Isosorbide dinitrate can be administered every 8 hours, tid (8 hour dosing gap), and every 6 hours but holding one dose (essentially tid). For many CHF patients, the problem of pharmacodynamic tolerance has promoted the application of time- or activity-targeted dosing. For example, chronic nitrate therapy for patients who are most symptomatic during the day should be interrupted or delayed during nighttime hours, and the opposite is proposed for the patient most troubled with paroxysmal nocturnal dyspnea and orthopnea.

Potential Undesirable Effects

Similar to the intravenous preparations, most side effects are related to vasoactivity; headaches, flushing, dizziness and hypotension are the most common adverse events and are usually best approached by downward dose adjustment. In my clinical experience, blurred vision and diarrhea are not uncommon during chronic nitrate therapy.[87]

Patients with elevated right heart (right atrial and central venous) pressures are most susceptible to pharmacodynamic resistance (lack of response) to nitrates.[36,88] Measures that reduce intravascular volume and right heart pressures (e.g., diuretics) can reestablish responsiveness to nitrates.

Pharmacodynamic tolerance (loss of drug response or effect with continuous or uninterrupted repeated dosing) is a major problem for chronic nitrate therapy, requiring the aforementioned modifications in dosing schedule to maintain effectiveness.[89–95] Basically, tolerance develops within a few hours of a rising or persistently elevated blood nitrate level. The mechanisms for this phenomenon have not been fully elucidated, although tolerance can be reversed by allowing blood nitrate levels to return toward baseline or to fall substantially. Other pharmacologic strategies (e.g., sulfhydryl donors) to eradicate nitrate tolerance have not yet produced consistent results or found their way into clinical relevance or practice.[89–95]

Hydralazine, Congeners, and the Hydralazine–Nitrate Combination

Although the cellular mechanisms of hydralazine are poorly understood, it is regarded as the prototypical direct-acting vasodilator. The molecular structure is depicted in Figure 44-5. Hydralazine is readily absorbed from the gastrointestinal tract, with peak plasma concentrations occurring at 30–60 minutes. Bioavailability is reduced to 10–30 percent because of first-pass extraction by the liver; 90 percent of circulating hydralazine is protein-bound. Eighty to ninety percent of administered hydralazine is eventually cleared and metabolized by the liver. The elimination half-life ranges from 0.5 to 2.0 hours and is prolonged in "slow acetylator" patients. Hydralazine pharmacokinetics do not appear to be substantially altered by CHF[96]; however, the results of these studies in human CHF have not been uniformly confirmatory.[97]

CLINICAL CARDIOVASCULAR PHARMACOLOGY

At the time the vasodilator concept gained attention as a management approach to CHF (middle to late 1970s), hydralazine had already earned a role as a vasodilator to treat systemic hypertension. It is therefore not surprising that hydralazine became one of the earliest orally administered vasodilating agents studied in human CHF.[83,84,98–104] In this clinical setting, hemodynamic studies consistently demonstrated that hydralazine reduces systemic and pulmonary vascular resistances and increases stroke volume and cardiac output (Fig. 44-6). The rise in stroke volume and cardiac output is largely secondary to "unloading" the failing ventricle of elevated afterload, but a reduction in mitral regurgitation and

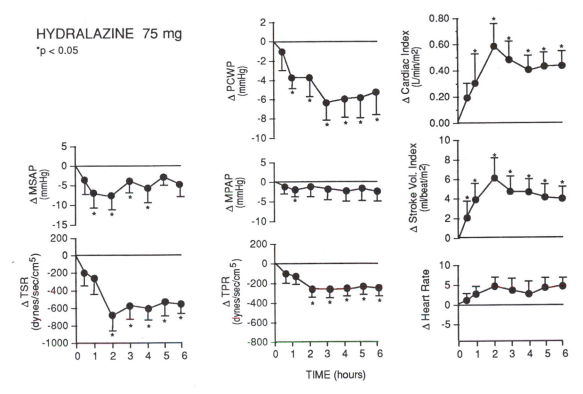

Fig. 44-6. Central hemodynamic effects of hydralazine in severe congestive heart failure ($n = 7$). The data are presented as mean change (Δ) from baseline ± standard error. MPAP, mean pulmonary artery pressure; MSAP, mean systemic arterial pressure; PCWP, mean pulmonary capillary wedge pressure; TPR, total pulmonary vascular resistance; TSR total systemic vascular resistance; Vol, volume. (Adapted from Leier et al.,[84] with permission.)

a mild positive inotropic effect may also contribute to the improvement in systolic performance.[104] Hydralazine can also lower ventricular filling pressures during CHF, probably via decreases in ventricular afterload and mitral regurgitation, because its venodilating effects are generally believed to be modest. As noted, hydralazine enhances the positive inotropic state of the ventricle,[104] an action that appears to be mediated through reflex activation of sympathetic tone and direct stimulation of myocytes.[105–107] These same mechanisms probably account for the disparate responses of aortic and conduit arteries versus systemic arterioles following hydralazine administration. The arteriolar-dilating effects of hydralazine in CHF are often accompanied by little change in characteristic aortic impedance and little change or a fall in aortic compliance.[108]

The central hemodynamic effects of the congeners dihydralazine and endralazine are generally comparable to those of hydralazine.[109,110] The addition of a nitrate preparation to hydralazine effects a greater reduction in ventricular filling pressures than those attained by hydralazine alone.[79,83,84,111,112]

In CHF, hydralazine reduces limb vascular resistance and increases overall limb blood flow propor-

tional to the increase in cardiac output.[84,102] The increase in limb flow, however, is not necessarily directed to "nutritive" vascular-capillary beds.[113,114] Similarly, renal vascular resistance decreases and renal blood flow increases following hydralazine, generally with little change or a modest improvement in renal function.[84,102,115–117] Hepatosplanchnic blood flow tends to rise with hydralazine in CHF, but the increase is proportionately less than that of concomitantly measured cardiac output.[102] The regional blood flow profile of the hydralazine–nitrate combination is similar to that just described for hydralazine alone.[84]

Most vasodilating agents decrease myocardial oxygen consumption in CHF. In contrast, hydralazine generally increases myocardial oxygen consumption, presumably because its positive inotropic properties and its tendency to augment heart rate and sympathetic nervous system tone exceed the beneficial energy-saving reduction in ventricular wall stress.[104,118–120] For CHF patients with normal coronary arteries, hydralazine effects an increase in coronary blood flow equal to or greater than the rise in myocardial oxygen demand.[119,120] For patients with occlusive coronary disease, coronary flow may not be able to match the increase in myocardial oxygen requirements. This circumstance is yet another reason to add a nitrate preparation to hydralazine when employed in the management of CHF.

CLINICAL INDICATIONS AND APPLICATION

Hydralazine as the Sole Vasodilator

Studies examining the effectiveness of chronic hydralazine therapy in CHF have been inadequate in study design (e.g., uncontrolled) or population size to confidently propose a definitive conclusion.[121–124] Nevertheless, hydralazine appears, from my experience, to be clinically effective as a sole vasodilator in several CHF-related scenarios. First, hydralazine via afterload reduction can effectively decrease the hemodynamic severity and clinical manifestations of aortic and mitral valvar regurgitation.[29,125–128] Second, hydralazine is one of the vasodilating agents employed for "tailored" vasodilator therapy to attain optimal hemodynamic augmentation and clinical improvement in patients with severe advanced CHF.[62,128] Finally, hydralazine is currently the most effective, orally administrable agent to improve and stabilize the typically tenuous clinical and hemodynamic status of the severe CHF patient during the withdrawal of intravenously administered cardiovascular support drugs (e.g., dobutamine, dopamine).[129] In this particular clinical setting, hypotension, systemic hypoperfusion, and cardiogenic near-shock/shock commonly threaten the smooth withdrawal of dobutamine or dopamine; with proper administration during the withdrawal phase, hydralazine generally maintains a reasonably stable hemodynamic status and, interestingly, often increases systemic blood pressure despite its vasodilating properties.[129] This beneficial response is likely mediated in this particular setting by hydralazine-induced positive inotropy and reversal of valvular regurgitation.

Although not yet adequately studied, the hydralazine congeners are likely to have similar clinical applications.[109,110,130]

Hydralazine–Nitrate Combination

The hydralazine–nitrate combination is often employed for the aforementioned conditions responsive to hydralazine alone. When feasible, it is reasonable to add a nitrate preparation to hydralazine therapy in patients with severe or symptomatic occlusive coronary artery disease.[131] In addition, the hydralazine–nitrate combination should be considered for its survival benefit in all symptomatic, systolic-dysfunc-

tion CHF patients who cannot tolerate ACE inhibitor therapy.[3] For most CHF patients, ACE inhibitors are preferred over the hydralazine–nitrate combination because of better tolerability and survival effects (V-HeFT II trial).[6] Albeit modest, chronic hydralazine–nitrate therapy was shown, in the same study, to improve exercise capacity compared to baseline and chronic ACE inhibitor therapy.[6]

Administration

With a generally accepted approach of starting at a low dose and advancing the dose as needed to attain the optimally tolerated and effective clinical endpoint(s), the usual chronic oral dose for hydralazine ranges from 50 to 150 mg q6–8h. Concomitantly administered nitrates may include isosorbide dinitrate (e.g., Isordil Tetradose) 20–60 mg q8h or q6h, perhaps withholding one dose daily to avert the possibility of tolerance; 2 percent nitroglycerin ointment at 0.5–2.0 inches q8h or q6h, withholding one dose; or isosorbide 5-mononitrate at 10–30 mg bid (i.e., q8h, withholding one dose).

When applied to the withdrawal of dobutamine (or dopamine) from patients with severe, dobutamine-dependent CHF, hydralazine is usually started as the sole unloading agent at an oral dose of 25 mg q6h and advanced every 6–12 hours as dobutamine is being gradually withdrawn.[129] Once dobutamine is fully withdrawn and the patient is reasonably stable (typically on hydralazine, a diuretic and digitalis) nitrates or an ACE inhibitor can then be added at a low dose and advanced as tolerated and needed.

Potentially Undesirable Effects

The spectrum and frequency of side effects of hydralazine are greater than those of most other CHF therapies. Problems related to vasoactive properties such as headaches, flushing, hypotension, and reflex tachycardia are not uncommon and are usually approached by measures directed at maintaining an adequate intravascular volume or by downward adjustment of dose. Gastrointestinal symptoms (e.g., nausea, abdominal discomfort, dysgeusia, diarrhea) are not uncommon and occur anytime during the course of therapy. Because of its positive inotropic properties and potential for evoking systemic hypotension and reflex tachycardia, hydralazine must be used with caution as the sole vasodilator in patients with extensive occlusive coronary artery disease; it is clinically reasonable to add a nitrate preparation in this setting. Arthralgia and other lupus-like symptoms are relatively uncommon (1–4 percent of patients) side effects of hydralazine therapy in CHF, even with the repeated high doses often employed.

Although the side effects of chronic nitrate dosing must be considered part of the adverse effect profile during long-term hydralazine–nitrate therapy, most of the undesirable events appear to be secondary to the hydralazine; obviously, it depends considerably on the doses of each drug used in the combination. Of 186 CHF patients receiving the hydralazine–isosorbide dinitrate combination in the V-HeFT I trial, 36 (about 19 percent) experienced side effects compared to 11 of 273 (4 percent) patients treated with placebo.[3] Headache and dizziness were the most common drug-induced complaints, present in all 36 (19 percent) of the hydralazine–nitrate group. Seven (4 percent) noted gastrointestinal symptoms and six (3 percent) experienced arthralgia or other rheumatoid or lupus-like symptoms.[3] Most of the adverse effects experienced by CHF patients treated with the hydralazine–nitrate combination (target daily dose of 300 mg for hydralazine and 160 mg for isosorbide dinitrate) in the V-HeFT II trial abated by simply reducing the dose.[6] This treatment limb accounted for headaches in 21 percent, excessive fatigue in 16 percent, nausea in 10 percent, arthralgia in 6 percent, palpitations in 5 percent, and symptomatic hypotension, nasal congestion, rash, and dysgeusia in 3–4 percent each.[6]

Other Considerations

MINOXIDIL

The clinical cardiovascular pharmacology of minoxidil, a direct-acting arterial/arteriolar vasodilator, is remarkably similar to that of hydralazine.[132–136] Hence, this antihypertensive agent was studied in CHF patients by Franciosa and colleagues,[137] employing a blinded, randomized placebo-controlled trial covering 3 months of therapy. With the exception of ejection fraction, which rose from 26.6 ± 17.7 percent to 42.7 ± 22.3 percent, all other clinical and laboratory parameters showed either no change or frank deterioration during minoxidil treatment compared to placebo; these parameters included clinical symptoms and signs of CHF, diuretic requirements, exercise capacity, and maximal oxygen consumption.[137] Minoxidil also appears to augment undesirable neurohormonal responses and levels (plasma renin activity and norepinephrine) in CHF.[136]

FLOSEQUINAN

A quinoline molecule, flosequinan dilates arterial/arteriolar and venous vasculature and appears to have modest positive inotropic and chronotropic properties.[138–140] Its early appeal resided in the fact that its venodilating effects gave, in contrast to those of hydralazine, a more "balanced" reduction of both preload and afterload. Hemodynamic studies in human CHF indicated that the responses to flosequinan are similar to combination hydralazine–nitrates[141–143]; and blinded, controlled trials showed that flosequinan generally improved symptoms and augmented exercise performance (exercise duration, maximal oxygen consumption, and anaerobic threshold).[144–147] These beneficial effects occurred irrespective of whether patients were concomitantly taking an ACE inhibitor. Unfortunately, a large multicenter trial (PROFILE) comparing the survival of CHF patients on standard CHF therapy treated long term with flosequinan 75 or 100 mg or with placebo showed that flosequinan at 100 mg caused a significant increase in mortality.[148] Shortly thereafter, the drug was withdrawn from further clinical investigation in humans. Whether the mild positive chronotropic or inotropic effects, modest phosphodiesterase inhibiting properties, nonideal neurohormonal profile, or potential arrhythmogenicity of flosequinan provoked this undesirable result remains conjecture.

ENDOGENOUS VASODILATION

The generally modest impact of formulated synthetic vasodilating molecules (e.g., hydralazine, flosequinan) on the clinical course of heart failure and the recent unfolding of the many mysteries of cell biology have directed the focus of "vasodilators for heart failure" toward endogenous vascular substances and mechanisms; basically, strategies are being developed to increase the levels of circulating vasodilating substances, augment vasoreactivity to endogenous or administered vasodilators, or block the influence of endogenous vasoconstrictors. Continuous, prolonged infusions of prostacyclin (epoprostenol) for severe CHF elicit favorable central hemodynamic responses and augment exercise capacity; however, the enthusiasm for this approach has been tempered by an undesirable effect on survival.[149] Preliminary reports suggest that endopeptidase inhibitors may be effective in the management of CHF by elevating circulating atrial natriuretic peptide.[150–152] Vascular responsiveness to endogenous and exogenous vasodilating substances, known to be impaired in CHF, may improve with low dose nitrate therapy via augmentation of endothelium-dependent vasodilation.[153] Blockade of the powerful endogenous vasoconstricting substances angiotensin II and endothelin, also holds promise for the future management of CHF.[154,155]

REFERENCES

1. Burch GE: Evidence for increased venous tone in chronic congestive heart failure. Arch Intern Med 1956;98:750–766

2. Gould L, Zahir M, Ettinger S: Phentolamine and cardiovascular performance. Br Heart J 1969;31:154–162

3. Cohn JN, Archibald DG, Ziesche S et al: Effect of vasodilator therapy on mortality in chronic congestive heart failure. Results of a Veterans Administration Cooperative Study. N Engl J Med 1986;314:1547–1552

4. Franciosa JA, Guiha NH, Limas CJ, Rodriguera E, Cohn JN: Improved ventricular function during nitroprusside infusion in acute myocardial infarction. Lancet 1972;1:650–654

5. Cohn JN, Franciosa JA: Vasodilator therapy of cardiac failure. N Engl J Med 1977;297:27–31, 254–258

6. Cohn JN, Johnson G, Ziesche S et al: A comparison of enalapril with hydralazine-isosorbide dinitrate in the treatment of chronic congestive heart failure. N Engl J Med 1991;325:303–310

7. Tsai SC, Adamik R, Manganiello VC, Moss J: Effects of nitroprusside and nitroglycerin on cGMP content and PGI$_2$ formation in aorta and vena cava. Biochem Pharmacol 1989;38:61–65

8. Ignarro LJ, Lippton H, Edwards JC et al: Mechanism of vascular smooth muscle relaxation by organic nitrates, nitrites, nitroprusside and nitric oxide. Evidence for the involvement of S-nitrosothiols as active intermediates. J Pharmacol Exp Ther 1981;218:739–749

9. Morcillio E, Reid PR, Dubin N, Ghodgaonkar R, Pitt B: Myocardial prostaglandin E release by nitroglycerin and modification by indomethacin. Am J Cardiol 1980;45:53–57

10. Levin RI, Jaffe EA, Weksler BB, Tack-Goldman K: Nitroglycerin stimulates synthesis of prostacyclin by cultured human endothelial cells. J Clin Invest 1981;67:762–769

11. DeCaterina R, Dorso CR, Tack-Goldman K, Weksler BB: Nitrates and endothelial prostacyclin production. Studies in vitro. Circulation 1985;71:176–182

12. Armstrong PW, Armstrong JA, Marks GS: Pharmacokinetic-hemodynamic studies of intravenous nitroglycerin in congestive heart failure. Circulation 1980;62:160–166

13. Armstrong PW, Armstrong JA, Marks GS: Blood levels after sublingual nitroglycerin. Circulation 1979;59:585–589

14. Armstrong PW, Moffat JA, Marks GS: Arterial-venous nitroglycerin gradient during intravenous infusion in man. Circulation 1982;66:1273–1276

15. Fung HL: Pharmacokinetic determinants of nitrate action. Am J Med 1984;76:22–26

16. Mason DT, Braunwald E: The effects of nitroglycerin and amyl nitrite on arteriolar and venous tone in the human forearm. Circulation 1965;32:755–765

17. Leier CV, Bambach D, Thompson MJ et al: Central and regional hemodynamic effects of intravenous isosorbide dinitrate, nitroglycerin, and nitroprusside in patients with congestive heart failure. Am J Cardiol 1981;48:1115–1123

18. Flaherty JT, Reid PR, Kelly DT et al: Intravenous

19. Armstrong PW, Walker DC, Burton JR, Parker JO: Vasodilator therapy in acute myocardial infarction. A comparison of sodium nitroprusside and nitroglycerin. Circulation 1975;52:1118–1122

20. Flaherty JT, Come PC, Baird MG et al: Effects of intravenous nitroglycerin on left ventricular function and ST segment changes in acute myocardial infarction. Br Heart J 1976;38:612–621

21. Ludbrook PR, Byrne JD, Kurnik PB, McKnight RC: Influence of reduction of preload and afterload by nitroglycerin on left ventricular diastolic pressure-volume relation and relaxation in man. Circulation 1977;56:937–943

22. Baxter RH, Tait CM, McGuinness JB: Vasodilator therapy in acute myocardial infarction. Use of sublingual isosorbide dinitrate. Br Heart J 1977;39:1067–1070

23. Bussmann WD, Schupp D: Effect of sublingual nitroglycerin in emergency treatment of severe pulmonary edema. Am J Cardiol 1978;41:931–936

24. Cintron GB, Glasser SP, Weston BA et al: Effect of intravenous isosorbide dinitrate versus nitroglycerin on elevated pulmonary arterial wedge pressure during acute myocardial infarction. Am J Cardiol 1988;61:21–25

25. Lavine SJ, Campbell CA, Held AC, Johnson V: Effect of nitroglycerin-induced reduction of left ventricular filling pressure on diastolic filling in acute dilated heart failure. J Am Coll Cardiol 1989;14:223–241

26. Gold HK, Leinbach RC, Sanders CA: Use of sublingual nitroglycerin in congestive failure following acute myocardial infarction. Circulation 1972;46:839–845

27. Elkayam U, Roth A, Kumar A et al: Hemodynamic and volumetric effects of venodilation with nitroglycerin in chronic mitral regurgitation. Am J Cardiol 1987;60:1106–1111

28. Delius W, Enghoff E: Studies of the central and peripheral hemodynamic effects of amyl nitrate in patients with aortic insufficiency. Circulation 1970;42:787–796

29. Stevenson LW, Bellil D, Grover-McKay M et al: Effects of afterload reduction (diuretics and vasodilators) on left ventricular volume and mitral regurgitation in severe congestive heart failure secondary to ischemic or idiopathic dilated cardiomyopathy. Am J Cardiol 1987;60:654–658

30. DeMarco T, Chatterjee K, Rouleau JL, Parmley WW: Abnormal coronary hemodynamics and myocardial energetics in patients with chronic heart failure caused by ischemic heart disease and dilated cardiomyopathy. Am Heart J 1988;115:809–815

31. Unverferth DV, Magorien RD, Lewis RP, Leier CV: The role of subendocardial ischemia in perpetuating myocardial failure in patients with nonischemic congestive cardiomyopathy. Am Heart J 1983;105:176–179

32. Dupuis J, Lalonde G, Lebeau R, Bichet D, Rouleau JL: Sustained beneficial effect of a seventy-two hour intravenous infusion of nitroglycerin in patients with severe chronic congestive heart failure. Am Heart J 1990;120:625–637

33. Gibson GR, Hunter JB, Raabe DS, Manjoney DL, Ittleman FP: Methemoglobin produced by high-dose in-

nitroglycerin in acute myocardial infarction. Circulation 1975;51:132–139

travenous nitroglycerin. Ann Intern Med 1982;96: 615–616

34. Kaplan KJ, Taber M, Teagarden JR, Parker M, Davidson R: Association of methemoglobinemia and intravenous nitroglycerin administration. Am J Cardiol 1985;55:181–183

35. Saxon SA, Silverman ME: Effects of continuous infusion of intravenous nitroglycerin administration. Am J Cardiol 1985;56:461–464

36. Magrini F, Niarchos AP: Ineffectiveness of sublingual nitroglycerin in acute left ventricular failure in the presence of massive peripheral edema. Am J Cardiol 1980;45:841–847

37. Elkayam U, Kulick D, McIntosh N et al: Incidence of early tolerance to hemodynamic effects of continuous infusion of nitroglycerin in patients with coronary artery disease and heart failure. Circulation 1987;76: 577–584

38. Dupuis J, Lalonde G, Lemieux R, Rouleau JL: Tolerance to intravenous nitroglycerin in patients with congestive heart failure. Role of increased intravenous volume, neurohormonal activation, and lack of prevention with N-acetylcysteine. J Am Coll Cardiol 1990;16:923–931

39. Schlant RC, Tsagaris TS, Robertson RJ: Studies on the acute cardiovascular effects of intravenous sodium nitroprusside. Am J Cardiol 1962;9:51–59

40. Schulz V: Clinical pharmacokinetics of nitroprusside, cyanide, thiosulphate and thiocyanate. Clin Pharmacokinet 1984;9:239–251

41. Haas GJ, Leier CV: Vasodilators. pp. 400–453. In Hosenpud JD, Greenberg BH (eds): Congestive Heart Failure. Springer-Verlag, New York, 1994

42. Cogan JJ, Humphreys MH, Carlson CJ, Benowitz NL, Rapaport E: Acute vasodilator therapy increases renal clearance of digoxin in patients with congestive heart failure. Circulation 1980;64:973–976

43. Brodie BR, Grossman W, Mann T, McLaurin LP: Effects of sodium nitroprusside on left ventricular diastolic pressure-volume relations. J Clin Invest 1977; 59:59–68

44. Masuyama T, St. Goar FG, Alderman EL, Popp RL: Effects of nitroprusside on transmitral flow velocity patterns in extreme heart failure. A combined hemodynamic and Doppler echocardiographic study of varying loading conditions. J Am Coll Cardiol 1990; 16:1175–1185

45. Guiha NH, Cohn JN, Mikulic E, Franciosa JA, Limas CJ: Treatment of refractory heart failure with infusion of nitroprusside. N Engl J Med 1974;291: 587–592

46. Franciosa JA, Silverstein SR: Hemodynamic effects of nitroprusside and furosemide in left ventricular failure. Clin Pharmacol Ther 1982;32:62–69

47. Pepine CJ, Nichols WW, Curry RC Jr, Conti CR: Aortic input impedance during nitroprusside infusion. J Clin Invest 1979;64:643–654

48. Yin FC, Guzman PA, Brin KP et al: Effect of nitroprusside on hydraulic vascular loads of the right and left ventricle of patients with heart failure. Circulation 1983;67:1330–1339

49. Konstam MA, Weiland DS, Conlon TP et al: Hemodynamic correlates of left ventricular versus right ventricular radionuclide volumetric responses to vasodilator therapy in congestive heart failure secondary to ischemic or dilated cardiomyopathy. Am J Cardiol 1987;59:1131–1137

50. Cogan JJ, Humphreys MH, Carlson CJ, Rapaport E: Renal effects of nitroprusside and hydralazine in patients with congestive heart failure. Circulation 1980;61:316–323

51. Chatterjee K, Parmley WW, Ganz W et al: Hemodynamic and metabolic responses to vasodilator therapy in acute myocardial infarction. Circulation 1973; 48:1183–1193

52. Miller RR, Vismara LA, Zelis R, Amsterdam EA, Mason DT: Clinical use of sodium nitroprusside in chronic ischemic heart disease. Circulation 1975;51: 328–386

53. Cohn JN, Mathew KJ, Franciosa JA, Snow JA: Chronic vasodilator therapy in the management of cardiogenic shock and intractable left ventricular failure. Ann Intern Med 1974;81:777–780

54. Awan NA, Miller RR, Vera Z, Mason DT: Reduction of ST segment elevation with infusion of nitroprusside in patients with acute myocardial infarction. Am J Cardiol 1976;38:435–439

55. Chatterjee K, Swan JH, Kaushik US, Jobin G, Magnusson P: Effects of vasodilator therapy in acute myocardial infarction on short-term and late prognosis. Circulation 1976;53:797–802

56. Leier CV, Magorien RD, Boudoulas H et al: The effect of vasodilator therapy on systolic and diastolic time intervals in congestive heart failure. Chest 1982;81: 723–729

57. Chiariello M, Gold HK, Leinbach RC, Davis MA, Maroko PR: Comparison between the effects of nitroprusside and nitroglycerin on ischemic injury during acute myocardial infarction. Circulation 1976;54: 766–773

58. Mann T, Cohn PF, Holman BL et al: Effect of nitroprusside on regional myocardial blood flow in coronary artery disease. Circulation 1978;57:732–738

59. Leier CV: Acute inotropic support. Intravenously administered positive inotropic drugs. pp. 63–105. In Leier CV (ed): Cardiotonic Drugs. Marcel Dekker, New York, 1991

60. Miller RR, Awan NA, Joye JA et al: Combined dopamine and nitroprusside therapy in congestive heart failure. Circulation 1977;55:881–884

61. Keung EC, Ribner HS, Schwartz W, Sonnenblick EH, LeJemtel TH: Effects of combined dopamine and nitroprusside therapy in patients with severe pump failure and hypotension complicating acute myocardial infarction. J Cardiovasc Pharmacol 1980;2: 113–119

62. Stevenson LW, Dracup KA, Tillisch JH: Efficacy of medical therapy tailored for severe congestive heart failure in patients transferred for urgent cardiac transplantation. Am J Cardiol 1989;63:461–464

63. Reid GM, Muther RS: Nitroprusside-induced acute azotemia. Am J Nephrol 1987;7:313–315

64. Packer M, Miller J, Medina N, Gorlin R, Herman JV: Rebound hemodynamic events after the abrupt withdrawal of nitroprusside in patients with severe chronic heart failure. N Engl J Med 1979;301: 1193–1197

65. Vesey CJ, Cole PV: Blood cyanide and thiocyanate concentrations produced by long-term therapy with sodium nitroprusside. Br J Anaesth 1985;57:148–155

66. Norris JC, Hume AS: In vivo release of cyanide from sodium nitroprusside. Br J Anaesth 1987;59:236–239

67. Bencowitz HZ, LeWinter MM, Wagner PD: Effect of sodium nitroprusside on ventilation-perfusion mismatching in heart failure. J Am Coll Cardiol 1984;4: 918–922

68. Pierpont G, Hale KA, Franciosa JA, Cohn JN: Effects of vasodilators on pulmonary hemodynamics and gas exchange in left ventricular failure. Am Heart J 1980; 99:208–216

69. Mookerjee S, Keighley JF, Warner RA, Bowser MA, Obeid AI: Hemodynamic ventilatory and blood gas changes during infusion of nitroferricyanide: studies in patients with congestive heart failure. Chest 1977; 72:273–278

70. Mehta J, Mehta P: Platelet function studies in heart disease. Enhanced platelet aggregate formation activity in congestive heart failure. Inhibition by sodium nitroprusside. Circulation 1979;60:497–503

71. Franciosa JA, Mikulic E, Cohn JN, Jose E, Fabie A: Hemodynamic and metabolic effects of isosorbide dinitrate in chronic congestive heart failure. Am Heart J 1975;90:346–352

72. Gray R, Chatterjee K, Ganz W, Forrester JS, Swan HJ: Hemodynamic and metabolic effects of isosorbide dinitrate in chronic congestive heart failure. Am Heart J 1975;90:346–352

73. Mantle JA, Russell RO, Moraski RE, Rackley CE: Isosorbide dinitrate for the relief of severe heart failure after myocardial infarction. Am J Cardiol 1976;37: 263–268

74. Taylor WR, Forrester JS, Magnusson P et al: Hemodynamic effects of nitroglycerin ointment in congestive heart failure. Am J Cardiol 1976;38:469–473

75. Franciosa JA, Blank RC, Cohn JN: Nitrate effects on cardiac output and left ventricular outflow resistance in chronic congestive heart failure. Am J Med 1978; 64:207–213

76. Gomes JAC, Carambas CR, Moran HE et al: The effect of isosorbide dinitrate on left ventricular size, wall stress, and left ventricular function in chronic refractory heart failure. Am J Med 1978;65:794–802

77. Franciosa JA, Cohn JN: Effect of isosorbide dinitrate on response to submaximal and maximal exercise in patients with congestive heart failure. Am J Cardiol 1979;43:1009–1014

78. Franciosa JA, Goldsmith SR, Cohn JN: Contrasting immediate and long-term effect of isosorbide dinitrate on exercise capacity in congestive heart failure. Am J Med 1980;69:559–566

79. Massie BM, Kramer B, Shen E, Haughom F: Vasodilator treatment with isosorbide dinitrate and hydralazine in chronic heart failure. Br Heart J 1981;45: 376–384

80. Leier CV, Huss P, Magorien RD, Unverferth DV: Improved exercise capacity and differing arterial and venous tolerance during chronic isosorbide dinitrate. Circulation 1983;67:817–822

81. Jordan RA, Seth L, Henry A, Wilen MM, Franciosa JA: Dose requirements and hemodynamic effects of transdermal requirements and hemodynamic effects of transdermal nitroglycerin compared with placebo in patients with congestive heart failure. Circulation 1985;71:980–986

82. Debbas N, Woodings D, Marks C et al: Dose-ranging study of isosorbide-5-mononitrate in chronic congestive heart failure treated with diuretics and angiotensin-converting enzyme inhibitor. Am J Cardiol 1988; 61:28E–30E

83. Massie B, Chatterjee K, Werner J et al: Hemodynamic advantage of combined administration of hydralazine orally and nitrates non-parenterally in the vasodilator therapy of chronic heart failure. Am J Cardiol 1977;40:794–801

84. Leier CV, Magorien RD, Desch CE, Thompson MJ, Unverferth DV: Hydralazine and isosorbide dinitrate: Comparative central and regional hemodynamic effects when administered alone or in combination. Circulation 1981;63:102–109

85. McDonald KM, Francis GS, Matthews J et al: Long-term oral nitrate therapy prevents chronic ventricular remodeling in the dog. J Am Coll Cardiol 1993; 21:514–522

86. Hoelzer M, Schaal SF, Leier CV: Electrophysiologic and antiarrhythmic effects of nitroglycerin in man. J Cardiovasc Pharmacol 1981;3:917–923

87. Dengel ME, Weber PA, Leier CV: Transient myopia following isosorbide dinitrate. Ann Ophthalmol 1983; 15:1156–1158

88. Kulick D, Roth A, McIntosh N, Rahimtoola SH, Elkayam U: Resistance to isosorbide dinitrate in patients with severe chronic heart failure. Incidence and attempt at hemodynamic prediction. J Am Coll Cardiol 1988;12:1023–1028

89. Leier CV: Nitrate tolerance. Am Heart J 1985;110: 224–232

90. Packer M, Lee WH, Kessler PD et al: Prevention and reversal of nitrate tolerance in patients with congestive heart failure. N Engl J Med 1987;317:799–804

91. Parker JO, Farrell B, Lahey KA, Rose BF: Nitrate tolerance. The lack of effect of N-acetylcysteine. Circulation 1987;76:572–576

92. Dakak N, Makhoul N, Flugelman MY et al: Failure of captopril to prevent nitrate tolerance in congestive heart failure secondary to coronary artery disease. Am J Cardiol 1990;66:608–613

93. Dupuis J, LaLonde G, Bichet D, Rouleau J: Captopril does not prevent nitroglycerin tolerance in heart failure. Can J Cardiol 1990;6:281–286

94. Katz RJ, Levy WS, Buff L, Wasserman AG: Prevention of nitrate tolerance with angiotensin converting enzyme inhibitors. Circulation 1991;83:1271–1277

95. Levy WS, Katz RJ, Wasserman AG: Methionine restores the venodilative response to nitroglycerin after the development of tolerance. J Am Coll Cardiol 1991; 17:474–479

96. Crawford MH, Ludden TM, Kennedy GT: Determinants of systemic availability of oral hydralazine in heart failure. Clin Pharmacol Ther 1985;38:538–543

97. Hanson A, Johansson BW, Wernersson B, Wahlander LA: Pharmacokinetics of hydralazine in chronic heart failure. Eur J Clin Pharmacol 1983;25:467–473

98. Chatterjee K, Parmley WW, Massie B et al: Oral hydralazine therapy for chronic heart failure. Circulation 1976;54:879–884

99. Franciosa JA, Pierpont G, Cohn JN: Hemodynamic improvement after oral hydralazine in left ventricular failure. Ann Intern Med 1977;86:388–393

100. Chatterjee K, Ports TA, Arnold S, Brundage B, Parmley WW: Comparison of hemodynamic effects of oral hydralazine and prazosin hydrochloride in patients

with chronic congestive heart failure. Br Heart J 1979;42:657–663

101. Fitchett DH, Neto JAM, Oakley CM, Goodwin JF: Hydralazine in the management of left ventricular failure. Am J Cardiol 1979;44:303–309

102. Magorien RD, Triffon DW, Desch CE et al: Prazosin and hydralazine in congestive heart failure. Regional hemodynamic effects in relation to dose. Ann Intern Med 1981;95:5–13

103. Packer M, Meller J, Medina N, Gorlin R, Herman MV: Hemodynamic evaluation of hydralazine dosage in refractory heart failure. Clin Pharmacol Ther 1980;27:337–346

104. Leier CV, Desch CE, Magorien RD et al: Positive inotropic effects of hydralazine in human subjects. Comparison with prazosin in the setting of congestive heart failure. Am J Cardiol 1980;46:1039–1044

105. McLean AJ, Barron K, duSouich P et al: Interaction of hydralazine and hydrazone derivatives with contractile mechanisms in rabbit aortic smooth muscle. J Pharmacol Exp Ther 1978;205:418–425

106. Daly P, Rouleau JL, Cousineau D, Burgess JH, Chatterjee K: Effects of captopril and a combination of hydralazine and isosorbide dinitrate on myocardial sympathetic tone in patients with severe heart failure. Br Heart J 1986;56:152–157

107. Elkayam U, Roth A, Hsueh W et al: Neurohumoral consequences of vasodilator therapy with hydralazine and nifedipine in severe congestive heart failure. Am Heart J 1986;111:1130–1138

108. Binkley PF, Van Fossen DB, Haas GJ, Cody RJ, Leier CV: Persistence of abnormal ventriculoarterial coupling and decreased conduit vessel compliance despite peripheral vasodilation with hydralazine and nitroglycerin in congestive heart failure [abstract]. J Am Coll Cardiol 1994;23:338A

109. Morand P, Lavigne G, Masson D, Latour F, Alison D: Treatment of severe chronic cardiac insufficiency with dihydralazine; short- and median-term results. Arch Mal Coeur 1979;72:268–275

110. Quyyumi AA, Wagstaff D, Evans TR: Acute hemodynamic effects of endralazine. A new vasodilator for chronic refractory congestive heart failure. Am J Cardiol 1983;51:1353–1357

111. Massie B, Chatterjee K, Werner J et al: Hemodynamic advantage of combined administration of hydralazine orally and nitrates non-parenterally in the vasodilator therapy of chronic heart failure. Am J Cardiol 1977;40:794–801

112. Massie BM, Kramer B, Shen E, Haughom F: Vasodilator treatment with isosorbide dinitrate and hydralazine in chronic heart failure. Br Heart J 1981;45:376–384

113. Wilson JR, Hoyt RW, Ferraro N, Janicki JS, Weber KT: Effect of hydralazine on nutritive flow to working canine gracilis skeletal muscle. J Am Coll Cardiol 1984;4:529–534

114. Wilson JR, Martin JL, Ferraro N, Lueber KT: Effect of hydralazine on perfusion and metabolism in the leg during upright bicycle exercise in patients with heart failure. Circulation 1983;68:425–432

115. Elkayam U, Weber L, Campses VM, Massry SG, Rahimtoola SH: Renal hemodynamics effects of vasodilation with nifedipine and hydralazine in patients with heart failure. J Am Coll Cardiol 1984;4:1261–1267

116. Pierpont GL, Brown DC, Franciosa JA, Cohn JN: Effect of hydralazine on renal failure in patients with congestive heart failure. Circulation 1980;61:323–327

117. Cogan JJ, Humphreys MH, Carlson CH, Benowitz NL, Rapaport E: Acute vasodilator therapy increases renal clearance of digoxin in patients with congestive heart failure. Circulation 1981;64:973–976

118. Rouleau JL, Chatterjee K, Benge W, Parmley WW, Hiramatsu B: Alterations in left ventricular function and coronary hemodynamics with captopril, hydralazine, and prazosin in chronic ischemic heart failure, a comparative study. Circulation 1982;65:671–678

119. Magorien RD, Brown GP, Unverferth DV et al: Effects of hydralazine on coronary blood flow and myocardial energetics in congestive heart failure. Circulation 1982;65:528–533

120. Magorien RD, Unverferth DV, Brown GP, Leier CV: Dobutamine and hydralazine. Comparative influences of positive inotropy and vasodilation on coronary blood flow and myocardial energetics in nonischemic congestive heart failure. J Am Coll Cardiol 1983;1:499–505

121. Chatterjee K, Ports TA, Brundage BH et al: Oral hydralazine in chronic heart failure. Sustained beneficial hemodynamic effects. Ann Intern Med 1980;92:600–604

122. Franciosa JA, Weber KT, Levine TB et al: Hydralazine in the long-term treatment of chronic heart failure. Lack of difference from placebo. Am Heart J 1982;104:587–594

123. Magorien RD, Unverferth DV, Leier CV: Hydralazine therapy in chronic congestive heart failure. Sustained central and regional hemodynamic responses. Am J Med 1984;77:267–274

124. Conradson TB, Ryden L, Ahlmark G et al: Clinical efficacy of hydralazine in chronic heart failure. One year double-blind placebo-controlled study. Am Heart J 1984;108:1001–1006

125. Slosky DA, Hindman MC, Peter RH, Wallace AG: Effects of oral hydralazine on rest and exercise hemodynamics in patients with aortic or mitral regurgitation and left ventricular dysfunction. Clin Cardiol 1981;4:162–167

126. Stevenson LW, Brunker RC, Belil D et al: Afterload reduction with vasodilators and diuretics decreases mitral regurgitation during upright exercise in advanced heart failure. J Am Coll Cardiol 1990;15:174–180

127. Dumesnil JG, Tran K, Dagenais GR: Beneficial long-term effects of hydralazine in aortic regurgitation. Arch Intern Med 1990;150:757–760

128. Hamilton MA, Stevenson LW, Child JS et al: Sustained reductions in valvular regurgitation and atrial volumes with tailored vasodilator therapy in advanced congestive heart failure secondary to dilated cardiomyopathy. Am J Cardiol 1991;67:259–263

129. Binkley PF, Starling RC, Hammer DF, Leier CV: Usefulness of hydralazine to withdraw from dobutamine in severe congestive heart failure. Am J Cardiol 1991;69:1103–1106

130. Quyyami AA, Wagstaff D, Evans TR: Long-term effects of endralazine, a new arteriolar vasodilator at rest and during exercise capacity in chronic congestive heart failure. Am J Cardiol 1984;54:1020–1024

131. Packer M, Meller J, Medina N, Yushak M, Gorlin R. Provocation of myocardial ischemic events during

initiation of vasodilator therapy for severe chronic heart failure. Clinical and hemodynamic evaluation of 52 consecutive patients with ischemic cardiomyopathy. Am J Cardiol 1981;48:939–946

132. Packer M, Meller J, Medina N, Yushak M: Sustained effectiveness of minoxidil in heart failure after development of tolerance to other vasodilator drugs. Am J Cardiol 1981;48:375–379

133. Franciosa JA, Cohn JN: Effects of minoxidil on hemodynamics in patients with congestive heart failure. Circulation 1981;48:375–379

134. McKay CR, Chatterjee K, Ports TA, Holly AN, Parmley WW: Minoxidil therapy in chronic congestive heart failure. Am Heart J 1982;104:575–580

135. Nathan M, Rubin SA, Seimienczuk D, Swan HJC: Effects of acute and chronic minoxidil administration on rest and exercise hemodynamics and clinical status in patients with severe, chronic heart failure. Am J Cardiol 1982;50:960–966

136. Markham RV, Gilmore A, Pettinger WA et al: Central and regional hemodynamic effects and neurohumoral consequences of minoxidil in severe congestive heart failure and comparison to hydralazine and nitroprusside. Am J Cardiol 1983;52:774–781

137. Franciosa JA, Jordan RA, Wilen MM, Leddy CL: Minoxidil in patients with chronic left heart failure. Contrasting hemodynamic and clinical effects in a controlled trial. Circulation 1984;70:63–68

138. Sim MF, Yates DB, Parkinson R, Cooling MJ: Cardiovascular effects of the novel arteriovenous dilator agent, flosequinan, in conscious dogs and cats. Br J Pharmacol 1988;94:371–380

139. Flaotico R, Haertlein BJ, Lakas-Weiss CS, Salata JJ, Tobia AJ: Positive inotropic and hemodynamic properties of flosequinan, a new vasodilator, and a sulfone metabolite. J Cardiovasc Pharmacol 1989;14: 412–418

140. Yates DB: Pharmacology of flosequinan. Am Heart J 1991;121:974–983

141. Kessler PD, Packer M: Hemodynamic effects of BTS 49465, a new long-acting systemic vasodilator drug, in patients with severe congestive heart failure. Am Heart J 1987;113:137–143

142. Crowley AH, Wynne RD, Stainer K et al: Flosequinan in heart failure. Acute haemodynamic and longer term symptomatic effects. BMJ 1988;207:169–173

143. Haas GJ, Binkley PF, Carpenter JA, Leier CV: Central and regional hemodynamic effects of flosequinan for congestive heart failure. Am J Cardiol 1989;63: 1354–1359

144. Haas GJ, Binkley PF, Leier CV: Chronic vasodilator therapy with flosequinan in congestive heart failure. Clin Cardiol 1990;13:414–420

145. Elborn JS, Stanford CF, Nicholls DP: Effect of flosequinan on exercise capacity and symptoms in severe heart failure. Br Heart J 1989;61:331–335

146. Massie BM, Berk MR, Brozena SC et al: Can further benefit be achieved by adding flosequinan to patient with congestive heart failure who remain symptomatic on diuretic, digoxin, and an angiotensin converting enzyme inhibitor? Circulation 1993;88:492–501

147. Packer M, Narahara KA, Elkayam U et al., and the principal investigators of the REFLECT Study: J Am Coll Cardiol 1993;22:65–72

148. Packer M, Rouleau J, Swedberg K et al: Effect of flosequinan on survival in chronic heart failure [abstract]. Circulation, Suppl. I 1993;88:301

149. Sueta CA, Gheorghiade M, Adams KF et al: Safety and efficacy of epoprostenol in patients with severe congestive heart failure. Am J Cardiol 1995;75: 34A–43A

150. Northridge DB, Jardine AG, Findlay IN et al: Inhibition of metabolism of atrial natriuretic factor causes diuresis and natriuresis in chronic heart failure. Am J Hypertens 1990;3:682

151. Munzel T, Kerz S, Holtz J et al: Neurohormonal inhibition and hemodynamic unloading during prolonged inhibition of ANF degradation in patients with severe chronic heart failure. Circulation 1992;86:1089

152. Eisner D, Muntze A, Kroner EP, Riegger GA: Effectiveness of endopeptidase inhibition (landoxatril) in congestive heart failure. Am J Cardiol 1992;70:494

153. Schwarz M, Katz SD, Demopoulos L et al: Enhancement of endothelium-dependent vasodilation by low-dose nitroglycerin in patients with congestive heart failure. Circulation 1994;89:1609–1614

154. Crozier I, Ikram H, Awan N et al: Losartan in heart failure. Hemodynamic effects and tolerability. Circulation 1995;91:691–697

155. Teerlink JR, Loffler BM, Hess P et al: Role of endothelin in the maintenance of blood pressure in conscious rats with chronic heart failure. Acute effects of the endothelin receptor antagonist Ro 47-0203 (Bosentan). Circulation 1994;90:2510–2518

45 Drugs for Heart Failure That Interfere with the Renin-Angiotensin System

Milton Packer

One of the most important advances in the management of chronic heart failure has been the development of therapeutic agents that inhibit the renin-angiotensin system. Interference with this system—specifically with the use of angiotensin-converting enzyme (ACE) inhibitors—has produced important hemodynamic, symptomatic, and prognostic benefits in patients with left ventricular dysfunction; and the clinical effects of ACE inhibitors have been superior to those seen with most other therapeutic interventions for heart failure. As a result, these drugs have been evaluated more extensively and their role in therapeutics has been defined more thoroughly than nearly any other pharmacologic intervention in cardiovascular medicine.

The development of drugs that interfere with the renin-angiotensin system is principally based on the hypothesis that the most important pathophysiologic abnormality of heart failure is activation of endogenous neurohormonal systems.[1] Neurohormonal activation occurs early in the development of heart failure[2]; circulating levels of neurohormonal factors are increased in proportion to the severity of the disease[3]; and patients with the highest levels of neurohormonal factors have the most unfavorable prognosis.[4,5] These observations have led to the belief that activation of the renin-angiotensin system has a major influence on the clinical status of patients with heart failure and plays an important role in determining the rate of progression of the underlying disease. Angiotensin II can exert adverse effects on the circulation, directly and indirectly[6,7]; and interference with its formation or actions can ameliorate the pathophysiologic abnormalities of heart failure

and can retard progression of disease in experimental models of left ventricular systolic dysfunction.[7–9]

This chapter reviews the pathophysiologic basis of and clinical results with drugs that interfere with the renin-angiotensin system. This Chapter will review the available data on ACE inhibitors and in addition briefly discuss the underlying rationale and the clinical effects of other agents that interfere with this important neurohormonal system (i.e., the renin inhibitors and angiotensin II receptor antagonists).

RENIN–ANGIOTENSIN SYSTEM IN HEART FAILURE

The observation that the kidneys produce renin in patients with heart failure was first made nearly 50 years ago,[10] but it was not until the late 1970s that clinical evidence emerged that angiotensin II contribute importantly to the pathophysiology of the syndrome.[11] For most of the last 50 years, the relation between circulating levels of renin and angiotensin and their physiologic actions was defined by the assumption that these factors interacted and exerted their effects primarily within the circulation. Accordingly, physicians believed that renin (synthesized largely by the kidneys) acted on angiotensinogen (produced largely by the liver) to form angiotensin I. Angiotensin I was then converted (by an action of the vascular endothelium) to angiotensin II, which then circulated in the plasma and interacted with cell-surface receptors to exert a constrictor effect on the peripheral circulation. Viewed in this fashion, any drug that interfered with the renin-angiotensin system (at any point in the cascade) would be expected to act primarily as a peripheral vasodilator drug.

Our concepts of the renin-angiotensin system have changed dramatically, however, as a result of progress in the fields of molecular and cellular biology. It is now widely recognized that the major interactions and effects of the renin-angiotensin system may not occur in the circulation but in the tissues. All of the components required for the production of angiotensin II are found within the tissues,[12,13] although it remains unclear whether these components exist as a result of local production or because of uptake of these components from the plasma. In any case, tissue (rather than circulating) levels of renin and angiotensin II may be the primary determinant of the activity of the renin-angiotensin system.[13] Furthermore, it is now recognized that angiotensin II may exert its principal biologic effects on the tissues of many organs rather than on just the blood vessels. Although angiotensin II has vasoconstrictor effects, it acts primarily as a regulator of growth and death for both myocytes and nonmyocytes.[14-17] Indeed, it seems probable that, from a teleologic viewpoint, the molecular and cellular actions of angiotensin II represent its primordial functions, and that its actions within the circulation are a recent (and less important) evolutionary development.

These observations suggest that, although activation of the renin-angiotensin system in heart failure was first described by measuring various components of the system within the plasma, assessment of its activity within tissues may be a more relevant way of delineating its importance in this disorder. For example, viewed from the perspective of the circulation, plasma renin activity is increased following an acute myocardial injury but then is suppressed for long periods until the syndrome of heart failure is well advanced.[18-20] However, viewed from the perspective of the tissues, tissue renin and ACE activity is not only increased following the cardiac insult but remains elevated in the heart and kidneys, at a time when circulating levels of renin and angiotensin II have returned to normal.[18-20] Indeed, in experimental models of heart failure, inhibition of plasma ACE exerts few clinical benefits, whereas inhibition of tissue ACE inhibits the development of cardiac hypertrophy and reduces the risk of death.[21]

How then can a physician assess the activity of the renin-angiotensin system in an individual patient with heart failure? Although we might be tempted to answer this question by determining if the plasma levels of renin activity and angiotensin II fall outside the "normal range," the range of normal values for renin activity and angiotensin II—established in hy-pertensive patients who were taking no medications and who were in sodium balance[22]—is difficult to apply to patients with chronic heart failure, who are commonly in a salt-retaining state despite treatment with diuretic drugs. Alternatively, although we might be tempted to assess the degree of angiotensin dependence by observing the immediate hypotensive response to the administration of an angiotensin II antagonist, low levels of angiotensin II may exert a prolonged pressor effect that is reversed by long-term (but not short-term) angiotensin II inhibition.[23] Thus until a clinical method becomes available for evaluating the activity of renin and angiotensin II in the tissues of patients, physicians would be best advised to assume that this system is activated in all patients with heart failure.

Whether angiotensin II exerts its principal actions in plasma or tissues, the effects of this hormone are mediated through its actions on the two classes of angiotensin II receptors, type 1 and type 2. The type 1 receptor mediates all of the known actions of the hormone, including its effects on growth and its constrictor effects on blood vessels.[24] In contrast, the actions of the type 2 receptor remain uncertain, although it is the most common subtype in the human heart. Evidence suggests that the type 2 receptor inhibits cell proliferation and may facilitate the occurrence of apoptosis (programmed cell death),[17,25] a process that has been implicated in the progression of heart failure.[26,27] Type 2 receptors are markedly up-regulated in the border zone of infarcted hearts, where they may mediate the initiation and progression of ventricular remodeling.[28] This mechanism may explain why selective interference with type 1 receptors fails to ameliorate the process of ventricular remodeling in experimental models of the disease.[29,30]

AGENTS THAT INTERFERE WITH THE RENIN–ANGIOTENSIN SYSTEM

Three types of agents that interfere with the renin-angiotensin system have been developed for the treatment of heart failure. Renin antagonists act by inhibiting the active site of renin, which is responsible for its ability to convert angiotensinogen to angiotensin I. ACE inhibitors act by inhibiting the enzyme responsible for the conversion of angiotensin I to angiotensin II. Finally, angiotensin receptor antagonists block the interaction of angiotensin with its receptors, usually the type 1 receptor. By far, most of the experience with these agents in heart failure has been with the ACE inhibitors, but it is of historical interest that the earliest pharmacologic approaches to interfering with the renin-angiotensin system targeted renin and the angiotensin receptor. β-Blockers (which inhibit the release of renin) were first used for the treatment of heart failure during the mid-1970s.[31] At that same time, angiotensin II receptor antagonists were used to treat heart failure,[11] even though the specific antagonist used (saralasin) also had agonist effects on the angiotensin II receptor.

ACE Inhibitors

Although pharmacologists have developed a number of distinct ways to inhibit the angiotensin-converting enzyme, ACE inhibitors are generally similar to each other in their therapeutic profile. Yet it remains unclear whether the benefits of these drugs can be entirely explained by their ability to suppress the formation of angiotensin II. The angiotensin-converting enzyme is identical to kininase II, the enzyme responsible for the degradation of kinins; thus ACE inhibition enhances the actions of kinins in the tissues and augments kinin-mediated prostaglandin synthesis.[32,33] As a result, ACE inhibition causes peripheral vasodilation, not only by blocking the formation of angiotensin II but enhancing kinin-mediated effects on blood vessels.[34,35] Similarly, ACE inhibition may improve diastolic function not only by inhibiting the adverse effects of angiotensin II on ventricular relaxation but also by enhancing the favorable effects of kinins on diastolic performance.[36,37] Finally, ACE inhibition may prevent the progressive loss of myocardial cells, not only by interfering with the toxic effects of angiotensin II but by enhancing kinin-mediated synthesis of the enzyme constituitive nitric oxide synthase (cNOS),[38] which can block the process of apoptosis. Indeed, evidence suggests that kinin potentiation may be even more important than angiotensin suppression in mediating the effects of ACE inhibitors. In experimental models of heart failure, ACE inhibitors exert favorable effects on ventricular remodeling that are not seen with angiotensin II receptor antagonists, and this advantage of ACE inhibitors is abolished by the co-administration of kinin antagonists.[29,39] Furthermore, in the clinical setting, the hemodynamic and prognostic benefits of ACE inhibitors appear to be attenuated by the co-administration of aspirin, which blocks kinin-mediated prostaglandin synthesis.[40,41]

The concept that the primary action of ACE inhibitors may be through their effects on kinins is supported by observations that ACE inhibitors may not produce effective long-term suppression of angiotensin II formation. When treatment with an ACE inhibitor is initiated, even small doses can decrease circulating levels of angiotensin II to low levels.[42,43] However, during long-term treatment, progressive larger doses of the ACE inhibitor may be needed to maintain the suppression of angiotensin II. This escape may occur because the use of ACE inhibitors is accompanied by reactive increases in plasma renin activity and circulating angiotensin I, which may require increasingly intense ACE inhibition to maintain an effective block.[44,45] Alternatively, in the presence of an ACE inhibitor, angiotensin II may be formed by alternate pathways (e.g., via chymase) that are not blocked by ACE inhibitors.[46,47] Although the importance of the chymase pathway remains unclear,[48] the failure of ACE inhibitors to produce sustained suppression of angiotensin II levels has provided a rationale for the development of angiotensin II receptor antagonists for the treatment of chronic heart failure.

Angiotensin II Receptor Antagonists

Angiotensin II receptor antagonists were developed based on the belief that interference with the renin-angiotensin system at its most distal site would provide the most effective and specific blockade of this important neurohormonal system. Furthermore, because angiotensin II receptor antagonists do not inhibit kininase, their use would not be associated with any of the adverse effects of ACE inhibitors that have been attributed to the accumulation of kinins. However, these apparent advantages of angiotensin II receptor antagonists should be balanced against the potential disadvantages of these drugs. First, insofar as kinins are important for mediating the benefits of ACE inhibitors,[30,39] angiotensin II receptor antagonists would be expected to be less effective than ACE inhibitors.[29,30] Second, most angiotensin II receptor antagonists are competitive in nature, and so their ability to block the receptor may be overcome by the reactive increases in angiotensin II that occur following blockade of the renin-angiotensin system at a distal site. Third, most angiotensin II receptor antagonists act selectively to block the type 1 receptor but do not interfere with the type 2 receptor. Insofar as the type 2 receptor may mediate the adverse effects of angiotensin on ventricular remodeling,[17,25] selective type 1 receptor antagonists may be limited in their ability to prevent the structural changes in the failing heart that are critical to the progression of the disease.[29,30]

CLINICAL EFFECTS OF ACE INHIBITORS IN HEART FAILURE

The two most critical pathophysiologic abnormalities of heart failure are (1) the abnormal hemodynamic conditions within the heart and peripheral circulation and (2) the activation of neurohormonal systems. Unlike most other drugs for heart failure (positive inotropic agents and direct-acting vasodilators), ACE inhibitors address both of these central pathophysiologic derangements.

Hemodynamic and Neurohormonal Effects

All ACE inhibitors produce favorable hemodynamic effects in patients with chronic heart failure. Contrary to conventional wisdom, the benefits of these drugs do not derive principally from their ability to enhance cardiac output but are related to their ability to produce sustained decreases in left ventricular filling pressure at rest and during exercise.[49,50] This effect on the distending pressures within the ventricle not only leads to a favorable effect on symptoms in the near term but may decrease the degree of ventricular remodeling that characterizes the progression of heart failure in the long term. Interestingly, the reduction in ventricular pressures and dimensions by ACE inhibitors may not be directly related to the suppression of angiotensin II formation. Angiotensin II has minimal constrictor effect on peripheral veins,[51,52] and so its suppression would not be expected to enhance venous capacitance and reduce ventricular distending pressures. However, peripheral venodilation would be expected as a result of the ability of ACE inhibitors to reduce circulating norepinephrine and increase the accumulation of local kinins.[34,35] Experimental data suggest that the increase in local kinins may be the more important factor, as the favorable effects of ACE inhibitors on ventricular distending pressures and remodeling are not fully shared by angiotensin II antagonists and are blocked by the co-administration of a bradykinin antagonist.[29,39,53]

What then are the hemodynamic benefits that derive from the suppression of angiotensin II? Available evidence suggests that the decline in circulating angiotensin II to low levels is responsible for the marked decrease in systemic vascular resistance that accompanies the administration of ACE inhibitors.[53] However, unlike direct-acting vasodilators, the dilatation of arterial resistance vessels does not result in large increases in cardiac output or left ventricular ejection fraction. This may occur because

ACE inhibitors exert a negative inotropic effect on the failing heart[54] (as a result of withdrawal of the cardiostimulatory actions of angiotensin II) and because ACE inhibitors exert minimal dilatory effects on the pulmonary vasculature[55] (because angiotensin II is not a potent pulmonary vasoconstrictor[51]). The nondilated pulmonary circuit acts to limit any increase in left ventricular systolic performance that might otherwise be expected to accompany a fall in systemic vascular resistance. The failure of cardiac output to increase while arterial resistance decreases may explain why hypotension occurs more frequently with ACE inhibitors than with other vasodilator drugs.

The limited ability of ACE inhibitors to increase cardiac output during short-term therapy might at first glance appear to be make these agents less attractive than other drugs for heart failure, but such a view overemphasizes the importance of the acute hemodynamic effects of therapeutic agents for heart failure. Although many peripheral vasodilators and positive inotropic drugs produce initial hemodynamic effects more impressive than those of ACE inhibitors, these effects are not necessarily sustained or beneficial. Tolerance is a major problem with many peripheral vasodilators but is an uncommon occurrence with ACE inhibitors,[50] perhaps because ACE inhibitors diminish rather than activate endogenous neurohormonal mechanisms. In fact, the long-term response to ACE inhibitors in many patients may exceed that seen during initiation of treatment. Even the complete lack of any discernible short-term effect does not preclude long-term benefits in many patients.[50,56] Furthermore, even if the hemodynamic effects are sustained during long-term treatment, this response is not necessarily accompanied by favorable effects on the clinical outcome of patients. Some positive inotropic agents and peripheral vasodilators produce long-term hemodynamic benefits but fail to improve symptoms or exercise tolerance and may enhance morbidity and mortality.[57,58] Indeed, observations indicate that the neurohormonal (rather than the hemodynamic) effects of drugs may be the primary determinant of their clinical and prognostic benefits in heart failure.[1] If so, there appears to be no reason to perform invasive hemodynamic measurements during the initiation of therapy with an ACE inhibitor in patients with chronic heart failure.

The ACE inhibitors produce a variety of neurohormonal benefits in patients with heart failure. Not only does the use of these drugs interfere with the formation of angiotensin II, but their long-term administration is accompanied by a decrease in circulating levels of other vasoconstrictor hormones (e.g., norepinephrine, vasopressin, and endothelin).[59,60] Furthermore, ACE inhibitors appear to potentiate the actions of many vasodilator systems that oppose the actions of the vasoconstrictor mechanisms (e.g., bradykinin, enkephalins, prostaglandins, and nitric oxide).[61] Finally, ACE inhibitors restore the depressed parasympathetic tone of patients with chronic heart failure toward normal.[62] It is not known whether these effects reflect a direct action of ACE inhibitors or are the expected responses to any intervention that improves the overall state of heart failure. However, it should be noted that these neurohormonal benefits are not characteristic of most drugs that have been developed for use in chronic heart failure.

Effect of ACE Inhibitors on Symptoms and Exercise Tolerance

The ACE inhibitors have been shown in double-blind, placebo-controlled trials to produce a variety of clinical benefits in patients with chronic heart failure.[63-73] Dyspnea is relieved; exercise tolerance is prolonged; and the need for hospitalization and emergency care for worsening heart failure is reduced. These favorable effects are seen in patients with mild, moderate, or severe symptoms, regardless of whether they are treated with digitalis.[64,74] However, ACE inhibitors should not be used as a substitute for diuretics in patients with a history of fluid retention, because diuretics are needed to maintain sodium balance and prevent the development of peripheral and pulmonary edema.[75] Nevertheless, ACE inhibitors may reduce the need for large doses of diuretics and potassium supplements and may attenuate many of the adverse metabolic and electrophysiologic effects of aggressive diuretic therapy (i.e., hypokalemia, hyponatremia, and ventricular arrhythmias).

Studies of ACE inhibitors indicates that the clinical benefits of these drugs may not become apparent until treatment is continued for many weeks. This pattern differs from the experience with positive inotropic drugs, which produce immediate hemodynamic and symptomatic benefits when administered intravenously. Although symptoms may be dramatically ameliorated during the first 48 hours of therapy with an ACE inhibitor in some patients, this pattern is uncommon. In most patients the improvement in clinical status following therapy with an ACE inhibitor is delayed for at least 2–4 weeks and often more.[64] This delay is probably related to the time required to realize the favorable biologic effects of antagonizing the actions of endogenous neurohormonal systems. In this regard, it is noteworthy that the clinical

benefits of other neurohormonal antagonists (e.g., β-adrenergic blockers) are also delayed during long-term therapy.[76] In all, approximately 60–65 percent of patients with severe heart failure treated with an ACE inhibitor experience an improvement in symptoms with the drug.[50,64]

Effect of ACE Inhibitors on Morbidity and Mortality

Early evidence that ACE inhibitors may enhance survival of patients with congestive heart failure was first derived from studies in experimental models of the disease. In dogs with tachycardia-induced heart failure, captopril attenuated the progressive increase in systemic vascular resistance that accompanied the onset of left ventricular dysfunction.[7] In rats with left ventricular dysfunction produced by an experimental myocardial infarction, captopril reduced the progressive increase in left ventricular dimensions and diastolic pressures that followed the initial insult to the myocardium[77] and, by doing so, prolonged survival.[78] Finally, captopril reduced the frequency of ventricular arrhythmias induced by experimental coronary reperfusion, in part because of the drug's ability to decrease the outpouring of myocardial catecholamines that are responsible for the creation of the arrhythmogenic state.[79]

These experimental data have been supported by the results of survival studies in patients with chronic heart failure. Long-term treatment with a variety of ACE inhibitors has been shown to reduce mortality regardless of the severity or etiology of the disease or the use of concomitant medications.[80-82] Specifically, ACE inhibitors prolong life in patients with mild, moderate, and severe symptoms; in patients with or without coronary artery disease; and in patients who are and are not receiving digitalis.[80-82] Significant long-term benefits have also been seen in patients with left ventricular systolic dysfunction who have survived a recent myocardial infarction.[83-86] The ability of ACE inhibitors to reduce mortality has been confirmed using various ACE inhibitors and was greater than those achieved with other vasodilators.[87] However, the magnitude (but not the presence) of a survival effect may be related to the severity of symptoms or left ventricular systolic dysfunction. Specifically, ACE inhibitors reduce mortality by approximately 25–30 percent in patients with class III–IV symptoms or in patients with a left ventricular ejection fraction less than 25 percent, whereas the magnitude of benefit declines to approximately 10–15 percent for patients with milder symptoms or degrees of ventricular impairment.[80-82]

In addition to these effects on mortality alone, patients also reduce the risk of clinical progression. Long-term therapy with ACE inhibitors attenuates the process of left ventricular remodeling that characterizes the progression of heart failure.[88,89] Furthermore, prolonged therapy with these drugs reduces the risk of worsening heart failure and diminishes the frequency of hospitalizations for heart failure or other cardiovascular reasons.[81–83] In patients with left ventricular dysfunction due to ischemic heart disease, ACE inhibitors decrease the risk of recurrent myocardial infarction and unstable angina.[83,90] The mechanisms responsible for the reduction in the risk of major ischemic events is unclear, as ACE inhibitors do not exert direct antiischemic or antianginal effects.

The mechanisms responsible for the reduction in overall mortality also remain uncertain. In some trials the decrease in the risk of death has been attributed entirely to a reduction in death due to progressive heart failure; the investigators were not able to discern any decrease in the incidence of sudden death in patients.[81] However, the traditional classification of mortality relies heavily on the symptomatic status of the patient immediately before his or her demise. The death of a patient with dyspnea at rest is considered to be secondary to progressive heart failure, whereas a death may be classified as sudden only if the symptomatic patient had improved during therapy and remained clinically improved until the time of death. Because ACE inhibitors produce symptomatic improvement more frequently than placebo, deaths among patients treated with an ACE inhibitor are more likely to be classified as sudden (when compared with placebo). The uncertainty of any conclusions about the mode of death is underscored by the findings of other studies, in which the improvement in survival was related primarily to a reduction in sudden death and not to a reduction in death due to progressive heart failure.[86,87] To make matters more complicated, ACE inhibitors can reduce the risk of recurrent myocardial infarction in patients with underlying ischemic heart disease, and this benefit may contribute to the reduction in sudden death seen in some studies.[83,90]

CLINICAL USE OF ACE INHIBITORS IN HEART FAILURE

The established benefits of ACE inhibitors in patients with heart failure lead to two important questions: Which patients should be treated with an ACE inhibitor? How should ACE inhibitors be used in these patients?

Who Should Be Treated with an ACE Inhibitor?

Although many patients with chronic heart failure improve symptomatically during long-term treatment with a converting enzyme inhibitor, it is difficult to predict the response to these drugs short of a therapeutic trial. Neither the pretreatment hemodynamic state nor the plasma renin activity accurately presages the long-term effects of treatment. Among all of the variables that have been examined, only two pretreatment variables have predicted the clinical efficacy of converting enzyme inhibitors: renal function and mean right atrial pressure.[91] In patients who have both a mean right atrial pressure of more than 12 mmHg and a serum creatinine concentration of more than 1.5 mg/dl, only 35 percent improve symptomatically. In contrast, if values for the two variables are low, nearly 85 percent show sustained benefits. These observations support the findings of experimental studies suggesting that both volume expansion and nephrectomy independently attenuate the hemodynamic response to ACE inhibitors.

However, ACE inhibitors should not be withheld even in patients with heart failure who have a low likelihood of experiencing symptomatic improvement. Although the demonstration that ACE inhibitors can ameliorate the symptoms of heart failure supports their utility, such studies provide little insight as to which patients with heart failure should receive these drugs and when during the course of the heart failure they should be used. If the ACE inhibitors were simply palliative treatment, they would be reserved as a therapeutic option for patients with end-stage disease and refractory symptoms. Because the ACE inhibitors can favorably alter the natural history of heart failure, the likelihood of clinical improvement in an individual patient has become a secondary issue, as it is possible for a patient to experience prognostic benefits in the absence of symptomatic benefits. In fact, the ability of ACE inhibitors to prolong life has emerged as the most powerful rationale for their widespread use, even if the magnitude of benefit in an individual patient can be expected to be small. Simply put, the available data do not allow physicians to justify withholding ACE inhibitors from any patient with heart failure who can tolerate treatment with the drug.

When considering which patients are candidates for an ACE inhibitor, physicians should recognize that many patients who are at high risk of side effects can benefit from long-term therapy with these drugs. Some physicians routinely avoid the use of ACE inhibitors in some groups of patients (e.g., those with low pretreatment blood pressure or mildly impaired renal function), whom they perceive to be at high risk of experiencing intolerance with treatment. Others readily discontinue the use of ACE inhibitors when the blood pressure falls further or if renal function deteriorates to a mild degree. Yet the available data indicate that such patients derive as much benefit from the use of ACE inhibitors as patients who are perceived to be at low risk. Patients with low baseline blood pressures and those who experience further decreases in blood pressure respond as well to ACE inhibitors as those in whom blood pressure is not a source of concern. Similarly, in controlled studies evaluating survival, patients with renal insufficiency before treatment or who show worsening renal function during treatment show as great a reduction in mortality with ACE inhibitors as those in whom renal function remains within normal limits before or during treatment. Hence strategies that avoid the use of ACE inhibitors in selected groups may deprive many patients of the symptomatic and prognostic benefits of these drugs.

How Should ACE Inhibitors Be Used?

Treatment with ACE inhibitors is generally initiated with small doses that are rapidly increased into the therapeutic range within 1–4 weeks. The full therapeutic effect may not become apparent for 2–3 months.

How should the benefits of ACE inhibitors be measured during this time? A number of quantitative measures have been suggested as a means of following the clinical course of patients with heart failure treated with ACE inhibitors, but there appears to be no reliable method of doing so other than by asking the patients how they feel. Noninvasive tests of left ventricular function (echocardiography or nuclear ventriculography) are not sufficiently sensitive to detect significant changes in cardiac performance with confidence; little change in cardiac performance may be seen even in patients who experience marked symptomatic improvement. Although exercise tolerance provides an objective measure of efficacy in patients with heart failure who participate in placebo-controlled studies, the duration of exercise is greatly influenced by the motivation the patient and the physician and this measure cannot be used reliably in an uncontrolled clinical setting. Most importantly,

therapy should be continued indefinitely regardless of whether the patient appears to respond symptomatically because of the likelihood (as emphasized earlier) that the drug can provide prognostic benefits even in the absence of any effect on symptoms or exercise tolerance.

What dose of an ACE inhibitor is needed to produce optimal benefits in patients with chronic heart failure? Nearly all of the controlled trials that have shown these agents can prolong life have employed large doses of the drugs (150–300 mg daily of captopril, 20–40 mg daily of enalapril, or 20 mg daily of lisinopril).[80–83] Nevertheless, these drugs are usually prescribed in the clinical setting at much lower doses (e.g., captopril 25–50 mg daily and enalapril and lisinopril 2.5–5.0 mg daily)—doses that are similar to those recommended for the initiation, rather than maintenance, of therapy. These low doses are popular among physicians because they produce symptomatic benefits in some patients and are believed to be as effective (and better tolerated) than higher doses. However, numerous studies have suggested that high doses of ACE inhibitors are more effective than low doses. In an open-label study with captopril, high doses (more than 75 mg daily) produced a more favorable effect on functional capacity than low doses (less than 75 mg daily).[92] In a double-blind study with quinapril, exercise capacity improved more in patients randomly assigned to 40 mg daily than in patients treated with 10 mg daily.[73] In two double-blind studies with enalapril, patients assigned to high doses (15–20 mg twice daily) experienced greater hemodynamic, neurohormonal, and symptomatic benefits and fewer cardiovascular events than those assigned to 2.5–5.0 mg twice daily.[93,94] Of note, in these four studies the frequency of side effects seen in patients treated with large doses was similar to that in patients treated with low doses. Finally, in an experimental model of heart failure that is exquisitely sensitive to converting enzyme inhibition, high doses of lisinopril were superior to low doses of lisinopril for prolonging life.[21] Taken collectively, these experiences suggest that physicians should prescribe ACE inhibitors at the target doses used in clinical trials; lower doses should be prescribed only if the target doses in an individual patient cannot be tolerated.

Even if optimal doses of ACE inhibitors are prescribed for the treatment of heart failure, the full benefits of therapy may not be realized because of the use of concomitant medications, most importantly the use of aspirin. Aspirin is widely used in patients with heart failure, either to reduce the risk of recurrent myocardial ischemic events in patients with coronary artery disease or to decrease the frequency of systemic embolic events in patients with normal coronary arteries, although the data supporting these uses are not compelling. Nevertheless, the use of aspirin has been shown to attenuate the hemodynamic actions of ACE inhibitors in patients with heart failure,[40] possibly because aspirin reduces the effects of kinins, which appear to play an important role in mediating the favorable effects of ACE inhibitors in this disorder. Indeed, in large multicenter trials, the concomitant use of aspirin was associated with a loss of the survival benefits of captopril and enalapril and caused marked attenuation of the benefits of these drugs on cardiovascular morbidity.[41] These data (together with the lack of data supporting the use of aspirin) suggest that physicians should reevaluate the use of aspirin in all patients with heart failure who are receiving ACE inhibitors.

ADVERSE EFFECTS OF ACE INHIBITORS IN HEART FAILURE

The adverse effects of ACE inhibitors can largely be attributed to the two principal pharmacologic actions of these drugs: (1) those related to the effects of angiotensin suppression; and (2) those related to the effects of kinin potentiation.

Adverse Effects Related to Angiotensin Suppression

The three principal adverse effects related to angiotensin suppression are hypotension, functional renal insufficiency, and potassium retention. Hypotension occurs as a result of the loss of the vasoconstrictor effect of angiotensin on the systemic vasculature[43] and may be potentiated by the lack of a pulmonary vasodilator effect.[55] Functional renal insufficiency results from the loss of angiotensin's vasoconstrictor effect on the efferent (postglomerular) arteriole and may be potentiated by a decrease in renal perfusion pressure.[95] Potassium retention may result from loss of the stimulatory effect of angiotensin on aldosterone secretion and may be potentiated by deterioration in renal function or by administration of potassium supplements.[96]

SYMPTOMATIC HYPOTENSION

The most common adverse effect of ACE inhibition in patients with severe heart failure is systemic hypotension. Blood pressure declines in nearly every patient treated with an ACE inhibitor, but these decreases (although occasionally marked) usually do not produce symptoms. Hypotension is only a concern if it is accompanied by dizziness, blurred vision, or syncope; such events may occur at any time during the course of treatment but are seen most frequently during the first 24 hours of therapy. Patients with the most marked activation of the renin-angiotensin system are most likely to experience early hypotensive reactions; such patients can be identified clinically by the presence of marked hyponatremia (serum sodium concentration less than 130 mmol/L)[97] or by the recent occurrence of a rapid diuresis. In such individuals, ACE inhibition should be initiated cautiously and in small doses (6.25 mg of captopril or 2.5 mg of enalapril); attempts to decrease dependence of the patient on the renin-angiotensin system by withholding diuretics for 1–2 days may enhance the margin of safety. Should symptomatic hypotension occur with first doses, it may not recur with repeated administration of the same doses of the drug; however, it is prudent under such circumstances to reduce the level of angiotensin dependence (i.e., reducing doses of diuretics, liberalization of dietary salt, or both). Most patients who experience early symptomatic hypotension remain excellent candidates for long-term ACE inhibition if appropriate measures are taken to minimize recurrent hypotensive reactions.

FUNCTIONAL RENAL INSUFFICIENCY

In states characterized by reduced renal perfusion, glomerular filtration is critically dependent on angiotensin II-mediated efferent arteriolar vasoconstriction[95]; under such circumstances, ACE inhibition may cause functional renal insufficiency.[98] Because the decline in glomerular filtration is related to the withdrawal of angiotensin II, it is not surprising that the risk of azotemia is highest in patients who are most dependent on the renin-angiotensin system for the support of renal homeostasis (class IV hypotensive or hyponatremic patients).[99] Functional renal insufficiency develops in 25–50 percent of patients with severe (class IIIB–IV) heart failure but in only 5–15 percent of patients with moderate (class II–III) heart failure. It should be noted that in patients who are at risk, functional renal insufficiency may occur even with small doses of ACE inhibitors; thus these side effects (once apparent) are often not responsive to a reduction in dose of the ACE inhibitor. The development of azotemia can usually be ameliorated by reducing the dose of concomitantly administered diuretic and thus can generally be managed without the need to withdraw treatment.

POTASSIUM RETENTION

Hyperkalemia can occur during ACE inhibition in patients with chronic heart failure and may be sufficiently severe to cause cardiac conduction disturbances.[96] Such events usually occur in patients in whom renal function deteriorates or who are taking oral potassium supplements, either in the form of prescribed potassium salts or as over-the-counter salt substitutes. Diabetes also increases the risk of hyperkalemia. Because ACE inhibition attenuates potassium loss by interfering with the stimulation of aldosterone synthesis, it is usually not necessary to administer potassium supplements to patients taking an ACE inhibitor, except when high doses of diuretics are required. Similarly, to minimize problems with hyperkalemia, potassium-sparing diuretics (e.g., spironolactone) should rarely be administered together with ACE inhibitors.

Adverse Effects Related to Kinin Accumulation

The most common adverse effects of ACE inhibitors related to kinin accumulation include cough and angioneurotic edema. Cough has been a particularly striking side effect of ACE inhibitors, occurring in as many as 5–25 percent of patients.[100] The cough is invariably nonproductive and is characteristically accompanied by a persistent and annoying "tickle" in the back of the throat. It usually appears within the first several months of therapy, disappears within 1–2 weeks of discontinuing treatment and recurs within days of rechallenge. In a patient with suspected "ACE inhibitor cough," other causes for cough should always be considered (particularly pulmonary congestion). Most episodes of cough in patients receiving an ACE inhibitor are not related to use of the ACE inhibitor; therefore physicians who attribute every cough in a patient receiving an ACE inhibitor to treatment with the drug deprive many patients of the benefits of these agents.

The diagnosis of "ACE inhibitor cough" should be made only after other causes of cough have been excluded and after the physician confirms that the cough disappears following withdrawal of the drug, recurs after rechallenge with the same drug, and recurs after rechallenge with another ACE inhibitor (the cough is related to the common action of all ACE inhibitors). A therapeutic trial of vigorous diuretic therapy may be needed to exclude pulmonary congestion as the cause of the cough. The cough is occasionally ameliorated by a reduction in the dose of the ACE inhibitor or by the use of cromolyn sodium,[101] but most frequently it requires withdrawal of the ACE inhibitor and use of alternative medications (e.g., angiotensin II receptor antagonists).

Angioneurotic edema occurs rarely (less than 1 percent risk) with any ACE inhibitor; and because its occurrence may be life-threatening, the clinical suspicion of such a reaction in an individual justifies avoidance of all ACE inhibitors for the lifetime of the patient. Angioneurotic edema appears to be more frequent in blacks.

Other Adverse Reactions

Rash and dysgeusia are not related to kinin accumulation but are probably related to the sulfhydryl moiety of some ACE inhibitors, occurring in about 3–5 percent of patients treated with captopril but in fewer than 1 percent of the patients treated with nonsulfhydryl ACE inhibitors. Both the rash and the dysgeusia may disappear despite continued therapy and may not recur on rechallenge with the drug.

Although the occurrence of leukopenia and proteinuria were raised as concerns when ACE inhibitors were first introduced into clinical practice, these side effects occur rarely and almost exclusively in patients with specific underlying diseases (e.g., collagen vascular diseases).

EFFECTS OF RENIN INHIBITORS AND ANGIOTENSIN RECEPTOR ANTAGONISTS

An alternative approach to inhibiting the actions of angiotensin II in patients with heart failure is the use of drugs that target components of the renin-angiotensin cascade other than the angiotensin-converting enzyme. Pharmacologic agents that inhibit the active site of renin or block the angiotensin II receptor have been developed and have been evaluated in patients with heart failure. Experience with these agents for treatment of this disorder is limited, however, and none of the drugs has been approved for the management of heart failure by the U.S. Food and Drug Administration. These new approaches offer several potential advantages over ACE inhibitors, but it seems unlikely that these drugs will replace ACE inhibitors as an established therapy for heart failure.

Angiotensin II Receptor Antagonists

Angiotensin II receptor antagonists were developed based on the premise that interference with the renin-angiotensin system without inhibition of kininase would be associated with all of the benefits of ACE inhibitors but without any of their adverse reactions.[102] The premise was largely based on the belief that all of the benefits of ACE inhibitors were related to the suppression of angiotensin II formation and that the side effects were related to the accumulation of kinins. As our knowledge of the pathophysiology of heart failure has advanced, the potential advantages of angiotensin II receptor antagonists (compared with ACE inhibitors) seem less likely. Most of the side effects of ACE inhibitors in heart failure are related to the suppression of angiotensin II formation, whereas many of the benefits of ACE inhibitors can be explained by the accumulation of kinins (both discussed earlier in this chapter). Furthermore, most angiotensin II receptor antagonists act selectively to block the type 1 receptor but do not interfere with the type 2 receptor, which may mediate the adverse effects of angiotensin on ventricular remodeling.[28-30]

Nevertheless, angiotensin II receptor antagonists (specifically losartan) have been evaluated for the treatment of heart failure, although experience to date is limited. In a single-dose, short-term hemodynamic study,[103] losartan produced dose-dependent hemodynamic benefits similar to those reported with ACE inhibitors up to a dose of 25 mg. Larger doses of losartan did not produce greater hemodynamic effects, possibly because these larger doses were associated with reactive increases in both plasma renin activity and angiotensin II. The latter may have acted to overcome the competitive blockade produced by the drug. These favorable hemodynamic effects of losartan were shown to be sustained after 8 weeks of treatment in a large multicenter study, but the circulatory benefits were not necessarily translated into an improvement in the clinical status of patients.[104]

Indeed, there have been no placebo-controlled trials demonstrating the symptomatic benefits of losartan or any angiotensin II receptor antagonist in patients with chronic heart failure. The only clinical study to date compared losartan and enalapril with a placebo group; but in the absence of a valid control group, the results of this trial are difficult to interpret.[105] Of note, however, was the observation in this study that the expected effects of ACE inhibition on potassium and renal function were less marked with losartan than with enalapril. Whether this finding represents a safety advantage of losartan or an indication that losartan produces less inhibition of the renin-angiotensin system (and less benefit) remains to be seen. Several large-scale studies comparing angiotensin II receptor antagonists and ACE inhibitors are presently being planned or are in progress.[106]

Until these trials are completed, it seems appropri-ate to reserve the use of angiotensin II receptor antagonists to patients with chronic heart failure who cannot tolerate treatment with an ACE inhibitor because of side effects related to the generation of kinins (cough, angioneurotic edema). Consideration should also be given in the future to adding angiotensin II antagonists to the treatment regimen of patients with heart failure already receiving ACE inhibitors in the hope that the receptor antagonists might block the actions of angiotensin formed by non-ACE-dependent pathways.[46]

Renin Inhibitors

Agents that inhibit the active site of renin have been developed for the treatment of hypertension,[107] but experience with these drugs in patients with heart failure is limited. In experimental and clinical studies, renin inhibition produced short-term hemodynamic effects similar to those seen with ACE inhibition,[108-112] but no long-term hemodynamic or clinical studies have been carried out to date.

REFERENCES

1. Packer M: The neurohormonal hypothesis. A theory to explain the mechanism of disease progression in heart failure. J Am Coll Cardiol 20:248, 1992
2. Francis GS, Benedict C, Johnstone DE et al: Comparison of neuroendocrine activation in patients with left ventricular dysfunction with and without congestive heart failure. A substudy of the Studies of Left Ventricular Dysfunction (SOLVD). Circulation 82:1724, 1990
3. Thomas JA, Marks BH: Plasma norepinephrine in congestive heart failure. Am J Cardiol 41:233, 1978
4. Cohn JN, Levine TB, Olivari MT et al: Plasma norepinephrine as a guide to prognosis in patients with chronic congestive heart failure. N Engl J Med 311:819, 1984
5. Swedberg K, Eneroth P, Kjekshus J, Wilhelmsen L: Hormones regulating cardiovascular function in patients with severe congestive heart failure and their relation to mortality. CONSENSUS trial study group. Circulation 82:1730, 1990
6. Tan L-B, Jalil JE, Pick R, Janicki JS, Weber KT: Cardiac myocyte necrosis induced by angiotensin II. Circ Res 69:1185, 1991
7. Riegger GAJ, Liebau G, Holzsehuh M et al: Role of the renin-angiotensin system in the development of congestive heart failure in the dog assessed by chronic converting-enzyme blockade. Am J Cardiol 53:614, 1984
8. Sabbah HN, Shimoyama H, Kono T et al: Effects of long-term monotherapy with enalapril, metoprolol, and digoxin on the progression of left ventricular dysfunction and dilation in dogs with reduced ejection fraction. Circulation 89:2852, 1994
9. McDonald KM, Rector T, Carlyle PF, Francis GS, Cohn JN: Angiotensin-converting enzyme inhibition and beta-adrenoceptor blockade regress established

ventricular remodeling in a canine model of discrete myocardial damage. J Am Coll Cardiol 24:1762, 1994

10. Merrill AJ, Morrison JL, Brannon ES: Concentration of renin in renal venous blood in patients with chronic heart failure. Am J Med 1:468, 1946

11. Turini GA, Brunner HR, Ferguson RR, Riviera JL, Gavras H: Congestive heart failure in normotensive man. Haemodynamics, renin and angiotensin-II blockade. Br Heart J 40:1134, 1978

12. Falkenhahn M, Franke F, Bohle RM et al: Cellular distribution of angiotensin-converting enzyme after myocardial infarction. Hypertension 25:219, 1995

13. Pieruzzi F, Abassi ZA, Keiser HR: Expression of renin-angiotensin system components in the heart, kidneys, and lungs of rats with experimental heart failure. Circulation 92:3105, 1995

14. Bruckschlegel G, Holmer SR, Jandeleit K et al: Blockade of the renin-angiotensin system in cardiac pressure-overload hypertrophy in rats. Hypertension 25:250, 1995

15. Farivar RS, Crawford DC, Chobanian AV, Brecher P: Effect of angiotensin II blockade on the fibroproliferative response to phenylephrine in the rat heart. Hypertension 25:809, 1995

16. Sung CP, Arleth AJ, Storer BL, Ohlstein EH: Angiotensin type 1 receptors mediate smooth muscle proliferation and endothelin biosynthesis in rat vascular smooth muscle. J Pharmacol Exp Ther 271:429, 1994

17. Yamada T, Horiuchi M, Dzau VJ: Angiotensin II type 2 receptor mediates programmed cell death. Proc Natl Acad Sci USA 93:156, 1996

18. Hirsch AT, Talsness CE, Schunkert H, Paul M, Dzau VJ: Tissue-specific activation of cardiac angiotensin converting enzyme in experimental heart failure. Circ Res 69:475, 1991

19. Schunkert H, Ingelfinger JR, Hirsch AT et al: Evidence for tissue-specific activation of renal angiotensinogen mRNA expression in chronic stable experimental heart failure. J Clin Invest 90:1523, 1992

20. Schunkert H, Tang S, Litwin SE et al: Regulation of intrarenal and circulating renin-angiotensin systems in severe heart failure in the rat. Cardiovasc Res 27:731, 1993

21. Wollert KC, Studer R, von Bulow B, Drexler H: Survival after myocardial infarction in the rat. Role of tissue angiotensin-converting enzyme inhibition. Circulation 90:2457, 1994

22. Brunner HR, Laragh JH, Baer L et al: Essential hypertension. Renin and aldosterone, heart attack and stroke. N Engl J Med 286:441, 1972

23. Riegger AJC, Lever AF, Millar JA et al: Correction of renal hypertension in the rat by prolonged infusion of angiotensin II inhibitors. Lancet 2:1317, 1977

24. Regitz-Zagrosek V, Neuss M, Holzmeister J, Fleck E: Use of angiotensin II antagonists in human heart failure. Function of the subtype 1 receptor. J Hypertens Suppl 13:63, 1995

25. Stoll M, Stecklings UM, Paul M et al: The angiotensin AT2-receptor mediates inhibition of cell proliferation in coronary endothelial cells. J Clin Invest 95:651, 1995

26. Sharov VG, Sabbah HN, Shimoyama H et al: Evidence of cardiocyte apoptosis in myocardium of dogs with chronic heart failure. Am J Pathol 148:141, 1996

27. Bing OH: Hypothesis. Apoptosis may be a mechanism for the transition to heart failure with chronic pressure overload. J Mol Cell Cardiol 26:943, 1995

28. Nio Y, Matsubara H, Marusawa S, Kanasaki M, Inada M: Regulation of gene transcription of angiotensin II receptor subtypes in myocardial infarction. J Clin Invest 95:46, 1995

29. McDonald KM, Garr M, Carlyle PF et al: Relative effects of alpha-1-adrenoceptor blockade, converting enzyme inhibitor therapy, and angiotensin II subtype 1 receptor blockade on ventricular remodeling in the dog. Circulation 90:3034, 1994

30. Stauss M, Zhu YC, Redlich T et al: Angiotensin-converting enzyme inhibition in infarct-induced heart failure in rats. Bradykinin versus angiotensin II. J Cardiovasc Risk 1:255, 1994

31. Waagstein F, Hjalmarson A, Varnauskas E, Wallentin I: Effect of chronic beta-adrenergic receptor blockade in congestive cardiomyopathy. Br Heart J 37:1022, 1975

32. Murthy VS, Waldron TL, Goldberg ME: The mechanism of bradykinin potentiation after inhibition of angiotensin-converting enzyme by SQ 14,225 in conscious rabbits. Circ Res, suppl. I 43:40, 1978

33. Ruocco NA Jr, Bergelson BA, Yu TK, Gavras I, Gavras H: Augmentation of coronary blood flow by ACE inhibition. Role of angiotensin and bradykinin. Clin Exp Hypertens 17:1059, 1995

34. Katz SD, Schwarz M, Yuen J, Golberger M, LeJemtel TH: Enalaprilat mediates peripheral vasodilation by endothelium-dependent mechanisms. Circulation, suppl. I 86:49, 1992

35. Auch-Schwelk W, Duske E, Calus M et al: Endothelium-mediated vasodilation during ACE inhibition. Eur Heart J, suppl. C 16:59, 1995

36. Friedrich SP, Lorell BH, Rousseau MF et al: Intracardiac angiotensin-converting enzyme inhibition improves diastolic function in patients with left ventricular hypertrophy due to aortic stenosis. Circulation 90:2761, 1994

37. Anning PB, Grocott-Mason RM, Lewis MJ, Shah AM: Enhancement of left ventricular relaxation in the isolated heart by an angiotensin-converting enzyme inhibitor. Circulation 92:2660, 1995

38. Buckley BJ, Mirza Z, Whorton AR: Regulation of Ca^{2+}-dependent nitric oxide synthase in bovine aortic endothelial cells. Am J Physiol 269:C757, 1995

39. McDonald KM, Mock J, D'Aloia A et al: Bradykinin antagonism inhibits the antigrowth effect of converting enzyme inhibition in the dog myocardium after discrete transmural myocardial necrosis. Circulation 91:2043, 1995

40. Hall D, Zeitler H, Rudolph W: Counteraction of the vasodilator effects of enalapril by aspirin in severe heart failure. J Am Coll Cardiol 20:1549, 1992

41. Al-Khadra AS, Salem DN, Rand WM et al: Effect of anti-platelet agents on survival in patients with left ventricular systolic dysfunction. Circulation, suppl. I 92:665, 1995

42. Cleland J, Semple P, Hodsman P et al: Angiotensin II levels, hemodynamics, and sympathoadrenal function after low-dose captopril in heart failure. Am J Med 77:880, 1984

43. Cleland JGF, Dargie HJ, McAlpine H et al: Severe hypotension after first dose of enalapril in heart failure. BMJ 291:1309, 1985

44. Helin K, Tikkanen I, Hohenthal U, Fyhrquist F: Inhi-

bition of either angiotensin-converting enzyme or neutral endopeptidase induces both enzymes. Eur J Pharmacol 264:135, 1994

45. Cleland JGF, Poole-Wilson PA: ACE inhibitors for heart failure. A question of dose. Br Heart J, suppl. 72:106, 1994

46. Urata H, Strobel F, Ganten D: Widespread distribution of human chymase. J Hypertens 12:S17, 1994

47. Morgan K: Diverse factors influencing angiotensin metabolism during ACE inhibition. Insights from molecular biology and genetic studies. Br Heart J suppl. 72:3, 1994

48. Zisman LS, Abraham WT, Meixell GE et al: Angiotensin II formation in the intact human heart. Predominance of the angiotensin-converting enzyme pathway. J Clin Invest 96:1490, 1995

49. Masse BM, Kramer BL, Topic, N: Long-term captopril therapy for chronic congestive heart failure. Am J Cardiol 53:1316, 1984.

50. Packer M, Medina N, Yushak M et al: Hemodynamic patterns of response during long-term captopril therapy for severe chronic heart failure. Circulation 68:803, 1983

51. Rose JC, Kot P, Cohn JN et al: Comparison of effects of angiotensin and norepinephrine on pulmonary circulation, systemic arteries and veins, and systemic vascular capacity in the dog. Circulation 25:247, 1962

52. DePasquale NP, Burch GE: Effect of angiotensin II on the intact forearm veins of man. Circ Res 13:239, 1963

53. Trippodo NC, Panchal BC, Fox M: Repression of angiotensin II and potentiation of bradykinin contribute to the synergistic effects of dual metalloprotease inhibition in heart failure. J Pharmacol Exp Ther 272:619, 1995

54. Foult JM, Tavolaro O, Anthony I et al: Direct myocardial and coronary effects of enalaprilat in patients with dilated cardiomyopathy. Assessment by a bilateral intracoronary infusion technique. Circulation 77:337, 1988

55. Packer M, Lee WH, Medina N et al: Hemodynamic and clinical significance of the pulmonary vascular response to long-term captopril therapy in patients with severe chronic heart failure. J Am Coll Cardiol 6:635, 1985

56. Massie BM, Kramer BL, Topic N: Lack of relationship between short-term hemodynamic effects of captopril and subsequent clinical responses. Circulation 69:1135, 1984

57. Packer M, Carver JR, Rodeheffer RJ et al: Effect of oral milrinone on mortality in severe chronic heart failure. N Engl J Med 325:1468, 1991

58. Packer M, Rouleau J, Swedberg K et al: Effect of flosequinan on survival in chronic heart failure. Preliminary results of the PROFILE study. Circulation, suppl. I 88:301, 1993

59. Cody RJ, Franklin KW, Kulger J et al: Sympathetic responsiveness and plasma norepinephrine during therapy of chronic congestive heart failure with captopril. Am J Med 72:791, 1982

60. Mettauer B, Rouleau JL, Bichet D et al: Differential long-term intrarenal and neurohormonal effects of captopril and prazosin in patients with chronic heart failure. Importance of initial plasma renin activity. Circulation 73:492, 1987

61. Warren JB, Loi RK: Captopril increases skin micro-

vascular blood flow secondary to bradykinin, nitric oxide, and prostaglandins. FASEB J 9:411, 1995

62. Flapan AD, Nolan J, Neilson JM, Ewing DJ: Effect of captopril on cardiac parasympathetic activity in chronic cardiac failure secondary to coronary artery disease. Am J Cardiol 69:532, 1992

63. Kramer BL, Massie BM, Topic N: Controlled trial of captopril in chronic heart failure. A rest and exercise hemodynamic study. Circulation 67:807, 1983

64. Captopril Multicenter Research Group: A placebo controlled trial of captopril in refractory chronic congestive heart failure. J Am Coll Cardiol 2:755, 1983

65. Sharpe DN, Murphy J, Coxon R et al: Enalapril in patients with chronic heart failure. A placebo-controlled, randomized, double-blind study. Circulation 70:271, 1984

66. Franciosa JA, Wilen MM, Jordan RA: Effects of enalapril, a new angiotensin-converting enzyme inhibitor, in a controlled trial in heart failure. J Am Coll Cardiol 5:101, 1985

67. Creager MA, Massie BM, Faxon DP et al: Acute and long-term effects of enalapril on the cardiovascular response to exercise and exercise tolerance in patients with congestive heart failure. J Am Coll Cardiol 6:163, 1985

68. Cleland JGF, Dargie JH, Hodsman GP et al: Captopril in heart failure. A double-blind controlled trial. Br Heart J 52:530, 1984

69. Cleland JGF, Dargie HJ, Ball SG et al: Effects of enalapril in heart failure. A double-blind study of effects on exercise performance, renal function, hormones, and metabolic state. Br Heart J 54:305, 1985

70. Cowley AJ, Rowley JM, Stainer KL et al: Captopril therapy for heart failure. A placebo-controlled study. Lancet 2:730, 1982

71. Pflugfelder PW, Baird MG, Tonkon MJ, DiBianco R, Pitt B: Clinical consequences of angiotensin-converting enzyme inhibitor withdrawal in chronic heart failure. A double-blind, placebo-controlled study of quinapril. The Quinapril Heart Failure Trial Investigators. J Am Coll Cardiol 22:1557, 1993

72. Chalmers JP, West MJ, Cyran J et al: Placebo-controlled study of lisinopril in congestive heart failure. A multicentre study. J Cardiovasc Pharmacol, suppl. 3 9:89, 1987

73. Riegger GAJ: Effects of quinapril on exercise tolerance testing in patients with mild to moderate congestive heart failure. Eur Heart J 12:705, 1991

74. Captopril-Digoxin Multicenter Research Group: Comparative effects of captopril and digoxin in patients with mild to moderate heart failure. JAMA 259:539, 1988

75. Richardson A, Bayliss J, Scriven A et al: Double-blind comparison of captopril alone against frusemide plus amiloride in mild heart failure. Lancet 2:709, 1987

76. Hall SA, Cigarroa CG, Marcoux L et al: Time course of improvement in left ventricular function, mass and geometry in patients with congestive heart failure treated with beta-adrenergic blockade. J Am Coll Cardiol 25:1154, 1995

77. Pfeffer JM, Pfeffer MA, Braunwald E: Influence of chronic captopril therapy on the infarcted left ventricle of the rat. Circ Res 57:84, 1985

78. Pfeffer MA, Pfeffer JM, Steinberg C et al: Survival after an experimental myocardial infarction. Benefi-

cial effects of long-term therapy with captopril. Circulation 72:406, 1985

79. Van Gilst WH, de Graeff PA, Wesseling H, et al: Reduction in reperfusion arrhythmias in the ischemic isolated rat heart by angiotensin converting enzyme inhibitors. A comparison of captopril, enalapril and HOE 498. J Cardiovasc Pharmacol 8:722, 1986

80. CONSENSUS Trial Study Group: Effects of enalapril on mortality in severe congestive heart failure. Results of the Cooperative North Scandinavian Enalapril Survival Study. N Engl J Med 316:1429, 1987

81. SOLVD Investigators: Effect of enalapril on survival in patients with reduced left ventricular ejection fractions and congestive heart failure. N Engl J Med 325:293, 1991

82. SOLVD Investigators: Effect of enalapril on mortality and the development of heart failure in asymptomatic patients with reduced left ventricular ejection fractions. N Engl J Med 327:685, 1992

83. Pfeffer MA, Braunwald E, Moye LA et al: Effect of captopril on mortality and morbidity in patients with left ventricular dysfunction after myocardial infarction. Results of the Survival and Ventricular Enlargement Trial. N Engl J Med 327:669, 1992

84. Gruppo Italiano per lo Studio della Sopravvivenza nell'infarcto Miocardico (GISSI–3). Effects of lisinopril and transdermal glyceryl trinitrate singly and together on 6-week mortality and ventricular function after acute myocardial infarction. Lancet 343:1115, 1994

85. Acute Infarction Ramipril Efficacy (AIRE) Study Investigators: Effect of ramipril on mortality and morbidity of survivors of acute myocardial infarction with clinical evidence of heart failure. Lancet 342:821, 1992

86. Kober L, Torp-Perdersen C, Carlsen JE et al: A clinical trial of the angiotensin-converting enzyme inhibitor trandolapril in patients with left ventricular dysfunction after myocardial infarction. N Engl J Med 333:1670, 1995

87. Cohn JN, Johnson G, Ziesche S et al: A comparison of enalapril with hydralazine-isosorbide dinitrate in the treatment of chronic congestive heart failure. N Engl J Med 325:303, 1991

88. Pfeffer MA, Lamas GA, Vaughn DE et al: Effect of captopril on progressive ventricular dilatation after anterior myocardial infarction. N Engl J Med 319:80, 1988

89. Sharpe N, Murphy J, Smith H et al: Treatment of patients with symptomless left ventricular dysfunction after myocardial infarction. Lancet 1:255, 1988

90. Yusuf S, Pepine CJ, Garces C et al: Effect of enalapril on myocardial infarction and unstable angina in patients with low ejection fractions. Lancet 340:1173, 1992

91. Packer M, Lee WH, Medina N, Yushak M, Kessler P: Identification of patients with severe heart failure most likely to fail long-term therapy with converting enzyme inhibitors. J Am Coll Cardiol 7:181A, 1986

92. Pacher R, Globits S, Bergler-Klein J et al: Clinical and neurohumoral response of patients with severe congestive heart failure treated with two different captopril dosages. Eur Heart J 14:273, 1993

93. Vagelos R, Nejedly M, Willson K, Yee YG, Fowler M: Comparison of low versus high dose enalapril ther-

apy for patients with severe congestive heart failure [abstract]. J Am Coll Cardiol 17:275A, 1991

94. Pacher R, Stanek B, Berger R et al: Low versus high dose enalapril in severe heart failure [abstract]. Eur Heart J 16:152, 1995

95. Packer M, Lee WH, Kessler PD: Preservation of glomerular filtration rate in human heart failure by activation of the renin-angiotensin system. Circulation 74:766, 1986

96. Packer M, Lee WH, Medina N, Yushak M: Identification of patients with heart failure at risk of potassium retention during converting-enzyme inhibition. Circulation, suppl. IV 76:273, 1987

97. Packer M, Medina N, Yushak M: Relationship between serum sodium concentration and the hemodynamic and clinical responses to converting-enzyme inhibition in severe heart failure. J Am Coll Cardiol 3:1035, 1984

98. Packer M, Lee WH, Medina N et al: Functional renal insufficiency during long-term therapy with captopril or enalapril for severe chronic heart failure. Ann Intern Med 106:346, 1987

99. Packer M, Lee WH, Kessler PD et al: Identification of hyponatremia as a risk factor for the development of functional renal insufficiency during converting-enzyme inhibition in severe chronic heart failure. J Am Coll Cardiol 10:837, 1987

100. Ravid D, Lishner M, Lang R, Ravid M: Angiotensin-converting enzyme inhibitors and cough. A prospective evaluation in hypertension and in congestive heart failure. J Clin Pharmacol 34:1116, 1994

101. Hargreaves MR, Benson MK: Inhaled sodium cromoglycate in angiotensin-converting enzyme inhibition cough. Lancet 345:13, 1995

102. Chang PI, Pitt B: Theoretical basis for the use of angiotensin II antagonists in the treatment of heart failure. Cardiologia, suppl. 1 39:409, 1994

103. Gottlieb SS, Dickstein K, Fleck E et al: Hemodynamic and neurohormonal effects of the angiotensin II antagonist losartan in patients with congestive heart failure. Circulation 88:1602, 1993

104. Crozier I, Ikram H, Awan N et al: Losartan in heart failure. Hemodynamic effects and tolerability. Circulation 91:691, 1995

105. Dickstein K, Chang P, Willenheimer R et al: Comparison of the effects of losartan and enalapril on clinical status and exercise performance in patients with moderate or severe chronic heart failure. J Am Coll Cardiol 26:438, 1995

106. Pitt B, Chang P, Timmermans PB: Angiotensin II receptor antagonists in heart failure. Rationale and design of the evaluation of losartan in the elderly (ELITE) trial. Cardiovasc Drug Ther 9:693, 1995

107. Kleinert HD: Renin inhibition. Cardiovasc Drug Ther 9:645, 1995

108. Sweet CS, Ludden CT, Frederick CM, Bush LR, Ribeiro LG: Comparative hemodynamic effects of MK-422, a converting-enzyme inhibitor, and a renin inhibitor in dogs with acute left ventricular failure. J Cardiovasc Pharmacol 6:1067, 1984

109. Fitzpatrick MA, Rademaker MT, Frampton CM et al: Hemodynamic and hormonal effects of renin inhibition in ovine heart failure. Am J Physiol 258:H1625, 1990

110. Mento PF, Maita ME, Murphy WR, Holt WF, Wilkes BM: Comparison of angiotensin converting enzyme

and renin inhibition in rats following myocardial infarction. J Cardiovasc Pharmacol 21:791, 1993

111. Neuberg GW, Kukin ML, Penn J et al: Hemodynamic effects of renin inhibition by enalkiren in chronic congestive heart failure. Am J Cardiol 67: 63, 1991

112. Kiowski W, Beerman J, Rickenbacher P et al: Angiotensinergic versus nonangiotensinergic hemodynamic effects of converting enzyme inhibition in patients with chronic heart failure. Assessment by acute renin and converting-enzyme inhibition. Circulation 90:2748, 1994

46 Positive Inotropic Therapy

Arthur M. Feldman
Barry M. Massie

Patients with dilated cardiomyopathies often exhibit both systolic and diastolic dysfunction, but it is systolic dysfunction that is the most consistent feature and the predominant pathophysiologic derangement in most patients. The resulting impairment of left ventricular pump function is ultimately responsible for the primary symptoms and signs of congestive heart failure: shortness of breath, exercise intolerance, fatigue, multiple organ dysfunction, and edema. Therefore intuitively patients with systolic dysfunction should benefit from pharmacologic agents that augment the contractility, or inotropic state, of the myocardium. Theoretically, this benefit should be reflected not only in improved symptom status but in stabilization of the progressive clinical course of dilated cardiomyopathy, as one mechanism of progression is the vicious cycle of increased wall stress begetting further left ventricular dilatation and dysfunction. Indeed, inotropic agents could be beneficial not only by supporting pump function but also by decreasing both adrenergic drive[1] and renin-angiotensin activation.[2]

Investigators have also raised cogent arguments that inotropic agents might be deleterious to the failing heart by inducing arrhythmias, adversely affecting myocardial energetics, impairing cardiac relaxation, and accelerating the progression of cardiac disease.[3–7] These arguments have to a large extent been stimulated by and gained support from the results of several clinical trials of inotropic agents, which have demonstrated adverse, rather than favorable, outcomes.[7–11] On the other hand, studies have suggested potential benefits of certain inotropic agents in patients with chronic congestive heart failure, and these agents remain a mainstay in the treatment of patients in the critical care environment.[12–14] Indeed, it is likely that this controversy will be resolved only when the mechanistic differences between agents that produce the same physiologic response—that is, increased contractility—are clarified and the differing clinical impact of this intervention in patients with differing etiologies and severity of cardiomyopathy are better understood.

In Chapter 43 Kelly et al. review the pharmacology and therapeutic usage of the oldest class of positive inotropic agents, the digitalis glycosides. Perhaps the controversy surrounding the use of inotropic agents in the management of patients with congestive failure is best exemplified by the fact that during the more than 200 years since Withering's discovery of the benefits of the foxglove plant only three additional inotropic agents have been approved for use in the management of patients with congestive heart failure in the United States, all of which are parenteral drugs used primarily for short-term therapy. In this chapter we discuss the pharmacology and therapeutic utility of the approved intravenous inotropic agents for managing patients with both acute and chronic heart failure. We also review the results of recent trials with a variety of oral inotropic agents and discuss the potential future role of this class of medications.

CLASSIFICATION OF INOTROPIC AGENTS

Part of the confusion regarding the use and evaluation of inotropic agents has come from the fact that they are generally viewed in the generic sense. That is, all inotropes are considered to produce the same physiologic outcome and clinical effects, whether beneficial or adverse. As we have improved our understanding of excitation-contraction coupling in both normal and failing human heart, we have gained a better understanding of how various agents can augment cardiac contractility.[15] Figure 46-1 illustrates the many pathways that have been shown to be important in regulating contractility.[16] It has become increasingly obvious that different inotropic agents not only have different mechanisms of action, they are also likely to have different short- and long-term benefits. In addition, designer agents have been developed that target selected proteins within the excitation-contraction pathway to selectively augment cardiac contractility. Historically, most discussions of inotropic drugs have primarily differentiated them by their route of administration into intravenous and oral agents. Such a classification system provides the clinician with no understanding of the mechanisms of action of these agents or insight into potential differences in clinical responses.

Therefore we have proposed a classification system that categorizes inotropic agents according to their mechanisms of action (Table 46-1).[16] Class I agents are those that augment intracellular levels of cyclic adenosine monophosphate (cAMP). Class II agents augment contractility by affecting ion pumps or channels. Class III agents enhance contractility by modulating intracellular calcium regulation.

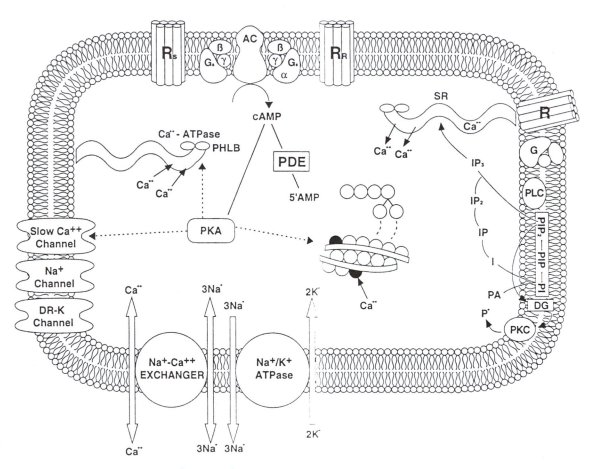

Fig. 46-1. Biochemical pathways important in regulation of cardiac contractility. AC-adenylyl cyclase; ATP, adenosine triphosphate; cAMP, cyclic adenosine monophosphate; DG, diacylglycerol; DR, delayed rectifier; G, guanine nucleotide-binding regulatory proteins that may stimulate (αG_S) or inhibit (αG_I) adenylyl cyclase; I, inositol; IP, inositol phosphate; IP_2, inositol diphosphate; IP_3, inositol triphosphate; PDE, phosphodiesterase; PHLB, phospholamban; PI, phosphatidylinositol; PIP, phosphatidylinositol 4-phosphate; PIP_2, phosphatidylinositol 4,5-biphosphate; PKA, protein kinase A; PKC, protein kinase C; PLC, phospholipase C; R, sarcolemmal receptor; R_R, inhibitory receptor; R_S, stimulatory receptor; SR, sarcoplasmic reticulum; Tn, troponin. (From Feldman,[16] with permission.)

Table 46-1. Classes of Inotropic Agents by Mechanism of Action

Class	Definition
I	Agents that increase intracellular cyclic adenosine monophosphate (cAMP) β-Adrenergic agonists Phosphodiesterase inhibitors
II	Agents that affect sarcolemmal ions pumps/channels Digoxin
III	Agents that modulate intracellular calcium mechanisms by Release of sarcoplasmic reticulum calcium (IP$_3$) Increased sensitization of the contractile proteins to calcium
IV	Drugs having multiple mechanisms of action Pimobendan Vesnarinone

Abbreviation: IP$_3$, inositol triphosphate.
(From Feldman,[16] with permission.)

Class IV agents increase myocardial contractility through multiple pathways. Although this classification system allows the physician to correlate the basic physiology of cardiac contractility with the action of selected inotropic drugs and helps to clarify the potential synergistic effects of some inotropic agents, it does have some limitations. This classification system does not suggest that some classes of inotropic agents might be more effective than others, nor does it imply that potential beneficial effects are shared by all members of a given class. Furthermore, as we have learned from evaluations of several new investigational agents, the advantageous or deleterious actions of various inotropic agents may be more a function of their ancillary properties or of the dose administered than of their specific inotropic mechanism.[13,14] However, a classification system does provide a framework for understanding the potential benefits and limitations of the traditional agents and allows us to better categorize the increasing numbers of new investigational drugs.

INOTROPIC AGENTS THAT INCREASE cAMP

The heart is often referred to as an "adrenergic" organ because this signaling pathway in ventricular myocardium mediates the most rapid and powerful enhancement modulation of cardiac contractility. Endogenous neurohormones released from sympa-

thetic nerve terminals are perceived, processed, and amplified by a transmembrane signaling system located within the cardiac sarcolemma.[17] This transduction system consists of membrane-bound receptors, the effector enzyme adenylyl cyclase, and members of a family of guanine nucleotide-binding transduction proteins (G proteins). In the heart the stimulatory guanine nucleotide-binding protein G$_S$ couples β-adrenergic receptors, histamine receptors,[18] and vasoactive intestinal peptide receptors[19] with activation of adenylyl cyclase. In contrast, the inhibitory guanine nucleotide-binding regulatory protein G$_I$ couples inhibitory receptors including muscarinic receptors[20] and adenosine receptors[21] with inhibition of the effector enzyme. Activation of adenylyl cyclase results in synthesis of the intracellular second messenger cAMP. Once synthesized, cAMP activates a cAMP-dependent protein kinase (or is alternatively metabolized by phosphodiesterase to inactivate 5'-AMP) with subsequent phosphorylation of a group of cellular proteins including the slow inward-gated calcium channel, the sarcoplasmic reticulum protein phospholamban, troponin I, and transacting regulatory proteins within the nucleus. In combination, these interactions result in enhanced contractility and relaxation.

The potential importance of agents that could augment cardiac contractility by stimulating the adrenergic nervous system was demonstrated in studies from the 1960s that first recognized that patients with congestive failure had a diminished response to adrenergic stimulation.[14] Subsequent studies, described in detail in Chapter 9, demonstrated that the diminished response to adrenergic stimulation was due to down-regulation of the β_1-adrenergic receptor, uncoupling of the β_2-adrenergic receptor from adenylyl cyclase, and an increase in the functional activity of the G$_I$ inhibitory protein.[22] With these pathophysiologic mechanisms in mind it was hypothesized that the inotropic state could be enhanced by increasing the levels of intracellular cAMP by either activating adrenergic receptors or inhibiting the metabolism of cAMP by the phosphodiesterase enzyme. Therefore a substantial number of oral adrenergic agonists were evaluated for the treatment of congestive heart failure; none proved consistently effective with long-term use.[7–9,23,24] Most disturbingly, a multicenter trial utilizing the long-term administration of the partial β-adrenergic agonist xamoterol was discontinued because of a substantial increase in mortality in xamoterol-treated patients (Fig. 46-2).[10] Several hypotheses were proposed to explain this unexpected finding: (1) desensitization of the β-adrenergic pathway; (2) arrhythmogenic effects of cAMP; and (3) direct cardiotoxic effects of cAMP.[4,6,7,25]

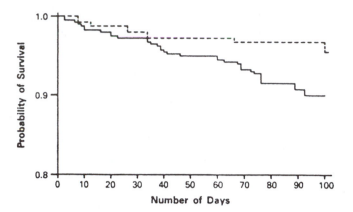

Fig. 46-2. Three-month survival probabilities from the xamoterol heart failure trial, showing increased mortality with xamoteral. Broken line, placebo ($n = 164$); solid lines, xamoterol ($n = 352$); $P = 0.02$; hazard ratio 2.54 (confidence interval 1.06 to 6.08). (From Xamoterol in Severe Heart Failure Study Group,[10] with permission.)

Which of these, if any, may have been operating remains unclear.

Despite the disappointing effects of the oral adrenergic agonists in managing patients with chronic congestive failure, intravenous adrenergic agonists have become a standard of therapy for short-term management of patients with acute or severely decompensated congestive heart failure syndromes. An enlarging body of evidence suggests that long-term use of dobutamine may also be beneficial.

Dobutamine

During the early 1960s through the mid-1970s, patients with cardiogenic shock were treated with the adrenergic agonists isoproterenol or norepinephrine. Unfortunately, isoproterenol, a nonselective β-agonist, did not prove useful for management of patients with cardiogenic shock or severe congestive heart failure because of associated tachycardia, arrhythmias, and peripheral vasodilation.[26] Norepinephrine efficacy was limited by tachycardia, arrhythmias, and vasoconstriction. However, in 1975 Tuttle nd Mills[27] modified the amino-terminal end of isoproterenol, resulting in the development of the inotropic agent dobutamine. In contrast to isoproterenol, dobutamine was not associated with tachycardia, arrhythmias, or substantial peripheral vasodilatation and maintained its potent inotropic properties. Although initially thought to be β_1 selective, it is now recognized that dobutamine can stimulate both α_1- and β_2-adrenergic receptors as well.[28] It is interesting that dobutamine elicits such a potent inotropic effect independent of a change in heart rate.[29] It has

been suggested that this unique property of dobutamine may come as a result of mixing the two stereoisomers of dobutamine, the presence of heightened autonomic drive in patients with heart failure, or the contribution of activation of α-receptors and their inotropic actions.[29–31] In the vasculature, dobutamine activates both β_2- and α_1-adrenergic receptors, thereby having a balanced effect on peripheral vascular resistance.

A major advantage of dobutamine in the critical care setting is its short half-life, in large part because of its rapid clearance due to metabolism by catechol-o-methyl-transferase.[32] This short half-life facilitates the treatment of clinically unstable patients, as in most cases the drug is metabolized or eliminated within 10–12 minutes after interruption of an intravenous infusion. Dobutamine is administered intravenously starting at 2–3 $\mu g \cdot kg^{-1} \cdot min^{-1}$ with 1–2 $\mu g \cdot kg^{-1} \cdot min^{-1}$ increases in dosage every 10–30 minutes until an appropriate hemodynamic effect has been obtained. There is a direct and linear correlation between dobutamine dose, plasma concentration, and hemodynamic response.[33] Because the onset of activity is rapid, peak effects can be obtained in a short time. Toxicity with dobutamine is relatively rare, although it may include production of tachycardia, arrhythmias, headaches, anxiety, tremors, and excessive changes in blood pressure. Dobutamine should be used with care in patients with a history of hypertension. In addition, it has been reported that patients with atrial fibrillation may experience increased ventricular response due to increased atrioventricular (AV) conduction while receiving dobutamine.[34]

There is a clear consensus that dobutamine is useful for *short-term management* of patients with cardiac decompensation and signs and symptoms of congestive heart failure.[35] In a variety of clinical settings, including decompensation of chronic congestive heart failure, acute myocarditis, or acute myocardial infarction, the use of dobutamine has been associated with an increase in stroke volume and cardiac output as well as a reduction in ventricular filling pressures.[36–41] Although dobutamine effectively increases cardiac contractility, it also increases oxygen demand. Indeed, at higher doses the increase in oxygen demand may well offset the improvement in cardiac contractility.[42] In a recent study using positron emission tomography (PET)-derived ^{11}C-acetate kinetics to determine the effects of dobutamine on oxidative metabolism and its effects on myocardial efficiency in patients with dilated cardiomyopathy, it was found that despite an increase in myocardial oxygen consumption dobutamine led to an increase in the work–metabolic index in patients with heart failure.[43] In addition, dobutamine reduced systemic vascular resistance and mitral regurgitation, suggesting that in this group of patients it had an important vasodilating action in addition to its inotropic affects. Finally, although it is generally assumed that the major efficacy of dobutamine comes from improving left ventricular performance, improved left atrial contributions to ventricular filling may also play a role in the beneficial effects of dobutamine.[44]

Although there is general agreement regarding the role of dobutamine in the short-term management of patients with congestive heart failure, the *chronic use of dobutamine* has been far more controversial. Early after the development of dobutamine, it was hypothesized that long-term use might be associated with further down-regulation of β-adrenergic receptors and rapid development of tolerance. Indeed, in 1980 Unverferth et al.[45] demonstrated that the hemodynamic effects of dobutamine were reduced by as much as 50 percent after 96 hours of continuous infusion. They suggested that the development of tolerance could be attenuated easily by increasing the infusion rates. Even short-term infusions were associated with hemodynamic and metabolic improvements, as patients exhibited increases in serum sodium concentrations, reductions in blood urea nitrogen and creatinine, and interestingly a rise in the creatine phosphate/ATP ratio.[46] Although it was recognized that sustained adrenergic stimulation could induce a decrease in adrenergic receptor density, it could also be hypothesized that improved pump function might result in a decrease in endogenous catecholamine release with subsequent up-regulation of receptor density and long-term improvement in hemodynamic responsiveness. Supporting the latter hypothesis, Colucci et al.[1] demonstrated that when dobutamine was administered into the coronary artery of patients with chronic congestive heart failure there was a substantial decrease in coronary sinus norepinephrine levels, which was postulated to be a result of reduced adrenergic drive following improvement in myocardial performance. Further support for the potential long-term benefits of dobutamine came from the finding that β-adrenergic receptor density was higher in patients awaiting transplantation who were receiving high doses of intravenous dobutamine for prolonged periods when compared with patients receiving low doses of dobutamine for relatively shorter times.[47]

Unfortunately, clinical information regarding long-term continuous use of dobutamine comes from small clinical trials or anecdotal information. Pickworth[48] reviewed existing literature on the chronic infusion of dobutamine and concluded that although it lessened symptoms of congestive heart failure, improved symptom classification, enhanced exercise tolerance, and increased left ventricular ejection fraction, it did not improve survival in most patients. In fact, the review cautioned that although dobutamine administration could contribute to an improvement in quality of life, it was arrhythmogenic and could cause sudden death. In contrast, in several publications, Miller and colleagues described their use of outpatient dobutamine for the therapy of refractory congestive heart failure and for patients awaiting heart transplantation. In their experience, intravenous inotropic therapy could be used safely in an outpatient setting to maintain a clinically compensated heart failure state while reducing the expenses associated with the prolonged time in an intensive care unit setting.[49,50] Their protocol for outpatient therapy included documentation of hemodynamic benefit in response to low doses of dobutamine, Holter recordings obtained both before and 2 days after the initiation of infusion to examine the arrhythmogenic potential of the dobutamine and its safety in the outpatient setting, and exclusion of any patients who demonstrated symptomatic sustained ventricular tachycardia during therapy or who had a history of sudden cardiac death caused by ventricular fibrillation in the absence of an internal defibrillator prior to institution of therapy. All patients were seen frequently after being begun on chronic infusions, and efforts were made to wean the patients to as low a dose as possible. Serum electrolytes, renal function, and adequacy of anticoagulation therapy were monitored weekly. This experience reported by Miller and colleagues was consistent with the experience of the heart failure treatment program at the University of Alabama at Birmingham, where only a single unexpected death was reported in a series of 120 patients receiving chronic administration of dobutamine at home (R. Bourge, personal communication).

Equally controversial is the use of *intermittent dobutamine* for management of patients with chronic congestive failure. In 1980 Unverferth and coworkers first demonstrated that the beneficial effects of a 72-hour infusion of dobutamine in patients with chronic congestive heart failure persisted for up to 4 weeks in a substantial number of patients after discontinuation of therapy.[35] Interestingly, this prolonged benefit of a 3-day infusion of dobutamine was associated with beneficial changes in both the ultrastructure and biochemistry of the myocardium.[45,46] Subsequently, Applefeld and colleagues were the first to test the potential benefits of intermittent outpatient dobutamine therapy in a small group of patients with chronic and irremediable congestive failure.[51] They found that intermittent therapy was beneficial in terms of both quality of life and hemodynamic performance. Indeed, comparable results have been seen in experimental animals with heart failure.[52] Unfortunately, enthusiasm for intermittent dobutamine therapy was diminished when a clinical trial randomizing patients to either intermittent dobutamine therapy or traditional therapy was discontinued prematurely because of increased early mortality in the dobutamine-treated patients.[53] However, this study did not use a rigorous protocol to minimize the risks of dobutamine administration: (1) electrolyte levels were not routinely monitored; (2) high dobutamine doses were utilized throughout the study; and (3) dobutamine concentrations were not titrated for intrastudy changes in body weight. Despite concerns regarding the use of intermittent dobutamine for treating patients with congestive heart failure, a substantial number of centers have effectively utilized this type of therapy to treat patients with heart failure, although clinical trials demonstrating beneficial affects of intermittent dobutamine in large populations are not available.[54,55]

Dopamine

Dopamine is a second adrenergic agonist that activates the β_1-adrenergic receptor, increases cardiac contractility, and has minimal effects on heart rate or blood pressure.[56–58] In contrast to dobutamine, dopamine has complex pharmacologic effects. At low doses (infusion rates of 0.5–2.0 $\mu g \cdot kg^{-1} \cdot min^{-1}$) dopamine acts primarily on dopamine receptors[59,60]; at infusion rates above 5.0 $\mu g \cdot kg^{-1} \cdot min^{-1}$ dopamine affects the β_1-adrenergic receptor and at slightly higher concentrations the α-adrenergic receptors. Because of the narrow threshold between activation of the β_1-adrenergic receptors and the peripheral α-adrenergic receptors, the net effect of higher doses of dopamine is potent peripheral vasoconstriction. At lower doses of dopamine activation of the dopaminergic receptors, found in the vascular smooth muscle of the renal, mesenteric, coronary, and cerebral arterial vessels,[61,62] results in improved diuresis and natriuresis. Dopamine is therefore of particular benefit at low dose in patients in whom it is difficult to achieve adequate diuresis with diuretics alone. Dopamine is also of great benefit for patients with abdominal pain secondary to mesenteric artery hypoperfusion. Alternatively, at high doses dopamine is the agent of choice for patients with cardiogenic shock associated with low peripheral vascular resistance.

Because of the clinical benefits elicited by dopamine in patients with congestive heart failure, efforts were made to develop orally active dopaminergic agonists. In addition, the design of these dopaminergic agonists took advantage of enhanced understanding of the diversity of the dopamine receptors. Dopamine receptors can be divided into two subfamilies: DA1 or DA1-like receptors and the DA2 or DA2-like receptors. The DA1-like receptors resemble β-adrenergic receptors in that they are encoded by intronless genes and contain seven membrane-spanning motifs. The DA2-like receptor genes contain introns in their coding regions but have a similar molecular configuration.[63] The DA1 receptor effects vasodilatation as described for dopamine. The DA2-like receptors are mainly localized in neuronal tissues and when activated result in decreased norepinephrine release and an increase in dopamine synthesis and release. In addition, DA2-like receptors inhibit angiotensin II-induced aldosterone secretion.[64]

With these pharmacologic properties in mind, an orally active dopaminergic agonist, ibopamine, was developed that had as its active metabolite epinine N-methyldopamine, which stimulates both DA1 and DA2 receptors.[65] Early clinical trials with ibopamine in Europe and Japan indicated that it was well tolerated and safe, and it appeared to have beneficial effects.[66–69] Indeed, the use of ibopamine was associated with a significant increase in cardiac index, stroke volume, and stroke work indices, with a concomitant reduction in systemic vascular resistance and no significant change in mean arterial pressure or heart rate. Ibopamine's effects on plasma norepinephrine were somewhat equivocal, however. The Dutch Digoxin-Ibopamine Multicenter Trial (DIMT) demonstrated that ibopamine and digoxin inhibit neurohormonal activation in patients with mild to moderate chronic heart failure.[70] However, ibopamine was effective only in patients with relatively preserved left ventricular function in terms of improving exercise time. Neither ambulatory arrhythmias nor mortality were significantly affected by either agent, although the study was too small to exclude a survival effect. Based on experience from a relatively large number of small clinical trials, investigators hypothesized that ibopamine would be beneficial in patients with congestive heart failure when administered chronically.[71]

Therefore in order to assess the long-term effects of ibopamine and more importantly its effects on morbidity and mortality, the PRIME-II study in Europe was designed to examine survival in patients with New York Heart Association (NYHA) class III or IV symptoms who had been hospitalized for heart failure or who manifested symptoms at rest within the prior 2 months, despite background therapy with angiotensin-converting enzyme (ACE) inhibitors in addition to diuretics and optional digoxin. PRIME-II was discontinued by its Data and Safety Monitoring Committee at the end of 1995 because of excess mortality in the ibopamine group. At that time, 1906 patients had been randomized in 165 centers, and 232 of 953 (24.3 percent) of the actively treated versus 193 of 953 (20.3 percent) of the placebo patients had died—a 20 percent increase in mortality ($P = 0.017$).[72] Of note is that the excess mortality was observed primarily in patients with class IV symptoms (34.9 percent versus 26.2 percent). Perhaps the most surprising finding was the significant interaction between ibopamine and concomitant amiodarone therapy, with 59 of 209 (28.2 percent) of patients receiving amiodarone and ibopamine dying versus 39 of 246 (15.9 percent) of patients on amiodarone and placebo. The mechanism of this interaction is uncertain, and it is possible that amiodarone therapy may have been a marker for patients at risk for ibopamine-induced arrhythmias. Indeed, the mechanism for the adverse overall result is unclear. One must wonder whether the mild inotropic actions of ibopamine were responsible for its deleterious effects with chronic use, or whether its lack of long-term potency as an anti-adrenergic agent was responsible for the disappointing results. Other reports have identified myocardial dopaminergic receptors, and the functional significance of the activation of these receptors remains undefined. In any case, the role of ibopamine, which is registered in several European countries, is uncertain.

Phosphodiesterase Inhibitors

Because of the marked potency of increased levels of cAMP in augmenting contractility, pharmacologic agents were developed that could increase intracellular cAMP levels by interacting with components of the receptor G protein adenylyl cyclase pathway distal to the β-adrenergic receptor. The first of such agents was forskolin, an extract of the Indian coleus plant that augments intracellular cAMP concentrations through effects on both the G stimulatory protein and adenylyl cyclase.[73] Unfortunately, this agent had no clinical applicability because of a poor side effect profile, nonspecific effects, and a marked positive chronotropic effect.[74] A second group of agents that was developed to increase intracellular concentrations of cAMP were those that inhibited the metabolism of cAMP by the phosphodiesterase

(PDE) enzyme. Amrinone, a bipyridine derivative that was shown to exert positive inotropic as well as potent vasodilatory effects, was the first PDE inhibitor studied.[75–77] In patients with congestive heart failure the intravenous administration of amrinone produced an increase in cardiac index, a decrease in left ventricular end-diastolic pressure, and a decrease in pulmonary capillary wedge pressure without changing either heart rate or mean aortic pressure.[78]

That inhibition of PDE-III, the myocardial enzyme, and resulting increase in intracellular cAMP concentrations was responsible in part for the inotropic properties of amrinone was demonstrated by a group of in vitro studies.[79–81] As would be expected with increased intracellular availability of cAMP, amrinone positively affected both contraction and relaxation, with marked augmentation of calcium release and reuptake by the sarcoplasmic reticulum.[82,83] These potent inotropic properties could be attenuated by treatment with calcium channel blockers or by exposure to low extracellular calcium concentrations.[83,84]

In patients with congestive heart failure, amrinone increased left ventricular contractility in association with a reduction in left ventricular filling pressure and systemic arterial pressure.[85] Investigators have suggested that these hemodynamic effects of amrinone may be predominantly due to its potent vasodilatory properties.[86–88]

Several lines of evidence support a positive inotropic action for PDE inhibitors. Low dose, intracoronary infusion of milrinone, a close congener of amrinone, increased myocardial contractility indices without producing peripheral vasodilation.[89] Studies in which left ventricular end-ejection pressure–volume relations were obtained during treatment with another PDE inhibitor, enoximone, demonstrated a shift upward and to the left, supporting a positive inotropic effect. Enoximone was also associated with a potent vasodilatory effect, and one-third of patients receiving the inotropic agent showed no inotropic responsiveness.[90] Interestingly, when papillary muscle preparations from patients with end-stage heart failure were exposed to increasing doses of the PDE inhibitor milrinone, there was no substantial contractile response.[91] However, when the same heart preparations were pretreated with forskolin to augment basal adenylyl cyclase activity and increase cAMP production, there was a robust response to milrinone, comparable to that seen in nonfailing human hearts. Because it is well recognized that failing human hearts are unable to produce normal quantities of cAMP because of abnormalities in receptor–G protein–adenylyl cyclase coupling, it has been postulated that the inotropic effectiveness of a PDE inhibitor is limited by the intracellular levels of cAMP.

Although approved for therapy in the United States for intravenous use in patients with congestive heart failure, amrinone has limited applications. Rich et al. demonstrated that in elderly patients dobutamine was as effective as amrinone for increasing cardiac contractility in patients with acute decompensation.[92] Of greater concern regarding the use of amrinone in patients with chronic failure is its clinical pharmacologic profile. First, there are important genetically determined differences in the rate of acetylation, a primary pathway of amrinone metabolism, resulting in marked differences in plasma concentrations after a single intravenous dose of amrinone in rapid or slow acetylator groups.[93] Additionally, amrinone is associated with serious adverse affects, including abdominal pain, nausea and vomiting, jaundice, myositis, pulmonary infiltrates, and polyarteritis.[94] Because of the long half-life of amrinone, the side effects and untoward hemodynamic effects can be long-lasting.[95] Finally and importantly, amrinone has been associated with a significant risk of thrombocytopenia.[96,97] Indeed in a report on the administration of amrinone to children after cardiac surgery, there was a nearly 50 percent incidence of thrombocytopenia.[98] Lastly, in the current economic environment, amrinone is substantially more expensive than dobutamine with no obvious benefits except in a group of patients who are dobutamine resistant (discussed below).

The early investigations with intravenous amrinone led to the development of a family of orally and intravenously administered inotropic agents, including amrinone, milrinone, enoximone, and indolidan. The long-term oral administration of amrinone in patients with chronic congestive failure was not associated with beneficial effects.[99,100] In at least one study the use of amrinone was associated with a suggestion of increased mortality.[95] Similarly, the oral administration of milrinone,[101] enoximone,[102] and indolidan failed to show beneficial effects with long-term administration. Indeed, the large multicenter Prospective Randomized Milrinone Survival Evaluation (PROMISE) trial was stopped prematurely because of a substantial increase in mortality among the patients randomized to receive milrinone (Fig. 46-3).[11] Although it has been proposed that lower concentrations of PDE inhibitors might prove beneficial without the mortality consequences,[16,103,104] no orally active PDE inhibitor is presently approved for clinical therapy in the United States.

The intravenous formulation of the bipyridine PDE inhibitor milrinone has been approved for patients with congestive heart failure. Milrinone has several advantages when compared with amrinone: a lower incidence of toxicity and no drug-associated thrombocytopenia. Short-term infusion results in a fall in end-diastolic pressure, whereas longer infu-

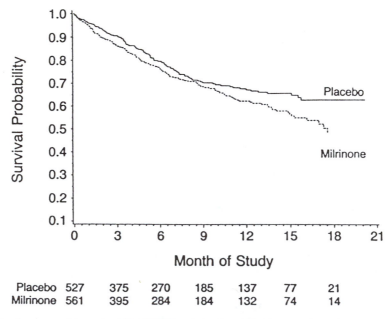

	0	3	6	9	12	15	18
Placebo	527	375	270	185	137	77	21
Milrinone	561	395	284	184	132	74	14

Fig. 46-3. Survival curves from the PROMISE trial, showing that milrinone therapy was associated with a 28 percent increase in mortality compared to the placebo group ($P = 0.038$). The number of patients at risk are shown at the bottom of the figure. (From Packer et al.,[11] with permission.)

sions produce sustained reductions in pulmonary capillary wedge pressure and right atrial pressure, accompanied by an increase in cardiac index. In addition, as would be expected from its vasodilatory properties, there was a sustained fall in systemic vascular resistance.[105] Similar results were seen in a multicenter baseline controlled phase III efficacy and safety trial in 189 patients in the United States[106] and in a concurrent European trial in 40 patients.[107] It was interesting, however, that in both of these clinical trials patients were noted to have asymptomatic ventricular arrhythmias. Indeed in 3 of 40 patients in the European study, the problem of increased ventricular tachycardia was deemed significant.

Although milrinone certainly has attractive properties for intravenous management of patients with acute congestive heart failure, it provides an important example where the economics of pharmacologic therapy play a role in evaluating the "best" therapeutic options. The cost of milrinone is nearly eightfold higher than that of dobutamine, yet there is no evidence to suggest that milrinone is any more effective in improving pump function in patients with cardiac decompensation. Even in those patients in whom the vasodilatory effects of milrinone might be therapeutically important, the combined use of dobutamine and either nitroprusside or intravenous nitroglycerin are equally affective. Furthermore, the ability to rapidly titrate the balance between the inotropic properties of dobutamine and the vasodilatory properties of nitroprusside or intravenous nitroglycerin provide a clinical and therapeutic benefit in critically ill heart failure patients with both low cardiac output and hemodynamic instability. It should be noted that anecdotal reports have described patients who are unresponsive to dobutamine but do respond effectively to intravenous milrinone.[108] Alternatively, we have cared for several patients who were transferred to our hospital with decompensated heart failure on milrinone therapy who did well after being gradually weaned from milrinone to dobutamine, presumably because they were intolerant of the substantial peripheral vasodilatory and decreased afterload. Therefore this discussion does not imply that there is no role for milrinone in the management of patients with decompensated heart failure but, rather, that therapy with dobutamine or potentially with dobutamine and intravenous nitroglycerin in combination is preferable as first-line therapy because of the marked differential in cost and the ability to more easily titrate pharmacologic effects.

An intriguing pharmacologic regimen has been the simultaneous use of dobutamine and a PDE inhibitor in bridging patients with severe cardiac decompensation to either heart transplantation or other surgical intervention. This combination therapy is based on the hypothesis that the combined use of these two drugs is pharmacologically synergistic. The administration of dobutamine effects an increase in intracellular cAMP production by the receptor–G protein–adenylyl cyclase signal transduction complex, whereas co-administration of a PDE inhibitor attenuates the metabolism of these relatively modest levels of cAMP, resulting in augmented cardiac contractility. This hypothesis is supported by studies in animals with experimentally induced heart failure,[109] studies utilizing isolated human papillary muscle preparations,[110] and clinical trials in patients with congestive failure.[111,112]

INVESTIGATIONAL INOTROPIC AGENTS

Since the mid-1970s a large array of pharmaceutical agents have been evaluated for management of patients with chronic or acute congestive heart failure. As discussed above, many of these agents that have as their primary mechanism of action enhanced contractility are mediated by increased production of cAMP. Unfortunately, although these medications can improve hemodynamic indices and clinical status over the short term, they have failed to produce sustained clinical improvements; and several have increased the mortality rate. As a result, digoxin remains as the only orally active inotropic agent approved for therapy in patients with congestive heart failure. More recently, other approaches to increasing myocardial contractility have been investigated. They have been reviewed and are also discussed in Chapter 55.[15,16] They include drugs that activate or inhibit selected ion channels, agents that increase the sensitivity of the contractile proteins to calcium, and agents that combine one or more of these mechanisms with relatively weak PDE inhibition.

Drugs Having Effects on Calcium Handling or Calcium Sensitivity

Because many of the deleterious effects of the positive inotropic agents investigated thus far have been ascribed to their effects of increasing intracellular cAMP or cytosolic calcium, an attractive mechanism of action is to increase the sensitivity of the contractile proteins to calcium.[15,113] The most extensively studied medication with this action is pimobendan. As expected from an agent that enhances calcium sensitivity, pimobendan shifts the calcium–force relation upward and to the left.[113–115] This calcium-sensitizing property is related to an increase in the affinity of troponin C for calcium.[15,113,115,116] Interestingly, myocardium obtained from explanted hearts of patients undergoing transplantation exhibits the same increase in calcium sensitivity of the contractile apparatus to calcium when treated with pimobendan.[117] However, it is also clear that pimobendan inhibits myocardial PDE-III and shares many of the pharmacologic properties of milrinone at physiologic concentrations.[113,117]

Pimobendan has been subjected to several clinical studies in heart failure patients already receiving diuretics, digoxin, and ACE inhibitors. In a pilot short-term study of 52 patients, acute administration of pimobendan at doses of 2.5, 5.0, and 10.0 mg produced dose-dependent increases in cardiac index pulmonary capillary wedge pressure.[118] During a 4-week follow-up period, doses of 2.5 and 5.0 mg bid increased exercise duration and peak oxygen uptake.

A larger 12-week double-blind placebo-controlled study of pimobendan (2.5, 5.0, and 10.0 mg daily, in two doses) confirmed these findings and highlighted the importance of evaluating a range of doses when evaluating positive inotropic agents.[119] The primary endpoints were exercise tolerance and quality of life. The 5 mg dose of pimobendan significantly increased exercise duration, oxygen uptake, and quality of life, as assessed by the Minnesota Living with Heart Failure Questionnaire (Fig. 46-4). Interestingly, these benefits were not seen with the 2.5 and 10.0 mg doses. Nonetheless, these results are striking, particularly considering that they were found in patients

receiving digoxin. A larger study examined the effects of the 2.5 and 5.0 mg total daily doses in 317 patients with NYHA class II and III heart failure followed for a minimum of 24 weeks.[120] A modest increase in exercise tolerance (mean 30 seconds) was seen in the 5 mg group, but pimobendan was also associated with a higher risk of death (19 deaths per 100 years at risk compared with 11 in the placebo group). Although this difference did not achieve statistical significance, it raises concern about the benefit/risk ratio of pimobendan, which is amplified by the narrow therapeutic window of this agent. Whether this adverse trend in mortality is related to PDE inhibition or is generic to potent positive inotropic agents remains unresolved.

Investigations continue with calcium-sensitizing agents, with the goal of developing an agent in which this mechanism of action is dissociated from PDE inhibition.[113] Experimental data suggest that a new compound, levosimendan, may have more selectivity at clinically relevant concentrations. Levosimendan increases calcium sensitivity of the contractile proteins by calcium-dependent binding of the drug to troponin C.[121,122] Of note is that although levosimendan has selective PDE-III inhibitory effects it does not increase the transmembrane Ca^{2+} current at pharmacologically relevant concentrations, nor does it increase cAMP at low concentrations.[122] Somewhat against a dissociation between the calcium-sensitizing and PDE-inhibiting effects, however, is the finding that this agent does not slow relaxation.[123]

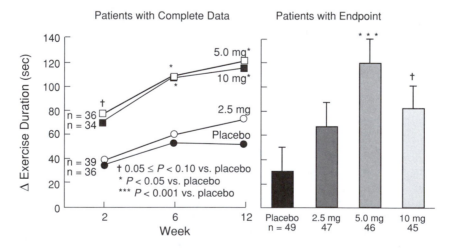

Fig. 46-4. Changes in exercise duration in a controlled trial of pimobendan, at the endpoint (right panel) and over time for patients with data at every time point (left panel). Exercise duration in the placebo group increased by only 29.6 seconds over the 12-week study. The 5 mg/day dose of pimobendan produced a significant increase of 121.6 seconds ($P < 0.001$ versus placebo). The 10 mg/day group produced a smaller increase of 81.1 seconds ($P = 0.05$). Over the 12-week study, only the 5- and 10-mg doses demonstrated a significant increase in exercise duration that was significantly increased compared with placebo at weeks 6 and 12. (From Kubo et al.,[13] with permission.)

Levosimendan is just beginning to enter clinical studies.[124]

Vesnarinone

Vesnarinone is a synthetic quinolinone derivative that received early interest because of the finding that it increases myocardial contractility in open-chest dog models without having a chronotropic effect or increasing myocardial oxygen consumption.[125,126] In contrast to other types of inotropic agents, including adrenergic agonists, calcium modulators, and PDE inhibitors, vesnarinone was found to prolong the action potential and slow the heart rate.[127,128] Subsequent studies showed that vesnarinone was a prototypical class IV inotropic agent; that is, it affects cardiac contractility through multiple mechanisms of action.[16] Originally, three distinct mechanisms of action were hypothesized to be responsible for the inotropic properties of vesnarinone: (1) a decrease in the delayed outward and inward rectifying potassium current[129]; (2) an ability to prolong the opening time of the sodium channel[130,131]; and (3) an inhibitory effect on PDE-III.[132] One report has suggested that the sodium channel effects are unimportant in the inotropic properties of vesnarinone, and that in both animal and human myocytes vesnarinone increases the current through L-type calcium channels.[133] It may therefore be the opposing effects—a decrease in the delayed outward and inward rectifying potassium currents and an increase in the inward calcium current—that are responsible for the antitachycardiac properties of vesnarinone in experimental animal models.[134] Interestingly, the electrophysiologic effects of vesnarinone are similar of those of the class 3 antiarrhythmic sotalol.[135]

Several investigators have classified vesnarinone as PDE inhibitor; this is an oversimplification that results in confusion in understanding the novel properties of this agent. Traditional PDE inhibitors shorten the action potential and increase the heart rate.[136–138] In contrast, vesnarinone prolongs the action potential, slows the heart rate, and has only modest vasodilatory effects. Furthermore, whereas traditional PDE inhibitors are unable pharmacologically to distinguish the two isoforms of cyclic guanosine monophosphate (cGMP)-inhibited PDE, vesnarinone is able to distinguish the two forms present in human tissue and therefore has a novel pharmacologic profile.[139]

Perhaps the most intriguing aspect of vesnarinone is its ability to inhibit the production of the proinflammatory cytokines, including tumor necrosis factor (TNFα) and interleukin-6 (IL-6) expression.[140,141] These proinflammatory cytokines are important in the cellular amplification of the immune response, as they recruit additional lymphocytes, monocytes, and other cell types to the site of antigen recognition and promote their differentiation.[142–144] Only recently has the potential role of cytokines in cardiac disease been recognized. Previously, it was thought that immune-mediated myocardial injury may be associated with persistence of infiltrating immune cells and factors in the myocardium.[145,146] It is now being recognized that the proinflammatory cytokines may play a role in the genesis of heart failure even in the absence of obvious myocardial inflammation. In 1990 Levine and coworkers first recognized that levels of TNF were elevated in patients with end-stage heart failure and cachexia.[147] Other studies have demonstrated that in the adult myocyte TNF exerts a concentration- and time-dependent negative inotropic effect that is reversible upon removal of the cytokine.[148] TNF has also been shown to diminish myocardial function in experimental models[149–151] and humans.[152,153] TNF has been implicated in the pathogenesis of a variety of cardiac diseases, including acute viral myocarditis,[154] cardiac allograft rejection,[155] and myocardial infarction.[156,157] Perhaps the most substantive evidence suggesting a role for proinflammatory cytokines in cardiac disease comes from studies by Torre-Amione et al.,[158] which demonstrated the presence of both TNFα mRNA and protein in the hearts of patients with congestive failure but not in nonfailing control hearts. In addition, these investigators demonstrated the presence of TNFα receptors and TNFα mRNA in both failing and nonfailing human hearts. Furthermore, patients with congestive heart failure appear to shed TNF receptors into the circulating plasma. Therefore the failing human heart can both make TNFα and respond to TNFα in an autocrine and paracrine fashion through the presence of local TNF receptors. Thus inhibition of TNF expression may play a critically important role in modulating the development of congestive heart failure.

The clinical development of vesnarinone began in Japan in 1986, with the demonstration that cardiovascular hemodynamics were improved after both acute and short-term administration.[159,160] As was seen in the earlier animal studies, these changes were not associated with alterations in either heart rate or systolic blood pressure, although mild vasodilatation was observed.[141] Early phase II trials in the United States demonstrated only modest effects,[161,162] although subsequent investigations with vesnarinone suggested that these early results might have been explained by the inclusion of patients with only modest levels of heart failure and because of the relatively short period of therapy. An initial randomized placebo-controlled trial in 76 patients with symptomatic heart failure and ejection fractions less than 30 percent demonstrated a significant decrease in the endpoint of mortality or major cardiovascular morbidity.[163] Additionally, vesnarinone was associated with an improvement in the quality of life and a small but not physiologic improvement in exercise capacity.

Based on this early randomized trial, a phase III randomly allocated, double-blind, placebo-controlled trial was begun in 1989.[14] All patients were symptomatic with primarily class III heart failure and had ejection fractions of less than 30 percent. In addition, they were receiving concomitant therapy with digoxin and an ACE inhibitor. Patients were initially randomized to receive either 60 mg of vesnarinone, 120 mg of vesnarinone, or placebo. The 120 mg group was discontinued early during the course of the study because it was associated with a substantial increase in mortality. Indeed, after 250 patients had been enrolled, there were 16 deaths in the high dose group, 6 deaths in the placebo group, and 3 among patients taking 60 mg of vesnarinone. Thereafter patients were randomly assigned only to the 60 mg dose (239 patients) or placebo (238 patients). The final result demonstrated a striking beneficial effect of this dose of vesnarinone. Only 26 of 239 (10.9 percent) patients receiving vesnarinone compared to 50 of 238 (21.0 percent) on placebo died or experienced severe wors-

ening of heart failure during the 6-month follow-up period (a 50 percent reduction in risk; $P = 0.003$) (Fig. 46-5). Similarly, there was a 62 percent reduction in all-cause mortality. This dramatic result was unexpected, given both the prior experience with positive inotropic agents and the magnitude of the beneficial effect. The U.S. Food and Drug Administration, therefore, requested additional long-term survival data, particularly in patients with NYHA class IV heart failure, and more information about the optimal dose.

These results were consistent with a phase III trial in Japan.[164] This study raised several interesting questions about vesnarinone and inotropes in general. Many inotropic agents appear to have toxicity at high doses, as pointed out earlier in the chapter. In the case of vesnarinone, however, it seems that the toxicity at a high dose was due to an increase in arrhythmogenicity rather than to an increase in inotropy. In a group of patients receiving either placebo or 60 mg of vesnarinone, mortality was equally attributable to pump failure or sudden death in the two groups. Among the patients who died while on high dose vesnarinone, most of the deaths were sudden, suggesting that high dose vesnarinone is associated with proarrhythmic effects. In addition, there was a close relation between mortality and hypokalemia in patients receiving vesnarinone (unpublished observations), further suggesting the arrhythmogenicity of 120 mg vesnarinone.

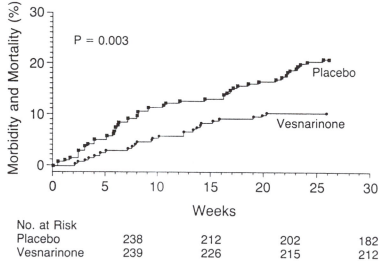

Fig. 46-5. Effect of vesnarinone 60 mg/day on the combined endpoint of death and severe decompensation of heart failure. There was a 50 percent reduction in events (26 versus 50, $P < 0.003$) with vesnarinone over the 6-month period of the study. A higher dose, 120 mg/day, increased mortality, indicating a narrow therapeutic window for this agent. The values below the figure are the numbers of patients in each group who were at risk at base-line and after each 8-week period. Subsequent results from the much larger VEST trial failed to demonstrate the same benefit, and the group receiving 60 mg of vesnarinone exhibited a 26 percent *increase* in all cause mortality. (From Feldman et al.,[14] with permission.)

Several investigators have suggested that the beneficial effects of vesnarinone might not be due to its inotropic properties, and therefore the drug should not be classified as an inotropic agent. There is now unambiguous evidence that vesnarinone has inotropic properties. Asanoi et al.[165] first demonstrated that vesnarinone shifted the pressure–volume relation upward and to the left with a marked improvement in patients who had been treated for at least 4 weeks. Furthermore, after a single 240 mg bolus in patients with chronic heart failure and elevated filling pressures, vesnarinone improves cardiac hemodynamics (J. E. Strobech and A. M. Feldman, unpublished observations). Finally, using a recently validated index equal to the ratio of left ventricular maximal ventricular power divided by the square of end-diastolic volume (power$_{nx}$/edv^2),[166] we were able to demonstrate that vesnarinone 60 mg/day produce a positive inotropic and lowered the afterload.[167]

The major side effects associated with the use of vesnarinone in the United States has been neutropenia, which occurred in fewer than 2 percent of patients in multicenter trials.[168] In all cases the neutropenia has been reversible, although there have been deaths among patients hospitalized for their neutropenia. Importantly, all cases of neutropenia have occurred within the first 16 weeks of therapy, necessitating only a defined period of monitoring the white blood cell count.

Based on the results of Japanese and U.S. studies, it was thought that several important questions regarding the use of vesnarinone in the therapy of patients with congestive heart failure had to be resolved: (1) Would the substantial improvements in survival that were observed at 6 months persist with long-term therapy? (2) What was the optimal dose of vesnarinone (i.e., might a lower dose such as 30 mg/day have the same survival benefits with lower toxicity)? (3) Would the benefits demonstrated in earlier clinical trials be applicable to populations underrepresented in those studies particularly in women, elderly individuals, and patients with the most severe degrees of heart failure)? To answer these important questions, the Vesnarinone Evaluation of Survival Trial (VEST) was conducted in 3800 patients in nearly 200 centers throughout the United States. However, preliminary analysis of the study results by the Data Safety and Monitoring Committee demonstrated that vesnarinone *increased* all cause mortality compared to placebo. Mortality was 26 percent higher at the 60 mg dose ($P = 0.007$).[169] However, analysis of the extensive data base generated by this study has only begun, and it will be very important to determine whether symptomatic improvement occurred in any patient subset within this study.

CONCLUSIONS

The armamentarium of inotropic agents in the United States today is limited. As was discussed in Chapter 43, digoxin continues to have a role in the management of patients with congestive heart failure, even though its effect on survival is neutral. However, based on data from trials with beta-adrenoceptor agonists, amrinone, milrinone, and ibopamine, the role of chronic oral inotropic therapy with other classes of drugs remains in doubt. It is noteworthy that each of these agents associated with an adverse effect increases intracellular cyclic AMP, either by stimulating its production (sympathetic agonists) or by inhibiting its metabolism (the phosphodiesterase inhibitors). Whether agents which increase contractility by other mechanisms will have an acceptable benefit to risk ratio remains unresolved, but the experience with vesnarinone and, to a lesser extent, with pimobendan, both of which are agents with other mechanisms of action but which also inhibit phosphodiesterase, indicates the need to proceed with such approaches very cautiously.

In contrast to the chronic use of positive inotropic drugs, the role of acute parenteral therapy is apparent. Four such intravenous agents are used commonly in patients with acute and decompensated heart failure—dobutamine, dopamine, amrinone, and milrinone. Each of these agents has a role in the management of patients with congestive heart failure, although the long-term use by chronic infusion or intermittent infusion of inotropic agents in patients with chronic congestive heart failure remains controversial. Meanwhile, because of the continued relevance of inotropic support to the therapy of congestive heart failure, additional agents are in the early developmental stages, but the level of evidence for efficacy and safety which will be required will be high given the adverse results with chronic positive inotropic agents thus far.

REFERENCES

1. Colucci WS, Denniss AR, Leatherman GF et al: Intracoronary infusion of dobutamine to patients with and without severe congestive heart failure. Dose-response relationships, correlation with circulating catecholamines, and effect of phosphodiesterase inhibition. J Clin Invest 1988;81:1103–1110

2. Covit AB, Schaer GL, Sealey NJ et al: Suppression of the renin-angiotensin system by intravenous digoxin in chronic congestive heart failure. Am J Med 1983;75:445–447

3. Katz AM: Potential deleterious effects of inotropic agents in the therapy of chronic heart failure. Circulation, suppl. III 1986;73:184–190

4. Lubbe WF, Podzuweit T, Opie LH: Potential arrhythmogenic role of cyclic adenosine monophosphate (AMP) and cytosolic calcium overload. Implications for prophylactic effects of beta-blockers in myocardial infarction and proarrhythmic effects of phosphodiesterase inhibitors. J Am Coll Cardiol 1992;19: 1622–1633

5. Packer M, Medina N, Yushak M: Hemodynamic and clinical limitation of long-term inotropic therapy with amrinone in patients with severe chronic heart failure. Circulation, 1984;70:1038–1047

6. Scholtz H, Meyer W: Phosphodiesterase-inhibiting properties of newer inotropic agents. Circulation suppl. III 1986;73:99–106

7. Packer M, Leier CV: Survival in congestive heart failure during treatment with drugs with positive inotropic actions. Circulation, suppl. IV 1987;75:55–63

8. Furberg CD, Yusuf S: Effect of drug therapy on survival in chronic congestive heart failure. Am J Cardiol suppl. 1988;62:41–45

9. Cody RJ: Do positive inotropic agents adversely affect the survival of patients with chronic congestive heart failure? J Am Coll Cardiol 1988;12:559–569

10. Xamoterol in Severe Heart Failure Study Group: Xamoterol in severe heart failure. Lancet 1990;336:1–6

11. Packer M, Carver JR, Rodeheffer RJ, et al: Effect of oral milrinone on mortality in severe chronic heart failure. N Engl J Med 1991;325:1468–1475

12. Notterman DA: Inotropic agents catecholamines, digoxin, amrinone. Crit Care Clin 1991;7:583–613

13. Kubo SH, Gollub S, Bourge R et al: Beneficial effects of pimobendan on exercise tolerance and quality of life in patients with heart failure. Results of a multicenter trial. Circulation 1992;85:942–949

14. Feldman AM, Bristow MR, Parmley WW et al: Effects of vesnarinone on morbidity and mortality in patients with heart failure. Vesnarinone Study Group. N Engl J Med 1993;29:149–155

15. Endoh M: The effects of various drugs on the myocardial inotropic response. Gen Pharmacol 1995;26:1–31

16. Feldman AM: Classification of positive inotropic agents. J Am Coll Cardiol 1993;22:1233–1237

17. Feldman AM: Modulation of adrenergic receptors and G-transduction proteins in failing human ventricular myocardium. Circulation, suppl. IV 1993;87: 27–34

18. Bristow MR, Cubicciotti R, Ginsburg R et al: Histamine-mediated adenylate cyclase stimulation in human myocardium. Mol Pharmacol 1982;21: 671–679

19. Christophe J, Waelbrocet M, Chatelain P, Robberecht P: Heart receptors for VIP, PHI, and secretin are able to activate adenylate cyclase and to mediate inotropic and chronotropic effects. Species variations and physiopathology. Peptides 1984;5:341–353

20. Hazeki O, Vi M: Modification by islet-activating protein of receptor-mediated regulation of cyclic AMP accumulation in isolated rat heart cells. J Biol Chem 1981;256:2856–2862

21. Hershberger RE, Feldman AM, Bristow MR: α-Adenosine receptor inhibition of adenylate cyclase in failing and nonfailing human ventricular myocardium. Circulation 1991;83:1343–1351

22. Robishaw JD, Foster KA: Role of G proteins in the regulation of the cardiovascular system. Annu Rev Physiol 1989;51:229–1244

23. Lambertz H, Meyer J, Erbel R: Long-term hemodynamic effects of prealterol in patients with congestive heart failure. Circulation 1984;69:298–305

24. Colucci WS, Alexander RW, Williams GH et al: Decreased lymphocyte beta-adrenergic-receptor density in patients with heart failure and tolerance to the beta-adrenergic agonist pirbuterol. N Engl J Med 1981;305:185–190

25. Packer M. Pathophysiological mechanisms underlying the effects of β-adrenergic agonists and antagonists on functional capacity and survival in chronic heart failure. Circulation, suppl. I 1990;82:77–88

26. Smith JH, Oriol A, Morch J et al: Hemodynamic studies in cardiogenic shock. Treatment with isoproterenol and metaraminol. Circulation 1967;35: 1084–1091

27. Tuttle RR, Mills J: Dobutamine. Development of a new catecholamine to selectively increase cardiac contractility. Circ Res 1975;36:185–196

28. Ruffolo RR, Spradin TA, Pollock GD et al: α- and β-adrenergic effects of the stereoisomers of dobutamine. J Pharmacol Exp Ther 1981;219:447–452

29. Ruffolo RR Jr: The mechanism of action of dobutamine [Letter]. Ann Intern Med 1984;100:313

30. Schumann HJ, Wagner J, Knorr A et al: Demonstration in human atrial preparations of α-adrenoceptors mediating positive inotropic effects. Naunyn Schmiedebergs Arch Pharmacol 1978;302:333–336

31. Lawless CE, Loeb HS: Dobutamine. A Ten-Year Review. NCM Publishers, New York, 1989

32. Jewitt D, Birkhead J, Mitchell A et al: Clinical cardiovascular pharmacology of dobutamine. A selective inotropic catecholamine. Lancet 1974;2:363–367

33. Leier CV, Unverferth DV, Kates RE: The relationship between plasma dobutamine concentrations and cardiovascular responses in cardiac failure. Am J Med 1979;66:238–242

34. Bianchi C, Diaz R, Gonzales C, Beregovich J: Effects of dobutamine on atrioventricular conduction. Am Heart J 1975;90:474–478

35. Unverferth DV, Magorien RD, Lewis RP, Leier CV: Long-term benefit of dobutamine in patients with congestive cardiomyopathy. Am Heart J 1980;100: 622–630

36. Beregovich J, Bianchi C, D'Angelo R et al: Haemodynamic effects of a new inotropic agent (dobutamine) in chronic cardiac failure. Br Heart J 1975;37: 629–634

37. Akhtar N, Mikulic E, Cohn JN, Chaudry MH: Hemodynamic effect of dobutamine in patients with severe heart failure. Am J Cardiol 1975;36:202–205

38. Leier CV, Webel J, Buch CA: The cardiovascular effects of the continuous infusion of dobutamine in patients with severe cardiac failure. Circulation 1977; 56:468–472

39. Bendersky R, Chatterjee K, Parmley WW et al: Dobutamine in chronic ischemic heart failure. Alterations in left ventricular function and coronary hemodynamics. Am J Cardiol 1981;48:554–558

40. Pozen RG, DiBianco R, Katz RJ et al: Myocardial metabolic and hemodynamic effects of dobutamine in heart failure complicating coronary artery disease. Circulation 1981;63:1279–1285

41. Meyer SL, Curry GC, Donsky MS et al: Influence of dobutamine on hemodynamics and coronary blood flow in patients with and without coronary artery disease. Am J Cardiol 1976;38:103–108

42. Teboul JL, Graini L, Boujdaria R et al: Cardiac index vs oxygen-derived parameters for rational use of dobutamine in patients with congestive heart failure. Chest 1993;103:81–85

43. Beanlands RSB, Bach DS, Raylman R et al: Acute effects of dobutamine on myocardial oxygen consumption and cardiac efficiency measure using carbon-11 acetate kinetics in patients with dilated cardiomyopathy. J Am Coll Cardiol 1993;22:1389–1398

44. Kono T, Sabbah HM, Rosman H et al: Divergent effects of intravenous dobutamine and nitroprusside on left atrial contribution to ventricular filling in dogs with chronic heart failure. Am Heart J 1994;127:874–880

45. Unverferth DV, Blanford M, Kates RE, Leier VI: Tolerance to dobutamine after a 72-hour continuous infusion. Am J Med 1980;69:262–266

46. Unverferth DV, Magorien RD, Altschuld R et al: The hemodynamic and metabolic advantages gained by a three-day infusion of dobutamine in patients with congestive cardiomyopathy. Am Heart J 1983;106:29–34

47. Bristow MR, Port JD, Hershberger RE, Gilbert EM, Feldman AM: The β-adrenergic receptor–adenylate cyclase complex as a target for therapeutic intervention in heart failure. Eur Heart J 1989;10:45–54

48. Pickworth KK: Long-term dobutamine therapy for refractory congestive heart failure. Clin Pharmacokinet 1992;11:618–624

49. Miller LW, Merkle EJ, Jennison SH: Outpatient use of dobutamine to support patients awaiting heart transplantation. J Heart Lung Trans 1994;13:S126–S129

50. Miller LW: Outpatient dobutamine for refractory congestive heart failure. Advantages, techniques, and results. J Heart Lung Trans 1991;10:482–487

51. Applefeld MM, Newman KA, Grove WR et al: Intermittent continuous outpatient dobutamine infusion in the management of congestive heart failure. Am J Cardiol 1983;51:455–458

52. Schoemaker RG, Debets JJM, Struyker-Boudier HAI, Smits JFM: Two weeks of intermittent dobutamine therapy restores cardiac performance and inotropic responsiveness in conscious rats with heart failure. J Cardiovasc Pharmacol 1991;17:949–956

53. Dies F, Krell MJ, Whitlow P et al: Intermittent dobutamine in ambulatory out-patients with chronic cardiac failure [abstract]. Circulation, suppl. II 1986;74:138

54. Krell MJ, Kline EM, Bates ER et al: Intermittent ambulatory dobutamine therapy in patients with severe congestive heart failure. Am Heart J 1986;112:787–791

55. Collins JA, Skidmore MA, Melvin DB, Engel PJ: Home intravenous dobutamine therapy in patients awaiting heart transplantation. J Heart Transplant 1990;9:205–208

56. Goldberg LI: Cardiovascular and renal actions of dopamine. Potential clinical application. Pharmacol Rev 1972;241:1–29

57. Goldberg LI, Volkman PH, Kohli JD: A comparison of the vascular dopamine receptor with other dopamine receptors. Annu Rev Pharmacol Toxicol 1978;18:57–79

58. Goldberg LI, Rajfer SI: Dopamine receptors. Applications in clinical cardiology. Circulation 1985;72:245–248

59. Rajfer SI, Goldberg LI: Dopamine in the treatment of heart failure. Eur Heart J, suppl. D 1982;3:103–106

60. Goldberg LI, Hsieh Y, Resnekov L; Newer catecholamines for treatment of heart failure and shock. An update on dopamine and a first look at dobutamine. Prog Cardiovasc Dis 1977;19:327–340

61. Lockhandwala MF, Barrett RJ: Cardiovascular dopamine receptors. Physiological pharmaceutical and therapeutic implications. J Auton Pharmacol 1982;2:189–215

62. Goldberg LI, Glock D, Kohli JD, Barnett A: Separation of peripheral dopamine receptors by a selective DA$_1$ antagonist, SCH 23390. Hypertension, suppl. I 1984;6:25–30

63. Civelli O, Bunzow JR, Grandy DK: Molecular diversity of the dopamine receptors. Annu Rev Pharmacol Toxicol 1993;32:281–307

64. Drake CR Jr, Carey RM: Dopamine modulates sodium-dependent aldosterone responses to angiotensin II in humans. Hypertension, suppl. I 1984;6:119–123

65. Rajfer SI, Rossen JD, Douglas FL, Goldberg LI, Karrison T: Effects of long-term therapy with oral ibopamine on resting hemodynamics and exercise capacity in patients with heart failure. Relationship to the generation of N-methyldopamine and to plasma norepinephrine levels. Circulation 1986;73:740–748

66. Caponnetto S, Terrachini V, Canale C et al: Long-term treatment of congestive heart failure with oral ibopamine: effects of rhythm disorders and neurohormonal alterations. Cardiology, suppl. 5 1990;77:43–48

67. Dei Cas L, Metra M, Nodari S, Riva S, Manca C: Lack of tolerance development during chornic ibopamine administration to patients with congestive heart failure. Cardiovasc Drugs Ther 1988;2:221–229

68. Dei Cas L, Metra M, Nodari S, Vilioli O: Efficacy of ibopamine treatment in patients with advanced heart failure. Purpose of a new therapeutic schema with multiple daily administrations. Cardiovasc Pharmacol, suppl. 8 1988;14:111–117

69. Itoh H, Taniguchi K, Tsajibayashi R, Koike A, Sato Y: Hemodynamic effects and pharmacokinetics of long-term therapy with ibopamine in patients with chronic heart failure. Cardiology 1992;80:356–360

70. Van Veldhuisen DJ, Man in't Veld AJ, Dunselman PH et al: Double-blind placebo-controlled study of ibopamine and digoxin in patients with mild to moderate heart failure. Results of the Dutch Ibopamine Multicenter Trial (DIMT). J Am Coll Cardiol 1993;22:1564–1573

71. Metra M, DeiCas L: Clinical efficacy of ibopamine in patients with chronic heart failure. Clin Cardiol, suppl. I 1995;18:22–31

72. Results of the PRIME-II trial. Presented at the Scientific sessions of the American College of Cardiology, Orlando, March 1996

73. Daly JW: Forskolin, adenylate cyclase, and cell physiology. An overview. Adv Cyclic Nucleotide Protein Phosphorylation Res 1984;17:81–89

74. Linderer T, Biamino G, Bruggemann T et al: Hemodynamic effects of forskolin, a new drug with combined positive inotropic and vasodilating properties [abstract]. J Am Coll Cardiol 1984;3:562

75. Blinks JR, Olsen JB, Jewell BR, Braveny P: Influence of caffeine and other methylxanthines on mechanical properties of isolated mammalian heart muscle. Evidence for a dual mechanism of action. Circ Res 1972; 30:367–392

76. Alousi AA, Farah AE, Lesher GY, Opalka CJ Jr: Cardiotonic activity of amrinone-WIN 40680 [5-amino-3,4'bipyridin-6(1H)-one]. Circ Res 1979;45: 666–677

77. Millard RW, Dube G, Grupp G et al: Direct vasodilator and positive inotropic actions of amrinone. J Mol Cell Cardiol 1980;12:647–652

78. Benotti JR, Grossman W, Braunwald E et al: Hemodynamic assessment of amrinone. N Engl J Med 1978;299:1373–1377

79. Endoh M, Yamashita S, Taira N: Positive inotropic effect of amrinone in relation to cyclic nucleotide metabolism in the canine ventricular muscle. J Pharmacol Exp Ther 1982;221:775–783

80. Kariya T, Willia LJ, Dage RC: Biochemical studies on the mechanism of cardiotonic activity of MDL 17,043. J Cardiovasc Pharmacol 1982;4:509–514

81. Bristow MR, Ginsburg R, Strosberg A et al: Cardiovascular pharmacology and inotropic potential of forskolin in the human heart. J Clin Invest 1984;74: 212–223

82. Gaide MS, Fitterman WS, Wiggins JR et al: Amrinone relaxes potassium-induced contracture of failing right ventricular muscle of cats. J Cardiovasc Pharmacol 1983;5:335–340

83. Adams HR, Rhody J, Sutko JL: Amrinone activates K+-depolarized atrial and ventricular myocardium of guinea pigs. Circ Res 1982;51:662–665

84. Kondo N, Shibata S, Kodama I, Yamada K: Electrical and mechanical effects of amrinone on isolated guinea pig ventricular muscle. J Cardiovasc Pharmacol 1983;5:903–912

85. LeJemtel TH, Keung E, Sonnenblick EH et al: Amrinone. A new non-glycosidic, non-adrenergic cardiotonic agent effective in the treatment of intractable myocardial failure in man. Circulation 1979;59: 1098–1004

86. Wilmshurst PT, Thompson DS, Juul SM et al: Comparison of the effects of amrinone and sodium nitroprusside on haemodynamics, contractility, and myocardial metabolism in patients with cardiac failure due to coronary artery disease and dilated cardiomyopathy. Br Heart J 1984;52:38–48

87. Firth B, Ratner AV, Grassman ED et al: Assessment of the inotropic and vasodilator effects of amrinone versus isoproterenol. Am J Cardiol 1984;54: 1331–1336

88. Franciosa JA: Intravenous amrinone: an advance or a wrong step? Ann Intern Med 1985;102:399–400

89. Ludmer PL, Wright RF, Arnold JM et al: Separation of the direct myocardial and vasodilator activities of milrinone administered by an intracoronary infusion technique. Circulation 1986;73:130–137

90. Installe E, DeCoster P, Gonzalez M et al: Comparison between the positive inotropic effects of enoximone, a cardiac phosphodiesterase III inhibitor, and dobutamine in patients with moderate to severe congestive heart failure. Eur Heart J 1991;12:985–993

91. Feldman MA, Copelas L, Gwathmey JK et al: Deficient production of cyclic AMP. Pharmacologic evidence of an important cause of contractile dysfunction in patients with end-stage heart failure. Circulation 1987;75:331–339

92. Rich MW, Woods WL, Davila-Roman VG et al: A randomized comparison of intravenous amrinone versus dobutamine in older patients with decompensated congestive heart failure. J Am Geriatr Soc 1995;443: 271–274

93. Hamilson RA, Kowalsky SF, Wright EM et al: Effect of the acetylator phenotype on amrinone pharmacokinetics. Clin Pharmacol Ther 1986;40:615–619

94. Wilmshurst PT, Webb-Peploe MM: Side effects of amrinone therapy. Br Heart J 1983;49:447–451

95. Kullberg MP, Freeman GB, Biddlecome C et al: Amrinone metabolism. Clin Pharmacol Ther 1981;29: 394–401

96. Ansell J, Tiarks C, McCue J et al: Amrinone-induced thrombocytopenia. Arch Intern Med 1984;144: 949–952

97. Kinney EL, Ballard JO, Carlin B, Zelis R: Amrinone-mediated thrombocytopenia. Scand J Haematol 1983;31:376–380

98. Ross MP, Allen-Webb EM, Pappas JB, McGough EC: Amrinone-associated thrombocytopenia. Pharmacokinetic analysis. Clin Pharmacol Ther 1993;53: 661–667

99. DiBianco R, Shebetai R, Silverman BD et al: Oral amrinone for the treatment of chronic congestive heart failure. Results of a multicenter randomized double-blind and placebo-controlled withdrawal study. J Am Coll Cardiol 1984;4:855–66

100. Massie B, Bourassa M, DiBianco R et al: Long-term oral administration of amrinone for congestive heart failure. Lack of efficacy in a multicenter controlled trial. Circulation 1985;71:963–971

101. DiBianco R, Shabetai R, Kostuk W et al: A comparison of oral milrinone digoxin and their combination in the treatment of patients with chronic heart failure. N Engl J Med 1989;320:677–683

102. Uretsky BF, Jessup M, Konstam MA et al: Multicenter trial of oral enoximone in patients with moderate to moderately severe congestive heart failure. Lack of benefit compared with placebo. Circulation 1990; 82:774–780

103. Seino Y, Takano T, Hayakawa H et al: Hemodynamic effects and pharmacokinetics of oral milrinone for short-term support in acute heart failure. Cardiology 1995;86:34–40

104. Packer M: Positive inotropic agents for chronic heart failure. A new perspective. Heart Failure 1993;9:136

105. Braunwald E: Intravenous milrinone. Therapeutic responses in heart failure. Am Heart J 1991;121: 1937–1938

106. Anderson JL: Hemodynamic and clinical benefits with intravenous milrinone in severe chronic heart failure. Results of a multicenter study in the United States. Am Heart J 1991;121:1956–1964

107. Klocke RK, Mager G, Kux A et al: Effects of a twenty-four hour milrinone infusion in patients with severe heart failure and cardiogenic shock as a function of

the hemodynamic initial condition. Am Heart J 1991; 121:1965–1973

108. Watson DM, Sherry KM, Weston GA: Milrinone, a bridge to heart transplantation. Anaesthesia 1991; 46:285–287

109. Buser PT, Auffermann W, Wu ST, et al: Dobutamine potentiates amrinone's beneficial effects in moderate but not in advanced heart failure. Circ Res 1990;66: 747–53

110. Feldman AM, Bristow MR: The β-adrenergic pathway in the failing human heart. Implications for inotropic therapy, Cardiology, suppl. 1 1990;77:1–32

111. Gage J, Rutman H, Lucido D, LeJemtel TH: Additive effects of dobutamine and amrinone on myocardial contractility and ventricular performance in patients with severe heart failure. Circulation 1986;74: 367–373

112. Uretsky BF, Lawless CE, Verbalis JG et al: Combined therapy with dobutamine and amrinone in severe heart failure. Chest 1987;92:657–662

113. Hagemeijer F: Calcium sensitization with pimobendan. Pharmacology, haemodynamic improvement, and sudden death in patients with chronic congestive heart failure. Eur Heart J 1993;14:551–566

114. Fitton A, Brogden RN: Pimobendan. A review of its pharmcology and therapeutic potential in congestive heart failure. Drugs Aging 1994;4:417–441

115. Fujino K, Sperelakis N, Solaro RJ: Sensitization of dog and guinea pig heart myofilaments to calcium activation and the inotropic effect of pimobendan. Comparison with milrinone. Circ Res 1988;63: 911–922

116. Solaro RJ, Fujino K, Sperelakis N: The positive inotropic effect of pimobendan involves stereospecific increases in the calcium sensitivity of cardiac myofilaments. J Cardiovasc Pharmacol, suppl. 2 1989;14: 7–12

117. Böhm M, Morano I, Pieske B et al: Contribution of cAMP-phosphodiesterase inhibition and sensitization of the contractile proteins for calcium to the inotropic effect of pimobendan in the failing human heart. Circ Res 1991;68:689–701

118. Katz SD, Kubo SH, Jessup M et al: A multicenter, randomized, double-blind, placebo-controlled trial of pimobendan, a new cardiotonic and vasodilator agent, in patients with severe congestive heart failure. Am Heart J 1992;123:95–103

119. Kubo SH, Gollub S, Bourge R et al: Beneficial effects of pimobendan on exercise tolerance and quality of life in patients with heart failure. Circulation 1992; 85:942–949

120. Just H, Hjalmarsson A, Remme WJ et al: Pimobendan in congestive heart failure. Results of the PICO trial [abstract]. Circulation, suppl. I 1995;92:722

121. Pollesello P, Ovaska M, Kaivola J et al: Binding of a new Ca^{2+}-sensitizer, levosimendan, to recombinant human cardiac troponin C. A molecular modelling, fluorescence probe and proton nuclear magnetic resonance study. J Biol Chem 1994;269:28584–28589

122. Edes I, Kiss E, Kitada Y et al: Effects of levosimendan, a cardiotonic agent targeted to troponin C, on cardiac function and on phosphorylation and Ca^{2+} sensitivity of cardiac myofibrils and sarcoplasmic reticulum in guinea-pig heart. Circ Res 1995;77: 107–113

123. Haikala H, Nissinen E, Etemadzadeh E et al: Tropo-

nin C-mediated calcium sensitization induced by levosimendan does not impair relaxation. J Cardiovasc Pharmacol 1995;25:794–801

124. Sundberg S, Lilleberg J, Nieminen MS, Lehtonen L: Hemodynamic and neurohumoral effects of levosimendan, a new calcium sensitizer, at rest and during exercise in healthy men. Am J Cardiol 1995;75: 1061–1066

125. Yamashita S, Hosokawa T, Kojima M et al: In vitro and in vivo studies of 3,4-dihydro-6-[4-(3,4-dimethoxybenzoyl)-1-piperazinyl]-2(1H)-quinolinone) on myocardial oxygen consumption in dogs with ischemic heart failure. Jpn Circ J 1986;50:659–666

126. Hori M, Inoue M, Tamai J et al: Beneficial effect of OPC-8212 (3,4-dihydro-6-[4-(3,4-dimethoxybenzoyl)-1-piperazinyl]-2(1H)-quinolinone) on myocardial oxygen consumption in dogs with ischemic heart failure. Jpn Circ J 1986;50:659–666

127. Grupp G, Grupp IL, Newman G, Schwartz A: Effects of a new positive inotropic agent, 3,4-dihydro-6-[4-(3,4-dimethoxybenzoyl)-1-piperaznyl]-2(1H)-quinolinone (OPC-8212) and its solvent sulfolane on isolated heart preparation of the rat, guinea pig, and dog. Arzneimittelforschung 1984;34:359–363

128. Schwartz A, Wallick ET, Lee SW et al: Studies on the mechanism of action of 3,4-dihydro-6-[4-(3,4-dimethoxybenzoyl]-1-piperazinyl]-2(1H)-quinolinone (OPC-8212), a new positive inotropic drug. Enzyme activities and Ca^{2+} transport processes of sarcolemma and intracellular organelles. Arzneimittelforschung 1984;34:384–389

129. Iijima R, Taira N: Membrane current changes responsible for the positive inotropic effect of OPC-8212, a new positive inotropic agent, in single ventricular cells of the guinea pig heart. J Pharmacol Exp Ther 1987;240:657–662

130. Lathrop DA, Schwartz A: Electro-mechanical effects of 3,4-dihydro-6-[4-(3,4-dimethoxybenzoyl)-1-piperazinyl]-2(1H)-quinolinone (OPC-8212), a new positive inotropic agent. Arzneimittelforschung 1984;34: 371–375

131. Rapundalo ST, Lathrop DA, Harrison SA et al: Cyclic AMP-dependent and cyclic-AMP-independent actions of a novel cardiotonic agent, OPC-8212. Naunyn Schmiedebergs Arch Pharmacol 1988;338:692–698

132. Yatani A, Imoto Y, Schwartz A, Brown AM: New positive inotropic agents OPC-8212 modulates single Ca^{2+} channels in ventricular myocytes of guinea pig. J Cardiovasc Pharmacol 1989;13:812–819

133. Lathrop DA, Nanasi PP, Schwartz A, Varro A: Ionic basis for OPC-8212-induced increase in action potential duration in isolated rabbit, guinea pit and human ventricular myocytes. Eur J Pharmacol 1993;240: 127–137

134. Yanagisawa R, Ishii K, Taira N: Anti-tachycardiac effect of OPC-8212, a novel cardiotonic agent, on tachycardiac responses of guinea pig isolated right atria to isoproterenol and histamine. J Cardiovasc Pharmacol 1987;1:47–54

135. Lathrop DA, Varro A, Schwartz A: Rate-dependent electrophysiologic effects of OPC-8212. Comparison to sotalol. Eur J Pharmacol 1989;164:487–496

136. Alousi AA, Stankus GP, Stuart JC, Walton LH: Characterization of the cardiotonic effects of milrinone, a new and potent cardiac bypyridine, on isolated tis-

sues from several animal species. J Cardiovasc Pharmacol 1983;5:804–811

137. Dage RC, Roebel LE, Hsieh CP et al: Cardiovascular properties of a new cardiotonic agent. MDL 17,043 (1,3-dihydro-4-methyl-5-[4-(methyltio)-benoyl]-2H-imidazol-2-one]. J Cardiovasc Pharmacol 1982;4: 500–508

138. Farah AE, Alousi AA: New cardiotonic agents. A search for digitalis substitute. Life Sci 1978;22: 1139–1147

139. Masuoka H, Ito M, Sugioka M et al: Two isoforms of cGMP-inhibited cyclic nucleotide phosphodiesterase in human tissues distinguished by their responses to vesnarinone, a new cardiotonic agent. Biochem Biophys Res Commun 1993;190:412–417

140. Matsumori A, Shioi T, Yamada T, Matsui S, Sasayama S: Vesnarinone, a new inotropic agent, inhibits cytokine production by stimulated human blood from patients with heart failure. Circulation 1994;89: 955–958

141. Matsui S, Matsumori A, Sasayama S: Vesnarinone prolongs survival and reduces lethality in a murine model of lethal endotoxemia. Life Sci 1994;55: 1735–1741

142. Kurnich J, McCluskey R: Perspective on cell mediated immunity in vivo. In: Lymphokines and the Immune Response. CRC Press, Boca Raton, FL, 1989

143. Gajewski TF, Schell SR, Nau G, Fitch FW: Regulation of T-cell activation. Differences among T-cell subsets. Immunol Rev 1989;111:79–110

144. Nathan CF: Secretory products of macrophages. J Clin Invest 1987;79:319–326

145. Maisch B, Deeg P, Liebau G, Kochsiek K: Diagnostic relevance of humoral and cytotoxic immune reactions in primary and secondary dilated cardiomyopathy. Am J Cardiol 1983;52:1072–1078

146. Forbes RD, Guttmann RD: Pathogenetic studies of cardiac allograft rejection using inbred rat models. Immunol Rev 1984;77:5–29

147. Levine B, Kalman J, Mayer L, Fillit AM, Packer M: Elevated circulating levels of tumor necrosis factor in severe chronic heart failure. N Engl J Med 1990; 323:236–241

148. Yokoyama T, Vaca L, Rossen RD et al: Cellular basis for the negative inotropic effects of tumor necrosis factor-alpha in the adult mammalian heart. J Clin Invest 1993;92:2303–2312

149. Finkel MS, Oddis CV, Jacobs TD et al: Negative inotropic effects of cytokines on the heart mediated by nitric oxide. Science 1992;257:387–389

150. Natanson C, Eichenholz PW, Danner RL et al: Endotoxin and tumor necrosis factor challenges in dogs simulate the cardiovascular profile of human septic shock. J Exp Med 1989;169:823–832

151. Eichenholtz PW, Eichacker PQ, Hoffman WD et al: Tumor necrosis factor challenges in canines. Patterns of cardiovascular dysfunction. Am J Physiol 1992; 263:H668–H675

152. Suffredini AF, Fromm RE, Parker MM et al: The cardiovascular response of normal humans to the administration of endotoxin. N Engl J Med 1989;321: 280–287

153. Blick M, Sherwin SA, Rosenblum M, Gutterman J: Phase I study of recombinant tumor necrosis factor in cancer patients. Cancer Res 1987;47:2986–2989

154. Smith SC, Allen PM: Neutralization of endogenous tumor necrosis factor ameliorates the severity of myosin-induced myocarditis. Circ Res 1992;70: 856–863

155. Arbustini EM, Grasso M, Diegoli M et al: Expression of tumor necrosis factor in human acute cardiac rejection. An immunohistochemical and immunoblotting study. Am J Pathol 1991;139:709–715

156. Maury CPJ, Teppo AM: Circulating tumor necrosis factor-alpha (cachetin) in myocardial infarction. J Intern Med 1989;225:333–336

157. Lefer AM, Tsao P, Aoki N, Palladino MA Jr: Mediation of cardioprotection by transforming growth factor-beta. Science 1990;249:61–64

158. Torre-Amione G, Kapadia S, Lee J et al: Tumor necrosis factor-α and tumor necrosis factor receptors in the failing human heart. Circulation 1995;92:1487–1493

159. Inoue M, Kim BH, Hori M et al: Oral OPC-8212 for the treatment of congestive heart failure. Hemodynamic improvement and increased exercise capacity. Heart Vessels 1986;2:166–171

160. Sasayama S, Inoue M, Asanoi H et al: Acute hemodynamic effects of a new inotropic agent, OPC-8212, on severe congestive heart failure. Heart Vessels 1986; 2:23–28

161. Feldman AM, Becker LC, Llewellyn MP, Baughman KL: Evaluation of a new inotropic agent, OPC-8212, in patients with dilated cardiomyopathy and heart failure. Am Heart J 1988;116:771–777

162. Kubo SH, Rector TS, Strobeck JE, Cohn JN: OPC-8212 in the treatment of congestive heart failure. Results of a pilot study. Cardiovasc Drug Ther 1988;2: 653–60

163. Feldman AM, Baughman KL, Lee WK et al: Usefulness of OPC-8212, a quinolinone derivative, for chronic congestive heart failure in patients with ischemic heart disease or idiopathic dilated cardiomyopathy. Am J Cardiol 1991;68:1203–1210

164. Asanoi H, Sasayama S, Kameyama T et al: Sustained inotropic effects of a new cardiotonic agent. OPC-8212 in patients with chronic heart failure. Clin Cardiol 1989;12:133–138

165. Asanoi H, Sasayama S, Iushi K, Kameyama T: Acute hemodynamic effects of a new inotropic agent (OPC-8212) in patients with congestive heart failure. J Am Coll Cardiol 1987;9:865–871

166. Kass DA, Van Anden E, Becker L et al: Dose-dependence of chronic positive inotropic effect of vesnarinone in patients with dilated cardiomyopathy. Am J Cardiol (in press, 1996)

167. Sharir T, Feldman MD, Haber H et al: Ventricular systolic assessment in patients with dilated cardiomyopathy by preload-adjusted maximal power, validation and noninvasive application. Circulation 1994;89:2045–2053

168. Feldman AM, Pepine CJ, Bristow MR et al: Incidence of vesnarinone-induced neutropenia. The US experience [abstract]. Circulation, suppl. I 1993;88:1301

169. Otsuka America, PNC: Letter to VEST Investigators, July 29, 1996.

47 *β*-Adrenoceptor Antagonists

Bert Andersson
Karl Swedberg

Since the first *β*-adrenergic antagonist was synthesized in 1957, these drugs have become one of the most important therapeutic tools in cardiovascular medicine. The negative inotropic effect and potential capability of inducing congestive heart failure in susceptible individuals were recognized early.[1,3] Congestive heart failure has been considered a contraindication for *β*-blockade, and there has been a widespread reluctance to change this opinion.

Diuretics, vasodilators, and angiotensin-converting enzyme (ACE) inhibitors are drugs that counteract pathophysiologic effects of congestive heart failure, such as increased intravascular volume, increased vasoconstriction, and activation of the renin-angiotensin system. In addition to *β*-blockers, there have been few attempts to modulate the increased sympathetic drive. During the early 1970s it was discovered that *β*-blockers were useful in the setting of an acute myocardial infarction, even in patients who were severely compromised. Waagstein and coworkers observed dramatic improvement following administration of an intravenous *β*-blocker in patients with acute myocardial infarction, tachycardia, and pulmonary edema.[4] This observation gave rise to the hypothesis that *β*-blockers might be beneficial to patients with congestive heart failure and an adversely high heart rate.

The first report on *β*-blockers used as therapy for heart failure, presented in 1975, was received with skepticism.[5] The Göteborg group presented several reports on patients with idiopathic dilated cardiomyopathy (IDCM) treated in open protocol studies.[6-10] Two other reports failed to reproduce the results in short-term studies.[11,12] Ten years after the original observation, the results were reproduced in two randomized placebo-controlled long-term studies.[13,14] Many studies have now been published on the subject,[15] and most major scientific meetings in cardiology have sessions dealing with *β*-blockers and heart failure. The first major trial was reported in 1993, the Metoprolol in Dilated Cardiomyopathy (MDC) trial,[16] and in 1994 another trial was reported, the Cardiac Insufficiency Bisoprolol Study (CIBIS).[17] More recently, a group of studies employing carvedilol have been presented. Collectively, these studies provide the largest experience with a single *β*-blocker. The intention with this chapter is to review the results of *β*-blocker studies performed on patients with congestive heart failure and to present potential mechanisms behind the effect of *β*-blockers in heart failure.

SYMPATHETIC NERVOUS SYSTEM AS A TARGET FOR THERAPY

Norepinephrine, the sympathetic neurotransmitter, binds to *β*-receptors on the cellular membrane, predominantly to the β_1-receptor. Through binding to the receptor, the hormone activates membrane-bound adenylate cyclase. This enzyme catalyzes conversion of adenosine triphosphate (ATP) to cyclic adenosine monophosphate (cAMP), which in turn acts as an intracellular second messenger on protein kinase, which transfers phosphate groups to calcium channel proteins. The result is an increase in calcium influx in response to membrane depolarization and an increased rate of contraction and relaxation. A contemporary overview of the β-adrenergic pathway has been reported by Bristow.[18]

Reduced myocardial contractility, which is a hallmark of congestive heart failure, has been the target for research and therapeutic interventions for decades. Several positive inotropic drugs have been developed with pharmacologic action on the sympathetic receptors and on subcellular enzymes. Short-term administration of sympathomimetics and phosphodiesterase inhibitors to patients with congestive heart failure often produces dramatic hemodynamic improvement.[19,20] However, all long-term studies with positive inotropic agents other than digotoxin

have failed, and many have shown increased mortality with treatment.[21–23]

SHORT–TERM EFFECTS OF β–BLOCKERS

The effects of β-blocker treatment are paradoxical,[24] and there are striking differences between short-term and long-term effects (Table 47-1). In some of the first β-blocker studies it was proposed that diastolic alterations were present during the first weeks of treatment.[5,8,9] Later studies have thrown some light on the mechanisms possibly involved in the process. In a combined invasive and noninvasive study, the effect of intravenous metoprolol was studied in 54 patients

Table 47-1. Short-Term and Long-Term Effects of β-Blockers on Congestive Heart Failure

Parameter	Short term		Long term	
	Effects	Refs.	Effects	Refs.
Heart rate	↓	25,[a] 26,[b] 27[c]	↓ ↑	26,[b] 27,[c] 29,[c] 30[a] 30,[a] 31[a]
Systolic blood pressure	↓	25, 28,[a] 26,[b] 27[c]	– ↓	27[c] 26[b]
Stroke volume index	–	25, 26,[b] 27[c] 28,[a]	↑	26,[b] 30,[a] 31[c]
Stroke work index	–	27[c]	↑	27,[c] 29,[c] 30,[a] 31[c]
Ejection fraction	– –	25,[a] 26[b] 26[b]	↑ –	26,[b] 27,[c] 30[a] 29,[c] 30,[a] 31[c]
Systemic vascular resistance	↓	27[c]	↓	26,[b] 27[c]
Ventriculoarterial coupling	–	28[a]	nr	nr
Left ventricular maximum dP/dt	↓	28[a]	↑	31,[c] 32,[a] 33[a]
Left ventricular end-diastolic volume	–	25,[a] 28[a]	↓	29,[c] 32,[a] 34[c]
Left ventricular end-diastolic pressure	– ↓	25[a] 26[b]	↓	31[c]
Pulmonary capillary wedge pressure	–	27,[c] 28[a]	↓	26,[b] 29,[c] 30[a]
E wave deceleration time	nr	—	↑	35[a]
Peak filling rate	↓	25,[a] 28[a]	–	—
Chamber stiffness	–	28[a]	–	31[c]
Left ventricular isovolumic relaxation	↑	28[a]	↓ –	31[c] 32[a]
Arterial norepinephrine	↑ nr	25[a] nr	↓ nr	29,[c] 30[a] 31[c]
Myocardial oxygen consumption	↓	25[a]	– ↓	30,[a] 31[b] 32[a]
Myocardial norepinephrine spillover	–	25[a]	–	30[a]
Myocardial lactate extraction	↑	25[a]	↑	30[a]

Abbreviations: ↑ increase; ↓ decrease; — unchanged; nr, no results.
[a] Metoprolol.
[b] Carvedilol.
[c] Bucindolol.

with congestive heart failure due to various causes.[25] Heart rate was reduced within a few minutes, accompanied by a somewhat slower decline in systolic blood pressure. There was a reflex increase in sympathetic nervous discharge as reflected by increased levels of norepinephrine and epinephrine. Cardiac output was decreased because of the fall in heart rate, whereas stroke volumes and filling pressures were unchanged. Metoprolol induced a decrease in myocardial oxygen consumption. The increase in left ventricular volume that is common in ischemic heart disease after acute β-blocker administration was not apparent in these patients with heart failure. Diastolic filling volumes were redistributed to late diastole, suggesting a less restrictive filling pattern. In a study by Ikram et al. acebutolol produced signs of reduced contractility with unchanged filling pressures.[36] Propranolol was less well tolerated in a study by Shanes et al.[37] Haber et al. demonstrated the similar effects of short-term metoprolol and propranolol, with signs of decreased contractility and afterload and no change in passive left ventricular diastolic stiffness.[28] Preservation of passive diastolic function and ventriculoarterial coupling was suggested to explain why β-blockers are well tolerated by patients with congestive heart failure. Carvedilol, a nonselective β-blocker with concurrent α-blocking properties, produced less reduction in heart rate and cardiac index and a fall in pulmonary capillary wedge pressure.[26]

During initiation of treatment the positive effects on myocardial metabolism must be balanced against the negative effects on systemic flow. Severely decompensated patients may not tolerate the initial depression of myocardial function produced by β-blockade and therefore β-blockade must be instituted gradually over several weeks, waiting for myocardial function to recover. A titration scheme developed by Waagstein et al. starting with metoprolol 5 mg bid with weekly increments up to 50 mg tid over 6 weeks, has been used in a number of trials and is adequate in most cases.[10] Metoprolol 5 mg tablets are not generally available, and a quarter of the 50 mg tablets has been used by some investigators.

The experience of β-blocker treatments is that the poorer the left ventricular function, the slower must be the titration. In preliminary reports it has been suggested that β-blockers with vasodilating properties, such as cervedilol and bucindolol, have better initial tolerance, and the titration may be less cautious.[38,39] Afterload reduction was suggested to be beneficial in counteracting the negative inotropic effect. However, there have not been any consistent differences regarding tolerability in larger trials. In the MDC trial, intolerance to metoprolol was reported in 4 percent of 417 cases with IDCM.[16] Five percent of 215 bucindolol-treated patients in five trials were intolerant.[27,29,31,40,41] These tolerability figures are not significantly different from those reported from ACE inhibitor trials.

LONG–TERM HEMODYNAMIC EFFECTS

Heart rate reduction is induced by β-blockers and is maintained during long-term treatment.[16,17,42] There is a gradual recovery of myocardial performance over 6–12 months, mostly reported as an increase in ejection fraction. Left ventricular filling pressure is reduced, with an increase in stroke volumes, cardiac output, and stroke work index.[16] Metoprolol treatment causes an increase in systemic blood pressure, probably due to the increase in stroke volumes, but without alterations of systemic vascular resistance.[30] These positive effects expressing increased myocardial efficiency have been achieved with unchanged or decreased myocardial oxygen consumption.[30,32,43] In addition to an increase in ejection fraction, vasodilating β-blockers such as bucindolol cause short-term and long-term vasodilation and reduced filling pressures. Systemic blood pressure did not increase during bucindolol treatment.[27]

FUNCTIONAL CAPACITY

Exercise capacity has been found to improve after metoprolol treatment, and hemodynamics during submaximal supine exercise have been similarly improved.[16,30] In contrast, Bristow and coworkers found bucindolol to cause clear suppression of heart rate response to exercise, which was interpreted as due to more potent β-blockade and simultaneous β_1 and β_2-blockade.[34] The attenuated chronotropic response was suggested to be responsible for the lack of increase in exercise performance. So far no convincing study shows an increased exercise capacity after carvedilol treatment of congestive heart failure.[44] Labetalol—another compound with β-blocking and vasodilator capacity—has been shown to increase exercise performance in a small study.[45] Several studies have demonstrated functional improvement following β-blockade treatment, expressed as an increase in New York Heart Association (NYHA) classification following treatment with metoprolol[16,42] and bucindolol.[27,31] Metoprolol and bisoprolol have been associated with a decrease in the rate of hospitalization and, furthermore, to improve subjective quality of life.[16]

ADRENERGIC β–RECEPTORS AND CATECHOLAMINES

As a consequence of increased sympathetic nerve discharge in heart failure, there is an increase in myocardial norepinephrine spillover[46,47] and simultaneous depletion of myocardial norepinephrine stores.[48] In response to the increased noradrenergic sympathetic discharge in congestive heart failure,[46,49] the adrenergic β_1-receptors are down-regulated and rendered less responsive to endogenous and pharmacologic stimulation.[50,51] There may be a transmural heterogeneity in the receptor down-regulation.[52]

Metoprolol treatment has been reported to cause up-regulation of β-receptors,[10,33] which would decrease the need for sympathetic stimulation. Bucindolol and carvedilol improve cardiac function in a similar way, but without up-regulation of the β-receptors.[53] The effects on up-regulation are predominantly on the β_1-receptors, although it has been suggested that β_1-blockade also sensitizes β_2-receptors.[54,55] Even though β_1-receptor up-regulation may not be necessary for myocardial recovery in the resting state, it may be of importance for increased exercise capacity. An increased inotropic response following long-term metoprolol treatment was shown by Heilbrun et al.[33] Exercise-induced release of epinephrine may also be responsible for the increased contractile response by action on β_2-receptors.

Activation of the sympathetic nervous system is a well known feature of congestive heart failure and is associated with poor prognosis.[56] Although there is no evidence to suggest a toxic effect of norepinephrine in physiologic concentrations, catecholamines have several actions that might be deleterious in congestive heart failure. An increase in contractility and heart rate enhances myocardial oxygen consumption and energy expenditure[57–59] and increases the risk of arrhythmias.[60] It is currently considered important to modulate the activated neurohormonal systems in congestive heart failure in order to achieve a good long-term response.[61,62] Although the effect of β-blockers on neurohormones has not yet been evaluated in any large trial, several smaller studies have shown a reduction in peripheral norepinephrine levels following treatment with metoprolol[30,43,63] or bucindolol.[27,29]

EFFECTS IN PATIENTS WITH CONGESTIVE HEART FAILURE SECONDARY TO ISCHEMIC HEART DISEASE

Most studies with β-blockers in patients with heart failure have been performed on those with IDCM. Although well recognized by every cardiologist, they account for only 10 percent of all heart failure cases.[64] The largest group comprises patients with congestive heart failure secondary to ischemic heart disease.[65–67] Several large randomized trials aiming to reduce mortality after acute myocardial infarction have reported beneficial effects in patients with mild to moderate heart failure.[68–70] Patients with severe heart failure were excluded before randomization in all these studies. β-Blockers have been used in studies that included patients with chronic ischemic heart disease, and a less beneficial effect was demonstrated in some of these studies compared with the effect on IDCM.[29,43] A randomized, placebo-controlled trial by Fisher et al. demonstrated a clear positive effect in 25 of 50 patients with ischemic cardiomyopathy.[42]

EFFECTS ON SURVIVAL

Although one of the first reports on the beneficial effects of β-blockers in congestive heart failure reported an improvement in survival compared to historical controls,[6] this result has not been confirmed by a large randomized survival study. The MDC trial was the first major placebo-controlled study.[16] This study was performed in 383 patients with IDCM with the primary objective of studying the effect of metoprolol on a combined endpoint consisting of all-cause mortality and the need for heart transplantation. There was a borderline significant effect of metoprolol on the combined endpoint, as expressed by a 34 percent risk reduction (95 percent confidence interval -6 to 62 percent; $P = 0.058$) (Fig. 47-1). The entire effect was achieved on the need for heart transplantation (19 patients in the placebo group and 2 patients in the metoprolol group; $P = 0.0001$). There was no difference in deaths between the two groups. In addition to the decrease in the number of patients progressing to transplant candidacy, metoprolol produced a noteworthy decrease in hospitalizations for heart failure and other evidence of deterioration and a significant increase in left ventricular ejection fraction. Thus metoprolol appeared to attenuate or reverse the progression of left ventricular dysfunction but showed no beneficial effect on the incidence of sudden death, which in part may have been due to the more frequent use of cardiac transplantation in the placebo group.

The second major placebo-controlled trial (CIBIS trial) included 641 patients with various causes of heart failure and compared bisoprolol and placebo.[17] There was a 20 percent nonsignificant reduction in mortality in the total group of patients. In the subgroup of patients without previous myocardial infarction there was a positive effect of bisoprolol on mortality [42 deaths in 187 patients (23 percent) in the placebo group and 18 deaths among 151 patients (12 percent) in the bisoprolol group; $P = 0.01$]; biso-

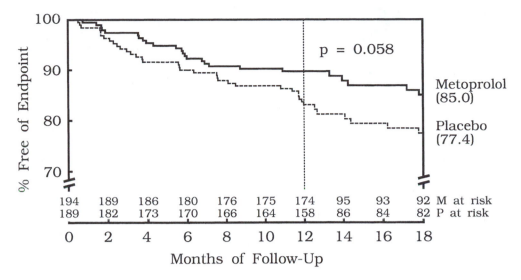

Fig. 47-1. Likelihood of reaching a primary endpoint (death or need for heart transplantation) in the MDC study. A total of 211 patients were followed for 12 months and 172 for 18 months. (From Waagstein et al.,[16] with permission.)

prolol had no effect in patients with a history of myocardial infarction (Fig. 47-2). The group of patients with IDCM was included in the group without myocardial infarction, and the positive effect on mortality is consistent with that reported in other studies demonstrating beneficial effects of β-blockers in this group of patients. In the context of postmyocardial infarction, the lack of effect in the ischemic group is of course surprising. The discrepancy between the two groups in the CIBIS trial could not be explained from the results of the study. Possible reasons for a different effect of β-blocker treatment in ischemic heart disease versus IDCM are discussed below. A confounding factor in the CIBIS trial was that antiarrhythmic therapy was used in 20 percent of patients, including amiodarone. In one study this drug has been shown to exert a positive effect on survival of patients with heart failure.[71] The CIBIS and the MDC trials had low mortality rates, leaving these studies without enough power to clearly state any effects or lack of effects on mortality. These results indicate that modern heart failure treatment has improved survival for IDCM patients, compared with earlier reports.[64,72]

Four studies conducted with carvedilol, a nonselective β-blocker with weak α-blocking properties, have been pooled in a prospectively planned survival analysis.[73] Each of these studies had similar entrance criteria, including a total of 1094 patients with primarily NYHA class II and III congestive heart failure and left ventricular ejection fractions of 0.35 or less who were undergoing therapy with ACE inhibitors and diuretics, as well as digoxin and vasodilators in

many cases. These patients were stratified into groups with severe limitation (6-minute walk distance < 150 meters),[74] a group with mild symptoms (6 minute walk distance > 450 meters),[75] and an intermediate group.[76,77] Patients were challenged with carvedilol 6.25 mg bid for 2 weeks, and only those patients who could tolerate this dose (approximately 90 percent) were randomized. Patients were followed for 6 months (a small group of patients with mild disease were continued up to 12 months), and pooled data for deaths and hospitalizations were analyzed.[73,77] The still ongoing studies of mild and severe heart failure patients were terminated before their scheduled completion by the Data and Safety Monitoring Board because of the excessive mortality in the placebo group.

The carvedilol-treated patients had a strikingly lower mortality rate (3.0 percent versus 7.8 percent); the relative risk was 0.33 by log-rank analysis (95 percent confidence limit 0.19–0.58). Of interest was that the mortality was reduced among patients with both ischemic and nonischemic cardiomyopathy, in contrast to the CIBIS experience. Although these findings are impressive, this pooled-data analysis is limited by the small number of events (n = 53) and the small number of severe heart failure patients, as the ability to perform a 6-minute walk test was an entry requirement. Furthermore, the premature study termination and the short duration of follow-up increase the possibility that these findings may have occurred by chance. More persuasive was a consistent reduction in hospitalizations in the carvedilol arms of each

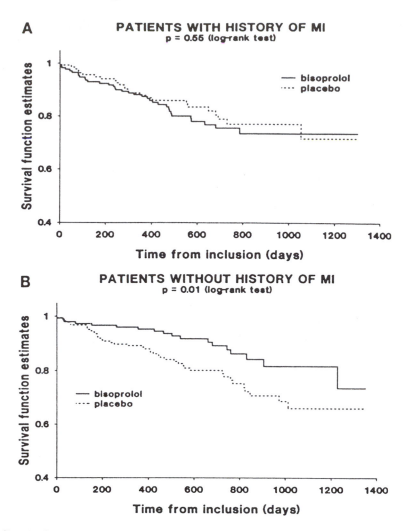

Fig. 47-2. **(A)** Survival curves (Kaplan-Meier) in CIBIS patients with a history of myocardial infarction ($n = 303$): 25 of 134 patients died receiving placebo, and 35 of 169 died receiving bisoprolol. **(B)** Survival curves (Kaplan-Meier) in CIBIS patients without a history of myocardial infarction ($n = 339$): 42 of 187 patients died receiving placebo, and 18 of 151 died receiving bisoprolol. (From CIBIS Investigators and Committees,[17] with permission.)

of the four studies.[73,78] Overall, there were 38 percent fewer hospitalizations for all cardiovascular causes (95 percent confidence interval 14.9–54.2 percent; $P = 0.003$) and a 47 percent reduction in heart failure hospitalizations (95 percent confidence interval 13.5–67.3 percent; $P = 0.011$). A dose-dependent effect on mortality was observed in one study.[76]

VARIOUS β–ADRENERGIC BLOCKERS

Although most studies have used metoprolol, other β-blockers such as labetalol, alprenolol, bucindolol, and carvedilol have produced similar effects regarding improvement in ejection fraction. Hence this ef-

fect on cardiac function appears to be a class effect, and selectivity or nonselectivity does not seem to be of importance. The improvement in exercise capacity may be related to either β_1-selectivity or to the ability to increase β_1-receptor sensitivity, as this effect has been observed after metoprolol treatment but not after bucindolol or carvedilol therapy. It has been proposed, but not confirmed in any published studies, that a simultaneous blockade of β_1- and β_2-receptors might be important for preventing lethal arrhythmias. Nebivolol is a new β_1-selective antagonist with a weak vasodilator effect. Only a few studies have been performed in heart failure patients, some demonstrating positive effects.[79,80] β-Blockers with agonist properties, such as xamoterol, are probably similar to other positive inotropic drugs and have been associated with poor long-term results.[81]

POSSIBLE MECHANISMS BEHIND THE EFFECTS FROM β-BLOCKERS

The pathophysiologic background of the improvement in cardiac function during β-blocker therapy is still not fully understood. Several potential mechanisms may explain why β-blockers are beneficial to patients with congestive heart failure.

1. The clinically most obvious of the possible positive effects is the reduction in heart rate. Heart rate is reduced immediately after initiation of β-blockade,[25] and the heart frequency remains attenuated during long-term treatment.[16,17] Increased heart rate is associated with poor survival,[82] and tachycardia per se may precipitate heart failure resembling IDCM.[83,84] In studies on myocardial preparations it has been demonstrated that peak contractile force in the failing myocardium occurred at much lower heart rates than in normal myocardium.[85] Similar conclusions have been drawn from the results in intact hearts.[86] Therefore there is experimental evidence supporting the idea that lowering the heart rate may increase the efficacy of the failing heart.

2. Decreased heart rate is associated with a prolongation of diastole, which intuitively would be beneficial to the failing heart. High heart rate and congestive heart failure are associated with a restrictive filling pattern in which the major portion of the diastolic volume fills the left ventricle early during diastole.[87,88] This pattern may be recognized by a dip–plateau sign in the left ventricular pressure tracing, an increase in peak filling rate on radionuclide angiography, or as a short E wave deceleration time on transmitral Doppler recordings. The latter observation has been associated with poor prognosis in patients with congestive heart failure.[89–91] β-Blockade treatment has been found to increase deceleration time and late diastolic filling.[25,35] In a state of increased wall stress, owing to dilatation and elevated filling pressure, a short diastolic filling time may further impede myocardial perfusion, and a lower heart rate might improve myocardial perfusion.[52,92–94]

3. It has been known for years that it is possible to affect myocardial metabolism by moderating myocardial substrate delivery. An isoproterenol-induced increase in myocardial oxygen consumption has been prevented by the inhibition of lipolysis.[95] Infusion of triglycerides was associated with a depression of myocardial infarction in the ischemic dog heart, which could be reversed by infusion of glucose and insulin.[96] Catecholamines increase lipolysis, which is suppressed by β-blockade.[97,98] Therefore, on both experimental and theoretic grounds it is possible that β-blocker treatment may beneficially affect myocardial metabolism by altering substrate delivery and by favoring carbohydrate metabolism. This hypothesis is supported by the fact that myocardial oxygen consumption was reduced by intravenous metoprolol, even when the heart rate was kept at a constant, high rate by atrial pacing.[25] Furthermore, patients with IDCM and myocardial lactate production at rest, which might suggest myocardial ischemia, turned myocardial metabolism into lactate extraction during long-term metoprolol treatment[30,32] (Fig. 47-3). Carbohydrate metabolism is

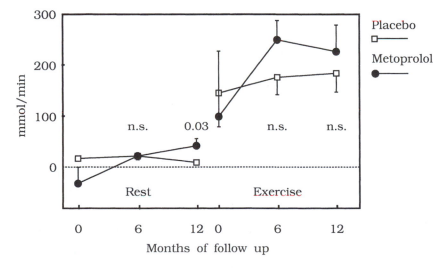

Fig. 47-3. Effects on net myocardial lactate release at rest and during supine bicycle submaximal exercise. *P* values denote intergroup comparison by analysis of variance from baseline to 6 and 12 months of follow-up. Data are mean values ± SEM. *Circles*, metoprolol; *squares*, placebo. (From Andersson et al.,[30] with permission.)

more energy-efficient with less oxygen consumption per ATP molecule produced. Using ^{31}P magnetic resonance spectroscopy, restoration of high energy metabolism was demonstrated following β-blockade.[99]

4. Chronic β-blockade reduces the effect of sympathetic stimulation and circulating catecholamines. Although there are only a few reports on the effect on circulating neurohormones, long-term treatment has been associated with a decrease in peripheral norepinephrine levels[27,29,30,43] and an increase in myocardial norepinephrine stores.[100] Up-regulation of β_1-receptors increases the responsiveness for catecholamine stimulation, which has been found after long-term metoprolol treatment.[10,33] Despite similar improvement in the resting ejection fraction, carvedilol and bucindolol have not been found to increase β-receptor density,[101] which may explain why these two β-blockers lack the ability to increase exercise capacity in patients with congestive heart failure.[34] Whether the up-regulation of β-receptors is detrimental or beneficial for survival is unknown.

5. Severe congestive heart failure is associated with disturbances in immunologic function,[102] and it has been found that β-blockade may induce an increase in T-suppressor and natural killer cells.[103] This effect was suggested to be due to blockade of sympathetic-induced changes in immunologic function. The cause of IDCM is still unknown, but autoimmunity has been proposed to be a possible mechanism behind myocardial deterioration. There is evidence that at least some IDCM patients express β_1-receptor antibodies, some of which may be physiologically active and have β-agonist function.[104–106] β-Blockers may have a role in the blockade of these agonist-like antibodies.

RESPONDERS TO β–BLOCKER TREATMENT

No studies have provided convincing information about which patients benefit from β-blockade treatment. It has been suggested that an elevated heart rate and high levels of catecholamines imply a possible good response to β-blockers (F. Waagstein, personal communication).[17,42] Furthermore, certain types of myocardial fibrosis may be predictive of unresponsiveness to β-blockade.[107] In an open study on patients with ischemic cardiomyopathy, regional wall motion improved in severely akinetic segments and was unchanged in normally contracting segments, although the therapeutic response was attenuated in patients in whom 50 percent or more of the left ventricle was akinetic.[108] These results may imply different effects of β-blockers for ischemic cardiomyopathy and IDCM and perhaps give some explanation for previous findings of a poorer response in patients with ischemic cardiomyopathy than in those with IDCM.[17,29,43] The β-receptor pathways have been found to differ with these two cardiomyopathies.[109] Thus it may be necessary to have a sufficient amount of viable myocardium to be able to respond to β-blockade. Severely decompensated patients should be stabilized on conventional treatment with diuretics, ACE inhibitors, and digitalis before β-blockers are initiated. Even patients in NYHA functional class IV may improve after β-blockade, but the risk of treatment failure is higher in severely deconditioned patients and those with terminal congestive heart failure.

UNANSWERED QUESTIONS

The first important question that remains to be answered is whether β-blockers could be used for heart failure other than that due to IDCM. Second, the ultimate survival study using β-blockers for congestive heart failure has not yet been performed.[110] Studies using bucindolol bisoprolol, metoprolol and carvedilol are in progress.

CONCLUSION

There are sufficient data to suggest that β-blockers may be used in patients with IDCM. These drugs are safe, improve cardiac function and quality of life, and produce no long-term adverse effects. It remains to be elucidated whether the concept of β-blockade could be expanded for use with other types of congestive heart failure. β-Blockers have a pharmacologic profile that fit well in the current theories of congestive heart failure treatment, in which modulation of neurohormones is considered essential for long-term success.

REFERENCES

1. Greenblatt DJ, Koch-Weser J: Adverse reactions to propranolol in hospitalized patients. Am Heart J 1973;86:478
2. Sloand EM, Thompson BT: Propranolol-induced pulmonary edema and shock in a patient with pheochromocytoma. Arch Intern Med 1984;144:173
3. Julian DG: Can beta blockers be safely used in patients with recent myocardial infarction who also have congestive heart failure. Circulation, suppl. I 1983;67:91
4. Waagstein F, Hjalmarson Å, Wasir HS: Apex cardiogram and systolic time intervals in acute myocardial

infarction and effects of practolol. Br Heart J 1974; 36:1109

5. Waagstein F, Hjalmarson Å, Varnauskas E, Wallentin I: Effect of chronic beta-adrenergic receptor blockade in congestive cardiomyopathy. Br Heart J 1975; 37:1022

6. Swedberg K, Waagstein F, Hjalmarson Å, Wallentin I: Prolongation of survival in congestive cardiomyopathy by beta-receptor blockade. Lancet 1979;30:1374

7. Waagstein F, Hjalmarson Å, Swedberg K, Wallentin I: Beta-blockers in dilated cardiomyopathies. They work. Eur Heart J, suppl. A 1983;4:173

8. Swedberg K, Hjalmarson Å, Waagstein F, Wallentin I: Beneficial effects of long-term beta-blockade in congestive cardiomyopathy. Br Heart J 1980;44:117

9. Swedberg K, Hjalmarson Å, Waagstein F, Wallentin I: Adverse effects of beta-blockade withdrawal in patients with congestive cardiomyopathy. Br Heart J 1980;44:134

10. Waagstein F, Caidahl K, Wallentin I et al: Long-term *β*-blockade in dilated cardiomyopathy. Effects of short- and long-term metoprolol treatment followed by withdrawal and readministration of metoprolol. Circulation 1989;80:551

11. Currie PJ, Kelly MJ, McKenzie A et al: Oral beta-adrenergic blockade with metoprolol in chronic severe dilated cardiomyopathy. J Am Coll Cardiol 1984; 3:203

12. Ikram H, Fitzpatrick D: Double-blind trial of chronic oral beta blockade in congestive cardiomyopathy. Lancet 1981;1:490

13. Engelmeier RS, O'Connell JB, Walsh R et al: Improvement in symptoms and exercise tolerance by metoprolol in patients with dilated cardiomyopathy. A double-blind, randomized, placebo-controlled trial. Circulation 1985;72:536

14. Anderson JL, Lutz JR, Gilbert EM et al: A randomized trial of low-dose beta-blockade therapy for idiopathic dilated cardiomyopathy. Am J Cardiol 1985; 55:471

15. Doughty RN, MacMahon S, Sharpe N: Beta-blockers in heart failure: promising or proved? J Am Coll Cardiol 1994;23:814

16. Waagstein F, Bristow MR, Swedberg K et al: Beneficial effects of metoprolol in idiopathic dilated cardiomyopathy. Lancet 1993;342:1441

17. CIBIS Investigators and Committees: A randomized trial of *β*-blockade in heart failure. The Cardiac Insufficiency Bisoprolol Study (CIBIS). Circulation 1994;90:1765

18. Bristow MR: Changes in myocardial and vascular receptors in heart failure. J Am Coll Cardiol, suppl. A, 1993;22:61

19. Baim DS, McDowell AV, Cherniles J et al: Evaluation of a new bipyridine inotropic agent—milrinone—in patients with severe congestive heart failure. N Engl J Med 1983;309:748

20. Colucci WS, Wright RF, Braunwald E: New positive inotropic agents in the treatment of congestive heart failure. Part II. N Engl J Med 1986;314:349

21. DiBianco R, Shabetai R, Kostuk W et al: A comparison of oral milrinone, digoxin, and their combination in the treatment of patients with chronic heart failure. N Engl J Med 1989;320:677

22. Uretsky BF, Jessup M, Konstam MA et al: Multicenter trial of oral enoximone in patients with moderate to moderately severe congestive heart failure. Circulation 1990;82:774

23. Feldman AM, Bristow MR, Parmley WW et al: Effects of vesnarinone on morbidity and mortality in patients with heart failure. N Engl J Med 1993;329:149

24. Eichhorn EJ: The paradox of *β*-adrenergic blockade for the management of congestive heart failure. Am J Med 1992;92:527

25. Andersson B, Lomsky M, Waagstein F: The link between acute haemodynamic adrenergic beta-blockade and long-term effects in patients with heart failure. Eur Heart J 1993;14:1375

26. DasGupta P, Lahiri A: Can intravenous *β*-blockade predict long-term hemodynamic benefit in chronic congestive heart failure secondary to ischemic heart disease? J Cardiovasc Pharmacol, suppl. 1 1992;19: S62

27. Gilbert EM, Anderson JL, Deitchman D et al: Long-term *β*-blocker vasodilator therapy improves cardiac function in idiopathic dilated cardiomyopathy. A double-blind, randomized study of bucindolol versus placebo. Am J Med 1990;88:223

28. Haber HL, Simek CL, Gimple LW et al: Why do patients with congestive heart failure tolerate the initiation of beta-blocker therapy. Circulation 1993;88: 1610

29. Woodley SL, Gilbert EM, Anderson JL et al: *β*-Blockade with bucindolol in heart failure caused by ischemic versus idiopathic dilated cardiomyopathy. Circulation 1991;84:2426

30. Andersson B, Hamm C, Persson S et al: Improved exercise hemodynamic status in dilated cardiomyopathy after beta-adrenergic blockade treatment. J Am Coll Cardiol 1994;23:1397

31. Eichhorn EJ, Bedotto JB, Malloy CR et al: Effect of *β*-adrenergic blockade on myocardial function and energetics in congestive heart failure. Circulation 1990;82:473

32. Eichhorn EJ, Heesch CM, Barnett JH et al: Effect of metoprolol on myocardial function and energetics in patients with nonischemic dilated cardiomyopathy. A randomized, double-blind, placebo-controlled study. J Am Coll Cardiol 1994;24:1310

33. Heilbrunn SM, Shah P, Bristow MR et al: Increased *β*-receptor density and improved hemodynamic response to catecholamine stimulation during long-term metoprolol therapy in heart failure from dilated cardiomyopathy. Circulation 1989;79:483

34. Bristow MR, O'Connell JB, Gilbert EM et al: Dose-response of chronic *β*-blocker treatment in heart failure from either idiopathic dilated or ischemic cardiomyopathy. Circulation 1994;89:1632

35. Andersson B, Caidahl K, diLenarda A, et al: Changes in diastolic filling patterns induced by long-term beta-adrenergic blockade in patients with idiopathic dilated cardiomyopathy. Circulation 1996;94:673

36. Ikram H, Chan W, Bennett SI, Bones PJ: Haemodynamic effects of acute beta-adrenergic receptor blockade in congestive cardiomyopathy. Br Heart J 1979; 42:311

37. Shanes JG, Wolfkiel C, Ghali J et al: Acute hemodynamic effects of pindolol and propranolol in patients with dilated cardiomyopathy. Relevance of intrinsic sympathomimetic activity. Am Heart J 1988;116: 1268

38. Fowler MB: Beta-blockers in heart failure. Potential of carvedilol. J Hum Hypertens 1993;7:S62
39. Eichhorn EJ: Effects of bucindolol in heart failure. Am J Cardiol 1993;71:65C
40. Pollock SG, Lystash J, Tedesco C et al: Usefulness of bucindolol in congestive heart failure. Am J Cardiol 1990;66:603
41. Anderson JL, Gilbert EM, O'Connell JB et al: Long-term (2 year) beneficial effects of beta-adrenergic blockade with bucindolol in patients with idiopathic dilated cardiomyopathy. J Am Coll Cardiol 1991;17:1373
42. Fisher ML, Gottlieb SS, Plotnick GD et al: Beneficial effects of metoprolol in heart failure associated with coronary artery disease. A randomized trial. J Am Coll Cardiol 1994;23:943
43. Andersson B, Blomström-Lundqvist C, Hedner T, Waagstein F: Exercise hemodynamics and myocardial metabolism during long-term beta-adrenergic blockade in severe heart failure. J Am Coll Cardiol 1991;18:1059
44. Das Gupta P, Broadhurst P, Raftery EB, Lahiri A: Value of carvedilol in congestive heart failure secondary to coronary artery disease. Am J Cardiol 1990;66:1118
45. Leung W-H, Lau C-P, Wong C-K et al: Improvement in exercise performance and hemodynamics by labetalol in patients with idiopathic dilated cardiomyopathy. Am Heart J 1990;119:884
46. Swedberg K, Viquerat C, Rouleau J-L et al: Comparison of myocardial catecholamine balance in chronic congestive heart failure and in angina pectoris without failure. Am J Cardiol 1984;54:783
47. Meredith IT, Eisenhofer G, Lambert GW et al: Cardiac sympathetic nervous activity in congestive heart failure. Evidence for increased neuronal norepinephrine release and preserved neuronal uptake. Circulation 1993;88:136
48. Chidsey CA, Braunwald E, Morrow AG: Catecholamine excretion and cardiac stores of norepinephrine in congestive heart failure. Am J Med 1965;59:442
49. Hasking GJ, Esler MD, Jennings GL et al: Norepinephrine spillover to plasma in patients with congestive heart failure. Evidence of increased overall and cardiorenal sympathetic nervous activity. Circulation 1986;73:615
50. Brodde O-E, Schüler S, Kretsch R et al: Regional distribution of β-adrenoceptors in the human heart. Coexistence of functional β_1- and β_2-adrenoceptors in both atria and ventricles in severe congestive cardiomyopathy. J Cardiovasc Pharmacol 1986;8:1235
51. Bristow MR, Ginsburg R, Umanis V et al: β_1- and β_2-adrenergic receptor subpopulations in failing and non-failing human ventricular myocardium. Coupling of both receptor subtypes to muscle contraction and selective β_1-receptor downregulation in heart failure. Circ Res 1986;59:297
52. Beau SL, Saffitz JE: Transmural heterogeneity of norepinephrine uptake in failing human hearts. J Am Coll Cardiol 1994;23:579
53. Bristow MR: Pathophysiologic and pharmacologic rationales for clinical management of chronic heart failure with beta-blocking agents. Am J Cardiol 1993;71:C12
54. Hall JA, Kaumann AJ, Brown MJ: Selective β_1-adrenoceptor blockade enhances positive inotropic responses to endogenous catecholamines mediated through β_2-adrenoceptors in human atrial myocardium. Circ Res 1990;66:1610
55. Motomura S, Deighton NM, Zerkowski H-R et al: Chronic β_1-adrenoceptor antagonist treatment sensitizes β_2-adrenoceptors, but desensitizes M_2-muscarin receptors in the human right atrium. Br J Pharmacol 1990;101:363
56. Cohn JN, Levine TB, Olivari MT et al: Plasma norepinephrine as a guide to prognosis in patients with chronic congestive heart failure. N Engl J Med 1984;311:819
57. Simons M, Downing SE: Coronary vasoconstriction and catecholamine cardiomyopathy. Am Heart J 1985;109:297
58. Wahr DW, Swedberg K, Rabbino M et al: Intravenous and oral prenaltorol in congestive heart failure. Effects on systemic and coronary hemodynamics and myocardial catecholamine balance. Am J Med 1984;76:999
59. Hasenfuss G, Holubarsch C, Blanchard EM et al: Influence of isoproterenol on myocardial energetics. Experimental and clinical investigation. Basic Res Cardiol, suppl. 1 1989;84:147
60. Cleland JGF, Dargie HJ: Arrhythmias, catecholamines and electrolytes. Am J Cardiol 1988;62:55A
61. Swedberg K, Eneroth P, Kjekshus D et al: Effects of enalapril and neuroendocrine activation on prognosis in severe congestive heart failure (follow-up of the CONSENSUS trial). Am J Cardiol 1990;66:40D
62. Swedberg K, Eneroth P, Kjekshus J et al: Hormones regulating cardiovascular function in patients with severe congestive heart failure and their relation to mortality. Circulation 1990;82:1730
63. Nemanich JW, Veith RC, Abrass IB, Stratton JR: Effects of metoprolol on rest and exercise cardiac function and plasma catecholamines in chronic congestive heart failure secondary to ischemic or idiopathic cardiomyopathy. Am J Cardiol 1990;66:843
64. Andersson B, Caidahl K, Waagstein F: Idiopathic dilated cardiomyopathy among Swedish patients with congestive heart failure. Eur Heart J 1995;16:53
65. Andersson B, Waagstein F: Spectrum and outcome of congestive heart failure in a hospitalized population. Am Heart J 1993;126:632
66. Kannel WB, Belanger AJ: Epidemiology of heart failure. Am Heart J 1991;121:951
67. Kannel WB, Pinsky J: Trends in cardiac failure. Incidence and causes over three decades in the Framingham study. J Am Coll Cardiol, suppl. A 1991;17:87
68. Norwegian Multicenter Study Group: Timolol-induced reduction in mortality and refinfarction in patients surviving acute myocardial infarction. N Engl J Med 1981;304:801
69. MIAMI Trial Researchers: Metoprolol in acute myocardial infarction (MIAMI). A randomised placebo-controlled international trial. Eur Heart J 1985;6:199
70. Chadda K, Goldstein S, Byington R, Curb JD: Effect of propranolol after acute myocardial infarction in patients with congestive heart failure. Circulation 1986;73:503
71. Doval HC, Nul DR, Grancelli HO et al: Randomised trial of low-dose amiodarone in severe congestive heart failure. Lancet 1994;344:493
72. Sugrue DD, Rodeheffer RJ, Codd MB et al: The clini-

cal course of idiopathic dilated cardiomyopathy. Ann Intern Med 1992;117:117

73. Packer M, Bristow MR, Cohn JN et al: Effect of carvedilol on morbidity and mortality in chronic heart failure. N Eng J Med 1996;334:1349

74. Cohn JN, Fowler MB, Bristow MA et al: Effect of carvedilol in severe chronic heart failure [abstract]. J Am Coll Cardiol, suppl. A 1996;27:169A

75. Colucci WS, Packer M, Bristow MR et al: Carvedilol inhibits clinical progression in patients with mild heart failure [abstract]. Circulation, suppl. I 1995;92:395

76. Bristow MR, Gilbert EM, Abraham WT et al: Multicenter oral carvedilol heart failure assessment (MOCHA) [abstract]. A six-month dose-response evaluation in class II–IV patients. Circulation, suppl. I 1995;92:142

77. Packer M, Colucci WS, Sackner-Bernstein J et al: Prospective randomized evaluation of carvedilol on symptoms and exercise tolerance in chronic heart failure. Results of the PRECISE trial [abstract]. Circulation, suppl. I 1995;92:143

78. Fowler MB, Gilbert EM, Cohn JN et al: Effects of carvedilol on cardiovascular hospitalizations in patients with chronic heart failure [abstract]. J Am Coll Cardiol, suppl. A 1996;27:169A

79. Brune S, Schmidt T, Tebbe U, Kreuzer H: Hemodynamic effects of nebivolol at rest and on exertion in patients with heart failure. Angiology 1990;41:696

80. Wisenbaugh T, Katz I, Davis J et al: Long-term (3-month) effects of a new beta-blocker (nebivolol) on cardiac performance in dilated cardiomyopathy. J Am Coll Cardiol 1993;21:1094

81. Xamoterol In Severe Heart Failure Study Group: Xamoterol in severe heart failure. Lancet 1990;336:1

82. Kjekshus J: Heart rate reduction. A mechanism of benefit? Eur Heart J, suppl. I, 1987;8:115

83. Grant SCD, Bennett DH: Cardiomyopathy secondary to sinus tachycardia. Int J Cardiol 1993;40:173

84. Tomita M, Spinale FG, Crawford FA, Zile MR: Changes in left ventricular volume, mass, and function during the development and regression of supraventricular tachycardia-induced cardiomyopathy. Circulation 1991;83:635

85. Mulieri LA, Hasenfuss G, Leavitt B et al: Altered myocardial force-frequency relation in human heart failure. Circulation 1992;85:1743

86. Hasenfuss G, Holubarsch C, Hermann H-P et al: Influence of the force-frequency relationship on haemodynamics and left ventricular function in patients with non-failing hearts and in patients with dilated cardiomyopathy. Eur Heart J 1994;15:164

87. Lavine SJ, Krishnaswami V, Levinson M, Shaver JA: Effect of heart rate alterations produced by atrial pacing on the pattern of diastolic filling in normal subjects. Am J Cardiol 1988;62:1098

88. Lavine SJ, Krishnaswami V, Shreiner DP, Amidi M: Left ventricular diastolic filling in patients with left ventricular dysfunction. Int J Cardiol 1985;8:423

89. Werner GS, Schaefer C, Dirks R et al: Prognostic value of Doppler echocardiographic assessment of left ventricular filling in idiopathic dilated cardiomyopathy. Am J Cardiol 1994;73:792

90. Shen WF, Tribouilloy C, Rey JL et al: Prognostic significance of Doppler-derived left ventricular diastolic filling variables in dilated cardiomyopathy. Am Heart J 1992;124:1524

91. Pinamonti B, Di Lenarda A, Sinagra G et al: Restrictive left ventricular filling pattern in dilated cardiomyopathy assessed by Doppler echocardiography. Clinical, echocardiographic and hemodynamic correlations and prognostic implications. J Am Coll Cardiol 1993;22:808

92. Boudoulas H, Rittgers SE, Lewis RP et al: Changes in diastolic time with various pharmacologic agents. Circulation 1979;60:164

93. Ferro G, Duilio C, Spinelli L et al: Effects of beta blockade on the relation between heart rate and ventricular diastolic perfusion time during exercise in systemic hypertension. Am J Cardiol 1991;68:1101

94. Ferro G, Spinelli L, Duilio C: Diastolic perfusion time and stress-induced myocardial ischemia. Circulation 1991;84:388

95. Kjekshus JD, Mjøs OD: Effect of free fatty acids on myocardial function and metabolism in the ischemic dog heart. J Clin Invest 1972;51:1767

96. Mjøs OD: Effects of inhibition of lipolysis on myocardial oxygen consumption in the presence of isoproterenol. J Clin Invest 1971;50:1869

97. Simonsen S, Kjekshus K: The effect of free fatty acids on myocardial oxygen consumption during atrial pacing and catecholamine infusion in man. Circulation 1978;58:484

98. Ihlen H, Simonsen S, Welzel D: Effects of adrenaline on myocardial oxygen consumption during selective and non-selective beta-adrenoceptor blockade comparison of atenolol and pindolol. Eur J Clin Pharmacol 1984;27:29

99. Neubauer S, Krahe T, Schindler R et al: P-31 magnetic resonance spectroscopy in dilated cardiomyopathy and coronary artery disease. Altered cardiac high-energy phosphate metabolism in heart failure. Circulation 1992;86:1810

100. Yamamoto T, Furutani Y, Katayama K et al: A case of dilated cardiomyopathy in which the effect of beta-blocker therapy was clearly demonstrated by ^{123}I-MIBG scintigraphy. Respir Circ 1994;42:989

101. Gilbert EM, Olsen SL, Renlund DG, Bristow MR: Beta-adrenergic receptor regulation and left ventricular function in idiopathic dilated cardiomyopathy. Am J Cardiol 1993;71:C23

102. Hwang S, Harris TJ, Wilson NW, Maisel AS: Immune function in patients with chronic stable congestive heart failure. Am Heart J 1993;125:1651

103. Maisel AS: Beneficial effects of metoprolol treatment in congestive heart failure. Reversal of sympathetic-induced alterations of immunologic function. Circulation 1994;90:1774

104. Limas CJ, Limas C, Kubo SH, Olivari MT: Anti-beta-receptor antibodies in human dilated cardiomyopathy and correlation with HLA-DR antigens. Am J Cardiol 1990;65:483

105. Magnusson Y, Marullo S, Höyer S et al: Mapping of a functional autoimmune epitope on the β_1-adrenergic receptor in patients with idiopathic dilated cardiomyopathy. J Clin Invest 1990;86:1658

106. Magnusson Y, Wallukat G, Waagstein F et al: Autoimmunity in idiopathic dilated cardiomyopathy. Characterization of antibodies against the β_1-adrenoceptor with positive chronotropic effect. Circulation 1994;89:2760

107. Yamada T, Fukunami M, Ohmori M et al: Which subgroup of patients with dilated cardiomyopathy

would benefit from long-term beta-blocker therapy? A histologic viewpoint. J Am Coll Cardiol 1993;21: 628

108. Andersson B, Caidahl K, Waagstein F: Recovery from left ventricular asynergy in ischemic cardiomyopathy following long-term beta blockade treatment. Cardiology 1994;85:14

109. Bristow MR, Anderson FL, Port JD et al: Differences in β-adrenergic neuroeffector mechanisms in ischemic versus idiopathic dilated cardiomyopathy. Circulation 1991;84:1024

110. Domanski MJ, Eichhorn EJ: Beta blockade in congestive heart failure. The need for a definitive study. Am J Cardiol 1994;73:597

48 Calcium Channel Blockers

Uri Elkayam
Konstantinos Vlachonassios
William Frishman

The calcium channel blockers (CCBs) are a heterogeneous group of drugs with widely variable effects on heart muscle, sinus node function, atrioventricular (AV) conduction, peripheral blood vessels, and coronary circulation.[1] Nine of these drugs—nifedipine, nicardipine, nimodipine, felodipine, isradipine, amlodipine, verapamil, diltiazem, bepridil—are approved in the United States for clinical use.[2] Although these drugs are mainly used for the treatment of hypertension and ischemic heart disease, there has been a strong interest and increasing experience in the use of CCBs in patients with congestive heart failure (CHF).

PHYSIOLOGIC BACKGROUND

Calcium ions play a fundamental role in the activation of cardiovascular cells. An influx of calcium ions into the cell through specific ion channels is essential for myocardial contraction, vascular smooth muscle relaxation, and function of the pacemaker tissueses of the heart. The blockage of calcium-mediated electromechanical coupling in contractile tissue in blood vessels and the heart results in arterial dilatation of the peripheral and coronary circulation and depression of myocardial contractility.[3,4] This negative inotropic effect of CCBs differentiates them from other coronary vasodilators, such as nitroglycerin and papaverine, which have little if any direct myocardial

activity. The effect of some CCBs on transmembrane influx of calcium can also depress sinoatrial and atrioventricular nodal function and is responsible for the successful use of some of these drugs for the treatment of supraventricular arrhythmias.[2] Because pathologic accumulation of calcium in the myocardium seems to be responsible for impaired relaxation, the use of CCBs has been demonstrated in experimental and human studies to improve myocardial diastolic function.[5]

CHEMICAL STRUCTURE AND PHARMACODYNAMICS

Structure of Calcium Channel Blockers

The structures of some of the available calcium channel blockers are shown in Figure 48-1. Nifedipine is a dihydropyridine derivative that is lipophilic and is inactivated by light.[1] Nicardipine, amlodipine, felodipine, isradipine, and nimodipine are also dihydropyridine derivatives, similar in structure to nifedipine. Diltiazem is a benzothiazepine derivative that is structurally unrelated to other vasodilators. Verapamil has some structural similarity to papaverine. Mibefradil (RO-5967), a drug now being evaluated in clinical trials, is from a new chemical class of benzimidazolyl-substituted tetraline derivatives.[2] Bepridil,

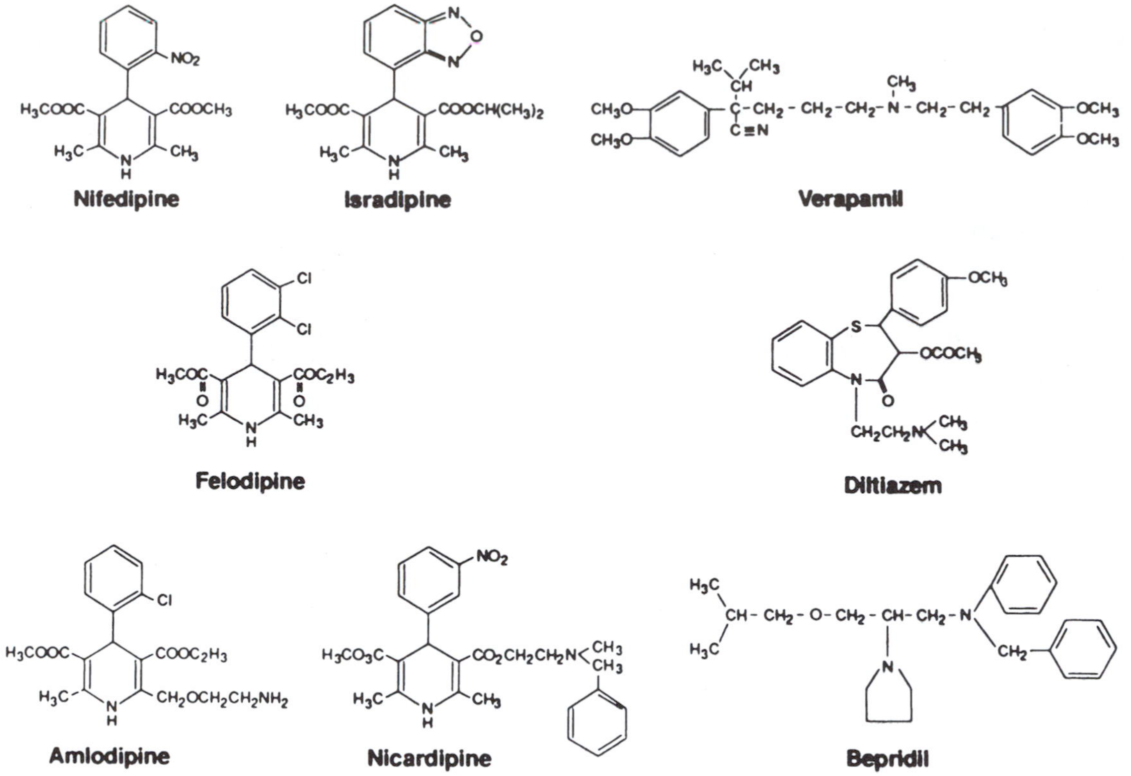

Fig. 48-1. Chemical structures of diltiazem (a benzothiazepine derivative), nifedipine, felodipine, isradipine, amlodipine, nicardipine (dihydropyridine derivatives), verapamil (structurally similar to papaverine), and bepridil (structure unlike other cardioactive drugs). (From Frishman,[1] with permission.)

which is currently available for treatment of angina pectoris, is not related chemically to any other CCB.[3]

Calcium Conducting Channels

The calcium conducting channels, located in the cell membrane, are formed from proteins functioning as ion-selective pores and allowing the influx of Ca^{2+} ions.[4] The Ca^{2+} channels are subdivided into two major subgroups according to their location and primary function: (1) voltage-activated, transsarcoluminal channels, which allow influx of Ca^{2+} ions across the cell membrane; and (2) Ca^{2+} release channels of the sarcoplasmic reticulum, which facilitate the exit of Ca^{2+} ions from the sarcoplasmic reticulum into the cell. The voltage-activated calcium conducting channels are further subdivided into six main types, labeled L, T, N, P, Q, and R.[5] The N, P, Q, and R type Ca^{2+} channels are found in neurons and play a role in neurotransmitter release. The P-type Ca^{2+} channels are predominantly found in cerebellar Purkinje cells. The L-type Ca^{2+} channels are found in skeletal, cardiac, and vascular muscle and have a large ion-carrying capacity. They remain open for a relatively long time because of their slow inactivation. The function

of the L-type channel is to admit the substantial amount of calcium ions required for initiation of contraction by way of calcium-induced calcium release from the sarcoplasmic reticulum. The T-type channels are activated at more negative potentials than the L-type and have a more rapid rate of inactivation. These channels are found in the vascular smooth muscle cells and the myocardium predominantly in atrial cells.[4,5] The common and most important characteristic of all calcium channel blockers is their ability to inhibit the inward flow of charge-bearing calcium ions selectively when the calcium ion channels become permeable. All calcium antagonists block the L-type channels, and mibefradil blocks the T-type channels as well.

Classification of Calcium Antagonists

Calcium channel blockers have been divided into first and second generation antagonists.[1,6] Verapamil, nifedipine, and diltiazem are considered first generation CCBs, and other dihydropyridine derivatives, developed later, have been called second generation CCBs. The later agents have greater tissue selectivity, with a predominant effect on blood vessels and less cardiodepressant action, and some have a longer duration of action. The CCBs can also be classified according to the voltage-gated channel with which they interact. Most of the available antagonists, including verapamil, diltiazem, nifedipine, and the other dihydropyridines, interact exclusively with the L-type Ca^{2+} channels. Mibefradil is the only agent that blocks both L- and T-type voltage-operated Ca^{2+} channels[7] and therefore forms a new class of CCB.

Bepridil also has unique properties. It possesses all the characteristics of the traditional calcium antagonists but in addition seems to affect the sodium channels (fast channels) and possibly the potassium channels, producing a quinidine-like effect.

PHARMACOKINETICS

Although classified together, CCBs demonstrate substantial differences in their pharmacokinetic properties[1] (Table 48-1). These variations in completeness of gastrointestinal absorption, amount of first-pass hepatic metabolism, protein binding, extent of distribution in the body, and pharmacologic

Table 48-1. Pharmacokinetics of the Calcium Channel Blockers and Sustained-Release Preparations

Agent	Trade Name	Absorption (%)	Bio-availability (%)[a]	Protein Binding (%)	Volume of Distribution (L/kg)	$t_{1/2}\beta$ (hr)	Clearance (ml·min⁻¹· kg⁻¹)	Time to Peak Plasma Concentration (h)
Diltiazem	Cardizem	> 90	35–60	78	5.0	4.1–5.6	15	2–3
Diltiazem SR	Cardizem SR	> 90	35–60	78	5.0	5–7	15	6–11
Diltiazem IV	Cardizem							
Diltiazem CD	Cardizem CD	> 95	40	70–80	5.0	5–8	15	10–14
Diltiazem XR	Dilacor XR	> 95	40	70–80	5.0	5–10	15	4–6
Verapamil	Calan, Isoptin	> 90	10–20	90	4.3	6 ± 4 IV 8 ± 6 PO	13 ± 7	1–2
Verapamil SR	Calan SR, Isoptin SR Verelan	> 90 > 90	10–20 20–35	90 90	4.3 162–380 L	4.5–12.0 12	13 ± 7	1–2 7–9
Nifedipine	Procardia, Adalat	> 90	65	90	1.32	≈5	500–600	0.5
Nifedipine CC	Adalat CC	> 90	84–89	92–98	1.32	—	500–600	2.0–2.5
Nifedipine GITS	Procardia XL	> 90	85	> 95	1.32	3.8–16.9	500–600	6 to plateau
Nicardipine	Cardene	> 90	≈30	> 90	0.66	≈1 IV 1–2 PO	14	0.5–2.0
Nicardipine SR	Cardene SR	> 90	35	> 95		8.6	0.6	1–4 immed.
Nicardipine IV	Cardene		100	> 90	9.3			
Amlodipine	Norvasc	> 90	60–65	> 95	21	35–45	7	6–12
Isradipine	Dynacirc	90–95	17	97	2.9	8.8	10	1.5
Felodipine ER	Plendil	> 95	15–25	> 99	10	15.1 ± 2.6	12	2.5–5.0
Bepridil	Vascor	> 90	≈60	> 95	80	33		5.3
Nimodipine	Nimotop	> 90	13	> 95	0.94	8–9		0.6

SR, Sustained release; IV, intravenous; CD, XR, CC, XL, extended release; PO, oral; GITS, gastrointestinal therapeutic system.
[a] Extraction ratio.
(From Frishman,[1] with permission.)

actions of the various metabolites may influence the clinical usefulness of these drugs in patients.[1]

Because many of the CCBs are relatively short-acting, a variety of sustained-release delivery systems have been developed: diffusion type (diltiazem, verapamil), bioerosion (diltiazem, nifedipine, nicardipine), osmosis (nifedipine), and diffusion-erosion (felodipine).[1] Clinical trials are now in progress evaluating verapamil, isradipine, and nicardipine as once-daily therapies with the gastrointestinal therapeutic system formulation (osmosis). Nisoldipine is also being evaluated as a once-daily therapy in the coat-core formulation.

RATIONALE FOR THE USE OF CALCIUM CHANNEL BLOCKERS

The rationale for the use of CCBs to treat heart failure is multifactorial. These drugs have a strong arteriolar dilator effect, leading to a reduction of systemic vascular resistance and thus left ventricular afterload. Drugs with similar hemodynamic effects, such as hydralazine, when used in combination with isosorbide dinitrate were shown to improve exercise tolerance and ejection fraction and improve survival in patients with mild to moderate heart failure.[8,9] Most of the available CCBs have a substantial antiischemic effect, and many are used effectively to treat myocardial ischemia.[2] Because coronary artery disease is the underlying cause of chronic CHF in 60–70 percent of patients with CHF,[8–11] it is not surprising that CCBs are considered by many clinicians a viable therapeutic option. The favorable effect of CCBs on left ventricular relaxation may lead to improvement of diastolic dysfunction,[12] an important cause of heart failure symptoms, even in patients with documented left ventricular systolic dysfunction.[13] In addition, the prevention of calcium ion entry into myocardial cells was reported to prevent the development of alcohol-mediated cardiac dysfunction in hamster myocardium and could have a similar protective effect in humans.[14]

CLINICAL EXPERIENCE WITH CALCIUM ANTAGONISTS

First Generation CCBs

NIFEDIPINE

Because of the powerful vasodilator effect of nifedipine a strong interest has been shown in using this drug as an unloading agent to treat heart failure.

Initial evaluations by several investigators[15–21] showed hemodynamic improvement after single-dose administration of nifedipine given either orally or sublingually in patients with acute or chronic heart failure. Most of these data were reported as a mean group response and demonstrated a reduction in systemic vascular resistance and mean blood pressure, with augmentation of cardiac output and stroke volume. Lack of change in both right and left ventricular filling pressures in most studies[13] verified the predominant arteriolar and negligible venous effects of the drug.

Although the initial experience with the use of nifedipine during heart failure led some investigators to conclude that the negative inotropic effect of nifedipine could be offset by its vasodilatory effect,[15–22] further evaluation in larger groups of patients demonstrated the clinical relevance of the cardiodepressant effect of the drug.[23–26] Comparison of nifedipine with nitroprusside demonstrated a smaller augmentation in cardiac output and a larger decrease in systemic blood pressure with nifedipine despite a similar reduction in systemic vascular resistance.[27] These hemodynamic changes were associated with a decrease in the first derivative of left ventricular pressure (dP/dt).[28] Similarly, a comparison of change in hemodynamic indices of left ventricular systolic function in the same patients with heart failure following a similar reduction in systemic vascular resistance with hydralazine and nifedipine resulted in a significantly smaller augmentation of stroke volume, cardiac output, and left ventricular stroke work index with nifedipine.[29] These results demonstrated the clinical relevance of its negative inotropic effect. Further evaluation of the hemodynamic profile of nifedipine in two large series of patients showed acute hemodynamic and clinical deterioration after a single dose of 20–50 mg in 19 and 29 percent of the patients, respectively.[23,30] Hemodynamic response could not be predicted from baseline hemodynamic data and the left ventricular ejection fraction in one study.[23] In the second study,[30] hemodynamic deterioration was associated with higher baseline levels of plasma renin activity and mean right atrial pressure and a lower serum sodium concentration. In addition, a strong relation was found between an unfavorable acute hemodynamic response to nifedipine and long-term mortality, supporting a hypothesis that hemodynamic deterioration after nifedipine administration was more likely to occur in patients with more severe heart failure.

The acute neurohormonal effects of nifedipine in patients with CHF were evaluated in two studies. Prida et al.[31] demonstrated significant activation of the renin system following administration of 10 mg oral nifedipine. This change in plasma renin activity was, however, not associated with an increase in aldosterone level. Similar findings were reported by Elkayam et al.[32] and were most likely due to inhibition of calcium-mediated secretion of aldosterone in the renal macula densa.

The long-term effect of nifedipine in patients with heart failure due to left ventricular systolic dysfunction was evaluated several years ago in two randomized trials. In the first study, Agostoni et al.[33] compared, in a double-blind, crossover design, the effect of captopril (50 mg three times daily) and nifedipine (20 mg three times daily) given for 8 weeks each to 18 patients with dilated cardiomyopathy who were optimally treated with digitalis and diuretic drugs. This study demonstrated symptomatic and functional improvement and enhancement of exercise tolerance with captopril but not with nifedipine. In this study, nifedipine initially resulted in a reduction in systemic vascular resistance that led to augmentation of cardiac output and a small reduction in left ventricular filling pressure. After prolonged treatment, however, cardiac output returned to baseline values, and pulmonary artery wedge pressure increased substantially accompanied by worsening heart failure symptoms in some patients. In a second study, Elkayam et al.[34] compared the effect of long-term administration (8 weeks) of isosorbide dinitrate (40 mg four times daily), nifedipine (20 mg four times daily), and their combination in patients with mild to moderate chronic heart failure. This study demonstrated a significantly higher incidence of heart failure worsening, necessitating an increase in diuretic dosage, hospitalization, or both in patients treated with nifedipine either alone or in combination with isosorbide dinitrate (Table 48-2). Hospitalization was required for 24 percent of patients during nifedi-

pine therapy and for 26 percent during nifedipine–isosorbide dinitrate combination therapy in compared to 0 percent during isosorbide dinitrate therapy alone. The total number of episodes of CHF worsening were 9 during nifedipine therapy, 3 during isosorbide dinitrate therapy, and 21 during nifedipine–isosorbide dinitrate combination therapy. Premature discontinuation of drug administration because of clinical deterioration or other side effects occurred in 29 percent of patients during nifedipine therapy, in 5 percent during isosorbide dinitrate therapy ($P = 0.05$ versus nifedipine), and in 19 percent during combination therapy. In summary, despite a strong vasodilatory effect, numerous studies have demonstrated an unfavorable effect of nifedipine on hemodynamic and clinical status in patients with CHF due to left ventricular systolic dysfunction.

DILTIAZEM

The unfavorable results reported with the use of nifedipine in patients with chronic heart failure led to the attempts to use diltiazem, a first-generation calcium antagonist with a lesser myocardial depressant effect.[35] Hemodynamic evaluation of this agent in patients with severe chronic heart failure demonstrated either no change or improvement in hemodynamic profile[36–38] and no change in plasma renin activity and catecholamines.[39] In comparison with nifedipine, use of diltiazem was associated with a significantly smaller incidence of hemodynamic and symptomatic deterioration.[38,39] Another report demonstrated the safe and effective use of intravenous diltiazem for heart rate control in patients with atrial fibrillation and left ventricular systolic dysfunction.[40] However, occasional reports of hemodynamic deterioration in patients receiving oral diltia-

Table 48-2. Episodes of Hospitalizations and Increase in Diuretic Drugs for Worsening Congestive Heart Failure

Treatment[a]	Patients (no.)			CHF episodes (no.)
	Hospitalizations	Increase in diuretic dose	Total	
NIF, 8 weeks (n = 21)	5*	3	8	9**
ISDN (n = 20)	0	3	3	3
NIF + ISDN (n = 23)	6*	2	8	21***

Abbreviations: NIF, nifedipine; ISDN, isosorbide dinitrate; CHF, congestive heart failure.
[a] Isosorbide dinitrates (ISDN) alone and nifedipine plus ISDN were given to patients with NYHA class II and III heart failure. All patients were also treated with digoxin and diuretics.
* $P < 0.05$ versus ISDN; ** $P < 0.001$ versus ISDN; *** $P < 0.01$ versus NIF.
(From Elkayam et al.,[34] with permission.)

zem[38,39,41] provided the first indication of a potential hazard of this drug.

The chronic use of diltiazem in patients with CHF resulted in conflicting findings. In 1989 Figulla et al.[42] reported on a prospective study using diltiazem (60–90 mg three times daily) in 22 patients with dilated cardiomyopathy in addition to conventional therapy with digitalis, diuretic drugs, and vasodilators. Outcome was compared with historical control data from 25 patients with chronic heart failure receiving conventional therapy alone. The mean survival of the control group was 29 months, and no patient treated with diltiazem died over a mean follow-up period of 15.4 months. In addition, a significant improvement in clinical status and left ventricular function was reported in the diltiazem group but not in the control group. Although the investigators suggested a beneficial effect of adjunctive diltiazem treatment for dilated cardiomyopathy, the uncontrolled design of the trial and the small number of patients in both arms severely limited the scientific and clinical value of the study.

In contrast to this study, the Multicenter Diltiazem Postinfarction Trial[43] was conducted in a large number of patients and in a prospective, randomized, placebo-controlled fashion. This study evaluated the effect of chronic diltiazem therapy (240 mg/day) initiated 3–15 days after the onset of myocardial infarction on mortality and reinfarction in 1237 patients and compared it to the effect of placebo in 1232 similar patients. In 490 patients with evidence of pulmonary congestion on the chest roentgenogram, diltiazem was associated with an increased incidence of cardiac events (Fig. 48-2). A similar pattern was observed with respect to depressed radionuclide ejection fraction and anterolateral Q wave infarction. In contrast, among 1909 patients without pulmonary congestion, diltiazem therapy resulted in a lower incidence of cardiac events. In a further evaluation of the development of congestive heart failure in this study, Goldstein et al.[44] showed that patients with pulmonary congestion, anterolateral Q wave infarction or reduced ejection fraction (less than 40 percent) at baseline were more likely to develop chronic heart failure during follow-up when compared to patients without these markers of left ventricular dysfunction. Furthermore, the likelihood of developing CHF with diltiazem was inversely related to the degree of left ventricular systolic dysfunction (Fig. 48-3). This trial conclusively demonstrated the hazard involved with the use of diltiazem in patients with left ventricular systolic dysfunction due to coronary artery disease and myocardial infarction.

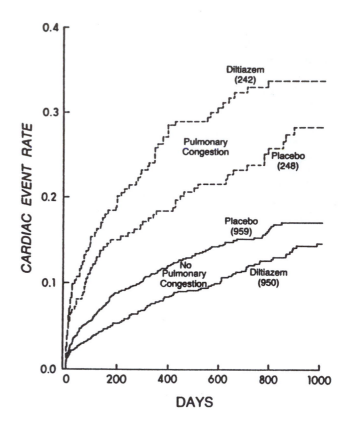

Fig. 48-2. Cumulative rate of first recurrent cardiac events on diltiazem and placebo in patients with and without chest radiographic evidence of pulmonary congestion. (From Multicenter Diltiazem Postinfarction Trial Research Group,[43] with permission.)

VERAPAMIL

Experience related to the use of verapamil during heart failure is limited because of the known negative inotropic effect of the drug and the warning by the manufacturer concerning the risk of developing heart failure.[45] In a small study, Ferlinz and Gallo[46] demonstrated symptomatic deterioration in 4 of 10 patients with CHF on long-term verapamil therapy despite acute hemodynamic improvement.

The Danish study on the effect of verapamil on death or reinfarction[47] in survivors of acute myocardial infarction may provide some indirect but useful information regarding the effect of this calcium antagonist in patients with chronic heart failure. This multicenter double-blind, placebo-controlled study evaluated verapamil (120 mg three times daily) versus placebo in patients 7–15 days after their myocardial infarction. At a mean follow-up time of 16 months, verapamil had caused a significant reduction of mortality and cardiac events in patients without, but not in patients with, chronic heart failure (Fig. 48-4). The exclusion criteria for this study included heart failure not controlled with furosemide

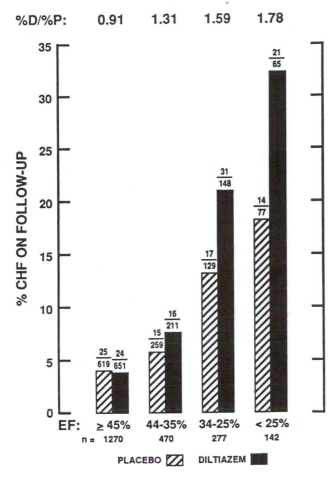

%D/%P: 0.91   1.31   1.59   1.78

Fig. 48-3. Relation between the percent of patients receiving diltiazem (D, *black bars*) or placebo (P, *hatched bars*) developing new or worsened congestive heart failure (CHF) during long-term follow-up. The number of patients with CHF is shown as the numerator and the total number in each ejection fraction (EF) group is shown as the denominator above each bar. (From Goldstein et al.,[44] with permission.)

($\leq$ 160 mg/day), which resulted in exclusion of 13 percent of the patients. Although the investigators concluded that in contrast to diltiazem verapamil had no detrimental effect in patients with heart failure, one cannot exclude the possibility that the favorable effect of verapamil reported in patients without heart failure was offset by the myocardial depressant effect of the drug in patients with heart failure.

Second Generation CCBs

NISOLDIPINE

In a study of the hemodynamic and neurohumoral effects of nisoldipine[48] in 17 patients with New York Heart Association (NYHA) functional class II–IV

CHF, the drug decreased systemic vascular resistance and mean systemic arterial pressure and increased stroke volume and left ventricular ejection fraction at rest and during exercise, and it reduced exercise values of left ventricular filling pressure. Intravenous infusion of nisoldipine demonstrated a coronary vasodilatory effect, leading to increased resting coronary sinus blood flow and decreased resting and exercise coronary vascular resistance. The systemic hemodynamic benefits were maintained during oral administration of nisoldipine for 4 weeks. Baseline group mean values of plasma norepinephrine and renin were elevated and did not change during chronic therapy, although a reduction of sympathetic activity was noted in patients who showed hemodynamic improvement. A similar hemodynamic effect of nisoldipine was demonstrated by other investigators.[49,50] A further evaluation of chronic administration (2 months) of nisoldipine in patients with CHF,[49] however, resulted in hospitali-

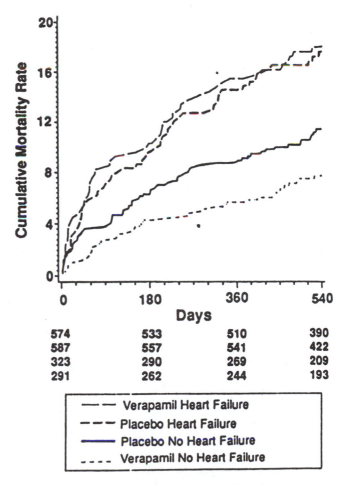

Fig. 48-4. Cumulative cardiac event rate on verapamil and placebo in patients with and without heart failure. (From Danish Study Group on Verapamil in Myocardial Infarction,[47] with permission.)

zation of 70 percent of the patients because of worsening heart failure despite initial improvement of the hemodynamic profile. This disappointing clinical effect was attributed to neurohumoral activation induced by the therapy.[51]

Del Cas et al.[52] studied the acute and chronic effects of nisoldipine on resting and exercise hemodynamics, neurohumoral parameters, and functional capacity in 14 patients with mild to moderate heart failure. Nisoldipine therapy (20 mg PO) was associated with a reduction in blood pressure and systemic vascular resistance and an increase in cardiac index at rest and during exercise. Left ventricular filling pressures were also improved by nisoldipine at peak exercise. Hemodynamic effects of the drug were preserved following chronic therapy. Despite these hemodynamic improvements, there were no significant changes in exercise duration or peak oxygen consumption after either acute or chronic nisoldipine therapy. Evaluation of the nisoldipine effect on neurohormones in this study showed a slight but significant increase in plasma norepinephrine levels at rest but not at peak exercise. No significant changes were observed in plasma renin activity or aldosterone levels.

Haitas et al.[53] compared the acute hemodynamic effects of intravenous nisoldipine and hydralazine in nine patients with moderate to severe CHF due to coronary artery disease. Both agents reduced left ventricular preload and afterload and increased cardiac output. The effects of hydralazine were greater and longer-lasting, however, and resulted in the development of hypotension in two patients and angina in the other two.

Two other studies have evaluated the effect of nisoldipine in patients with heart failure following myocardial infarction. In a double-blind study Lewis et al.[54] compared the effect of nisoldipine and placebo given for 8 weeks each on exercise performance in 19 patients with moderate to severe heart failure following myocardial infarction. At the end of the 8-week period, the peak estimated workload, the rate of perceived exertion, and to a lesser degree the duration of treadmill exercise increased in patients receiving nisoldipine compared with those receiving placebo. There was no change in peak double product, suggesting that myocardial oxygen demand was not altered. The resting left ventricular ejection fraction measured using radionuclide ventriculography was also unchanged in the two groups after 8 weeks. In a second study, Eichstaedt[55] compared the effect of nisoldipine (20 mg daily) and β-acetyldigoxin (0.3 mg daily) on the left ventricular ejection fraction in patients with left ventricular dysfunction and heart failure due to multiple myocardial infarctions. Patients were studied at rest and during exercise. β-Acetyldigoxin was superior to nisoldipine in terms of

improving left ventricular function in a subgroup of patients with moderately decreased ejection fraction (20–33 percent). However, in a subgroup of patients with an ejection fraction of less than 25 percent nisoldipine was associated with a significant increase in ejection fraction (4.0 percent at rest and 5.4 percent during exercise), whereas β-acetyldigoxin did not improve left ventricular function in this group of patients.

In summary, the available information demonstrates a strong vasodilatory effect of nisoldipine in patients with CHF resulting in decreased left ventricular afterload and leading to augmentation of cardiac output and left ventricular ejection fraction in some patients. These changes, however, result in either no or small changes in exercise capacity. Despite initial hemodynamic improvement, clinical deterioration may occur, indicating a potential risk associated with a chronic use of nisoldipine in patients with chronic CHF.

NICARDIPINE

Evaluation of the effect of nicardipine in small groups of patients with CHF suggested favorable acute and short-term effects. Ryman et al. evaluated the effect of 1 week of therapy with oral nicardipine (30 mg three times daily) at rest and during exercise on hemodynamics, oxygen consumption, and catecholamine levels in 10 patients with severe CHF.[56] Therapy resulted in a decrease in systemic vascular resistance and pulmonary artery wedge pressure and an increase in cardiac index at rest and during exercise. Plasma norepinephrine concentrations did not change.

In another study, intravenous nicardipine (10 mg) resulted in acute and short-term improvement in left ventricular performance in patients with mild to moderate CHF.[57,58] The same investigators[59] reported significant improvements in ejection fraction, cardiac output, and peak filling rate assessed by radionuclide ventriculography acutely after intravenous nicardipine administration and after 4 weeks of long-term oral therapy (20–40 mg three times daily) in patients with CHF due to ischemic heart disease, suggesting a beneficial effect of nicardipine on left ventricular systolic and diastolic function.

Gheorghiade et al.[60] evaluated the long-term effect of nicardipine (20–30 mg q8h) given over 4 months in patients with chronic CHF treated with standard CHF drug therapy including angiotensin-converting enzyme (ACE) inhibitors. In this study, adjunctive therapy with nicardipine resulted in clinical worsening in 60 percent of the patients compared to only 20 percent of patients receiving placebo ($P = 0.06$). Concomitant use of captopril did not prevent neurohormonal activation (renin increased from 7 ± 6 to 22 ± 28 ng $\cdot$ ml^{-1} $\cdot$ h^{-1}; $P < 0.05$).

In summary, despite reported favorable effects of nicardipine on the hemodynamic profile and systolic and diastolic left ventricular function, long-term administration of this drug may result in significant clinical deterioration in patients with chronic CHF.

FELODIPINE

Felodipine was reported to have negligible negative inotropic effects and high selectivity to smooth muscle.[61] The short-term administration of felodipine in patients with CHF during the resting state resulted in a reduction in systemic vascular resistance and blood pressure along with elevated left ventricular filling pressure and an increase in cardiac output.[62–65] Studies examining the long-term effects of felodipine in chronic CHF have demonstrated hemodynamic benefits similar to those seen during short-term administration.[66–69] Dunselman et al.[67] examined the long-term hemodynamic effects of felodipine in 23 patients with moderate to severe (NYHA class III) CHF who were already on a regimen of digoxin and diuretics. At the end of an 8-week treatment period, those receiving felodipine (versus placebo) were found to have a modest increase in stroke volume and cardiac output and a reduction in systemic vascular resistance. Similar results were obtained by Kassis and Amtrop,[68,69] who reported a reduction in left ventricular afterload, improvement in left ventricular systolic function during felodipine therapy, and normalization of abnormal baroreflex control of peripheral circulation.

Several studies analyzing the effect of long-term administration of felodipine on cardiovascular hemodynamics during exercise demonstrated that felodipine mediated a decrease in vascular resistance and an increase in cardiac output during moderate exercise with a variable effect on pulmonary artery wedge pressure.[70,71]

In a double-blind study, Dunselman et al.[67] compared the effects of enalapril and felodipine on cardiopulmonary exercise in patients with NYHA class III CHF secondary to coronary artery disease. These investigators found an improvement in aerobic capacity and exercise duration after 16 weeks of enalapril (10 mg twice daily) in 11 patients but not in 9 patients receiving felodipine therapy (10 mg twice daily).

The largest experience with the use of felodipine in patients with heart failure has been provided by the V-HeFT III study.[72] This study enrolled 451 male patients with heart failure and exercise tolerance limited by dyspnea or fatigue who were treated with diuretics and enalapril. The mean age was 63 years; the etiology of CHF was coronary artery disease in 52 percent of the patients; the mean ejection fraction

was 30 percent; and the mean treadmill exercise time was 568 seconds. These patients were randomized to receive either felodipine 5 mg bid or placebo. The study demonstrated no difference between felodipine and placebo in terms of mortality in patients with or without coronary artery disease, although its power to detect differences was small due to the small number of events. Similarly, felodipine did not have an effect on peak exercise capacity at 12 weeks after randomization, and there was a trend toward a higher rate of worsening CHF in the initial 12 weeks in the felodipine group. Plasma norepinephrine was elevated at baseline (515 ± 257 pg/ml) and demonstrated a similar rise in the felodipine and placebo groups (26 and 24 pg/ml, respectively). The plasma atrial natriuretic peptide (ANP) level was 128 ± 107 pg/ml at baseline and was reduced by felodipine 4.0 pg/ml, whereas it increased in the placebo group 27 pg/ml ($P = 0.014$). Based on these results, the investigators of the V-HeFT III study concluded that felodipine, when used as adjunctive therapy to ACE inhibitors and diuretics in patients with CHF, may exert a sustained favorable effect on ANP, possibly due to its hemodynamic effect; but it does not influence either mortality or exercise tolerance in this patient population.

In summary, the overall available information suggests a beneficial hemodynamic effect of felodipine, another vasoselective CCB of the dihydropyridine group, in patients with chronic CHF. However, there is no evidence that these hemodynamic changes can lead to clinical improvement or reduced mortality.

Felodipine in 252 patients conducted in the U.K. found similar results. No improvement in exercise therapy was noted, and a total of 18 patients developed worsening CHF or chest pain on felodipine, compared to 3 on placebo.[74]

NILVADIPINE

Limited information is available regarding the effect of nilvadipine, a new dihydropyridine used for heart failure. Evaluation of the acute hemodynamic effects revealed significant reductions in systemic vascular resistance, blood pressure, pulmonary artery pressure, and pulmonary capillary wedge pressure. In addition, an increase in cardiac index, stroke volume, stroke work, and forearm blood flow without a change in right atrial pressure have been reported.[73,75]

ISRADIPINE

The acute hemodynamic effects of isradipine were evaluated in a group of 12 patients with severe CHF by Greenberg et al.[76] When compared with placebo, isradipine decreased systemic vascular resistance and increased stroke volume and cardiac index. The heart rate and pulmonary artery wedge pressure did not change significantly. The hemodynamic improvement was associated with relief of symptoms in six of the seven patients treated chronically with isradipine.

NITRENDIPINE

Nitrendipine at a single dose of 10–20 mg decreased systemic vascular resistance and increased cardiac index in eight patients with CHF (NYHA class III or IV).[77] Pulmonary artery wedge pressure decreased, but venous capacitance did not change. The improvement in left ventricular function was associated with a decrease in plasma renin and norepinephrine levels.

Third Generation Calcium Antagonists

AMLODIPINE

A multicenter study[78] randomized 142 patients with CHF to either placebo ($n = 49$) or amlodipine 5 mg ($n = 48$) or 10 mg/day ($n = 45$) for 12 weeks while standard CHF therapy was kept constant. Amlodipine was found to produce a dose-dependent increase in cardiac index ($P = 0.02$) and decreases in systemic and pulmonary resistance ($P = 0.06$ and 0.01, respectively) without change in the left ventricular filling pressure. These hemodynamic changes were seen with 10 mg but not with 5 mg. In contrast, 5 mg of amlodipine but not 10 mg was reported to improve quality of life ($P = 0.01$) and health perception (P

$= 0.05$), and it reduced the number of days confined to bed ($P = 0.03$).

Another study by Packer et al. evaluated the effect of amlodipine (10 mg/day) on exercise tolerance, CHF score, and plasma catecholamines in 186 patients with a left ventricular ejection fraction of less than 40 percent and moderate to severe symptoms of heart failure.[79] All patients received diuretics and digitalis, and 80 percent were also treated with ACE inhibitors. The results of the study demonstrated a significantly larger improvement in exercise time (62 $\pm$ 17 versus 22 $\pm$ 13 seconds; $P < 0.05$) and a reduction in CHF symptoms and signs (55 versus 29 percent; $P < 0.05$) with 4 months of amlodipine treatment compared to placebo. These favorable changes were associated with a significant reduction in the serum norepinephrine level in the amlodipine group.

Based on these encouraging results, the Prospective Randomized Amlodipine Survival Evaluation (PRAISE) was designed and conducted.[80] This study evaluated the effect of chronic treatment with amlodipine 10 mg/day in addition to background therapy with digitalis, diuretics, and ACE inhibitors on morbidity and mortality in patients with chronic severe (NYHA class III[b]–IV) CHF (Fig. 48-5). The study was prospectively designed to evaluate separately the effect of therapy in patients with ischemic and nonischemic cardiomyopathy. A total of 1153 patients were randomized and were followed for 6–33 months (median 14.5 months). Of the patients, 732 were diagnosed as having ischemic and 421 patients nonischemic dilated cardiomyopathy (NIDCM). The results of the study (Table 48-3) demonstrated an identical effect on the combined endpoint of mortality and morbidity in the subgroup of patients with ischemic cardiomyopathy (45.4 percent for placebo

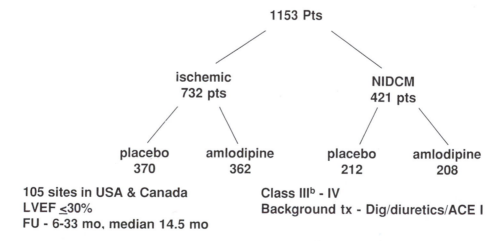

Fig. 48-5. Patients information of the PRAISE (prospective, randomized, amlodipine survival evaluation) study.

Table 48-3. PRAISE Results

Parameter	Percent		Relative risk	P
	Amlodipine	Placebo		
All events				
All patients ($n = 1153$)	38.9	42.3	0.91	0.300
CAD ($n = 732$)	45.3	45.4	1.04	0.731
CM ($n = 421$)	27.8	36.8	0.69	0.029
Mortality				
All patients	33.3	38.3	0.84	0.082
CAD	40.1	40.3	1.02	0.846
CM	21.5	34.9	0.55	0.001

Abbreviations: CAD, coronary artery disease; CM, cardiomyopathy.

and 45.3 percent for amlodipine; $P = 0.741$). In contrast, there was a significant reduction in the combined endpoint in the group of patients with NIDCM (36.8 versus 27.8 percent; $P = 0.034$). Even more impressive were the mortality results. All-cause mortality was lower in the patients with NIDCM treated with amlodipine (34.9 versus 21.5 percent; $P < 0.001$) but not in patients with ischemic cardiomyopathy (40.1 versus 40.3 percent; $P = 0.871$). The primary conclusion from the PRAISE study is that for the first time a calcium antagonist has been proved safe and well tolerated in patients with clinical heart failure and severe left ventricular dysfunction. The finding of a 45 percent reduction in mortality in patients with NIDCM is intriguing and makes amlodipine a reasonable adjunctive agent for patients of this type who remain symptomatic despite treatment with diuretics, ACE inhibitors, and digoxin. However, additional data are required to support more widespread use in NIDCM. PRAISE-2, which is now under way, will address this issue.

Other Calcium Antagonists

BEPRIDIL

Bepridil is a long-acting calcium antagonist chemically unrelated to the dihydropyridines or to other calcium antagonists. Several trials have demonstrated the efficacy of this drug as an antianginal agent.[81–83] The administration of intravenous bepridil resulted in a significant negative inotropic effect in patients with normal left ventricular function.[84,85]

Josephson et al.[86] studied the acute hemodynamic effects of intravenous bepridil in patients with impaired left ventricular function (less than 46 percent) and coronary artery disease. After the administration of either 2 or 4 mg/kg, a significant increase in

pulmonary capillary wedge pressure (PCWP) and a significant decrease in cardiac index, left ventricular dP/dt, and ejection fraction were noted. No data on chronic effects of oral bepridil in patients with CHF are available at the present time.

MIBEFRADIL (RO 40-5967)

Mibefradil, a chemically novel calcium antagonist, substituted tetraline derivative, and the only calcium antagonist able to block both L- and T-type voltage-operated calcium channels. Animal experiments comparing equipotent doses of mibefradil, verapamil, and diltiazem failed to show a negative inotropic effect with mibefradil.[87,88] Studies have shown the effectiveness and safety of mibefradil 25–150 mg given up to 28 days in patients with chronic stable angina and hypertension.[89] Two studies have evaluated the effect of mibefradil in patients with impaired left ventricular (LV) function. In the first study, hemodynamic effect of a single intravenous mibefradil dose was evaluated in 24 patients with an LV ejection fraction less than 40 percent and 26 patients with an LV ejection fraction more than 40 percent. Mibefradil administration resulted in a fall in arterial pressure, heart rate, LV end-systolic pressure and end-diastolic volume, systolic and diastolic wall stress, and peripheral vascular resistance. There was no change in LV end-diastolic pressure or in cardiac output or LV ejection fraction. A decrease in cardiac contractility was found in one patient. There was no clinical deterioration noted, and plasma norepinephrine remained stable.

A second study examined the safety of mibefradil at doses of 6.25, 12.5, 25, 50, and 100 mg PO for 8 days to patients with ischemic cardiomyopathy and NYHA class II–III CHF with a LV ejection fraction less than 40 percent. This study demonstrated that mibefradil was well tolerated.[89]

Based on the above preliminary findings suggesting a potent vasodilatory and antiischemic effect in addition to negative chronotropic effect and lack of effect on contractility and neurohormonal profile, a large study has been designed to evaluate the efficacy of this drug for treatment of chronic CHF (MACH I: Mortality Assessment of Congestive Heart Failure). This study, presently ongoing, was designed as a multicenter, double-blind, placebo-controlled study randomizing patients with chronic CHF, NYHA classes II–IV, LV ejection fraction less than 35 percent, and an echocardiographic LV end diastolic dimension of 60 mm or more who are symptomatic on optimal doses of loop diuretics and ACE inhibitors. The randomization goal is 2050 patients, and the objective of the study is to assess the effect of mibefradil on exercise duration, cardiovascular morbidity, and mortality. Recruitment to the MACH-1 study was scheduled to be completed in 1996 and the follow-up in 1998.

nary artery disease. Furthermore, this study demonstrated a substantial reduction in mortality in patients with CHF due to nonischemic cardiomyopathy and provided a strong indication for a potential therapeutic benefit of amlodipine when added to standard CHF therapy in this patient population. No clear explanation is available at the present time regarding the reason for the deleterious effect demonstrated with some of the dihydropyrides and the contrasting benefit seen with amlodipine.

Finally, more information will become available in the next several years regarding the safety and efficacy of other CCBs for treatment of CHF. The PRAISE II study will provide further information regarding the therapeutic role of amlodipine in patients with nonischemic dilated cardiomyopathy. In addition, the MACH-I study is evaluating the effect of mibefradil, the only CCB capable of blocking both L- and T-type Ca^{2+} channels, on morbidity and mortality in patients with chronic CHF.

CONCLUSION

A considerable effort has been made since the early 1980s to evaluate the safety and efficacy of CCBs for treatment of patients with chronic CHF. Available studies have provided strong evidence for a potential detrimental effect of the first generation calcium antagonists in patients with CHF, indicating the need for great caution when these drugs are used in patients with significant depression of left ventricular systolic function. A number of second generation CCBs have demonstrated a strong vasodilatory effect and favorable hemodynamic action but failed to show a similar improvement in exercise capacity, morbidity, or mortality. Moreover, drugs such as nicardipine and nisoldipine have resulted in a detrimental effect in some patients and therefore cannot be considered safe when used in patients with moderate to severe heart failure. Available information from the V-HeFT III study demonstrate the lack of an unfavorable effect of felodipine on exercise tolerance in patients with chronic heart failure. Although the mortality rate was similar in the felodipine and placebo groups, because of the relatively small number of patients in this study no clear conclusion can be drawn regarding the effect of felodipine on mortality in patients with CHF.

An encouraging signal regarding a potential role of CCBs for treatment of chronic heart failure has been provided by the PRAISE study. This prospective large scale study demonstrated the safety of amlodipine, a long-acting dihydropyridine derivative, when used in patients with heart failure due to coro-

REFERENCES

1. Frishman WH: Current status of calcium channel blockers. Curr Probl Cardiol 1994;14:637–688
2. Veniant M, Clozel JP, Hess P et al: Hemodynamic profile of Ro 40-5967 in conscious rats. Comparison with diltiazem, verapamil and amlodipine. J Cardiovasc Pharmacol, suppl. 10 1991;18:55–58
3. Benet LZ: Pharmacokinetics and metabolism of bepridil. Am J Cardiol 1985;55:8C–13C
4. Nayler WG: The voltage-activated, calcium antagonist-sensitive calcium channels. Their structure, composition and calcium antagonist binding sites. p. 23–36. In: Amlodipine. Springer-Verlag, Berlin 1993
5. Tsien RW: Molecular biology of calcium channels and structural determinants of key functions presented in the symposium: a new class of calcium antagonists. From molecular biology to clinical benefit. XVIIth Congress of the European Society of Cardiology, Amsterdam, August 1995
6. Nyeler WG: The chemistry of the calcium antagonists. pp. 36–44. In Nyeler WG (ed): Amlodipine. Spring-Verlag, Berlin, 1993
7. Mishra SK, Hermjmeyer K: Selective inhibition of T-type Ca^+ channels by Ro 40-5967. Circ Res 1994;75:144–148
8. Cohn JN, Archibald DG, Ziesche S et al: Effect of vasodilator therapy on mortality in chronic congestive heart failure. Results of a Veterans Administration cooperative study (V-HeFT). N Engl J Med 1986;314:1547–1552
9. Cohn JN, Johnson G, Ziesche S et al: A comparison of enalapril with hydralazine-isosorbide dinitrate in the treatment of chronic congestive heart failure. N Engl J Med 1991;325:303–310
10. SOLVD Investigators: Effect of enalapril on survival in patients with reduced left ventricular ejection frac-

tions and congestive heart failure. N Engl J Med 1991;
325:293–302

11. Packer M, Carver JR, Rodeheffer RJ et al: Effect of oral milrinone on mortality in severe chronic heart failure. N Engl J Med 1991;325:1468–1475

12. Lahiri A, Rodrigues EA, Carboni GP, Raftery EB: Effects of long-term treatment with calcium antagonists on left ventricular diastolic function in stable angina and heart failure. Circulation, suppl. III 1990;81:130–138

13. Zile MR: Diastolic dysfunction: detection, consequences and treatment. Part 2. Diagnosis and treatment of diastolic dysfunction. Mod Concepts Cardiovasc Dis 1990;59:1

14. Garrett JS, Wikman-Coffelt J, Sievers R, Finkbliner WE, Parmley WW: Verapamil prevents the development of alcoholic dysfunction in hamster myocardium. J Am Coll Cardiol 1987;9:1326–1331

15. Low RI, Takeda P, Mason DT, DeMaria AN: The effects of calcium channel blocking agents on cardiovascular function. Am J Cardiol 1982;49:547–553

16. Klugmann S, Salvi A, Camerini F: Hemodynamic effects of nifedipine in heart failure. Br Heart J 1980; 43:440–446

17. Matsumoto S, Ito T, Sada T et al: Hemodynamic effects of nifedipine in congestive heart failure. Am J Cardiol 1980;46:476–480

18. Ludbrook PA, Tiefenbrun AJ, Sobel BE: Influence of nifedipine on left ventricular systolic and diastolic function. Relationship to manifestations of ischemia and congestive failure. Am J Med 1981;71:683–692

19. Magorien RD, Leier CV, Kolibash AJ, Barbush TJ, Unverferth DV: Beneficial effects of nifedipine on rest and exercise myocardial energetics in patients with congestive heart failure. Circulation 1984;70:884–890

20. Hof RP: Comparison of cardiodepressant and vasodilator effects of PN 200-110 (isradipine), nifedipine and diltiazem in anesthetized rabbits. Am J Cardiol, suppl. 1987;59:37B–42B

21. Miller AB, Conetta DA, Bass TA: Sublingual nifedipine. Acute effects in severe chronic congestive heart failure secondary to idiopathic diseased cardiomyopathy. Am J Cardiol 1985;55:1359–1362

22. Millard RW, Lathrop DA, Grupp G et al: Differential cardiovascular effects of calcium-channel blocking agents. Potential mechanisms. Am J Cardiol 1982;49:499–506

23. Elkayam U, Weber L, McKay C, Rahimtoola SH: Spectrum of acute hemodynamic effects of nifedipine in severe congestive heart failure. Am J Cardiol 1985;56:560–568

24. Elkayam U, Weber L, Torkan B, Berman D, Rahimtoola SH: Acute hemodynamic effect of oral nifedipine in severe chronic congestive heart failure. Am J Cardiol 1983;52:1041–1054

25. Fleckenstein A: Specific pharmacology of calcium in myocardium, cardiac pacemakers and smooth muscle. Annu Rev Pharmacol Toxicol 1977;17:149–166

26. Gillmer DJ, Kark P: Pulmonary edema precipitated by nifedipine. BMJ 1980;280:1420–1421

27. Elkayam U, Weber L, Torkan B, McKay CR, Rahimtoola SH: Comparison of hemodynamic response to nifedipine and nitroprusside in severe chronic congestive heart failure. Am J Cardiol 1984;53:1321–1325

28. Fifer MA, Colucci WS, Lorell BH, Jaski BE, Barry WH: Inotropic vascular and neuroendocrine effects of nifedipine and nitroprusside in severe chronic congestive heart failure. Am J Cardiol 1984;53:1321–1325

29. Elkayam U, Weber L, McKay CR, Rahimtoola SH: Differences in hemodynamic response to vasodilation due to calcium antagonism with nifedipine and direct-acting agonism with hydralazine in chronic congestive heart failure. Am J Cardiol 1984;54:126–131

30. Packer M, Lee WH, Medina N et al: Prognostic importance of the immediate hemodynamic response to nifedipine in patients with severe left ventricular dysfunction. J Am Coll Cardiol 1987;10:1303–1311

31. Prida XE, Kubo SH, Largh JH, Cody RJ: Evaluation of calcium-mediated vasoconstriction in chronic congestive heart failure. Am J Med 1983;75:795–800

32. Elkayam U, Roth A, Hsueh W et al: Neurohumoral consequences of vasodilator therapy with hydralazine and nifedipine in severe congestive heart failure. Am Heart J 1986;111:1130–1138

33. Agostoni PG, De Cesare N, Doria E et al: Afterload reduction. A comparison of captopril and nifedipine in dilated cardiomyopathy. Br Heart J 1986;55:391–399

34. Elkayam U, Amin J, Mehra A et al: A prospective, randomized, double-blind, crossover study to compare the efficacy and safety of chronic nifedipine therapy with that of isosorbide dinitrate and their combination in the treatment of chronic congestive heart failure. Circulation 1990;82:1954–1961

35. Henry PD: Comparative pharmacology of calcium antagonists. Nifedipine, verapamil and diltiazem. Am J Cardiol 1980;46:1047–1058

36. Walsh RW, Porter CB, Starling MR, O'Rourke RA: Beneficial effects of intravenous and oral diltiazem in severe congestive heart failure. J Am Coll Cardiol 1984;3:1044–1050

37. Charlap S, Frishman WH: Calcium antagonists and heart failure. Med Clin North Am 1989;73:339–359

38. Packer M, Lee WH, Medina Y, Yushak M: Comparative negative inotropic effects of nifedipine and diltiazem in patients with severe left ventricular dysfunction [abstract]. Circulation, suppl. III 1985;72:275

39. Kulick DL, McIntosh N, Campese VM et al: Central and renal hemodynamic effects and hormonal response to diltiazem in severe congestive heart failure. Am J Cardiol 1987;59:1138–1143

40. Heywood JT, Graham B, Marais GE, Jutzy KR: Effects of intravenous diltiazem on rapid atrial fibrillation accompanied by congestive heart failure. Am J Cardiol 1991;67:1150–1152

41. Roth A, Harrison E, Mitani G et al: Efficacy and safety of medium and high-dose diltiazem alone and in combination with digoxin for heart rate control at rest and during exercise in patients with chronic atrial fibrillation. Circulation 1986;73:316–324

42. Figulla HR, Rechenberg JV, Wiegand V, Soballa R, Kreuzer H: Beneficial effects of long-term diltiazem treatment in dilated cardiomyopathy. J Am Coll Cardiol 1989;13:653–658

43. Multicenter Diltiazem Postinfarction Trial Research Group: The effect of diltiazem on mortality and reinfarction after myocardial infarction. N Engl J Med 1988;319:385–392

44. Goldstein RE, Boccuzzi SJ, Cruess D, Nattel S: Diltiazem increases late-onset congestive heart failure in

postinfarction patients with early reduction in ejection fraction. Circulation 1991;83:52–60

45. Physicians Desk Reference. 47th Ed. p. 2250. Medical Economics, Montvale, NJ, 1993

46. Ferlinz J, Gallo CT: Responses of patients in heart failure to long-term oral verapamil administration [abstract]. Circulation, suppl. II 1984;70:305

47. Danish Study Group on Verapamil in Myocardial Infarction. Secondary prevention with verapamil after myocardial infarction. Am J Cardiol 1990;66:331–401

48. Kiowski W, Erne P, Pfisterer M, Beuhler FR, Burkart F: Arterial vasodilator, systemic and coronary hemodynamic effects of nisoldipine in congestive heart failure secondary to ischemic or dilated cardiomyopathy. Am J Cardiol 1987;59:1118

49. Minderjahn KP, Hanrath P, Bleifeld W: The influence of nisoldipine on rest and exercise hemodynamics of the left ventricle in chronic left heart insufficiency. Z Kardiol, suppl. 1 1983;72:83

50. Thier W, Roewer N, Minderjahn KP, Hanrath P, Bliefeld W: Hemodynamic effect of nisoldipine in chronic congestive heart failure [abstract]. J Am Coll Cardiol 1986;3:479

51. Barjon JN, Rouleau JL, Bichet D, Juneau C, De Champlain J: Chronic renal and neurohumoral effects of the calcium-entry blocker nisoldipine in patients with congestive heart failure. J Am Coll Cardiol 1987;9: 622–630

52. Del Cas L, Metra M, Ferrari R, Visioli O: Acute and chronic hemodynamic effects of the dihydropyridine calcium antagonist nisoldipine on resting and exercise hemodynamics, neurohumoral parameters and functional capacity of patients with chronic heart failure. Cardiovasc Drugs Ther 1993;7:103–110

53. Haitas B, Meyer TE, Angel ME, Reef E: Comparative haemodynamic effects of intravenous nisoldipine and hydralazine in congestive heart failure. Br J Clin Pharmacol 1990;29:366–368

54. Lewis BS, Makhoul N, Merdler A et al: Effect of nisoldipine on exercise performance in heart failure following myocardial infarction. Cardiology 1991;79:39–45

55. Eichstaedt H: Effects of calcium antagonists in patients with coronary disease and heart failure. Left ventricular function following nisoldipine measured by radionuclide ventriculography. J Cardiovasc Pharmacol, suppl. 5 1992;29:50–54

56. Ryman KS, Kubo SH, Lystash J, Stone G, Cody RJ: Effects of nicardipine on rest and exercise hemodynamics in chronic congestive heart failure. Am J Cardiol 1986;58:583–588

57. Lahiri A, Robinson CW, Kohli RS, Carvana MP, Raftery EB: Acute and chronic effects of nicardipine on systolic and diastolic left ventricular performance in patients with heart failure. A pilot study. Clin Cardiol 1986;9:257–261

58. Lahiri A, Robinson CW, Tovey J et al: Intravenous nicardipine in patients with chronic congestive heart failure. A nuclear stethoscope study. Postgrad Med J, suppl. 4 1984;69:35–38

59. Lahiri A, Rodrigues EA, Carboni GP, Raferty EB: Effects of long-term treatment with calcium antagonists on left ventricular diastolic function in stable angina and heart failure. Circulation, suppl. III 1990;81: 130–138

60. Gheorghiade M, Hall V, Goldberg D, Levine TB, Goldstein S: Long-term clinical and neurohormonal effects of nicardipine in patients with severe heart failure on maintenance therapy with angiotensin converting enzyme inhibitors [abstract]. J Am Coll Cardiol, suppl. A 1991;17:274A

61. Ljung B: Vascular selectivity of felodipine. Drugs, suppl. 2 1985;29:46–58

62. Timmis AD, Campbell S, Monaghan MJ, Walker L, Jewitt DE: Acute and metabolic effects of felodipine in congestive heart failure. Br Heart J 1984;51:445–451

63. Emanuelsson H, Hjalmarson A, Holmberg S, Waagstein F: Acute hemodynamic effects of felodipine in congestive heart failure. Eur J Clin Pharmacol 1985; 28:489–493

64. Tweddel AC, Hutton I: Felodipine in ventricular dysfunction. Eur Heart J 1986;7:54–60

65. Binetti G, Pancaldi S, Giovanelli N et al: Hemodynamic effects of felodipine in congestive heart failure. Cardiovasc Drugs Ther 1987;1:161–167

66. Agostini P, Doria E, Riva S, Polese A: Acute and chronic efficacy of felodipine in congestive heart failure. Int J Cardiol 1991;30:89–95

67. Dunselman PHJM, Kuntze CEE, Van Bruggen A et al: Efficacy of felodipine in congestive heart failure. Eur Heart J 1989;10:354–364

68. Kassis E, Amtrop O: Cardiovascular and neurohumoral postural responses and baroreceptor abnormalities during a course of adjunctive vasodilatory therapy with felodipine for congestive heart failure. Circulation 1987;75:1204–1213

69. Kassis E, Amtrop O: Long-term clinical, hemodynamic, angiographic and neurohumoral responses to vasodilation with felodipine in patients with chronic congestive heart failure. J Cardiovasc Pharmacol 1990;15:347–352

70. Tan LB, Murray RG, Little WA: Felodipine in patients with chronic heart failure. Discrepant haemodynamic and clinical effects. Br Heart J 1987;58:122–128

71. Timmis AD, Smyth P, Kenny JF, Campbell S, Jewitt DE: Effects of vasodilator treatment with felodipine on hemodynamic responses to treadmill exercise in congestive heart failure. Br Heart J 1984;52:314–320

72. Cohn JN, Ziesche SM, Loss LE et al: Effect of felodipine on short-term exercise and neurohormone and long-term mortality in heart failure. Results of V-HeFT III. Circulation (in press)

73. Ohtsuka M, Ono T, Hoiro J et al: Comparison of the cardiovascular effect of FR34235, a new dihydropyridine, with other calcium antagonists. J Cardiovasc Pharmacol 1983;5:1074–1082

74. Littler WA, Sheridan DJ: Placebo controlled trial of felodipine in patients with mild to moderate heart failure. Br Heart J 1995;428–433

75. Sato H, Ikenouchi H, Aoyagi T et al: Acute hemodynamic effects of nilvadipine, a new calcium channel blocker, in patients with congestive heart failure. J Cardiovasc Pharmacol 1990;15:317–322

76. Greenberg B, Siemienczuk D, Broudy D: Hemodynamic effects of PN 200-110 in congestive heart failure. Am J Cardiol 1987;59:70B–74B

77. Olivari MT, Levine TB, Cohn JN: Acute hemodynamic effects of nitrendipine in congestive heart failure. J Cardiovasc Pharmacol suppl. 7 1984;6:S1002–1005

78. Smith WB, De Abate AC, Gollub SB et al: Beneficial long-term hemodynamic and clinical effects of amlodi-

pine in chronic heart failure. Results of a multicenter randomized, double-blind, placebo-controlled, dose-ranging study. Circulation, suppl. I 1994;90:602

79. Packer M, Nicod P, Khandheria BR et al: Randomized, multicenter, double-blind, placebo-controlled evaluation of amlodipine in patients with mild-to-moderate heart failure [abstract]. J Am Coll Cardiol 1991;17:274A

80. Packer M: PRAISE. Presented in the 44th Annual Scientific Session of the American College of Cardiology, New Orleans, 1995

81. DiBianci R, Alpert J, Katz RJ et al: Bepridil for chronic stable angina pectoris. Results of a prospective multicenter, placebo-controlled, dose-ranging study in 77 patients. Am J Cardiol 1984;53:35–41

82. Hill JA, O'Brien JT, Scott E, Conti CR, Pepine CJ: Effects of bepridil on exercise tolerance in chronic stable angina. A double-blind, randomized, placebo-controlled, crossover trial. Am J Cardiol 1984;53:679–683

83. Singh BN: Safety profile of bepridil determined from clinical trials in chronic stable angina in the United States. Am J Cardiol, suppl. 11 1992;69:68D–74D

84. Alpert JS, Benotti JR, Brady PM et al: Hemodynamic effects of intravenous bepridil in patients with normal left ventricular function. Am J Cardiol, suppl. 7 1985;55:20C–24C

85. Tamari I, Borer JS, Moses JW et al: Hemodynamic assessment of intravenous bepridil administration in ischemic heart disease. Am J Cardiol, suppl. 7 1985;55:25C–29C

86. Josephson MA, Mody T, Coyle K, Singh BN: Effects on hemodynamics and left ventricular ejection fraction of intravenous bepridil for impaired left ventricular function secondary to coronary artery disease. Am J Cardiol 1987;60:44–49

87. Clozel JP, Banken L, Osterrieder W: Effects of Ro 40-5967, a novel calcium antagonist, on myocardial function during ischemia induced by lowering coronary perfusion pressure in dogs. Comparison with verapamil. J Cardiovasc Pharmacol 1989;14:715–721

88. Ezzaher A, Bouonani NEH, So JB, Hittinger L, Crozatier B: Increased negative inotropic effect of calcium channel blockers in the hypertrophied and failing rabbit heart. J Pharmacol Exp Ther 1991;257:466–471

89. Investigational Drug Brochure Ro 40-5967 (calcium antagonist), January 1992 and addendum to the Investigational Drug Brochure (4th Version, January 1992) of Ro 40-5967 (calcium antagonist), January 1993

Management of Arrhythmias in Patients with Heart Failure: Evaluation and Treatment with Drugs and Devices

49

Jaswinder S. Gill

A. John Camm

Arrhythmias of ventricular origin are frequently found with heart failure and are commonly thought to be the cause of death from this condition. Data from the Framingham Study demonstrated that 55 percent of men and 24 percent of women died within 4 years of developing heart failure, a prognosis that is worse than for many of the common malignant neoplasms. Of these deaths, 40–50 percent were considered sudden.[1] The large-scale studies of angiotensin-converting enzyme (ACE) inhibitors during heart failure demonstrate that as heart failure severity increases the risk of sudden death also rises, being 8–14 percent in patients with New York Heart Association (NYHA) functional class II and III during a follow-up of 2–3 years, whereas this figure is observed over 1 year in patients with class III–IV failure. Most of the studies that address this problem deal with heart failure due to ischemic heart disease and dilated cardiomyopathy as a single condition. However, it is unclear whether the underlying substrate, the frequency and type of arrhythmia, and the ultimate outcome of the arrhythmia are similar for the two major etiologies of heart failure.

RISK OF ARRHYTHMIA DURING HEART FAILURE

Patients with congestive heart failure have a high incidence of complex ventricular arrhythmias, 80 percent having frequent ventricular premature beats and 50 percent demonstrating nonsustained ventricular tachycardia on Holter monitoring. Mortality for such patients is 30–50 percent per year, with half of the deaths being classified as sudden.[2-8] In most studies sudden cardiac death has been defined as unexpected death from circulatory failure within 1 hour of the onset of symptoms in a patient with left ventricular dysfunction whose heart failure symptoms have remained stable or improved over the previous 2–4 weeks and in whom another cause for circulatory collapse cannot be identified clinically. This definition attempts to exclude patients for whom death is sudden but characterized by progressively worsening failure and the death due to an identifiable cause, such as pulmonary embolism or acute myocardial infarction.

Several systematic studies have been conducted to examine the cause of sudden death in patients with left ventricular dysfunction. The terminal event, thought to be ventricular tachycardia or ventricular fibrillation, was indeed identified in a proportion of patients with heart failure due to ischemic heart disease. Such patients demonstrate a high frequency of complex ventricular ectopy, and around half with severe ventricular dysfunction demonstrate nonsustained ventricular tachycardia. In patients with complex arrhythmias on ambulatory monitoring, however, left ventricular function is the most powerful predictor of sudden cardiac death.[9-11] Deterioration of left ventricular function is marked by increasingly frequent, complex ventricular arrhythmias and an increased incidence of sudden cardiac death. However, there is also a high incidence of bradyarrhythmias and electromechanical dissociation as the terminal event.[12,13] Occasionally rapid supraventricular rhythms can precipitate fatal or near-fatal ventricular arrhythmia.[14]

Several groups of investigators have addressed the question of factors that can predict the risk of sudden death in patients with heart failure. It appears that factors related to neurohumoral activation in response to the heart failure and the degree of heart failure are more strongly related to the risk of sudden cardiac death than electrophysiologic features of the arrhythmia. Left ventricular ejection fraction is the major most predictive variable,[15,16] though hyponatremia, pulmonary capillary wedge pressure, pulmonary artery pressure, and right atrial pressure have some contribution. The presence of atrial fibrillation,[17] a history of syncope,[18] and ventricular arrhythmias are also valuable additional factors in risk prediction. There is some suggestion that patients with heart failure secondary to ischemic heart disease have a poorer survival than those with dilated cardiomyopathy.[19] The particular value of electrophysiologic measurements in risk stratification are discussed later in the chapter.

VENTRICULAR ARRHYTHMIAS DURING HEART FAILURE

Ventricular Tachycardia

Sustained monomorphic ventricular tachycardia (VT) occurs in approximately 9 percent of patients with advanced heart failure referred for cardiac transplantation.[20] In patients with ischemic heart failure there is considerable evidence that these tachycardias have reentrant mechanisms based on scarring within the myocardium, and there is a high rate of inducibility by programmed electrical stimulation.[21] With dilated cardiomyopathy, sustained monomorphic VT is rare and not easily provocable by programmed electrical stimulation; and the mechanism is likely to be triggered automaticity as well as reentry.[22] Occasionally, bundle branch reentry is the cause of sustained VT in patients with dilated cardiomyopathy and is easily treated by ablation of the right bundle branch.[23] An episode of sustained VT identifies patients who are at high risk for arrhythmia recurrences and sudden cardiac death.[24] Patients with hemodynamically tolerated VT have a lower risk of death than patients in whom the arrhythmia is not well tolerated. Furthermore, patients who suffer cardiac arrest due to VT have a substantial risk of recurrent cardiac arrest, even if the arrhythmia inducible at electrophysiology study

is suppressed with antiarrhythmic drugs.[25] In patients with dilated cardiomyopathy there is also a high risk of sudden death if the patient presents with VT. Poll et al. reported that in all of 13 patients presenting with sustained monomorphic VT could be induced at electrophysiology study; and on follow-up four died suddenly.[26] In the study of Brembilla-Perrot et al. sustained monomorphic VT was induced in 8 of 11 patients with dilated cardiomyopathy who presented with this arrhythmia. There was a 60 percent recurrence rate of sudden cardiac death or VT in patients with nonsuppressible VT but 20 percent in those with suppressable VT.[27] These data also suggest that if VT is suppressible the risk of sudden cardiac death is reduced.

Sustained Polymorphic Ventricular Tachycardia/Torsade de Pointes

Sustained polymorphic VT and torsade de pointes generally occur in the presence of precipitating factors, such as acute ischemia, QT prolongation, or digitalis toxicity. Torsade de pointes in particular is associated with diuretic-induced hypokalemia and hypomagnesemia and antiarrhythmic drug therapy. Torsade de pointes occurs in approximately 1.4 percent of patients with cardiac arrest secondary to heart failure and is associated with an increased risk of sudden death despite attempts to remove precipitating factors.[28]

Ventricular Fibrillation

Ventricular fibrillation (VF) generally occurs in the presence of acute myocardial ischemia or severe myocardial dysfunction. In some instances, VF occurs in the presence of decompensated heart failure. At electrophysiologic study, VT is inducible in approximately 32 percent of patients, and VF is induced in 16 percent.[29] The risk of further recurrences is high in patients with one cardiac arrest and depressed ventricular function, justifying the use of intensive treatment.

RISK STRATIFICATION IN PATIENTS WITH HEART FAILURE

Although the major factors related to risk of death in patients with heart failure are neurohumoral factors and the degree of impairment of left ventricular function, factors related to electrophysiology also contribute to risk stratification. They include the presence of ventricular ectopic activity, results of programmed electrical stimulation, and the presence of late potentials on the signal-averaged electrocardiogram (ECG).

Ventricular Ectopic Activity

Ventricular ectopic activity is almost universally found on Holter recordings in patients with heart failure. Ventricular ectopic beats occur in 70–95 percent of patients, and nonsustained VT is found in 20–80 percent.[3,5,30] It is well recognized that in patients with ischemic heart disease the frequency and complexity of ventricular ectopic beats is related to the degree of left ventricular impairment, and the latter is the single most important prognostic indicator. However, the presence of ectopic beats provides additional independent prognostic information, which has formed the basis of prognostication in patients after myocardial infarction.[31,32] This relation between ventricular ectopic beats and mortality is present in patients treated with thrombolytics as well as those managed during the prethrombolysis era.[33] Data from the GISSI study suggest that in patients with a left ventricular ejection fraction of 0.35 or less the presence of 10 or more ectopic ventricular beats per hour or complex ventricular ectopy was associated with a 2.1 to 2.4-fold increase in the risk of sudden cardiac death.

With nonischemic cardiomyopathy, ventricular ectopy is again common and has been related to mortality in several studies,[5,34] although other reports do not confirm these findings.[35] Similarly, there is no consistent relation between the frequency and severity of the ventricular ectopic beats and the degree of impairment of left ventricular function.[5,34]

Programmed Electrical Stimulation

In patients who have a sustained ventricular arrhythmia following myocardial infarction, sustained monomorphic VT can be induced in more than 90 percent of patients.[36] The initiation of polymorphic VT or VF is nonspecific and does not confer any prognostic information.[37] The possibility of inducing VT increases with decreasing left ventricular function.[38] The authors of this report also demonstrated that patients with inducible VT have a 19 percent risk of sudden death, whereas in the group without inducible VT there is only a 3 percent risk. Patients with depressed ventricular function and inducible sustained VT have a higher risk of spontaneous VT than those who do not have inducible VT.[39] Patients who are noninducible, however, are still at substantial risk of sudden death (26 percent at 1 year).[40]

In patients with dilated cardiomyopathy of nonischemic origin who have suffered an eipsode of sustained VT, electrophysiologic study is of limited value for predicting sudden cardiac death, as discussed in the previous section.

Signal-Averaged Electrocardiography

The occurrence of late potentials on the signal-averaged ECG in patients after myocardial infarction is associated with the presence of inducible VT and an increased incidence of arrhythmic events such as sudden cardiac death or spontaneous sustained VT.[41] This test provides additional and independent information but is of low positive predictive value.[42] Various methods of analysis of the signal-averaged ECG have been developed, but it is unclear whether they improve the predictive accuracy of signal averaging in patients after myocardial infarction.[43,44]

Patients with nonischemic dilated cardiomyopathy and sustained VT have a high prevalence of late potentials (up to 80 percent).[45] The presence of positive late potentials in patients with no sustained VT is variable among studies and does not seem to relate to the occurrence of sudden cardiac death in most.[46,47] Again, several methods of analysis are being applied to the signal-averaged ECG data, and their value is not yet clear.

ANTIARRHYTHMIC DRUG THERAPY IN PATIENTS WITH HEART FAILURE

The use of antiarrhythmic drugs in patients with heart failure is beset with problems. The first, and usually most troublesome, is the depression of ventricular function by antiarrhythmic drugs, leading to an exacerbation of heart failure. The only drugs that appear to be free of this problem are quinidine and amiodarone. All the class 1 drugs and sotalol depress the cardiac index and elevate the intracardiac filling pressure.[48] The exception appears to be quinidine, which acutely does not appear to depress cardiac function.[49] The second problem is proarrhythmia, which is exacerbation of an existing arrhythmia or precipitation of a new arrhythmia. Proarrhythmic effects are more likely to be seen in patients with impaired left ventricular function.[50] Drugs can precipitate sustained VT or VF or exacerbate nonsustained VT, particularly if they have a marked effect on slowing cardiac conduction.[51] Some antiarrhythmic drugs have a potent effect on lengthening the QT interval and can precipitate torsade de pointes. The results of the CAST study, which demonstrated an increase in mortality in patients with ventricular premature contractions (VPCs) following myocardial infarction treated with class 1c drugs have produced a reluctance to use class 1 drugs in patients with underlying cardiac disease.[52] Class 2 drugs β-adrenoceptor blockers, are contraindicated in patients with impaired left ventricular function and are therefore not generally used; this issue is addressed below. Attention has therefore been focused on class 3 drugs, particularly amiodarone.

Amiodarone has a number of advantages, including a lack of an adverse effect on ventricular function, a potent effect on arrhythmogenesis without excessive slowing of conduction, and antiarrhythmic actions in the atrium (preventing atrial fibrillation) and the ventricle. The use of amiodarone in patients with heart failure suggests that there may be some effect on preventing arrhythmic death. Hamer et al.[53] studied patients with heart failure but no sustained ventricular arrhythmia. Over 6 months patients treated with amiodarone had suppression of nonsustained VT, and only one died suddenly, whereas four of the placebo-treated group died suddenly. Such data and the promising results achieved with amiodarone following myocardial infarction[54–56] led to large controlled studies examining the value of amiodarone on preventing sudden cardiac death in patients with congestive cardiac failure.

In the GESICA study, 516 patients on optimal standard therapy for cardiac failure were randomized to amiodarone 300 mg daily or standard therapy. There were 87 deaths in the amiodarone-treated group compared to 106 in the control group [28 percent risk reduction, confidence interval (CI) 4–45 percent, $P = 0.02$]. The reduction in deaths was due to an improvement in the rates of sudden death and death due to worsening heart failure (Fig. 49-1).[57] The results from another study have not been as promising. Singh et al.[58] examined the use of amiodarone in patients with congestive cardiac failure and asymptomatic ventricular arrhythmias. Patients ($n = 674$) with 10 or more ventricular premature beats per hour were randomized to amiodarone (400 mg daily maintenence dose) or placebo. There was no significant difference in overall mortality between the groups; and, in particular, sudden cardiac mortality did not differ (Fig. 49-2). There was a trend to a reduction in mortality among the patients with nonischemic cardiomyopathy who received the drug and the much greater proportion of these patients in GESICA is probably the most likely explanation for the difference of these 2 trials.[58a]

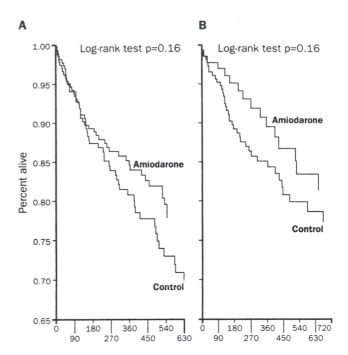

Fig. 49-1. Cumulative survival curves for **(A)** death from progressive heart failure and **(B)** sudden death, demonstrating the improved survival of the amiodarone-treated group in comparison to controls. (From Doval et al.,[57] with permission.)

Two studies have been specifically directed to study the efficacy of amiodarone in the prevention of sudden cardiac death (SCD) and malignant ventricular arrhythmias in patients after myocardial infarction who are stratified into the high risk group. The first of these studies is the European Myocardial Infarct Amiodarone Trial (EMIAT).[59] Patients with acute myocardial infarction 5–21 days previously, aged 18–75 years, an ejection fraction less than 40 percent, and ventricular ectopic beats on Holter monitoring were randomized to receive amiodarone or placebo. The patients were followed, with the endpoints of the study being total mortality, total cardiac mortality, arrhythmic death, and arrhythmic death together with resuscitated SCD. The results of this study have just been announced. There was no difference in total mortality or cardiac mortality between the amiodarone and placebo arms, but there was a reduction in the arrhythmic deaths and arrhythmic death together with resuscitated SCD. Relative risk for arrhythmic deaths and resuscitated SCD was 0.5 on an intention-to-treat analysis. The second study on this theme is the Canadian Amiodarone Myocardial Infarction Arrhythmia Trial (CAMIAT).[60] Again patients with myocardial infarction 6–45 days previously and the ECG demonstrating 10 or more ventricular ectopic beats or nonsustained VT of more

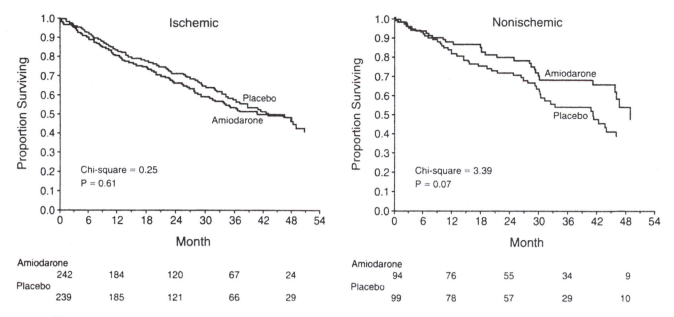

Fig. 49-2. Kaplan-Meier survival curves in patients with ischemic and nonischemic cardiomyopathy treated with amiodarone or placebo. There is a trend toward a beneficial effect of amiodarone in patients with nonischemic cardiomyopathy, whereas none is seen in the ischemic group. (From Singh et al.,[58] with permission.)

than three beats were randomized to amiodarone or placebo. The primary endpoint was arrhythmic death, with a secondary endpoint of total mortality. The results of this study have also just been announced. There was a 32.6% reduction in arrhythmic death, 27.4% reduction in cardiac death, and 21.0% reduction in all-cause mortality. Despite the differences in design of these two studies, the results suggest that arrhythmic mortality may be reduced by the use of amiodarone in patients after myocardial infarction who demonstrated an adverse risk profile for SCD.

Interest in the β-adrenoceptor blocking drugs for the treatment of patients with congestive cardiac failure has been rekindled by the emergence of agents with peripheral vasodilating properties, as well as β-adrenoceptor blocking actions on the myocardium. One report[61] described a dramatic reduction in mortality in patients with NYHA class II–IV congestive cardiac failure. Altogether 1052 patients were randomized to receive carvedilol (a vasodilating β-adrenoceptor blocker) or placebo. After 25 months mortality was 8.2 percent in the placebo group and 2.9 percent in the carvedilol-treated group (67 percent reduction). The benefit appears to reflect both a reduction in deaths due to progressive heart failure and to sudden death.

The use of ACE inhibitors in patients with congestive heart failure to alleviate symptoms and improve prognosis has been a major advance. Some of the large placebo-controlled studies have shown a reduc-

tion in sudden death among patients treated with ACE inhibitors.[62,63] Furthermore, the latter report demonstrated that the ACE inhibitor enalapril decreased the occurrence of baseline ventricular tachycardia at 3 months and the emergence of new ventricular tachycardia at 1 and 2 years.[64] These data raise the possibility that ACE inhibitors may have a direct antiarrhythmic effect in patients with congestive cardiac failure. However, this hypothesis has been difficult to prove and has not been supported by the much larger SOLVD trials.[64a] It has been reviewed by Pahor et al.[65]

PACEMAKER THERAPY IN CONGESTIVE HEART FAILURE

Symptomatic and clinical improvements using a pacemaker have been documented in patients with idiopathic dilated cardiomyopathy and end-stage heart failure.[66,67] Such improvements in the clinical state have also been reported in patients with congestive heart failure secondary to coronary artery disease.[68] It is interesting to note that the best improvements were obtained with short atrioventricular (AV) delays. In the study of Brecker et al.[69] maximal improvements in cardiac output were achieved with AV delays of 31 ms but were seen with delays as little as 6 ms. The mechanism proposed for this improvement was, first, that effectively by losing the atrial filling the inappropriate increase in preload was diminished and the heart would function on a more beneficial part of the Frank-Starling curve. Furthermore, mitral incompetence, which frequently occurs in patients in congestive heart failure paced with long AV intervals, is reduced, augmenting cardiac output. Whether these acute hemodynamic and clinical improvements are translated onto long-term benefits in survival and freedom from malignant arrhythmias remains unknown. Certainly, improvement in the size of the ventricular chambers and avoidance of bradycardia and asystole suggest that malignant ventricular arrhythmias and asytole could be avoided. In the study of Hochleitner et al.[70] 17 patients with critical congestive heart failure from idiopathic dilated cardiomyopathy were treated with dual chamber pacemakers programmed to short AV delays. The median survival time in these severely ill patients was 22 months. During this period, four patients received donor hearts, and nine experienced sudden death at home without a defined cause (Fig. 49-3). These data suggest that although there may be clinical improvements in the state of the patient the tendency to sudden, presumed arrhythmogenic death may not be avoided. One study suggested that the use of VDD pacing with short AV intervals did not improve the hemodynamic state of the patient, and indeed there was a decrease in stroke index with short AV delays. Nevertheless in patients with mitral regurgitation, the degree of regurgitation could be reduced with a consequent improve-

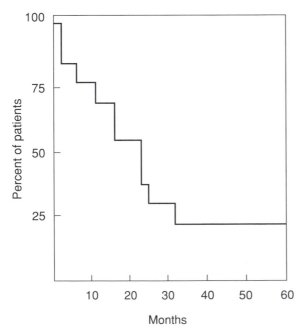

Fig. 49-3. Cumulative survival after DDD pacing for congestive heart failure during a 5-year follow-up. Four patients who received donor hearts are not included. (From Hochleitner et al.,[70] with permission.)

ment in forward flow. However, the ultimate benefits to the patient from pacing are being questioned.

IMPLANTABLE CARDIOVERTOR DEFIBRILLATORS IN CONGESTIVE HEART FAILURE

Early studies with implantable cardiovertor defibrillators (ICDs) demonstrated the efficacy of this device for termination of VF or VT. Comparisons of cohorts with historical controls suggest that this device reduces sudden death among patients who have been resuscitated from VF or hemodynamically unstable VT. Therefore it has been suggested that the use of an ICD may be of value in patients with congestive heart failure, where patients are at high risk of malignant ventricular arrhythmia and sudden cardiac death.

A number of questions must be addressed before the value of implantable defibrillators can be considered. First, can adequate defibrillation thresholds be achieved in patients with congestive heart failure? Data from animal studies demonstrate that the energy required for defibrillation increases as the left ventricular mass increases.[71,72] Thus if defibrillation thresholds were unacceptably high, ICDs would not be usable in patients with congestive heart failure. Several studies suggest that although there is a relation between the left ventricular ejection fraction and the defibrillation threshold, the magnitude of this effect is small. Kelley et al.[73] and Troupe et al.[74] found no relation between the defibrillation threshold and the left ventricular ejection fraction using epicardial electrodes, although an effect was observed by Leitch and Yee.[75] Similarly, the thresholds were not significantly related to the ejection fraction in the patients with endocardial systems who have been studied.[76] Thus if seems likely that the heart can be defibrillated adequately in patients with congestive heart failure.

Second, the question of whether patients with congestive heart failure are likely to have a greater mortality and morbidity during the operative procedure is important. The induction of ventricular fibrillation during defibrillation threshold testing impairs myocardial perfusion and can lead to a negative effect on myocardial contractility. Repeated inductions may result in hemodynamic deterioration and increased perioperative mortality. There is certainly some evidence that patients with impaired left ventricular ejection fractions fare less well at implantation of a defibrillator, but almost all of these data are with epicardial systems requiring a thoracotomy. Kim et al[77] reported that of 22 patients with ejection fractions below 30 percent who underwent ICF implantation 2 died during the perioperative period, whereas there was no mortality in the group of 24 patients who had ejection fractions above this value. Similarly, Jeevanaudam et al. reported that among 16 patients undergoing ICD implantation as a bridge to transplantation, 2 patients could not be discharged from hospital because of hemodynamic deterioration and the need for inotropic support.[78] The use of nonthoracotomy lead systems could reduce or remove at least some of this additional risk.

The third question that must be addressed is the effect of the ICD on the overall mortality of patients who have severely impaired cardiac function. By preventing sudden arrhythmic death, the ICD may merely prolong survival, allowing death to occur by progressive heart failure. Thus the gain in mean survival and the quality of survival may be so small that it is effectively negligible[79], thus the ICD could be expensive therapy for little net gain.

The fourth area of concern is whether the ICD can prevent death among patients with severely impaired ventricular function. The patient may develop incessant arrhythmia that cannot be effectively treated by the ICD or electromechanical dissociation where pacing therapy is ineffective. It appears from the data available that although the death rates from sudden cardiac death can be lowered by the use of ICDs (around 20 percent) total mortality remains substantial (around 30–40 percent).[80,81] Nevertheless there are considerable data that ICDs can prolong survival even in patients with severely depressed cardiac function. A study examining the time to first delivery of therapy with symptoms noted that 50 percent of patients with ejection fractions below 25 percent had a shock within 1 year, and 40 percent survived more than 3 years; those with better ejection fractions were less likely to receive a shock within the first year (40 percent), and more survived 3 years.[82]

CURRENT ICD TRIALS IN PATIENTS WITH IMPAIRED LEFT VENTRICULAR FUNCTION

Several controlled trials are now in progress or in the early planning stages to address the areas of concern noted above and evaluate whether the ICD is effective and cost-effective therapy in patients with impaired left ventricular function and congestive cardiac failure.

Secondary Prevention Trials

CARDIAC ARREST STUDY HAMBURG

The Cardiac Arrest Study Hamburg (CASH) compares ICDs versus drugs in the survivors of cardiac arrest. The patients would have suffered failed sudden death, with documented VT or VF unrelated to acute myocardial infarction. Patients are entered into the study within 3 months of the cardiac arrest, and those who demonstrate evidence of severe ischemia are revascularized. Subjects are randomized to receive either amiodarone 400–600 mg daily, metoprolol 12.5–300.0 mg daily, or ICD. The fourth limb of the study (propafenone 450–900 mg daily) was stopped because of its associated high mortality. The endpoints are total mortality, recurrence of cardiac arrest, and recurrence of ventricular tachycardia or new arrhythmias. This study includes many patients with impaired left ventricular function; and although this problem is not included in the specific endpoints of the study, it will be possible to examine the influence of the different treatment limbs on patients with impaired left ventricular function.

ANTIARRHYTHMICS VERSUS IMPLANTABLE DEFIBRILLATORS

The purpose of the Antiarrhythmics Versus Implantable Defibrillators (AVID) implantation versus two drugs known to improve survival in patients with primary ventricular arrhythmias. Patients presenting with primary VF, sustained VT with syncope, sustained VT with an ejection fraction of 40 percent or less, or sustained VT with blood pressure less than 80 mmHg and an ejection fraction of 40 percent or less who are less than 6 months from the primary event will be randomized. They will be subjected to an ICD or drug therapy, which will be sotalol, monitored by electrophysiologic study or Holter monitoring, or empiric amiodarone. The primary endpoints are total mortality; secondary endpoints are the cost benefits, mode of death, quality of life, and surgical morbidity.

CANADIAN IMPLANTABLE DEFIBRILLATOR STUDY

The Canadian Implantable Defibrillator Study (CIDS) compares survival of patients with malignant ventricular arrhythmias treated with either ICD or empiric amiodarone. Patients randomized will include those with VF, sustained VT and an ejection fraction of 35 percent or less, syncope with VT, or VT inducible at electrophysiologic study. They will receive either an ICD or amiodarone 300 mg daily. The endpoints are arrhythmic mortality and any deaths within 3 days of ICD implantation.

COMMENT

All the above studies are secondary prevention trials with use of the ICD in patients who have already suffered at least one arrhythmic event. A number of studies are in progress to examine patients who are at high risk of malignant arrhythmias but in whom no event has yet occurred.

Prophylactic Trials in Coronary Artery Disease

Two studies have been designed to examine the effectiveness of ICD implantation in patients after myocardial infarction who are defined at high risk of arrhythmic death. The risk stratification parameters used to identify these patients include the following.

1. History of complicated course of acute myocardial infarction, including pulmonary edema and heart failure
2. Left ventricular dysfunction [left ventricular ejection fraction (LVEF) less than 40 percent]
3. Complex ventricular ectopic beats, especially nonsustained VT on Holter monitoring
4. Positive signal-averaged ECG
5. Reduced heart rate variability
6. Depressed baroreceptor sensitivity

MULTICENTER AUTOMATIC DEFIBRILLATOR IMPLANTATION TRIAL

The primary hypothesis of the Multicenter Automatic Defibrillator Implantation Trial (MADIT) was that implantation of an ICD in high risk patients results in significant reduction in death when compared to the best conventional therapy, which is decided by the investigator. Secondary aims of MADIT were to evaluate the effect of ICDs on the first cardiac event, compare actual survival versus hypothetical survival in the ICD limb, assess operative morbidity

and mortality, and study the possible additive beneficial or detrimental effects of antiarrhythmic drug therapy when combined with ICD treatment.

The design of this trial is illustrated in (Fig. 49–4). Patients with evidence of a Q wave myocardial infarction and an ejection fraction of 35 percent or less were assessed for evidence of nonsustained VT by Holter monitoring and for inducibility at programmed ventricular stimulation of drug therapy. Patients were required to suffer hemodynamic compromise with the induced VT and these were then treated with procainamide (or quinidine, if intolerant to procainamide). If they were still inducible they were randomized to implantation of ICD or conventional therapy, which is selected by the managing physician. It has just been announced that this trial has been terminated prior to completion because of a favorable outcome in the ICD limb of the study. Most of the patients in the "conventional" arm were taking antiarrhythmic drugs such as amiodarone.

However, further details of the results are required in order to apply them to clinical practice. In particular, the effect of the requirement for failure of procainamide suppression and the type of antiarrhythmic therapy selected need to be assessed.

MULTICENTER UNSUSTAINED TACHYCARDIA TRIAL

The Multicenter Unsustained Tachycardia Trial (MUSTT) is not a direct study of the efficacy of the ICD, but device therapy is included in one of the limbs, offering an opportunity to examine the usefulness of ICD implantation. The primary hypothesis is that electrophysiologic (EP)-guided therapy can reduce sudden arrhythmic death or spontaneous episodes of sustained VT. Additional aims are quantiti-

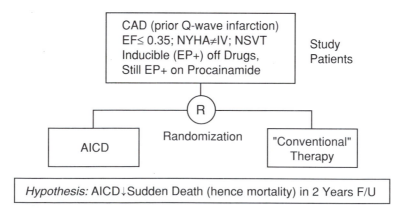

Fig. 49-4. Design of the Multicenter Automatic Defibrillator Implantation Trial (MADIT). CAD, coronary artery disease; EF, ejection fraction; NYHA, New York Heart Association; NSVT, nonsustained ventricular tachycardia; EP, electrophysiologic study; AICD, automatic implantable cardiovertor defibrillator; F/U, follow-up.

fication of sudden cardiac death risk in untreated patients with an LVEF of less than 40 percent with nonsustained VT who are inducible to sustained VT and confirmation of the low risk of sudden cardiac death in patients not inducible to sustained VT.

Patients with coronary artery disease, an LVEF or 40 percent or less, and non sustained VT (with or without a positive signal-averaged ECG) receive programmed electrical stimulation. Those who are not inducible are simply subjected to follow-up. Patients who are inducible are randomized to EP-guided therapy or to no antiarrhythmic therapy. The EP-guided group is further subdivided into patients who are drug responders (who are followed on the appropriate drug) and nondrug responders (who undergo ICD implantation). MUSTT has a minimum follow-up of 2 years for 900 patients and will have an 80 percent power to detect a 33 percent reduction in incidence of arrhythmic events with a type 1 error of 0.05 percent or less.

CABG Patch Trial

In patients with established cardiac ischemia, coronary revascularization can reduce mortality. In patients with a depressed LVEF, there may still be a 20–30 percent incidence of sudden cardiac death, which does not appear to be avoided by coronary revascularization. These patients form a large and important group in whom implantation of an ICD at the time of revascularization may prevent further mortality.

The hypothesis being tested in the CAGB Patch Trial is that implantation of an ICD in patients with established coronary artery disease can decrease the incidence of sudden cardiac death and symptomatic sustained VT. The criteria for entry into the study are as follows.

1. Male or female patients less than 80 years of age
2. Scheduled for coronary artery bypass grafting (CABG)
3. LVEF less than 36 percent
4. Filtered QRS duration more than 114 ms on signal-averaged ECG
5. Patient and physician consent

Patients have CABG as required and are then randomly assigned to receive an ICD or just have the bypass operation completed. Patients are then regularly followed by the study group who collaborate with the managing physician. Primary endpoints for the study are total mortality and serious arrhythmic recurrences. The trial will randomized around 1000 patients, and results are expected by the end of 1997.

CARDIOMYOPATHY TRIAL

Patients with dilated cardiomyopathy have a high incidence of sudden cardiac death, and there are few predictors of serious arrhythmias apart from the degree of left ventricular impairment. Implantation of a prophylactic ICD would therefore potentially be of value for extending the life of these patients or serving as a bridge to transplantation. Patients aged between 18 and 70 years with dilated cardiomyopathy with an LVEF of 30 percent or less and symptomatic heart failure (NYHA class II or III) are included in the Cardiomyopathy Trial. Subjects should not have had symptomatic ventricular arrhythmias prior to entry to the study. The significant exclusion criteria include the diagnosis known for more than 9 months, the presence of significant coronary artery disease, and if heart transplantation is expected within 6 months. Patients with class I or IV heart failure are also excluded. Subjects are randomized to receive an ICD or not receive a device. They are and followed for the primary endpoints, which are mortality and occurrence of serious arrhythmia.

DEFIBRILLATORS AS A BRIDGE TO TRANSPLANTATION STUDY

The Defibrillators as a Bridge to Transplantation (DEFIBRILLAT) study is currently in the planning stages. It will randomize patients with congestive heart failure awaiting cardiac transplantation to implantation of an ICD or not. The primary endpoint is mortality or serious cardiac arrhythmia.

COMMENT

All these studies have been set up during the era of thoracotomy and epicardial systems, with a procedural mortality much greater than that seen with the modern transvenous systems, which can be implanted in the pectoral position. A new study, SCDHeFT, about to start in the United States, compares empiric amiodarone, placebo (in a double-blind fashion), and an implanted pectoral transvenous ICD for patients with conventionally treated class 2 or 3 heart failure. The patients should have ejection fractions of 35 percent or less and no ventricular arrhythmia. The results of this exciting study are keenly awaited.

CONCLUSIONS

An enormous amount has been learned about the risks of impaired cardiac function resulting in congestive cardiac failure. The factors that can help to risk-stratify individuals with congestive cardiac failure have been extensively explored, and new treatment modalities have resulted in major and dramatic improvements in survival. The problem of sudden cardiac death in patients with heart failure persists, however, and advances in this area have perhaps not been so clear as those for the treatment of pump failure. Several treatment modalities hold considerable promise, and ongoing large-scale studies will provide at least some answers in this area.

REFERENCES

1. Kannel WB, Plehn JF, Cupples LA: Cardiac failure and sudden death in the Framingham study. Am Heart J 1988;115:869–875
2. Franciosa JA: Survival in men with severe chronic left ventricular failure due to either coronary artery disease or idiopathic dilated cardiomyopathy. Am J Cardiol 1983;51:831–836
3. Wilson JR, Schwartz JS, St. John Sutton M et al: Prognosis in severe heart failure. Relationship to hemodynamic measurement and ventricular ectopic activity. J Am Coll Cardiol 1983;2:403–410
4. Holmes J, Kubo S, Cody R, Kligfield P: Arrhythmias in ischemic and nonischemic dilated cardiomyopathy. Prediction of mortality by ambulatory electrocardiography. Am J Cardiol 1985;55:146–151
5. Meinertz TE, Hofmann T, Kasper W et al: Significance of ventricular arrhythmias in idiopathic cardiomyopathy. Am J Cardiol 1984;53:902–907
6. Von Olshausen K, Schafer A, Mehmel HC et al: Ventricular arrhythmia in dilated cardiomyopathy. Br Heart J 1984;51:195–201
7. Unverferth DV, Magorieu RD, Moeschberger MI et al: Factors influencing one-year mortality of dilated cardiomyopathy. Am J Cardiol 1984;54:147–152
8. Fuster V, Gersh BJ, Guiliani ER et al: The natural history of idiopathic dilated cardiomyopathy. Am J Cardiol 1981;47:525–531
9. Follansbee WP, Michelson EL, Morganroth: Non-sustained ventricular tachycardia in ambulatory patients: characteristics and association with sudden cardiac death. Ann Intern Med 1980;92:741–747
10. Schulze RA Jr, Strauss HW, Pitt B: Sudden death in the year following myocardial infarction. Relation of ventricular premature contractions in the late hospital phase and left ventricular ejection fraction. Am J Med 1977;62:192–199
11. Bigger TJ Jr, Fleiss JL, Kleiger R et al: The relationship between ventricular arrhythmias, left ventricular dysfunction and mortality in the two years after myocardial infarction. Circulation 1984;69:250–258
12. Stevenson WG, Stevenson LW, Middlekauff HR, Saxon LA: Sudden death prevention in patients with advanced ventricular dysfunction. Circulation 1993;88:2593–2561
13. Luu M, Stevenson WG, Stevenson LW et al: Diverse mechanisms of unexpected cardiac arrest in advanced heart failure. Circulation 1989;80:1675–1680
14. Wang Y, Scheinman MM, Chein WW et al: Patients with supraventricular tachycardia presenting with aborted sudden death. Incidence, mechanism and long-term follow-up. J Am Coll Cardiol 1991;18:1711–1719
15. Rockman HA, Juneau C, Chatterjee K, Rouleau JL: Long-term predictors of sudden and low output death in chronic congestive heart failure secondary to coronary artery disease. Am J Cardiol 1989;64:1344–1348
16. Romeo F, Pelliccia F, Cianfrocca C et al: Predictors of sudden death in idiopathic dilated cardiomyopathy. Am J Cardiol 1989;63:138–140
17. Middlekauff HR, Stevenson WG, Stevenson LW: Prognostic significance of atrial fibrillation in advanced heart failure. A study of 390 patients. Circulation 1991;84:40–48
18. Middlekauff HR, Stevenson WG, Stevenson LW, Saxon LA: Syncope in advanced heart failure. High risk of sudden death regardless of syncope origin. J Am Coll Cardiol 1993;21:110–116
19. Gradman A, Deedwania P, Cody R et al: Predictors of total mortality and sudden death in mild to moderate heart failure. J Am Coll Cardiol 1989;14:564–570
20. Keogh AM, Baron DW, Hickie JB: Prognostic guidelines in patients with dilated or ischemic dilated cardiomyopathy assessed for cardiac transplantation. Am J Cardiol 1990;65:903–908
21. De Bakker JMT, Van Capelle FJL et al: Re-entry as a cause of ventricular tachycardia in patients with chronic ischemic heart disease. Electrophysiologic and anatomic correlation. Circulation 1988;77:589–606
22. Milner PG, DiMarco JP, Lermann BB: Electrophysiological evaluation of sustained ventricular tachyarrhythmias in idiopathic dilated cardiomyopathy. PACE 1988;11:562–568
23. Tchou P, Jazzayeri M, Denker S et al: Transcatheter electrical ablation of right bundle branch. A method of treating macroreentrant ventricular tachycardia attributed to bundle branch re-entry. J Am Coll Cardiol 1986;78:246–257
24. Constantin L, Martins JB, Kienzle MG et al: Induced sustained ventricular tachycardia in nonischemic dilated cardiomyopathy. Dependence on clinical presentation and response to antiarrhythmic agents. PACE 1989;12:776–783
25. Poole JE, Mathisen TI, Kudenchuk et al: Long-term outcome in patients who survive out of hospital ventricular fibrillation and undergo electrophysiologic studies. Evaluation by electrophysiologic subgroups. J Am Coll Cardiol 1990;16:657–656
26. Poll DS, Marchlinski FE, Buxton AE, Josephson ME: Usefulness of programmed electrical stimulation in idiopathic dilated cardiomyopathy. Am J Cardiol 1986;58:992–997
27. Brembilla-Perrot B, Donetti J, Terrier de la Chaise A et al: Diagnostic value of ventricular stimulation in patients with idiopathic dilated cardiomyopathy. Am Heart J 1991;121:1124–1131
28. Stevenson WG, Middlekauff HM, Stevenson LW et al: Significance of aborted cardiac arrest and sustained ventricular tachycardia in patients referred for treatment therapy of advanced heart failure. Am Heart J 1992;124:123–130
29. Poole JE, Mathisen TL, Kudenchuk PJ et al: Long-term outcome in patients who survive out of hospital ventricular fibrillation and undergo electrophysiologic studies. Evaluation by electrophysiologic subgroups. J Am Coll Cardiol 1990;12:982–988

30. Massie BM, Conway M: Survival of patients with congestive heart failure: post, present, and future prospects. Circulation, suppl. IV 1987;75:11–19

31. Bigger JT, Fleiss JL, Kleiger R et al: The relationship among ventricular arrhythmias, left ventricular dysfunction, and mortality in the 2 years after myocardial infarction. Circulation 1984;69:250–258

32. Hallstrom AP, Bigger JT, Doen D et al: Prognostic significance of ventricular premature depolarizations measured 1 year after myocardial infarction in patients in the early postinfarction asymptomatic ventricular arrhythmia. J Am Coll Cardiol 1992;20:259–264

33. Maggioni AP, Zuanetti G, Franzosi G et al: Prevalence and prognostic significance of ventricular arrhythmias after acute myocardial infarction in the fibrinolytic era. Circulation 1993;87:312–322

34. De Maria R, Gavazzi A, Caroli A et al: Ventricular arrhythmias in dilated cardiomyopathy as an independent prognostic hallmark. Am J Cardiol 1992;69:1451–1457

35. Olshausen KV, Stein V, Schwartz F et al: Long-term prognostic significance of ventricular arrhythmias in idiopathic dilated cardiomyopathy. Am J Cardiol 1984;53:146–151

36. Stevenson WG, Weiss JN, Wiener I, Nademanee K: Slow conduction in the infarct scar. Relevance to occurrence, detection and ablation of ventricular reentry curcuits resulting from myocardial infarction. Am Heart J 1989;117:454–467

37. Denniss AR, Richards DA, Cody DV et al: Prognostic significance of ventricular tachycardia and fibrillation induced at programmed stimulation and delayed potentials detected on the signal averaged electrocardiogram of survivors of acute myocardial infarction. Circulation 1968;74:741–745

38. Bourke JP, Richards DAB, Ross DL et al: Routine programmed electrical stimulation in survivors of acute myocardial infarction for prediction of spontaneous ventricular tachyarrhythmias during follow-up results, optimal stimulation protocol and cost-effective screening. J Am Coll Cardiol 1991;18:780–788

39. Wilber DJ, Olshanksky B, Moran JF, Scanlon PJ: Electrophysiological testing and nonsustained ventricular tachycardia. Use and limitations in patients with coronary artery disease and impaired ventricular function. Circulation 1990;82:350–358

40. Stevenson WG, Stevenson LW, Weiss J, Tillisch JH: Inducible ventricular arrhythmias and sudden death during vasodilator therapy of severe heart failure. Am Heart J 1988;116:1447–1454

41. McClements BM, Adgey AAJ: Value of signal-averaged electrocardiography, radionuclide, Holter monitoring and clinical variables for prediction of arrhythmic events in survivors of acute myocardial infarction in the thrombolytic era. J Am Coll Cardiol 1993;21:1419–1427

42. Buckingham TA, Ghosh S, Homan SM et al: Independent value of signal averaged electrocardiography and left ventricular function in identifying patients with sustained ventricular tachycardia with coronary artery disease. Am J Cardiol 1987;159:568–571

43. Kulakowaki P, Malik M, Poloniecki J et al: Frequency versus time domain analysis of signal-averaged electrocardiograms. II. Identification of patients with ventricular tachycardia after myocardial infarction. J Am Coll Cardiol 1992;20:135–140

44. Kelen GJ, Henkin R, Stares AM et al: Spectral turbulence analysis of the signal-averaged electrocardiogram and its predictive accuracy for sustained monomorphic ventricular tachycardia. Am J Cardiol 1991;7:965–969

45. Denereaz D, Zimmerman M, Adamec R: Significance of ventricular late potentials in non-ischemic dilated cardiomyopathy. Eur Heart J 1992;14:895–901

46. Meinertz T, Treese N, Kasper W et al: Determinents of prognosis in idiopathic dilated cardiomyopathy. Am J Cardiol 1985;56:337

47. Ohnishi Y, Inoue T, Fukuzaki H: Value of the signal-averaged electrocardiogram as a predictor of sudden death in myocardial infarction and dilated cardiomyopathy. Jpn Circ J 1990;54:127–136

48. Packer M: Haemodynamic consequences of antiarrhythmic drug therapy in patients with chronic congestive heart failure. J Cardiovasc Electrophysiol 1991;25:240–247

49. Crawford MH, White DH, O' Rourke RA: Effects of oral quinidine on left ventricular performance in normal subjects and patients with congestive cardiomyopathy. Am J Cardiol 1979;44:714–718

50. Pratt CM, Eaton T, Francis M et al: The inverse relationship between baseline left ventricular ejection fraction and outcome of antiarrhythmic therapy. A dangerous imbalance in the risk-benefit ratio. Am Heart J 1989;118:433–440

51. Stanton MS, Prystowsky EN, Fineberg NA et al: Arrhythmogenic effects of antiarrhythmic drugs. A study of 506 patients treated for ventricular tachycardia of fibrillation. J Am Coll Cardiol 1989;14:209–215

52. Cardiac Arrhythmia Suppression Trial (CAST) Investigators: Preliminary report. Effect of encainide and flecainide on mortality in a randomized trial of arrhythmia suppression after myocardial infarction. N Engl J Med 1989;321:406–410

53. Hamer AWF, Arkles LB, John JA: Beneficial effects of low dose amiodarone in patients with congestive cardiac failure. A placebo-controlled trial. J Am Coll Cardiol 1989;14:1768–1774

54. Cairnes JA, Connolly SJ, Gent M, Roberts R: Post-myocardial infarction mortality in patients with ventricular premature depolarisations. Canadian Amiodarone Myocardial Infarction Arrhythmia Trial pilot study. Circulation 1991;84:550–557

55. Burkart F, Pfisterer M, Kiowski W et al: Effect of antiarrhythmic therapy on mortality in survivors of myocardial infarction with asymptomatic comples ventricular arrhythmias. Basel Antiarrhythmia Study of Infarct Survival (BASIS). J Am Coll Cardiol 1990;16:1171–1178

56. Ceremuzynski L, Kleczar E, Krzeminska-Pakula M et al: Effect of amiodarone on mortality after myocardial infarction. A double-blind placebo-controlled, pilot study. J Am Coll Cardiol 1992;20:1056–1062

57. Doval HC, Nul DR, Grancelli HO et al: Randomised trial of low-dose amiodarone in severe congestive heart failure. Lancet 1994;344:493–498

58. Singh SN, Fletcher RD, Fisher SG et al: Amiodarone in patients with congestive heart failure and asymptomatic ventricular arrhythmia. N Engl J Med 1995;333:77–82

58a. Massie BM, Fisher SG, Radford M et al: Effect of amiodarone on clinical status and left ventricular function in patients with congestive heart failure. Circulation 1996;93:2128–2134

59. EMIAT Investigators: The European Myocardial Infarct Amiodarone Trial (EMIAT). Am J Cardiol 1993; 72:95F–98F

60. CAMIAT Investigators: Canadian Amiodarone Myocardial Infarction Arrhythmia Trial (CAMIAT). Rationale and protocol. Am J Cardiol 1993;72:87F–84F

61. Packer M, Bristow MR, Cohn J et al: Effect of carvedilol on morbidity and mortality in patients with chronic heart failure. Circulation, suppl. I 1995;92:142

62. Newman TJ, Maskin CS, Dennick LG et al: Effects of captopril on survival in patients with heart failure. N Engl J Med 1996;331:1344–1355

63. Cohn JN, Johnson G, Ziesche S et al: A comparison of enalapril with hydralazine-isosorbide dinitrate in the treatment of chronic congestive heart failure. N Engl J Med 1991;325:303–310

64. Fletcher RD, Cintron GB, Johnson G et al: Enalapril decreases prevalence of ventricular tachycardia in patients with chronic congestive heart failure. Circulation, suppl. VI 1993;87:49–55

64a. The SOLVD Investigators: Effect of enalapril on survival in patients with reduced left ventricular ejection fractures and congestive heart failure. N Engl J Med 1991;325:293–302

65. Pahor M, Gambassi G, Carbonin P: Antiarrhythmic effects of ACE inhibitors. A matter of faith or reality? Cardiovasc Res 1994;28:173–182

66. Hochleitner H, Hortnagl H, Fridrich L et al: Usefulness of physiologic dual-chamber pacing in drug-resistant idiopathic cardiomyopathy. Am J Cardiol 1992; 70:1320–1325

67. Kataoka H: Hemodynamic effect of physiological dual chamber pacing in a patient with end-stage dilated cardiomyopathy. PACE 1991;14:1330–1335

68. Auricchio A, Sommariva L, Salo RW, Scarfuri A, Chiariello L: Improvement of cardiac function in patients with severe congestive heart failure and coronary artery disease by dual chamber pacing with shortened AV delay. PACE 1993;16:2034–2043

69. Brecker SJD, Xiao HB, Sparrow J, Gibson DG: Effects of dual-chamber pacing with short atrioventricular delay in dilated cardiomyopathy. Lancet 1992;340: 1308–1312

70. Hochleitner M, Hortnagl H, Hortnagl H, Fridrich L, Gschnitzner F: Long-term efficacy of physiologic dual-chamber pacing in the treatment of end-stage idiopathic dilated cardiomyopathy. Am J Cardiol 1992;70: 1320–1325

71. Chapman PD, Sagar KB, Wetherbee JN, Troup PJ: Relationship of left ventricular mass to defibrillation threshold for the implantable defibrillator. A combined clinical and animal study. Am Heart J 1987;114: 274–278

72. Dorian P, Wang MJ: Defibrillation current and impedance are determinants of defibrillation energy requirements. PACE 1988;11:1960–2001

73. Kelly PA, Cannom DS, Garan H et al: The automatic implantable cardioverter-defibrillator. Efficacy, complications and survival in patients with malignant ventricular arrhythmias. J Am Coll Cardiol 1988;11: 1278–1286

74. Troupe PJ, Chapman PD, Olinger GN, Kleinman LH: The implantable defibrillation. Relation of defibrillation lead configuration and clinical variables to defibrillation threshold. J Am Coll Cardiol 1985;6: 1315–1321

75. Leitch JW, Yee R: Predictors of defibrillation efficacy in patients undergoing epicardial defibrillator implantation. J Am Coll Cardiol 1993;21:1632–1637

76. Bardy GH, Hofer B, Johnson G et al: Implantable transvenous cardioverter-defibrillators. Circulation 1993;87:1152–1168

77. Kim SG, Fisher JD, Choue CW et al: Influence of left ventricular function on outcome of patients treated with implantable defibrillators. Circulation 1992;85: 1304–1310

78. Jeevanandam V, Bielefld MR, Auteri JS et al: The implantable defibrillator. An electronic bridge to cardiac transplantation. Circulation, suppl. II 1991;86: 276–279

79. Kim SG: Implantable defibrillator therapy. Does it really prolong life? How can we prove it? Am J Cardiol 1993;71:1213–1218

80. Akhtar M, Avitall B, Jazayeri M et al: Role of implantable cardiovertor defibrillator therapy in the management of high risk patients. Circulation, suppl. I 1992; 85:131–139

81. Mehta D, Saksena S, Krol RB: Survival of implantable cardiovertor defibrillator recipients. Role of left ventricular function and its relationship to device use. Am Heart J 1992;124:1608–1614

82. Levine JH, Mellits ED, Baumgardner RA et al: Predictors of first discharge and subsequent survival in patients with automatic implantable cardiovertor defibrillators. Circulation 1991;84:558–566

50 Anticoagulants and Antiplatelet Agents

John G. F. Cleland

Thromboembolic events are among the most potentially catastrophic complications of heart failure and are not uncommon. Nonetheless, the question of whether to use prophylactic anticoagulant or antithrombotic therapy in these patients remains unresolved and virtually unstudied.

Currently aspirin is one of the most widely prescribed agents among patients with heart failure, yet there is little evidence that it is effective and some indication that it may adversely affect their hemodynamics and prognosis. Although there is more evidence that anticoagulants may be beneficial to heart failure patients, it comes from clinical trials with major design flaws[1-3] and populations quite different from current patient populations. Prescription databases in the United Kingdom suggest that fewer than 0.5 percent of patients with heart failure receive anticoagulants. A survey of British cardiologists suggested that only 3 percent used anticoagulants routinely for heart failure patients without contraindications.[4] It is likely that anticoagulants are used more liberally in the United States, but they were not frequently used in the large clinical trials (Table 50-1).

Although antiplatelet and anticoagulant agents have been widely advocated in the past, current European and American guidelines clearly state that no recommendation to use either group of agents can be made on the basis of current data.[5-7] This judgment applies equally to patients with and without coronary disease as the cause of heart failure. The American guideline specifically suggested that "a randomized controlled trial is greatly needed to evaluate the effectiveness of antiplatelet therapy, low dose anticoagulation, and full anticoagulation" and stated that until then both "anticoagulation and antiplatelet therapy should be discouraged for patients in sinus rhythm."[7] A joint UK–US trial has already started to compare warfarin, aspirin, and no antithrombotic therapy in a randomized prospective open-label mortality study.[8]

RATIONALE FOR USE OF ANTITHROMBOTIC AGENTS FOR HEART FAILURE

The goals of antithrombotic therapy for heart failure, like other treatments, is to maintain quality of life and prolong survival. Because thromboembolic events can interfere with both objectives, their prevention is a reasonable therapeutic goal unless it entails excess risk or unwarranted cost.

An important issue in this regard is the frequency of clinically important thromboembolism. Clinical trials have shown that cerebrovascular events may now be relatively uncommon in patients with heart failure, although early clinical trials[1-3] suggested that stroke was a common mode of death of patients with heart failure (Table 50-2).[9-16] This difference may reflect the changing etiology of heart failure, better management of atrial fibrillation, or lower rates of recognition due to the lower autopsy rates in recent studies. Indeed, one study using magnetic resonance imaging has suggested a high incidence of occult cerebral infarction associated with cortical atrophy among patients with moderately severe [median New York Heart Association (NYHA) class III and ejection fraction 28 percent] dilated cardiomyop-

Table 50-1. Use of Antiplatelet and Anticoagulant Agents in Heart Failure Trials

Trial	No. of pts.	Mean age (years)	Atrial fibrillation (%)	Antiplatelet agents (%)	Anticoagulants (%)
V-HeFT-I	632	58	15	13[a]	13 (31)[b]
CONSENSUS	253	71	50	?	33.5
V-HeFT-II	804	61	15	27[a]	21 (41)[b]
SOLVD Treatment	2569	61	10	34	16
Prevention	4228	59	4	54	12

[a] Reported as a percentage of patient-years exposure; corresponding figures for anticoagulants were 14 and 12 percent in V-HeFT-I and V-HeFT-II, respectively.
[b] In patients with atrial fibrillation.

athy.[17] Cortical atrophy correlated with impairment in cognitive test performance. Thus cerebral injury may occur commonly and insidiously and might have serious adverse effects on the quality of life.

Clinically recognized peripheral embolism, excluding cerebral embolism, is uncommon in studies of heart failure. In the past, pulmonary embolism was a common mode of death in hospitalized patients,[1–3] but it is less frequently recognized now. Whether this reduction reflects shorter periods of enforced bed rest, the use of heparin prophylaxis for deep venous thrombosis, or poorer current recognition related to low autopsy rates is unclear. Older series frequently atributed sudden death to pulmonary embolism found at postmortem examination but not recognized during life. The current fashion, supported by less solid evidence, is that sudden death is usually arrhythmic in patients with heart failure.

The lack of evidence that cerebral, peripheral, or pulmonary embolic events are currently a major contributor to morbidity and mortality in patients with heart failure is one reason why anticoagulants are not used more widely. However, there are alternative reasons to use antithrombotic agents. Myocardial infarction is not infrequent in patients with heart failure due to coronary disease, contributes to progression of ventricular dysfunction and symptoms, and is attended by a subsequent mortality rate of about 70 percent at 3 months.[18] There are data on the effect of both antiplatelet and anticoagulant agents on recurrent infarction and death after an initial infarct, although the evidence for benefit is less conclusive and more controversial than is often appreciated.[8,19]

Recurrent infarction precedes death in about 20 percent of patients with heart failure due to coronary disease and an even higher proportion of deaths

Table 50-2. Incidence of Embolic Events in Landmark Studies of Heart Failure

Trial and NYHA Class	No. of pts	Follow-up (years)	AF (%)	CVA (%)	PTE (%)	Other (%)	Total (%)
V-HeFT-I (NYHA II-III)	632	2.3	15	4.1 (1.8)	0.8	0.8	5.7 (2.5)
CONSENSUS (NYHA III-IV)	**253**	**0.5**	**50**	**2.3[a] (4.6)**	**?**	**?**	**?**
V-HeFT-II (NYHA II-III)	804	2.6	15	4.7 (1.8)	0.7	0.2	5.6 (2.2)
SOLVD—combined (NYHA I-III)	6797	3.3	6	3.8 (1.2)	0.7	1.1	5.6 (1.7)
AIRE (post-MI)	1986	1.3	?	2.7 (2.1)	?	?	?
PROMISE (NYHA III-IV)	**1088**	**0.5**	**?**	**4.0 (3.5)**	**?**	**?**	**?**

Abbreviations: AF, atrial fibrillation; CVA, cerebral vascular accident; PTE, peripheral thromboembolism.
Rows in boldface type identify the two studies of patients with the most severe heart failure; they also have the highest annual incidence of stroke.
The SAVE study was not included as has not reported a stroke rate.
The numbers in parentheses represent the calculated annual risk, except for the PROMISE study where it is the reported annual rate of strokes.
[a] Only fatal strokes were reported, which may be only one-third of the total rate of stroke.

among those who also have angina.[18] Coronary thrombosis is a frequent postmortem finding in patients dying suddenly,[20,21] and sudden death accounts for half or more of all deaths during heart failure. Trials suggest 30–50 percent lower mortality among patients with coronary disease and heart failure who undergo revascularization, a procedure that may minimize the effects of coronary occlusion.[22] This fact further supports the view that coronary vascular events are an important contributor to prognosis in patients with heart failure.

Although the frequency of peripheral thromboembolic events may be lower than previously thought, they are still likely to be an important source of morbidity and mortality in the heart failure population and may be responsible for many sudden deaths. It is more certain that warfarin, rather than aspirin, has the potential to reduce stroke, pulmonary embolism, and myocardial infarction.[19]

THROMBOTIC SUBSTRATE OF HEART FAILURE

A variety of factors associated with heart failure predispose to thrombosis, including the classic triad of vascular pathology, increased coagulability, and impaired flow (Table 50-3).

Endothelium

Endothelial dysfunction is a loose but often used term for a wide range of abnormalities, although it is most popularly applied to the endothelium's capacity to synthesize nitric oxide. Endothelial production of nitric oxide and prostacyclin may be important to reducing platelet adhesion and activation; if there is deficient production it could result in an increased tendency to thrombosis.[23,24] However, published evidence is conflicting on whether endothelial nitric oxide production is impaired during heart failure. Indeed the greater vasoconstriction in patients with heart failure than in normal subjects after the administration of L-NMMA, an inhibitor of nitric oxide synthesis, suggests that the basal activity of this vasodilator may be increased.[25] Similarly, inhibitors of prostaglandin synthesis cause vasoconstriction during heart failure, most notably in patients with severe heart failure and hyponatremia.[26] Thus, if anything, there appears to be up-regulation of endothelial defense mechanisms against thrombosis in patients with heart failure. This point is noteworthy, as aspirin may potentially interfere with increased prostacyclin production during heart failure.

The endothelium is the site of production of von Willebrand factor, the plasma concentrations of which are elevated in patients with heart failure.[27,28] Plasma concentrations of von Willebrand factor have been related to those of endothelin-1,[28] another endothelial product that is increased during heart failure. Both endothelin-1 and von Willebrand factor correlate with pulmonary vascular resistance during heart failure, suggesting a link between endothelial function and hemodynamic state.[27,29] Both endothelin-1 and von Willebrand factor could promote hemostasis.[30]

Similarly, other endothelial products, such as endogenous tissue plasminogen activator (tPA) and prothrombotic plasminogen activator inhibitor (PAI-1), are probably increased during heart failure.[31,32]

In summary, the available evidence points to endothelial hyperactivity rather than impairment. Both endothelial promoters and antagonists of coagulation are increased, and it appears important not to inadvertently alter this balance adversely.

Atheroma

Endothelial characteristics and function are not likely to be uniform in patients with heart failure. Endothelial heterogeneity is well recognized in the presence of atherosclerotic disease. Areas affected by atherosclerosis fail to produce nitric oxide and prostacyclin in response to the usual stimuli, resulting in inappropriate vasoconstriction and increased thrombotic potential. Ulcerated atheromatous plaques may be denuded of endothelium and be particularly vulnerable to thrombosis. It is likely that cata-

Table 50-3. Factors Contributing to Altered Thromboembolic Risk in Heart Failure

Parameter	Changes in heart failure
Vessel or chamber wall	Altered endothelial function, (e.g. nitric oxide, prostacyclin, von Willebrand factor, endothelin)
	Atheroma
Coagulability	Platelet activation
	Thrombin activation
	Increased fibrinolysis
Flow	Increased plasma viscosity
	Low cardiac output
	Cardiac chamber volume and shape
	Atrial fibrillation

strophic vascular events are related more to these areas of the vessel wall.

Coagulability

Several studies have shown that patients with heart failure have increased plasma concentrations of β-thromboglobulin, a marker of platelet activation.[25,33] Increased plasma concentrations of fibrinopeptide A and thrombin–antithrombin III (TAT) complexes, markers of the action of thrombin on fibrinogen, have also been demonstrated.[34] Plasma concentrations of endothelial procoagulant (vWf and PAI-1) and fibrinolytic factors (tPA) or products (D-dimer) are also increased during heart failure.[28,31–34]

Increased fibrinolysis in patients with heart failure is a result of increased fibrin formation and reflects the need to balance production and clearance of fibrin. Treatment with anticoagulants should reduce fibrin deposition; secondarily, the rate of fibrinolysis should fall. This reaction has been demonstrated[35,36] with warfarin, reducing not only TAT but also D-dimer concentrations.

Patients with atrial fibrillation and heart failure are at particularly high risk for thromboembolism, but it does not appear to be due to great changes in hemostatic factors.[36] The risk of left atrial thrombus developing does not appear to be related to increased fibrinogen or plasma viscosity in patients with dilated cardiomyopathy, although rheologic markers do correlate with the appearance of spontaneous echocardiographic contrast.[37,38] Cardioversion or anticoagulation can reduce D-dimer levels in this setting,[36] suggesting that altered flow is the primary factor. Hemostatic abnormalities may not be apparent in patients with heart failure and well preserved left ventricular systolic function in the absence of atrial fibrillation.[36]

It is unclear to what extent disturbance of hemostatic factors in heart failure patients reflects sluggish blood flow in cardiac chambers or blood vessels, abnormal endothelial activity, or neuroendocrine activation.[28] Angiotensin II increases plasma concentrations of PAI-1, and bradykinin increases those of tPA, the latter at least in the presence of an angiotensin-converting enzyme (ACE) inhibitor.[31,39] ACE inhibitors reduce plasma levels of tPA and may have beneficial effects on platelet aggregation.[39] The importance of the effects of ACE inhibitors on vascular events and their ability to correct disordered hemostasis is just beginning to be explored.[40]

In summary, hypercoagulability in patients with heart failure is balanced by an increase in fibrinolysis. Elevations of endogenous inhibitors of plasminogen, as may occur in a circadian fashion or under the influence of angiotensin II, could trigger vascular occlusion. Similarly, increased platelet activation may be held in check by increased endothelial prostacyclin production. Care must be taken not to impair those endogenous factors holding the thrombotic process in check.

Blood Flow and Viscosity

Blood flow depends on the size of the vessel or chamber, the shape and function of the cardiac chambers,[41] the resistance in the vascular bed, and the viscosity of blood. Peripheral blood flow may be normal at rest until heart failure is advanced, and it may not play a major role in thrombosis risk until the condition is advanced.

Plasma viscosity is increased in heart failure due to an increase in fibrinogen.[28] The hematocrit is not markedly different in heart failure and control subjects. Increased whole blood viscosity can be explained by increases in plasma viscosity. The importance of changes in viscosity to changes in flow has not been explored in heart failure.

Chamber Volume and Shape

It is generally thought that patients with atrial fibrillation, those with severe left ventricular dysfunction, and those with large left atrial size are at an increased risk of thromboembolic events.[41,42] However, the data are conflicting or inadequate to confirm some of these assumptions. The atrial appendages, sites of the most marked blood stasis, are particularly prone to the development of thrombus.

Several investigators have suggested that left ventricular thrombus is related to the severity of ventricular dysfunction in patients with dilated cardiomyopathy, but this idea has not been confirmed in groups of patients with a heterogeneous etiology for ventricular dysfunction.[43,44] Patients with ventricular thrombus are probably at increased risk of vascular events, although agreement is far from universal.[43,45,46] The V-HeFT studies suggested that those patients with the lowest ejection fraction and exercise performance were at greatest risk of embolism, but neither factor was sufficiently discriminating to be of clinical use.[12] Data were recorded at baseline, but the events may have occurred years later and ventricular dysfunction and heart failure may have progressed, weakening any relation between clinical status, cardiac structure, and outcome. The incidence of stroke is much higher in studies of patients with end-stage heart failure, such as CONSENSUS and PROMISE.

Atrial Fibrillation

Atrial fibrillation is a common and important aspect of heart failure (Table 50-2).[10–16] The landmark trials probably underestimate the proportion of patients with heart failure and atrial fibrillation for at least three reasons. First, it is difficult to estimate the ejection fraction in the presence of atrial fibrillation, and these patients may be excluded from studies with entry criteria based on this measurement. Trials such as CONSENSUS, which did not require an ejection fraction for entry, recruited a higher proportion of patients with atrial fibrillation. Second, atrial fibrillation is more frequent among elderly patients with heart failure. Again the CONSENSUS study, where the mean age of the patients was 71 years, had a much higher frequency of atrial fibrillation. Lastly, atrial fibrillation may be more common in heart failure patients with normal systolic function, and these patients were excluded from most of the trials.

In a multivariate analysis of the Stroke Prevention Fibrillation (SPAF) study, uncontrolled heart failure was the single most powerful clinical marker of additional risk for thromboembolism in patients with atrial fibrillation (Table 50-4), although the association with chronic well controlled heart failure was weaker.[47] An interaction between heart failure and atrial fibrillation on thromboembolic risk has not been clearly demonstrated in other studies of atrial fibrillation. In studies of heart failure, atrial fibrillation has not been associated with a greater risk of stroke, although this finding probably reflects the greater likelihood of the patients having been treated with warfarin.[12,48] Patients with atrial fibrillation and heart failure may be at an increased risk of sudden death, and they have had a worse overall prognosis in some but not all studies[48,49] (Table 50-5).

Ventricular or Atrial Thrombus

Echocardiographic studies have suggested that a substantial number of patients with heart failure have left ventricular mural thrombi. Ciaccheri et al. demonstrated that 14 of 126 (11%) of patients with dilated cardiomyopathy had thrombus demonstrated at least once on serial echocardiography (more than 1000 examinations had been performed over 41 months).[50] Patients with thrombi were given anticoagulants, and none had an embolic episode. The rate of embolism in the patients without thrombi was 1.4 per 100 patient-years. It is not clear whether the result reflects the low embolic potential of ventricular thrombus or the efficacy of anticoagulants. Nandra et al.[51] reported similar results. Katz et al.[52] found left ventricular thrombi in 50 percent of patients with NYHA class III heart failure, and these patients had an embolic rate of 5.3 per 100 patient-years of follow-up—more than three times the risk of the general heart failure population studied. No embolus occurred among those without echocardiographic evidence of thrombus over 2 years of follow-up. Roberts et al., in a pathologic study,[53] noted that 60 percent of patients with left ventricular thrombus had evidence of systemic embolism.

Transesophageal echocardiography has demonstrated that 10 percent or more of patients with

Table 50-4. Thromboembolic Risk in Placebo Groups of Randomized Studies on Atrial Fibrillation

Study	No. of pts.	Age (years)	Patient subset	Event rate per year (%)	Relative risk
AFASAK	336	74	All cases	6	
			Prior MI	14	2.5
SPAF	568	67	All cases	6	
			HF any	10	1.9
			HF severe	18	3.2
BAATAF	208	68	All cases	3	NA
CAFA	191	68	All cases	5	NA
SPINAF	265	67	All cases	4	NA
EAFT[a]	378	70	All cases	19	NA

Abbreviations: MI, myocardial infarction; HF, heart failure; NA, not available.
[a] EAFT was a secondary prevention study in patients who already had had a stroke.

Table 50-5. Relation Between Atrial Fibrillation, Stroke, and Death in Studies of Heart Failure

Study	Incidence (%)			
	Stroke	Thromboembolism	Death	P
V-HeFT[12]				
No AF	5.0	5.6	48	
AF	3.0	3.4	37	NS
Katz[52]				
No AF				
AF				
Middlekauf[48]				
No AF	?	6.0	29	0 <
AF	?	8.0	48	0.01

atrial fibrillation have an atrial thrombus, and its is likely that it is even more frequent in those who also have heart failure.[38] The prevalence of atrial thrombus in patients with heart failure in sinus rhythm is unknown.

The embolic potential of ventricular and atrial thrombus remains controversial; sessile thrombus may rarely cause embolism, but the risk from thrombus that is mobile or protrudes into the ventricular cavity may be higher.[54] As freshly formed thrombus is most likely to embolize, serial echocardiography may be limited in its potential to detect a threatening thrombus.[55,56] Indeed some have suggested that urgent heparin therapy is required in any patient with atrial fibrillation, as oral anticoagulation is too slow.[57]

USE OF ASPIRIN

There is no evidence that aspirin as a single agent is of any use for preventing embolic events associated with heart failure or other conditions. The principal indication for the use of aspirin in heart failure patients is for its potential to reduce coronary vascular events, if such benefit could be shown in this population. Evidence in this regard is conflicting, and this question assumes particular importance in heart failure patients because of the potential for aspirin to interfere with the beneficial effects of ACE inhibitors. Therefore this subject must be reviewed in some depth.

Aspirin for Ischemic Heart Disease

The most common underlying cause of heart failure in patients under the age of 75 years in industrialized societies is ischemic heart disease.[58] The Aspirin

Trialists have suggested that the benefits of aspirin in patients with coronary artery disease were "extraordinarily definitely established" based on a meta-analysis[59,60] including the ISIS-2 study, a study that lasted only 35 days and which was conducted in patients who had suffered an acute myocardial infarction. ISIS-2 is the only trial of aspirin to show a significant reduction in mortality among patients with ischemic heart disease.

The disparity between ISIS-2 and the other postinfarction trials suggests that the benefits of aspirin regarding mortality may be confined to the period immediately following myocardial infarction, a view supported by several long-term trials.[61–64] The later the patients were randomized after infarction, the less positive were the results of the trials. Similarly, this discordance raises the question of whether postinfarction aspirin therapy should be continued long term or reserved for the first few weeks after myocardial infarction.

Six substantial trials[63–68] initiated the use of aspirin more than 1 month after infarction. The GAMIS trial lost about one-third of patients to follow-up and should be discounted as a valid study. Aspirin did not reduce mortality in the remaining five studies. Even the effect on vascular deaths was small (Table 50-6), compared for instance to the effect of ACE inhibitors or β-blockers after infarction.[19,69] Data from the two remaining long-term studies[61,62] that recruited patients within 1 month of infarction showed a mortality of those on aspirin at 152 (10.4%) versus 192 on placebo (12.8%) (P = NS) over an average follow-up of 1 year, suggesting that 24 lives were saved per 1000 patient-years of treatment. Scrutiny of the mortality curves of these two studies supports the view that the benefits of aspirin may be confined to the first 2–3 months after myocardial infarction. Aspirin did appear to reduce the incidence of nonfa-

Table 50-6. Effects of Aspirin on Mortality in Late-Initiation Long-Term Studies After Myocardial Infarction

Treatment (5 studies)	Total deaths (no.)	Vascular deaths (no.)	Nonvascular deaths (no.)	Nonfatal myocardial infarction (no.)	Nonfatal stroke (no.)
Controls (n = 5667)	494 (8.72%)	434 (7.66%)	60 (1.06%)	457 (8.06%)	109 (1.92%)
Aspirin (n = 6880)	602 (8.75%)	513 (7.46%)	89 (1.29%)	426 (6.19%)	82 (1.19%)
Events prevented per 1000 treated	−0.3	+2.0	−2.3	+18.7	+7.3
Events prevented per year per 1000 treated	−0.1	+0.7	−0.8	+6.2	+2.4

Numbers are taken from the 1988 meta-analysis.[4] Negative numbers indicate an excess of events in aspirin-treated groups. Average duration of trials was approximately 3 years. Note that the numbers randomized to the aspirin and control groups were unequal.

tal stroke and nonfatal myocardial infarction. The effect of aspirin on morbidity alone might support its long-term use, but again the effect on nonfatal events was not large.

The AMIS and PARIS-II[64,65] trials both reported the influence of baseline characteristics on outcome (Table 50-7). The AMIS trial, the largest aspirin study ever conducted in terms of patient-years exposure, showed a trend to increased mortality with aspirin in most subgroups studied. Differences in baseline characteristics may have biased the AMIS study against aspirin, but the failure of aspirin to show significant benefit even among groups stratified for risk does not support this conjecture.[65] The PARIS-II trial showed an overall trend to benefit with aspirin, but the trend was in the opposite direction among patients with heart failure or major ventricular dysfunction. Long-term use of aspirin in patients with coronary disease and well preserved ventricular function is supported by data from the Swedish SAPAT study where only patients with angina but not myocardial infarction were studied.[70] Overall these data suggest that long-term aspirin may indeed be helpful in patients with well preserved ventricular function but possibly harmful in high risk patients with major ventricular damage. Most of the long-term studies of aspirin used doses in excess of 900 mg/day, with 300 mg/day being the lowest dose

Table 50-7. Effects of Aspirin on Mortality in Patients With and Without Evidence of Heart Failure After Myocardial Infarction

Condition	PARIS II (%)		AMIS (%)	
	Placebo	Aspirin	Placebo	Aspirin
Total mortality	7.3 (114/1565)	7.1 (111/1565)	9.7 (219/2267)	10.9 (246/2267)
Heart failure				
Absent	NA	NA	7.8	7.9
Present	NA	NA	21.2	23.7
NYHA				
Class I	5.8	4.9	7.3	8.6
Class II	8.9	9.4	14.3	14.3
First infarct	6.2	5.9	8.1	9.2
> One infarct	13.5	13.5	19.6	19.2
Digoxin				
No	6.3	5.5	7.4	8.1
Yes	13.7	15.6	21.0	20.8

Abbreviations: NYHA, New York Heart Association; NA, not available.
NB: NYHA class I was attributed to all patients after myocardial infarction who did not exhibit features of heart failure.

used.[59,60] Although these higher doses may have produced adverse effects that possibly obscured a benefit of aspirin at the lower doses used today, there are no data to show a long-term benefit from aspirin at such low doses. Comparative trials in patients at risk of stroke have not shown any major difference in benefit or harm with doses ranging from 75 to 1200 mg/day,[65,66] but neither do the studies conducted with lower doses of aspirin show a clear reduction in coronary events in this population when compared to a placebo.[71,72]

Although aspirin appears inexpensive, treating the side effects may not be. Patients taking aspirin are at a fourfold increased risk of gastrointestinal hemorrhage.[73] Aspirin may account for one-third of all major gastrointestinal hemorrhage in subjects over 60 years of age[74] (those most likely to have heart failure). Currently for every 1000 patients taking aspirin, about two each year have a major gastrointestinal bleed, leading to death in 10 percent of cases.[73,74] A considerably greater number of patients have aspirin-induced dyspepsia. Prophylaxis and treatment of dyspepsia with H_2-antagonists or omeprazole and hospital management of hemorrhage is expensive. Several of the long-term aspirin trials also noted that patients taking high dose aspirin had higher serum urea and uric acid levels.[64,65] As renal function is often precarious in patients with heart failure, this point is of some concern. The effect of low doses of aspirin on renal function in large long-term trials is unknown.

Evidence for Aspirin Benefit from Large Heart Failure Trials

There is no evidence that aspirin has an effect on mortality in patients with heart failure because the issue has not been addressed. The V-HeFT studies suggest a reduction in thromboembolic events, not including myocardial infarction, with aspirin; but this study was not a randomized comparison.[12] Retrospective analysis of the SOLVD and PROMISE trials showed that strokes were no less common in patients with heart failure who were taking aspirin.[15,16]

Interaction Between Aspirin and ACE Inhibitors?

All the long-term studies on the effects of aspirin on mortality after infarction were conducted before treatment with ACE inhibitors was commonplace. The question of a potentially harmful interaction between ACE inhibitors and aspirin was raised by the SOLVD study finding that among those taking aspirin enalapril produced no benefit in terms on mortality.[75,75a] When the same issue was examined in post-infarction ACE inhibitor trials, there was a trend toward less benefit from ACE inhibition among those taking aspirin, with the exception of the SAVE trial.[69,76] Even the SAVE trial showed a trend toward less benefit on the combined morbidity and mortality outcome among those taking captopril and aspirin.[77] Although an interaction between aspirin and enalapril on mortality in the SOLVD trial was observed, there was no evidence of an adverse interaction between aspirin and enalapril in terms of recurrent coronary events. It should be noted that the interaction observed are with baseline therapy.[18]

Aspirin inhibits the production of prostaglandins. The prostaglandins are a diverse group of compounds; some are vasodilators and antithrombotic (e.g., prostacyclin), and others are vasoconstrictors and prothrombotic (e.g., thromboxanes). Production of vasodilator prostaglandins appears to be an important counterregulatory pathway in patients with heart failure,[26] reflecting extensive dysfunctional endothelium. Plasma concentrations of vasodilator prostaglandins are increased proportional to activation of the renin-angiotensin system and the serum sodium concentration.[26] Thus the response of prostaglandin synthetic pathways to inhibitors in patients with heart failure may be different from that in patients with coronary artery disease and good ventricular function.

The overall effect of ACE inhibitors on prostaglandin synthesis and platelet aggregability remains controversial, but aspirin and ACE inhibitors could exert similar effects in a number of ways. ACE inhibitors may reduce the degradation of bradykinin and thereby enhance production of prostaglandins.[78] Angiotensin II can also stimulate the production of vasodilator prostaglandins; and ACE inhibition, by reducing angiotensin II production, could also theoretically reduce renal prostaglandin synthesis.[79,80] ACE inhibitors may also reduce production of thromboxanes, much the same as aspirin.[81] Platelet activation generates angiotensin II, which may enhance local vasoconstriction, although it is not clear if this sequence can be prevented by ACE inhibitors.[82] Angiotensin II may, in turn, enhance thromboxane-induced arterial contraction.[83].

Administration of indomethacin to patients with heart failure results in vasoconstriction and a fall in cardiac output, renal blood flow, and glomerular filtration rate.[26,84] Effects are more prominent among patients with hyponatremia.[26] High doses of aspirin cause urinary sodium retention, but it is not known if low doses exert similar effects on salt and water metabolism in patients with heart failure.[85] Inhibition of prostaglandin synthesis may cause hyponatremia,[86] an ominous prognostic sign for heart failure.[87] Several studies have addressed the interaction of aspirin and other inhibitors of prostaglandin synthesis on cardiovascular function in patients with heart failure. Although the results are conflicting, there is sufficient evidence of an adverse interaction to give rise to concern, even though an adverse renal or hemodynamic effect of aspirin in doses lower than 300 mg/day has not been demonstrated.[8,87–92]

Baur et al.[80] studied the effects of aspirin and enalapril on urinary excretion of prostaglandin metabolites. Their data suggest that enalapril and aspirin have similar effects on thromboxane metabolism, which supports the view that the lack of mortality benefit with ACE inhibition in patients taking aspirin may be due to a common mechanism. Jeserich et al,[9a] came to similar conclusions.

Conclusions

There are no data to support the use of aspirin in heart failure populations. Usage is subject to the terms and conditions of the subscription and License Agreement and the applicable Copyright and intellectual property protection as dictated by the appropriate laws of your country and/or International Convention. It is possible that aspirin does exert long-term benefit in patients with well preserved ventricular function, but the increased importance of vasodilator prostaglandins may render aspirin harmful to patients with heart failure. The possibility of an interaction with ACE inhibitors is worrisome, and further research is urgently required. At this time data do not support the use of aspirin in heart failure patients, except perhaps those with active or unstable angina or cerebrovascular disease.

USE OF WARFARIN IN HEART FAILURE

Warfarin can potentially reduce both embolic events and coronary vascular occlusion. The most important embolic events are cerebrovascular and pulmonary emboli. Although the former are usually evident and frequently catastrophic, the latter may be inapparent but lethal. In the older series, pulmonary emboli were found in 40 percent of autopsied patients dying in hospital[93] but detected during life in fewer than 5 percent.[94]

Controlled Trials of Anticoagulants

Three randomized controlled trials (Table 50-8) of anticoagulation in patients with heart failure have been reported.[1–3] All were open-label, used days of the week or admission ward to randomize patients (no longer an accepted practice), and included at

Table 50-8. Controlled Trials of Anticoagulants During Heart Failure

Study	No. of subjects	Deaths (no.)	SCD (no.)	PTE (no.)	CVA (no.)	TEE (no.)
Harvey & Finch[1]						
Controls	100	17	?	15	?	16
A/C	80	9	?	2	?	3
Anderson & Hull[2]						
Controls	150	20	4	9	0	12[b]
A/C	147	11	1	3	0	3
Griffith et al.[3]						
Controls	165	31	6	5	7	19[c]
A/C	300	29	2	4	4	8
Total						
Controls	415	68 (16%)	10+	29 (7%)	7+	47 (11%)
A/C	527	49 (9%)	3+	9 (2%)	4+	14 (3%)

Abbreviations: A/C, anticoagulated patients; SCD, sudden cardiac death; PTE, peripheral thromboembolism; CVA, cerebral vascular accident; TEE, thromboembolic events.

[a] 138 Patients with rheumatic heart disease who showed marked benefit have been excluded (see Table 50-9).
[b] Includes one myocardial infarction and two mesenteric infarcts.
[c] Includes five myocardial infarcts, one peripheral embolism, and one mesenteric embolism.

Table 50-9. Effect of Anticoagulants According to the Etiology of Heart Failure

Etiology	Total pts. (NO/AC)	Sinus rhythm (NO/AC)	Deaths (NO/AC)	Sudden death (NO/AC)	MI (NO/AC)	CVA (NO/AC)	PTE (NO/AC)
Rheumatic	138	45	16/6	6/1	1/0	5/1	7/1
HBP	226	178	12/17	2/2	0/0	5/2	2/3
CAD	153	99	9/7	2/0	2/0	0/2	3/1
HBP + CAD	54	27	7/3	2/0	3/0	2/0	0/0
Misc.	32	30	3/2	0/0	0/0	0/0	0/0
Total	213/390	134/229	47/35 22%/9%	13/4 6%/2%	6/0 3%/0	12/5 6%/2%	12/5 6%/2%

Abbreviations: NO/AC, no treatment/anticoagulation; MI, myocardial infarction; CVA, cerebral vascular accident; PTE, peripheral thromboembolism; HBP, hypertension; CAD, coronary artery disease.

Patients were given treatment according to the ward to which they were allocated. Follow-up was for the duration of hospital admission only, in general was 4–14 days.

(Data from Griffith et al.[3])

least some patients with rheumatic heart disease. Follow-up was only for the duration of the hospital admission. Nonetheless these studies, conducted more than 40 years ago, remain the best evidence available to support the use of warfarin during heart failure.

The three trials suggested that anticoagulants could reduce in-hospital mortality by approximately 25 percent and reduce pulmonary embolism or sudden otherwise unexplained cardiac death by 60 percent. Reductions in stroke were less clear-cut; nevertheless there was a dramatic reduction in total thromboembolic events. Benefit may not have been uniform across subgroups (Table 50-9). The study by Griffith et al.[3] suggested that patients with hypertension as the sole cause of heart failure might experience increased mortality on warfarin, perhaps reflecting the difficulty of controlling hypertension, assuming that it was attempted during the 1940s. Currently, control of hypertension is advised prior to treatment with anticoagulants to reduce the risk of cerebral hemorrhage.

Uncontrolled Trials of Anticoagulants During Heart Failure

More than a dozen uncontrolled trials have described the effects of anticoagulation on thromboembolic events during heart failure.[12,15,17,44,50,95–103] Kyrle et al. reported that 38 patients with heart failure and a history of thromboembolism had no further thromboembolic events over the subsequent year while taking anticoagulants but that four of five patients who had stopped anticoagulants had another event.[44] Several other small observational studies suggested that anticoagulants are highly effective in preventing embolic events.[97,102] Yokota et als. results were less impressive.[103] Middlekauf et al.[48] and retrospective analyses of the V-HeFT[12] and SOLVD[15] studies suggested no reduction in thromboembolic events during anticoagulation. In contrast, retrospective analysis of the PROMISE trial suggested that among patients with an ejection fraction below 20 percent warfarin reduced the risk of stroke from 3.3 percent to 0.6 percent ($P < 0.05$), with the most marked benefit occurring in patients without an ischemic etiology.[16] There was a trend to benefit with warfarin among all subgroups reported. However, these data must be used with caution because they have been published only in abstract form. A report from the CONSENSUS study (personal communication) and SOLVD also suggest a marked reduction in mortality with the use of warfarin.[97]

Observational studies are confounded by the problem that high risk patients may receive the more aggressive treatment, biasing the result against active therapy. For instance, in the V-HeFT and SOLVD studies patients with atrial fibrillation were more likely to be receiving warfarin. No doubt the same was the case for patients with prior embolic episodes. It is impossible to correct reliably for such biases. Several of the studies suggesting benefit compared retrospective case controls with current treatment and are therefore flawed.

Controlled Trials of Warfarin for Atrial Fibrillation

It is outside the scope of the present review to discuss the evidence for anticoagulation or antithrombolic therapy in patients with atrial fibrillation. Numerous trials have confirmed such benefit, and it is most prominent in patients with associated cardiovascular disease.[42,47,104–112] Although debate continues over the relative value of treatment of warfarin and aspirin,[110–112] patients with heart failure are likely to have a better outcome with the former agent.

Controlled Trials of Warfarin After Myocardial Infarction

Five long-term trials comparing warfarin with an untreated control group (two trials) or placebo (three trials) have been reported.[19] The reduction in relative risk of reinfarction varied from 25 to 60 percent (47 percent in the largest study), the reduction in stroke ranged from 39 to 55 percent, and the relative risk of death range from 10 to 33 percent. No subgroup analysis is available to determine if benefit was different in patients with and without heart failure. Comparative trials of aspirin and warfarin after myocardial infarction have suggested no substantial difference in outcome.[19]

Cost of Warfarin

Superficially the cost of warfarin appears modest. However, once the costs of monitoring and side effects are taken into account, warfarin is a less attractive option.[113,114] The risk of serious bleeding is 0.6–1.5 percent per annum; around 5 percent of patients may expect a major bleeding episode, 20 percent of which are fatal. Because of the potential for fluctuating hepatic function, bleeding complications are likely to be more frequent in patients with moderate to severe heart failure. The need for frequent monitoring has financial implications for the patient (in terms of traveling, time off work, and so on) and an adverse effect on the quality of life.[113]

On the other hand, unlike aspirin, there is no evidence of an interaction with ACE inhibitors. Warfarin was associated with a strikingly better outcome in the CONSENSUS study. ACE inhibitors could have synergistic effects with warfarin on coagulation by altering the balance of procoagulant and fibrinolytic effects.

Conclusions

Experience with warfarin in heart failure patients is conflicting. Neither U.S. nor European guidelines on heart failure recommend routine anticoagulation. However, in patients who have atrial fibrillation or who have suffered an embolic event, randomized clinical trials strongly support the use of anticoagulants. A substantial clinical trial is required to demonstrate efficacy before extending recommendations to other groups of patients. It is possible that mini-dose warfarin (1–2 mg/day) is as effective as higher doses, though the evidence of benefit is scant and conflicting.[115,116] If a low-dose strategy was effective it would make treatment with warfarin less expensive and safer.

CONCLUSION

Thromboembolic complications are an important source of mortality and morbidity in heart failure patients, although their incidence is much lower than previously thought. The benefits of aspirin and warfarin are unproved in patients with heart failure regardless of the etiology, although patients with atrial fibrillation should receive warfarin, as should those who have already shown a propensity for embolization.

The potential for an interaction between ACE inhibitors and aspirin is of particular concern. At present the benefits of routine aspirin used long term after infarction remain unproved and may even be harmful in patients with heart failure. In contrast, the benefits of ACE inhibitors in patients with heart failure are well established. Therefore if the clinician is concerned about the potential interaction of aspirin and an ACE inhibitor in patients with postinfarction ventricular dysfunction or heart failure, it seems preferable to stop the aspirin rather than the ACE inhibitor. Warfarin could be used as an alternative to aspirin, although the benefits of warfarin during heart failure remain to be established. The best solution in the absence of adequate clinical data is to carry out a randomized clinical trial.

ACKNOWLEDGMENTS

This work was supported by the British Heart Foundation.

REFERENCES

1. Harvey WP, Finch CA: Dicumarol prophylaxis of thromboembolic disease in congestive heart failure. N Engl J Med 1950;242:208–211

2. Anderson GM, Hull E: The effect of dicumarol upon the mortality and incidence of thromboembolic complications in congestive heart failure. Am Heart J 1950;39:697–702

3. Griffith GC, Stragnell R, Levinson DC, Moore FJ, Ware AG: A study of the beneficial effects of anticoagulant therapy in congestive heart failure. Ann Intern Med 1952;37:867–887

4. Cleland JGF, Sbarouni E, Oakley CM et al: Prophylaxis against thrombo-embolic events. Results of a survey of British Cardiologists [abstract]. Br Heart J 1993;69:P51

5. Konstam MA, Dracup K for the Agency for Health Care Policy and Research: Heart Failure. Evaluation and Care of Patient with Left Ventricular Systolic Dysfunction. Clinical Practice Guideline No. 11. US Department of Health and Human Services

6. Guidelines for the Treatment of Heart Failure. The Working Group of the European Society of Cardiology. Eur Heart J (in press)

7. Baker DW, Wright RF: Management of heart failure. IV. Anticoagulation for patients with heart failure due to left ventricular systolic dysfunction. JAMA 1994;272:1614–1618

8. Cleland JGF, Bulpitt CJ, Falk RH et al: Is aspirin safe for patients with heart failure? Br Heart J 1995; 74:215–219

9. CONSENSUS Trial Study Group: Effects of enalapril on mortality in severe congestive heart failure. Results of the Cooperative North Scandinavian Enalapril Survival Study (CONSENSUS). N Engl J Med 1987;316:1429–1435

9a. Jeserich M, Pape L, Just H et al: Effect of long-term angiotensin-converting enzyme inhibition on vascular function in patients with chronic congestive heart failure. Am J Cardiol 1995;76:1079–1081

10. Cohn JN, Archibald DG, Ziesche S et al: Effect of vasodilator therapy on mortality in chronic congestive heart failure. Results of a Veterans Administration Cooperative Study. N Engl J Med 1986;314: 1547–1552

11. Cohn JN, Johnson G, Ziesche S et al: A comparison of enalapril with hydralazine-isosorbide dinitrate in the treatment of chronic congestive heart failure. N Engl J Med 1991;325:303–310

12. Dunkman WB, Johnson GR, Carson PE et al: Incidence of thromboembolic events in congestive heart failure. Circulation, suppl. VI 1993;87:94–101

13. SOLVD Investigators: Effect of enalapril on survival in patients with reduced left ventricular ejection fractions and congestive heart failure. N Engl J Med 1991;325:293–302

14. SOLVD Investigators: Effect of enalapril on mortality and the development of heart failure in asymptomatic patients with reduced left ventricular ejection fractions. N Engl J Med 1992;327:685–691

15. Cohn JN, Benedict CR, LeJemtel TH et al: Risk of thromboembolism in left ventricular dysfunction. SOLVD [abstract]. Circulation, suppl. I 1992;86:252

16. Falk R, Pollack A, Tandon PK, Packer M: The effect of warfarin on prevalence of stroke in severe heart failure [abstract]. J Am Coll Cardiol, suppl. A 1993; 21:218A

17. Schmidt R, Fazekas F, Offenbacher H, Dusleag J, Lechner H: Brain magnetic resonance imaging and neuropsychological evaluation of patients with idiopathic dilated cardiomyopathy. Stroke 1991;22: 195–199

18. Yusuf S, Pepine CJ, Garces C et al: Effect of enalapril on myocardial infarction and unstable angina in patients with low ejection fractions. Lancet 1992;240: 1173–1178

19. Cleland JGF, McMurray J, Ray S: Overview of post-infarction trials. In: Cleland JGF (ed) Prevention Strategies After Myocardial Infarction. Sci Press 1994;37–73

20. Davies MJ, Thomas A: Thrombosis and acute coronary artery lesions in sudden cardiac death. N Engl J Med 1984;310:1137–1140

21. Friedman M, Manwaring JH, Rosenman RH et al: Instantaneous and sudden deaths. Clinical hological differentiation in coronary artery disease. JAMA 1973;225:1319–1328

22. Hausmann H, Ennker J, Topp H et al: Coronary artery bypass grafting and heart transplantation in end-stage coronary artery disease. A comparison of hemodynamic improvement and ventricular function. J Card Surg 1994;9:77–84

23. Yang Z, Arnet U, Bauer E et al: Thrombin-induced endothelium-dependent inhibition and direct activation of platelet-vessel wall interaction. Role of prostacyclin, nitric oxide, and thromboxane A-2. Circulation 1994;89:2266–2272

24. Kawa C: Pathogenesis of acute myocardial infarction. Novel regulatory systems of bioactive substances in the vessel wall. Circulation 1994;90:1033–1043

25. Habib F, Dutka D, Crossman D, Oakley CM, Cleland JGF: Enhanced basal nitric oxide production in heart failure. Another failed counter-regulatory vasodilator mechanism? Lancet 1994;344:371–373

26. Dzau VJ, Packer M, Lilly LS et al: Prostaglandins in severe congestive heart failure. Relation to activation of the renin-angiotensin system and hyponatremia. N Engl J Med 1984;310:347–352

27. Penny WF, Weinstein M, Salzman EW, Ware JA: Correlation of circulating von Willebrand factor levels with cardiovascular hemodynamics. Circulation 1991;83:1630–1636

28. Sbarouni E, Bradshaw A, Andreotti F et al: Relationship between hemostatic abnormalities and neuroendocrine activity in heart failure. Am Heart J 1994; 127:607–612

29. Cody RJ, Haas GJ, Binkley PF, Capters Q, Kelley R: Plasma endothelin correlates with the extent of pulmonary hypertension in patients with chronic congestive heart failure. Circulation 1992;85: 504–509

30. Ohlstein EH, Gaboury CL, Conlin PR, Lippton H: Endothelin and platelet function. Thromb Res 1990;57: 967–974

31. Ridker PM, Gaboury CL, Conlin PR et al: Stimulation of plasminogen activator inhibitor in vivo by infusion of angiotensin II. Evidence of a potential interaction between the renin-angiotensin system and fibrinolytic function. Circulation 1993;87:1969–1973

32. Keber I, Keber D, Stegnar M, Vene N: Tissue plasminogen activator release in chronic venous hypertension due to heart failure. Thromb Haemost 1992; 68:321–324

33. Jafri SM, Ozawa T, Mammen E et al: Platelet function, thrombin and fibrinolytic activity in patients with heart failure. Eur Heart J 1993;14:205–214

34. Siostrzonek P, Koppensteiner R, Kreiner G et al: Abnormal blood rheology in idiopathic dilated cardiomyopathy. Am J Cardiol 1992;69:1497–1499

35. Takano K, Iino K, Ibayashi S et al: Hypercoagulable state under low-intensity warfarin anticoagulation assessed with hemostatic markers in cardiac disorders. Am J Cardiol 1994;74:935–939

36. Lip YH: A Study of Thrombogenesis in Atrial Fibrillation and Left Ventricular Dysfunction. MD thesis (Glasgow), 1995

37. Siostrzonek P, Koppensteiner R, Gossinger HD et al: Hemodynamic and hemorheologic determinants of left atrial thrombus formation in patients with idiopathic dilated cardiomyopathy. Am Heart J 1993; 125:430–435

38. Black IW, Chesterman CN, Hopkins AP et al: Hematologic correlates left atrial spontaneous echo contrast and thromboembolism in nonvalvular atrial fibrillation. J Am Coll Cardiol 1993;21:451–457

39. Vaughan DE: Thrombotic effects of angiotensin. J Myocard Isch, suppl. 1 1995;7:44–49

40. Timmis AD, Pitt B: Effects of ACE inhibitors on coronary atherosclerosis and restenosis. Br Heart J, suppl. 1994;72:57–60

41. Fatkin D, Kelly RP, Fenely MP: Relations between left atrial appendage blood flow velocity, spontaneous echocardiographic contrast and thromboembolic risk in vivo. J Am Coll Cardiol 1994;23:961–969

42. Stroke Prevention in Atrial Fibrillation Investigators: Predictors of thromboembolism in atrial fibrillation. II. Echocardiographic features of patients at risk. Ann Intern Med 1992;116:6–12

43. Stratton JR, Resnick AD: Increased embolic risk in patients with left ventricular thrombi. Circulation 1987;75:1004–1011

44. Kyrle PA, Koringer C, Gossiner H et al: Prevention of arterial and pulmonary embolism by oral anticoagulants in patients with dilated cardiomyopathy. Thromb Haemost 1985;54:521–523

45. Stratton JR, Nemanich JW, Johannessen KA, Resnick AD: Fate of left ventricular thrombi in patients with remote myocardial infarction and idiopathic cardiomyopathy. Circulation 1988;78:1388–1393

46. Falk RH, Foster E, Coats MH: Ventricular thrombi and thromboembolism in dilated cardiomyopathy. A prospective follow-up study. Am Heart J 1992;123: 136–142

47. Stroke Prevention in Atrial Fibrillation Investigators: Predictors of thromboembolism in atrial fibrillation. I. Clinical features of patients at risk. Ann Intern Med 1992;116:1–5

48. Middlekauf HR, Stevenson WG, Stevenson LW: Prognostic significance of atrial fibrillation in advanced heart failure. A study of 390 patients. Circulation 1991;84:40–48

49. Carson PE, Johnson GR, Dunkman B et al: The influence of atrial fibrillation on prognosis in mild to moderate heart failure. The V-HeFT studies. Circulation, suppl. VI 1993;87:102–110

50. Ciaccheri M, Castelli G, Cecchi F et al: Lack of correlation between intracavity thrombosis detected by cross-sectional echocardiography and systemic emboli in patients with dilated cardiomyopathy. Br Heart J 1989;62:26–29

51. Nandra CS, Dick CD, Herzog CA, Asinger RW: Left ventricular thrombi in dilated cardiomyopathy.

52. Katz SD, Marantz PR, Biasucci L et al: Low incidence of stroke in ambulatory patients with heart failure. A prospective study. Am Heart J 1993;26:141–146

53. Roberts WC, Siegel RJ, McManus BM: Idiopathic dilated cardiomyopathy. Analysis of 152 necropsy patients. J Am Coll Cardiol 1987;60:1340–1355

54. Gutterman DD: Characterization of the acute left ventricular thrombus. Hermit or nomad? J Am Coll Cardiol 1989;12:565–566

55. Missault L, Jordaens L, Gheeraert P, Adang L, Clement D: Embolic stroke after unanticoagulated cardioversion despite prior exclusion of atrial thrombi by transesophageal echocardiography. Eur Heart J 1994;15:1279–1280

56. Black IW, Fatkin D, Sagar KB et al: Exclusion of atrial thrombus by transesophageal echocardiography does not preclude embolism after cardioversion of atrial fibrillation. A multicenter study. Circulation 1994;89:2509–2513

57. De Keyser J, Herroelen L: Strokes soon after oral anti-coagulant therapy in patients with atrial fibrillation [letter]. Lancet 1991;338:1158

58. Garg R, Yusuf S: Epidemiology of congestive heart failure. In Barnett DB, Pouleur H, Francis GS (eds): Congestive Heart Failure. Marcel Dekker, New York, 1993

59. Antiplatelet Trialists' Collaboration: Secondary prevention of vascular disease by prolonged antiplatelet treatment. BMJ 1988;296:320–331

60. Antiplatelet Trialists' Collaboration: Collaborative overview of randomized trials of antiplatelet therapy. I. Prevention of death, myocardial infarction, and stroke by prolonged antiplatelet therapy in various categories of patients. BMJ 1994;308:81–106

61. Elwood PC, Sweetnam PM: Aspirin and secondary mortality after myocardial infarction. Lancet 1979;2: 1313–1315

62. Elwood PC, Cochrane AL, Burr ML et al: A randomized controlled trial of acetylsalicylic acid in the secondary prevention of mortality from myocardial infarction. BMJ 1974;1:436–440

63. Persantine-Aspirin Reinfarction Study (PARIS) Research Group: Persantine and aspirin in coronary heart disease. Circulation 1980;62:449–462

64. Klimt CR, Kratterud GL, Stamler J, Meier P: The Persantine-Aspirin Reinfarction Study. Part II. Secondary coronary prevention with persantine and aspirin. J Am Coll Cardiol 1986;7:251–269

65. Aspirin Myocardial Infarction Study Research Group: A randomized, controlled trial of aspirin in persons recovered from myocardial infarction. JAMA 1980;243:661–668

66. Coronary Drug Project Research Group: Aspirin in coronary heart disease. Circulation, suppl. V 1980; 62:59–62

67. Breddin K, Loew D, Lechner K, Oberla K, Walter E: The German-Austrian Aspirin Trial. A comparison of acetylsalicylic acid, placebo and phenoprocoumon in secondary prevention of myocardial infarction. Circulation, suppl. V 1980;62:67–71

68. Vogel G, Fischer C, Huyke R: Prevention of reinfarction with acetylsalicylic acid. pp. 123–128. In Breddin K, Lowe D, Oberla K, Dorndorf W, Marx R (eds): Prophylaxis of Venous, Peripheral, Cardiac and

Course following diagnosis and anti-coagulation [abstract]. J Am Coll Cardiol, suppl. A 1993;21:102A

Cerebral Vascular Diseases with Acetylsalicylic Acid. Schattauer Verlag, Stuttgart, 1981

69. Cleland JGF: ACE inhibitors for myocardial infarction. How should they be used? Eur Heart J 1995;16: 153–159

70. Jull-Moller S, Edvardsson N, Jahnmatz B et al: Double-blind trial of aspirin in primary prevention of myocardial infarction in patients with stable chronic angina pectoris. Lancet 1992;340:1421–1425

71. Boysen G, Soelberg-Sorensen P, Juhler M et al: Danish very-low-dose aspirin after carotid endarterectomy trial. Stroke 1988;19:1211–1215

72. SALT Collaborative Group: Swedish Aspirin Low-Dose Trial (SALT) of 75 mg aspirin as secondary prophylaxis after cerebrovascular ischaemic events. Lancet 1991;338:1345–1349

73. Sze PC, Reitman D, Pincus MM, Sacks HS, Chalmers TC: Antiplatelet agents in the secondary prevention of stroke. Meta-analysis of the randomized control trials. Stroke 1988;19:436–442

74. Faulkner G, Prichard P, Somerville K, Langman MJS: Aspirin and bleeding peptic ulcers in the elderly. BMJ 1988;297:1311–1313

75. Al-Khadra AS, Salem DN, Rand WM et al: Effect of antiplatelet agents on survival in patients with left ventricular systolic dysfunction [abstract]. Circulation, suppl. I 1995;I665–I666

75a. Cleland JGF, Poole-Wilson PA: Is aspirin safe in heart failure? More data [abstract]. Heart 1996;75: 426–427

76. Nguyen KN, Aursnes I, Snappin S, Kjekshus J: Antagonism between enalapril and aspirin: subgroup analysis of the Cooperative New Scandinavian Enalapril Survival Study II (CONSENSUS II). J Am Coll Cardiol suppl. A 1995;25:23A

77. Pfeffer MA, Braunwald E, Moye LA et al: Effect of captopril on mortality and morbidity in patients with left ventricular dysfunction after myocardial infarction. N Engl J Med 1992;327:669–677

78. Zusman RM: Effects of converting-enzyme inhibitors on the renin-angiotensin aldosterone, bradykinin, and arachidonic-acid–prostaglandin systems. Correlation of chemical structure and biological activity. Am J Kidney Dis 1987;10:13–23

79. Shebuski RJ, Aitken JW: Angiotensin II stimulation of renal prostaglandin synthesis elevates circulating prostacyclin in the dog. J Cardiovasc Pharmacol 1980;2:667–672

80. Baur LHB, Schipperheyn JJ, Van der Laarse A et al: Combining salicylate and enalapril in patients with coronary artery disease and heart failure. Br Heart J 1995;73:227–236

81. Lin L, Nasjletti A: Role of endothelium-derived prostanoid in angiotensin-induced vasoconstriction. Hypertension 1991;18:158–164

82. Ferri C, DeAngelis C, DelPorto MA et al. Blood platelets and angiotensin II. Angiotensin II release after platelet aggregation. J Hypertens suppl. 1988;6: 69–71

83. Birkebaek NH, Vejby-Christensen H, Jakobsen P, Winther K: The effect of nifedipine and captopril on platelet activation and prostanoid production in essential hypertension. J Hypertens suppl. 1988;6: 378–380

84. Gottlieb SS, Robinson S, Kritchen CM, Fisher ML: Renal response to indomethacin in congestive heart failure secondary to ischemic or idiopathic dilated cardiomyopathy. Am J Cardiol 1992;70:890–893

85. Riegger GAJ, Kahles HW, Elsner D, Dromer EP, Kochsiek K: Effects of acetylsalicylic acid on renal function in patients with chronic heart failure. Am J Med 1991;90:571–575

86. Clive DM, Stoff JS: Renal syndromes associated with nonsteroidal antiinflammatory drugs. N Engl J Med 1984;310:563–571

87. Cleland JGF, Dargie HJ, Ford I: Mortality in heart failure. Clinical variables of prognostic value. Br Heart J 1987;58:572–582

88. Hall D, Zeitler H, Rudolph W: Counteraction of the vasodilator effects of enalapril by aspirin in severe heart failure. J Am Coll Cardiol 1992;20:1549–1555

89. Nishimura H, Kubo S, Ueyama M, Kubota J, Kawamura K: Peripheral hemodynamic effects of captopril in patients with congestive heart failure. Am Heart J 1989;117:100–105

90. Van Wijngaarden J, Smit AJ, de Graeff PA et al: Effects of acetylsalicylic acid on peripheral haemodynamics in patients with chronic heart failure treated with ACE inhibitors. J Cardiovasc Pharmacol 1994; 23:240–245

91. Schwartz D, Kornowski R, Lehrman H et al: Combined effect of captopril and aspirin in renal hemodynamics in elderly patients with congestive heart failure. Cardiology 1992;81:334–339

92. Townsend JN, Lote CJ, Littler WA, Davies MK: Randomized double blind study of the effect of pretreatment with indomethacin on the central and peripheral haemodynamic responses to captopril in severe heart failure [abstract]. Eur Heart J, suppl. 1993;14: 463

93. Kinsey D, White P: Fever in congestive heart failure. Arch Intern Med 1940;65:163–170

94. Hines L, Hunt J: Pulmonary infarction in heart disease. Ann Intern Med 1941;15:644–647

95. Wishart JH, Chapman CB: Dicumarol therapy in congestive heart failure. N Engl J Med 1948;239: 701–704

96. Diaz RA, Obaasohan A, Oakley CM: Prediction of outcome in dilated cardiomyopathy. Br Heart J 1987;58: 393–399

97. Al-Khadra AS, Salem DN, Rand WM et al: Effect of warfarin anti-coagulation on survival in patients with left ventricular systolic dysfunction [abstract]. J Am Coll Cardiol, suppl. A 1996;27:142a

98. Massumi RA, Rios JG, Gooch AS et al: Primary myocardial disease. A report of fifty cases and a review of the subject. Circulation 1965;31:19–41

99. Hatle L, Orjavik O, Storstein O: Chronic myocardial disease. Clinical picture related to long-term prognosis. Acta Med Scand 1976;199:399–405

100. Gottdiener JS, Gay JH, Van Voorhees L, DiBanco R, Fletcher RD: Frequency and embolic potential of left ventricular thrombus in dilated cardiomyopathy. Assessment by 2-dimensional echocardiography. Am J Cardiol 1983;52:1281–1285

101. Segal JP, Stapleton JF, McClellan JR, Walter BR, Harvey WP: Idiopathic cardiomyopathy. Clinical features, prognosis and therapy. Curr Probl Cardiol 1978;3:1–49

102. Fuster V, Gersh BJ, Giuliani ER et al: The natural

history of idiopathic dilated cardiomyopathy. Am J Cardiol 1981;47:525–531

103. Yokota Y, Kawanishi H, Hayakawa M et al: Cardiac thrombus in dilated cardiomyopathy. Relationship between left ventricular pathophysiology and left ventricular thrombus. Jpn Heart J 1989;30:1–11

104. Peterson P, Godtfredsen J, Andersen B, Boysen G, Andersen ED: Placebo controlled randomized trial of warfarin and aspirin for prevention of thromboembolic complications in chronic atrial fibrillation. The Copenhagen AFASAK study. Lancet 1989;1:175–179

105. Ezekowitz MD, Bridgers SL, James KE et al: The Veterans Affairs SPINAF Investigators. Warfarin in the prevention of stroke associated with nonrheumatic atrial fibrillation. N Engl J Med 1992;327: 1406–1412

106. Connolly SJ, Laupacis A, Gent M et al: Canadian Atrial Fibrillation Anti-coagulation Study. J Am Coll Cardiol 1991;18:349–355

107. Boston Area Anticoagulation Trial for Atrial Fibrillation Investigators: The effect of low-dose warfarin on the risk of stroke in patients with nonrheumatic atrial fibrillation. N Engl J Med 1990;323:1505–1511

108. Stroke Prevention in Atrial Fibrillation Investigators: Stroke prevention in atrial fibrillation study. Final results. Circulation 1991;84:527–539

109. European Atrial Fibrillation Trial Study Group: Secondary prevention in nonrheumatic atrial fibrillation after transient ischaemic attack or minor stroke. Lancet 1993;342:1255–1262

110. Stroke Prevention in Atrial Fibrillation Investigators: Warfarin versus aspirin for prevention of thromboembolism in atrial fibrillation. Stroke prevention in atrial fibrillation II study. Lancet 1994;343: 687–691

111. Laupacis A, Boysen G, Connelly S et al: Risk factors for stroke and efficacy of antithrombotic therapy in atrial fibrillation. Analysis of pooled data from five randomized controlled trials. Arch Intern Med 1994; 154:1449–1457

112. Albers GW: Atrial fibrillation and stroke. Three new studies, three remaining questions. Arch Intern Med 1994;154:1443–1448

113. Hirsh J: Influence of low-intensity warfarin treatment on patient's perception of quality of life. Arch Intern Med 1991;151:1921–1922

114. Forfar JC: a 7 year analysis of hemorrhage in patients on long-term anticoagulant treatment. Br Heart J 1979;42:128–132

115. Fordyce MJF, Baker AS, Staddon GE: Efficacy of fixed minidose warfarin prophylaxis in total hip replacement. BMJ 1991;303:219–220

116. Bern MM, Lokich JJ, Wallach SR et al: Very low doses of warfarin can prevent thrombosis in central venous catheters. A randomized prospective trial. Ann Intern Med 1990;112:423–428

51 Surgery for Chronic Heart Failure

Arie Blitz
Frank Scholl
Hillel Laks

Despite improvements in the medical management of heart failure, most patients have a progressive downhill course that results in death. Patients with ischemic cardiomyopathy (ICM) or valvar heart disease generally have reduced survival compared to those with idiopathic dilated cardiomyopathy.

With the improved results of heart transplantation there has been a tendency to refer patients with heart failure and end-stage heart disease for transplantation. Due to the limited number of donors, however, only 2340 heart transplants were performed in 1994, whereas 2933 were listed at the end of 1994; 730 patients died while waiting. Hence patients with heart failure referred to a transplant center must be carefully screened to evaluate whether other types of surgery could be of benefit. The largest group are those with ICM for whom coronary revascularization or endoaneurysmorrhaphy might be feasible. Patients with end-stage valve disease may also be candidates for valve replacement or repair.

The decision-making for these groups is difficult. One must compare the increased risk of the surgical procedure and its long-term survival with the early mortality and long-term survival after transplantation. In addition, one must consider the risk to the patient while waiting on the transplant list.

ISCHEMIC HEART DISEASE

Coronary artery disease (CAD) has overtaken hypertension as the leading cause of heart failure in the Western world.[1–3] The medical treatment of acute myocardial infarction (MI) has improved substantially, so that since 1980 mortality from an acute MI has declined by more than 30 percent.[4] This has had the inadvertent consequence of allowing more patients with severe infarctions to survive their infarct and yet go on to develop some of the late complications of CAD, including ICM.[5,6]

Ischemic Cardiomyopathy

Burch and associates coined the term "ischemic cardiomyopathy" to refer to patients possessing the cardinal features of ventricular dysfunction, diffuse fibrosis of the ventricular myocardium, and coronary artery disease.[7] Although the outlook for these patients was dismal, several developments have improved their management and outcome: better understanding of its pathophysiology, improvements in medical therapy, advances in diagnostic technology, and enhanced surgical options and techniques.

ETIOLOGY AND PATHOPHYSIOLOGY

Myocardial infarctions that singly or cumulatively involve a substantial portion of the left ventricle in most cases eventually culminate in ventricular dysfunction and heart failure. Kannel and colleagues reported on men 35–80 years of age who survived an acute MI in the Framingham Study. They found that the prevalence of heart failure was only 2 percent at

30 days but increased to 14 percent at 5 years and 22 percent at 10 years. Hence long after the acute event is over, the effect of MI on ventricular function continues to evolve.[8]

The pathophysiology of the postinfarction ventricle is complex.[9] Remodeling involves distinct changes in both the infarcted myocardium and the remote viable myocardium. Weisman and colleagues have shown that, early after infarction, infarct expansion occurs as a result of both myocyte stretch and slippage.[10] A similar phenomenon occurs in the remote viable myocardium. The cumulative effect is such that thinning and lengthening of myocardium predominates during the early period after an acute MI (hours to months). Gradually, as the ventricle enlarges wall stress increases, and cellular hypertrophy and other changes in the noninfarcted myocardium have important effects on left ventricular shape and performance. This compensatory hypertrophy may or may not normalize wall stress, depending on the size of the initial infarct. If wall stress remains elevated, further ventricular enlargement occurs, ultimately resulting in a poorly functioning ventricle.[9] Fueling this process are additional infarctions occurring over the course of time, which are due in part to progressive CAD and in part to increasing left ventricular wall stress. The ultimate result is a heart that is poorly contractile and consists of an admixture of viable myocardium and scar tissue (i.e., the cardiomyopathic heart).

Between the extremes of viable and scarred myocardium exist regions of viable myocardium that Rahimtoola has characterized as "hibernating."[11] Hibernating myocardium is viable tissue that exhibits reduced function so myocardial energy demands do not outstrip myocardial energy supply. Hence these regions have perfusion that is sufficient to maintain myocardial viability but insufficient for normal myocardial function. This situation is in contradistinction to regions of infarcted tissue, where an inadequate blood supply has rendered the tissue nonviable and scarred.[11]

Numerous studies have supported the existence of hibernating myocardium.[12–18] The significance of hibernating myocardium lies in the reversibility of its functional abnormalities if blood supply can be restored. The concept of hibernating myocardium has thus provided a springboard for the development of techniques for its detection and quantification, as well as for determining how much hibernating myocardium needs to be present before a surgical benefit can be appreciated.

PRESENTATION AND DIAGNOSIS

Patients with ischemic cardiomyopathy may be asymptomatic or may present with angina or symptoms of failure. Findings on studies include evidence of prior myocardial infarction on electrocardiogram (ECG) more than 75 percent of cases, with cardiomegaly and pulmonary congestion on chest roentgenography.[19–23] Echocardiography is useful for evaluating ejection fraction, segmental contractile function, and exclusion of valvar disease. Cardiac catheterization is critical for delineation of coronary artery disease, evaluation of segmental contractile function, and measurement of intracardiac pressures.

A variety of techniques are available for the detection of hibernating myocardium and its differentiation from infarcted myocardium. Markers of reversible ischemia have included anginal response to nitrates,[24,25] redistribution or reinjection thallium scanning,[26] extrasystolic[27] or inotrope-induced[28–30] potentiation of ventricular contraction, and positron emission tomography (PET).[13–18,31–34] The PET scan has emerged as the gold standard because it assesses viability directly rather than having to depend on indirect markers, such as blood flow and function. Regions of scar appear as matched defects of perfusion and metabolism, whereas regions of hibernating myocardium appear as a mismatched pattern (i.e., a perfusion defect with relatively preserved or enhanced glucose metabolism).

The average reported positive and negative predictive accuracies for PET regarding improvement in regional contractility after revascularization are both approximately 83 percent when pooling the results from clinical studies.[13–18,32–35] In addition, the extent of mismatch predicts postrevascularization improvement of the left ventricular ejection fraction (EF),[13,16,34,36,37] relief of heart failure symptoms,[31,38,39] and improved survival.[38,39] Because of these advantages of PET, it is used for patients being considered for transplantation, who might benefit from revascularization instead.[18,40,41]

NATURAL HISTORY OF ISCHEMIC CARDIOMYOPATHY

The natural history of patients with ischemic cardiomyopathy is dismal. Data from the Coronary Artery Surgery Study (CASS) registry reveals that although patients with an EF below 35 percent were not part of the randomized protocol, their 5-year survival on medical treatment was only 54 percent. In the subgroup of patients with more severe ventricular dysfunction (EF less than 25 percent), the 5-year survival was only 41 percent.[42] Long-term follow-up of these patients (with a median follow-up of 12 years), revealed a 12-year survival of only 21 percent for patients with EF values below 35 percent, compared to 54 percent survival in patients with EF values between 35 and 50 percent.[43]

A review of several series published since the early 1970s on the survival of patients with ICM corroborates the poor outcome of medically treated patients.[44–50] Keeping in mind the retrospective nature and inherent heterogeneity of these studies, the average 1- and 5-year survivals across these studies are approximately 61 and 27 percent, respectively. There is a trend in the more recent studies (i.e., after 1984) for an increasing prominence of congestive failure and a decreasing prominence of angina as a clinical presentation. This change is due in part to (1) the realization that ischemia may be silent and (2) the improved surgical results in these high risk patients. It is also important to recognize that survival on medical therapy has improved since many of these reports.

INDICATIONS FOR SURGERY

Ever since publication of the CASS trial, it has been recognized that patients with low EFs have the greatest survival benefits, relative to medical therapy, from revascularization.[42,51] Five-year survivals in the medical and surgical groups (EF less than 35 percent) were 54 and 68 percent, respectively ($P = 0.0007$).[42] In patients with an EF below 25 percent, the 5-year mortalities were 41 and 62 percent, respectively ($P = 0.0056$). For patients with preoperative angina, these values were 39 percent and 62 percent for the medical and surgical groups, respectively ($P = 0.0006$). However, for patients without angina who presented with preoperative heart failure, the values were 23 percent for both patient groups, and there was no apparent symptomatic improvement. These results led the CASS group to conclude that in patients with clinical ischemia survival improvements were greatest among patients with lower EFs, but that patients with predominant heart failure symptoms did not benefit from revascularization.

More recently the operative mortality rate has been reduced to less than 10 percent in most series[19,42,48,52–59] due to improved myocardial protection and perioperative management. The improved results have resulted in the extended use of revascularization in the subgroup of patients with heart failure.[60–63] As a result, currently about 7 percent of coronary artery bypass graft (CABG) procedures in the United States are performed on patients with heart failure, and half of these patients have severe heart failure with a New York Health Association (NYHA) functional class of III or IV.[64]

Table 51-1 lists the features of series published over the last 15 years on almost 2000 patients with ICM who underwent revascularization. Averaging the means for the studies, the average age was 60 years (range 55–67 years), mean EF was 21 percent (range 16–25 percent), females comprised 12 percent (range 0–24 percent), prior MI was present in 90 percent (range 75–100 percent), patients with preoperative angina was found in 84 percent (range 23–100 percent), and preoperative heart failure was present in 47 percent (range 0–100 percent). Table 51-1 also lists the operative mortalities and actuarial survivals. The overall mean operative mortality is 8.5 percent (range 0–37 percent). Etiologies for operative mortality consist primarily of postoperative low cardiac output syndrome and malignant ventricular arrhythmias. Mean 1- and 5-year actuarial survivals were 81 percent (range 38–94 percent) and 63 percent (range 53–79 percent), respectively. Late deaths are predominantly either sudden or due to worsening heart failure.

Risk factors for early mortality in ICM patients include low EF,[75] heart failure,[56,76] redo operations, urgency of operation,[54] left ventricular dilatation,[40] high left ventricular end-diastolic pressure (LVEDP),[44] ventricular arrhythmias,[74] absence of angina, older age,[74] and poor target vessels.[74] Risk factors for decreased late survival include low EF,[61,77] high LVEDP,[61] heart failure,[56,77] incomplete revascularization,[56] and concomitant peripheral vascular disease.[61] These factors must be assessed preoperatively in patients being considered for revascularization. In some cases the preoperative status may be improved, as in the case of active acute ischemia or severe failure treated with preoperative insertion of an intraaortic balloon pump (IABP). Postoperatively, selected patients may have improved long-term survival with automatic implantable cardioverter defibrillator (AICD) placement.

Most studies that have compared preoperative to postoperative functional status or ventricular function have documented improvements in these parameters. Table 51-1 compares the preoperative and postoperative NYHA status and EFs of survivors in the series over 15 years. For the seven studies where NYHA was measured preoperatively *and* postoperatively, mean NYHA class improved by approximately 40 percent (range 27–69 percent). NYHA status was significantly improved in five of these studies and unimproved in one; no statistical value was given for the remaining study. For the 10 studies that compared preoperative to postoperative EF, the mean EF increased by approximately 48 percent (range 29–78

Table 51-1. Ischemic Cardiomyopathy:

First Author	Year of Publication	Years of Study	No. of Pts.	Mean Age (years)	Female (%)	Prior MI (%)	Angina (%)	CHF Symptoms (%)	EF Cutoff (%)	Mean EF (%)	Mean No. of Diseased Vessels
Kennedy[65]											
EF 20–30%	1981	1975–1978	92	na	na	na	na	na	20–30	na	na
EF <20%	1981	1975–1978	15	na	na	na	na	na	<20	na	na
Hochberg[66]	1983	1976–1982	41	na	na	na	100	na	<20	na	na
Balu[67]	1988	1974–1982	32	na	na	na	na	0	<25	na	na
Kron[55]	1989	1983–1988	39	63	21	na	56	67	≤20	18	na
Wong[20]	1990	1986–1989	22	55	0	100	96	50	<30	25	2.9
Louie[40]	1991	1984–1990	22	56	5	na	23	100	<30	23	na
Christakis[54]	1992	1982–1990	487	na	15	na	100	na	≤20	na	na
Goor[68]	1992	1978–1985	45	na	4	na	na	22	<30	na	na
Luciani[50]	1993	1985–1993	49	60	6	na	67	23	<30	23	3.1
Van Trigt[60]	1993	1981–1991	118	na	na	na	100	58*	≤25	21	na
Elefteriades[19]	1993	1986–1992	83	67	17	75	49	52	≤30	25	na
Lansman[21]	1993	1986–1990	42	65	24	98	100	64	≤20	16	na
Milano[61]	1993	1981–1991	118	na	11	na	100	58	<25	21	na
Olsen[22]	1993	1988–1991	31	57	10	87	100	0	≤30	20	na
Gill[71]	1994	1981–1985	166	59	15	na	82	42	≤30	na	na
Hausmann[72]	1994	1986–1992	265	59	15	na	100	na	<30	24	na
Jegaden[73]	1994	1970–1990	61	na	na	na	96	na	<30	na	3.0
Langenburg[74]	1995	1983–1993	96	63	18	na	91	100	≤25	20	na
Mickleborough[23]	1995	1982–1993	79	59	13	92	91	35	<20	18	na

Abbreviations: na, not available; MI, myocrdial infarction; CHF, chronic heart failure; EF, ejection fraction; LM, left mean.

percent). All of these EF improvements were statistically significant.

It is of note that good results have been obtained in series that have included a mix of patients with heart failure and angina of varying severity. For example, the Duke group reported the results of isolated CABG in 118 patients with an EF of 25 percent or less.[61] Class III or IV heart failure was present in 58 percent of their patients. Operative mortality was 11 percent. Actuarial survivals at 1 and 5 years were 77.2 and 57.5 percent, respectively (mean follow-up of 27 months) and was better than the estimated survival with medical therapy alone. Survivors experienced significant improvement in angina class ($P < 0.0001$), congestive failure class ($P < 0.0001$), and follow-up EF ($P < 0.005$). The data from this report are encouraging in light of the fact that more than half of the patients had severe heart failure, and yet operative and late survivals are comparable to those reported in other series including fewer patients with preoperative heart failure.

Wechsler and Junod examined the experience of two medical centers with revascularizing patients with preoperative heart failure but included patients with high EFs.[64] At one of these centers, 62 percent of the patients with significant heart failure had an EF less than 40 percent, and 30 percent had higher EFs. Operative mortality in patients with NYHA III or IV heart failure for the two centers was 6.5 and 10.4 percent, respectively. Actuarial survival at 3 years was approximately 72 percent for patients in

NYHA III or IV failure compared to approximately 81 percent for patients with NYHA I or II failure in the overall group. Because of the heterogeneity of the patients with respect to their ventricular function, it is difficult to compare these numbers to studies comprised predominantly of patients with severe ventricular dysfunction.

A series made up exclusively of patients with severe left ventricular dysfunction and heart failure was reported by Langenburg and colleagues.[74] They retrospectively reviewed their experience with 96 patients, all of whom had heart failure and EFs of 25 percent or less and who underwent isolated, nonemergent CABG from 1983 to 1993. The early mortality rate was 8 percent. Increased age and poor vessel quality were the only significant predictors of poor outcome. Thus it appears that satisfactory early mortality rates can be obtained in patients with ICM and heart failure. It is unclear, however, what the severity of heart failure was in this study, so the results are of questionable applicability to patients who would be considered transplant candidates.

UCLA Clinical Results and Operative Technique

Our group has attempted to define the role of coronary revascularization in the population of patients with severe heart failure who are potential candidates for transplantation. Our criteria for revascularization in patients with ICM stem from our early

Patient Characteristics and Results

LM Disease (%)	Hospital Mortality (%)	Mean Follow-up (months)	Actuarial Survival (years)					NYHA Classification			Ejection Fraction		
			1	2	3	4	5	Mean Preop	Mean Postop	P	Mean Preop	Mean Postop	Mean Change (%)
na	4.4	na	na	na	na	na	na	na	na	na	na	na	na
na	6.7	na	na	na	na	na	na	na	na	na	na	na	na
na	37.0	na	38	23	15	na	na	na	na	na	na	na	na
na	0	na	89	84	84	75	61	na	na	na	na	na	na
na	2.6	21	88	83	83	na	na	na	na	na	18.7	26.0	39
na	9.1	24	72	72	na	na	na	na	na	na	25.0	na	na
na	13.6	12	72	72	72	na	na	3.9	1.2	<0.05	23.0	36.0	57
20.0	9.8	na	na	na	na	na	na	na	na	na	na	na	na
6.7	9.0	na	na	na	na	na	71	na	na	na	na	na	na
na	14.0	26	85	83	83	79	79	3.7	2.6	<0.05	23.0	41.0	78
na	11.0	27	77	68	65	60	58	na	na	na	21.0	27.0	29
na	8.4	22	87	87	80	na	na	2.8	1.8	<0.01	24.6	33.2	35
20.0	4.8	34	88	75	68	62	53	3.4	1.8	<0.0001	15.7	22.6	44
na	11.0	27	77	72	68	60	58	2.4	1.8	<0.0001	21.0	27.0	29
26.0	9.7	na	90	na	na	na	na	na	na	na	23.0	35.0	52
16.9	1.8	57	90	83	77	68	64	na	na	na	na	na	na
na	7.6	24	89	88	87	86	na	2.5	1.8	na	23.8	38.1	60
na	11.0	82	na	na	na	na	55	na	na	na	na	na	na
na	8.3	na	na	na	na	na	na	na	na	na	20.0	na	na
13.0	3.8	44	94	82	78	74	68	1.9	1.9	na	18.0	na	na

experience,[40] which revealed improved outcome in patients meeting the following criteria: EF 20 percent or more, left ventricular end-diastolic dimension (LVEDD) less than 70 to 75 mm or LVEDD index less than 40 to 44 mm/m^2, good targets in at least two major regions, and reversible ischemia seen by PET scan in at least two regions. These criteria are not rigid, however; and occasional ICM patients not meeting all of these criteria but considered otherwise a relatively good risk are assigned to CABG.

A retrospective review was performed on all patients with ICM who underwent either revascularization (CABG) or were listed for heart transplantation at the UCLA Medical Center during the period from January 1984 to January 1995.[41] We restricted the analysis to patients with advanced ICM having an EF of 30 percent or less with significant coronary artery disease (more than 70 percent stenosis of at least one major vessel) documented by cardiac catheterization. Patients were excluded from consideration if they were in cardiogenic shock, if they were experiencing an acute MI preoperatively, or if they underwent concomitant surgery for valvar disease or left ventricular aneurysm. The 120 remaining patients after exclusions were designated the OC (overall CABG) group. A subgroup was identified that included patients who were either accepted as transplant candidates by our program ($n = 24$) or were judged by reviewers blinded to the patients' identification and subsequent clinical course to be suitable candidates for transplantation ($n = 32$).

These 56 patients were designated the ACT (acceptable candidates for transplantation) group. Most of these patients had undergone PET studies or other imaging studies indicating the presence of viable myocardium. During this same period, 398 patients with ischemic cardiomyopathy were listed for transplantation, and 237 patients were ultimately transplanted (TXP group). Available data on these patients were used for making comparisons with either CABG group.

All of our patients with ICM undergoing revascularization have Swan-Ganz catheters placed either preoperatively or preinduction to enhance perioperative management. In more than half of these patients, intraaortic balloon pump (IABP) devices were inserted for therapeutic (refractory unstable angina, hemodynamic compromise during induction, or difficulty weaning from cardiopulmonary bypass) or prophylactic (anticipation of difficulties during induction or weaning) indications. Coronary bypass grafting is performed on cardiopulmonary bypass with moderate hypothermia (28°C). Our regimen of myocardial protection includes blood cardioplegia, with cold induction for patients who are not acutely ischemic, cold maintenance, and warm reperfusion with leukocyte-depleted, modified, substrate-enhanced blood cardioplegia. A combination of antegrade cardioplegia via the aortic root or vein grafts and retrograde cardioplegia via the coronary sinus is administered. Complete revascularization is the aim in all cases and is substantiated in our series by the mean of 3.9 grafts per patient. Internal mammory artery (IMA) grafts are performed whenever feasible. Both proximal and distal anastomoses are performed during a single period of aortic cross-clamping, and antegrade cardioplegia is administered via the vein grafts. Left ventricular venting is used selectively in cases where ventricular distension is a concern. In patients who have a history of malignant ventricular dysrhythmias and positive electrophysiologic studies, automatic implantable cardiac defibrillators (AICDs) are placed.

Early mortalities for the three groups were similar (7.5 percent in the OC group, 7.1 percent in the ACT group, and 7 percent in the TXP group). Neither the OC nor the ACT survival curves was significantly different from that of the TXP patients. For patients in the OC group, mean NYHA class improved from 3.0 to 1.6 postoperatively ($P < 0.0001$) in patients who had preoperative heart failure. Mean Canadian Cardiovascular Society (CCS) class improved from 3.4 to 1.1 ($P < 0.0001$) in patients with preoperative angina. The mean EF improved from 26 percent to 33 percent ($P < 0.0001$). For patients in the ACT group the mean NYHA class improved from 3.2 to 1.6 postoperatively ($P < 0.0001$) in patients who had preoperative heart failure. The mean CCS class improved from 3.5 to 1.2 ($P < 0.0001$) for patients with preoperative angina. The mean EF improved from 24 percent to 30 percent ($P = 0.0001$). For patients in the TXP group the mean NYHA class improved from 3.5 to 1.2 postoperatively ($P < 0.0001$), and the mean EF fraction improved from 21 percent to 60 percent ($P < 0.0001$). Postoperative NYHA class and EF were significantly better in the transplanted patients than in either revascularization group.

These findings indicate that, regardless of which CABG group was compared to the TXP group, both early and late mortalities were comparable. In addition, actuarial survival, whether from the date of operation or the date of assignment, was at least as good, if not better, in the CABG patients than in the transplanted patients. Furthermore, symptom improvement was substantial, with most patients on follow-up expressing satisfaction with their functional state.

SUMMARY

Revascularization is an effective mode of therapy for patients with ICM, provided reversible areas of ischemia are demonstrable, adequate targets are available, and ventricular dysfunction is not too severely depressed. Revascularization should be considered complementary to transplantation in the management of the challenging group of patients with severe heart failure. Revascularization can be performed with acceptable operative mortality and good long-term survival, even in patients with severe heart failure preoperatively.

Revascularization benefits these patients in two ways: It recruits hibernating muscle, and it protects normal myocardium from future ischemic events. The former results in improved myocardial function and symptom class postoperatively, and the latter allows for increased late survival.

Left Ventricular Aneurysm

ETIOLOGY

Left ventricular aneurysm (LVA) is the most common mechanical complication of acute myocardial infarction, reportedly occurring in approximately 15 percent (range 3–38 percent) of patients.[78–82] These aneurysms arise from the progressive expansion of previously infarcted myocardium, resulting in a thin-walled fibrous scar over the course of several months. Patients with poor collateral flow from adjacent coronary arteries are thought to be at increased risk for aneurysm formation.[83–86]

Not all akinetic or dyskinetic scars are ventricular aneurysms. Nonaneurysmal infarcts are distinguished by the absence of a discrete border zone, the presence of trabeculation on the inner surface, the presence of a thicker wall partly composed of myocardium, nonadherence to overlying pericardium, and the absence of thrombus.[87] Unfortunately, this distinction is not always clear.[88] Angiographically, LVAs are defined as an area of the left ventricle protruding from the expected outline of the ventricular chamber and displaying either akinesis or dyskinesis.[89] Acute LVAs are typically dyskinetic, and chronic aneurysms are typically akinetic due to the presence of mature organized scar tissue. Most (about 90 percent) of LVAs result from occlusions of the proximal left anterior descending artery (LAD), leading to aneurysms in the anteroapical region.

PATHOPHYSIOLOGY

Infarct expansion and aneurysm formation compromise ventricular function and have adverse effects on remote myocardium. By Laplace's law, the remaining left ventricle is under increased wall tension, thereby decreasing the perfusion of the underlying myocardium and concomitantly increasing oxygen demand. This unfavorable situation results in further ischemia, dysfunction, and dilatation.[90–92]

Aneurysms, when dyskinetic, also waste contractile energy and stroke volume.[93,94]

PRESENTATION AND DIAGNOSIS

Although angina is the most common presenting symptom in patients with LVAs, aneurysms are also one of the leading causes of heart failure in patients with CAD.[84] Their presentation is generally subacute or chronic. Angina is usually due to associated CAD of vessels supplying viable myocardium. In many instances, however, failure symptoms predominate or coexist, particularly with large aneurysms. In addition, chronic aneurysms can present with ventricular dysrhythmias or systemic embolization.[95] Table 51-2 summarizes the preoperative data from surgical series published since 1980.[95–134] Pooling the results from these studies reveals that angina was present in an average of 73 percent (range 40–98 percent) of patients, and heart failure was present in an average of 59 percent (range 23–100 percent) of patients undergoing LVA repair.

NATURAL HISTORY

The prognosis of medically treated patients with LVA is poor, with mortality ranging from 12 to 88 percent at 5 years,[79,80,109,135–139] although these deaths are often not directly related to the LVA. Survival among medically treated patients depends on how the aneurysm is defined. For early functionally defined LVAs the prognosis is dismal, with a 1-year survival ranging from 50 to 60 percent.[140,141] In patients with anatomically defined LVAs, survival depends greatly on the symptom status. Asymptomatic patients have a 10-year survival of 90 percent versus 46 percent for symptomatic patients.[140,141] The CASS registry reported a 4-year survival of 71 percent.[142] Patients with a dyskinetic LVA had a 54 percent 5-year survival, and patients with decreased myocardial function in the surrounding myocardium had a 36 percent 5-year survival.[139] In addition, patients with large aneurysms at presentation have a worse prognosis.

OPERATIVE INDICATIONS, TECHNIQUES, RESULTS

The indications for aneurysmectomy include heart failure, angina, recurrent ventricular tachycardia, and thromboembolism.[143] In patients with failure, LVA resection can improve both systolic and diastolic ventricular function and can alleviate symptoms of heart failure.[105,110,113] In addition, resection of the aneurysm results in increased stroke work index

without increasing LVEDP during exercise.[133] As is the case for ICM, the presence of heart failure decreases both early and late survival in comparison to other indications. It is unclear, however, whether survival is improved by surgery. Data from the CASS study show improved survival for patients with more extensive LV dysfunction or higher LVEDP.[113] Improved survival of these patients compared with those given medical therapy has been confirmed by others as well.[110] However, Louagie and colleagues did not find a survival benefit in surgically treated patients, although functional outcome was improved by surgery.[115] More recently, Dor et al. showed that patients with an EF of less than 30 percent frequent ventricular arrhythmias, and large ventricular volumes benefited the most from aneurysm resection.[134]

Some authors recommend LV aneurysmectomy even for asymptomatic patients, particularly those with high filling pressures, worsening LV enlargement, or a decreasing EF.[137,144] Nevertheless, there is no evidence to date that surgery in asymptomatic patients improves survival in this group of patients. Transplantation is indicated in those end-stage cases where the remaining ventricular segments are severely impaired, particularly if there are poor targets in these remaining areas.

Table 51-2 also summarizes the results of surgical treatment of LVAs. Problems arise here, as elsewhere, when trying to compare heterogeneous studies that employed variable definitions of LVA and included heterogeneous groups of patients and surgical procedures. Most (an average of 78 percent across studies) underwent concomitant revascularization at the time of aneurysm repair. Overall these studies reveal an early mortality rate of about 8.4 percent (range 0–30 percent). Average actuarial survival across the studies is 88 percent (range 80–99 percent) at 1 year and 73 percent (range 58–97 percent) at 5 years.

Aneurysmectomy can be performed with the aorta cross-clamped and the heart under cardioplegic arrest or with the aorta unclamped and the heart beating or fibrillating.[137] Specific operative techniques include either linear or patch repair.[125] The latter may include endoaneurysmorrhaphy as part of the technique.[145,146] With this technique a patch is placed within the ventricular cavity excluding both the septal area of scarring and the aneurysm. Other innovations include the method of Dor in which a purse-string suture is placed within the left ventricle to reduce the LV size and to exclude both the LVA and the adjacent, scarred ventricular septum. The main advantage of the endoaneurysmorrhaphy method is that it excludes all of the scarred tissue from the ventricular cavity, which allows greater re-

Table 51-2. Left Ventricular Aneurysmectomy: Patient Characteristics and Results

First Author	Year of Publication	Years of Study	No. of Pts.	Mean Age (years)	Patients with Anterior LVA (%)	Patients with Angina (%)	Patients with Heart Failure (%)	Mean Total EF (%)	Mean Preop NYHA Class	Patients with 3-V CAD (%)	EM (%)	Actuarial Survival by Year (%) 1	2	3	4	5	6
Frank[96]	1980	1969–1979	135	51	92	na	na	38	na	30	9.6	88	87	82	81	77	na
Froelich[97]	1980	1977–1978	18	59	100	83	89	na	3.6	na	0.0	na	na	na	na	na	na
Jones[98]	1981	1974–1979	74	56	74	na	23	35	na	50	2.7	94	93	90	na	na	na
Reddy[99]	1981	1958–1979	1572	55	74	na	na	na	na	na	11.0	na	na	na	na	na	na
Otterstad[100]	1981	na	26	55	100	na	85	37	3.1	15	25.0	na	na	na	na	na	na
Rittenhouse[101]	1982	1974–1980	104	57	100	78	38	na	3.0	44	7.7	89	86	82	77	74	74
Brawley[102]	1983	1975–1980	84	53	100	na	57	na	na	na	19.0	na	na	na	na	na	na
Kiefer[103]	1983	1977–1981	42	56	100	na	95	na	3.2	na	11.9	na	na	na	na	na	na
Barrat-Boyes[95]	1984	1969–1981	145	54	na	63	48	na	na	50	15.0	71	67	59	56	49	48
Novick[104]	1984	1970–1982	67	53	96	84	48	na	3.4	46	8.9	88	82	77	76	70	66
Olearchyk[105]	1984	1971–1980	244	55	91	98	26	na	3.2	34	10.6	89	na	71	69	81	66
Skinner[106]	1984	1974–1977	41	52	90	73	34	na	na	51	12.0	86	77	76	74	69	na
Gonzales-Santos[107]	1985	1979–1983	119	53	94	na	77	35	na	26	5.9	80	77	76	74	76	na
Keenan[108]	1985	1973–1983	100	56	86	40	75	na	na	na	7.0	85	81	75	74	68	58
Taylor[109]	1985	na	14	52	100	86	100	29	3.1	79	7.1	na	na	na	na	na	na
Yabe[110]	1985	1978–1980	16	52	89	na	na	na	na	35	7.1	99	98	98	98	97	na
Akins[111]	1986	1977–1984	100	57	93*	88	54	37	3.1	na	2.0	na	na	na	na	na	na
Cohen[112]	1986	1978–1979	12	na	na	50	25	na	na	na	8.3	83	81	76	74	63	61
Faxon[113]	1986	1974–1979	238	58	na	87	31	na	na	38	na	na	na	na	na	na	na
Marks[114]	1986	1980–1984	37	58	95	60	35	35	2.9	38	30.0	87	82	75	69	70	58
Louagie[115]	1989	1979–1985	49	55	100	48	100	31	na	27	8.2	na	na	na	na	na	na
Palatianos[116]	1988	1980–1987	40	59	85	na	38	36	na	43	7.3	88	82	77	71	69	na
Vauthey[117]	1988	1970–1985	246	57	84	71	60	na	na	na	8.0	na	na	na	na	na	na
Cosgrove[118]	1989	1984–1987	212	59	na	na	43	36	3.3	46	8.0	na	na	na	na	na	na
Mangschau[119]	1989	1984–1986	14	54	na	na	100	24	3.3	28	6.8	na	na	na	na	na	na
Komeda[120]	1992	1978–1989	336	56	83	90	48	na	2.3	76	13.0	89	88	86	84	84	78
Couper[121]	1990	1971–1988	303	57	89	92	65	34	na	54	5.0	81	73	67	63	58	52
Baciewicz[122]	1991	1974–1986	298	57	na	na	79	35	na	52	4.8	92	92	90	89	85	82
DiDonato[123]	1992	1988–1989	35	55	100	na	23	39	1.8	na	5.6	na	na	na	na	na	82
Kesler[125a]	1992	1984–1989	40	58	100	na	na	36	na	na	4.5	na	83	na	na	na	na
Kesler[125b]	1992	1984–1989	22	60	100	na	na	28	2.3	25	0.0	100	86	na	na	na	na
Iguidbashian[126]	1993	na	4	75	na	na	na	35	na	56	4.1	100	100	91	na	na	na
Salati[127]	1993	1988–1991	48	57	100	na	na	39	na	56	6.7	86	80	70	64	64	na
Elefteriades[124]	1993	1986–1992	75	65	88	na	44	25	3.0	62	na	na	na	na	na	na	na
Prates[128]	1993	na	13	53	na	na	na	na	na	54	8.0	na	na	na	na	na	na
Jakob[129a]	1993	1985–1989	25	59	96	na	na	35	2.6	54	0.0	na	na	na	66	na	na
Jakob[129c]	1993	1985–1989	27	61	96	na	na	35	2.7	54	5.7	na	na	na	na	na	na
Oxelbark[130]	1993	1985–1988	70	56	100	na	100	na	3.2	54	3.3	na	na	na	na	na	na
Mills[92]	1993	1987–1991	61	57	86	na	na	na	na	na	3.0	88	86	84	82	80	na
Mickleborough[131]	1994	1982–1992	92	58	90	75	63	23	3.0	na	23.0	80	75	60	60	60	75
Stahle[132d]	1994	1970–1989	26	61	na	54	100	na	3.5	15.4	8.1	99	92	88	85	82	75
Stahle[132e]	1994	1970–1989	198	57	na	83	100	na	3.1	47	0.0	na	na	na	na	na	na
Kawachi[133]	1994	na	8	50	100	63	88	27	3.1	na	na	na	na	na	na	na	na
Dor[134]	1995	1988–1993	171	57	97	85	57	36	2.6	25	6.2	na	na	na	na	na	na

Abbreviations: CAD, coronary artery disease; EF, ejection fraction; LVA, left ventricular aneurysm; NYHA, New York Heart Association, EM-early mortality.
a Patients undergoing linear closure of aneurysmectomy.
b Patients undergoing circular closure of aneurysmectomy.
c Patients undergoing Dor closure of aneurysmectomy.
d Patients undergoing LVA alone.
e Patients undergoing LVA with concomitant CABG.

covery of the EF and near-normal LV volumes.[147-150] Mickleborough and colleagues have shown that tailored scar excision to allow removal of nonfunctioning ventricular wall—while still utilizing a linear closure technique—results in low operative mortality, objective evidence of LV functional improvement, symptomatic relief, and excellent long-term survival.[131]

Brawley et al. found that the presence or absence of occlusive disease in the arteries supplying the LV lateral wall is an important determinant of the mortality rate associated with resection of anterior apical LVAs in patients with severe congestive heart failure.[151] Revascularization should be performed in most cases and should include vessels supplying the aneurysm. Stahle and colleagues reviewed the outcome of 303 consecutive patients operated on for LVA. Early mortality was 23 percent in patients who underwent aneurysm resection alone and 8.1 percent in cases of aneurysm resection with CABG. In addition, several authors have found improved survival in patients undergoing IMA grafting at the time of aneurysm repair.[117,132] If patients have concomitant ischemic mitral regurgitation, the valve can be either repaired or replaced via the ventriculotomy at the time of aneurysm repair. Recalcitrant arrhythmias are treated by concomitant endocardial resection or cryoablation after mapping or by automatic implantable cardiac defibrillator insertion.

Although the effect of aneurysmectomy on long-term survival is controversial, symptomatic improvement is generally noted.[108,115,152-154] Several studies have also documented an improvement in indices of LV function,[110,130,155-157] but it is not a uniform finding.[97] Improvements in LV function are most notable for patients presenting with failure.[116] Increased postoperative function appears to be related to improved inferior wall motion.[158]

Burton and colleagues found that patients whose primary symptom was angina exhibit significantly higher overall survival rates (actuarial 5-year survival 75 percent) than those undergoing operation because of heart failure (actuarial 5-year survival 52 percent) or ventricular tachyarrhythmias (actuarial 5-year survival 57 percent).[159] The improved survival in patients presenting with angina in contrast to heart failure has been corroborated by others.[104]

Mangschau and colleagues examined their surgical experience with 26 patients who had LVAs and symptoms of heart failure. Of these patients,[14] underwent resection, and 12 were accepted for transplantation. The latter group tended to have a worse preoperative functional status and ventricular dysfunction than the former. Operative mortality rates were not significantly different between the two

Table 51-3. Risk Factors for Early Mortality Following Left Ventricular Aneurysm Resection

Advanced age[118,122,160,161,162]

Resting LV dysfunction[101,103,104,121,159,160,162-164]

Mitral regurgitation[159]

Heart failure[95,101,104,118,121,132,159-164]

Decreased CO or CI[159,161,165-167]

Elevated LVEDP[103,104,162]

Impaired septal systolic function[167]

Poor contractile segment wall motion[101,103,159,162]

Emergent operation[104,118,121]

Left main disease[118]

Resection of akinetic scar[121]

Extent and severity of CAD[95]

No concomitant revascularization[104]

Incomplete revascularization[122,162]

Preoperative ventricular arrhythmias[96,104,121]

Abbreviations: LV, left ventricular; CO, CI, cardiac output and input; LVEDP, LV end-diastolic pressure; CAD, coronary artery disease.

groups. Functional status ($P < 0.004$) and the LV ejection fraction (LVEF) ($P < 0.05$) improved after aneurysm resection, whereas hemodynamic values remained unchanged. Factors favoring transplantation over revascularization were an LVEF of less than 25 percent, mitral insufficiency, and right ventricular dysfunction.[119]

Risk factors for early mortality after LVA resection are listed in Table 51-3. Risk factors for late death include the presence of heart failure,[104,159] advanced age,[122,160] anterior aneurysm,[160] systemic hypertension,[122] significant left main coronary artery narrowing,[122] significant right coronary artery narrowing,[95] incomplete revascularization,[95] poor function of the contractile ventricular segments,[95,161,163] and emergent operation status.[122]

SUMMARY

Repair of LVAs can be accomplished with acceptable morbidity and mortality. Most series report improved survival in comparison to medical therapy. Indications include heart failure, angina, arrhythmias, and thromboembolism. Operative risk is increased in patients who present with heart failure or arrhythmias as the predominant indication for surgery. Complete revascularization should accompany resection in most instances. Good functional status and long-term survival is obtained in most patients postoperatively. Evidence of very poor LV function or significant right ventricular dysfunction is an indication that the patient might be better served by heart transplantation.

VALVULAR HEART DISEASE

The objectives of valve surgery are to prolong survival, ameliorate symptoms, and prevent progressive LV dysfunction. The optimal timing of surgical intervention for valvar disease is often controversial and depends on the particular lesion. It represents a balance between the goal of preserving LV function and minimizing symptoms on the one hand and the early morbidity and mortality associated with surgery and the long-term sequelae of prosthetic valves and anticoagulation on the other. The increasing use and improving results of valve repair procedures have shifted this balance somewhat toward earlier intervention, as has the use of balloon valvuloplasty for mitral stenosis. Unfortunately, the benefit of balloon aortic valvuloplasty in adults with calcific aortic stenosis have been short-lived, and therefore this procedure is generally reserved for patients for whom surgery is not an option, usually because of noncardiac considerations.

This chapter touches briefly on each of the valve lesions that commonly present with or induce heart failure in adults. However, the issues related to stenotic valve disease are generally more straightforward than those with regurgitant lesions, so the emphasis is on the latter. Mitral regurgitation, in particular, can occur as a complication of heart failure of other etiologies and can itself increase the symptoms and accelerate its progression.

Mitral Stenosis

ETIOLOGY AND PATHOLOGY

Most cases of mitral stenosis arise as a result of chronic rheumatic heart disease.

PATHOPHYSIOLOGY

With increasing severity of the stenotic lesion, the left atrium has to maintain higher filling pressures to maintain adequate forward flow. The presence of left atrial hypertension eventually leads to pulmonary edema and progressive left atrial enlargement. Dyspnea is markedly exacerbated by exercise, as the pressure gradient is proportional to the square of the

blood flow across the valve.[168] Because flow is limited to diastole, situations that increase the flow per beat or shorten the duration of diastole increase the transvalvar gradient and increase dyspnea. As the disease process progresses, the patient may develop pulmonary hypertension, atrial fibrillation, or both. In most patients LV function is maintained because the ventricle is underloaded rather than overloaded. Less frequently, LV dysfunction may result from further scarring of the mitral apparatus or scarring of the left ventricle secondary to the chronically reduced coronary perfusion.[169–171]

PRESENTATION AND DIAGNOSIS

Except in the setting of high output states, such as pregnancy, symptoms from mitral stenosis usually do not appear until the mitral valve area is reduced by more than 50 percent, to 2 cm² or even much smaller. Typically, the appearance of symptoms follows the occurrence of rheumatic fever by about 10–20 years. The earliest symptom usually is dyspnea on exertion. As the stenotic process progresses, the patient notes increasing dyspnea with lesser activity, eventually accompanied by paroxysmal nocturnal dyspnea and orthopnea. The onset of rapid atrial fibrillation markedly reduces diastolic filling time and often abruptly precipitates pulmonary edema. Patients with mitral stenosis can alternatively present with hemoptysis, bronchitis, or embolic stroke.[172]

Echocardiography is pivotal to the diagnosis and management of patients with mitral stenosis. It can assess the extent of disease, left atrial size, the coexistence of mitral regurgitation and other valvular pathology, and LV function. Transesophageal echocardiography provides better visualization of the mitral valve and is required to recognize thrombus in the left atrium. The transvalvular gradient, mitral valve area, and pulmonary artery pressure can be estimated. Finally, echocardiography can be especially useful for determining the need for mitral valve replacement versus repair by demonstrating the degree of calcification and regurgitation. Cardiac catheterization is rarely needed to determine the severity of mitral stenosis but may be helpful for quantifying regurgitation, which if more than mild excludes balloon valvuloplasty. Coronary angiography is indicated in older patients or those with multiple risk factors or chest pain. Importantly, about 25 percent of patients over age 40 with mitral stenosis and without angina have significant CAD.[173]

INDICATIONS FOR SURGERY

Because LV function is usually maintained in mitral stenosis and life-threatening arrhythmias are uncommon, the primary indication for valve surgery is alleviation of symptoms. Less commonly, hemoptysis or evidence of pulmonary hypertension precipitates earlier intervention. Embolization despite adequate anticoagulation is another indication for surgery, particularly if commissurotomy is feasible.

COMMISSUROTOMY

In a patient with indications for intervention, the choices are as follows: closed or open commissurotomy, percutaneous transmitral valvotomy, or mitral valve replacement. Closed commissurotomy has for the most part been replaced by open valvotomy in most centers. Nevertheless, closed commissurotomy is still practiced in many areas of the world.

Closed commissurotomy (CC) is feasible only in selected patients who have isolated stenosis with pliable noncalcified valves, minimal mitral regurgitation, and no atrial clot. Operative mortality is generally low (0–3 percent), and long-term survival is high (70–80 percent at 10–12 years), although most patients in published series are young and good risk.[174–178] Reoperations, primarily for valve replacement, are required in a substantial number of patients, but often not for 10 years or more.

Open mitral commissurotomy (OC) is currently the preferred practice at most centers.[179] The main advantages of OC over closed commissurotomy are that it allows direct visualization of the mitral valvular apparatus, precise incision of the commissures, debridement of calcium, separation of fused chordae, and repair of associated lesions. Furthermore, it may result in a lower incidence of embolization than for the closed technique, as thrombus can be directly visualized and removed. Excellent results have been obtained in most series reporting on OC, with the operative mortality ranging from 0 to 4 percent in most recent series.[178–182] Ten-year survival usually exceeds 80–90 percent, and most patients obtain substantial, long-lasting symptom relief.

Since its introduction by Lock and colleagues in 1985, percutaneous mitral valvuloplasty has proved to be a safe, effective procedure for mitral stenosis.[182–196] In fact, of all valvular lesions, mitral stenosis is the one most amenable to successful balloon valvuloplasty. Most patients experience doubling of the mitral valve area.[172] Patients must be selected judiciously, with all of the exclusions mentioned for CC pertaining to this procedure as well.[197] Patients particularly suited for balloon valvuloplasty are those at the extremes of age and pregnant women. Most patients eventually experience restenosis, but some may never require another operation and others can undergo operation under safer circumstances. The reoperation rate is related to the adequacy of the initial procedure.

MITRAL VALVE REPLACEMENT

Mitral valve replacement is reserved for patients whose valves are distorted with involvement of the valve apparatus or are heavily calcified and those with more than mild mitral regurgitation. A bioprosthetic or mechanical prosthesis may be used. Although there are many gray areas about which type of prosthetic valve is most appropriate, several generalizations can be made regarding the decision to replace a valve with a mechanical prosthesis versus a bioprosthesis. For young adults (under age 65–70 years) and particularly children, mechanical valves are preferred for their proved durability. Elderly patients (age more than 70 years) and patients considered at high risk for thromboembolism or hemorrhage should receive a bioprosthesis if they are not in atrial fibrillation. If a woman of childbearing age desires children, she should receive a bioprosthesis because of the risks of anticoagulation should she become pregnant. Other factors swaying a decision toward a mechanical valve include the presence of chronic atrial fibrillation or other indications for lifelong anticoagulation or the presence of a small annular size, which would require a low-profile mechanical prosthesis for improved hemodynamics. Currently, the breakdown between mechanical and bioprosthetic valve use is about 65/35 percent in the U.S. market.[198]

The Society of Thoracic Surgeons database of mitral valve replacements (MVRs) includes data from more than 650 institutions in the United States for the period 1991–1993.[199] The average operative mortality of the 3625 patients undergoing MVR was 5.3 percent. The mortality rate of the subgroup of patients undergoing primary elective MVR was 3.4 percent. Mortality rate was higher for emergent and repeat operations. Operative mortality was also higher for older patients, with a rate of 1.2 percent for patients less than 50 years of age and 6.6 percent for patients between 70 and 80 years. Concomitant CABG was similarly associated with a higher mortality rate of 13.4 percent; females had a higher mortality rate than men for most groups. For patients undergoing primary MVR, the operative morbidities included 6 percent reoperation, 4 percent stroke, 3 percent renal failure, 6 percent prolonged mechanical ventilation (more than 5 days). If patients underwent concomitant CABG, these morbidity rates were increased by more than 50 percent.

Mitral Regurgitation

ETIOLOGY

Mitral regurgitation (MR) results from a variety of causes, but the most common entities resulting in chronic MR are myxomatous degenerative disease, rheumatic heart disease, and ischemia. Formerly, chronic rheumatic heart disease was the most common cause of acquired mitral valve abnormalities, but myxomatous degeneration (floppy mitral valve) has supplanted it as the leading cause of MR in recent years.[200–202] MR can arise from disease of any one or more of its four basic components: annulus, leaflets, chordae, and papillary muscle.

PATHOPHYSIOLOGY

The pathophysiology of chronic MR, regardless of its underlying etiology, begins with volume overload of the left ventricle. In an attempt to sustain its forward output, the left ventricle dilates so that more volume is ejected with each contraction by the Frank-Starling mechanism.[203,204] The relative proportion of forward and regurgitant flows is determined by the aortic pressure, left atrial pressure, and regurgitant orifice size. Chronic MR eventually leads to left atrial dilatation, accompanied by stretching of the left atrial muscle fibers and fibrosis, which sets the stage for subsequent atrial fibrillation. If the process is allowed to continue unchecked, pulmonary hypertension and right heart failure occur.

Load-dependent indices of LV function such as the EF are unreliable in patients with MR, because the EF overestimates cardiac contractility to the extent that a normal EF may imply impaired contractility. Hence load-independent indices are preferable, but in patients who are asymptomatic the end-systolic dimension appears to be a good parameter to follow if the afterload (arterial blood pressure) remains relatively constant.[204] Several studies indicate that there is depressed myocardial contractility in patients with volume overload from chronic MR.[205–207]

PRESENTATION AND DIAGNOSIS

The presentation of these patients may range from the asymptomatic state to florid heart failure. The echocardiogram is indispensable for their diagnosis and management. The nature of the valve pathology can often be determined, MR can be quantified and localized, its etiology determined, pulmonary artery pressures can be estimated, and critical information about cardiac function and chamber dimensions is obtained. Cardiac catheterization allows one to determine the severity of the MR and the left- and right-sided pressures; it can also quantitate ejection and regurgitant fractions. In addition, coronary angiography should be performed in patients older than 40 years of age or with other indications.

NATURAL HISTORY

The natural history of chronic MR is marked by a long asymptomatic phase eventually culminating in heart failure. Survival depends on the etiology, the severity of the clinical findings, and the degree of LV dysfunction at presentation. Overall, patients with chronic MR have an expected 5-year survival of about 80 percent and a 10-year survival of about 60 percent.[208–210] In the group of patients who are symptomatic, the 5-year survival drops to 45 percent.[210–212] The worst survival is observed in patients with severe symptoms (NYHA III–IV) and decreased ventricular function.[211]

INDICATIONS FOR SURGERY

The appropriate timing of surgical intervention for chronic MR is controversial because of the varied etiology of MR and the often narrow window between onset of symptoms or LV dysfunction and progression to irreversible damage. Indications for valvar surgery have evolved as clinicians try to pinpoint the period at which the patient's symptoms are progressing but prior to the establishment of irreversible LL dysfunction. Patients with severe irreversible ventricular dysfunction—with an EF under 30 percent and an LVEDD over 75 mm—are better served by heart transplantation.

Indications for surgery for chronic mitral insufficiency include NYHA class III–IV symptoms, lesser symptoms with deteriorating LV function, and subacute endocarditis. Of supreme importance is the close follow-up of patients in the second group (i.e., those with minimal symptoms but deteriorating LV function).[213] Most authors advocate operating when indices of ventricular dysfunction reach critical values, even in the apparent absence of symptoms.[214] If it is clear from the echocardiogram that repair rather than replacement can be accomplished, we prefer to proceed with valve repair even in the absence of symptoms or significant LV dysfunction in patients with severe MR and without associated risk factors. In any event, the more aggressive the recommendation, in general, the greater is the emphasis on valve repair versus replacement. As for the management of other valvar disease, the availability of interventions that show improved clinical results over valve replacement results in interventions in patients with lesser symptomatology.

Treatment Options

Surgical options include mitral valve replacement or repair. Replacement can be performed with a mechanical prosthesis or a bioprosthesis. Whatever the type of prosthesis utilized, it has been shown that preservation of as much of the subvalvar apparatus as is possible results in superior LV function postoperatively and reduces surgical risk.[215–225] Kaul and colleagues showed a significant improvement in actuarial survival at 10 years in patients with MR and severe preoperative LV dysfunction (LVEF less than 25 percent) who had preservation of the mitral subvalvar support at the time of valve replacement (70 percent versus 48 percent, $P < 0.01$).[223]

Although restoration of a competent atrioventricular valve in patients with severe MR results in a decrease in global LVEF due to increased afterload, it is associated with an increase in the forward stroke volume. This concept was illustrated by Crawford et al. in 1990, who showed a mean decrease in LVEF from 56 percent to 45 percent ($P < 0.001$) following mitral valve replacement for MR that was accompanied by an increase in the forward stroke/end-diastolic volume ratio from 0.32 to 0.45 ($P < 0.01$).[226]

Mitral valve repair has several advantages over replacement. It results in superior preservation of LV function due to maintenance of LV geometry. In most series the morbidity and mortality are lower than for replacement, although patient selection may be the important factor here.[215,221,227–236] Repair techniques are durable, there is a much lower risk of endocarditis and thromboembolism, and LV rupture is avoided. In addition, the cost is about one-third the cost of a replacement, owing largely to the cost of the artificial valve in the latter.[237,238] Successful repair is more likely when the MR is due to myxomatous and ischemic disease, rather than other etiologies.[239,240] Currently, there is approximately a 1 to 2 percent failure rate per year for mitral valve repair.[241]

A review of the recent literature on mitral valve repair and replacement for MR is represented in Tables 51-4 and 51-5, respectively. In general, the populations operated on for repair have had less severe disease, but several conclusions are warranted: (1) In appropriately selected patients, the results from

mitral valve repair are comparable or superior to those for replacement; (2) mitral valve repair results in better post-operative LV function; (3) repair is associated with a lower risk of thromboembolism and endocarditis; (4) it is less expensive; (5) mitral valve replacement is indicated for patients with severe calcification of the mitral valve apparatus or otherwise nonreconstructible disease; (6) results for ischemic MR are inferior to those obtained for other etiologies for MR.

Mitral repair techniques may also be useful in patients who develop annular dilatation from cardiomyopathy. In a series of 11 patients with cardiomyopathy all in NYHA functional class II or IV with severe MR and a mean LVEF of 16 percent (range 9–25 percent), Bolling et al. obtained excellent results with flexible ring mitral annuloplasty with or without coronary artery grafting. There were no operative deaths, and the 1-year actuarial survival was 75 percent. At a mean of 8 months of follow-up all patients were in NYHA class I or II.[254]

In a review of our series at the UCLA Medical Center, from 1982 to 1995 a total of 185 patients underwent repair of the mitral valve for acquired mitral regurgitation. The mean age at the time of repair was 62.2 years (range 20–89 years). Etiology of mitral disease was as follows; degenerative 61 percent, ischemic 31 percent, rheumatic 2 percent, endocarditis 5 percent, and other 0.5 percent. A review of preoperative NYHA classes showed 10 percent of patients in functional class I, 23 percent in class II, and 68 percent of patients in class III or IV heart failure. Operative mortality was 3.2 percent, with an actuarial survival at 5 years of 76 percent. Patients had a 5-year freedom from reoperation of 94 percent. At last follow-up, 90 percent of patients were in NYHA class I or II. Of the patients requiring reoperation, two underwent rerepair and five underwent mitral valve replacement.

Risk factors for operative mortality include increased age,[261–263] NYHA class III or IV,[217,220,261,264] associated coronary artery disease,[217,263] increased LVEDP,[220,264] increased PCWP,[220,226,263] increased RVEDP,[220] LV end-systolic volume index greater than 60 ml/m^2,[220,226,264] LV end-diastolic volume index greater than 100 ml/m^2,[206,220,226] EF at rest less than 40 percent,[220,227,261] end-systolic dimension greater than 2.6 cm/m^2,[265] fractional shortening less than 31 percent[209,265] end-systolic wall stress index greater than 195 mmHg.[265,266]

The place of transplantation in patients with severe MR and severe LV impairment is not clear. Generally, patients with an EF less than 25 percent and an LVEDD more than 75 mm have been referred for

Table 51-4. Valve Repair for Mitral Regurgitation: Patient Characteristics and Results

First Author	Year of Publication	Years of Study	No. of Patients	Mean Age (Years)	Patients with Atrial Fibrillation (%)	Mean EF	Mean NYHA Class	Patients with NYHA Class III or IV (%)	Etiology	Hospital Mortality (%)	Actuarial Survival by Year (%)			
											1	3	5	8
Craver[242]	1990	1984–1988	65	61	na	57	na	na	I-8%, R-8%, D-78%, E-6%	1.5	93	84	na	na
Deloche[243]	1990	1972–1979	195	49	na	na	2.9	97	I-4%, R-38%, D-58%, O-4%	5.3	98	97	96	93
Hendren[244]	1991	1985–1989	65	66	na	na	3.3	na	I-100%	9.2	na	63	63	na
Kawachi (a)[245a]	1991	1975–1988	43	51	51	68	2.2	na	na	2.3	97	97	93	91
Krause[246]	1991	1985–1990	63	68	na	na	na	44	I-47%, R-10%, D-41%, E-2%	3.0	na	na	na	na
Michel[221]	1991	1972–1990	155	51	28	60	na	61	R-17%, D-65%, E-14%, C-2%, O-2%	1.3	97	94	88	85
Kenny[247]	1992	1985–1991	100	66	na	46	na	80	I-7%, R-15%, D-67%, E-8%, C-1%	1.0	94	na	na	na
Okita (a)[248]	1992	na	16	51	na	66	na	na	R-13%, D-56%, E-6%, C-25%	na	na	na	na	na
David[231]	1993	1981–1992	184	57	34	na	na	71	D-100%	0.54	97	95	91	88
Gorton[249]	1993	1991–1992	21	65	na	na	na	90	I-33%, R-5%, D-62%	5.0	na	na	na	na
Akins (a)[250]	1994	1985–1992	133	65	na	54	2.8	58	I-16%, D-84%	3.0	na	na	na	na
Azar[251]	1994	1984–1992	50	74	28	46	na	na	I-56%, R-12%, D-14%, E-6%, P-22%	6.0	86	77	74	na
Cohn[252]	1994	1984–1993	219	63	38	na	na	77	D-100%	2.3	98	93	86	na
Oury (a)[253]	1994	1986–1990	87	na	na	na	na	na	I-100%	7.0	83	60	60	na
Bolling[254]	1995	1993–1994	16	64	na	18	3.9	100	Dilated cardiomyopathy 100%	0	75	na	na	na
Okada (b)[255]	1995	1987–1993	11	54	na	na	na	18	D-100%	0	na	na	na	na
Okada (c)[255]	1995	1987–1993	15	51	na	na	na	20	D-100%	0	na	na	na	na
Perier[256]	1995	1990–1993	4	26	na	na	2.3	25	C-100%	0	100	100	na	na

Abbreviations: na, not available; EF, ejection fraction; NYHA, New York Heart Association; I, ischemic etiology; R, rheumatic etiology; D, degenerative etiology; E, endocarditis etiology; C, congenital etiology; O, other etiology; P, leaflet prolapse.

[a] Subgroup of larger study.
[b] Patients undergoing repair with Carpentier ring.
[c] Patients undergoing repair with Duran ring.
[d] Etiologies not mutually exclusive.

Table 51-5. Valve Replacement for Mitral Regurgitation: Patient Characteristics and Results

First Author	Year of Publication	Years of Study	No. of Pts.	Mean Age (years)	Mean EF	Mean NYHA	Patients in NYHA Class III or IV (%)	Etiology	% Hospital Mortality	Actuarial Survival by Year (%)			
										1	3	5	10
Cohn[215a]	1990	1988–1990	52	62	57	na	na	I-4%, R-29%, D-53%, E-14%	6	na	na	na	na
Craver[242]	1990	1984–1988	65	60	57	na	na	na	5	90	86	82	na
Crawford[226]	1990	na	48	57	56	na	na	na	na	na	na	na	na
Acar[257a]	1991	1970–1990	139	na	55	na	na	na	na	na	na	na	na
Kawachi[245]	1991	1975–1988	48	50	64	2.7	na	na	8	89	87	82	48
Reed[258]	1991	1979–1987	176	57	na	na	na	na	5	82	73	64	na
Kaul[223b,c]	1992	na	12	66	20	3.2	na	D-100%	16	77	70	70	70
Kaul[223d]	1992	na	10	58	32	2.5	na	D-100%	0	90	90	90	90
Kaul[223b,d]	1992	na	19	59	22	3.1	na	D-100%	22	73	61	46	46
Okita[248c]	1992	na	22	49	63	na	na	R-54%, D-32%, E-14%	0	100	100	100	na
Okita[248d]	1992	na	28	45	57	na	na	R-61%, D-28%, E-11%	na	95	95	90	na
Akins[250a]	1994	1985–1992	130	67	56	2.9	65	I-9%, D-91%	12	na	na	na	na
David[259]	1994	na	18	na	na	na	na	I-100%	22	na	na	74	na
Oury[253a]	1994	1986–1990	82	na	na	na	na	I-100%	13	77	65	60	na

Abbreviations: See Table 51-4.
[a] Subgroup of larger study.
[b] Severe LV dysfunction.
[c] Group undergoing valve replacement with chordal preservation.
[d] Group undergoing valve replacement without chordal preservation.

transplantation at our center, as these patients are at high risk not only for operative intervention but also for progressive LV dysfunction and late mortality after conventional mitral valve replacement. The point cannot be overstressed: One should make every effort to refer patients for early operation before LV function deteriorates irreversibly.

ISCHEMIC MITRAL REGURGITATION

About 3 to 25 percent of cases of MR are caused by ischemia.[200,267–269] Papillary muscle dysfunction or rupture causing mitral regurgitation may result from coronary artery disease. Ischemia without infarction or with partial infarction results in dysfunction of the papillary muscle, whereas a complete infarction may result in rupture of the papillary muscle. The posteromedial papillary muscle is more commonly involved because of the solitary blood supply provided by the posterior descending artery; hence papillary muscle dysfunction is more commonly associated with inferior wall myocardial in-

farctions. The anterior papillary muscle has a dual supply from both the circumflex and left anterior descending arteries.[227,270] The mechanism in cases of dysfunction arises from failure of the leaflets to coapt during systole because the papillary muscle or its contiguous myocardium fails to contract adequately. There is evidence to suggest that papillary muscle dysfunction is not sufficient to cause the degree of clinical MR that is seen. In addition, overlying abnormalities of ventricular contraction must coexist.[271,272]

In a study comparing mitral valve repair to replacement in patients with ischemic MR, Rankin et al. showed improved operative survival with repair.[273] However, more recent evidence points out that in this subset of high risk patients valve replacement with a bioprosthesis and chordal sparing techniques may be the most prudent course of action. In most patients a prosthetic valve lasts their expected life-span, as most of these patients are elderly, and the risk of reoperation for failed reconstruction would be unacceptable. Oury et al. found an equal operative and 5-year survival in patients undergoing valve repair and replacement using a bioprosthesis and chordal sparing for ischemic MR.[253]

Numerous studies have confirmed the increased short- and long-term mortality among patients with ischemic MR undergoing operation compared to that for patients with other MR etiologies. Additionally, in a study by Karp et al. comparing patients who underwent concomitant mitral valve replacement and CABG, the survival was better in patients undergoing the replacement for nonischemic causes.[274]

Aortic Stenosis

ETIOLOGY

Over the past few decades the etiology of aortic stenosis (AS) has evolved to reflect a decreasing incidence of rheumatic heart disease and an aging population. The mean age at presentation was 48 years prior to the 1960s, whereas more recent experience reveals a mean age of 61 years.[275] Senile calcific AS, currently the most common etiology, is due to the progressive sclerosis, thickening, and calcification of congenitally bicuspid aortic valves.

PATHOPHYSIOLOGY

Aortic stenosis causes significant obstruction to aortic outflow, resulting in pressure overload of the left ventricle. Concentric hypertrophy results, with eventual increases in LVEDP and pulmonary venous pressure. LV dilatation and heart failure then ensue if the AS is left uncorrected. Concentric hypertrophy has adverse consequences for both myocardial oxygen supply and demand. The hypertrophy results in elevated wall stress, which increases oxygen demand, and decreased subendocardial blood flow, which decreases oxygen delivery. As a result, patients with AS may have angina even in the absence of CAD.

PRESENTATION AND DIAGNOSIS

The three major symptoms of AS are angina, dyspnea on exertion, and syncope. Angina is the most common presenting symptom, occurring in 50–70 percent of patients.[87] The classic triad of angina, syncope, and dyspnea on exertion is present in approximately one-third of presenting patients.

Echocardiography enables measurement of the transvalvar gradient and calculation of the aortic valve area (AVA). Peak gradients of more than 60 mmHg and mean gradients of 50 mmHg are suggestive of severe AS.[238] Patients presenting with AS over the age of 40 should also undergo cardiac catheterization, with measurement of left- and right-sided pressures, coronary arteriography, ejection fraction, and gradients. Severe AS is defined by an AVA of less than 0.75 cm^2 or an AVA index less than 0.45 cm^2/m^2.

One must recognize that in the failing ventricle even a high grade lesion may not result in a high peak systolic gradient, as the ventricle may not be able to generate a high pressure. Low aortic valve gradients in high grade stenoses have been show to be predictive of undiagnosed coronary disease.[276] Also, coexistent aortic regurgitation may overestimate the degree of AS because the AVA calculation is flow-dependent.

NATURAL HISTORY

Asymptomatic patients with AS may remain asymptomatic for many years. Seventy percent of patients with moderate AS (AVA 0.7–1.2 cm^2) remain free of complications at 4 years.[277,278] Patients with severe AS, however, develop symptoms 1.5–2.0 years after diagnosis.[278] The natural history of AS, once symptomatic, is dismal; the average life expectancy of medically treated patients is 3–5 years after the onset of angina, 3 years after the onset of syncope, and less than 2 years after the onset of heart failure.[279] Most medically treated patients die within 5 years of the diagnosis. Actuarial survival of medically treated patients was 38 percent at 5 years and 20 percent at 10 years in one series.[208]

A prospective study of patients over 62 years of age with severe unoperated valvar AS, congestive heart failure as defined by clinical examination, and chest radiograph showed 100 percent mortality at a mean follow-up of 13 months (range 2–24 months) in patients with an EF less than 50 percent and 90 percent at a mean follow-up of 19 months (range 2–36 months) in patients with an EF more than 50 percent.[280]

Chizner and colleagues found that half of the patients with symptomatic moderate or severe AS were dead at 2 years, and half of these deaths were sudden.[281] Patients with even moderate AS are at significant risk for death from the AS or are candidates for valve replacement.[277] Sudden death, most likely due to arrhythmias, may occur in asymptomatic or symptomatic patients but is relatively infrequent in the former.[278,281,282]

INDICATIONS FOR SURGERY

Patients with symptomatic AS should undergo surgical correction. Even asymptomatic patients who are on digoxin or diuretic treatment for CHF should be operated on early, as it is likely these medications are masking the extent of LV dysfunction and have been associated with poorer long-term survival after aortic valve replacement (AVR).[283] Early operation before cardiac function impairment improves the operative results.[284] For asymptomatic patients with critical AS (AVA less than 0.75 cm^2 or AVA index less than 0.45 cm^2/m^2), patients should be followed for the development of symptoms and operative correction performed when symptoms appear.[238] The risk of surgery (3–5 percent operative mortality) is higher than the risk of sudden death (1–2 percent) in medically treated asymptomatic patients.

Because most patients with AS are elderly, caution should be advised when following these patients. AS can progress rapidly in the elderly, so these patients must be followed closely. Elderly patients tend to be offered valve replacement at a later stage of disease, often with more advanced LV failure, and a higher early mortality and frequency of postoperative low cardiac output state.[285]

Patients with low transvalvar pressure gradients and severe ventricular impairment are at a high operative risk, with a reported perioperative mortality rate of 33 percent. However, these patients should still be considered candidates for AVR, as survivors often show significant functional improvement, and the prognosis with medical treatment is dismal.[286] The EF may take several months to improve. In addition, AVR does not preclude these patients from undergoing heart transplantation in the case of a failed operation. Patients with lesser degrees of AS with ICM may be candidates for transplantation rather than replacement.

TREATMENT OPTIONS

The interventional options for patients with AS include balloon valvuloplasty, aortic valve repair, and aortic valve replacement. Balloon valvuloplasty of the stenotic aortic valve relieves the stenosis by causing aortic wall expansion at the commissures and cracking cusps and sinus calcium.[238] In most cases the AVA is mildly increased, and peak gradient decreases. Unlike valvuloplasty for mitral stenosis, however, this technique has not been successful for long-term relief of AS. Restenosis occurs relatively rapidly: 50–75 percent experience restenosis within 9 months.[287,288] In one series only 32 percent of patients undergoing balloon valvuloplasty for AS had long-lasting symptomatic improvement during a mean follow-up of 20 months.[289] Thus current indications for balloon valvuloplasty are limited to inoperability due to advanced age or co-morbid disease, cardiogenic shock, poor LV function with a low gradient

and small AVA ("AVR test"), and the need for noncardiac surgery.[238]

Aortic valve replacement has been, and continues to be, the primary modality for treatment for AS. Table 51-6 lists the demographic features of patients who underwent AVR for AS over a 10-year period.[284–286,290–296] The overall mean age was 70 years (range 59–82 years), mean peak valve gradient was 71 mmHg (range 22–103 mmHg), females comprised 41 percent (range 16–73 percent), those with preoperative heart failure 83 percent (range 68–100 percent), those with preoperative angina 65 percent (range 8–100 percent), those with preoperative syncope 30 percent (range 0–46 percent).

Operative data are also listed in Table 53-6. Overall, the patients undergoing associated CABG comprised 27 percent (range 0–100 percent). The average percent of mechanical valves placed was 58 percent (range 0–98 percent), and the average percent of bioprosthetic valves placed in these studies was 42 percent (range 2–100 percent). The mean operative mortality was 4.3 percent (range 2.2–6.5 percent). Mean 1- and 5-year actuarial survivals were 80 percent (range 59–92 percent) and 70.2 percent (range 51–86 percent), respectively. According to the Society of Thoracic Surgeons national cardiac surgery database, the contributing centers performed 7958 isolated AVRs and 6549 AVRs and CABGs for aortic valve disease from January 1993 to June 1994.[297] Overall operative mortality for isolated AVR was 4.2 percent. Operative mortality for primary isolated elective AVR was 3.1 percent. Patients undergoing AVR with concomitant CABG had an overall operative mortality of 7.5 percent, with 5.4 percent mortality for patients undergoing primary elective operation. Operative mortalities by NYHA class in the patients undergoing primary isolated AVR were 2 percent, 1.9 percent, 3.8 percent, and 8 percent for NYHA class I, II, III, and IV, respectively. Risk by EF was analyzed using a cut-off of 50 percent, and risk by LVEDP was analyzed with a cut-off of 15 mmHg; there was no difference noted in operative risk between groups in either case. Groups with more severe ventricular dysfunction, however, were not analyzed separately.

Due to the significant risks associated with prosthetic valve material and anticoagulation, an interest in aortic valve repair has been rekindled. Duran pioneered the application of reconstructive techniques on the aortic valve.[298] Some series have shown good early results with repair in patients with AS, with late restenosis expected and more likely in patients with rheumatic and congenital AS than in patients with senile AS. The actuarial freedom from aortic valve-related symptoms in patients with

Table 51-6. AVR for Aortic Stenosis:

First Author	Years of Study	No. of Patients	Mean Age (years)	% Female	Mean Peak Valve Gradient	Patients with CHF Symptoms	Mean NYHA Class	Patients with NYHA Class III or IV (%)	Patients with Angina
Craven[290]	1975–1987	1168	na	na	na	na	na	na	na
Deleuze[284]	1981–1989	60	82	55	62	78	3.1	68	72
Lund[276a]	1975–1986	122	60	31	103	84	2.6	63	87
Lund[276b]	1975–1986	55	64	16	77	84	2.9	87	96
Lund[276c]	1975–1986	28	66	18	92	75	2.8	79	100
Lund[276d]	1975–1986	307	59	34	96	88	2.7	65	47
Azariades[292e]	1972–1989	na	na	na	na	na	na	na	na
Azariades[292f]	1972–1989	na	na	na	na	na	na	na	na
Culliford[293]	1976–1988	71	82	55	66	68	na	91	8.4
Lund[283]	1965–1986	690	59	29	96	71	2.8	71	65
Olsson[285g]	1981–1989	44	82	73	na	88	na	86	67
Olsson[285h]	1981–1989	83	70	70	na	91	na	36	80
Brogan[286]	1988–1992	18	68	17	22	100	na	100	39
Morris[295i]	1983–1990	783	70	35	na	na	na	na	na
Logeais[296]	1976–1993	675	79	60	34	90	2.8	na	50

Abbreviations: AI, aortic insufficiency; CHF, congestive heart failure; NYHA, New York Heart Association.

[a] Patient group with no CAD by angiography.
[b] Patient group with CAD who underwent CABG and AVR.
[c] Patient group with CAD who did not undergo CABG with AVR.
[d] Patient group who did not undergo angiography.
[e] Patient group with AVR + CABG.
[f] Patient group with AVR only.
[g] patient group >80 years of age.
[h] Patient group 65–70 years of age.
[i] Patient group with isolated AI, in larger study.
[j] Aortic valve repair for AS.

senile AS was reported to be 87 percent at 7 years in one series.[299] In selected patients aortic valve repair may prolong the progression to severe AS and alleviate symptoms associated with AS. Patients with senile, congenital, and rheumatic disease may be candidates for aortic valve repair. Decalcification and commissurotomy are the main techniques used to repair stenotic aortic valves. Shapira in 1990 reported a 96 percent rate of successful valve repair for all patients, with an associated 24 percent incidence of restenosis for a mean follow-up of 64 months.[299]

Aortic Regurgitation

ETIOLOGY

Chronic aortic regurgitation (AI) can be due to processes that affect either the leaflets or the aortic wall itself. Paralleling the decrease in rheumatic AS has been the decline of rheumatic AI. Other causes of chronic AI include aortic root dilatation, leading to cusp prolapse. In most cases the etiology is unclear, but in some instances it occurs secondary to medial degeneration, as seen in Marfan syndrome. Also, chronic AI can result during the healing phase of endocarditis.[238]

PATHOPHYSIOLOGY

Chronic AI results in volume and pressure overload of the left ventricle. The regurgitation leads to LV dilatation to compensate for the increased volume. The left ventricle also hypertrophies to accommodate the increased systolic wall stress. The pathogenesis of eccentric LV hypertrophy from volume overload in which chamber size and wall thickness are well balanced gradually gives way over a period of years to LV dilatation and systolic dysfunction. If the AI continues unchecked, the left ventricle reaches a critical volume at which cardiac function begins to deteriorate, LVEDP increases, and EF decreases. As the LVEDP rises, it may diminish the degree of regurgitation, as the difference between the aortic and LV diastolic pressures diminishes. Once the stage is reached that there is diminished pulse pressure in the setting of AI with elevated aortic diastolic pres-

Patient Characteristics and Results

Patients with Syncope Symptoms (%)	Patients Undergoing Associated CABG (%)	Patients Undergoing Isolated Valve Procedure (%)	Patients Undergoing Mechanical (m) vs. Biopresthetic (b) AVR (%)	% 30 Day Mortality	Mean Follow-up (years)	Actuarial Survival %			
						1	3	5	10
na	34	66	na	6	na	na	na	na	na
27	8	90	m-0, b-100	28	na	65	61	61	na
34	0	100	m-97, b-3	4	na	92	89	86	86
35	100	0	m-96, b-4	4	na	89	82	68	61
46	0	100	m-96, b-4	18	na	78	71	51	51
39	0	100	m-97, b-3	9	na	na	na	81	60
na	na	na	na	na	na	83	70	70	34
na	na	na	na	na	na	59	59	59	41
0	51	49	m-8, b-92	13	2.2	84	82	na	na
39	8	92	m-98, b-2	9	6.5	86	80	76	60
44	22	na	na	14	na	na	na	na	na
25	29	na	na	4	na	na	na	na	na
17	28	92	na	33	na	na	na	na	na
na	55	45	m-27, b-73	3	4.2	na	na	80	na
22.4	12	80	m-6.4, b-94	12	na	na	na	na	na
				6	5.3	na	na	na	na

sures, LV function has deteriorated significantly and perhaps irreversibly.[238]

PRESENTATION AND DIAGNOSIS

Patients may be asymptomatic, inasmuch as there is a long asymptomatic phase of chronic AI even in the setting of dramatic physical findings. Alternatively, the patients may present with symptoms of heart failure and, more rarely, syncope, ventricular arrhythmias, sudden death, or angina. As in the case in AS, angina does not necessarily imply the coexistence of CAD; often there is an imbalance between oxygen supply and demand in the absence of CAD. Coronary disease occurs in about 20 percent of patients.

Diagnosis by two-dimensional echocardiography and color flow Doppler echocardiography is useful for confirming the diagnosis. It can ascertain the degree of AI, end-systolic and end-diastolic measurements, and EF. Cardiac catheterization provides both left- and right-sided pressures, and can likewise assess the degree of AI and the EF. As in patients with AS, coronary arteriography is indicated in patients over

40 years of age and in those with significant risk factors for CAD.

NATURAL HISTORY

As mentioned before, a long latency period may be present with chronic AI, so patients may be asymptomatic for many years. Asymptomatic patients with mild to moderate AI have a 90 percent 10-year survival, whereas those with moderate to severe AI have a 50 percent 10-year survival. Symptomatic patients have a significantly worse prognosis. Average survival for patients with angina is 5 years and in those with heart failure 2 years. Fewer than 5 percent of patients with class III or IV symptoms upon presentation are alive at 10 years.[300]

INDICATIONS FOR SURGERY

The indications for surgery in the asymptomatic patient with moderate to severe AI are controversial. In general, they have a favorable natural history. Unfortunately, the asymptomatic patient may insidiously develop significant LV dysfunction. Asymp-

Table 51-7. AVR for Aortic Regurgitation:

First Author	Years of Study	No. of Patients	Mean Age (years)	% Female	Mean EF	Mean LVEDD	Mean LVESD	Patients with CHF Symptoms (%)
Bonow[302]	1976–1983	80	44	19	37	75	58	85
Carabello[311]	1980–1987	14	na	na	na	na	35	43
Pugliese[312]	1979–1985	89	47	na	na	na	na	89
Okamura[313]	1976–1988	18	na	na	47	72	54	78
Okamura[313]	1976–1988	23	na	na	58	64	47	na
Morris[295a]	1983–1990	111	61	25	50	na	na	na
Shigenobu[314b]	1974–1991	55	44	44	60	56	na	51
Shigenobu[314c]	1974–1991	32	51	19	58	63	na	50
Shigenobu[314d]	1974–1991	14	38	36	59	54	na	57

Abbreviations: CHF, congestive heart failure; EF, ejection fraction; LVEDD, left ventricular end-diastolic dimension; LVESD, left ventricular end-systolic dimension; NYHA, New York Heart Association.
[a] Subgroup of larger study.
[b] Subgroup undergoing valve replacement for rheumatic disease.
[c] Subgroup undergoing valve replacement for degenerative disease.
[d] Subgroup undergoing valve replacement for Marfan disease.
[e] Aortic valve repair.

tomatic patients develop symptoms of moderate severity at a rate of approximately 5–6 percent per year.[301] The patient with significant preoperative LV systolic dysfunction is at higher risk for development of postoperative CHF within 5 years. In addition, a small proportion (about 4 percent) of minimally symptomatic patients with LV dysfunction die suddenly. Patients with evidence of long-standing LV dysfunction or poor exercise tolerance preoperatively make up a high risk group and were shown to have poorer 5-year survival by Bonow et al. in 1985.[302] Likewise patients with good exercise tolerance or brief duration of LV dysfunction preoperatively were shown to have greater reduction in LVEDD and greater improvement in EF postoperatively.[303] Patients who are asymptomatic or mildly symptomatic should be treated medically but followed closely for any evidence of worsening LV systolic function or symptoms. Asymptomatic patients with evidence of worsening LV function should proceed to operation. Development of minimal symptoms perceived by the patient as a modest decrease in functional capacity may be an important indicator of impending ventricular dysfunction and a poor operative outcome after AVR. It may go unnoticed by the physician or be considered normal functional capacity and be missed without close follow-up. Patients with these minimal symptoms were also found to be at risk of sudden death.[301]

Predictors of irreversible LV dysfunction have been sought by authors in several series.[213] The end-systolic volume index (ESVI) is often considered the best predictor of post-operative outcomes and LV function. Unfortunately, the ESVI is afterload-dependent. Some have suggested using the end-systolic stress (ESS)/end-systolic volume index, which is more independent (though not completely) of afterload. The critical value of ESS/ESVI appears to be 2.9, with those patients having higher values standing a good chance of LV function improving postoperatively.[304] Patients meeting criteria for irreversible LV dysfunction should undergo transplantation rather than a valve operation.

Currently accepted indications for aortic valve surgery in patients with AI include symptoms of angina or heart failure, the presence of acute severe AI or endocarditis, and asymptomatic patients with indices indicating worsening ventricular function.[213,238,305,306] However, the role of prophylactic operation in the asymptomatic patient with normal resting ventricular function remains controversial.[301]

Treatment Options

Aortic valve replacement has been standard therapy for the treatment of severe AI. Concomitant aortic root enlargement requires either the addition of supracoronary grafting or insertion of a valved conduit.

The options for valve replacement include mechanical valves, bioprosthetic valves, and biologic valves. A variety of mechanical valves are currently avail-

Patient Characteristics and Results

Patients in NYHA Class III or IV (%)	Patients Undergoing Isolated Valve Procedure (%)	Patients Undergoing Mechanical (m) vs. Bioprosthetic (b) AVR (%)	% 30-Day Mortality	Mean Follow-up (years)	Actuarial Survival (%)			
					1	3	5	10
85	95	m-50, b-50	4	3.8	91	88	83	73
43	100	na	0	1.9	na	na	na	na
89	100	m-100, b-0	5.6	5.2	na	na	na	na
78	100	m-100, b-0	17	na	78	60	49	12
na	100	m-100, b-0	0	na	88	88	78	72
na	65	m-44, b-56	4	na	na	na	80	81
51	na	m-100, b-0	0	na	na	na	98	99
50	na	m-100, b-0	0	na	na	na	84	85
57	na	m-100, b-0	21	na	na	na	85	86

able, and an excellent discussion of their relative merits and disadvantages can be found in the review by Akins.[198] Bioprostheses included porcine valves (either ring or freehand) and bovine pericardium valves. These tissue valves are more resistant to thromboembolism and endocarditis than the mechanical valves, but their durability is compromised by a greater incidence of structural deterioration.

Kawachi and Tokunaga compared the outcome of their patients receiving mechanical valves versus those receiving bioprostheses.[307] Freedom from reoperation was 95 percent per patient-year of follow-up for mechanical valves and 75 percent per patient-year for bioprostheses. Ten-year actuarial survival for patients receiving mechanical valves was 74 percent and for patients receiving bioprostheses 77 percent. Freedom from thromboembolism, structural failure, and endocarditis for mechanical valves was 77, 100, and 96 percent, respectively, and 94, 83, and 88 percent, respectively, for bioprostheses. This study confirms that mechanical prostheses are more durable but are associated with higher thromboembolic rates.

Increasingly popular valve replacement options include the use of biologic valves, which include either aortic homografts or pulmonary autografts (Ross procedure). Initial results with aortic homografts were disheartening, as most patients required reoperation by 10 years.[308] With the change in sterilization and preservation methodology to current cryopreservation techniques, 10-year reoperation-free survival is now about 85–90 percent. The improved durability is thought to be secondary to the preserved viability of fibroblasts.[309]

Pulmonary autograft replacement of the aortic valve was initially performed by Ross and colleagues in 1967. With this operation the patient's own pulmonic valve is used to replace the diseased aortic valve, and either a pulmonic or aortic homograft is used to replace the patient's pulmonic valve. The technique has proved durable, with 48 percent of patients being free from reoperation for valve failure at 19 years of follow-up.[310]

Overall, the expected durability of the valve replacement options for aortic valve disease are essentially lifelong for the mechanical valves, 10–12 years for the bioprosthetic valves in patients over age 35 years, 15–20 years for homografts, and 20–25 years for pulmonary autografts. In patients with severe failure and LV impairment, the added cross-clamp time and operative complexity associated with the use of biologic valves usually makes them a second choice to mechanical valves or bioprostheses.

Table 51-7 lists the demographic features and operative data of patients who underwent aortic valve replacement for AI for several series.[295,302,311–314] Averaging the means for the studies, the overall mean age was 48 years (range 38–61 years), mean EF was 52 percent (range 37–60 percent), 29% were females (range 19–44 percent), and 65 percent (range 43–89 percent) had preoperative heart failure. Overall, 6 percent (range 0–35 percent) underwent associated CABG. The average proportional mechanical valves placed was 87 percent (range 44–100 percent), and the average proportion of bioprosthetic valves placed in these studies was 13 percent (range 0–56 percent). Table 53-7 also lists the operative mortalities and actuarial survivals. Overall mean operative mortality is 5.7 percent (range 0–21 percent). Mean 1- and 5-year actuarial survivals were 86 percent (range 78–91 percent) and 80 percent (range 49–98 percent), respectively. Operative mortality for AVR in patients with AI is somewhat higher than for AS, averaging about 5 percent. Risk factors for operative mortality include NYHA class III or IV, age over 65, cardiothoracic ratio over 0.65, and hemodynamic evidence of systolic dysfunction (EF less than 45 percent, cross-sectional area index of 20 cm^2/m^2, CI less than 2.2 L/min/m^2, ESD more than 55 mm, and ESVI more than 200 ml/m^2).[238,315]

About 80 percent of patients report symptomatic improvement following AVR. Carabello and colleagues found that mean NYHA class improved from 2.42 preoperatively to 1.42 postoperatively.[311] Indices of LV function also improve with surgery. In the same study, the mean EF improved from 45 percent to 60 percent. Another study showed that the mean resting EF improved from 43 percent to 56 percent, and the mean exercise EF increased from 36 percent to 51 percent operatively.[303] Both LVEDD operatively[303,316] and LVESD[313] improve with AVR for AI. The most important predictor of long-term survival is the patient's preoperative systolic function. Once evidence of severe LV dilatation and depressed systolic function (LVESD more than 55 mm or LVESVI more than 200 ml/m^2) intervenes, only half of the patients have improved EFs postoperatively.

There has been renewed interest in aortic valve repair techniques. The success of techniques of mitral valve repair have led to similar interest in the repair of the diseased aortic valve. Although follow-up data are limited, aortic valve repair has been shown to be a safe and effective method of alleviating the symptoms of AI, especially in young patients and women of childbearing years. Repair of the aortic valve is technically more complex than that of the mitral valve, and so the techniques may take longer to evolve. In addition, the developments in mitral valve repair have outpaced those in aortic valve repair owing in part to the smaller margin of error allowable when repairing the latter.[317]

Repairs done with annuloplasty and triangular resection of prolapsed leaflets have shown good results on early follow-up, with no significant gradient across the repaired valve.[318] In addition, the mean NYHA class improved from 2.43 to 1.07, and the degree of AI improved from a mean of 3.4 to 0.6. Duran et al.[321] showed that in a large series composed primarily of patients with rheumatic disease, leaflet extension combined with other techniques of valvuloplasty has proved reliable, with good results at 4 years and a low (6.5 percent) rate of reoperation. Patients in that series had an improvement in the degree of AI from a mean score of 2.29 preoperatively to 1.19 postoperatively. One caveat is the fact that the overall experience with aortic valve repair tends to be with young patients with less co-morbid disease and a lower incidence of heart failure than in patients undergoing AVR.[239,298,317–321]

CONCLUSION

The major surgically remediable causes of chronic heart failure discussed here include ischemic cardiomyopathy, left ventricular aneurysm, and valvar heart disease. For all these disease states, the critical issues include determining which patients should be offered operation and, if so, which type of operation. In addition, we need to determine if irreversible disease is present and identify important risk factors for poor outcome in order to define patients who would perhaps be better served by alternative therapies including heart transplantation. Numerous instruments are currently available to evaluate the extent of reversibility, and further advances and refinements are expected.

REFERENCES

1. McKee P, Castelli W, McNamara P, Kannel W: The natural history of congestive heart failure. The Framingham study. N Engl J Med, 1971;285:1441–1446
2. Applefeld M: Chronic congestive heart failure. Where have we been? Am J Med, (suppl. 2B) 1986;80:73–77
3. Sutton GC: Epidemiologic aspects of heart failure. Am Heart J 1990;120:1538–1540
4. O'Connell J, Bristow M: Economic impact of heart failure in the United States. Time for a different approach. J Heart Lung Transplant, suppl. 1994;13: S107–S112
5. Ho K, Anderson K, Kannel W, Grossman W et al: Circulation 1993;88:107–115
6. Kannel W, Belanger A: Epidemiology of heart failure. Am Heart J 1991;121:951–957
7. Burch G, Giles T, Colcolough M: Ischemic cardiomyopathy. Am Heart J 1970;79:291–292
8. Kannel W, Sorlie P, McNamara P: Prognosis after initial myocardial infarction. The Framingham study. Am J Cardiol 1979;44:53–59
9. Rumberger J: Ventricular dilatation and remodeling after myocardial infarction. Mayo Clin Proc 1994;69: 664–674

10. Weisman HF, Bush DE, Mannisi JA, et al: Cellular mechanisms of myocardial infarct expansion. Circulation 1988;78:186–201

11. Rahimtoola SH: The hibernating myocardium [see comments]. Am Heart J 1989;117:211–221

12. DiCarli MF, Asgarzadie F, Schelbert H et al: Quantitative relation between myocardial viability and improvement in heart failure symptoms in patients with ischemic cardiomyopathy. Circulation 1995;92:3436–3444

13. Tillisch J, Brunken R, Marshall R: Reversibility of cardiac wall-motion abnormalities predicted by positron emission tomography. N Engl J Med 1986;314:884–888

14. Tamaki N, Yonekura Y, Yamashita K et al: Relation of change in wall motion and glucose metabolism after coronary artery bypass grafting—assessment with positron emission tomography. Jpn Circ J 1991;55:923–929

15. Carrel T, Jenni R, Haubold-Reuter S et al: Improvement of severely reduced left ventricular function after surgical revascularization in patients with preoperative myocardial infarction. Eur J Cardiothorac Surg 1992;6:479–484

16. Lucignani G, Paolini G, Landoni C et al: Presurgical identification of hibernating myocardium by combined use of technetium-99m hexakis 2-methoxyisobutylisonitrile single photon emission tomography and fluorine-18 fluoro-2-deoxy-D-glucose positron emission tomography in patients with coronary artery disease. Eur J Nucl Med 1992;19:874–881

17. Marwick TH, MacIntyre WJ, Lafont A et al: Metabolic responses of hibernating and infarcted myocardium to revascularization. A follow-up study of regional perfusion, function, and metabolism. Circulation 1992;85:1347–1353

18. Maddahi J, Blitz A, Phelps M, Laks H: The use of positron emission tomography imaging in the management of patients with ischemic cardiomyopathy. Ad Cardiac Surg 1996;7:163–188

19. Elefteriades JA, Tolis G Jr, Levi E et al: Coronary artery bypass grafting in severe left ventricular dysfunction. Excellent survival with improved ejection fraction and functional state. J Am Coll Cardiol 1993;22:1411–1117

20. Wong JW, Tong MC, Ong KK: Coronary artery bypass in patients with impaired left ventricular function. Ann Acad Med Singapore 1990;19:34–36

21. Lansman SL, Cohen M, Galla JD et al: Coronary bypass with ejection fraction of 0.20 or less using centigrade cardioplegia. Long-term follow-up. Ann Thorac Surg 1993;56:480–485; discussion 485–486

22. Olsen P, Kassis E, Niebuhr-Jorgensen U: Coronary artery bypass surgery in patients with severe left ventricular dysfunction. Thorac Cardiovasc Surg 1993;41:118–120

23. Mickleborough L, Maruyama H, Takagi Y et al: Results of revascularization in patients with severe left ventricular dysfunction. Circulation suppl. II 1995;92:73–79

24. Cohen M, Charney R, Hershman R et al: Reversal of chronic ischemic myocardial dysfunction after transluminal coronary angioplasty. J Am Coll Cardiol 1988;12:1193–1198

25. Helfant R, Pine R, Meister S et al: Nitroglycerin to unmask reversible asynergy. Correlation with post coronary bypass ventriculography. Circulation 1974;50:108–112

26. Bonow RO, Dilsizian V: Thallium 201 for assessment of myocardial viability [see comments]. Semin Nucl Med 1991;21:230–241

27. Dyke S, Cohn P, Gorlin R, Sonnenblick E: Detection of residual myocardial function in coronary artery disease using post-extrasystolic potentiation. Circulation 1974;50:694–699

28. Charney R, Schwinger M, Chun J et al: Dobutamine echocardiography and resting-redistribution thallium-201 scintigraphy predicts recovery of hibernating myocardium after coronary revascularization. Am Heart J 1994;128:864–869

29. Nesto RW, Cohn L, Collins J et al: Inotropic contractile reserve: a useful predictor of increased 5 year survival and improved post operative left ventricular function in patients with coronary artery disease and reduced ejection fraction. Am J Cardiol 1982;50:39–46

30. Scognamiglio R, Fasoli G, Ponchia A, Volta SD: Detection of an irreversible myocardial damage in heart failure. Circulation, suppl. II 1991;84:563

31. Di Carli MF, Asgarzadie F, Schelbert HR et al: Quantitative relation between myocardial viability and improvement in heart failure symptoms after revascularization in patients with ischemic cardiomyopathy. Circulation 1995;92:3436–3444

32. Tamaki N, Yonekura Y, Yamashita K: Positron emission tomography using fluorine-18-deoxyglucose in evaluation of coronary artery bypass grafting. Am J Cardiol 1989;64:860–865

33. Gropler R, Siegel B, Sampathkumaran K: Dependence of recovery of contractile function on maintenance of oxidative metabolism after myocardial infarction. J Am Cardiol 1992;19:989–997

34. Paolini G, Lucignani G, Zuccari M et al: Identification and revascularization of hibernating myocardium in angina-free patients with left ventricular dysfunction. Eur J Cardiothorac Surg 1994;8:139–144

35. Gropler R, Geltman E, Sampathkumaran K: Comparison of carbon-11-acetate with fluorine-18-fluorodeoxyglucose for delineating viable myocardium by positron emission tomography. J Am Coll Cardiol 1993;22:1587–1597

36. Besozzi M, Brown M, Hubner K: Retrospective post therapy evaluation of cardiac function in 208 coronary artery disease patients evaluated by positron emission tomography [abstract]. J Nucl Med 1992;33:885

37. Depre C, Melin J, Vanoverschelde J: Assessment of myocardial viability after bypass surgery by pre-operative PET flow-metabolism measurements and ultrastructural analysis of myocardial biopsies [abstract]. Circulation, suppl. 1 1993;88:199

38. Eitzman D, Al-Aouar Z, Kanter H: Clinical outcome of patients with advanced coronary artery disease after viability studies with positron emission tomography. J Am Coll Cardiol 1992;20:559–565

39. Di Carli MF, Davidson M, Little R et al: Value of metabolic imaging with positron emission tomography for evaluating prognosis in patients with coronary artery disease and left ventricular dysfunction. Am J Cardiol 1994;73:527–533

40. Louie HW, Laks H, Milgalter E et al: Ischemic cardiomyopathy. Criteria for coronary revascularization

and cardiac transplantation. Circulation, suppl. III 1991;84:290–295

41. Blitz A, Laks H, Drinkwater D et al: Revascularization versus transplantation for ischemic cardiomyopathy. Ann Thorac Surg (1996, in press)

42. Alderman E, Fisher L, Litwin P et al: Results of coronary artery surgery in patients with poor left ventricular function (CASS). Circulation 1983;68:785–795

43. Emond M, Mock MB, Davis KB et al: Long-term survival of medically treated patients in the Coronary Artery Surgery Study (CASS) Registry. Circulation 1994;90:2645–2657

44. Yatteau RF, Peter RH, Behar VS et al: Ischemic cardiomyopathy. The myopathy of coronary artery disease. Natural history and results of medical versus surgical treatment. Am J Cardiol 1974;34:520–525

45. Manley J, King J, Zeft J et al: The "bad" left ventricle; results of coronary surgery and effect on later survival. J Thorac Cardiovasc Surg 1976;72:841–848

46. Zubiate P, Kay J, Mendez A: Myocardial revascularization for the patient with drastic impairment of function of the left ventricle. J Thorac Cardiovasc Surg 1977;73:84–86

47. Castaner A, Betriu A, Sanz G et al: Natural history of severe left ventricular dysfunction after myocardial infarction. Chest 1984;85:744–750

48. Faulkner S, Stoney W, Alford W et al: Ischemic cardiomyopathy. Medical versus surgical treatment. J Thorac Cardiovasc Surg 1977;74:77–82

49. Harris PJ, Lee KL, Harrell Jr FE et al: Outcome in medically treated coronary artery disease. Ischemic events: nonfatal infarction and death. Circulation 1980;62:718–726

50. Luciani GB, Faggian G, Razzolini R et al: Severe ischemic left ventricular failure. Coronary operation or heart transplantation? Ann Thorac Surg 1993;55: 719–723

51. Killip T, Passamani E, Davis K et al: A randomized trial of coronary bypass surgery. Eight years followup and survival in patients with reduced ejection fraction. Circulation, suppl. V 1985;72:102–109

52. Pigott J, Kouchoukos N, Oberman A, Cutter G: Late results of surgical and medical therapy for patients with coronary artery disease and depressed left ventricular function. J Am Coll Cardiol 1985;5: 1036–1045

53. Dreyfus G, Duboc D, Blasco A et al: Coronary surgery can be an alternative to heart transplantation in selected patients with end-stage ischemic heart disease. Eur J Cardiothorac Surg, 1993;7:482–487; discussion 488

54. Christakis G, Weisel R, Fremes S et al: Coronary artery bypass grafting in patients with poor ventricular function. J Thorac Cardiovasc Surg 1992;103: 1083–1092

55. Kron IL, Flanagan TL, Blackbourne LH et al: Coronary revascularization rather than cardiac transplantation for chronic ischemic cardiomyopathy. Ann Surg 1989;210:348–352; discussion 352–354

56. Tyras DH, Kaiser GC, Barner HB et al: Global left ventricular impairment and myocardial revascularization: determinants of survival. Ann Thorac Surg 1984;37:47–51

57. Freeman WK, Schaff HV, O'Brien PC et al: Cardiac surgery in the octogenarian: perioperative outcome

58. Coles JG, Del Campo C, Ahmed SN et al: Improved long-term survival following myocardial revascularization in patients with severe left ventricular dysfunction. J Thorac Cardiovasc Surg 1981;81:846–850

59. Pryor D, FH Jr, Rankin J et al: The changing survival benefits of coronary revascularization over time. Circulation suppl. V 1987;76:13–21

60. Van Trigt P: Ischemic cardiomyopathy. The role of coronary artery bypass. Coron Artery Dis 1993;4: 707–712

61. Milano CA, White WD, Smith LR et al: Coronary artery bypass in patients with severely depressed ventricular function. Ann Thorac Surg 1993;56:487–493

62. Bounous E, Mark D, Pollock B et al: Surgical survival benefits for coronary disease patients with left ventricular dysfunction. Circulation suppl. I 1988;78: 151–157

63. Califf R, Harrell F, Lee K et al: The evolution of medical and surgical therapy for coronary artery disease. A 15-year experience. JAMA 1989;261:2077–2086

64. Wechsler AS, Junod FL: Coronary bypass grafting in patients with chronic congestive heart failure. Circulation 1989;79:92–96

65. Kennedy JW, Kaiser GC, Fisher LD et al: Clinical and angiographic predictors of operative mortality from the collaborative study in coronary artery surgery (CASS). Circulation 1981;63:793–802

66. Hochberg M, Parsonnet V, Gielchinsky I, Hussain S: Coronary artery bypass grafting in patients with ejection fractions below forty percent. Early and late results in 466 patients. J Thorac Cardiovasc Surg 1983;86:519–527

67. Balu V, Szmedra L, Dean D, Bhayana J: Long-term survival of patients with low ejection fraction. Texas Heart Inst J, 1988;15:44–48

68. Goor DA, Golan M, Bar-El Y et al: Synergism between infarct-borne left ventricular dysfunction and cardiomegaly in increasing the risk of coronary bypass surgery. J Thorac Cardiovasc Surg 1992;104: 983–989

69. Luciani GB, Faggian G, Mazzucco A et al: Myocardial revascularization in ischemic cardiomyopathy. A way for better donor heart allocation. Transplant Proc 1993;25:3173–3174

70. Olsen PS, Kassis E, Niebuhr-Jorgensen U: Coronary artery bypass surgery in patients with severe left-ventricular dysfunction. Thorac Cardiovasc Surg 1993;41:118–120

71. Gill IS, Loop FD, Kramer J et al: Primary isolated coronary artery bypass in left ventricular dysfunction. Survival and predictors of survival. Can J Cardiol 1994;10:923–926

72. Hausmann H, Ennker J, Topp H et al: Coronary artery bypass grafting and heart transplantation in end-stage coronary artery disease. A comparison of hemodynamic improvement and ventricular function. J Card Surg 1994;9:77–84

73. Jegaden O, de Gevigney G, Montagna P et al: Late survival up to 20 years after isolated coronary bypass surgery using internal mammary artery in patients with severe left ventricular dysfunction. J Cardiovasc Surg (Torino) 1994;35:129–134

74. Langenburg SE, Buchanan SA, Blackbourne LH et al: Predicting survival after coronary revascariza-

tion for ischemic cardiomyopathy. Ann Thorac Surg 1995;60:1193–1196; discussion 1196–1197

75. Kay G, Sun G, Aoki A, Prejean C: Influence of ejection fraction on hospital mortality, morbidity, and costs for CABG patients. Ann Thorac Surg 1995;60: 1640–1651

76. Spencer FC, Green GE, Tice DA et al: Coronary artery bypass grafts for congestive heart failure. A report of experiences with 40 patients. J Thorac Cardiovasc Surg 1971;62:529–542

77. Gill IS, Loop FD, Kramer J et al: Primary isolated coronary artery bypass in left ventricular dysfunction. Survival and predictors of survival. Can J Cardiol 1994;10:923–926

78. DePace NL, Dowinsky S, Untereker W et al: Giant inferior wall left ventricular aneurysm. Am Heart J 1990;119:400–402

79. Dubnow M, Burchell H, Titus J: Postinfarction ventricular aneurysm. A clinicomorphologic and electro-cardiographic study of 80 cases. Am Heart J 1965; 70:753–760

80. Schlichter J, Hellerstein H, Katz L: Aneurysm of the heart. A correlative study of one hundred and two proved cases. Medicine 1954;33:43–75

81. Arvan S, Badillo P: Contractile properties of the left ventricle with aneurysm. Am J Cardiol 1985;55: 338–341

82. Nagle RE, Williams DO: Proceedings. Natural history of ventricular aneurysm without surgical treatment. Br Heart J 1974;36:1037

83. Banka V, Bodenheimer M, Helfant R: Determinants of reversible asynergy. Effect of pathologic Q waves, coronary collaterals, and anatomic location. Circulation 1974;50:714

84. Cheng TO: Incidence of ventricular aneurysm in coronary artery disease. An angiographic appraisal. Am J Med 1971;50:340–355

85. Hirai T, Fujita M, Nakajima H et al: Importance of collateral circulation for prevention of left ventricular aneurysm formation in acute myocardial infarction. Circulation 1989;79:791–796

86. Forman MB, Collins HW, Kopelman HA et al: Determinants of left ventricular aneurysm formation after anterior myocardial infarction. A clinical and angiographic study. J Am Coll Cardiol 1986;8:1256–1262

87. Kirklin J, Barratt-Boyes B: Cardiac surgery. In: Kirklin J, Barratt-Boyes B (eds) Cardiac Surgery. 2nd ed. Vol. 1. Churchill Livingstone, New York, 1993

88. Buehler DL, Stinson EB, Oyer PE, Shumway NE: Surgical treatment of aneurysms of the inferior left ventricular wall. J Thorac Cardiovasc Surg 1979;78: 74–78

89. Salati M, Di Biasi P, Paje A et al: Functional results of left ventricular reconstruction. Ann Thorac Surg 1993;56:316–322

90. Kitamura S, Kay J, Krohn B et al: Geometric and functional abnormalities of the left ventricle with a chronic localized noncontractile area. Am J Cardiol 1973;31:701–707

91. Klein MD, Herman MV, Gorlin R: A hemodynamic study of left ventricular aneurysm. Circulation 1967; 35:614–630

92. Mills NL, Everson CT, Hockmuth DR: Technical advances in the treatment of left ventricular aneurysm. Ann Thorac Surg 1993;55:792–800

93. Jan K: Distribution of myocardial stress and its influence on coronary blood flow. J Biomech 1985;18: 815–820

94. Streeter D, Vaishnav R, Pater D et al: Stress distribution in the canine left ventricle during diastole and systole. Biophys J 1970;10:345–363

95. Barratt-Boyes BG, White HD, Agnew TM et al: The results of surgical treatment of left ventricular aneurysms. An assessment of the risk factors affecting early and late mortality. J Thorac Cardiovasc Surg 1984;87:87–98

96. Frank G, Klein H, Bednarska E et al: Results after resection of postinfarction left ventricular aneurysms. Thorac Cardiovasc Surg 1980;28:423–427

97. Froehlich RT, Falsetti HL, Doty DB, Marcus ML: Prospective study of surgery for left ventricular aneurysm. Am J Cardiol 1980;45:923–931

98. Jones EL, Craver JM, Hurst JW et al: Influence of left ventricular aneurysm on survival following the coronary bypass operation. Ann Surg 1981;193: 733–742

99. Reddy S, Cooley D, Duncan J, Norman J: Left ventricular aneurysm. Twenty-year surgical experience with 1572 patients at the Texas Heart Institute. Bull Texas Heart Inst 1981;8:165–186

100. Otterstad JE, Christensen O, Levorstad K, Nitter-Hauge S: Long-term results after left ventricular aneurysmectomy. Br Heart J 1981;45:427–433

101. Rittenhouse EA, Sauvage LR, Mansfield PB et al: Results of combined left ventricular aneurysmectomy and coronary artery bypass: 1974 to 1980. Am J Surg 1982;143:575–578

102. Brawley RK, Magovern Jr GJ, Gott VL et al: Left ventricular aneurysmectomy. Factors influencing postoperative results. J Thorac Cardiovasc Surg 1983;85:712–717

103. Kiefer SK, Flaker GC, Martin RH, Curtis JJ: Clinical improvement after ventricular aneurysm repair. Prediction by angiographic and hemodynamic variables. J Am Coll Cardiol 1983;2:30–37

104. Novick RJ, Stefaniszyn HJ, Morin JE et al: Surgery for postinfarction left ventricular aneurysm. Prognosis and long-term follow-up. Can J Surg 1984;27: 161–167

105. Olearchyk AS, Lemole GM, Spagna PM: Left ventricular aneurysm. Ten years' experience in surgical treatment of 244 cases. Improved clinical status, hemodynamics, and long-term longevity. J Thorac Cardiovasc Surg 1984;88:544–553

106. Skinner JR, Rasak C, Kongtahworn C et al: Natural history of surgically treated ventricular aneurysm. Ann Thorac Surg 1984;38:42–45

107. Gonzalez-Santos JM, Ennabli K, Galinanes M et al: Surgical treatment of the post-infarction left ventricular aneurysm. Factors influencing early and late results. Thorac Cardiovasc Surg 1985;33:86–93

108. Keenan DJ, Monro JL, Ross JK et al: Left ventricular aneurysm. The Wessex experience. Br Heart J 1985; 54:269–272

109. Taylor NC, Barber R, Crossland P et al: Does left ventricular aneurysmectomy improve ventricular function in patients undergoing coronary bypass surgery? Br Heart J 1985;54:145–152

110. Yabe Y, Yamashita T, Komatsu H et al: Study of left ventricular function and myocardial viability in patients with left ventricular aneurysm developed after

myocardial infarction. A comparative study of medical and surgical therapy. Jpn Heart J 1985;26:53–68

111. Akins CW: Resection of left ventricular aneurysm during hypothermic fibrillatory arrest without aortic occlusion. J Thorac Cardiovasc Surg 1986;91:610–618

112. Cohen DE, Vogel RA: Left ventricular aneurysm as a coronary risk factor independent of overall left ventricular function. Am Heart J 1986;111:23–30

113. Faxon DP, Myers WO, McCabe CH et al: The influence of surgery on the natural history of angiographically documented left ventricular aneurysm. The Coronary Artery Surgery Study. Circulation 1986;74:110–118

114. Marks C, Miller A, Yakirevich V, Vidne B: Surgical treatment of left ventricular aneurysms. Int Surg 1986;71:69–72

115. Louagie Y, Alouini T, Lesperance J, Pelletier LC: Left ventricular aneurysm with predominating congestive heart failure. A comparative study of medical and surgical treatment. J Thorac Cardiovasc Surg 1987;94:571–581

116. Palatianos GM, Craythorne CB, Schor JS, Bolooki H: Hemodynamic effects of radical left ventricular scar resection in patients with and without congestive heart failure. J Surg Res 1988;44:690–695

117. Vauthey JN, Berry DW, Snyder DW et al: Left ventricular aneurysm repair with myocardial revascularization. An analysis of 246 consecutive patients over 15 years. Ann Thorac Surg 1988;46:29–35

118. Cosgrove DM, Lytle BW, Taylor PC et al: Ventricular aneurysm resection. Trends in surgical risk. Circulation 1989;79:97–101

119. Mangschau A, Geiran O, Forfang K et al: Left ventricular aneurysm and severe cardiac dysfunction. Heart transplantation or aneurysm surgery? J Heart Transplant 1989;8:486–493

120. Komeda M, David TE, Malik A et al: Operative risks and long-term results of operation for left ventricular aneurysm. Ann Thorac Surg 1992;53:22–28; discussion 28–29

121. Couper GS, Bunton RW, Birjiniuk V et al: Relative risks of left ventricular aneurysmectomy in patients with akinetic scars versus true dyskinetic aneurysms. Circulation, suppl. IV 1990;82:248–256

122. Baciewicz PA, Weintraub WS, Jones EL et al: Late follow-up after repair of left ventricular aneurysm and (usually) associated coronary bypass grafting. Am J Cardiol 1991;68:193–200

123. Di Donato M, Barletta G, Maioli M et al: Early hemodynamic results of left ventricular reconstructive surgery for anterior wall left ventricular aneurysm. Am J Cardiol 1992;69:886–890

124. Elefteriades JA, Solomon LW, Salazar AM et al: Linear left ventricular aneurysmectomy. Modern imaging studies reveal improved morphology and function. Ann Thorac Surg 1993;56:242–250; discussion 251–252

125. Kesler K, Fiore A, Naunheim K et al: Anterior wall left ventricular aneurysm repair. A comparison of linear versus circular closure. J Thorac Cardiovasc Surg 1992;103:841–848

126. Iguidbashian JP, Follette DM, Contino JP et al: Pericardial patch repair of left ventricular aneurysm. Ann Thorac Surg 1993;55:1022–1024

127. Salati M, Di Biasi P, Paje A, Santoli C: Left ventricular geometry after endoventriculoplasty. Eur J Cardiothorac Surg 1993;7:574–578; discussion 579

128. Prates PR, Vitola D, Sant'anna JR et al: Surgical repair of ventricular aneurysms. Early results with Cooley's technique. Tex Heart Inst J 1993;20:19–22

129. Jakob HG, Zolch B, Schuster S et al: Endoventricular patch plasty improves results of LV aneurysmectomy. Eur J Cardiothorac Surg 1993;7:428–435; discussion 436

130. Oxelbark S, Mannting F, Ramstrom J et al: Surgery for chronic left ventricular aneurysm. Benefits and side effects. Scand J Thorac Cardiovasc Surg 1993;27:157–164

131. Mickleborough LL, Maruyama H, Liu P, Mohamed S: Results of left ventricular aneurysmectomy with a tailored scar excision and primary closure technique. J Thorac Cardiovasc Surg 1994;107:690–698

132. Stahle E, Bergstrom R, Nystrom SO et al: Surgical treatment of left ventricular aneurysm—assessment of risk factors for early and late mortality. Eur J Cardiothorac Surg 1994;8:67–73

133. Kawachi K, Kitamura S, Kawata T et al: Hemodynamic assessment during exercise after left ventricular aneurysmectomy. J Thorac Cardiovasc Surg 1994;107:178–183

134. Dor V, Sabatier M, Di Donato M et al: Late hemodynamic results after left ventricular patch repair associated with coronary grafting in patients with postinfarction akinetic or dyskinetic aneurysm of the left ventricle. J Thorac Cardiovasc Surg 1995;110:1291–1299; discussion 1300–1301

135. Cohen M, Packer M, Gorlin R: Indications for left ventricular aneurysmectomy. Circulation 1983;67:717–722

136. Proudfit W, Bruschke A, Sones F: Natural history of obstructive coronary artery disease. Ten year study of 601 nonsurgical cases. Prog Cardiovasc Dis 1978;21:53–78

137. Elefteriades J, Solomon L, Mickleborough L, Cooley D: Left ventricular aneurysmectomy in advanced left ventricular dysfunction. Cardiol Clin 1995;13:59–72

138. Grondin P, Kretz JG, Bical O et al: Natural history of saccular aneurysms of the left ventricle. J Thorac Cardiovasc Surg 1979;77:57–64

139. Bruschke A, Proudfit W, Sones F: Progress study of 590 consecutive nonsurgical cases of coronary disease followed 5–9 years. Circulation 1973;47:1147–1163

140. Visser CA, Kan G, Meltzer RS et al: Incidence, timing and prognostic value of left ventricular aneurysm formation after myocardial infarction. A prospective, serial echocardiographic study of 158 patients. Am J Cardiol 1986;57:729–732

141. Meizlish JL, Berger HJ, Plankey M et al: Functional left ventricular aneurysm formation after acute anterior transmural myocardial infarction. Incidence, natural history, and prognostic implications. N Engl J Med 1984;311:1001–1006

142. Faxon DP, Ryan TJ, Davis KB et al: Prognostic significance of angiographically documented left ventricular aneurysm from the Coronary Artery Surgery Study (CASS). Am J Cardiol 1982;50:157–164

143. Cheng TO: Cardiac failure in coronary heart disease. Am Heart J 1990;120:396–412

144. Guyton R: Discussion of Cooley DA, Frazier OH, Duncan JM, Reul GJ, Krajcer Z. Intracavitary repair of

ventricular aneurysm and regional dyskinesia. Ann Surg 1992;215:423

145. Cooley D: Ventricular endoaneurysmorrhaphy. Results of an improved method of repair. Texas Heart Inst J 1989;16:72–75

146. Cooley DA, Frazier OH, Duncan JM et al: Intracavitary repair of ventricular aneurysm and regional dyskinesia. Ann Surg 1992;215:417–423; discussion 423–424

147. Dor V, Saab M, Coste P et al: Left ventricular aneurysm: a new surgical approach. Thorac Cardiovasc Surg 1989;37:11–19

148. Jatene AD: Left ventricular aneurysmectomy. Resection or reconstruction. J Thorac Cardiovasc Surg 1985;89:321–331

149. Stoney WS, Alford WC Jr, Burrus GR, Thomas CS Jr: Repair of anteroseptal ventricular aneurysm. Ann Thorac Surg 1973;15:394–404

150. Rivera R, Delcan JL: Factors influencing better results in operation for postinfarction ventricular aneurysms. Ann Thorac Surg 1979;27:445–450

151. Brawley RK, Schaff H, Stevens R et al: Influence of coronary artery anatomy on survival following resection of left ventricular aneurysms and chronic infarcts. J Thorac Cardiovasc Surg 1977;73:120–128

152. Balu V, Hook N, Dean DC, Naughton J: Effect of left ventricular aneurysmectomy on exercise performance. Int J Cardiol 1984;5:210–213

153. Donaldson RM, Honey M, Balcon R et al: Surgical treatment of postinfarction left ventricular aneurysm in 32 patients. Br Heart J 1976;38:1223–1228

154. Fontan F: The prognostic value of pre-operative left ventricular performance in left ventricular resection. Thorac Cardiovasc Surg 1979;27:281–288

155. Dymond DS, Stephens JD, Stone DL et al: Combined exercise radionuclide and hemodynamic evaluation of left ventricular aneurysmectomy. Am Heart J 1982;104:977–987

156. Martin JL, Untereker WJ, Harken AH et al: Aneurysmectomy and endocardial resection for ventricular tachycardia. Favorable hemodynamic and antiarrhythmic results in patients with global left ventricular dysfunction. Am Heart J 1982;103:960–965

157. Shaw RC, Connors JP, Hieb BR et al: Postoperative investigation of left ventricular aneurysm resection. Circulation, suppl. II 1977;56:7–11

158. Di Donato M, Barletta G, Maioli M et al: Early hemodynamic results of left ventricular reconstructive surgery for anterior wall left ventricular aneurysm. Am J Cardiol 1992;69:886–890

159. Burton NA, Stinson EB, Oyer PE, Shumway NE: Left ventricular aneurysm. Preoperative risk factors and long-term postoperative results. J Thorac Cardiovasc Surg 1979;77:65–75

160. Rizzoli G, Bellotto F, Gallucci V et al: Early and late determinants of survival after surgery of left ventricular aneurysm. Eur J Cardiothorac Surg 1988;2:265–272

161. Cooperman M, Stinson EB, Griepp RB, Shumway NE: Survival and function after left ventricular aneurysmectomy. J Thorac Cardiovasc Surg 1975;69:321–328

162. Bogers AJ, Hermans J, Dubois SV, Huysmans HA: Incremental risk factors for hospital mortality after postinfarction left ventricular aneurysmectomy. Eur J Cardiothorac Surg 1988;2:160–166

163. Marco JD, Kaiser GC, Barner HE et al: Left ventricular aneurysmectomy. Arch Surg 1976;111:419–422

164. Walker WE, Stoney WS, Alford WC Jr et al: Techniques and results of ventricular aneurysmectomy with emphasis on anteroseptal repair. J Thorac Cardiovasc Surg 1978;76:824–831

165. Moran JM, Scanlon PJ, Nemickas R, Pifarre R: Surgical treatment of postinfarction ventricular aneurysm. Ann Thorac Surg 1976;21:107–113

166. Swan H, Magnusson P, Buchbinder N et al: Aneurysm of the cardiac ventricle. Its management by medical and surgical intervention. West J Med 1978;129:26

167. Mullen DC, Posey L, Gabriel R et al: Prognostic considerations in the management of left ventricular aneurysms. Ann Thorac Surg 1977;23:455–460

168. Burckhardt D, Hoffmann A, Kiowski W: Treatment of mitral stenosis. Eur Heart J, suppl. B 1991;12:95–98

169. Bolen J, Lopes M, Harrison D, Alderman E: Analysis of left ventricular function in response to afterload changes in patients with mitral stenosis. Circulation 1975;52:894

170. Holzer JA, Karliner JS, Ra OR, Peterson KL: Quantitative angiographic analysis of the left ventricle in patients with isolated rheumatic mitral stenosis. Br Heart J 1973;35:497–502

171. Curry GC, Elliott LP, Ramsey HW: Quantitative left ventricular angiocardiographic findings in mitral stenosis. Detailed analysis of the anterolateral wall of the left ventricle. Am J Cardiol 1972;29:621–627

172. Rapaport E: Recognition and management of mitral stenosis. Heart Dis Stroke 1993;2:64–68

173. Mattina C, Green S, Tortolani A et al: Frequency of angiographically significant coronary arterial narrowing in mitral stenosis. Am J Cardiol 1986;57:802–805

174. Turi ZG, Reyes VP, Raju BS et al: Percutaneous balloon versus surgical closed commissurotomy for mitral stenosis. A prospective, randomized trial [see comments]. Circulation 1991;83:1179–1185

175. Patel JJ, Shama D, Mitha AS et al: Balloon valvuloplasty versus closed commissurotomy for pliable mitral stenosis. A prospective hemodynamic study. J Am Coll Cardiol 1991;18:1318–1322

176. Shrivastava S, Mathur A, Dev V et al: Comparison of immediate hemodynamic response to closed mitral commissurotomy, single-balloon, and double-balloon mitral valvuloplasty in rheumatic mitral stenosis. J Thorac Cardiovasc Surg 1992;104:1264–1267

177. Arora R, Nair M, Kalra GS et al: Immediate and long-term results of balloon and surgical closed mitral valvotomy. A randomized comparative study. Am Heart J 1993;125:1091–1094

178. Villanova C, Melacini P, Scognamiglio R et al: Long-term echocardiographic evaluation of closed and open mitral valvulotomy. Int J Cardiol 1993;38:315–321

179. Cohn LH, Allred EN, Cohn LA et al: Long-term results of open mitral valve reconstruction for mitral stenosis. Am J Cardiol 1985;55:731–734

180. Eguaras MG, Luque I, Montero A et al: A comparison of repair and replacement for mitral stenosis with partially calcified valve [see comments]. J Thorac Cardiovasc Surg 1990;100:161–166

181. Okita Y, Miki S, Ueda Y et al: Mitral valve replacement with maintenance of mitral annulopapillary muscle continuity in patients with mitral stenosis. J Thorac Cardiovasc Surg 1994;108:42–51

182. Reyes VP, Raju BS, Wynne J et al: Percutaneous balloon valvuloplasty compared with open surgical commissurotomy for mitral stenosis [see comments]. N Engl J Med 1994;331:961–967

183. Lock J, Khalilullah M, Shrivastava S et al: Percutaneous catheter commissurotomy in rheumatic mitral stenosis. N Engl J Med 1985;313:1515–1518

184. McKay R, Lock J, Safian R et al: Balloon dilatation of mitral stenosis in adult patients. Postmortem and percutaneous mitral valvuloplasty studies. J Am Coll Cardiol 1987;9:723–731

185. McKay C, Kawanishi D, Rahimtoola S: Catheter balloon valvuloplasty of the mitral valve in adults using a double-balloon technique. Early hemodynamic results. JAMA 1987;257:1753–1761

186. Palacios I, Block P, Brandi S et al: Percutaneous balloon valvotomy for patients with severe mitral stenosis. Circulation 1987;75:778–784

187. Block P, Palacios I, Block E et al: Late (two year) follow-up after percutaneous mitral valvotomy. Am J Cardiol 1992;69:537–541

188. Arora R, Kalra GS, Murty GS et al: Percutaneous transatrial mitral commissurotomy. Immediate and intermediate results. J Am Coll Cardiol 1994;23:1327–1332

189. Cohen DJ, Kuntz RE, Gordon SP et al: Predictors of long-term outcome after percutaneous balloon mitral valvuloplasty. N Engl J Med 1992;327:1329–1335

190. National Heart, Lung, and Blood Institute Balloon Valvuloplasty Registry Participants: Multicenter experience with balloon mitral commissurotomy. NHLBI Balloon Valvuloplasty Registry Report on immediate and 30-day follow-up results. Circulation 1992;85:448–461

191. Pan M, Medina A, Suarez de Lezo J et al: Factors determining late success after mitral balloon valvulotomy. Am J Cardiol 1993;71:1181–1185

192. Chen CR, Cheng TO, Chen JY et al: Long-term results of percutaneous mitral valvuloplasty with the Inoue balloon catheter. Am J Cardiol 1992;70:1445–1448

193. Vahanian A, Michel PL, Cormier B et al: Results of percutaneous mitral commissurotomy in 200 patients. Am J Cardiol 1989;63:847–852

194. Vahanian A, Michel PL, Cormier B et al: Immediate and mid-term results of percutaneous mitral commissurotomy. Eur Heart J suppl. B 1991;12:84–89

195. Vahanian A, Cormier B, Iung B: Percutaneous transvenous mitral commissurotomy using the Inoue balloon. International experience. Cathet Cardiovasc Diagn, suppl. 2 1994;2:8–15

196. Desideri A, Vanderperren O, Serra A et al: Long-term (9 to 33 months) echocardiographic follow-up after successful percutaneous mitral commissurotomy. Am J Cardiol 1992;69:1602–1606

197. Chen C, Wang X, Wang Y et al: Value of two-dimensional echocardiography in selecting patients and balloon sizes for percutaneous balloon mitral valvuloplasty. J Am Coll Cardiol 1989;14:1651–1658

198. Akins C: Results with mechanical cardiac valvular prostheses. Ann Thorac Surg 1995;60:1836–1844

199. Data analyses of the Society of Thoracic Surgeons National Cardiac Surgery database. Summit Medical, Minneapolis, 1995

200. Agozzino L, Falco A, de Vivo F et al: Surgical pathology of the mitral valve. Gross and histological study of 1288 surgically excised valves. Int J Cardiol 1992;37:79–89

201. Luxereau P, Dorent R, De Gevigney G et al: Aetiology of surgically treated mitral regurgitation. Eur Heart J, suppl. B 1991;12:2–4

202. Roberts WC: Morphologic features of the normal and abnormal mitral valve. Am J Cardiol 1983;51:1005–1028

203. Braunwald E: Mitral regurgitation. Physiologic, clinical and surgical considerations. N Engl J Med 1969;281:425–433

204. Eckberg DL, Gault JH, Bouchard RL et al: Mechanics of left ventricular contraction in chronic severe mitral regurgitation. Circulation 1973;47:1252–1259

205. Urabe Y, Mann DL, Kent RL et al: Cellular and ventricular contractile dysfunction in experimental canine mitral regurgitation. Circ Res 1992;70:131–147

206. Nakagawa M, Shirato K, Ohyama T et al: Left ventricular end-systolic stress-volume index ratio in aortic and mitral regurgitation with normal ejection fraction. Am Heart J 1990;120:892–901

207. Carabello BA, Nakano K, Corin W et al: Left ventricular function in experimental volume overload hypertrophy. Am J Physiol 1989;256:H974–H981

208. Rapaport E: Natural history of aortic and mitral valve disease. Am J Cardiol 1975;35:221–227

209. Levine H: Is valve surgery indicated in patients with severe mitral regurgitation even if they are asymptomatic? Cardiovasc Clin 1990;21:161–173

210. Gray R, Helfant R: Timing of surgery for valvular heart disease. Cardiovasc Clin 1991;21:209–215

211. Delahaye F, Delaye J, Ecochard R et al: Influence of associated valvular lesions on long-term prognosis of mitral stenosis. A 20-year follow-up of 202 patients. Eur Heart J, suppl. B 1991;12:77–80

212. Munoz S, Gallardo J, Diaz-Gorrin JR, Medina O: Influence of surgery on the natural history of rheumatic mitral and aortic valve disease. Am J Cardiol 1975;35:234–242

213. Assey ME, Spann JF Jr: Indications for heart valve replacement. Clin Cardiol 1990;13:81–88

214. Mudge GH Jr: Asymptomatic mitral regurgitation. When to operate? J Card Surg, suppl. 2 1994;9:248–251

215. Cohn LH, Couper GS, Kinchla NM, Collins JJ Jr: Decreased operative risk of surgical treatment of mitral regurgitation with or without coronary artery disease. J Am Coll Cardiol 1990;16:1575–1578

216. Sakai K, Nakano S, Taniguchi K et al: Global left ventricular performance and regional systolic function after suture annuloplasty for chronic mitral regurgitation. Circulation, suppl. II 1992;86:39–45

217. Lytle B: Impact of coronary artery disease on valvular heart surgery. Cardiol Clin 1991;9:301–314

218. Hansen DE, Cahill PD, DeCampli WM et al: Valvular-ventricular interaction. Importance of the mitral apparatus in canine left ventricular systolic performance. Circulation 1986;73:1310–1320

219. Ishihara K, Zile MR, Kanazawa S et al: Left ventricular mechanics and myocyte function after correction of experimental chronic mitral regurgitation by combined mitral valve replacement and preservation of the native mitral valve apparatus. Circulation, suppl. II 1992;86:16–25

220. Gray R, Helfant R: Timing of surgery for valvular heart disease. Cardiovasc Clin 1990;21:209–215

221. Michel PL, Iung B, Blanchard B et al: Long-term results of mitral valve repair for non-ischaemic mitral regurgitation. Eur Heart J, suppl. B 1991;12:39–43

222. Gaasch W, Zile M: Left ventricular function after surgical correction of chronic mitral regurgitation. Eur Heart J, suppl. B 1991;12:48–51

223. Kaul T, Ramsdale D, Meek D, Mercer JL: Mitral valve replacement in patients with severe mitral regurgitation and impaired left ventricular function. Int J Cardiol 1992;35:169–179

224. Rozich JD, Carabello BA, Usher BW et al: Mitral valve replacement with and without chordal preservation in patients with chronic mitral regurgitation. Mechanisms for differences in postoperative ejection performance. Circulation 1992;86:1718–1726

225. Ghosh PK, Shah S, Das A et al: Early evidence of beneficial effects of chordal preservation in mitral valve replacement on left ventricular dimensions. Eur J Cardiothorac Surg 1992;6:655–659

226. Crawford MH, Souchek J, Oprian CA et al: Determinants of survival and left ventricular performance after mitral valve replacement. Department of Veterans Affairs Cooperative Study on Valvular Heart Disease. Circulation 1990;81:1173–1181

227. Braunwald E: Heart Disease. A Textbook of Cardiovascular Medicine. pp. 1018–1092. Saunders, Philadelphia, 1992

228. Yacoub M, Halim M, Radley-Smith R et al: Surgical treatment of mitral regurgitation caused by floppy valves. Repair versus replacement. Circulation, suppl. II 1981;64:210–216

229. Adebo O, Ross J: Surgical treatment of ruptured mitral valve chordae. A comparison between mitral valve replacement and valve repair. Thorac Cardiovasc Surg 1984;32:139–142

230. Jebara VA, Dervanian P, Acar C et al: Mitral valve repair using Carpentier techniques in patients more than 70 years old. Early and late results. Circulation, suppl. II 1992;86:53–59

231. David TE, Armstrong S, Sun Z, Daniel L: Late results of mitral valve repair for mitral regurgitation due to degenerative disease. Ann Thorac Surg 1993;56:7–12; discussion 13–14

232. Bernal JM, Rabasa JM, Vilchez FG et al: Mitral valve repair in rheumatic disease. The flexible solution. Circulation 1993;88:1746–1753

233. Fernandez J, Joyce DH, Hirschfeld KJ et al: Valve-related events and valve-related mortality in 340 mitral valve repairs. A late phase follow-up study. Eur J Cardiothorac Surg 1993;7:263–270

234. Carpentier A, Chauvaud S, Fabiani JN et al: Reconstructive surgery of mitral valve incompetence: Ten-year appraisal. J Thorac Cardiovasc Surg 1980;79:338–348

235. Galloway AC, Colvin SB, Baumann FG et al: A comparison of mitral valve reconstruction with mitral valve replacement. Intermediate-term results. Ann Thorac Surg 1989;47:655–662

236. Sand ME, Naftel DC, Blackstone EH et al: A comparison of repair and replacement for mitral valve incompetence. J Thorac Cardiovasc Surg 1987;94:208–219

237. Currie PJ: Valvular heart disease. A correctable cause of congestive heart failure. Postgrad Med 1991;89:123–126, 131–136

238. Bojar M: Adult Cardiac Surgery. p. 56. Blackwell, Oxford. 1992

239. Duran CM, Gometza B, Balasundaram S, al Halees Z: A feasibility study of valve repair in rheumatic mitral regurgitation. Eur Heart J, suppl. B 1991;12:34–38

240. Loop F, Cosgrove D, Stewart W: Mitral valve repair for mitral insufficiency. Eur Heart J, suppl. B 1991;12:30–33

241. Cosgrove D, Stewart W: Mitral valvuloplasty. Curr Probl Cardiol 1989;14:359–415

242. Craver JM, Cohen C, Weintraub WS: Case-matched comparison of mitral valve replacement and repair. Ann Thorac Surg 1990;49:964–969

243. Deloche A, Jebara VA, Relland JY et al: Valve repair with Carpentier techniques. The second decade. J Thorac Cardiovasc Surg 1990;99:990–1001; discussion 1001–1002

244. Hendren WG, Nemec JJ, Lytle BW et al: Mitral valve repair for ischemic mitral insufficiency [see comments]. Ann Thorac Surg 1991;52:1246–1251; discussion 1251–1252

245. Kawachi Y, Oe M, Asou T et al: Comparative study between valve repair and replacement for mitral pure regurgitation—early and late postoperative results. Jpn Circ J 1991;55:443–452

246. Krause AH, Okies JE, Bigelow JC et al: Early experience with mitral valve reconstruction for mitral insufficiency. Am J Surg 1991;161:563–566

247. Kenny A, Fuller CA, Shapiro LM, Wells FC: Conservative surgery of the mitral valve. A report of the first 100 cases from one unit and one surgeon. Br Heart J 1992;68:505–509

248. Okita Y, Miki S, Kusuhara K et al: Analysis of left ventricular motion after mitral valve replacement with a technique of preservation of all chordae tendineae. Comparison with conventional mitral valve replacement or mitral valve repair. J Thorac Cardiovasc Surg 1992;104:786–795

249. Gorton ME, Piehler JM, Killen DA et al: Mitral valve repair using a flexible and adjustable annuloplasty ring. Ann Thorac Surg 1993;55:860–863

250. Akins CW, Hilgenberg AD, Buckley MJ et al: Mitral valve reconstruction versus replacement for degenerative or ischemic mitral regurgitation. Ann Thorac Surg 1994;58:668–675; discussion 675–676

251. Azar H, Szentpetery S: Mitral valve repair in patients over the age of 70 years. Eur J Cardiothorac Surg 1994;8:298–300

252. Cohn LH, Couper GS, Aranki SF et al: Long-term results of mitral valve reconstruction for regurgitation of the myxomatous mitral valve. J Thorac Cardiovasc Surg 1994;107:143–150; discussion 150–151

253. Oury JH, Cleveland JC, Duran CG, Angell WW: Ischemic mitral valve disease. Classification and systemic approach to management. J Card Surg, suppl. 1994;9:262–273

254. Bolling SF, Deeb GM, Brunsting LA, Bach DS: Early outcome of mitral valve reconstruction in patients with end-stage cardiomyopathy. J Thorac Cardiovasc Surg 1995;109:676–682; discussion 682–683

255. Okada Y, Shomura T, Yamaura Y, Yoshikawa J: Comparison of the Carpentier and Duran prosthetic rings used in mitral reconstruction. Ann Thorac Surg 1995;59:658–662; discussion 662–663

256. Perier P, Clausnizer B: Isolated cleft mitral valve: Valve reconstruction techniques. Ann Thorac Surg 1995;59:56–59

257. Acar J, Michel PL, Luxereau P et al: Indications for surgery in mitral regurgitation. Eur Heart J, suppl. B 1991;12:52–54

258. Reed D, Abbott RD, Smucker ML, Kaul S: Prediction of outcome after mitral valve replacement in patients with symptomatic chronic mitral regurgitation. The importance of left atrial size. Circulation 1991;84: 23–34

259. David TE: Techniques and results of mitral valve repair for ischemic mitral regurgitation. J Card Surg, suppl. 1994;9:274–277

260. Akins CW, Hilgenberg AD, Buckley MJ et al: Mitral valve reconstruction versus replacement for degenerative or ischemic mitral regurgitation. Multiplane transesophageal echocardiography: our initial experience. Ann Thorac Surg 1994;58:668–675; discussion 675–676

261. Acar J, Michel P, Luxereau P et al: Indications for surgery in mitral regurgitation. Eur Heart J, suppl. B 1991;12:52–54

262. Kelbaek H: An improved noninvasive method for measurement of cardiac output and evaluation of left-sided cardiac valve incompetence. Angiology 1989;40: 458–463

263. Nair CK, Biddle WP, Kaneshige A et al: Ten-year experience with mitral valve replacement in the elderly. Am Heart J 1992;124:154–159

264. Von Herwerden L, Tjan D, Tijssen J et al: Determinants of survival after surgery for mitral valve regurgitation in patients with and without coronary artery disease. Eur J Cardiothorac Surg 1990;4:329–336

265. Zile M, Gaasch W, Carroll J et al: Chronic mitral regurgitation. Predictive value of preoperative echocardiographic indices of left ventricular function and wall stress. J Am Coll Cardiol 1984;3:235–242

266. Fenster MS, Feldman MD: Mitral regurgitation. An overview. Curr Probl Cardiol 1995;20:193–280

267. Strong M, Brockman S: Mitral valve reconstruction. Cardiovasc Clin 1992;21:255–262

268. Rankin J, Hickey M, Smith L et al: Ischemic mitral regurgitation. Circulation, suppl. I 1989;79:116–121

269. Carabello BA: Preservation of left ventricular function in patients with mitral regurgitation. A realistic goal for the nineties [comment]. J Am Coll Cardiol 1990;15:564–565

270. LeFeuvre C, Metzger J, Lachurie M: Treatment of severe mitral regurgitation caused by ischemic papillary muscle dysfunction. Indications for coronary angioplasty. Am Heart J 1992;123:860–865

271. Kono T, Sabbah HN, Stein PD et al: Left ventricular shape as a determinant of functional mitral regurgitation in patients with severe heart failure secondary to either coronary artery disease or idiopathic dilated cardiomyopathy. Am J Cardiol 1991;68:355–359

272. Kono T, Sabbah HN, Rosman H et al: Left ventricular shape is the primary determinant of functional mitral regurgitation in heart failure. J Am Coll Cardiol 1992;20:1594–1598

273. Rankin JS, Feneley MP, Hickey MS et al: A clinical comparison of mitral valve repair versus valve replacement in ischemic mitral regurgitation. J Thorac Cardiovasc Surg 1988;95:165–177

274. Karp RB, Mills N, Edmunds LH Jr: Coronary artery bypass grafting in the presence of valvular disease. Circulation, suppl. I 1989;79:182–184

275. Stone PH: Management of the patient with asymp-

tomatic aortic stenosis. J Card Surg, suppl. 1994;9: 139–144

276. Lund O, Nielsen TT, Pilegaard HK et al: The influence of coronary artery disease and bypass grafting on early and late survival after valve replacement for aortic stenosis. J Thorac Cardiovasc Surg 1990;100: 327–337

277. Kennedy KD, Nishimura RA, Holmes DR Jr, Bailey KR: Natural history of moderate aortic stenosis. J Am Coll Cardiol 1991;17:313–319

278. Pellikka PA, Nishimura RA, Bailey KR, Tajik AJ: The natural history of adults with asymptomatic, hemodynamically significant aortic stenosis [see comments]. J Am Coll Cardiol 1990;15:1012–1017

279. Ross J Jr, Braunwald E: Aortic stenosis. Circulation, suppl. V 1968;38:61

280. Aronow WS, Ahn C, Kronzon I, Nanna M: Prognosis of congestive heart failure in patients aged > or = 62 years with unoperated severe valvular aortic stenosis. Am J Cardiol 1993;72:846–848

281. Chizner MA, Pearle DL, deLeon AC Jr: The natural history of aortic stenosis in adults. Am Heart J 1980; 99:419–424

282. Kelly TA, Rothbart RM, Cooper CM et al: Comparison of outcome of asymptomatic to symptomatic patients older than 20 years of age with valvular aortic stenosis. Am J Cardiol 1988;61:123–130

283. Lund O: Preoperative risk evaluation and stratification of long-term survival after valve replacement for aortic stenosis. Reasons for earlier operative intervention [see comments]. Circulation 1990;82: 124–139

284. Deleuze P, Loisance DY, Besnainou F et al: Severe aortic stenosis in octogenarians. Is operation an acceptable alternative? [see comments]. Ann Thorac Surg 1990;50:226–229

285. Olsson M, Granstrom L, Lindblom D et al: Aortic valve replacement in octogenarians with aortic stenosis. A case-control study. J Am Coll Cardiol 1992;20: 1512–1516

286. De Brogan WC, Grayburn PA, Lange RA, Hillis LD: Prognosis after valve replacement in patients with severe aortic stenosis and a low transvalvular pressure gradient. J Am Coll Cardiol 1993;21:1657–1660

287. Berland J, Cribier A, Savin T et al: Percutaneous balloon valvuloplasty in patients with severe aortic stenosis and low ejection fraction. Immediate results and 1-year follow-up. Circulation 1989;79:1189–1196

288. Davidson C, Harrison J, Leithe M et al: Failure of balloon aortic valvuloplasty to result in sustained clinical improvement in patients with depressed ventricular function. Am J Cardiol 1990;65:72–77

289. Legrand V, Beckers J, Fastrez M et al: Long-term follow-up of elderly patients with severe aortic stenosis treated by balloon aortic valvuloplasty. Importance of haemodynamic parameters before and after dilatation. Eur Heart J 1991;12:451–457

290. Craver JM, Weintraub WS, Jones EL et al: Predictors of mortality, complications, and length of stay in aortic valve replacement for aortic stenosis. Circulation, suppl. I 1988;78:85–90

291. Lund O, Pilegaard HK, Magnussen K et al: Long-term prosthesis-related and sudden cardiac-related complications after valve replacement for aortic stenosis. Ann Thorac Surg 1990;50:396–406

292. Azariades M, Fessler CL, Ahmad A, Starr A: Aortic

valve replacement in patients over 80 years of age. A comparative standard for balloon valvuloplasty. Eur J Cardiothorac Surg 1991;5:373–377

293. Culliford AT, Galloway AC, Colvin SB et al: Aortic valve replacement for aortic stenosis in persons aged 80 years and over. Am J Cardiol 1991;67:1256–1260

294. Lund O, Pilegaard H, Nielsen TT et al: Thirty-day mortality after valve replacement for aortic stenosis over the last 22 years. A multivariate risk stratification. Eur Heart J 1991;12:322–331

295. Morris JJ, Schaff HV, Mullany CJ et al: Determinants of survival and recovery of left ventricular function after aortic valve replacement. Ann Thorac Surg 1993;56:22–29; discussion 29–30

296. Logeais Y, Langanay T, Roussin R et al: Surgery for aortic stenosis in elderly patients. A study of surgical risk and predictive factors. Circulation 1994;90: 2891–2898

297. Data Analyses of the Society of Thoracic Surgeons National Cardiac Surgery Database, in The Fourth Year—January 1995. Summit Medical, Minneapolis, 1995

298. Duran CM: Present status of reconstructive surgery for aortic valve disease. J Card Surg 1993;8:443–452

299. Shapira N, Lemole GM, Fernandez J et al: Aortic valve repair for aortic stenosis in adults. Ann Thorac Surg 1990;50:110–120

300. Nishimura RA, McGoon MD, Schaff HV, Giuliani ER: Chronic aortic regurgitation: indications for operation—1988. Mayo Clin Proc 1988;63:270–280

301. Borer J, Kligfield P: Aortic regurgitation. Making management decisions. Am Coll Cardiol Curr J Rev 1995;4:30–32

302. Bonow RO, Picone AL, McIntosh CL et al: Survival and functional results after valve replacement for aortic regurgitation from 1976 to 1983. Impact of preoperative left ventricular function. Circulation 1985; 72:1244–1256

303. Bonow RO, Dodd JT, Maron BJ et al: Long-term serial changes in left ventricular function and reversal of ventricular dilatation after valve replacement for chronic aortic regurgitation. Circulation 1988;78: 1108–1120

304. Taniguchi K, Nakano S, Matsuda H et al: Timing of operation for aortic regurgitation. Relation to postoperative contractile state. Ann Thorac Surg 1990;50: 779–785

305. Assey M, Usher B, Hendrix G: Valvular heart disease. Use of invasive and noninvasive techniques in clinical decision-making. Part I. Aortic valve disease. Mod Concepts Cardiovasc Disease 1989;58:55–60

306. Barratt-Boyes B: The timing of operation in valvular insufficiency. J Cardiac Surg 1987;2:435–452

307. Kawachi Y, Tokunaga K: Preferability of bioprostheses for isolated aortic valve replacement—a comparative study between mechanical and bioprosthetic valves. Jpn Circ J 1990;54:137–145

308. Barratt-Boyes BG, Roche AH, Subramanyan R et al: Long-term follow-up of patients with the antibiotic-sterilized aortic homograft valve inserted freehand in the aortic position. Circulation 1987;75:768–777

309. O'Brien M, Stafford E, Gardner M et al: A comparison of aortic valve replacement with viable cryopreserved and fresh allograft valves, with a note on chromosomal studies. J Thorac Cardiovasc Surg 1987;94: 812–823

310. Matsuki O, Okita Y, Almeida RS et al: Two decades' experience with aortic valve replacement with pulmonary autograft. J Thorac Cardiovasc Surg 1988; 95:705–711

311. Carabello BA, Usher BW, Hendrix GH et al: Predictors of outcome for aortic valve replacement in patients with aortic regurgitation and left ventricular dysfunction. A change in the measuring stick. J Am Coll Cardiol 1987;10:991–997

312. Pugliese P, Negri A, Muneretto C et al: Aortic insufficiency. A multivariate analysis of incremental risk factors for operative mortality and functional results. J Cardiovasc Surg (Torino) 1990;31:213–219

313. Okamura K, Mitsui T, Hori M: Cross-sectional area index of left ventricular myocardium as a risk factor influencing early and late postoperative survival in aortic regurgitation. Clin Cardiol 1991;14:49–52

314. Shigenobu M, Sano S: The clinical and pathological features of isolated aortic regurgitation in relation to its etiology. Surg Today 1994;24:393–398

315. Okamura K, Mitsui T, Hori M: Cross-sectional area index of left ventricular myocardium as a risk factor influencing early and late postoperative survival in aortic regurgitation. Clin Cardiol 1991;14:49–52

316. Henry WL, Bonow RO, Borer JS et al: Evaluation of aortic valve replacement in patients with valvular aortic stenosis. Circulation 1980;61:814–825

317. Duran CM: Perspectives in reparative surgery for acquired valvular disease. Adv Card Surg 1993;4:1–23

318. Cosgrove DM, Rosenkranz ER, Hendren WG et al: Valvuloplasty for aortic insufficiency. J Thorac Cardiovasc Surg 1991;102:571–576; discussion 576–577

319. Duran CM, Gometza B, De Vol EB: Valve repair in rheumatic mitral disease. Circulation, suppl. III 1991;84:125–132

320. Duran C, Kumar N, Gometza B, Al Halees Z: Indications and limitations of aortic valve reconstruction. Ann Thorac Surg 1991;52:447–453; discussion 453–454

321. Duran CM, Gallo R, Prabhakar G et al: New prosthetic ring for aortic valve annuloplasty. Cardiovasc Surg 1993;1:166–171

Candidates for Heart Transplantation: Selection and Management

52

Lynne Warner Stevenson

Cardiac transplantation has evolved during the last 25 years from an experimental procedure with 25 percent 1-year survival rate to an accepted therapy with a survival rate of 80–85 percent at 1 year and 60–70 percent at 5 years.[1,2] To demonstrate the benefit of the procedure when it was still experimental, selection of early candidates identified those with the most obvious immediate compromise and the most favorable profile of other organ function and psychosocial adaptation. As transplantation became accepted as the best therapy for end-stage heart failure, endorsed by Medicare in 1986, the number of centers in the United States increased from 37 in 1984 to almost 200 in 1994.[1] The number of transplant centers worldwide exceeds 250. There have now been more than 30,000 heart transplants performed worldwide.[2]

Improving results have led to an ever-expanding pool of potential candidates who could benefit from the procedure. Current estimates of the potential candidates under 65 years of age range from 12,000 to 40,000 yearly in the United States, and these figures represent only a small fraction of the estimated 400,000 to 1 million patients with advanced heart failure in the United States. The steady increase in the number of patients listed for transplantation (Fig. 52-1) has not been matched by growth in the number of available donor hearts, which has remained between 2000 and 2500 over a recent 3-year period. Refinement of immunosuppression has diminished the negative impact of many conditions, such as diabetes or advanced age—once considered unacceptable risks for posttransplant complications. As contraindications have been relaxed, however, in-creasing scrutiny of listing practices has resulted, not only from the frequency of death on the lengthening waiting list, currently between 12 and 20 percent, but also from the surprising frequency of survival beyond 2 years, which suggests that some patients may have been listed prematurely.[3]

The same era that has seen the acceptance of cardiac transplantation has also seen dramatic evolution of medical therapy for heart failure, challenging previous assumptions about when left ventricular dysfunction becomes "end-stage." It can no longer be assumed that all patients with a particularly low ejection fraction require transplantation in order to survive with good quality of life. In addition to examination for contraindications, potential candidates should undergo rigorous evaluation for all potential therapies in order to identify those who will derive the greatest increment in quality and length of life from transplantation.

GENERAL APPROACH TO THE POTENTIAL CANDIDATE

Investigation of the cause of heart disease may suggest therapeutic options other than transplantation, facilitate estimation of prognosis, and occasionally identify diseases with other systemic effects that preclude transplantation. More than 90 percent of adults referred for transplantation have dilated heart failure due in almost equal proportion to coronary artery disease and nonischemic dilated cardiomyopathy. Fewer than 10 percent of patients carry other diagnoses, such as restrictive cardiomyopathy,

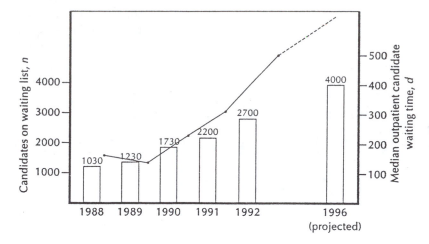

Fig. 52-1. There is an increasing number of patients on the waiting list for cardiac transplantation. The line indicates the median waiting time for outpatient candidates during the same years. The projected waiting list size and outpatient waiting time, derived from computer modeling of expected outcomes, are shown for 1996, assuming continuation of the current practice of listing twice as many new patients each month as undergo transplantation.[3] (Copyright © 1994 Curr Opin Cardiol, with permission.)

primary valvar disease, or congenital heart disease.[4] Although the general approach to the patient is similar regardless of etiology, most of the specific considerations discussed below apply to advanced heart failure (Table 52-1).

Reversible Ischemia and Valve Disease

All patients referred should undergo careful evaluation for potentially reversible causes of left ventricular dysfunction or clinical decompensation (Table 52-2). In some patients with low ejection fractions and coronary artery disease, major myocardial segments receiving inadequate coronary blood flow may improve following revascularization with coronary artery bypass grafting or catheter-based interventional procedures.[5] Angina or radionuclide evidence of reversible ischemia after exercise may not always be present. Glucose uptake in areas of low flow may

identify viable myocardium more reliably. Uncontrolled experiences suggest that extensive myocardial metabolic activity, left ventricular diastolic dimension less than 75 mm, and ejection fraction over 18 percent may identify patients more likely to improve.[6] In addition to technical feasibility of bypass grafting, the quality of the distal target vessels ap-

---

Table 52-1. Approach to the Potential Candidate for Heart Transplantation

Address potentially reversible components of heart failure
Tailor medical therapy to relieve congestion
Evaluate functional capacity and risk
Identify contraindications to transplantation
Determine candidacy for transplantation
Maintain and reevaluate

Table 52-2. Potentially Reversible Factors in Heart Failure

Intrinsic factors
    Extensive myocardial ischemia
    Recent onset cardiomyopathy
    Superimposed viral infection
    Alcohol or cocaine use
    Tachycardias
    Anemia
    Metabolic factors
        Thyroid disease
        Electrolyte disturbances
        Obesity
Factors of therapy
    Ineffective drug regimen
        Inadequate doses of vasodilators
        Incomplete diuresis
    Noncompliance with drug regimen with salt and
        fluid restriction
    Concomitant drug therapy causing
        Increased fluid retention
        Depressed contractility
    Deconditioning
        Perception of heart "failure"
        Deleterious prescription to reduce activity

pears critical. Chronic diabetes mellitus and multiple previous bypass operations may decrease the likelihood of a good postoperative outcome. It has been estimated from practice surveys that no more than 5 percent of potential candidates with coronary artery disease who have been referred from metropolitan areas to a transplant center are appropriate for revascularization.[7] The use of revascularization in the transplant population may increase, however, with the evolution of techniques for detecting candidates for revascularization and more widespread recognition of the potential value of this intervention, as well as changing reimbursement and practice patterns. There is even less information regarding valve replacement for mitral or aortic regurgitation in patients with markedly low ejection fractions. Although it has been well established that the risk of such procedures is increased even in patients with only modest impairment of left ventricular dysfunction, comparison of those risks to the risks of transplantation in some cases alters the balance in favor of such salvage operations. The preservation of left ventricular function with mitral valve repair, compared to valve replacement, may increase the number of candidates for this procedure.

If carefully selected, most patients can survive cardiac surgery even if they enter with a low ejection fraction. Those who survive often demonstrate gradual improvement or can at least be stabilized after discharge to undergo elective cardiac transplantation. There are few guarantees, however, for patients unable to be weaned from cardiopulmonary bypass. Short-term assist devices after surgical procedures

may allow time for sufficient improvement in myocardial function to allow discharge. Patients requiring mechanical assistance to bridge from postcardiotomy shock to transplantation have been reported to have poorer outcome than patients receiving a primary bridge.[8,9] Those surviving to transplantation have subsequent survival only slightly lower than those undergoing elective transplantation.

The decision between salvage surgery and transplantation should include consideration of the chances of death while awaiting transplantation, good outcome after other surgical procedures, surviving to emergency transplantation after postcardiotomy shock, and enjoying a good outcome after transplantation. Although few potential transplant candidates are appropriate for high risk cardiac surgery as an alternative, each such procedure affects not one but two patients and should be carefully considered prior to committing to transplantation.

Spontaneous Improvement of Cardiomyopathy

Patients with recent-onset cardiomyopathy without coronary artery disease improve spontaneously in almost 50 percent of cases presenting with less than 3 months of symptoms, regardless of whether histologic evidence of myocarditis is present. In patients with sufficient severity to cause referral for transplantation, major improvement defined as improvement of at least 0.15 in ejection fraction occurs in only 27 percent of patients, usually in those with the least hemodynamic compromise and less mitral regurgitation at the time of referral (Table 52-3).[10] Although overall survival for recent-onset cardiomyopathy is similar to that of more chronic nonischemic cardiomyopathy, it represents merging of the improved group with high survival and the unimproved group for which survival is particularly poor (Fig. 52-2). Occasionally, young patients present with a fulminant picture of acute cardiac and other organ failure, usually in association with a viral syndrome, and have up to 50 percent chance of recovering; but they may require high dose catecholamine or mechanical support for a period of days. Cardiomyopathy presenting within the last trimester of pregnancy or initial postpartum months may have a slightly higher chance of improvement than other recent-onset cardiomyopathy.[11]

Heavy alcohol consumption has been estimated to cause approximately 10 percent of cardiomyopathy in adults but is probably underrecognized.[12] Spontaneous improvement or even normalization is not uncommon if the patient discontinues drinking, especially if heart failure is not long-standing. The relatively common consumption of two drinks daily

Table 52-3. Improvement in Recent-Onset Cardiomyopathy After Referral for Transplant (<6 Months)

Parameter	Improved	Not Improved
No. of patients	13	36
Months of symptoms	1.2	3.2
NYHA class	3.1	3.7
Left ventricular ejection fraction (initial)	0.22	0.19
Left ventricular diastolic dimension (mm)	67	74
Mitral regurgitation (0–3)	1.3	2.0
Cardiac output (L/min)	5.2	3.6
Pulmonary capillary wedge pressure (mmHg)	16	24
Right atrial pressure (mmHg)	6	13
Serum sodium (mEq/L)	139	134

(From Steimle et al.,[10] with permission.)

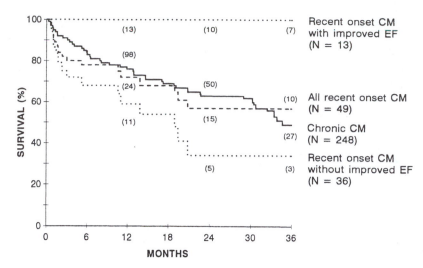

Fig. 52-2. Kaplan-Meier survival curves of 297 patients with primary dilated cardiomyopathy evaluated for cardiac transplantation. The survival of all 49 patients with recent-onset cardiomyopathy was not different from the survival of 248 cardiomyopathy patients with more than 6 months of symptoms. The survival for recent-onset cardiomyopathy patients whose ejection fraction later improved (top line) was 100 percent, compared to 36 percent for patients with recent-onset cardiomyopathy who did not demonstrate later improvement in ejection fraction. (From Steimle et al.,[10] with permission.)

may be sufficient to worsen heart failure in patients with other etiologies of left ventricular dysfunction. Patients with severe ischemic heart failure in whom ventricular function improves unexpectedly within the year after evaluation frequently admit later to previous heavy alcohol consumption. Absolute abstinence for at least 3–6 months should be observed prior to ultimate acceptance for transplantation to demonstrate both the irreversibility of decompensation and the patient's ability to avoid excessive alcohol consumption after transplantation.

Illicit drug use may contribute to cardiomyopathy. Cocaine use is well recognized to cause acute coronary syndromes but can also cause a chronic cardiomyopathy similar to that seen with pheochromocytoma. Use of anabolic steroids for body building has anecdotally been associated with cardiomyopathy, which improves following their discontinuation.

Tachycardia-Related Left Ventricular Dysfunction

Tachyarrhythmias can cause cardiomyopathy in otherwise normal hearts, but more often they aggravate left ventricular dysfunction due to other causes. Tachycardia-induced cardiomyopathy is most commonly recognized in children but has also been seen in adults with incessant or frequent supraventricular tachycardias or unrecognized ventricular tachycardias that are relatively slow and hemodynamically well tolerated. Evidence is emerging that

relatively modest elevations in heart rate may be poorly tolerated in the setting of ventricular dysfunction. Atrial fibrillation, which is present in approximately 20 percent of patients referred for transplantation, presents a major target for therapy. Adequate rate control is difficult to achieve in many patients with atrial fibrillation in the setting of heart failure, with ventricular rates often rising above 150 bpm with minimal exertion. Conversion to sinus rhythm or at least aggressive rate control are frequently associated not only with marked clinical improvement of a degree similar to that resulting from effective vasodilator therapy but also with marked improvement of ejection fraction beyond that resulting from standard medical therapy.[13] Amiodarone in relatively low doses facilitates cardioversion to sinus rhythm in up to 80 percent of heart failure patients, 70 percent of whom remain in sinus rhythm during the next year.[14] It is not clear whether the benefits result from restoration of atrioventricular synchrony or merely from prevention of excessive heart rates. Even when sinus rhythm cannot be maintained, amiodarone may be the safest adjunct to digoxin for rate control in this population. Patients in whom rate control cannot be achieved in persistent atrial fibrillation may be candidates for atrioventricular node ablation with pacemaker implantation.

Metabolic Disorders

Decompensation in heart failure occasionally results from metabolic abnormalities. Both hyperthyroidism and hyperthyroidism can decrease cardiac function, although function may not return completely to normal following effective thyroid therapy. Electrolyte abnormalities such as hypokalemia and hypocalcemia can depress myocardial contractility. The most common "metabolic" abnormality in heart failure is severe obesity, which has clearly been associated with depressed myocardial function that improves following dramatic weight loss.[15] Some patients may return to near-normal ventricular function. Almost all patients who have severe heart failure and obesity derive some clinical improvement from weight loss. This point must be emphasized to the patients who claim that weight loss is not possible due to their limited activity level. Weight loss is important to establish also because obesity is a major factor causing morbidity after transplantation.

Discontinuation of Potentially Deleterious Medications

Some patients continue to receive medications that often worsen heart failure. Administration of first generation calcium channel antagonists has been associated with worsening hemodynamic status and survival for patients with heart failure.[16] Usually prescribed for vasodilation, angina, or control of ventricular response in atrial fibrillation, these calcium channel blocking agents should be discontinued and replaced by other therapies in most patients with decompensation. The balance between vasodilation and the potentially adverse negative inotropic actions and neurohormonal activation may be more favorable with newer calcium channel antagonists such as amlodipine and felodipine. The former has proved safe in one large trial (PRAISE), and investigation with the latter continues.

Antiarrhythmic therapy is not only of uncertain value (see below) but has significant potential to worsen heart failure. Almost all such agents can depress contractility, especially class Ic drugs, disopyramide and sotalol. The use of β-blockers is beneficial in some patients with heart failure, but their effectiveness specifically in decompensated heart failure has not been demonstrated.[17] Early experience describes increased fluid retention when initiated too rapidly or in patients with clinical symptoms of congestion.[18] It is controversial whether β-blockers should be withdrawn in severely decompensated patients who have been maintained on these agents.

Inhibitors of prostaglandin synthesis, such as the nonsteroidal antiinflammatory drugs (NSAIDs), are frequently administered for minor musculoskeletal complaints or gout. Now that these agents can be obtained without prescription, it is even more important to ask patients specifically about them. Prostaglandin production helps to vasodilate the afferent renal arterioles in the face of increased sympathetic tone and decreased renal perfusion. Fluid retention and deterioration of renal function frequently accompany the use of prostaglandin inhibitors in heart failure. These agents, and even aspirin, may interfere with the response to angiotensin-converting enzyme (ACE) inhibitors (see Ch. 50).

TAILORED THERAPY PRIOR TO TRANSPLANTATION

Most patients referred for transplantation have not been aggressively managed, and often there is considerable room for clinical improvement. The summary of general recommendations regarding recipient guidelines in the Bethesda Conference on Cardiac Transplantation specifies that functional status should not be assessed until patients have undergone aggressive therapy with combinations of vasodilators and diuretic agents[19]: "Therapy should be adjusted until clinical congestion has been resolved or until further therapy has been repeatedly limited by severe or symptomatic hypotension (generally systolic blood pressure <80 mmHg) or marked azotemia. Patients should not be considered to have *refractory* hemodynamic decompensation until therapy with intravenous followed by oral vasodilators and diuretic agents has been pursued using continuous hemodynamic monitoring to approach hemodynamic goals."

At the time of referral to transplantation, most patients are already taking digoxin, diuretics, and ACE inhibitors, which have in some cases been reduced or stopped owing to hypotension. Although optimal doses of ACE inhibitors and other vasodilators have been validated in trials of mild to moderate heart failure, patients with severe heart failure demonstrate wide variation in the doses of vasodilators that are tolerated or effective. For all potential candidates, transplant evaluation provides a vital opportunity for simultaneous design of the medical regimen, which can often postpone the need for transplantation.

The first challenge is to recognize the volume overload characteristic of most patients with severe symptoms of congestion.[20] Although volume overload frequently exceeds 5 liters, rales are rare with chronic heart failure, and peripheral edema and ascites occur in only about 25 percent of these patients. Scrupulous attention must be paid to jugular venous distension and the symptom of orthopnea to detect volume overload. Previous therapy has often been

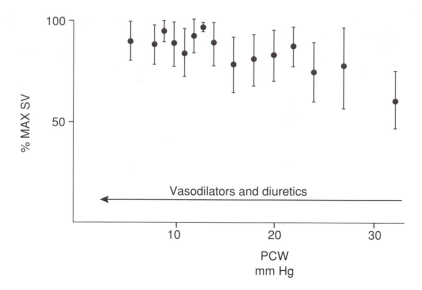

Fig. 52-3. Maintenance and improvement of stroke volume as pulmonary capillary wedge pressures were reduced with vasodilators and diuretics in 20 patients presenting for heart transplantation with an average initial ejection fraction of 18 percent pulmonary capillary wedge pressure of 30 mmHg, and cardiac index 1.9 L·min^{-1}· sqm^{-1}. Stroke volumes obtained at each pulmonary capillary wedge pressure were compared to the best stroke volume obtained under any loading conditions. (From Stevenson and Tillisch,[21] with permission.)

limited by concern that therapy to decrease volume status depresses cardiac output. Most patients with chronically dilated heart failure, however, can achieve their highest cardiac outputs with pulmonary capillary wedge pressures in the range of 15 mmHg (Fig. 52-3).[21] The 30–50 percent improvement of forward stroke volume frequently achieved with vasodilation and diuresis to lower filling pressures results largely from forward redistribution of mitral regurgitant flow, which can otherwise subtract more than 50 percent of the total ventricular stroke volume at rest and during exercise.[22]

Most patients with low ejection fractions can maintain hemodynamic compensation with empiric adjustment of vasodilators and diuretics and are unlikely to benefit from hemodynamic monitoring to more exact goals. These patients are generally considered to be too well for transplantation except for other indications such as refractory angina or arrhythmias. Some patients with mild resting hemodynamic abnormalities can undergo adjustment of vasodilators or diuretics guided by blood pressures and clinical signs. Those patients who are considered for transplantation because severe symptoms persist, however, should undergo invasive hemodynamic monitoring for further tailoring of therapy before transplantation is considered to be the only op-

tion.[19,23] Hemodynamic monitoring allows coupled optimization of both filling pressures and systemic vascular resistance by simultaneous diuretic and vasodilator therapy, which can rarely be achieved empirically once decompensation is severe (Table 52-4). Even though the degree of hemodynamic improvement may not correlate well with the degree of clinical impairment, those patients who do *not* improve hemodynamically are unlikely to improve clinically.[24]

The general indications for hemodynamic monitoring during adjustment of therapy are listed in Table 52-5. Establishment of optimal hemodynamic status is frequently easiest with intravenous agents. It is not clear whether initial therapy with intravenous nitroprusside or dobutamine merely facilitates subsequent titration of oral vasodilators or is necessary to improve the baseline to allow introduction of oral agents that would not otherwise have been tolerated or effective. In addition to allowing design of an effective chronic regimen, reduction of filling pressures during continuous hemodynamic monitoring over several days allows sustained reduction of filling pressures, which may demonstrate the reversibility of elevated pulmonary pressures that would otherwise have represented a contraindication to transplantation.

Table 52-4. Tailored Therapy for
Advanced Heart Failure

1. Measurement of baseline hemodynamics
2. Intravenous nitroprusside and diuretics tailored
to hemodynamic goals
    PCW ≤ 15 mmHg
    SVR ≤ 1200 dynes/s/cm^{-5}
    RA ≤ 8 mmHg
    SBP ≥ 80 mmHg
3. Definition of optimal hemodynamics by 24–48
hours
4. Titration of high-dose oral vasodilators as nitroprusside weaned (combinations of: captopril, isosorbide dinitrate, hydralazine as needed as alternative
or addition)
5. Monitored ambulation and diuretic adjustment
for 24–48 hours
6. Maintain digoxin levels 1.0–2.0 ng/dl if no contraindication
7. Detailed patient education
8. Flexible outpatient diuretic regimen including
metolazone as needed
9. Progressive walking program
10. Vigilant follow-up

Abbreviations: PCW, pulmonary capillary wedge pressure; SVR, systemic vascular resistance; RA, right atrial
pressure; SBP, systolic blood pressure.

Systematic application of tailored therapy to patients referred with class IV symptoms of heart failure leads to sustained improvement in filling pressures and cardiac output, functional class, and
exercise capacity.[25,26] In combination with patient

Table 52-5. Suggested Indications for
Invasive Monitoring of Hemodynamics
During Therapy for Congestion

Congestion with hypoperfusion suggested by
    Mental obtundation
    Pulse pressure <25%
    Declining renal function
    Hemodynamic intolerance to ACE inhibitors
        (likely when systolic blood pressure <90
        mmHg and serum sodium <133 mEq/L)

Congestion in the presence of
    Active ischemia
    Symptomatic ventricular arrhythmias
    Pulmonary disease
    Impaired baseline renal function

Congestion persisting or recurring despite
    ACE inhibitors as tolerated
    Combination high dose diuretics
    Sodium and water restriction

education, progressive exercise, and meticulous follow-up by an experienced multidisciplinary team,
this approach has been used in one study to reduce
the rehospitalization rate for heart failure by more
than 75 percent[26] and in another to decrease the average cost per patient by more than $1000.[27] Many
patients initially considering transplantation appreciate sufficient improvement to postpone transplantation, and patients found ineligible for transplantation are often discharged to an improved quality of
life even without a surgical option.

INDICATIONS FOR TRANSPLANTATION

Dilated Cardiomyopathy

Most candidates for transplantation have dilated
cardiomyopathies. After potentially reversible factors have been addressed and the medical regimen
has been optimized, patients are evaluated to estimate their prognosis, which forms the basis for the
decision of whether transplantation is indicated at
that time.[4,19] Although the extended prognosis of advanced heart failure treated medically remains
worse than that of transplantation, the inadequate
supply of donor organs, cost of posttransplant care,
and the finite life-span after transplantation require
that indications for transplantation be based on the
1- to 2-year prognosis.[3] Patients requiring continuing hospitalization for inotropic therapy of refractory
heart failure clearly have sufficient limitation of both
quality and length of life to justify transplantation
as soon as possible. The challenge arises when assessing indications and timing for transplantation of
ambulatory patients.

During the early days of transplantation, New
York Heart Association (NYHA) class IV symptoms
were necessary and sufficient indications for transplantation. These severe symptoms of heart failure,
characterized by dyspnea with any activity and often
at rest, almost always reflect severely elevated filling
pressures that can often be relieved through aggressive design of currently available medical therapies
as discussed above. Presentation with class IV symptoms is no longer an indication for transplantation
because such patients frequently respond to medical
therapy designed to normalize volume status and
systemic vascular resistance.[23] Indeed, survival of
patients presenting for transplantation with class IV

symptoms has improved steadily since the mid-1980s (Fig. 52-4).[28–30] Most of these patients remain free of the congestive symptoms typical of class IV failure. Although much better than often described by proponents of surgical therapies for heart failure, however, their survival as a group remains much worse than that after transplantation.[31] Further evaluation is necessary to distinguish patients who would do better with transplantation from those who can expect a similar 2-year survival without transplantation. Numerous risk factors have been proposed in this population (Table 52-6).

Although a left ventricular ejection fraction below 20–25 percent has been proposed as a risk factor for unacceptable early mortality and thus an indication for transplantation,[32] the ejection fraction alone is a poor predictor of individual prognosis due in part to errors in measurement and should not be used as an indication for transplantation. Even when initial class IV symptoms and an ejection fraction less than 25 percent are combined, the 2-year prognosis is not uniformly dismal, as evidence by a 45 percent survival without urgent transplantation.[31] Indeed, this figure underestimates the survival of this high risk group, as they can often be rescued by subsequent "urgent transplant."

Quantification of functional capacity using gas exchange analysis in heart failure patients provides a more objective endpoint for evaluation in therapeutic trials. In the first V-HeFT study, a peak oxygen consumption less than 14.5 ml·kg^{-1}·min^{-1} predicted

Table 52-6. Proposed Risk Factors in Potential Candidates for Cardiac Transplantation

Clinical factors
  Persistent class IV symptoms
  Coronary artery disease
  Rehospitalizations

Cardiac factors
  Ejection fraction <20%
  Poor right ventricular function
  Left ventricular diastolic dimension >75–80 mm
  Pulmonary capillary wedge pressure >16 or right atrial pressure >7 mmHg despite tailored therapy
  Cardiac index <2.0–2.5 L·min^{-1}·sq m^{-1}
  Severe mitral regurgitation
  Severe tricuspid regurgitation

Arrhythmia substrate
  History of syncope (SD)
  History of "secondary" cardiac arrest (SD)
  Atrial fibrillation
  Degree of ventricular ectopy
  Positive signal-averaged ECG

Systemic integration
  Low peak oxygen consumption
  Low serum sodium
  High plasma norepinephrine
  Low T$_3$/reverse T$_3$ ratio

Almost all potential risk factors become more positive in patients with more advanced disease, who are at higher risk for both sudden death and death during progressive hemodynamic decompensation. The factors that seem to identify a specific risk of sudden death are followed by (SD).

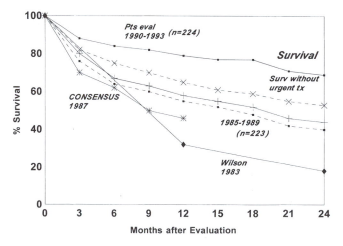

Fig. 52-4. Kaplan-Meier curves for survival (solid lines) and survival without urgent transplantation (dashed lines) for 447 patients referred with NYHA class IV symptoms of heart failure. All 447 patients underwent therapy tailored to hemodynamic goals as described in the text. Survival is compared to previously published survival for class IV heart failure in 1983[28] and 1987.[29]

worse survival in the group with an ejection fraction above 28 percent and the group with lower ejection fraction.[33] Experiences of Szlachcic et al. and Likoff et al. confirmed the measurement of peak oxygen consumption as an independent prognostic guide.[34,35] In an analysis of 114 potential transplant candidates, Mancini et al. provided initial validation of peak oxygen consumption as a criterion for transplant candidacy, suggesting 14 ml·kg^{-1}·min^{-1} on treadmill testing.[36] Other experience has identified values between 10 and 14 ml·kg^{-1}·min^{-1}.[37,38] Bicycle exercise testing may yield values of peak oxygen consumption 8–10 percent lower than those on a treadmill. Synthesis of the published experiences suggests that peak oxygen consumption may distinguish three general categories during heart failure: a peak oxygen consumption less than 10–12 ml·kg^{-1}·min^{-1} confers a particularly poor prognosis, with 1-year survival in the range of 50 percent, whereas peak oxygen consumption over 16–18 ml·kg^{-1}·min^{-1} identifies a group of patients with 2-year survival over 80 percent (Fig. 52-5). Definition of the best and worst groups leaves a middle group for which the prognosis must be further refined. Many risk factors have been proposed as aids in this stratification, but prospective multicenter analyses are required to determine which are useful and how they should be employed in decisions regarding acceptance and priority for transplantation (Table 52-6).

Although the survival benefit of cardiac transplantation is the easiest to predict, many patients are unwilling to accept the burdens of immunosuppression and endomyocardial biopsies unless a major improvement in quality of life is also expected. Quantification of functional capacity not only provides a valuable prognostic index but allows some estimates of potential clinical benefit. Because exercise capacity is limited by multiple cardiac and systemic factors, posttransplant patients may not show major improvement in exercise tolerance compared to stable patients with moderate to severe heart failure[39,40] (Fig. 52-6). Less easy to quantify is the perception of prolonged fatigue after exertion, which seems to be more prominent before transplantation. As for the consideration of survival, expected benefits for exercise capacity from transplantation can be considered major for patients with peak oxygen consumption below $10-12$ ml·kg^{-1}·min^{-1} and limited for patients with peak oxygen consumption over $16-18$ ml·kg^{-1}·min^{-1} in the absence of other major cardiac symptoms such as angina or arrhythmias.

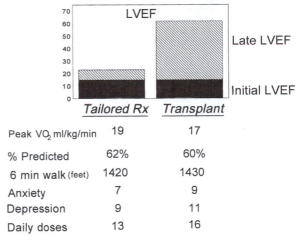

	Tailored Rx	Transplant
Peak VO$_2$ ml/kg/min	19	17
% Predicted	62%	60%
6 min walk (feet)	1420	1430
Anxiety	7	9
Depression	9	11
Daily doses	13	16

Fig. 52-6. Functional capacity of patients with heart failure stable at 1 month after evaluation, who then went on to transplantation or were not listed due to contraindications.[39] The 22 survivors 1 year after transplantation were compared to 20 survivors on medical therapy after an equivalent time. Left ventricular ejection fraction improved to normal in the transplant survivors, but peak oxygen consumption and 6-minute walk distance were not significantly different from patients on medical therapy. Anxiety and depression were equivalent (higher values = more impairment), as were the number of daily medication doses.

The current guidelines for indications for cardiac transplantation focus on functional capacity as reflecting the expected benefits in terms of quality of life and survival (Table 52-7).[19] Patients who cannot be rendered ambulatory due to heart failure are assumed to have peak oxygen consumption values close to resting levels ($3-4$ ml·kg^{-1}·min^{-1}) and do not require formal exercise testing. Functional capacity and prognosis are ideally assessed after sufficient time for demonstration of stability on an optimal medical regimen.[4] Patients who undergo substantial adjustment in their medical regimen, especially when associated with marked improvement in fluid or hemodynamic status, may continue to improve their exercise tolerance over a period of weeks to months. In contrast, patients without such responses are unlikely to increase their peak oxygen consumption.

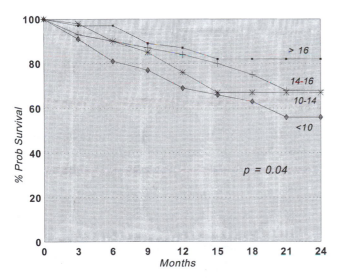

Fig. 52-5. Kaplan-Meier curves for survival without urgent transplantation in 330 patients undergoing cardiopulmonary exercise testing at the time of evaluation for cardiac transplantation. Patients are classified according to values of peak oxygen consumption obtained during incremental symptom-limited bicycle testing after a 6-minute warm-up period at 20 watts.[38]

Transplantation in Patients Without Dilated Cardiomyopathy

Although heart failure symptoms result from dilated heart failure with a low ejection fraction in more than 90 percent of the patients in the age range re-

Table 52-7. Selection Criteria for Benefits from Transplantation

Accepted indications for transplantation
    Maximal VO$_2$ <10 ml·kg^{-1}·min^{-1} with achievement of anaerobic metabolism
    Severe ischemia consistently limiting routine activity not amenable to bypass surgery or angioplasty
    Recurrent symptomatic ventricular arrhythmias refractory to all accepted therapeutic modalities

Probable indications for cardiac transplantation
    Maximal VO$_2$ <14 ml·kg^{-1}·min^{-1} and major limitation of the patient's daily activities
    Recurrent unstable ischemia not amenable to bypass or angioplasty
    Instability of fluid balance/renal function not due to patient noncompliance with regimen of weight monitoring, flexible use of diuretic drugs, and salt restriction

Inadequate indications for transplantation
    Ejection fraction ≤20%
    History of functional class III or IV symptoms of heart failure
    Previous ventricular arrhythmias
    Maximal VO$_2$ > 15 ml·kg^{-1}·min^{-1} without other indications

(Adapted from Mudge et al.,[19] with permission.)

ferred for transplantation, other conditions causing severe symptoms or limited life expectancy occasionally warrant transplantation (Table 52-7). Patients may also be referred with class IV symptoms of congestion due to restrictive disease, in which the ventricle is minimally dilated and the ejection fraction is in the range of 30–45 percent. Fluid balance can be difficult to maintain in such patients, who may be considered for transplantation after failure of a meticulous regimen of salt and fluid restriction and flexible diuretics including metolazone. Even in the absence of characteristic echocardiographic appearance, amyloidosis needs to be excluded by endomyocardial biopsy due to the frequent progression of amyloidosis in noncardiac organs as well as in the transplanted heart.[41] When restrictive disease with venous congestion has been present for many years, liver function should be carefully assessed because these patients are among the few who may develop irreversible "cardiac cirrhosis," which limits posttransplant outcome.

Hypertrophic cardiomyopathy rarely requires cardiac transplantation when still in the hypercontractile stage. Diuretics and agents that decrease contractility can generally control congestive symptoms. Myomectomy, mitral valve replacement, or a trial of dual-chamber pacing should be considered. In the patients in whom hypertrophic cardiomyopathy becomes "burned out," congestive symptoms and exercise intolerance may become severe with ejection fractions below 40 percent. Although the prognosis for these patients has not been well established, the clinical status suggests that quality of life and outcome can become sufficiently limited to warrant transplantation.

A small number of patients undergo transplantation for indications other than heart failure. Some patients without congestive symptoms may undergo transplantation to relieve angina when multiple revascularization procedures have been previously performed and no further attempts are feasible. Their ejection fractions are usually below 30 percent because those with better ejection fractions would almost always be candidates for bypass surgery even if arm veins or subdiaphragmatic arteries were required. Some patients may require transplantation primarily for recurrent discharges from automatic implantable defibrillators. Although these devices reduce the risk of death in such patients, they do not always restore effective cardiac rhythms in the presence of severe left ventricular dysfunction, and the quality of life can be rendered unacceptable. Unusual trauma or isolated intracardiac tumors are rare indications for transplantation.

CONTRAINDICATIONS TO TRANSPLANTATION

Associated Systemic Illness

Selection of candidates for transplantation includes a careful search for any noncardiac condition that limits life expectancy or increases the risk of complications from the procedure or from immunosuppression (Table 52-8). The ideal candidate is sick enough to need a transplant but sufficiently intact to expect a good result. Age remains a subject of controversy. Although highly selected older patients have good outcomes, large series consistently demonstrate decreased long-term survival in older recipients[42–44] (Fig. 52-7). Survival in the teenage recipient group is also decreased owing to a greater tendency to rejection and more frequent noncompliance with medical therapy. Potential candidates over age 60 are generally evaluated more carefully for evidence of diseases causing co-morbidity in this age group. Conditions that limit the potential for full rehabilitation are also relative contraindications but have led to suggestions of discrimination against the handicapped.

A search for the etiology of disease is important in

Table 52-8. Contraindications for Cardiac Transplantation

General eligibility

Absence of any noncardiac condition that would itself shorten life expectancy or increase the risk of death from rejection or from complications of immunosuppression, particularly infection

Specific contraindications

Over the upper age limit of 55–65 years (various programs)

Active infection

Active ulcer disease

Severe diabetes mellitus with end-organ damage

Severe peripheral vascular disease

Pulmonary function (FEV_1, FVC) <60%[a] or history of chronic bronchitis

Serum creatinine >2 mg/dl; creatinine clearance <50 ml/min[a]

Bilirubin >2.5 mg/dl, transaminases more than twice normal[a]

Pulmonary artery systolic pressure >60 mmHg[a]

Mean transpulmonary gradient >15 mmHg[a]

High risk of life-threatening noncompliance

Inability to make strong consistent commitment to transplantation program

Cognitive impairment severe enough to limit comprehension of medical regimen

Psychiatric instability severe enough to jeopardize incentive for adherence to long-term medical regimen

History of recurring alcohol or drug abuse

Failure to establish stable address or telephone number

Demonstration of repeated noncompliance with medication or follow-up

[a] May need to provide optimal hemodynamics with nitroprusside or dobutamine (or both) for 72 hours to determine reversibility of organ dysfunction caused by heart failure.

shortage of donor hearts, however, it is not feasible to collect systematic information about the results of transplantation in all conditions. As described by Copeland et al., selection must reflect "a combination of empirically derived contraindications with limited natural history and considerable common sense."[46]

Although diabetes mellitus is no longer an absolute contraindication for transplantation, worsening of control and progression of complications make diabetics less optimal candidates. In particular, glucose control can be difficult during times of high dose corticosteroid administration, and cyclosporin may accelerate the progression of nephropathy. Evidence of end-organ damage, such as peripheral neuropathy, proteinuria, retinopathy, and peripheral vascular disease, usually is a contraindication. Patients with juvenile-onset diabetes are generally excluded.

Organ transplant recipients are at increased risk of malignancy, presumably because immunosuppression allows more extensive replication of potentially oncogenic viruses and interferes with normal policing of malignant clones.[47] Lymphomas occur up to 40 times more frequently in transplant recipients. Transplantation is generally not performed in patients with neoplasms other than superficial skin lesions within the prior 3–5 years. Particular attention should be devoted to screening for recurrent disease in patients with tumors, such as breast cancer, with a high risk of late recurrence. Many patients have undergone successful transplantation, however, 5–10 years after successful therapy of lymphoma, which is often treated with cardiotoxic agents.

Pulmonary Vascular Disease and Dysfunction of Other Organs

When evaluating the pulmonary circulation and intrinsic pulmonary, renal, and hepatic function, it should be recognized that aggressive treatment of heart failure may improve all of these assessments (Table 52-8). Even evaluation of psychological function in some cases requires sustained improvement of central hemodynamics and cerebral perfusion.

Excessively elevated pulmonary vascular resistance is a major contraindication to transplantation. Pulmonary hypertension presents a major immediate risk to the vulnerable right ventricle, even if pulmonary pressures later decrease. Acute right heart failure is a major factor in early postoperative morbidity and mortality. The specific definitions for unacceptable pulmonary hypertension vary but generally include pulmonary vascular resistance, which should be reducible to below 240–300 dynes·s cm^{-5} and pulmonary artery systolic pressure, which

order to exclude patients with active rheumatologic disease, such as lupus erythematosus, rheumatoid arthritis, or scleroderma, which could cause continued disease after transplantation. Amyloidosis is a contraindication in most programs due to the tendency for systemic progression and recurrence in the allograft.[41] Transplantation for Chagas' disease is often followed by clinical reactivation of the disease following transplantation. The ability to suppress this recurrent disease remains controversial but is an important issue due to the high incidence in South America.[45]

Patients having major systemic conditions with the potential to persist or deteriorate on immunosuppression often inspire emotional debate among the transplant team, as some of these patients might do well after transplantation. Faced with the severe

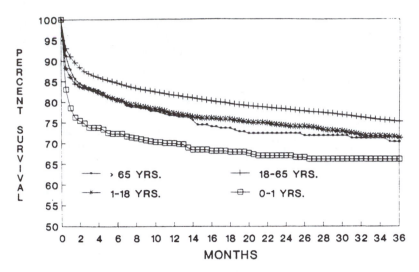

Fig. 52-7. Actuarial survival curves for heart transplant recipients according to age at the time of transplant. Patients undergoing transplantation between 18 and 65 years of age had the best survival; survival was lower for older and younger patients. (From Hosenpud et al.,[2] with permission.)

should be reducible to levels below 50–60 mmHg. The transpulmonary gradient (mean pulmonary artery systolic pressure minus mean pulmonary capillary wedge pressure) usually shows the least improvement during pharmacologic therapy and should be below 12–15 mmHg.[48] Intravenous nitroprusside is often titrated acutely to systemic blood pressure tolerance to demonstrate reversibility in the catheterization suite.[49] Patients with pulmonary capillary wedge pressures chronically over 25 mmHg, however, are most likely to demonstrate reversibility after sustained reductions in filling pressures over several days. Even if more acute reduc-

tions can be demonstrated, these patients are likely to benefit chronically from revision of their medical regimen under hemodynamic monitoring to maintain lower filling pressures and pulmonary artery pressures after discharge (Table 52-9). The rare patient whose pulmonary pressures remain severely elevated despite successful reduction of filling pressures presents significant perioperative risk. A brief trial of prostaglandin E_1 or nitric oxide may demonstrate reversibility and assist planning of a strategy for early postoperative management. For patients with irreversible pulmonary hypertension, heterotopic transplantation (in which the new heart is

Table 52-9. Preoperative Reversibility of Pulmonary Hypertension During Tailored Therapy[b] in 100 Transplant Recipients

Hypertension	Initial PAS >50 mmHg	Initial PVR >240 dynes/s/cm⁵	Initial TPG >15 mmHg
No	35% (6%)[a]	59% (9%)[a]	86% (7%)[a]
Yes	65% (8%)	41% (5%)	14% (7%)
If yes, reversible[b]	41% (3%)	25% (11%)	8% (17%)
Not reversible	24% (10%)	16% (0%)	6% (0%)

Abbreviations: PAS, pulmonary artery systolic pressure; PVR, pulmonary vascular resistance; TPG, transpulmonary gradient (mean pulmonary artery pressure minus pulmonary capillary wedge pressure).

Numbers in parentheses indicate 30-day mortality after transplantation. [a] Reproducibility of the posttransplant results may depend in part on the vigor with which pulmonary congestion is prevented preoperatively, the preservation and age of the donor heart, and early postoperative hemodynamic management.

[b] Reversibility determined after 72 hours of therapy tailored to reduce pulmonary capillary wedge pressure to 15 mmHg, followed in 5 percent of patients by a trial of prostaglandin E1, if necessary.

"piggy-backed" to the old heart) has been performed at times, but this procedure is associated with 1-month mortality of 25 percent compared to 10 percent and is now rarely performed.[50,51]

Patients with severe congestive symptoms should not undergo pulmonary function testing until after pulmonary capillary wedge pressures have been reduced to near-normal levels for at least 5 days and again later if repeated evaluation of results is still unacceptable. Both restrictive and obstructive patterns may be observed.[52] The general criteria have been at least 50–60 percent of predicted forced vital capacity and forced expired volume in 1 second. Most centers require cessation of smoking for at least 3 months before transplantation to reduce perioperative complications and to decrease the chance of postoperative resumption of smoking, which occurs frequently and may increase the risk of early graft coronary artery disease.[53] Random assay of urinary cotinine levels may help assess compliance with a nonsmoking program. A history of morning sputum production and chronic "smoker's cough" is a contraindication in some programs due to the high risk of later pulmonary infection during immunosuppression. Mild intrinsic asthma is generally not a contraindication, although systematic data have not been collected on posttransplant outcome.

Renal function is generally optimized by several days of inotropic infusions and may worsen transiently after aggressive diuresis even when systemic perfusion is maintained. Disproportionate elevation of blood urea nitrogen (BUN) is common. Creatinine clearance of at least 50 ml/min is preferred, but occasionally lower rates are accepted if clearly the result of acute decompensation, if accompanied by normal renal size on ultrasonography, and the absence of significant proteinuria. Patients with creatinine over 2 mg/dl or BUN over 50 mg/dl may be at particularly high risk for renal dysfunction during the early postoperative period. Early renal dysfunction in these patients may be mitigated by the use of antithymocyte globulins instead of cyclosporin for the first few days.

In contrast to renal function, hepatic function is generally optimized by establishing and maintaining low right-sided filling pressures with minimization of retrograde flow from tricuspid regurgitation. Although elevated bilirubin and alkaline phosphatase is the most common pattern, all patterns of abnormal liver chemistries have been observed. The rare elevation of transaminases into the thousands is usually the result of a recent period of critical hypoperfusion. This "shock liver" pattern should be allowed to recover during support with drugs or devices before transplantation is performed.

Compliance Issues

Noncompliance with medications and scheduled follow-up remains a major factor in rejection and mortality for all organ transplant recipients.[54,55] The psychological burdens of transplantation combined with mood swings during glucocorticoid therapy can precipitate lethal episodes of overt suicidal behavior or passive suicide attempts by missing immunosuppressive medications. Current alcohol or drug abuse is a contraindication. All psychiatric and social support factors are integrated into an assessment of the chances for long-term compliance. Relative weakness of either the patient or family support can be counterbalanced by strength in the other component. One of the many reasons an effective transplantation program cannot operate without an integrated heart failure program is the need for ongoing education and assessment of patients who would otherwise have been rejected on the basis of a previous record of noncompliance.[56]

EVALUATION PROCEDURES

Although the logical sequence of candidate evaluation should include the identification of indications prior to evaluation for contraindications, in practice the indications and contraindications are investigated concurrently. Placement of an indwelling pulmonary artery catheter often required for optimization of medical therapy also allows assessment of the pulmonary vascular resistance under optimal conditions. Patients referred on apparently optimal therapy prior to right heart catheterization for evaluation of pulmonary vascular resistance are occasionally found to have unexpectedly abnormal hemodynamics that present targets for further pharmacologic intervention. Patients who initially appear only slightly too well for transplantation, particularly those with active coronary artery disease or recent-onset cardiomyopathy, should in many cases undergo full evaluation in case they later develop rapid deterioration during which full evaluation for contraindications is not feasible.

Evaluation of a potential candidate seen first in critical condition remains a challenge. When the patient's organ function and cognition are acutely impaired, decisions regarding both operative risk and patient commitment are based on experienced guesswork and emotional bias. A common problem is the relatively young patient with a history of poor compliance or alcoholism in whom there is no time to test the commitment to reform. Peripheral vascular disease is often underdiagnosed during an urgent evaluation. Renal and hepatic dysfunction hoped to be reversible may become major impediments to postoperative recovery. Many patients in critical condition must be refused transplantation, with the cost of immediate disappointment eliminating the tragedy of prolonged postoperative misery prior to death. Dying patients who can be rescued by transplantation, however, are sometimes the most rewarding recipients, as they ultimately have the most to gain in terms of survival and quality of life. The increasing availability of mechanical support devices may allow many such patients to be stabilized until they satisfy both physiologic and psychological criteria for candidacy, following which the chance of favorable posttransplant outcome is enhanced (see below).

The general criteria for transplant candidacy are similar in the major transplant programs, although they differ occasionally regarding specific patients with several relative contraindications. Contraindications accepted by most centers are shown in Table 52-10.[7] In centers with a high volume of heart failure referral and aggressive medical therapy, approximately 50 percent of patients undergoing full evaluation are accepted for transplantation. The largest experience comes from the registry of the International Society of Heart and Lung Society, which identifies

---

Table 52-10. Consensus[a] on Candidate Selection Practice

Diseases that are or may be considered contraindications in the absence of other exclusions
    Amyloidosis
    Scleroderma
    Sarcoidosis
    Systemic lupus erythematosus
    Duchenne's muscular dystrophy
    Becker's muscular dystrophy
    Obesity (>125–150% ideal body weight)
    Chronic obstructive pulmonary disease (FEV$_1$ < 50% predicted)
    Active peptic ulcer disease
    Hypercoagulable state
Psychosocial conditions that are or may be considered contraindications
    Recent alcohol or cocaine abuse
    Current smoker
    Current incarceration
    Current noncompliance
    No permanent address
    No telephone
    Axis II psychiatric disorder
    No social support systems

   a Consensus reflects ≥70 percent of 48 major centers representing the United States (Medicare-approved centers), Canada, United Kingdom, and Australia.[7]

---

increased risk of posttransplant death in patients with older age, ejection fraction less than 11 percent, mechanical support while waiting, and female gender.[2,50] The Cardiac Transplant Working Group provided the first multivariate analysis of death, demonstrating older age, elevated serum creatinine, low cardiac output, and mechanical ventilation to be associated with worse survival; female gender was associated with more rejection but equivalent survival.[57] Examination of program attributes demonstrated the most important program factor in survival to be the previous experience of the transplant cardiologist, with contribution from the transplant nurse coordinator.[58]

MANAGEMENT ON THE WAITING LIST

The consensus conference on transplantation suggested that candidates should be seen monthly by the heart failure/transplant cardiologist at the center where the transplant is to be performed.[7] Assessment of postural vital signs, internal jugular venous pressure, and symptoms of orthopnea or dizziness allows further adjustment of diuretics and vasodilator doses if necessary. With more frequent clinic visits with candidates, the primary physician may need to take over the monitoring of electrolytes, renal function, and anticoagulation.

The major principles for management of transplant candidates are the same as those developed to decrease the need for transplantation and to optimize management of ineligible patients. Maintenance of minimal filling pressures not only relieves the congestive symptoms but reduces the pulmonary and hepatic congestion that contribute to pulmonary hypertension, prolonged intubation, coagulopathy, and hepatic dysfunction during the postoperative course. Patient participation includes restriction to 2 g or less of sodium and 2000 ml or less of fluid intake daily; daily weight diaries are kept that guide independent adjustment of diuretic doses. Medications indicated, considered, or probably contraindicated in potential transplant candidates are shown in Table 52-11.

Anticoagulation to prevent systemic and pulmonary emboli during heart failure is routine in some programs for all candidates with low ejection fractions. In other programs, anticoagulation has been reserved for patients with atrial fibrillation, previous embolic events, or mobile thrombi visualized on echocardiography or angiography. In 120 transplant candidates without any of these risk factors, the incidence of embolic events in the absence of

Table 52-11. Outpatient Therapies for Advanced Heart Failure

Routine use
  ACE inhibitors
  Digoxin
  Diuretics
  Nitrates
  Potassium
  Exercise
Selected use
  Anticoagulation
  Hydralazine
  Amiodarone
  β-Blockers
  Magnesium
  AICD
  Ultrafiltration
  Nocturnal oxygen
Detrimental
  Amrinone, milrinone
  Vesnarinone
  Ibopamine
  Flosequinan
  Prostacyclin infusion
  Diltiazem, nifedipine
  Type I antiarrhythmic agents
  NSAIDS
Under clinical investigation
  Carvedilol
  Home dobutamine: low dose
  Pimobendan
  Amlodipine
  AII receptor antagonist
  Coenzyme Q_{10}
  L-Carnitine
  Nocturnal CPAP

Abbreviations: AICD, automatic implantable cardioverter defibrillator; NSAIDs, nonsteroidal antiinflammatory agents; AII, angiotensin II; CPAP, continuous positive airway pressure

anticoagulation was 4 percent during a mean follow-up of 300 days.[59] The guidelines developed by the Agency for Health Care Policy and Research in the United States[60] do not at this time recommend routine anticoagulation for heart failure patients without such additional risk factors, particularly atrial fibrillation, which may be associated with a yearly risk as high as 18 percent. The risks of embolic events, which can cause tragic strokes and death, should be balanced against the risks of anticoagulation. The risk of hemorrhagic events is low when anticoagulation is monitored closely, which is particularly crucial during periods of hepatic congestion and adjustment of amiodarone doses. Perioperative bleeding is usually greater after warfarin therapy, even when vitamin K is administered prior to transplantation.

Sudden death occurs in 15–30 percent of patients awaiting transplantation.[61] The risk is increased in patients with syncope, which is an indication for admission and evaluation. Therapy for asymptomatic nonsustained ventricular tachycardia is not recommended unless the runs are relatively long and rapid. Type I antiarrhythmic agents may increase the chance of sudden death in heart failure patients. Therapy with amiodarone, when avoided in patients with unprotected conduction system disease, does not worsen survival and may improve left ventricular function and survival during severe heart failure.[62,63] In the GESICA trial with an overall mortality of 55 percent at 2 years, similar to ambulatory transplant candidates with a class IV history, mortality was decreased by 28 percent with amiodarone.[63] The discrepancy between this result and the negative result from the Veterans Administration trial of amiodarone has not yet been satisfactorily explained, although the severity of illness in the latter population was lower and the amiodarone dose was higher.[64] Postoperative pulmonary and hemodynamic problems attributed to prior amiodarone use have been described in other surgical populations but have rarely occurred after transplantation.[65]

As the waiting periods lengthen, criteria for transplant candidacy continue to evolve (Fig. 52-8). Deterioration leading to hospitalization until transplantation occurs most frequently during the first 6 months after evaluation, with a lower but persistent frequency thereafter. Hospitalization may be indicated to prevent imminent death from fatal arrhythmias or hemodynamic collapse or to prevent organ system deterioration, which would significantly increase the risk of transplantation. Progressive right heart failure and renal or hepatic dysfunction are indications for hospitalization even if the candidate finds them compatible with life at home. Patients whose condition renders them bedridden require hospitalization or help to increase their activity level. Although patients with the most severe compromise can expect the greatest improvement from transplantation, the preoperative condition is the most important determinant of postoperative outcome and should be optimized.

The escalating approach to the hospitalized patient includes hemodynamic monitoring to optimize loading conditions. If further support with low levels of dobutamine, dopamine, or phosphodiesterase inhibitors is needed to maintain the candidate until transplantation, continuous hemodynamic monitoring is not needed if fluid balance, renal function, and blood pressure can be maintained on stable doses of these agents. Advances to higher levels of support with additional agents should in many cases be

Patients for initial evaluation

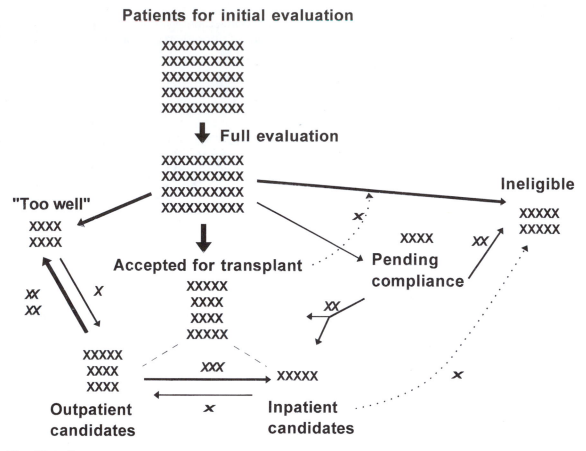

Fig. 52-8. Dynamic nature of candidacy and priority for heart transplantation. Patients may improve or deteriorate after the initial evaluation such that transplantation is deferred, accelerated, or contraindicated.

guided initially by hemodynamic measurements, but chronic maintenance of indwelling lines should be avoided owing to the risk of preoperative infection. Although the full agonists epinephrine and norepinephrine often increase cardiac output, the continued need for these agents is usually a trigger to consider mechanical assistance.

The indications for mechanical support continue to evolve. Hemodynamic criteria frequently suggested as indications for mechanical support have included cardiac index less than 2.0 L. min.$^{-1}$ sq m^{-1} pulmonary capillary wedge pressure more than 20 mmHg, systolic blood pressure less than 90 mmHg, and systemic vascular resistance more than 2100 dynes·s·cm^{566} which are typical of many patients who not only can be stabilized but discharged after adjustment of medical therapy. There is considerable discordance between clinical status and hemodynamic indices; but at the most severe end of the spectrum, mechanical support would generally be indicated for an inability to maintain a systolic blood pressure at 75–80 mmHg or more, a cardiac index of 1.5 L.$^{-1}$ sq m^{-1} and pulmonary venous saturation

of 50 percent or less on maximal pharmacologic support. Evidence of ongoing lactate production also indicates the need for aggressive intervention. On maximal therapy, more subtle trends of declining cardiac index and renal function are difficult to interpret, but they are at least as important as the absolute measured numbers.[67]

The benefit of intraaortic balloon counterpulsation is controversial for patients without coronary artery disease for whom mechanical support in some cases is provided directly with a left ventricular assist device. Patients demonstrating continued dependence on intraaortic balloon counterpulsation may eventually be considered for placement of a ventricular assist device, which allows ambulation and rehabilitation prior to transplantation. As of November 1993, a total of 180 Novacor devices and 157 HeartMate devices have been implanted in the United States.[68] Complications include infection, most commonly through the drive line, bleeding, and thromboemboli from the device. Thromboembolic events are less common with the HeartMate due to endothelialization of the titanium surface. Placement of left ventricular assist devices for bridging to transplantation is currently associated with an approximately 70 percent survival for transplantation, with most intervening deaths due to infection or coagulopathy. The good outcome after transplantation results from better preoperative status but in part also reflects death of the highest risk candidates during the period of mechanical support. In an uncontrolled trial of candidates with cardiac indices below 2 L·min^{-1}·sq m^{-1} on intravenous inotropic agents and intraaortic balloon supports, survival after transplantation was 90 percent for patients surviving with a left ventricular assist device until transplant compared to 70 percent for those compromised patients managed without a left ventricular assist device until transplantation (E. Rose, personal communication).

During the long waiting period, some patients able to remain at home demonstrate sufficient improvement to warrant removal from the active waiting list. The highest risk of death is during the early period after listing, after which some of the factors that led to deterioration before referral may resolve spontaneously and the benefits of optimized medical ther-

apy may be realized. The Bethesda Guidelines and the Consensus Conference emphasized the importance of periodic reevaluation. Suggested criteria for reevaluation include an assessment of clinical stability and demonstration of improved exercise capacity documented by gas exchange analysis (Table 52-12). In one study, 29 percent of ambulatory patients initially listed with peak oxygen consumption less than 14 ml·kg^{-1}·min^{-1} (average 11 ml·kg^{-1}·min^{-1}) demonstrated sufficient improvement for removal from the list, with a subsequent 2-year survival of 92 percent[69] (Fig. 52-9).

FUTURE OF CARDIAC TRANSPLANTATION

Advances in surgical techniques and immunosuppression for cardiac transplantation, in combination with the personal dedication of the early teams, have established transplantation as an effective therapy for patients with truly end-stage heart disease. Patients with an expected survival of less than 50 per-

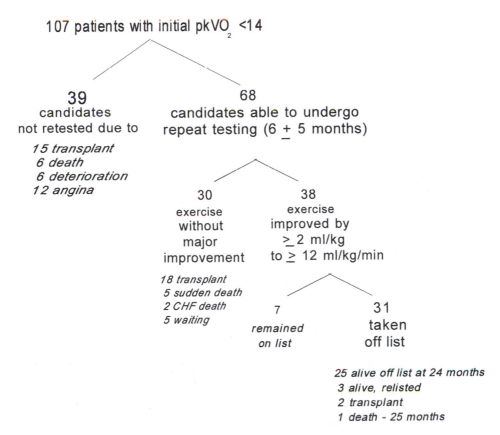

Fig. 52-9. Option and outcome of reevaluation of 107 ambulatory heart transplant candidates initially listed with a peak oxygen consumption of less than 14 ml·kg^{-1} min^{-1} (average 11 ml·kg^{-1} min^{-1}). Of the candidates originally listed, 29 percent were able to leave the transplant list after reevaluation, with overall survival over 90 percent at 2 years.

Table 52-12. Assessment of Clinical Stability

Clinical criteria
- Stable fluid balance without orthopnea, elevated jugular venous pressures, or other evidence of congestion on the flexible diuretic regimen
- Stable blood pressure with systolic at least 80 mmHg
- Stable serum sodium and renal function
- Absence of symptomatic ventricular arrhythmias
- Absence of frequent angina
- Absence of severe drug side effects
- Stable or improving activity level without dyspnea during self-care or one block exertion

Exercise criteria (if initial peak VO_2 < 14 ml·kg^{-1}·min^{-1})
- Improvement in peak oxygen consumption of ≥ 2 ml·kg^{-1}·min^{-1}
- Peak oxygen consumption ≥ 12 ml·kg^{-1}·min^{-1}

---

cent at 2 years can be offered a 60 percent chance of surviving 6 years and 35 percent chance of surviving 10 years on current transplantation protocols.[2] Quality of life is generally good, although fewer than 50 percent of patients return to full-time employment.[70]

The promise of transplantation, however, has not been fulfilled as originally conceived at the time of the first Bethesda conference on transplantation more than 25 years ago, when it was hoped that the supply of donor hearts would eventually be adequate for the number of candidates.[71] Transplantation can realistically be offered to few of the estimated 12,000–40,000 patients estimated to be potential candidates, because it is limited by the donor heart supply of only 2000–2500 each year. More than 70 percent of these hearts are currently being used for patients waiting in hospitals. Patients waiting at home can expect an average wait of 2 years and will soon be unlikely to ever receive a heart unless they deteriorate enough to require continued hospitalization.[3]

The development of left ventricular assist devices currently offers another chance for those hospitalized patients unlikely to survive unsupported until transplantation. Increasing experience and refinement of these devices suggests that some mechanically supported patients are able to resume a reasonable quality of life at home. Although now employed as a "bridge" to transplantation, such devices may themselves eventually prove to be a new route to extended function and survival.[68]

Perhaps the most important benefit gained from the development of transplantation and artificial support devices is the increased focus on the general problem of heart failure. Once considered to be a terminal disease with little response to therapy, heart failure is increasingly the target of extensive investigation and education. With greater emphasis on the recognition and therapy of left ventricular dysfunction in all stages, the proportion of patients needing cardiac transplantation should begin to decrease.

REFERENCES

1. O'Connell JB, Gunnar RM, Evans RW et al: Task Force 1. Organization of heart transplantation in the U.S. J Am Coll Cardiol 1993;22:8–14
2. Hosenpud JD, Novick RJ, Breen TJ, Daily OP: The registry of the International Society for Heart and Lung Transplantation. Eleventh official report—1994. J Heart Lung Transplant 1994;13:561–570
3. Stevenson LW, Warner SL, Steimle AE et al: The impending crisis awaiting cardiac transplantation. Modeling a solution based on selection. Circulation 1994;89:450–457
4. Stevenson LW, Miller L: Cardiac transplantation as therapy for heart failure. Curr Probl Cardiol 1991;16:219–305
5. Elefteriades JA, Tolis G, Levi E, Mills LK, Zaret BL: Coronary artery bypass grafting in severe left ventricular dysfunction. Excellent survival with improved ejection fraction and functional state. J Am Coll Cardiol 1993;22:1411–1417
6. Louie HW, Laks H, Milgalter E et al: Ischemic cardiomyopathy. Criteria for coronary revascularization and cardiac transplantation. Circulation, suppl. III 1991;84:290–295
7. Miller LW, Kubo SH, Young JB et al: Report of the consensus conference on candidate selection for cardiac transplantation. J Heart Lung Transplant 1995;14:562–571
8. Votapka TV, Pennington DG: Circulatory assist devices in congestive heart failure. Cardiol Clin 1994;12:143
9. Frazier OH, Rose EA, Macmanus Q et al: Multicenter clinical evaluation of the HearMate 1000IP left ventricular asist device. Ann Thorac Surg 1992;53:1080
10. Steimle AE, Stevenson LW, Fonarow GC, Hamilton MA, Moriguchi JD: Prediction of improvement in recent onsent cardiomyopathy after referral for heart transplantation. J Am Coll Cardiol 1994;23:553–559
11. O'Connell JB, Constanzo-Nordin MR, Subramanian R et al: Peripartum cardiomyopathy. Clinical, hemodynamic, histologic, and prognostic characteristics. J Am Coll Cardiol 1986;8:52–56
12. Regan TJ: Alcohol and the cardiovascular system. A review. JAMA 1991;264:377–381
13. Grogan M, Smith HC, Gersh BJ, Wood DW: Left ventricular dysfunction due to atrial fibrillation in patients initially believed to have idiopathic dilated cardiomyopathy. Am J Cardiol 1992;69:1570–1573
14. Middlekauff HR, Weiner I, Stevenson WG, Saxon LA, Stevenson LW: Low dose amiodarone for atrial fibrillation in advanced heart failure restores sinus rhythm

and improves functional capacity [abstract]. Circulation, Suppl. I 1992;86:808

15. Alexander JK: the cardiomyopathy of obesity. Prog Cardiovasc Dis 1985;27:325–334

16. Multicenter Diltiazem Postinfarction Trial Research Group: The effect of diltiazem on mortality and reinfarction after myocardial infarction. N Engl J Med 1988;319:385–392

17. Waagstein F, Bristow MR, Swedberg K et al: Beneficial effects of metoprolol in idiopathic dilated cardiomyopathy. Lancet 1993;42:1442–1446

18. Waagstein F, Caidahl K, Wallentin I, Bergh C-H, Hjalmarson A: Long-term beta-blockade in congestive cardiomyopathy. Effects of short- and long-term metoprolol treatment followed by withdrawal and readmission of metoprolol. Circulation 1989;80:551–563

19. Mudge GH, Goldstein S, Addonizio LJ et al: Task Force 3. Recipient guidelines/prioritization. J Am Coll Cardiol 1993;22:21–31

20. Stevenson LW, Perloff JK: The limited reliability of physical signs for the estimation of hemodynamics in chronic heart failure. JAMA 1989;261:884–888

21. Stevenson LW, Tillisch JH: Maintenance of cardiac output with normal filling pressures in dilated heart failure. Circulation 1986;74:1303–1308

22. Stevenson LW, Brunken RC, Belil D et al: Afterload reduction with vasodilators and diuretics decreases mitral valve regurgitation during upright exercise in advanced heart failure. J Am Coll Cardiol 1990;15:174–180

23. Stevenson LW: Tailored therapy before transplantation for treatment of advanced heart failure. Effective use of vasodilators and diuretics. Heart Lung Transplant 1991;10:468–476

24. Massie B, Ports T, Chatterjee K et al: Long-term vasodilator therapy for heart failure. Clinical response and its relationship to hemodynamic measurements. Circulation 1981;63:269–278

25. Steimle AE, Stevenson LW, Chelimsky-Fallick C, Fonarow GA, Tillisch JH: Prolonged maintenance of cardiac output with normal filling pressures during chronic therapy for advanced heart failure [abstract]. Circulation, suppl. I 1993;88:59

26. Fonarow GC, Stevenson LW, Walden JA et al: Impact of a comprehensive management program on the hospitalization rate for patients with advanced heart failure [abstract]. J Am Coll Cardiol 1995;25:264

27. Jessup MJ, Carver JR, Bumbaugh J, Kahm H: How much does cardiac transplantation cost? J Heart Lung Transplant 1994;13:S69

28. Wilson JR, Schwartz JS, St. John Sutton M et al: Prognosis in severe heart failure. Relation to hemodynamic measurements and ventricular ectopic activity. J Am Coll Cardiol 1983;2:403–410

29. CONSENSUS Trial Study Group: Effects of enalapril on mortality in severe congestive heart failure. Results of the Cooperative North Scandinavian Enalapril Survival Study. N Engl J Med 1987;316:1429–1435

30. Stevenson WG, Stevenson LW, Middlekauff HR et al: Results of major trials influence therapy and survival for patients with advanced heart failure [abstract]. Circulation, suppl. I 1994;90:380

31. Stevenson LW, Couper G, Natterson BJ et al: Target heart failure population for new therapies. Circulation 1995;92:II174–181

32. Keogh AM, Freund J, Baron DW, Hickie JB: Timing of transplantation in idiopathic dilated cardiomyopathy. Am J Cardiol 1988;61:418–422

33. Cohn J, Johnson G, Shabetai R et al: Ejection fraction, peak exercise oxygen consumption, cardiothoracic ratio, ventricular arrhythmias, and plasma norepinephrine as determinants of prognosis in heart failure. Circulation, suppl. VI 1993;87:5–16

34. Szlachcic J, Massie B, Kramer B, Topic N, Tubau J: Correlates and prognostic implication of exercise capacity in chronic congestive heart failure. Am J Cardiol 1985;55:1037–1042

35. Likoff M, Chandler S, Kay H: Clinical determinants of mortality in chronic congestive heart failure secondary to idiopathic dilated or ischemic cardiomyopathy. Am J Cardiol 1987;59:634–638

36. Mancini DM, Eisen H, Kussmaul W et al: Value of peak exercise oxygen consumption for optimal timing of cardiac transplantation in ambulatory patients with heart failure. Circulation 1991;83:778–786

37. Haywood GA, Rickenbacher PR, Trindade PT et al: Deaths in patients awaiting heart transplantation. The need to identify high risk category two patients. Circulation, suppl. I 1994;90:360

38. Stevenson LW, Steimle AE, Chelimsky-Fallick C et al: Outcomes predicted by peak oxygen consumption during evaluation of 333 patients with advanced heart failure [abstract]. Circulation, suppl. I 1993;88:94

39. Stevenson LW, Sietsema K, Tillisch JH et al: Exercise capacity for survivors of cardiac transplantation or sustained medical therapy for stable heart failure. Circulation [abstract]. 1990;81:78–85

40. Walden JA, Stevenson LW, Dracup K et al: Extended comparison of quality of life between stable heart failure patient and heart transplant recipients. J Heart Lung Transplant 1994;13:1109–1118

41. Hosenpud JD, DeMarco T, Frazier H et al: Progression of systemic disease and reduced long-term survival in patients with cardiac amyloidosis undergoing heart transplantation. Circulation, suppl. III 1991;84:338–343

42. Olivari MT, Antolick A, Kaye MP, Jamieson SW, Ring WS: Heart transplantation in elderly patients. J Heart Transplant 1988;7:258–264

43. Grattan MT, Moreno-Cabral CE, Starnes VA et al: Eight-year results of cyclosporine-treated patients with cardiac transplants. J Thorac Cardiovasc Surg 1990;99:500–509

44. Kaye MP: Registry of the International Society for Heart and Lung Transplantation. Tenth official report—1993. J Heart Lung Transplant 1993;12:541–548

45. Stolf NAG, Higushi L, Bocchi E et al: Heart transplantation in patients with Chagas' disease cardiomyopathy. J Heart Transplant 1987;5:307–312

46. Copeland JG, Emery RW, Levinson MM et al: Selection of patients for cardiac transplantation. Circulation 1987;75:2–9

47. Penn I: Cancers after cyclosporine therapy. Transplant Proc 1988;20:276–279

48. Erickson KW, Costanzo-Nordin MR, O'Sullivan EJ et al: Influence of preoperative transpulmonary gradient on late mortality after orthotopic heart transplantation. J Heart Transplant 1990;9:526–537

49. Costard-Jäckle A, Fowler MB: Influence of preoperative pulmonary artery pressure on mortality after heart transplantation. Testing of potential reversibil-

ity of pulmonary hypertension with nitroprusside is useful in defining a high risk group. J Am Coll Cardiol 1992;19:48–54

50. Kaye MP: The registry of the International Society for Heart and Lung Transplantation. Ninth official report. J Heart Lung Transplant 1992;599:11–20

51. Desruennes M, Muneretto C, Gandjbakhch I et al: Heterotopic heart transplantation. Current status in 1988. J Heart Transplant 1989;8:479–485

52. Wright RS, Levine MS, Bellamy PE et al: Ventilatory and diffusion abnormalities in potential heart-transplant recipients. Chest 1990;98:816–820

53. Radovancevic B, Poindexter S, Birovljev S et al: Risk factors for development of accelerated coronary artery disease in cardiac transplant recipients. Eur J Cardiothorac Surg 1990;4:309–312

54. Olbrisch ME, Levenson JL: Psychological evaluation of heart transplantation candidates. An international survey of process, criteria and outcomes. J Heart Lung Transplant 1991;10:948–955

55. Rodriguez MD, Colon A, Santiago-Delphin EA: Psychosocial profile of noncompliant patients. Transplant Proc 1991;23:1807–1809

56. Herrick CM, Mealey PC, Tischner LL, Holland CS: Combined heart failure-transplant program. Advantages in assessing medical compliance. J Heart Transplant 1987;6:141–145

57. Bourge RC, Naftal DC, Costanzo M et al: Risk factors for death after cardiac transplantation. A multi-institutional study. J Heart Lung Transplant 1993;12:549–562

58. Laffel GL, Barnett AI, Finkelstein S et al: The relation between experience and outcome in heart transplantation. N Engl J Med 1992;327:1220–1225

59. Natterson PD, Stevenson WG, Saxon LA, Middlekauff HR, Stevenson LW: Risk of arterial embolization in 224 patients awaiting cardiac transplantation. Am Heart J 1995;129:564–50

60. Konstam MA, Dracup K, Baker DW et al: Heart Failure. Evaluation and Care of Patients with Left-Ventricular Systolic Dysfunction. US Department of Health and Human Services, Rockville, MD, June 1994

61. Stevenson WG, Stevenson LW, Middlekauff HR, Saxon LA: Sudden death prevention in patient with advanced left ventricular dysfunction. Circulation 1993;88:2953–2961

62. Hamer AWF, Arkles LB, Johns JA: Beneficial effects of low dose amiodarone in patients with congestive heart failure. A placebo-controlled trial. J Am Coll Cardiol 1989;14:1768–1774

63. Doval HC, Nul DR, Grancello HO et al: Randomized trial of low-dose amiodarone in severe congestive heart failure. Lancet 1994;344:493–498

64. Singh SN, Fletcher RD, Fisher SG et al: Amiodarone in patients with congestive heart failure and asymptomatic ventricular arrhythmia. N Engl J Med 1995; 333:77–82

65. Chelimsky-Fallick C, Middlekauff HR, Stevenson WG et al: Amiodarone therapy does not compromise subsequent heart transplantation. J Am Coll Cardiol 1992; 20:1556–1561

66. Norman JC, Colley DA, Igo SR et al: Prognostic indices for survival during postcardiotomy intra-aortic balloon pumping. J Thorac Cardiovasc Surg 1977;74:709

67. Loisance DY, Deleuze PH, Houel R et al: Pharmacologic bridge to cardiac transplantation. Current limitations. Ann Thorac Surg 1993;55:310–313

68. McCarthy PM, Sabik JF: Implantable circulatory support devices as a bridge to heart transplantation. Semin Thorac Cardiovasc Surg 1994;6:174–180

69. Stevenson LW, Steimle AE, Fonarow G et al: Improvement in exercise capacity of candidates awaiting heart transplantation. J Am Coll Cardiol 1995;25:163–170

70. Evans RW: Executive Summary. The National Cooperative Transplantation Study. Report BHARC-100-91-020. Battelle Seattle Research Center, Seattle, June 1991

71. Moore FD (chairman): Fifth Bethesda conference report. Cardiac and other organ transplantation. Am J Cardiol 1968;22:896–912

53

Managing Heart Failure with Transplantation, Ventricular Assist Devices, and Cardiomyoplasty

James B. Young

Garrie J. Haas

Randall C. Starling

Heart failure is a complicated clinical syndrome and milieu. Impairment of cardiac pump function is the central difficulty, but it is important to remember that the syndrome is also characterized by profound perturbation of humoral, neurohumoral, and cytokine systems (particularly in patients with advanced, life-threatening heart failure). Altered cardiac filling dynamics, decreased forward blood flow with altered organ perfusion, and structural heart remodeling (hypertrophy and chamber dilation) account for the metabolic and humoral difficulties originally engendered by central pump dysfunction. Myocardial injury leading to heart failure can be caused by many distinct diseases, but medical therapies today focus mostly on attenuating background difficulties causing cardiac injury or interdicting effects of humoral perturbation. Though amelioration of peripheral physiologic abnormalities characteristic of the heart failure syndrome can dramatically alter prognosis, for truly changing the long-term outlook replacement of the malfunctioning pump is necessary. Indeed, few things are more impressive than observing the dramatic functional improvement of patients with advanced heart failure or cardiogenic shock after successful heart transplantation or mechanical ventricular assist device insertion. Time has proved that heart transplantation and, in certain circumstances, mechanical ventricular assist device implantation afford remarkable physiologic rehabilitation in selected patients. Though still fraught with challenging difficulties, these procedures are becoming well accepted. Symptomatic limitations directly related to heart failure's hemodynamic abnormalities improve substantially and often completely resolve. Indeed, in these patients, transplantation is vastly superior to any other therapy available to improve functional capacity and prolong life. As well, some types of mechanical assist devices can stabilize otherwise terminal patients long enough for organs to come available for transplantation. Not only can ventricular assist devices "bridge" patients to heart transplant from cardiogenic shock, they also improve the metabolic, humoral, and inflammatory abnormalities. One must realistically define outcomes that can be anticipated after cardiac transplantation and ventricular assist device insertion, frankly addressing the fact that cardiac allografts do not function entirely normally, and mechanical assist devices still have many difficulties. Finally, because of limitations in the availability of organ donors and the unknown potential of mechanical cardiac assist devices, other surgical options, such as dynamic cardiomyoplasty, continue to be evaluated. In this chapter attempt to put cardiac transplantation, mechanical ventricular assist device insertion, and dynamic cardiomyoplasty for treatment of advanced heart failure into reasonable clinical perspective.

HISTORICAL PERSPECTIVES

Few modern surgical procedures caused as much excitement, public interest, controversy, and dilemma as human heart transplantation and insertion of artificial hearts. Indeed, the history of cardiac transplantation and mechanical assist device development are closely intertwined. Interestingly, the concept of replacing a diseased heart to cure ailments is not new. Reference, though abstract, to receiving "a new heart" can be found in the Old Testament, dated to the sixth century BC, where the prophet Ezekiel is said to proclaim "a new heart also I will give you, and a new spirit will I put within you; and I will take away the stony heart out of your flesh, and I will give you a heart of flesh."[1] During the fourth century BC, legend has it that the erudite Chinese physician, Pien Chiao, exchanged hearts of two men to cure an unfavorable disequilibrium in their respective "energies," yin and yang.[2] Multiple chimeric Eastern and Western mythologic creatures portray unusual hybrids of man and beast that, combined, created mythical warring creatures of indomitable physique: the Eastern god Ganesha and Western mythologic beasts such as centaurs and minotaurs.[3]

Still, physicians and surgeons needed to gain insight into the pathophysiology of cardiac disease before effective medical and surgical therapeutics could be developed. It was only after detailed anatomic insight became available that the concept of organ swapping to improve diseased states emerged in rational fashion. Amazingly, it has been but 100 years since the earliest direct cardiac operations were performed. The German surgeon Ludwig Rehn became the first to suture a stab wound of the heart in 1896.[4] Experimental heart transplantation was performed shortly thereafter when Carrel and Guthrie, at the University of Chicago in 1905, transplanted the heart of a small puppy into the neck of a larger dog.[5] Carrel's group also performed kidney, ovarian, and testicular transplants with varying degrees of success.[6] Not only did these investigators demonstrate that successful vascular anastomoses could be performed but also that heterotopic cardiac transplant paradigms beat rhythmically for some time prior to stopping with what we now know is acute rejection.

Models of orthotopic cardiac transplants as well as autotransplants were used to study nuances of cardiac and circulatory neurohumoral control. Indeed Mann et al., persuing these issues in 1933, suggested that cardiac transplantation as a therapeutic modality was limited more by biologic effects than mechanical or operative challenges.[7] Early understanding of the humoral and cell-mediated immune system was rudimentary, but the power of "self" rec-

ognition was well understood. Indeed during the late Renaissance the great Bolognese surgeon, Gaspare Taglioccozzi, described with extraordinary accuracy first and second set rejection in his detailed accounting of failed "nose transplants."[8] Taglioccozzi had attempted to engraft the noses of slaves onto faces of several noblemen who had lost theirs for various ignominious reasons. Failure of the tissue swapping was characterized by a necrotizing inflammatory event, dramatically speeded up if the recipient had undergone a previous attempt at nose transplant. Only utilization of the patient's own tissue (rotating a tissue flap from the forehead subsequently popularized by the French master Carpue) was successful.[9] Because of work done during and shortly after World War II to understand the frustrating failure of skin grafts used to treat devastating blitzkrieg bomb burns, cell-mediated and humoral rejection were clarified, which gave greater understanding to the immunologic properties accounting for Taglioccozzi's failed operations.[10]

With the development and subsequent clinical use of cardiopulmonary bypass machinery in 1953, circulatory arrest with surgical correction of intracardiac abnormalities became possible.[11,12] During the 1960s surgical investigators had demonstrated that transplanted animal hearts could survive for as long as 1 year.[12] Interestingly, in 1964 the first well documented patient to undergo cardiac transplant received a primate heart rather than a human allograft.[13] Hardy et al., at University Hospital in Jackson, Mississippi, transplanted the heart of a chimpanzee into a 68-year-old man with diabetes mellitus, severe coronary artery disease, and diffuse peripheral vascular disease. The patient had developed cardiogenic shock due to an unstable ischemic syndrome, and emergency coronary bypass grafting surgery was attempted. After failing to wean the patient from cardiopulmonary bypass, cardiac transplantation, a procedure that had been contemplated by Hardy for some time, was attempted with the primate's heart. The graft was implanted satisfactorily, with the patient partially coming off cardiopulmonary bypass. However, the xenograft was not large enough to maintain circulation adequately for much more than 60 minutes. A subsequent landmark in cardiac transplantation occurred in 1966 when Lower transplanted a human cadaveric heart into a chimpanzee at the Medical College of Virginia, demonstrating that the organ was capable of maintaining adequate circulatory support for several hours.[11,12]

Several investigators, such as Shumway of Stanford University and Lower of the Medical College of Virginia were poised to perform human-to-human cardiac transplants when Barnard of Capetown, South Africa, performed the first one on December 3, 1967.[14] The patient survived 18 days, dying of *Pseudomonas* septicemia. Not only did this procedure shock the public, it stirred resentment in the medical and surgical professional communities and fueled bitter discussion regarding definition of an appropriate heart "donor," particularly with respect to the concept of brain death.[15] A rush to transplantation began, and 3 days after the Capetown procedure Kantrowitz et al. in New York transplanted the heart of an anencephalic infant into an 18-day-old child with a life-threatening congenital cardiac abnormality, but the infant survived for only a few hours.[16] Over the ensuing 12 months, 102 heart transplants were performed in 17 nations, with more than half of the procedures done in the United States.[11,12] Setbacks occurred repeatedly, and there were few long-term survivors. Major difficulties were rejection and overwhelming infection due to relatively crude immunosuppressive techniques (little different from protocols used today). Unrealistic expectations had been fostered, and because only 21 of the first 165 patients receiving transplants worldwide were still alive in 1971 most programs ceased performing these operations.[17,18] Indeed, only 35 percent of the transplant patients lived more than 3 months, with 10 percent survival at about 2 years.[17,18] With dogged persistence, the Stanford University heart transplant program eventually developed relatively successful immunosuppressive protocols; in particular, the ability to diagnose acute rejection by obtaining percutaneous, transvenous, endomyocardial biopsy specimens provided a dramatic boon to this procedure.[19] With the development of immunosuppressive regimens and, in particular, introduction of the potent and more selective agent cyclosporine during the early 1980s, cardiac transplantation began in earnest once again throughout the world.[18] It occurred in the setting of an already burgeoning renal transplant experience and emerging reports of successful liver, lung, and pancreas transplantation. None of these procedures were being performed in a clinical or scientific vacuum.

Mechanical circulatory assist device development paralleled the heart transplantation experience for several reasons. Not only were there concerns about the ability to attenuate rejection effectively after transplantation; the reality of a terribly inadequate heart donor pool became.[11,12,18] Furthermore, the long term outlook for a heart allograft was not known. Tactics to completely replace the heart with a mechanical system or temporarily sustain left heart circulation to attenuate difficulties while one awaited donor heart allocation emerged. Indeed, estimates today of the number of advanced heart failure patients in the United States alone who might benefit from some form of mechanical circulatory assistance are as high as 60,000, a figure open to much debate.[11,20,21] Importantly, the potential number of patients considered as mechanical assist candidates is likely large. For example, at any given time almost 4000 patients are awaiting heart transplantation, with only approximately 2500 donor organs coming available annually.[21]

Sporadic attempts at experimental extracorporeal solid organ perfusion and support began during the 1930s, with Carrel a pioneer.[5] The team of Carrel and Charles Lindbergh pursued development of a circulatory assist device (Lindbergh, the engineer–aviator–gadget man, was motivated by an ill sister-in-law who was dying of inoperable rheumatic mitral valve disease). In 1937 the Russian surgeon Demikhov allegedly replaced a dog's heart with two diaphragm pumps driven by an extracorporeal electric motor.[11,22] It was Gibbon in 1953, however, who ultimately demonstrated the feasibility of a heart–lung bypass pump oxygenator for total body perfusion such that "open heart" surgery could be successfully performed.[23]

Along a different line of research, intraaortic balloon pump counterpulsation was developed by Moulopoulos and Kolff in 1961[24] and clinically popularized by Kantrowitz's group.[25] This approach to supporting the failing circulation, though not dependent in the strictest of terms on direct mechanical flow augmentation, remains the most common form of mechanical assistance utilized in heart failure patients. It is limited, however, to those thought to have at least partially reversible left ventricular dysfunction. An isolated left ventricular assist device was first used successfully in 1963 at The Methodist Hospital and Baylor College of Medicine, in Houston, Texas. DeBakey and colleagues placed an externally powered, pneumatic ventricular assist pump into a young Mexican women with rheumatic mitral valve disease who was unable to be weaned from cardiopulmonary bypass after valve replacement surgery.[26,27] Conduits were placed in the left atrium and right axillary artery with the pump remaining extracorporeal. Ventricular function recovered sufficiently to allow removal of the device several days after its insertion, and the patient was successfully discharged from the hospital only to die in an automobile mishap several years later. This was the first demonstration that such a device could substantively contribute to support of the circulation for an extended time and provide an opportunity for native heart function to recover enough for device removal, a targeted indication for these machines even today.

Akutsu and Kolff reported the first experimental implantation of a total artificial heart in 1958.[28] Animal survival was always less than 24 hours, and it took some time before more reasonable success could be demonstrated in animal paradigms. Liotta, Cooley, and the Texas Heart Institute team, also in Houston, implanted the first orthotopic cardiac prosthesis in a patient in 1969.[11] The patient had advanced cardiac failure due to ischemic heart disease and was unable to be weaned from cardiopulmonary bypass after undergoing resection of a left ventricular aneurysm. Machine insertion was done with the idea that cardiac transplantation could ultimately be performed (a so-called bridge to transplant). The total artificial heart adequately supported the patient's circulation for 64 hours, until an appropriate donor allograft was obtained and implanted. Though the patient was successfully bridged to cardiac transplantation, he died of pneumonia 32 hours after the transplant. A second total artificial heart was implanted, again by the Texas Heart Institute team, in July 1981; and public interest became dramatically aroused in December 1982, when DeVries and associates implanted a Jarvick 7 100-ml pneumatic artificial heart into a patient at the University of Utah with no intention of bridging to cardiac transplant.[29] The patient, Dr. Barney Clark, survived for 112 days before dying of multiorgan failure. Between late 1984 and early 1985, three subsequent Jarvick 7 model implants were performed at Humana Hospital in Louisville, Kentucky, with one patient surviving a record 620 days.[11,12,29] A handful of additional "permanent" total artificial heart implants have been attempted worldwide, with all patients eventually dying of complications that included thrombosis, thromboembolism, and infection. Most centers implanted the total artificial heart as a bridge to transplant, with the registry of the International Society of Heart and Lung Transplantation reporting that about one-half of the approximately 100 devices inserted as bridge to transplantation between 1986 and 1989 were total artificial heart devices.

Virtually no total artificial hearts were used in this fashion during the 1990–1993 period, but there was great success when left ventricular assist devices were implanted.[30] The first ventricular assist device (in distinction to the total artificial heart) used to bridge a patient to transplant after "stone heart" syndrome during double valve replacement surgery was in 1978. A single-chambered, externally powered, pneumatic ventricular assist device supported the patient's circulation for 5 days prior to heart transplant.[11] The patient subsequently died of infection.

Multiple subsequent "bridging" procedures have now been successfully performed with two devices, the HeartMate (Thermo Cardiosystems, Woburn, MA) and Novacor (Baxter, Palo Alto, CA) systems, demonstrating a dramatic ability to attenuate cardiovascular collapse in the setting of severe advanced heart failure.[31] Other assist devices have also been used successfully to bridge patients to transplant. It is clear that this emerging technology is now well established, though still fraught with challenges and difficulties.[32] Proper utilization of ventricular assist devices and transplantation allow the greater likelihood of ameliorating disastrous heart failure conditions.[31–34]

PATTERNS OF CARDIAC TRANSPLANTATION

The latest registry report (1996) of the International Heart and Lung Transplantation Society now contains data on 34,326 heart transplants performed at 251 centers (as well as an additional 1954 combined heart–lung transplants reported from 105 centers) since 1982 (Fig. 53-1).[35] There was dramatic rise in the number of heart transplants done between 1983 and 1990 (increasing from fewer than 500 procedures to more than 3500 performed worldwide annually). Between the years 1993 and 1994 a plateau was reached with respect to numbers of procedures performed. Table 53-1 details characteristics of heart transplant recipients reported by the United Network of Organ Sharing (UNOS), which limits its database and analysis to procedures performed in the United States.[36] Though worldwide there has been a slight decline in total number of heart transplant procedures, in the United States between 1988 and 1994 there was a steady but small rise in the number done, increasing from 1676 in 1988 to 2340 in 1994.[36] Some subtle demographic changes are apparent, with slightly more patients in older age cohorts receiving transplants. Among the cohort aged 50 years or more, an increase from 51.4 percent of the procedures in 1988 to 57.5 percent in 1994 may be noted. Still, it is important to realize that more than half of the heart transplants performed during any given year were in individuals over age 50. Also interesting is the preponderance of men undergoing heart transplantation, though this percentage has fallen from 79.3 percent in 1988 to 76.1 percent in 1994. These figures pertain despite the fact that the prevalence of heart failure and advanced heart disease is only slightly less in women than men. A fairly constant rate of repeat heart transplantation was noted between 1988 and 1994, with only about 3 percent of the procedures being performed as a second go-

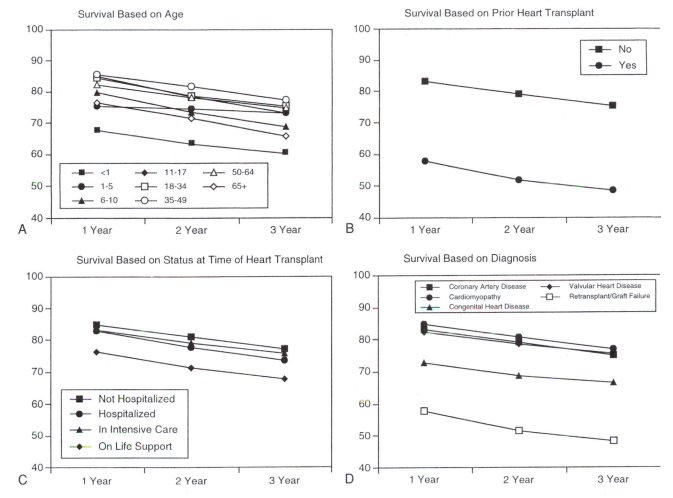

Fig. 53-1. Data from the latest Registry report with respect to (**A**) survival based on recipient age; (**B**) retransplant or primary procedure; (**C**) urgency of status based on acuity of illness; and (**D**) reason for heart failure development. As discussed in the text, old and young recipients and those undergoing a second transplant procedure seemingly have higher mortality. (Data extrapolated from United Network of Organ Sharing Analysis.[36])

around. Repeat heart transplantation is not as successful as the initial procedure. Great concern is raised as heart transplant recipients generally age more, with the demand for replacing failed allografts greatly increasing at the same time the number of patients listed for their first heart transplant continues to rise. Heterotopic heart transplantation was never performed frequently, but even so the incidence has fallen from 1.1 percent in 1988 to 0.2 percent in 1994.

Diseases treated with heart transplantation have changed slightly, with a gradual increase in the percent of patients given transplants for cardiomyopathy and a concomitant decrease in the number treated for coronary artery disease. Between 1988 and 1994 the percentage of patients receiving transplants for cardiomyopathy went from 36.6 to 56.2 percent, and the percentage of coronary artery dis-

ease patients fell from 50.4 to 30.8 percent. These data are different from those of other registries, however, with many centers having a preponderance of coronary artery disease patients in their transplant cohort. Indeed, in the Cardiac Transplant Research Database (CTRD) 50 percent of patients receiving hearts had ischemic heart disease and 36 percent dilated cardiomyopathy.[37–39]

Reflecting the pressure on donor organ allocation and increased number of patients awaiting heart transplantation is the illness acuity of those undergoing this procedure. In 1988 there were 42.2 percent of patients undergoing heart transplant who were not hospitalized at the time of donor allocation, whereas in 1994 only 38.3 percent of patients were called in from home while waiting to undergo the procedure.[36] Indeed in 1994 about 54% of patients receiving organs were hospitalized in an intensive

Table 53-1. Heart Transplant Recipient Characteristics: 1988–1994 (Year-End Data)

Parameter	1988	1989	1990	1991	1992	1993	1994
No. of recipients	1676	1705	2108	2125	2171	2297	2345
Age (%)							
<1	2.3	4.3	4.3	5.9	4.1	4.7	4.0
1–5	1.3	1.3	2.3	2.5	2.9	2.4	2.9
6–10	1.2	1.0	1.1	0.9	1.1	1.4	1.7
11–17	2.6	2.4	2.9	3.0	2.7	3.4	2.9
18–34	11.4	10.9	8.3	8.2	8.1	8.8	7.6
35–49	29.4	29.3	27.9	26.2	24.5	23.4	23.5
50–64	50.4	48.4	49.7	49.9	52.6	51.3	53.4
65+	1.4	2.4	3.4	3.4	3.9	4.5	4.1
Male (%)	79.3	79.8	78.6	77.2	76.7	78.5	76.1
Prior heart transplant (%)	2.7	2.5	2.6	3.0	2.9	3.2	2.9
Heterotopic (%)	1.1	0.8	0.7	0.7	0.6	0.3	0.2
Recipient descriptions (%)							
Hospitalized	14.4	6.7	8.2	6.6	8.2	5.5	2.6
ICU	26.0	24.8	30.0	23.8	22.2	22.1	5.2
ICU/life support	17.4	16.8	15.6	23.6	22.5	31.4	54.0
Not hospitalized	42.2	51.7	46.1	46.0	44.1	41.0	38.3
Diagnosis (%)							
Cardiomyopathy	36.6	37.2	36.5	42.3	44.0	43.0	56.2
CAD	50.4	47.7	49.0	40.8	40.7	41.5	30.8
Congenital	4.1	6.5	7.0	8.9	7.5	8.1	7.0
VHD	5.5	4.5	4.2	3.4	2.9	2.9	2.3
Heart transplant	2.7	2.4	2.6	2.9	2.9	3.1	2.2

Abbreviations: ICU, intensive care unit; CAD, coronary artery disease; VHD, valvular heart disease.
(Data from United Network of Organ Sharing Analysis.[36])

care unit and on life support systems, whereas only 17.4 percent in 1988 were given transplants while in this category.

WAITING LIST CHARACTERISTICS

Of the 42,778 patients listed on the UNOS waiting list November 1, 1995, there were 3383 (8 percent) awaiting hearts (Table 53-2). This number should be compared to the 30,378 patients (71 percent of the waiting list) hoping for kidneys.[40] This data should be put into the perspective of the number of cadaveric donors from which solid organs were recovered in the United States in 1993. Only 4845 such donors came available, with but 3925 of them suitable multiorgan donors (81 percent of the overall cadaveric donor pool). Of the suitable multiorgan donors, only 2437 became heart donors. Obviously, the number of candidates listed each year for cardiac transplantation does not begin to approximate the number of donors (Table 53-2). This fact may have lead to a trend to listing less ill patients for heart allocation in the hopes that they would survive longer waits. Death certificate analysis suggests that up to 16,000 pa-

tients annually might be candidates (if 55 years of age is used as the upper recipient age cutoff), but this number dramatically rises to more than 40,000 patients when individuals age 55–65 years are added to the recipient pool.[20] In contrast, when the most liberal estimates of donors are made, only 5,000–10,000 donor hearts are likely to become available.[18,21]

The disparity between donor availability and recipient need is dramatized by the increased waiting times noted recently. Table 53-2 demonstrates that the proportion of patients waiting longer than 12 months before receiving a donor heart rose from 12.5 percent in 1988 to 45.4 percent in 1994.[36] Despite that fact, the absolute percent of deaths on the UNOS heart transplant waiting list fell from 15.0 percent in 1988 to 11.4 percent in 1994, suggesting that patients may be listed earlier in their disease state or are receiving more effective treatment. With UNOS heart allocation schemes designed to distribute organs to sicker "status I" hospitalized patients in an intensive care unit and on "life support" (as documented in Table 53-1), a reasonable balance seems to have been struck, with patients going on the list earlier but receiving organs only when substantive,

Table 53-2. UNOS Heart Transplant Waiting List Characteristics: 1988–1994 (Year-End Data)

Parameter	1988	1989	1990	1991	1992	1993	1994	1995
No. of patients	1030	1320	1788	2267	2690	2834	2933	3383
Age (%)								
<1	0.6	0.5	1.2	1.1	1.2	0.9	0.8	NA
1–5	0.4	1.4	0.6	1.2	1.0	1.2	1.6	3.1 (0–5)
6–10	0.3	0.2	0.3	0.4	0.4	0.6	0.5	0.9
11–17	1.3	1.0	0.9	1.2	1.4	1.5	1.9	1.8
18–34	7.7	7.1	8.4	2.5	2.3	7.8	7.8	NA
35–49	35.3	32.6	32.0	30.2	29.2	28.5	28.2	35.4 (18–49)
50–64	52.2	55.0	53.1	54.7	55.3	55.0	55.1	54.6
65+	2.2	2.3	3.4	3.6	4.2	4.6	4.1	4.2
Male (%)	86.1	85.5	84.7	84.1	83.5	82.0	81.4	80.7
Time waiting (%)								
0–30 Days	19.3	15.9	13.2	10.9	8.7	9.2	9.0	NA
31–60 Days	12.4	11.9	9.7	9.7	8.2	6.7	6.9	NA
61–90 Days	11.3	10.2	8.2	8.5	7.2	5.3	5.7	NA
91–120 Days	7.3	7.4	7.6	7.1	6.5	5.4	5.1	NA
121–150 Days	7.4	6.0	6.2	6.0	5.6	5.4	3.9	NA
151–180 Days	7.2	5.0	5.9	6.1	5.2	3.9	3.5	NA
6–12 Months	22.6	23.1	28.7	24.6	26.8	21.9	20.6	NA
>1 Year	12.5	20.5	20.4	27.2	31.8	42.1	45.4	NA
Deaths (%)	15.0	14.1	13.1	14.5	13.1	12.2	11.4	NA

Abbreviation: NA, not available.
(Data from United Network of Organ Sharing Analysis.[36])

dramatic, life-threatening deterioration develops but sometimes requiring circulatory assist devices to keep them stable during the wait.[36] Other changes of interest include a decrement in the proportion of males awaiting heart transplantation (from 86.1 percent in 1988 to 80.7 percent in 1995) and a rise in the proportion of patients over 50 years of age on the list (from 54.4 percent in 1988 to 58.8 percent in 1995).

CARDIAC ALLOGRAFT DONOR

Not all solid-organ donors qualify as heart donors. Table 53-3 summarizes the demographics of U.S. heart donors.[36] The percent of male donors has fallen from 71.7 to 68.7 percent, and donors are generally older. In 1988 only 2.1 percent of the donor pool was older than 50 years with 8.9 percent in 1994 being this old. Indeed, more than one-third of all heart donors in 1994 were over the age of 35 compared to only one-fifth in 1988. Also, donor deaths due to motor vehicle accidents have decreased, from almost 40 percent to slightly under 30 percent, with a concomitant decrement in gunshot wounds (generally to the head) from 21.3 percent in 1988 to 4.7 percent in 1994. It is our perception that though slightly more donors are identified today they frequently are from

high risk subsets. Risk factors for cardiovascular disease are noted more frequently in today's donor pool, the incidence of multiorgan trauma is higher, and social difficulties such as drug use or risk factors for acquired immunodeficiency syndrome (AIDS) are noted more often. Though many organs taken from such donors work perfectly well, failure is more frequent.

Table 53-4 details observations necessary to diagnose brain death.[15,41–43] Essential is no evidence of cerebral cortex function plus complete absence of brain stem activity. Patients must be in a deep coma (unresponsive) without evidence of cerebral receptivity. Absence of brain stem activity is apparent when no light pupillary reflex, corneal reflex, extraocular reflex, gag reflex, cough reflex, and apnea (in the face of hypercarbia) are observed. The cause of death should be known, and there should be no concomitant hypothermia, hypotension, significant metabolic perturbation, drug intoxication, or substantive use of central nervous system depressants. These features should persist over time without change; and if appropriate clinical findings are present, ancillary or "confirmatory" tests are not mandatory. Electroencephalography, radionuclide cerebral blood flow imaging, or cerebral angiography may be used, however, to help clarify confusing presentations, alleviate a caregiver's anxiety about making a brain

Table 53-3. Heart Donor Characteristics: 1988–1994 (Year-End Data)

Parameter	1988	1989	1990	1991	1992	1993	1994
No. of donors	1785	1782	2168	2198	2247	2442	2527
Age, years (%)							
<1	1.5	3.3	3.1	4.2	2.9	3.4	2.9
1–5	1.7	2.1	3.1	3.5	3.8	3.2	3.5
6–10	2.2	1.6	1.8	2.2	2.9	2.4	2.1
11–17	17.7	15.3	14.9	15.0	16.5	18.6	18.0
18–34	55.6	53.0	51.2	48.2	42.7	42.9	40.2
35–49	19.2	21.4	22.2	22.2	24.5	21.0	24.4
50–64	2.0	3.1	3.7	4.6	6.5	7.8	8.2
65+	0.1	0.1	0	0.1	0.3	0.7	0.7
Male (%)	71.7	72.1	69.8	68.4	68.3	68.6	68.7
Cause of death (%)							
MVA	39.9	34.0	33.3	30.5	25.0	26.9	29.5
GSW/SW	21.3	22.1	21.3	22.7	24.6	23.2	4.7
CVA	20.6	23.4	23.2	24.5	26.6	25.7	28.0
Head trauma	10.3	12.0	12.8	11.5	13.5	12.7	27.9
Asphyxia	1.4	2.0	2.2	3.0	2.0	2.4	1.9
Drowning	0.4	0.3	0.6	0.7	0.9	0.8	0.3
Drug overdose	1.1	0.9	0.9	0.5	0.7	0.5	0.5
CV	0.7	0.6	0.6	0.7	0.5	0.9	0.8

Abbreviations: GSW, gunshot wound; SW, stab wound; MVA, motor vehicle accident; CVA, cerebral vascular accident; CV, cardiovascular.
(Data from United Network of Organ Sharing Analysis.[36])

Table 53-4. Brain Death Criteria

No evidence of cerebral cortex function
   No light-pupillary reflex (pupils "fixed")
   No corneal reflex
   No extraocular reflex (absence of "doll's eyes")
   No gag reflex
   No cough reflex
   No respirations during apnea test[a]
Irreversibility
   Cause of death known
   No concomitant hypothermia, hypotension, or significant metabolic perturbation
   No drug intoxication or significant central nervous system depressant use
   Observations persist over time (for adults: 6 hours with confirmatory tests, 12 hours without, and 24 hours in the setting of anoxic brain injury)
Ancillary confirmatory tests (not mandatory)
   Electroencephalogram
   Radio nuclide imaging
   Cerebral angiography

[a] Apnea test: preoxygenation with 100 percent FIO_2 for 10 minutes; disconnect ventilator, give O_2 at 8–12 L/min by tracheal cannula; observe for spontaneous respirations; obtain $PaCO_2$ after 10 minutes; if $PaCO_2$ >60 mmHg and no respirations have occurred, individual is apneic.

death diagnosis, or help shorten observation periods in some circumstances.

Allocation of specific donors to individuals on the heart transplant waiting list is based primarily on the severity of the patient's heart failure syndrome: status I versus status II, with status I defined as patients requiring cardiac or pulmonary assistance (or both) with a total artificial heart, left or right (or both) ventricular assist device or intraaortic balloon pump, or ventilator, or patients in an intensive care unit who require inotropic agents to maintain adequate cardiac output.[36,42] Additional factors bearing on allocation include length of time on the waiting list, recipient–donor size match, blood type compatibility, and distance of donor from recipient (anticipated ischemic time during organ harvest and implantation.[39] These are the primary factors taken into account by local organ procurement organizations in conjuction with UNOS when potential distribution lists are generated.[36] Obviously, many other issues play a critical role in the appropriate matchup of donors and recipients, such as the age of the donor versus that of the recipient, but these factors are not generally taken into account, a priori, by the UNOS allocation system.

Table 53-5 lists some suggested guidelines for acceptance of cardiac donors and focuses on the issue of benefit when a given organ donor is utilized in any

Table 53-5. Suggested Guidelines for Cardiac Donors

Age less than 55 years (older donors are sometimes acceptable)

Negative serologies for human immunodeficiency virus (HIV) and hepatitis (some hepatitis B or C positive donors may be acceptable)

No active severe systemic infection

No malignancy with a possibility of metastasis or other concerning co-morbid condition such as diabetes or collagen vascular disease of significance

No evidence of significant cardiac disease or trauma

Low probability of coronary atherosclerosis (donor coronary angiograms should be obtained in high risk settings)

Acceptable ventricular function without substantive cardiac trauma, without aggressive inotropic support (dopamine <10 ng/kg/min in most situations)

Blood type compatible with recipient

Negative prospectively performed cytotoxic T cell crossmatch for sensitized recipient

Donor body weight index between 75% and 125% of recipient's (size mismatch affected by recipient pulmonary hypertension; small donors might be acceptable heterotopic candidates)

Anticipated allograft ischemia times less than 4–5 hours

particular clinical setting versus the risk of allowing the patients to wait longer. Though a great deal of discussion has emerged regarding "marginal" donors, it is in fact a misnomer. Always, acceptance of an offered organ is based on carefully considered risk–benefit perspectives. It is unreasonable to assume that anyone would recommend the use of a donor organ if the likelihood of function failure was significant. Risks have now been defined by multicenter clinical trial experience, where the impact of various donor parameters can be isolated and objectively analyzed. These data allow an informed decision to be made such that fair recommendations can be given to patients. Optimal parameters generally include donor age less than 55 years, although older donors are perfectly satisfactory in many circumstances. Negative serologies for human immunodeficiency virus (HIV) and hepatitis, particularly active hepatitis, are important. Some hepatitis B- or C-positive donors may be acceptable. Donors should have no active, severe, systemic infection, particularly bacteremia or fungemia. Malignancies (excepting primary brain tumors) with the possibility of metastasis or other concerning co-morbid conditions such as diabetes mellitus or collagen vascular disease may create difficulties after transplant for the recipient.

Donors dying of primary brain tumors rarely create problems.

Complicating donor selection is the fact that brain death itself may create a milieu hostile to normal ventricular function. In young patients with no known history of cardiac disease and all other observations not particularly concerning (including a reasonably normal electrocardiogram), depressed ventricular function frequently is noted but is reversed after removal of the heart from the brain death milieu and subsequently reimplanted. Because brain death is "total brain death," acute interruption of the midbrain pituitary-based hormone axis is noted with a subsequent decrement in hormone release (particularly thyroid- and adrenal-stimulating hormones). Replacement of these hormones may be helpful. Differentiating between potentially irreversible ventricular dysfunction and those situations simply due to the brain death environment can be difficult, so a great deal of clinical experience is desirable.

Also important is that cardiac donors should be blood type-compatible with the recipient and preferably blood-type identical. If patients have preformed panel-reactive antibodies of significance prior to transplantation, a negative, prospectively performed cytotoxic T and B cell crossmatch is often sought. Donor body weight or mass index between 75 and 125 percent of the recipient's is desirable. Size mismatch decisions should be influenced by the presence of recipient pulmonary hypertension where large donors may be more desirable. Small donors may be acceptable when used in heterotopic biologic support pump fashion. Finally, as mentioned, anticipated allograft ischemic times less than 4–5 hours are important and desirable.

The relation of donor histocompatibility status (HLA) to that of the recipient is not generally determined prospectively, and therefore allocation schemes for hearts are not based on HLA matching criteria as they are for kidney transplantation. This does not mean that HLA match or mismatch plays no role in outcome after cardiac transplantation.[44,45] It has been shown that (using death due to allograft arteriopathy as a primary endpoint) patients with chronic, low grade inflammation manifested by consistently high endomyocardial biopsy scores and few episodes of mild degrees of rejection during surveillance biopsy have a worse HLA donor–recipient match.[45] Of specific importance seems to be the fact that complete HLA-A, HLA-B, or HLA-DR mismatch is associated with higher rejection rates and more allograft arteriopathy. Most heart transplants are performed in the setting of complete six antigen mismatch.

To exclude the single center bias when exploring

this tissue, HLA mismatch and other potential risk factors for rejection were analyzed in data from 27 institutions participating in the Cardiac Transplant Research Database between January 1, 1990 and June 30, 1992.[44] Complete HLA information on the A, B, and DR loci was available for both donor and recipient in 1190 cases. Only 6 percent of the patient population had zero, one, or two mismatches. Indeed, the mean number of mismatches overall in the group was 4.4 loci. Using parametric multivariable analysis, risk factors for first rejection and the time to first rejection included a younger patient age, female gender of both donor and recipient, number of HLA mismatches, and being an African American recipient. The few patients with zero, one, or two mismatches had 54 percent freedom from rejection at 1 year versus only 36 percent for patients with three or more HLA mismatches. Other donor-associated risk factors for death after cardiac transplantation in this same data set were older donor age, smaller donor body surface area (particularly when a female donor heart was placed in a large male patient), greater donor inotropic support, presence of donor diabetes mellitus, long ischemic times, diffuse donor heart wall motion abnormalities on preharvest echocardiography, and, for pediatric donors, death from causes other than closed head trauma.

OPERATIVE CONSIDERATIONS

Orthotopic heart transplantation is preferred to heterotopic procedures. In this operation the native heart is completely amputated and donor biatrial anastomoses performed with an end-to-end anastomosis of the aorta and pulmonary artery. This technique is the traditional one delineated early by the Stanford group.[46] One disadvantage of this procedure is that varying sizes of atrial cuffs, particularly for the right atrium, remain, and efficiency of atrial to ventricular electromechanical coupling is diminished.[47,48] Furthermore, bradyarrhythmias due to impaired recovery of donor sinus node function are frequently noted.[49] Bicaval anastomosis is helpful for alleviating some of these problems.[50] This technique has been associated with less bradycardia and lower right heart pressures early after transplant. Greater efficiency of atrioventricular electromechanical coupling is apparent, but the technique is more difficult to perform and prolongs the operating time. Additionally, narrowing of the superior vena cava or inferior vena cava anastomoses may be noted postoperatively, sometimes causing difficulty during a surveillance endomyocardial biopsy. In adequately sized donor hearts, bicaval anastomoses may be the preferred approach for performing orthotopic transplantation.

Heterotopic transplantation may have a therapeutic niche, but this operation is still infrequently performed.[51] With this procedure the native heart is left in place, and the donor heart is anastomosed in parallel fashion to the circulation with end-to-side aortic and pulmonary artery connections. There are variable degrees of contribution to the pulmonary and systemic circulation, and in some circumstances only right ventricular circulatory assist can be observed. Because mortality after this procedure is higher than after orthotopic heart transplants, heterotopic procedures have been unfairly maligned. This procedure was often performed in the setting of substantive pulmonary hypertension that would, all other circumstances being equal, exclude the patient as a transplant candidate (at least utilizing an orthotopic procedure). Also, heterotopic procedures were sometimes recommended when the donor heart was suspect, with the thought that it could be removed at some future time because the native heart theoretically is left functioning. Indeed, heterotopic transplantation could address situations where native heart function might be eventually restored, such as in cases of acute myocarditis. Also, when a donor is small in relation to a given recipient, or when ventricular arrhythmias may be the overwhelming difficulty, heterotopic transplantation might present an attractive alternative.[52] Still, heterotopic heart transplantation does not ameliorate anginal syndromes in the native heart, overcome problems caused by valvar insufficiency, or eliminate the requirement for full anticoagulation to prevent emboli from thrombosed native hearts. Interestingly, initial use of xenographic transplants will likely be in heterotopic positions.

OUTCOMES AFTER CARDIAC TRANSPLANTATION

Survival after heart transplantation is now reasonable when compared to the natural history of patients with severe, advanced, and end-stage heart failure. In the 1995 annual report of the United States Scientific Registry for Organ Transplantation (which included patients undergoing heart transplantation between October 1987 and December 1994) actuarial 1-year survival after heart transplant was 82.3 percent at 1 year and 74.4 percent at 3 years.[36] Figure 53-2B compares cardiac transplant patient survival at 1 year to cadaveric kidney, living related kidney, liver, pancreas, lung, and heart–lung transplantation. Also, two distinct eras, 1988 and 1993, are de-

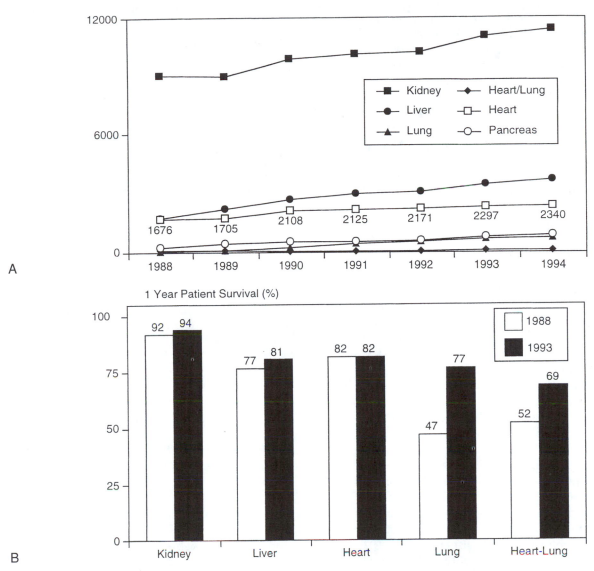

Fig. 53-2. Number of heart transplant procedures performed are put into perspective with other solid organ transplants. **(A)** Though a slight increase in the number of transplants is noted each year, it is not great. **(B)** Importantly, survival at the 1-year follow-up point is above 80 percent and has not changed substantially during the UNOS observation period. (Data extrapolated from United Network of Organ Sharing Analysis.[36])

tailed. No survival difference is noted for heart transplants between the two eras, both being equally good. Comparing hearts to other solid-organ transplants, success rates are excellent. UNOS data suggests that 3-year actuarial survival after heart transplant may be slightly higher among caucasians (75.4%) than African Americans (68.3 percent) or Hispanics (70.7 percent). Male recipients also have a slightly higher 3-year survival (75.2 percent) than female recipients (71.8 percent). Three-year survival for patients aged 1 year and less was 60.4 percent and for patients aged 65 or more 65.7 percent. The highest 3-year sur-

vival in the UNOS database was noted in the age group 35–49 years and was 77.3 percent.

The Cardiac Transplant Research Database group has given a great deal of insight into a number of broad outcome questions. Risk factors for death after heart transplantation were identified by analyzing the total primary heart transplant experience in 1719 consecutive primary transplants performed between January 1, 1990 and June 30, 1992.[37,39] Mean follow-up of survivors was 13.9 months, and actuarial survival was 85 percent at 1 year. By multivariable analysis, risk factors for death included younger recipient age ($P = 0.006$), older recipient age ($P = 0.005$), ventilator support at the time of transplantation ($P = 0.006$), higher pulmonary vascular resistance ($P = 0.02$), older donor age ($P < 0.0001$), smaller donor body surface area ($P = 0.003$), more donor inotropic support ($P = 0.01$), donor diabetes mellitus ($P = 0.01$), long ischemic time ($P = 0.003$), diffuse donor heart wall motion abnormalities by echocardiography ($P = 0.06$), and for pediatric donors death from causes other than closed head trauma ($P = 0.02$). In this analysis, the overall 30-day mortality rate was 7 percent but increased to 11 percent when donor age exceeded 50 years; it was 12 percent when inotropic support exceeded a dobutamine plus dopamine dosage of 20 μg·kg^{-1}·min^{-1} and 22 percent when diffuse echocardiographic wall motion abnormalities were detected in the donor heart. The interaction of donor risk factors with recipient characteristics was such that the heart of a smaller female donor given high dose inotropes and placed in a larger male recipient produced a predicted 30-day mortality of 26 percent, whereas the heart of a 25-year-old male donor given high dose inotropes with diffuse echocardiographic wall motion abnormalities and transplanted into a 50-year-old male recipient led to a predicted 30-day mortality of 17 percent. Another analysis, which focused solely on recipient characteristics and had fewer patients with a slightly shorter follow-up, demonstrated that the two most common causes of death overall were infection and early graft failure (accounting for 45 percent of the deaths). In addition to the above-mentioned risk factors, ventilator support at the time of transplantation ($P = 0.09$), abnormal renal function ($P = 0.1$), lower pretransplantation cardiac output ($P = 0.009$), higher pulmonary vascular resistance ($P = 0.006$), and donor and recipient not both blood type O ($P = 0.009$) were also identified as independent risk factors for death.[39] The recipient age effect was greatest in patients under 5 years of age (1-year survival rate 68 percent versus 85 percent for all others; $P = 0.002$). Patients aged 60 years and older had a 1-year survival of 81 percent. As mentioned, ventilator dependency at the time of transplantation was an adverse risk factor, with the 3-month survival in this group only 65 percent. Transplantation of a blood group O heart into a non-O recipient had a lower 1-year survival rate than did blood group O into an O blood type recipient (82 percent versus 88 percent survival; $P = 0.06$). The adverse effect of a longer ischemic time was most notable after 4 hours (1 month survival rate 71 percent for more than 4 hours of ischemia versus 85 percent for less than 4 hours; $P = 0.0003$).

These observations are concordant with other

Table 53-6. Factors Negatively Affecting Outcome After Cardiac Transplantation

Recipient age
Concomitant systemic illness
Infiltrative/inflammatory diseases (amyloid/sarcoid/lupus)
Irreversible pulmonary hypertension
Substantive parenchymal pulmonary disease
Acute pulmonary thromboembolism
Substantive symptomatic peripheral or cerebrovascular disease
Irreversible and significant renal or hepatic dysfunction
Active peptic ulcer disease
Symptomatic diverticulitis
Diabetes mellitus with end-organ damage
Obesity
Severe osteoporosis
Active infection
Coexistent malignant neoplasms
Psychosocial instability or substance abuse that likely will compromise outcome by adversely affecting compliance with treatment programs

large scale reports. Table 53-6 lists many factors thought to negatively affect outcome after cardiac transplantation. In addition to the issues already discussed, it is obvious that concomitant systemic illness adversely affects results. Of particular importance are reports indicating that patients with systemic infiltrative or inflammatory diseases such as amyloidosis or sarcoidosis fare less well if heart transplant is performed. Indeed, evidence suggests that some diseases, such as amyloid, rapidly recur in the transplanted heart.[43,53] Substantive parenchymal pulmonary disease in the form of severe chronic bronchitis or emphysema also creates difficulties. Obviously, patients with symptomatic peripheral or cerebrovascular disease have a compromised outcome, as might those with irreversible renal or hepatic dysfunction. Immunosuppressive agents, in particular cyclosporine, tacrolimus, and azathioprine, are toxic to the kidney and liver. Active peptic ulcer disease may be worsened after chronic steroid administration, and individuals with symptomatic diverticulitis are at risk of bowel perforation, with abdominal catastrophe masked by steroid administration. Though more controversial, some reports have suggested that obesity and severe osteoporosis are independent risk factors for poor outcomes. A major concern is patient and family compliance with medication administration, lack of cardiovascular risk factor attenuation, and rebellion against transplant center and physician recommendations.

All things considered, survival after cardiac transplantation far outstrips that noted in most patient cohorts with New York Heart Association (NYHA) class IV advanced heart failure. With improving pharmacotherapeutic protocols for cardiac transplantation, however, one must be extraordinarily careful to select those individuals who have the highest risk of death. Though initial reports suggested that 5-year survival after the development of symptomatic heart failure was less than 50 percent, subsequent clinical trial data suggest that much better survival rates can be achieved.[54,55] To gain maximum benefit from this procedure, patients should be severely symptomatic with virtually no likelihood of surviving 6–24 months.[43,53] Selection of patients is addressed in Chapter 51.

FUNCTION OF THE TRANSPLANTED HEART

Independent of long-term survival, heart transplantation affords a dramatic degree of rehabilitation, provided that patients were markedly symptomatic before surgery. Still, heart allografts do not function entirely normally.[48,56–59] Though exercise tolerance is less than might be expected, patients still have dramatic improvement in quality of life. Table 53-7 summarizes many important physiologic issues related to function of the transplanted heart. As previously suggested, after biatrial anastomosis orthotopic heart transplantation, variable portions of donor and recipient atria are present but not contracting synergistically. This situation leads to less atrial contribution to net stroke volume than normally would be expected.[60] Furthermore, ventricular diastolic pressure rises dramatically during exercise, and an overt restrictive hemodynamic pattern has been documented early after transplantation that usually resolves within days or weeks but can persist in a latent fashion much longer. This "stiff heart" syndrome is likely multifactorial and due to allograft rejection, denervation, and ischemic injury at the time of donor harvesting and subsequent implantation.[61]

An additional problem can be donor–recipient size mismatch.[62] Usually donors weigh 20–40 percent less than recipients. A significant negative correlation has been identified between the donor/recipient weight ratio and the resting heart rate, right atrial pressure, and pulmonary capillary wedge pressure at the 3-month posttransplant observation point.[62]

Denervation creates several changes that are inimicable to exercise hemodynamics.[63–65] For example, a characteristic of the transplanted heart is a

Table 53-7. Issues Related to Cardiac Allograft Function

Hemodynamics
    Donor/recipient atrial asynchrony
    Bicaval versus biatrial anastomosis
    Early restrictive physiology
    Late occult restrictive physiology

Allograft denervation
    Altered reflex control of peripheral vasoconstriction/dilation
    Altered Na^+/H_2O regulations via CNS-dependent vasopressin, renin, angiotensin, aldosterone secretion
    Absence of anginal syndrome during ischemia
    Absent vagus nerve control
    Rapid heart rate at rest
    Blunted heart rate response to exercise
    Loss of diurnal blood pressure fluctuation
    Hypersensitivity to circulating catecholamines
    Exaggerated response to acetylcholine

Altered humoral homeostatic feedback loops
    ANP secretion enhanced
    Elevated exercise circulating catecholamines
    Increased paracrine peptides (endothelin)
    Elevated exercise circulating catecholamines

Myocardial injury/maladaptation
    Organ preservation/recovery injury
    Operative complications
    Allograft rejection
    Cardiac allograft vasculopathy
    Hypertensive heart disease
    Ventricular hypertrophy

Donor-related issues
    Effect of brain death on cardiac function
    Donor/recipient size mismatch
    Age-related diastolic dysfunction
    Preexisting atherosclerosis
    Preexisting ventricular hypertrophy
    Preexisting cardiomyopathy
    Preexisting structural heart disease (e.g., atrial septal defect, anomalous coronary artery anatomy)

Abbreviations: CNS, central nervous system; ANP, atrial natriuretic peptide.

higher than normal resting heart rate (95–110 bpm versus 60–100 bpm in normals) and slower heart rate acceleration than normal during exercise. The afferent and efferent enervation, characteristic of donor heart cardiectomy and subsequent organ implantation, alters normal humoral homeostasis by impairing renin-angiotensin-aldosterone regulation, changing cardiac filling parameters, and abolishing normal diurnal variation in blood pressure.[66]

Generally the cardiac pressure–volume curves are shifted to the right in the orthotopic heart transplant population. Furthermore, many drugs utilized in the transplant patient (cyclosporine, for example) adversely affect renal perfusion and function.[48] This alteration of renal function contributes to altered posttransplant cardiac function.

In summary, the cardiac allograft is a denervated preparation that, in the absence of significant rejection, allograft vasculopathy, or severe hypertension, performs at rest similarly but not identically to a normal heart. Diastolic dysfunction is common early after cardiac transplantation and may recur at later stages in some patients, primarily due to cell-mediated rejection or hypertrophy and stiffening of the left ventricle. Significant allograft vasculopathy, thought to be a form of "chronic rejection," can also contribute to this difficulty. Cardiac reserve during exercise is usually reasonable but less than that seen in normals. Augmentation of cardiac performance during stress is related mostly to endogenous elevation of catecholamines and changes in ventricular loading parameters.

COMPLICATIONS AFTER HEART TRANSPLANTATION

Table 53-8 summarizes the most significant complications noted after heart transplant. Globally, they include the ever present specter of rejection, infec-

---

Table 53-8. Complications Noted After Heart Transplant

Allograft rejection
    "Humoral" rejection
    "Vascular" rejection
    "Cell-mediated" rejection
Infection
    Bacterial
    Viral
        Cytomegalovirus
        Hepatitis
        Herpes virus
Allograft arteriopathy
Malignancy
    Skin cancers
    Solid organ malignancies
    Posttransplant lymphoproliferative disorder
Immunosuppressive drug-related difficulties
    Nephrotoxicity
    Seizures
    Meningitis, encephalitis
    Hypertension
    Dyslipidemia
    Osteoporosis
    Obesity
    Cholelithiasis
    Cholestasis
    Pancreatitis
    Hirsutism
    Gingival hyperplasia

---

tion, arteriopathy, and immunosuppressive drug-related difficulties such as nephrotoxicity, hypertension, and dyslipidemia.

Allograft Rejection

As with any organ or tissue transplanted, allograft rejection is a difficulty that should be anticipated. Indeed, rejection was the rate-limiting factor to successful transplantation during the early era. Traditionally, cardiac rejection has been classified as hyperacute, acute, and chronic forms.[54,56,67] More recently, in an attempt to focus on mechanism, cardiac allograft rejection has been segregated into "cell-mediated" or "vascular-directed" (antibody-mediated) forms.[68,69] "Chronic rejection" traditionally has been referred to as the development of cardiac allograft arteriopathy.[54,56,70–73]

Critical to successful management of cardiac allograft recipients is the diagnosis and staging of rejection. The most commonly utilized grading schema for rejection is that of the International Society of Heart and Lung Transplantation (ISHLT) (Table 53-9).[67] This standardized endomyocardial biopsy grading scale starts with a grade 0 rejection score, which refers to a specimen with no significant abnormality, which is rarely seen. For grade 1A, only a small degree of focal perivascular or interstitial lymphocytic infiltrate is apparent, and no myocyte "damage" or

---

Table 53-9. ISHLT Standardized Endomyocardial Biopsy Grading Scheme

Grade	Criteria[a]
0	Normal myocardium
1A	Focal (perivascular or interstitial) lymphocytic infiltrate without myocyte necrosis
1B	Diffuse but sparse lymphocytic infiltrate without necrosis
2	One focus only of "aggressive" lymphocytic infiltrate, focal myocyte injury, or both
3A	Multifocal aggressive infiltrates, myocyte damage, or both
3B	Diffuse lymphocytic infiltrate with myocyte necrosis
4	Diffuse, aggressive, polymorphous infiltrate with necrosis (with or without edema, hemorrhage, vasculitis)

Abbreviation: ISHLT, International Society for Heart and Lung Transplantation.[67]

[a] Biopsy graded by worst infiltrate noted on at least three to five specimens reviewed.

"necrosis" can be seen. Grade 1B refers to a more diffuse but generally sparse infiltrate, without cellular damage or necrosis. Grade 2 defines a more aggressive infiltrate, and there may be one focal area of myocyte damage. Grade 3A describes a multifocal and aggressive infiltrate, and grade 3B refers to a diffuse multifocal and aggressive process invariably accompanied by myocyte necrosis. Grade 4 rejection is a diffuse and aggressive polymorphous infiltrate associated with vasculitis, hemorrhage, and necrosis. Though on occasion an intense lymphocytic infiltrate is noted in subendocardial regions but without significant extension deeper into the myocardium, it is not indicative of cardiac allograft rejection. This finding has been given the name "Quilty pattern," after the first patient noted to have these findings.

Shortcomings of the ISHLT standardized endomyocardial biopsy grading scheme include a lack of correlation to physiologic events, such as reduced ejection fraction or symptomatic left ventricular systolic dysfunction; and the presence of "vascular rejection" is not accounted for. Immunofluorescence studies have been suggested as important for diagnosing humoral or vascular rejection. Humoral rejection is characterized by the presence of antibodies having specificity for donor HLA class II antigens, which are located on the cardiac allograft endothelium. Vascular rejection may occur more frequently in patients receiving antilymphocytic antibody therapy early as rejection prophylaxis. It has also been noted that this form of rejection is associated with decreased long-term survival and more severe subsequent allograft arteriopathy.

The Cardiac Transplant Research Database has been evaluated with respect to populations at risk for rejection.[38,44] A total of 918 rejection episodes (defined by treatment with immunosuppressive therapy augmentation) in 911 patients who had undergone primary heart transplant between January 1, 1990 and July 1, 1991 were analyzed.[38] During a mean follow-up of 8.1 months (range 0–18 months), 54 percent of the patients had one or more rejection episodes that were treated. The mean cumulative number of rejection episodes per patient was 0.8 at 3 months, 1.10 at 6 months, and 1.3 at 12 months after transplant. By univariate analysis, female donor hearts and the use of induction therapy (both $P < 0.01$) were associated with greater cumulative rejection frequency. By multivariate analysiss, younger donor age and female donor gender were indepen-

Table 53-10. Immunosuppressive Agents

Drug	Mechanism	Toxicity	↑[CYC]	↓[CYC]
Cyclosporine	IL-2 blocked	HTN Renal Neurotoxicity Hirsutism Tremor	Erythromycin Ketoconazole Diltiazem Cimetidine Ciprofloxacin Grapefruit	Dilantin Phenobarbital Rifampin Cholestyramine Tegritol
Steroids	Lymphocytolytic ↓Ab/Ag interaction	Increased glucose HTN Osteoporosis Cataracts		

Azathioprine	Purine antimetabolite	Leukopenia
		Pancreatitis
		Stomatitis
		Hepatic
			(Allopurinol
			  potentiates
			  toxicity)	

Methotrexate	Folate analog Inhibits purine synthesis	Leukopenia Hepatitis Stomatitis		
Tacrolimus	IL-2↓	HTN Renal Neurotoxicity GI		
Mycophenolate	Inhibits purine synthesis	GI		
OKT$_3$, ALG, ATG	Opsonizes lymphocytes	Fever ARDS CNS		

Abbreviations: IL, interleukin; Ab/Ag, antibody/antigen; HTN, hypertension; GI, gastrointestinal; ARDS, adult respiratory distress syndrome; CNS, central nervous system; [CYC], cyclosporine concentration

dent risk factors for earlier-appearing rejection. Utilizing a multiple variable prediction analysis, there was an 85 percent probability of rejection at 1 month for a 50-year-old female recipient with a female donor and a 50 percent likelihood of rejection for a 50-year-old man with a male donor. Importantly, more than 40 percent of patients were free of rejection episodes during the first year after transplant during this era of modern immunosuppression, but younger recipient age and female donors were more frequently associated with earlier onset rejection.

Table 53-10 summarizes the immunosuppressive agents most frequently used after heart transplantation.[54,56,74] Generally, patients are given high dose steroids during the peritransplant period with concomitant cyclosporine and azathioprine administration. Triple immunosuppressive therapeutic protocols are designed to prevent rejection and decrease the toxicity of individual drugs. Induction cytolytic therapy with antilymphocyte globulin, antithymocyte globulin, or OKT3 monoclonal antibody is used in some programs routinely and, generally, when renal insufficiency creates high risk situations for cyclosporine therapy. Methotrexate is sometimes used as add-on or substitute therapy for chronic, refractory rejection. Tacrolimus is similar in action to cyclosporine, but less is known about proper dosing in the heart transplant setting. The beneficial effects and toxicity of tacrolimus and cyclosporine appear similar. The newest commercially available immunosuppressive drug is mycophenolic acid,[74] which inhibits purine synthesis. Its major side effects include gastroenterologic toxicity, but the agent is seemingly well tolerated and effective in renal transplant patients.

It is important to know the drugs that can either increase or decrease the blood concentration of cyclosporine or enhance the toxicity of azathioprine. Because azathioprine is a purine antimetabolite, allopurinol substantially increases this drug's toxicity. Erythromycin, ketoconazole, diltiazem, cimetidine, ciprofloxacin, and significant daily grapefruit juice consumption increase cyclosporine blood levels. It might increase renal toxicity, but on the other hand diltiazem and ketoconazole have been used to lower the requisite dose of daily cyclosporine required to maintain therapeutic and clinically effective drug concentrations. Dilantin, phenobarbital, rifampin, tegritol, and cholestyramine reduce cyclosporine blood levels. Problematic side effects of cyclosporine include hypertension, nephrotoxicity, seizures, tremor, hirsutism, and gingival hyperplasia. Azathioprine can produce leukopenia (or even pancytopenia), pancreatitis, stomatitis, and cholestatic jaundice. Steroids increase glucose levels, contribute to

Table 53-11. Tailored Immunotherapy: Clinical Considerations When Considering Immunomodulating Techniques
Time since transplant
Early (≤3 months)
Late (>3 months)
Immunologic status at time of transplant
Recipient sex
Donor sex
Presence of panel-reactive antibodies
Positive donor-specific crossmatch
HLA mismatch status
Recipient age
Rejection history
Endomyocardial biopsy score
ISHLT score
Presence of "vascular rejection"
Hemodynamic observations
Clinical signs of rejection
Fever
Heart failure
Infection status
Presence of active viral, fungal, protozoal, bacterial infections
Donor/recipient CMV status
End-organ function
Renal function
Hepatic function
Posttransplant lymphoproliferative disease

Abbreviations: HLA, human leukocyte antigen; ISHLT, International Society of Heart and Lung Transplantation; CMV, cytomegalovirus.

hypertension, and can adversely affect osteoporosis and cataract formation.

Though it is intuitive that tailored immunotherapy (Table 53-11) might be the best approach in patients after heart transplant, it is usually not the strategy taken. Rather, standard immunotherapeutic protocols are generally followed, with individuals treated according to "cookbook" algorithms driven by the endomyocardial biopsy score. It is important to consider other issues, however, such as the length of time since transplant, when considering treatment strategies. The hazard of rejection, for example, is vastly greater during the first 3 months after transplant than subsequently.[38] It makes sense to treat rejection more aggressively during the early postoperative period. Also, the immunologic status of the recipient at the time of transplant might bear on the need for more aggressive rejection prophylaxis or treatment. Recipient sex, donor sex, presence of panel reactive antibodies prior to transplantation, a positive donor lymphocyte specific crossmatch, and HLA mismatch status may dictate more or less aggressive treatment of biopsy-identified myocardial infiltrates. The rejection history is important as well. Certainly rejection in the face of hemodynamic compromise or clinical signs of ventricular dysfunction indicates more aggressive myocyte injury and portends a worse prognosis. The presence of active infection or posttransplant lymphoproliferative disorder might temper enthusiasm for an aggressive immunotherapeutic prescription.

Table 53-12 outlines a few strategies for addressing rejection. It should be emphasized that these therapeutic recommendations are simply guides, and individualization of treatment is mandatory if optimum long-term heart transplant results are to be seen. The most common ad hoc adjunctive immunotherapeutic protocols are short pulses of oral prednisone therapy (100 mg for three consecutive days) or parenteral methylprednisolone (1 g for 3 days). Cytolytic therapy with monoclonal anti-CD3 lymphocyte antibody (OKT3) or antithymocyte (ATG) or antilymphocyte (ALG) globulin is usually reserved for substantive refractory rejection episodes or episodes associated with hemodynamic compromise. Whenever any decision is made regarding rejection therapy, the toxicities of chronically administered drugs and optimization of triple drug therapeutic protocols become critical. Appropriate drug dosages are mandatory and consideration of each drug's potential toxicity necessary. Reasonable therapeutic levels have been defined for cyclosporine and tacrolimus that identify safe, clinically effective dosages.

Because of the risk, expense, and limitations of endomyocardial biopsy, noninvasive surveillance techniques have been pursued as surrogate markers of rejection. Several serologic markers of immune system activation and many imaging procedures evaluating myocardial perfusion or function give some insight into the course of rejection.[43] Serologic markers generally focus on the dynamics of inflammatory reactions, and myocardial function measurements are directed at detecting and quantifying the damaging effects of myocardial inflammation. However, all noninvasive techniques have limitations, and none has withstood the test of time or had the global expe-

Table 53-12. Treating Rejection

ISHLT Grade	Patient status	Treatment	
		Early (≤3 months)	Late (>3 months)
0	Stable	No changes	Consider↑ immunosuppression
IA	Stable	No changes	Adjust dose for toxicity
IB	Stable	No changes	Adjust dose for toxicity
II	Stable	No changes	Adjust dose for toxicity
	↑CVP; ↑PCWP; ↓EF; arrhythmias; or clinical signs	Increase dose of immunosuppressive to optimal levels Consider prednisone 100 mg PO × 3 days	
IIIA	Stable	Increase dose of immunosuppressive to optimal levels Prednisone 100 mg PO × 3 days	
	↑CVP; ↑PCWP; ↓EF; arrhythmias; or chemical signs	Methylprednisolone 1 g IV × 3 days Increase dose of immunosuppressive to optimal levels	
IIIB	Stable	Methylprednisolone, 1 g IV × 3 days Optimize immunosuppressive doses	Prednisone, 100 mg × 3 days
	↑CVP; ↑PCWP; ↓EF; arrhythmias; or clinical signs	Optimize immunosuppressive doses ALG, ATG, or OKT3 × 7–10 days	Methylprednisolone 1 g IV × 3 days
IV	Irrespective of findings	ALG, ATG, or OKT3 × 7–10 days	

Abbreviations: CVP, central venous pressure; PCWP, pulmonary capillary wedge pressure; EF, ejection fraction; IV, intravenous. See text for other abbreviations.

rience required to completely replace endomyocardial biopsy. Perhaps serial echocardiographic evaluation of patients and, in particular, assessment of left ventricular diastolic function using Doppler studies give the greatest insight into the dynamics of rejection. In reality, the most important information gleaned from serial rejection surveillance methods that focus on serologic measurements (including interleukins, circulating lymphocyte subsets, leukokine-activated leukocytes, and intracellular adhesion molecules) is the ability to delineate the long-term prognosis to some degree. Generally, markers of cellular inflammation that are increased chronically portend a worse prognosis. A variety of interleukins (ILs), such as soluble IL-2 receptor and intercellular adhesion molecules, have been related to long-term prognosis, but their use for the diagnosis of rejection is limited.

Infections

Infections, defined as significant episodes generally treated with intravenous antimicrobial therapy, were analyzed in the Cardiac Transplant Research Database.[74] An incidence of 0.5 infection per patient was observed during the follow-up period, which averaged 8.4 months after transplant. Despite the fact that 67 percent of patients were free from infection during this interval, 21 percent had one and 11 percent had more than one significant infection. Two peak periods for infection were identified. During the first 30 postoperative days nosocomial infections are prominent and seemingly related to indwelling catheters and drainage tubes. *Staphylococcus* species and gram-negative organisms are most frequent during this early period, in contrast to the second peak infection period (2–6 months postoperatively) when opportunistic infection such as cytomegalovirus, *Pneumocystis*, and fungi were more frequently noted. Toxoplasmosis was found within the first 20 days but more often developed approximately 3 months after transplant. There were few independent risk factors for infection following cardiac transplantation in this analysis, with the exception of mechanical ventilation at the time of transplant. All patients were at significant risk of infection because of the requirement for multiple aggressive immunotherapeutic protocols. In terms of serious infection, the lung has been the most common site, followed by blood, urine, and the gastrointestinal tract. Sternal wound infections are particularly problematic and account for 25 percent of the deaths due to infection overall. Fortunately, this difficulty occurred in only 7 percent of patients in this series. Induction cytolytic therapy was more frequently associated with significant subsequent viral infection, particularly cytomegalovirus.

Allograft Arteriopathy

Coronary artery disease developing de novo in a transplanted heart has sometimes been referred to as chronic rejection.[56,57] This form of coronary atherosclerosis is the leading cause of death after cardiac transplantation during long follow-up periods. After 5 years there appears to be an incidence of allograft arteriopathy ranging between 30 and 50 percent. Though annual coronary angiography has been the traditional method of diagnosing the problem, it is an insensitive approach.[70] Intravascular ultrasonography has been investigated and seems to be a promising, sensitive technique. Unfortunately, observation with routine annual intravascular ultrasonographic studies has proved frightening with respect to the high incidence and diffuseness of this difficulty. This procedure allows not only assessment of the luminal diameter but also a precise description of the appearance of the intima and media. Doppler flow probes can be inserted into the transplanted heart's coronary artery and the coronary flow reserve calculated, which is related to allograft arteriopathy. As might be anticipated, the histologic appearance of allograft arteriopathy is distinct from coronary artery disease in the nontransplant population. Diffuse, symmetric hyperplasia of smooth muscle cells and macrophages that have migrated into the expanded intima cause concentric rather than eccentric vessel involvement. Great lengths of the vessel are diseased. Although atheromatous plaque can be noted in the epicardial arteries of transplanted hearts, they are usually minimally calcified, are far more cellular, and contain an extraordinarily high quantity of cholesterol than native coronary artery disease lesions. Additonally, ulceration and thrombus formation are unusual in heart transplant patients until late in the disease.[71]

Allograft arteriopathy likely is a primary immune-mediated process enhanced by other co-morbid states, such as dyslipidemia, hypertension, and viral infection. Evidence supporting this hypothesis includes the fact that there is selective involvement of the allograft vascular bed with other native vessels being spared, the diffuse and concentric involvement of the entire coronary circulation including veins, and its occurrence in all age groups as well as the young posttransplant patient. The presence of measurable circulating HLA antibodies and immunohistochemical stains suggesting "vascular" rejection seem to portend significant subsequent allograft arteriopathy. Other risk factors for allograft arteriopathy include HLA mismatch (particularly at the DR locus), hypertriglyceridemia, obesity, and cytomegalovirus infection.[34] Inflammatory endothelial cell injury caused by the rejection process likely promotes regulator gene expression, which in the face of certain cytokines and growth factors stimulates smooth muscle cell proliferation, macrophage deposition, and atherosclerosis. Treatment of the difficulty is limited and generally revolves around the intensification of immunotherapy to reduce any inflammatory component of the process. Control of traditional atherosclerotic cardiovascular disease risk factors such as hypertension and dyslipidemia is likely also important. There has been some suggestion that routine prescription of diltiazem and pravastatin are protective. Newer immunotherapeutic agents, which inhibit smooth muscle cell proliferation and migration as well as being immunosuppressive (e.g., rapamycin and mycophenolic acid), may prove more protective. Other agents, such as low-molecular-weight heparin and the somatostatin analog angiopeptin (which inhibits insulin-like growth factor), are intriguing.

Malignancy

Malignant neoplasms after cardiac transplantation can present significant difficulty and, as after all solid-organ transplantation, are likely related to the intensity of immunosuppressive therapy. The predominant tumor associated with cyclosporine-based immunosuppression is the so-called posttransplant lymphoproliferative disorder, a non-Hodgkin's lymphoma. More than three-fourths of the cases are B cell subtypes, and unfortunately clonal analysis of immunoglobulin production does not predict subsequent therapeutic response. Many monoclonal tumors have regressed with a reduction in immunotherapy. Epstein-Barr virus may play a role in these malignancies, as genome footprints of this virus have been demonstrated by monoclonal antibody fluorescent staining techniques within the B cell proliferations. Primary infection with Epstein-Barr virus results in higher mortality. A controversial observation has been that the use of cytolytic therapy, particularly OKT3, in heart transplant recipients predisposes to these lymphoproliferative disorders.[54,56] Multiple variable analyses performed on more than 30 risk factors suggested that the use of more than 75 mg of OKT3 over 6 months is an independent predictor of the development of posttransplant lymphoproliferative disorder. Obviously, any patient receiving substantive immunosuppressive therapy is at risk of developing a malignancy. Patients with a history of malignant disorders should have these difficulties thoroughly excluded prior to transplant to eliminate the possibility of disease recurrence. Sun exposure in the setting of cyclosporine and azathioprine administration elicits a substantial increase in the incidence of both benign and malignant skin neoplasms.

Hypertension

Hypertension is a challenging complication of cardiac transplantation; and because allograft arteriopathy is a major difficulty after transplant, a great deal of attention is directed toward its control.[34] Obviously, many patients undergoing cardiac transplantation have preexistent hypertension, as coronary artery disease is a substantial cause of heart failure. Hypertension and coronary heart disease are obviously intimately linked. Data suggest that as many as 75 percent of patients treated with immunosuppressive protocols that include cyclosporine and prednisone become hypertensive. Because cyclosporine is nephrotoxic renal-based blood pressure elevation is likely. Furthermore, enervation of the heart abolishes normal diurnal variation of blood pressure, and it has been demonstrated that nocturnal hypertension is particularly linked to ventricular hypertrophy. Transient acute renal failure occurring within days or weeks of transplantation can contribute to fluid and solute retention, further worsening hypertension. Blood pressure can also be affected by more chronic renal insufficiency characterized by serum creatinine elevation, which sometimes persists for several weeks or even months after transplant. It does not appear that heart transplant patients are more or less likely than liver transplant or lung transplant recipients to develop renal insufficiency and failure related to cyclosporine therapy; and blood pressure control is sometimes difficult in these individuals.

Dyslipidemia

As many as 80 percent of heart transplant patients treated with triple drug immunosuppressive therapy protocols based on cyclosporine develop lipid abnormalities.[77–79] This point is particularly troublesome in view of the fact that elevated triglyceride levels and total cholesterol have been associated with accelerated allograft arteriopathy. The connection between dyslipidemia and native vessel atherosclerosis is obvious. Guidelines for lipid-lowering drug therapy originally formulated to optimize benefits of treatment while minimizing risks of therapy in nontransplant dyslipidemic populations do not address specific treatment needs of patients after transplantation. Compared to patients with native vessel coronary artery disease, the risk and benefits of lipid-lowering therapy remain incompletely defined. Concern with lipid-lowering drugs arose after initial reports detailed rhabdomyolysis in patients on high doses of statins in the face of cyclosporine therapy.[78] Subsequently, several studies have used lovastatin, simvastatin, or pravastatin and suggested that the overall incidence of rhabdomyolysis was, at best, only about 1 percent when low dose therapeutic routines were used. Importantly, one prospective randomized, nonblinded, single center clinical trial investigated the effects of pravastatin on patient outcomes after surgery.[80] As mentioned above, starting this drug within 2 weeks of the transplant produced a reduction in overall mortality and lower incidence of transplant arteriopathy as quantified by angiography and intracoronary ultrasonography at the 1-year anniversary cardiac catheterization. Indeed, pravastatin was even suggested to have an immunosuppressive effect, as rejection episodes were also diminished. This observation led some investigators to prescribed lipid-lowering drugs routinely after heart transplantation. More clinical trials are necessary to completely delineate the risks and benefits of this approach.

Future Developments in Cardiac Transplantation

Several new immunosuppressive drugs are being evaluated in solid-organ transplant recipients.[74] Limited information is available regarding the use of cyclosporine analogs in heart transplant recipients, although preliminary trials suggest that cyclosporines A and G have rejection rates that are similar but fewer renal and systemic complications.

Tacrolimus is a newly available macrolide antibiotic similar in action to cyclosporine (inhibiting the production of IL-2 and other lymphokines as well as preventing IL-2 receptor expression). It is seemingly associated with a lower incidence of hypertension, gingival hyperplasia, and hirsutism than cyclosporine.

Rapamycin is a macrolide antibiotic that decreases IL-2-driven T cell proliferation but not IL-2 production. Rapamycin can cause nephrotoxicity, hepatotoxicity, and glucose intolerance; but its toxicity overall may be lower than that of cyclosporine. This drug is currently being used in clinical trials after heart transplant.

Mycophenolate mofetil is an ester of mycophenolic acid and has been approved for use in kidney transplant recipients. It inhibits inosine monophosphate dehydrogenase in the guanine nucleotide synthesis pathway. Importantly, both rapamycin and mycophenolate mofetil inhibit smooth muscle cell growth and therefore might be beneficial by limiting allograft arteriopathy in addition to having effects on cell-mediated immunity.

Monoclonal antibodies are being pursued that lack the toxicity and nonspecificity of currently available preparations. Antibodies reacting with the TCR/CD3 complex and the CD4 molecule are being evaluated. Furthermore, monoclonal antibodies reacting with adhesion molecules and lymphokines, as well as antibodies reacting with antigen-presenting cells, may eventually prove valuable in cardiac transplant recipients.

Several immunosuppressive procedures are being evaluated, including total lymphoid irradiation. This maneuver may induce specific allograft tolerance when combined with immunosuppressive drug administration, but the timing and dose of the irradiation is not well characterized. Apheresis procedures are more common with improved machinery to effect fluid and cell separation. Therapeutic plasma exchange, nonspecific global antibody adsorption with staphylococcal protein A, and selective immunoadsorption have been studied, though incompletely, in cardiac transplant recipient populations. Even more recently, chemoinactivation photophoresis has piqued interest. This technique uses ex vivo ultraviolet A light inactivation of mononuclear cells obtained by leukopheresis after injection of 8-methoxypsoralen. The photomanipulated mononuclear cells are reinfused, and the mononuclear cell-bound psoralen seems to enhance suppressor T cell mechanisms by altering antigen presentation or cytokine expression kinetics.

LEFT VENTRICULAR ASSIST DEVICE FOR ADVANCED HEART FAILURE

Because of the disparity between the number of patients awaiting heart transplantation and donor organ availability, aggressive attempts to support the circulation mechanically have been used for years. Enthusiasm for permanent total artificial heart implantation as a bridge to heart transplantation rapidly abated when clinical outcomes after these procedures did not meet the unrealistically high expectations that had emerged. Bridging to heart transplant with left ventricular assist devices has, however, been more successful and better accepted. The combined registry for the clinical use of mechanical ventricular assist pumps and the total artificial heart, in conjunction with heart transplantation, now has more than 2000 patients in its database, covering the period 1985 through January 1994.[30] A total of 484 ventricular assist devices or total artificial hearts have been included. Between 1985 and 1988 a rather substantial increase in the number of implants inserted to "bridge" to transplant were undertaken, with about half of the implants in 1988 being total artificial heart devices. In contrast, for 1992 and 1993 no artificial hearts were included in this database! Nearly 70 percent of patients having ventricular assist devices or total artificial hearts subsequently underwent heart transplant, with 69 percent surviving to hospital discharge. Outcome statistics suggest that isolated left ventricular support systems are more successful than right or biventricular assistance and the total artificial heart. Within the grouping of left ventricular assist devices, no individual mode of support proved advantageous over others for transplantation or discharge rates. The 30-day mortality for all devices was approximately 36 percent and remains higher than that for orthotopic cardiac transplantation at similar time points of follow-up. Obviously, organ availability for these patients was limited. Isolated left ventricular support, however, had a 30-day mortality of only 9 percent, with similar improvement of 12- and 24-month survival.

Table 53-13 summarizes the number of mechanical ventricular assist devices employed as a bridge to transplantation in the ISHLT database, demonstrating that most patients, to date, have been supported for only short periods.[30] Still, it is important to note that several individuals remained on devices for periods approaching 1 year. Centrifugal support systems can be utilized for only short-term periods. Thromboembolism is commonplace when these devices are left in place longer than 2–3 weeks. Complications of left ventricular assist device insertion include significant bleeding or intravascular coagulopathy (43 percent of patients), infection (29 percent), renal insufficiency (23 percent), and thrombus or emboli (17 percent). Permanent implantation, without intention to "bridge" to transplant, of certain devices (e.g., the HeartMate vented electric system) is beginning to occur. As insight is gained into adverse events including infection, emboli, right ventricular dysfunction, and sustained ventricular arrhythmias after device insertion, solutions will emerge. Though existing left ventricular assist devices are appropriate therapy for patients dying of end-stage heart disease, many challenges exist; and unrealistic expectations should be avoided. Continued success with staged cardiac transplantation is anticipated, and prudent use of these devices will expand our end-stage heart failure treatment armamentarium.[32,34,81-83]

DYNAMIC CARDIOMYOPLASTY

Dynamic cardiomyoplasty is a much discussed operation, with a great deal of interest generated by several lay readership publications. The operation has been performed for more than a decade.[84-86] The procedure is theoretically designed to boost left ventricular systolic and diastolic function by wrapping, circumferentially, the left or right latissimus dorsi muscle around the heart. The muscle is dissected out from the posterior thorax and rotated carefully from

Table 53-13. Mechanical Ventricular Assist Devices as a "Bridge" to Transplantation

Support Type	n	Days Wait Mean ± SEM (range)	Transplanted n (%)	Discharged n (%)
LVAD	187	44 ± 5 (0–370)	138 (74)	125 (91)
CENT	23	8 ± 2 (1–29)	17 (74)	13 (77)
ELECT	76	46 ± 7 (0–370)	51 (67)	47 (92)
PNEUM	88	51 ± 7 (0–344)	70 (80)	65 (93)
RVAD	5	20 ± 17 (0–72)	2 (40)	0
BVAD	164	17 ± 2 (0–162)	113 (69)	77 (68)
TAH	191	23 ± 4 (0–438)	135 (71)	66 (49)
"Hybrid" BVAD	37	na	12 (32)	6 (50)
Total	584	na	400 (69)	274 (69)

Abbreviations: L, left; R, right; B, biventricular; VAD, ventricular assist device; TAH, total artificial heart; na, not available.
Combined registry for use of mechanical ventricular assist devices and the total artificial heart as bridge to transplant (ISHLT)[30]

the normal anatomic position into the chest, with great attention to preservation of the neurovascular pedicle. Critical to the success of this procedure is conversion of skeletal muscle performance from fatigable to fatigue-resistant myocytes with appropriate repetitive electrical pacemaker stimulation. Skeletal muscle is accustomed to working intermittently rather than continuously (as the heart does), and fatigability must be overcome if the contractile power of the latissimus dorsi shortening is to be translated into clinical benefit. The major breakthrough leading to increased interest in dynamic cardiomyoplasty was the demonstration that pulsed and entrained electrical stimulation of the skeletal muscle in regular fashion induced a more fatigue-resistant muscle. A cardiomyostimulating device has been developed (Cardiostim; Medtronic) and senses the R wave of the QRS complex, subsequently triggering latissimus dorsi contraction via a synchronized circuit. Because direct stimulation of skeletal muscle fibers requires high energy to induce contraction and might lead to tissue damage, an intramuscular electrode is woven through the latissimus dorsi muscle near the main nerve branch to deliver the stimulation impulse. This pacing system is then coupled to a sensing lead attached to the patient's left ventricle. Once conditioning of the muscle occurs, augmented contractility theoretically improves systolic performance. Diastolic buttressing of the ventricles by the muscle wrap also might induce favorable diastolic properties. It has been termed the girdling effect. Theoretically, cardiomyoplasty contributes to symptomatic improvement in heart failure patients with attenuation of many hemodynamic and circulatory abnormalities characteristic of heart failure.

It has been estimated that approximately 600 cardiomyoplasty procedures have been performed worldwide. A formal study of the Medtronic Cardiostem device in patients with heart failure is now ongoing and has enrolled well over 125 patients from 14 centers in Europe and America. In the Phase I feasibility study (performed between July 1985 and April 1991) the operation was suggested to be safe and the surgical procedure reproducible at multiple clinical sites. Importantly, dynamic cardiomyoplasty was noted to be less risky for patients in NYHA class III heart failure than those in class IV heart failure, where operative mortality exceeds 20 to 30 percent. Also this pilot study suggested that dynamic cardiomyoplasty improved the functional status of patients by approximately 80 percent irrespective of preoperative heart failure severity.

A Phase II clinical trial began in May 1991, concluding in the summer of 1994. A total of 360 Phase I and Phase II patients were enrolled by April 1993,

and procedure-related deaths (deaths occurring during the initial cardiomyoplasty procedure hospitalization) were noted in 36 percent of patients with NYHA class IV heart failure, in contrast to 16 percent of the class II patients. The overall rate of procedure-related deaths was 10 percent for Phase II patients entering the study after a center had completed 10 procedures. Survival at 2 years for NYHA class III patients was approximately 60 percent and about 40 percent for NYHA class IV patients. Of note is that comparable figures are often seen with medical therapy, raising some doubt about the value of this procedure. Deaths were generally cardiac-related (approximately 80 percent) and divided equally between worsening heart failure and suspected terminal arrhythmic events. Surviving patients generally demonstrated an improvement in exercise capacity and hemodynamics, with daily activity scores rising rather dramatically compared to a patient's preoperative evaluation. A retrospective analysis of factors associated with procedure-related mortality suggested that the risk associated with a low ejection fraction was not as great if the patient's peak VO_2 was higher. Likewise, a low peak VO_2 predicted less risk if the ejection fraction was higher. This experience shaped patient entry criteria for subsequent clinical trials evaluating this procedure and suggested that study inclusion be focused on adult heart failure patients with dilated cardiomyopathy or ischemic heart disease manifesting reduced exercise capacity but having peak VO_2 greater than 10 $ml \cdot kg^{-1} \cdot min^{-1}$. Additionally, an intact latissimus dorsi muscle with reasonable overall body muscle mass was critical. Additional factors making the operation unduly risky include pulmonary hypertension, poor pulmonary function studies with obstructive pulmonary disease, severe biventricular failure, preoperative dependence on intravenous inotropic medications, and intractable NYHA functional class IV heart failure symptomatology. Older age, prior sternotomy or thoracotomy, massive cardiomegaly, need for concomitant cardiac surgery, atrial fibrillation, low right ventricular ejection fraction, severe mitral regurgitation, and malignant arrhythmias (including those treated with implantable defibrillating devices) also predicted poor outcome and could be considered relative contraindications.

To place cardiomyoplasty into the perspective of clinical heart failure management strategies more definitively, a randomized clinical trial has been instituted in which outcomes after this procedure are being compared to aggressive medical management. NYHA class IV heart failure patients are excluded from this trial. Total mortality, exercise endpoints, quality of life scores, and congestive heart failure symptomatology are being evaluated. It is hoped that this objective, carefully performed clinical trial will better define the impact of this operation and help determine the characteristics of patients most likely to benefit from the procedure. Though the hypothesis of improved native heart energetics and function after dynamic cardiomyoplasty are intuitive and attractive, further clinical study is necessary.

CONCLUSION

The options of heart transplantation, mechanical ventricular assist device implantation, and cardiomyoplasty substantially broaden the advanced heart failure treatment spectrum. Performing the procedures clearly are effective in appropriately selected individuals, whereas the value of cardiomyoplasty does have contraindications. Realistic expectations must be delineated in order to utilize the described technology most appropriately.

REFERENCES

1. Ezekiel 36:26. p. 1283. In Ryrie CC (ed): The Ryrie Study Bible. Moody Press, Chicago, 1978
2. Kahan BD: Pien Chiao, the legendary exchange of hearts, traditional Chinese medicine, and the modern era of cyclosporine. Transplant Proc, suppl. 2 1988;20: 2–25
3. Cavendish R: Mythology. An Illustrated Encyclopedia. Razzoli Press, New York, 1980
4. Rehn L: Ueber peritrirende Herzwunden und Hertznaht. Arch Klin Chir 1897;55:315–320
5. Malinin TI: Remembering Alexis Carrel and Charles A. Lindbergh. Tex Heart Inst 1996;23:28–35
6. Carrel A, Guthrie CC: The transplantation of veins and organs. Am Med 1905;10:1101–1106
7. Mann FC, Priestley JT, Markowitz J et al: Transplantation of the infarct native heart. Arch Surg 1933;26: 219–28
8. Gnudi MT, Webster JP: The life and times of Gaspare Taglioccozzi; surgeon of Bollognese. Classics of Medicine Library, Birmingham, Al, 1989
9. Carpue JC: An account of two successful operations for restoring a lost nose from the integuments of the forehead. Classics of Medicine Library, Birmingham, Al, 1981
10. Silverstein AM: A History of Immunology. Academic Press, Harcourt, Brace, Jovanovich, New York, 1989
11. Cooley DA: A brief history of heart transplants and mechanical assist devices. pp. 5–15. In Frazier OH, Macris M, Radovancevic B (eds): Support and Replacement of the Failing Heart. Lippincott-Raven, Philadelphia, 1996
12. Cooper DKC: Orthotopic and heterotopic heart transplantation. Experimental development and early clinical experience. pp. 3–10. In Cooper DKC, Novitzky D (eds): The Transplantation and Replacement of Thoracic Organs. Kluwer, Boston, 1990
13. Hardy JD, Chanez CM, Kurras FE et al: Heart transplantation in man. Developmental studies and report of a case. JAMA 1964;188:1132–1137
14. Barnard CH: A human cardiac transplant. An interim report of a successful operation performed at Groote Schurr Hospital, Capetown. S Afr Med J 1967;41: 1271–1278
15. Arnold RM, Youngner SJ (eds): Special issue. Ethical, psychosocial, and public policy implications of procuring organs from non-heart beating cadavers. Kennedy Inst Ethics J 1993;3:103–278
16. Kantrowitz A, Haller JD, Joos H et al: Transplantation of the heart in an infant and an adult. Am J Cardiol 1968;22:782–790
17. Fox RC, Swazey JP: The Courage to Fail. A Social View of Organ Transplants and Dialysis. University of Chicago Press, Chicago, 1974
18. Fox RC, Swazey JP: Spare Parts. Organ Replacement in American Society. Oxford University Press, Oxford, 1992
19. Caves PK, Stinson EB, Graham AF et al: Percutaneous transvenous endomyocardial biopsy. JAMA 1973;225: 228–231
20. Evans RW, Manninen DL, Dong FB: The National Heart Transplantation Study: Final Report. Battelle Human Affairs Research Centers, Seattle, WA, 1991
21. Evans RW, Manninen DL, Garrison LP Jr et al: Donor availability as the primary determinant of the future of heart transplantation. JAMA 1986;255:1892
22. Shumakov VI: Iskusstvennoje Serdee. Izd Znanie, Moscow, 1975
23. Gibbon JH: The application of a mechanical heart and lung apparatus to cardiac surgery. Minn Med 1954; 37:171–176
24. Mouloopoulos SD, Topaz SR, Kolff WS: Extracorporeal assistance to the circulation and intraaortic balloon pumping. Trans Am Soc Artif Intern Organs 1962;8: 86–92
25. Kantrowitz A, Tjonneland S, Freed et al: Initial experience with intraaortic balloon pumping in cardiogenic shock. JAMA 1968;203:113–120
26. DeBakey ME, Liotta D, Hall CW: Left heart bypass using an implantable blood pump. pp. 223–233. In: Mechanical Devices to Assist the Failing Heart. Proceedings of a Conference Sponsored by the Committee in Trauma, September 1964. National Academy of Sciences–National Research Council, Washington, DC, 1966
27. Debakey ME: Left ventricular bypass pump for cardiac assistance. Clinical experience. Am J Cardiol 1971;27: 3–10
28. Akutsu T, Kolff WJ: Permanent substitutes for valves and heart. Trans Am Soc Artif Intern Organs 1958;4: 230–235
29. DeVries WC, Anderson JL, Joyce LD et al: Clinical use of the total artificial heart. N Engl J Med 1984;310: 273–280
30. Mehta SM, Avfiero TX, Pae WE et al: Combined registry for the clinical use of mechanical ventricular assist pumps and the total artificial heart in conjunction with heart transplantation. Sixth official report— 1994. J Heart Lung Transplant 1995;14:585–93
31. Frazier OH, Short HD, Wampler RK et al: Mechanical circulation support in the transplant patient. pp.

147–167. In Frazier OH, Macris M, Radovancevic B (eds): Support and Replacement of the Failing Heart. Lippincott-Raven, Philadelphia, 1996

32. McCarthy PM: HeartMate implantable left ventricular assist device. Bridge to transplantation and future applications. Ann Thorac Surg, suppl. 2 1995;59:46–51

33. McCarthy PM, Sabik J: Implantable circulatory support devices as a bridge to heart transplantation. Semin Thorac Surg 1991;6:174–80

34. McCarthy PM, James KB, Savage RM et al: Implantable left ventricular assist device. Approaching an alternative for end-stage heart failure. Circulation, suppl. II 1994;90:83–86

35. Hosenpud JD, Novick RJ, Breen TJ et al: The Registry of the International Society for Heart and Lung Transplantation. Twelfth official report—1994. J Heart Lung Transplant 1994;13:561–570

36. 1995 Annual Report of the US Scientific Registry of Transplant Recipients and the Organ Procurement and Transplantation Network—Transplant Data: 1988–1995. UNOS, Richmond, and the Division of Organ Transplantation, Bureau of Health Resources Development, Health Resources and Services Administration, US Department of Health and Human Services, Bethesda, 1995

37. Bourge RC, Naftel DC, Costanzo-Nordin MR et al: Pre-transplantation risk factors for death after heart transplantation. A multi-institutional study. J Heart Lung Transplant 1993;12:549

38. Kobashigawa JA, Kirklin JK, Naftel DC et al: Pre-transplantation risk factors for acute rejection after heart transplantation. A multi-institutional study. J Heart Lung Transplant 1993;12:355–366

39. Young JB, Naftel DC, Bourge RC et al: Matching the heart donor and heart transplant recipient. Clues for successful expansion of the donor pull. A multivariable, multi-institutional report. J Heart Lung Transplant 1994;13:353–65

40. UNOS Update 1995;11:54–55

41. O'Connell JB, Bourge RC, Costanzo-Nordin MR et al: Cardiac transplantation. Recipient selection, donor procurement, and medical follow-up. A statement for health professionals from the Committee on Cardiac Transplantation of the Council on Clinical Cardiology, American Heart Association. Circulation 1992;86:1061–1079

42. Baldwin JC, Anderson JL, Boucek MM et al: Task Force 2 (Bethesda conference—cardiac transplantation). Donor guidelines. J Am Coll Cardiol 1993;22:15

43. Costanzo MR, Augustine S, Bourge R et al: Selection and treatment of candidates for heart transplantation. A statement for health professionals from the Committee on Heart Failure and Cardiac Transplantation of the Council on Clinical Cardiology, American Heart Association. Circulation 1995;92:3593–3612

44. Jarcho J, Naftel DC, Shroyer TW et al: Influence of HLA mismatch on rejection after heart transplantation. A multiinstitutional study. J Heart Lung Transplant 1994;13:583–596

45. Pollack MS, Ballantyne CM, Payton-Ross C et al: HLA match and other immunological parameters in relation to survival, rejection severity, and accelerated coronary artery disease after heart transplant. Clin Transplant 1990;4:269

46. Stinson EB, Dong E, Schroeder J et al: Initial clinical experience with heart transplantation. Am J Cardiol 1968;22:791–803

47. Cresci S, Goldstein JA, Hiram C et al: Impaired left atrial function after heart transplantation. Disparate contribution of donor and recipient atrial components studied on-line with quantitative echocardiography. J Heart Lung Transplant 1995;14:647–653

48. Young JB, Winters WL Jr, Bourge R et al: Task Force 4 (Bethesda conference—heart transplantation). Function of the heart transplantation recipient. J Am Coll Cardiol 1993;22:31

49. Raghavan C, Maloney JD, Nitta J et al: Long-term follow-up of heart transplant recipients requiring permanent pacemakers. Transplant 1995;14:1081–1089

50. Leyh RG, Jahnke AW, Kraatz EG et al: Cardiovascular dynamics and dimensions after bicaval and standard cardiac transplantation. Ann Thorac Surg 1995;59:1495–1500

51. Desruennes M, Muneretto C, Gandjbakheh I et al: Heterotopic heart transplantation. Current status in 1988. J Heart Transplant 1989;8:479

52. Kotliar CD, Smart FW, Sekela ME et al: Heterotopic heart transplantation and native heart ventricular arrhythmias. Ann Thorac Surg 1991;51:987–991

53. Mudge GH, Goldstein S, Addonizio LJ et al: Twenty-fourth Bethesda conference: cardiac transplantation. Task Force 3. Recipient guidelines/prioritization. J Am Coll Cardiol 1993;22:21–31

54. Young JB: Contemporary management of patients with heart failure. Med Clin North Am 1995;79:1171–1190

55. Heart Failure. Evaluation and Care of Patients with Left-Ventricular Systolic Dysfunction. Clinical Practice Guideline. AHCPR publication 94–0612. Rockville, MD: US Dept of Health and Human Services, 1994

56. Miller LW: Long-term complications of cardiac transplantation. Prog Cardiovasc Dis 1991;32:229

57. Miller LW, Schlant RC, Kosbashigawa J et al: Task Force 5 (Bethesda conference—cardiac transplantation). Complications. J Am Coll Cardiol 1993;22:41

58. St. Goar FG, Gibbons R, Schnittger I et al: Left ventricular diastolic function. Doppler echocardiographic changes soon after cardiac transplantation. Circulation 1990;82:872–878

59. Stevenson LW, Sietsema K, Tillisch JH et al: Exercise capacity for survivors of cardiac transplantation or sustained medical therapy for heart failure. Circulation 1990;81:78–85

60. Schruder JJ, Vander Veen FH, Vander Velde ET et al: Beat to beat analysis of left ventricular pressure volume relation and stroke volume by conductance catheter and aortic model flow in cardiomyoplasty patients. Circulation 1995;91:2010–2017

61. Young JB, Leon CA, Short HD III et al: Evolution of hemodynamics after orthotopic heart and heart/lung transplantation. Early restrictive patterns persisting in occult fashion. J Heart Transplant 1987;6:34–43

62. Hosenpud JD, Pantely GA, Morton MJ et al: Relationship between recipient-donor body size matching and hemodynamics three months following cardiac transplantation. J Heart Transplant 1989;8:241–243

63. Gilmore JP, Daggett WN: Response of the chronic cardiac denervated dog to acute volume expansion. Am J Physiol 1966;210:509–512

64. Glazier JJ, Mullen GM, Johnson MR et al: Factors

associated with the development of persistently depressed cardiac output during the first year after cardiac transplantation. Clin Cardiol 1994;17:489–494

65. Parent R, Stanley P, Chartrand C: Long-term daily study of blood volume in cardiac auto-transplanted dogs. Eur Surg Res 1987;19:193–199

66. Scherrer U, Vissing SF, Morgan BJ et al: Cyclosporine induced sympathetic activation and hypertension after heart transplantation. N Engl J Med 1990;323: 693–699

67. Billingham ME, Cary NR, Hammond EH et al: A working foundation for the standardization of nomenclature in the diagnosis of heart and lung rejection. Heart Rejection Study Group. J Heart Transplant 1990;9: 587

68. Hammond EH, Yowell R, Nuwoda S et al: Vascular (humoral) rejection in heart transplantation. Pathologic observations and clinical implications. J Heart Transplant 1989;8:430

69. Hammond EH, Yowell RL, Price GD et al: Vascular rejection and its relationship to allograft coronary artery disease. J Heart Lung Transplant 1992;11:511

70. Miller LW, Wolford TL, Donohue TJ et al: Cardiac allograft vasculopathy. New insights from intravascular ultrasound and coronary flow measurements. Transplant Rev 1995;9:77–96

71. Johnson DE, Gao SZ, Schroeder JS et al: The spectrum of coronary artery pathologic findings in human cardiac allografts. J Heart Transplant 1989;8:349

72. Johnson MR: Transplant coronary disease. Non-immunologic risk factors. J Heart Lung Transplant 1992; 11:S124

73. Mills RM, Young JB: Evaluation for cardiac transplantation and follow-up of the cardiac transplant recipient. In: Pepine CJ, Hill JA, Lambert CR (eds) Diagnostic and Therapeutic Cardiac Catheterization. 2nd Ed. Williams & Wilkins, Baltimore (in press)

74. Costanzo-Nordin MR, Cooper DKC, Jessup M et al: Task Force 6 (Bethesda conference—cardiac transplantation). Future developments. J Am Coll Cardiol 1993;22:54

75. Lowry R, Young JB: Non-invasive techniques to determine cardiac allograft rejection. pp. 213–231. In Frazier OH, Radovancevic B (eds): Cardiac Transplantation and Mechanical Circulatory Support. Lippincott-Raven, Philadelphia, 1996

76. Miller LW, Naftel DC, Bourge RC et al: Infection following cardiac transplantation. A multi-institutional analysis. J Heart Lung Transplant 1992;2:192

77. Ballantyne CM, Podet EJ, Patsch WP et al: Effects of cyclosporine therapy on plasma lipoprotein levels. JAMA 1989;26:53

78. Ballantyne CM, Radovancevic B, Farmer JA et al: Hyperlipidemia after heart transplantation. Report of a 6-year experience with treatment recommendations. J Am Coll Cardiol 1992;19:1315

79. Kubo SH, Peters JR, Knutson KR et al: Factors influencing the development of hypercholesterolemia after heart transplantation. Am J Cardiol 1992;70:520

80. Kobashigawa JA, Katznelson S, Laks H et al: Effect of pravastatin on outcomes after cardiac transplantation. N Engl J Med 1995;333:621

81. McCarthy PM, Portner PM, Tobler HG et al: Clinical experience with the Novacor ventricular assist system. J Thorac Cardiovasc Surg 1991;102:578–587

82. McCarthy PM, Savage RM, Fraser CD et al: Hemodynamic and physiologic changes during support with an implantable left ventricular assist device. J Thorac Cardiovasc Surg 1995;109:109–115

83. Kormos RL, Murali S, Dew MA et al: Chronic mechanical circulatory support. Rehabilitation, low morbidity, and superior survival. Ann Thorac Surg 1994;57: 51–58

84. Lorusso R, Zogno M, LaCanna G et al: Dynamic cardiomyoplasty as an effective therapy for dilated cardiomyopathy. J Cardiovasc Surg 1993;8:177–183

85. McGovern JA, Furnary AP, Christlieb IY et al: Indications and risk analysis for clinical myoplasty. Semin Thorac Cardiovasc Surg 1991;3:145–148

86. Kass A, Baughman KL, Pak PH et al: Reverse remodeling from cardiomyoplasty and human heart failure. External constraint versus active assist. Circulation 1995;91:2314–2318

54 Management of Refractory Heart Failure

Kanu Chatterjee
Teresa De Marco

The approach to managing patients with chronic heart failure is discussed in Chapter 37 and in the chapters dealing with specific classes of therapeutic agents. In general, the treatment goals for the management of symptomatic patients with chronic heart failure due to left ventricular systolic dysfunction are to relieve symptoms, improve quality of life, enhance cardiac performance, and improve survival. It is now clear that optimal management of most patients includes two and in most cases, three medications.

Diuretic therapy is the most effective approach to symptoms related to fluid overload, including peripheral edema, hepatic congestion, and ascites. In addition, diuretics reduce symptoms of pulmonary congestion, such as exertional dyspnea, orthopnea, and paroxysmal dyspnea, even in patients without evidence of fluid retention.[1,2] Diuretic monotherapy, however, is generally inappropriate because of the resulting neurohormonal abnormalities and electrolyte imbalances.[3] Aggressive diuresis can cause further impairment of left ventricular ejection performance associated with a reduction in cardiac output due to inappropriate peripheral vasoconstriction, which increases left ventricular ejection impedance.[3,4]

The angiotensin-converting enzyme (ACE) inhibitors overcome these disadvantages of diuretic therapy, and these two agents are therefore usually employed in combination. In addition to counteracting the neurohormonal and electrolyte abnormalities induced by diuretics, ACE inhibitors prolong survival in patients with symptomatic heart failure and pre-vent the progression of left ventricular dysfunction and clinical symptomatology in patients with few or no symptoms of heart failure but significantly impaired left ventricular ejection fractions.[5–7] Other vasodilator regimens, such as the combination of hydralazine and isosorbide dinitrate, also improve prognosis in symptomatic heart failure patients,[8] but not as well as ACE inhibitors.[9]

The third limb of the "standard" three-drug regimen for symptomatic heart failure is digoxin. Although controversy has surrounded the use of digitalis therapy in patients with congestive heart failure who are in sinus rhythm, randomized, placebo-controlled studies in patients with well characterized symptomatic left ventricular systolic dysfunction have clarified the appropriate role of this agent. In two studies that employed randomized digoxin withdrawal (one with and one without background ACE inhibitor therapy), patients who received placebo experienced more symptomatic deterioration, poorer exercise tolerance, reduced functional class, and declining ejection fractions than those who continued on digoxin therapy.[10,11] Most importantly, the Digitalis Investigator Group (DIG) trial unequivocally demonstrated that digoxin has an overall neutral effect on survival in patients with heart failure but significantly reduces hospitalizations and deaths related to worsening heart failure. Based on these results, the role of digoxin appears to be primarily for symptom relief and prevention of clinical deterioration in patients who remain symptomatic despite optimal therapy with diuretics and ACE inhibitors.[12] Congestive heart failure is defined as refractory when symptomatic and clinical manifestations of heart failure persist or worsen despite adequate triple therapy. It must be emphasized that before refractory heart failure is diagnosed it is essential to determine if optimal triple therapy has been provided. It is necessary to use adequate doses of diuretics, digitalis, and ACE inhibitors or hydralazine and isosorbide dinitrate before an inadequate response to such a therapeutic regimen is established.

SIGNS AND SYMPTOMS OF REFRACTORY HEART FAILURE

Refractory heart failure is a clinical diagnosis and is based on the presence of progressively worsening or frequent exacerbations of symptoms of heart failure despite adequate triple therapy. Usually, patients complain of increased congestive symptoms, such as dyspnea at rest or on minimal exertion and orthopnea. The mechanisms of worsening dyspnea with chronic heart failure are not entirely clear, although, increasing left atrial and pulmonary venous pressures, excessive ventilatory response to exertion, and respiratory muscle dysfunction due to chronic underperfusion may be contributory.[13] Increasing fatigue, tiredness, and diminishing exercise capacity frequently accompany worsening dyspnea. The mechanisms of fatigue and impaired exercise tolerance during chronic heart failure are also poorly understood. The underperfusion of the skeletal muscles, neuroendocrine abnormalities including activation of the renin-angiotensin-aldosterone system, enhanced adrenergic activity, increased cytokine levels, and alterations in the structural and metabolic function of the skeletal muscles may be contributory.[14–16] Loss of skeletal muscle mass and cardiac cachexia are frequently observed in patients with refractory heart failure. Increased levels of cytokines, such as tumor necrosis factor and interleukins, have been implicated as one of the important mechanisms for cardiac cachexia.[17] Increasing peripheral edema and progressive hepatic enlargement causing right upper quadrant abdominal pain are other symptoms that may be present in patients with refractory heart failure. Increasing fatigue or worsening chest pain not associated with other symptoms are rare presentations of refractory heart failure.

The clinical signs of refractory heart failure are variable and similar to those in patients with decompensated heart failure. A laterally displaced and sustained left ventricular apical impulse indicating left ventricular enlargement with reduced ejection frac-

tion is almost always appreciated. Systemic arterial pulsus alternans with tachycardia, when present, provides further evidence for impaired left ventricular systolic function. A left ventricular S3 gallop and increased intensity of the pulmonic component of the second heart sound are frequently present and indicate increases in left ventricular end-diastolic and pulmonary artery pressure, respectively. Secondary mitral regurgitation evidenced by the presence of an early systole or a pansystolic murmur is frequently recognized. The physical findings indicative of right ventricular failure, such as elevated jugular venous pressure and right ventricular S3 gallop, are also present in most patients with refractory heart failure. Findings suggestive of tricuspid regurgitation such as a prominent V wave followed by a sharp Y descent and an early or a pansystolic murmur along the lower left sternal border that increases in intensity with inspiration and hepatic pulsation are present in many patients with end-stage refractory heart failure. Increasing peripheral edema and ascites and rapid weight gain are other signs of severe right heart failure. It must be recognized that the absence of findings of right heart failure does not exclude decompensated and refractory left heart failure. It is of interest that in many patients with documented marked elevation of pulmonary capillary wedge pressure (exceeding 25 mmHg) the clinical and radiologic signs of pulmonary venous congestion are absent.[18,19] The chest radiograph almost invariably reveals significant cardiomegaly, but radiologic findings of pulmonary venous hypertension and alveolar edema are conspicuously absent in many patients with refractory heart failure. Arterial pressure is variable in patients with refractory heart failure. Significant hypotension with a systolic blood pressure of 90 mmHg or less indicates an adverse prognosis.

DIAGNOSIS

During the initial evaluation of a patient with refractory heart failure it is desirable to investigate for the presence of secondary rectifiable causes (Table 54-1). Uncontrolled hypertension, intercurrent illnesses, unrecognized hyper- or hypothyroidism, electrolyte imbalances (particularly severe hyponatremia or hyperkalemia), and patient noncompliance are secondary causes of refractory heart failure. Inadequate diuretic and vasodilator therapy are also not uncommon, mitigatable causes. Atrial fibrillation with a rapid ventricular response is an important potential rectifiable cause. In patients with atrial fibrillation, it is desirable to determine the

Table 54-1. Potential Causes of Refractory Heart Failure

Suboptimal triple therapy
Noncompliance
Severe anemia
Chronic severe thyroid dysfunction
Alcohol consumption
Concomitant use of drugs that can depress cardiac function, increase blood pressure, and promote fluid retention
Worsening renal failure with electrolyte disorders
Treatment-induced progressive hypotension
Atrial fibrillation with rapid ventricular response
Frequent, nonsustained ventricular tachycardia
Overt or silent myocardial ischemia
Worsening mitral and tricuspid regurgitation

ventricular rate as well as the pulse rate because significant pulse deficits may exist in the presence of a rapid ventricular response. It is also important to inquire about new cardiac and noncardiac medications and changes in alcohol consumption, which may cause worsening heart failure. Some antiarrhythmic drugs, particularly types IA, IC, III (sotalol), and IV (calcium channel blockers), can cause substantial depression of cardiac function and worsening heart failure. Nonsteroidal antiinflammatory drugs (NSAIDs) also cause fluid retention, and they may increase systemic vascular resistance by inhibiting prostaglandin synthesis. Furthermore, NSAIDs attenuate the beneficial hemodynamic and neurohormonal effects of ACE inhibitors. Alcohol consumption can cause worsening congestive heart failure due to its cardiodepressant effects. In patients with coronary artery disease, myocardial ischemia is a potential mechanism for worsening congestive heart failure, and thus assessment for the presence and extent of hibernating myocardium is desirable as reperfusion therapy of the ischemic myocardium can potentially improve ventricular function and congestive heart failure.

During initial evaluation, it is also desirable to investigate for the adverse prognostic factors in patients with refractory heart failure.[20-25] Symptoms at rest [New York Heart Association (NYHA) class IV] and significant hypotension are important clinical predictors of adverse outcome. When hemodynamic monitoring is indicated (usually to assess the response to vasodilator and inotropic therapy), certain hemodynamic parameters obtained during hemodynamic monitoring may provide useful prognostic information. Persistently elevated pulmonary capillary wedge pressure exceeding 25 mmHg, markedly reduced left ventricular stroke work index usu-

ally less than 20 g-m/m^2, markedly elevated right atrial pressure, moderate to severe pulmonary hypertension, and increased pulmonary vascular resistance indicate a poor prognosis. Cardiopulmonary exercise testing can be performed in ambulatory patients; a markedly decreased exercise duration and a maximal oxygen consumption (VO$_2$max) of 14 ml·kg^{-1}·min^{-1} or less is associated with a poor prognosis.

Abnormalities of myocardial metabolic function, such as a markedly decreased coronary sinus venous oxygen content of less than 4 volumes percent, has been associated with enhanced mortality in patients with ischemic and those with nonischemic dilated cardiomyopathy.[24] The degree of fibrosis and myocyte loss determined in the biopsy specimens has also been used to assess prognosis of patients with heart failure; however, such invasive investigations, including assessment of myocardial metabolism, are seldom necessary in clinical practice. Several neurohormonal abnormalities have been associated with a poor prognosis in patients with heart failure.[26,27] Markedly elevated level of atrial natriuretic peptides, increased plasma renin activity, elevated angiotensin II and aldosterone levels, and increased levels of tumor necrosis factor and interleukins have been shown to indicate a poor prognosis in patients with severe heart failure. However, in clinical practice, the routine assessment of changes in neuroendocrine profile to evaluate prognosis is seldom necessary. Hyponatremia with serum sodium levels of 130 mEq/L or less and impaired renal function with increased levels of creatinine and blood urea nitrogen (BUN) are associated with a worse prognosis; and as these measurements can be easily performed, assessment of renal function and changes in electrolytes should be routine during the initial evaluation of patients with refractory heart failure.

THERAPEUTIC APPROACH

Once the diagnosis of refractory heart failure is established and reversible causes have been eliminated, several therapeutic options are considered for management of such patients. Patients with refractory heart failure should be considered for cardiac transplantation, as this approach is the only one that can substantially improve the long-term prognosis of such patients.[28] However, a large proportion of patients with refractory heart failure are not eligible for cardiac transplantation for a variety of reasons, including age and associated co-morbid disorders. Furthermore, most patients who are otherwise eligible and suitable candidates for cardiac transplantation cannot receive such therapy because of the paucity of donor hearts. Thus pharmacotherapy remains the only option for such patients. Cardiomyoplasty and other surgical procedures have been explored and are discussed elsewhere (see Ch. 53).

Combination Vasodilator Therapy

Addition of hydralazine and isosorbide dinitrate to digitalis, diuretics, and ACE inhibitors often improves systemic hemodynamics with a reduction in pulmonary capillary wedge and right atrial pressures and an increase in cardiac output.[29] In some patients there is also improvement in clinical status and exercise tolerance. The rationale for the combination therapy is that there is a greater potential to increase the left ventricular ejection fraction and improve exercise tolerance and VO$_2$max. In the Vasodilator Heart Failure Trial II (V-HeFT-II)[9] the magnitude of increase in left ventricular ejection fraction with hydralazine–isosorbide dinitrate combination was greater than that with enalapril. Similarly, the increase in exercise duration and VO$_2$max were also greater with hydralazine–isosorbide dinitrate than with enalapril. In clinical practice, when hydralazine and isosorbide dinitrate are added to ACE inhibitors, the initial doses of hydralazine and isosorbide dinitrate should be low, with the doses gradually increased to the maximum tolerable dose without producing hypotension. The initial dose of hydralazine is usually 25 mg four times a day, and the dose can be increased every second or third day until a maximum dose of 300 mg a day is administered. Most patients, particularly those with refractory heart failure and relative hypotension, cannot tolerate doses of hydralazine exceeding 200 mg a day. The initial dose of isosorbide dinitrate is usually 20 mg three or four times a day, and one can increase it up to 160 mg a day if tolerated. The major clinical problem of such a combination therapy of vasodilators and ACE inhibitors is hypotension and subsequently impaired renal function. The optimal combination therapy is best achieved with hemodynamic monitoring. However, in patients with adequate arterial pressure, combination therapy can be initiated without hemodynamic monitoring and in the outpatient setting, monitored by frequent clinical evaluation. Combining direct vasodilator therapy with ACE inhibitors does not, however, produce immediate clinical improvement, which may occur only after treatment for several weeks. It must be emphasized that a survival benefit has not been demonstrated with such combination therapy in patients with refractory heart failure.

Vasoselective Long-Acting Calcium Channel Blockers

Immediate-release dihydropyridines (e.g., nifedipine) and other calcium channel blockers (e.g., diltiazem) are generally contraindicated for the management of patients with congestive heart failure due to impaired left ventricular systolic function: These agents can cause worsening congestive heart failure and even increase mortality. Immediate-release short-acting nifedipine has been shown to cause deterioration in the clinical status and to increase the frequency of hospital admissions for treatment of worsening heart failure.[29,30] In the Multicenter Diltiazem Post-Infarction Trial[31] the incidence of adverse cardiac events including mortality was higher in patients with congestive heart failure or reduced left ventricular ejection fraction following treatment with diltiazem. These deleterious effects of the first generation calcium channel blockers during heart failure have been related to their more prominent negative inotropic effects and inappropriate activation of adrenergic systems.[32–34] The more vasoselective calcium channel blockers such as amlodipine and felodipine have been reported to have less negative inotropic effect and may not activate the adrenergic system because of their sustained, continuous pharmacodynamic effects. Amlodipine has been reported to improve exercise tolerance and clinical functional class in patients with chronic heart failure with background treatment with digitalis, diuretics, ACE inhibitors, or other vasodilators. A reduction in the circulating norepinephrine levels during long-term therapy with amlodipine compared to placebo has been also observed.[35] In the PRAISE trial[36] symptomatic patients with a left ventricular ejection fraction of 30 percent or less and with a background treatment of digitalis, diuretics, and ACE inhibitors were randomized to receive amlodipine or placebo. Mortality in the whole study population was not significantly different in the amlodipine and placebo groups. However, in the subset of patients with nonischemic dilated cardiomyopathy, there was a substantial reduction in mortality with addition of amlodipine to triple therapy. In these patients, the risk of sudden death was reduced by 38 percent and that of pump failure death by 45 percent. In patients with ischemic heart disease and pump failure, there were no differences in the overall mortality and sudden or pump failure deaths between amlodipine- and placebo-treated patients. Unfortunately, there was no evidence of improvement in functional class or clinical status in either ischemic or nonischemic cardiomyopathy.

The V-HeFT-III trial[37] involved symptomatic patients receiving diuretic and enalapril as background therapy and randomized to receive felodipine 5 mg twice daily or placebo. Approximately 50 percent of these patients had coronary artery disease, and the average ejection fraction of all patients was 30 percent. During follow-up averaging 540 days (range 90–1119 days) there was no difference between felodipine and placebo therapy in overall mortality or in mortality in the subgroups with or without coronary artery disease. Felodipine also did not exert a beneficial effect on clinical status or exercise tolerance, and there was a trend toward more worsening of heart failure during the initial 12 weeks of felodipine treatment. These preliminary data suggest that felodipine added to an ACE inhibitor in patients with congestive heart failure without overt myocardial ischemia does not exert a favorable effect on the course of heart failure and survival.

The results of these studies suggest that patients with cardiomyopathy already treated with digitalis, diuretics, and ACE inhibitors usually tolerate the newer vasoselective, long-acting calcium channel blockers, and therefore these drugs may be useful for treating concomitant angina or hypertension. In addition, patients with nonischemic dilated cardiomyopathy may derive a survival benefit with amlodipine. Relatively normotensive patients without resting tachycardia might be better candidates for combination therapy with a vasoselective calcium channel blocker and ACE inhibitors along with digitalis and diuretics. However, more clinical trials are required to identify the appropriate subset of patients with refractory heart failure suitable for such combination therapy.

β-Blocker Therapy

The rationale for β-adrenergic receptor blockade therapy is attenuation of the potential adverse effects of enhanced adrenergic activity accompanying heart failure on cardiac performance, myocardial energetics and metabolic function, peripheral vascular and ventricular remodeling, and progression of heart failure.[38–42] That systemic cardiac and renal adrenergic activity is significantly increased in patients with symptomatic heart failure has been amply demonstrated employing several techniques to assess adrenergic activity in these patients. Circulating norepinephrine levels are consistently increased, as a result not only of decreased clearance but also from increased spillover.[16,43,44] Net myocardial norepinephrine release and the spillover rate' are also substantially increased in patients with overt heart failure.[43,44] Muscle sympathetic nerve activity, a direct measure of sympathetic outflow, is also markedly increased during heart failure.[45] Decreased heart rate variability, a measure of autonomic tone also suggests an increase in sympathetic tone and a decrease in parasympathetic modulation.[46] The chronically heightened systemic and cardiac adrenergic activity can lead to myofibrillar degeneration, cardiomyopathy, and decreased survival. Chronic elevations of catecholamine may also contribute to decreased myocardial contractile performance through down-regulation of β-receptors and alterations of the G protein complex, which couples β-receptors to cyclic adenosine monophosphate (cAMP).[47,48] Furthermore, markedly increased norepinephrine levels (exceeding 650 pg/ml) have been reported to be associated with a poor prognosis in patients with symptomatic heart failure.[26,42]

A number of clinical studies have reported the beneficial effects of β-adrenergic blocking drugs on systemic hemodynamics, the left ventricular ejection fraction, and the contractile response.[49–52] Although acute intravenous administration of metoprolol decreases cardiac output and heart rate and increases the left ventricular end-diastolic pressure, chronic oral metoprolol therapy is associated with a substantial increase in cardiac output and stroke volume and a reduction in left ventricular end-diastolic pressure, suggesting improved left ventricular systolic function.[53] It is of interest that systolic blood pressure may not change or may even increase following chronic β-blocker therapy, and the calculated systemic vascular resistance may also decrease. As expected, the heart rate decreases significantly during maintenance chronic metoprolol treatment. The left ventricular contractile response to β-adrenergic agonist stimulation with dobutamine also increases following chronic β-blocker therapy.[50] In both uncontrolled and controlled studies, chronic β-blocker therapy with metoprolol has been reported to increase the left ventricular ejection fraction and decrease end-systolic volume with or without a significant change in left ventricular end-diastolic volume.[54,55] The newer β-adrenergic antagonists with additional vasodilator properties, such as bucindolol, bisoprolol, nebivolol, celiprolol, and carvedilol, have been reported to improve systemic hemodynamics and the left ventricular ejection fraction.[56–64] Like metoprolol, these newer β-adrenergic blocking agents can also decrease the end-systolic volume substantially with little or no change in left ventricular end-diastolic volume, resulting in an increase in the left ventricular ejection fraction. Furthermore, left ventricular mass also can decrease following chronic β-blocker therapy, suggesting their potential beneficial effects on ventricular remodeling and progression of heart failure.

The mechanisms for improvement of left ventricular function during chronic β-blocker therapy in patients with heart failure due to ischemic or nonischemic dilated cardiomyopathy are not entirely clear and are likely to be multifactorial. As the major determinant for the increased ejection fraction appears to be decreased end-systolic volume, an enhanced contractile response, a reduction in left ventricular ejection impedance, or both must be considered as potential hemodynamic mechanisms. In many clinical trials, a reduction in systemic vascular resistance has been observed following chronic β-blocker therapy; thus a reduction in left ventricular ejection impedance remains a potential mechanism for improved left ventricular ejection fraction. In some studies an increase in left ventricular contractile response has been documented, and up-regulation of the β-adrenergic receptors has been postulated as the potential mechanism.[53] Unlike the normal heart, in a failing heart an increase in heart rate is associated with decreased contractility—an inverse force–frequency relation.[65,66] A reduction in heart rate is a consistent response to chronic β-blocker therapy, so potential exists for improved contractility by partial attenuation of the inverse force–frequency relation in the failing heart. Furthermore, chronic β-blocker therapy may improve myocardial energetics and substrate utilization.[51] The reduction in heart rate during chronic β-blocker therapy is also likely to be associated with improved left ventricular filling, which may secondarily improve left ventricular systolic function. The changes in the abnormal neuroendocrine profile of heart failure during chronic β-blocker therapy are not consistent or predictable. In some studies a reduction in the circulating catecholamine levels has be observed, but in others there was no consistent change in systemic adrenergic activity.[54,67–69] The changes in plasma renin activity and the angiotensin II, vasopressin, and atrial natriuretic peptide levels have also been variable.[68] The changes in cardiac norepinephrine spillover rate appear to be related to the selectivity of the β-blocker used. With metoprolol, a relatively β-selective antagonist, cardiac norepinephrine spillover may increase, presumably owing to enhanced norepinephrine release from the prejunctional neuron, which is inhibited by a nonselective β-adrenergic blocking agent such as propranolol.[69] Thus the contribution of changes in the neuroendocrine profile to improving cardiac performance with β-blocker therapy remains uncertain.

A number of controlled prospective studies have provided evidence for the beneficial effects of chronic β-blocker therapy in improving clinical status, exercise tolerance, and quality of life.[52,54,55,57–59,64,68] The duration of submaximal exercise and the distance during 6-minute walk tests can substantially increase during chronic β-blocker therapy.[70] Such benefits have been observed with metoprolol and the newer β-adrenergic antagonists with vasodilator properties.[70–75] However, the improvement in exercise tolerance or left ventricular function has not been uniformly observed in all studies.[72] The impact of β-blocker therapy on the prognosis of patients with heart failure due to ischemic or nonischemic dilated cardiomyopathy has not been firmly established.[76] In a prospective randomized trial of propranolol versus placebo after myocardial infarction, propranolol decreased cardiovascular mortality and sudden death in patients who had congestive heart failure.[77] During the Cardiac Arrhythmia Suppression Trial (CAST),[78] in the subgroup of patients with an ejection fraction below 40 percent, the time to death or cardiac arrest was significantly prolonged with β-blocker therapy. In the Metoprolol in Dilated Cardiomyopathy (MDC) trial[79] 383 patients in NYHA functional class III and IV congestive heart failure were randomized to metoprolol or placebo. There was a 34 percent reduction in the risk of mortality and the need for transplantation in the metoprolol-treated patients, although this risk reduction was not statistically significant compared to placebo-treated patients. The reduction resulted entirely from a greater number of placebo-treated patients who needed cardiac transplantation, as mortality did not differ between the two groups. Metoprolol therapy was also associated with fewer hospitalizations and visits to the emergency department for treatment of exacerbation of congestive heart failure. In the CIBIS trial, bisoprolol, a β-adrenergic antagonist with vasodilatory properties, was used in patients with nonischemic and ischemic dilated cardiomyopathy. Although a beneficial effect of ameliorating symptoms of heart failure was observed, overall mortality remained unchanged with bisoprolol treatment.[80] Among patients with nonischemic dilated cardiomyopathy, however, there was a trend to improved survival.

More dramatic results have been reported with carvedilol, a β-adrenergic and α-adrenergic antagonist with vasodilating and antioxidant effects. Initially several small studies demonstrated that this agent improved the hemodynamic and clinical status of patients with congestive heart failure.[64] Subsequently, a series of multicenter studies were conducted in patients with mild, moderate, or severe heart failure with ejection fractions of 35 percent or less in which carvedilol or placebo was added to digitalis, a diuretic, and ACE inhibitors.[72–75] When these studies were analyzed together, a significant reduction in hospitalizations and mortality with carvedilol was observed. By intention-to-treat statistical analysis, mortality was 8.2 percent in the placebo group but only 2.9 percent in the carvedilol group. The mortality benefit was similar in patients in NYHA II or III–IV functional class. Furthermore, the decrease in the risk in mortality with carvedilol was similar among patient with ischemic heart disease and those with nonischemic dilated cardiomyopathy. Several points must be kept in mind when considering these favorable results. During the open-label titration period before randomization to carvedilol and placebo, a considerable number of patients could not tolerate carvedilol and were not eligible for randomization. Furthermore, only a relatively smaller number of patients with severe heart failure (NYHA class IV) and clinically unstable patients were randomized. Thus the survival benefit of carvedilol in truly refractory heart failure patients remains uncertain. Nevertheless, these studies do indicate that the patients already treated with digitalis, diuretics, and ACE inhibitors may benefit from addition of carvedilol, not only for improving clinical status and quality of life but also for improving survival. Whether similar benefits will occur with the use of other β-adrenergic blocking agents remains to be established.

The practical problems for institution of β-blocker therapy in patients with congestive heart failure should be considered. The introduction of β-blockers in patients with congestive heart failure may cause rapid deterioration of cardiac function and a rebound rise in plasma catecholamines.[81] Furthermore, a considerable proportion of patients (up to 27 percent) discontinue β-blocker therapy because of intolerance or lack of beneficial response.[82] It also must be appreciated that the improvement in symptoms, clinical class, and left ventricular ejection fraction does not occur immediately after institution of β-blocker therapy. The clinical experience suggests that a minimum of 4–6 weeks of treatment is necessary before any clinically relevant improvement is expected.[83] The initiation of treatment with standard or relatively larger dose of β-adrenergic blocking agents is almost invariably associated with clinical and hemodynamic deterioration. Therefore treatment should be begun with low doses of the β-adrenergic blocking drug and should be increased gradually to a maximum tolerable dose that produces a discernible hemodynamic response. The usual dose of metoprolol varies between 25 and 100 mg a day, that of bucindolol between 25–100 mg a day, and of carvedilol between 6.25 and 25.00 mg twice daily. It also needs to be appreciated that in clinical practice it is difficult

to determine which subsets of patients are likely to benefit from β-blocker therapy. In some studies it was suggested that patients with ischemic cardiomyopathy are unlikely to respond to β-blocker therapy in contrast to those with idiopathic dilated cardiomyopathy. In the carvedilol trial, however, patients with coronary artery disease and nonischemic dilated cardiomyopathy benefited equally.[72] It has been suggested that patients with higher systolic blood pressure and significantly impaired left ventricular diastolic function as evident from increased left ventricular end-diastolic pressure are more likely to benefit from β-blocker therapy.[84] Patients with a high baseline heart rate (probably reflecting higher baseline adrenergic activity) may also benefit more with β-blocker therapy than patients with relatively less activated adrenergic system.[68] Admittedly, more studies are required to identify patients most suitable for β-blocker therapy. Presently, patients with normal or slightly elevated arterial pressure and tachycardia and refractory to standard triple therapy appear to be the best candidates. Patients who are unstable and demonstrate evidence of rapid progressive deterioration in heart failure should not be considered for β-blocker therapy until they are stabilized.

Amiodarone for Refractory Heart Failure

Amiodarone, classified as a type III antiarrhythmic agent, has multiple pharmacodynamic properties.[85,86] It is primarily a potassium channel blocking agent, but it also blocks the sodium and calcium channels. It prolongs the effective refractory period of the action potential and increases the action potential duration. It also reduces the spontaneous phase IV depolarization, which might be the principal mechanism for reduction of the sinus rate. It reduces the conduction through the atrioventricular node. It nonspecifically blocks sympathetic tone, alters thyroid metabolism, and inhibits phospholipases and adenosine triphosphate (ATP)-sensitive potassium channels. The latter two properties may stabilize myocardial lipid membranes during ischemia and consequently modulate arrhythmogenesis.[86–89] Clinically, it is an effective agent for reducing the ventricular response during atrial flutter and fibrillation, preventing recurrence of supraventricular tachycardia (including atrial flutter and fibrillation), and suppressing nonsustained and sustained ventricular tachycardia.

In patients with chronic heart failure due to depressed left ventricular ejection fraction, amiodarone has also effectively controlled ventricular and supraventricular tachyarrhythmias. Amiodarone, however, in addition to its antiarrhythmic effect, exerts a direct negative inotropic effect; and it exerts vasodilatory and antiischemic effects. These varied pharmacologic actions make its effects in heart failure difficult to predict.

In uncontrolled studies, low dose amiodarone therapy in patients with chronic heart failure has been shown to improve left ventricular ejection fraction.[90,91] The mechanisms for this action remain unclear. Despite its negative inotropic effect and the potential for deterioration of cardiac performance, sometimes observed during intravenous or oral loading therapy, the left ventricular ejection fraction may improve during long-term chronic oral therapy.[92,93] It has been suggested that vasodilatation with amiodarone, which improves the left ventricular ejection fraction, may balance or overcome the deleterious effects resulting from its negative inotropic property. Its antiischemic effect may also be contributory to improving left ventricular function. As long term/low dose amiodarone therapy almost invariably results in a reduction in heart rate, partial correction of the decreased contractility associated with an inverse force–frequency relation in the failing heart may be an important contributory factor in improving the left ventricular ejection fraction in patients with heart failure. It must be appreciated, however, that the relation between changes in left ventricular ejection fraction and mortality during low dose amiodarone therapy remains controversial.[94]

The effects of amiodarone therapy on survival of patients with heart failure due to impaired left ventricular systolic function have been assessed in prospective studies, and variable results have been observed.[91,94–98] In the Veterans Administration (VA) Cooperative Study of amiodarone for congestive heart failure, low dose amiodarone therapy was not associated with an increase or a decrease in mortality or sudden death.[98] Lack of any significant survival benefit was observed irrespective of whether ventricular arrhythmias were suppressed. However, there was a significant reduction in the combined endpoint of cardiac deaths and hospitalizations in patients without evidence of coronary artery disease.[94]

In the GESICA trial,[97] another large multicenter trial of amiodarone in patients with heart failure, survival was significantly improved with amiodarone. This study differed from the VA trial in that the patients were sicker (NYHA class III or IV). Furthermore, in contrast to the VA study, most of the patients had nonischemic cardiomyopathy, and a substantial number of women were included. During

follow-up of approximately 24 months, there was a 36 percent reduction in the risk of mortality; the risks of reduction of heart failure death and sudden death were similar. In truly refractory class IV heart failure patients, particularly those requiring intermittent or long-term inotropic supportive therapy with either β-adrenergic agonist or phosphodiesterase inhibitors, addition of amiodarone appears to improve survival.[90]

The role of chronic low dose amiodarone therapy in improving survival of such patients cannot be established without more controlled studies, however. In certain subsets of patients with severe refractory heart failure, amiodarone has the potential to improve clinical status, cardiac performance, and survival. In the GESICA trial, an elevated initial baseline heart rate exceeding 90 bpm identified a subgroup of patients with a worse prognosis but with better benefit from the use of amiodarone treatment. In those patients in whom the heart rate decreased to fewer than 90 bpm with therapy, the survival benefit increased and persisted during the follow-up of 24 months.[99] In patients requiring long-term inotropic supportive therapy, amiodarone can potentially improve survival by reducing the risk of enhanced arrhythmogenic mortality associated with inotropic therapy. In patients with atrial fibrillation complicating severe congestive heart failure, amiodarone may be of particular benefit in decreasing ventricular response or maintaining sinus rhythm. Atrial fibrillation with rapid ventricular response occurs in approximately 20–30 percent of patients with severe chronic congestive heart failure and can cause deterioration of cardiac performance, hemodynamics, and clinical status.[100–103] Rapid ventricular responses, impair ventricular filling, decrease forward stroke volume and cardiac output, and increase left ventricular diastolic and pulmonary venous pressures.[104] Furthermore, a rapid ventricular rate may decrease ventricular contractile performance due to an inverse force–frequency relation in the failing heart.

In patients with depressed left ventricular systolic function with or without overt heart failure, antiarrhythmic drugs other than amiodarone are contraindicated because of their proarrhythmic effects and their potential to cause further deterioration of cardiac function. Type I antiarrhythmic drugs, such as quinidine, procainamide, and disopyramide, are contraindicated because of their proarrhythmic and negative inotropic effects. Type IB antiarrhythmic drugs, such as tocainide or mexilitine, are usually ineffective in controlling atrial or ventricular tachyarrhythmias. Type IC drugs, such as encainide and flecainide, enhance mortality owing to their proarrhythmic effects. The dose of the β-adrenergic blocking agents, which are required for treatment of supraventricular and ventricular tachyarrhythmias, is not usually tolerated by patients with overt heart failure and depressed left ventricular systolic function. Although sotalol appears equivalent to quinidine in terms of maintaining normal sinus rhythm and perhaps superior in terms of heart rate and symptom control if atrial fibrillation recurs in patients with left ventricular dysfunction but without overt heart failure, it has significant proarrhythmic and negative inotropic effects. The dose of sotalol is usually required to control arrhythmias is not tolerated by patients with symptomatic heart failure with depressed left ventricular ejection fraction. Thus amiodarone appears to be the drug of choice for appropriate management of patients with atrial fibrillation complicating congestive heart failure. In another subset of patients with significant resting sinus tachycardia who cannot tolerate adequate β-blocker therapy to control heart rate, amiodarone may be of benefit. It should be appreciated that suppression of sustained or nonsustained ventricular arrhythmias is not the principal indication for low dose amiodarone therapy, as there is no correlation between suppression of arrhythmias, changes in left ventricular function, and survival. Low dose amiodarone (200–300 mg/day) is well tolerated by patients with chronic heart failure, and the incidence of adverse effects is low. For example, the incidence of torsade de pointes is less than 1 percent.[105] Similarly, peripheral neuropathy and retinal degeneration, which are usually irreversible, are rarely encountered when low dose amiodarone is used. Abnormalities of liver function and thyroid function occur more frequently, however, and periodic assessment of liver and thyroid function should be considered in all patients on long-term amiodarone treatment.[106]

Nonpharmacologic Approaches to Arrhythmias

In some patients nonpharmacologic therapy may be necessary to control supraventricular tachycardia, atrial flutter, or fibrillation refractory to amiodarone therapy.[107–110] Incessant atrial tachycardia, paroxysmal, atrioventricular (AV) node reentry tachycardia, AV reentry tachycardia, and type I atrial flutter are amenable to radiofrequency ablation therapy. Complete AV nodal ablation requires pacemaker therapy, which can be associated with complications such as stroke and sudden death. Most sudden deaths occur in patients with severe (NYHA functional class III or IV) heart failure.[111] Several studies

have reported the hemodynamic benefits of AV node ablation as treatment for atrial fibrillation in patients with depressed left ventricular function.[112–116] Improvements in cardiac performance, including an increased ejection fraction, have been observed in up to 83 percent of patients with congestive heart failure treated by AV node ablation and pacemaker therapy.[116,117] However, pacemaker therapy may be associated with worsening mitral regurgitation. Compared to pharmacotherapy, radiofrequency AV node ablation as treatment for chronic atrial fibrillation is not associated with increased mortality.[118] Thus in selected patients with atrial fibrillation and a rapid ventricular response refractory to medical therapy, radiofrequency ablation of the AV node and pacemaker therapy may be of benefit.

Short-Term and Long-Term Catecholamine Treatment

Dobutamine, a predominantly β_1-receptor agonist with minor β_2- and α-adrenergic agonist property is the most frequently used adrenergic agent for treatment of refractory congestive heart failure. With doses of $1–10$ $\mu g \cdot kg^{-1} \cdot min^{-1}$ it produces an immediate increase in cardiac index and stroke volume index, decreases in systemic and pulmonary vascular resistances, and minimal changes in the heart rate and systemic blood pressure.[119] With larger doses of dobutamine, however, arterial pressure may fall owing to a marked reduction in systemic vascular resistance and an inadequate increase in cardiac output. These patients also tend to develop tachycardia. A marked increase in heart rate may be associated with a substantial increase in myocardial oxygen demand and impaired myocardial perfusion, which may be further compromised by a reduction in arterial perfusion pressure.

When refractory congestive heart failure is complicated by a low systemic blood pressure, dobutamine is generally combined with a vasopressor, such as dopamine or norepinephrine. Lower doses of dopamine, $0.5–2$ $\mu g \cdot kg^{-1} \cdot min^{-1}$, however, promote vasodilatation; and the combination of low dose dopamine and dobutamine may not correct hypotension.[29] With moderate doses of dopamine ($2–8$ $\mu g \cdot kg^{-1} \cdot min^{-1}$) there is activation of β_1-adrenergic receptors, which is associated with increased contractility. Higher doses of dopamine (exceeding $8–10$ $\mu g \cdot kg^{-1} \cdot min^{-1}$) activates the α-receptor, resulting in increased systemic vascular resistance and increased arterial pressure. Instead of dopamine, norepinephrine or phenylephrine, which are predominantly α-receptor agonists, can be used in combination with dobutamine to maintain arterial pressure and increase cardiac output concurrently. Occasionally it is necessary to add intravenous vasodilators such as sodium nitroprusside or nitroglycerin to optimize the hemodynamic improvements.

Although the hemodynamic effects of dobutamine are observed within a few minutes after starting its infusion, the beneficial hemodynamic changes can persist for days to weeks, even after its discontinuation following 24–72 hours of therapy.[120] The mechanisms of sustained hemodynamic benefits following short-term dobutamine infusion are not known, although improved mitochondrial function and conditioning effects have been proposed.[121] Intermittent low dose dobutamine infusion therapy has been employed for treatment of refractory heart failure. Such therapy in the outpatient minimizes exacerbation of congestive heart failure and reduces the frequency of readmission to intensive care units. Most patients receiving intermittent dobutamine therapy demonstrate an improvement in NYHA functional class, improved exercise tolerance, and occasionally improvement in quality of life.[122,123] However, intermittent dobutamine infusion therapy is associated with increased mortality, primarily due to an increase in the incidence of sudden death.[124] Thus intermittent dobutamine infusion therapy should be undertaken only when monitoring for ventricular arrhythmias is available.

Data with other catecholamines, particularly when used chronically, have not been favorable. Mortality rates were increased when xamoterol (an oral β_1-selective partial agonist) and ibopamine (an oral agent hydrolyzed to the dopaminergic agonist epinine) were utilized in patients with severe heart failure, although there was some evidence that these agents were beneficial in patients with mild symptoms.[125,126] Oral levodopa, which is converted to dopamine by aromatic amino acid decarboxylation, has been shown to improve hemodynamics, left ventricular function, and occasionally the clinical status of patients with severe heart failure.[127,128] The dose of levodopa that has been found to produce beneficial hemodynamic effects is large, 2 g three to four times daily; and these large doses are rarely tolerated owing to centrally mediated nausea and other abdominal symptoms, tremor, and ataxia. Thus the role of adrenergic agonists in the long-term management of patients with refractory heart failure remains unproved.

Phosphodiesterase Inhibitors

The phosphodiesterase inhibitors, also referred as inodilators, inhibit phosphodiesterase isoform III in cardiac and vascular tissues, which is associated with increased intracellular cAMP. Increased intracellular calcium concentration mediated by cAMP enhances the myocardial contractile force. Phosphodiesterase inhibitors also exert direct vasodilating effects on the peripheral vascular beds. The acute hemodynamic effects of phosphodiesterase inhibitors, such as amrinone, milrinone, and enoximone, whether given intravenously or orally, are characterized by increased cardiac index, decreased systemic vascular resistance, and decreased pulmonary capillary wedge pressure without a significant change in heart rate or mean arterial pressure.[129,130] There is also a substantial reduction in right atrial pressure and right ventricular diastolic pressure along with improved right ventricular performance. In addition, phosphodiesterase inhibitors may improve myocardial relaxation and left ventricular filling, which may contribute to improved systemic hemodynamics and left ventricular systolic performance. In general, these effects are achieved without an increase in myocardial oxygen consumption. However, they may induce primary coronary vasodilatation, which may shunt blood flow from the ischemic to the nonischemic myocardium in patients with coronary artery disease.

The phosphodiesterase inhibitors also can decrease pulmonary vascular resistance substantially and decrease pulmonary artery pressure in patients with postcapillary pulmonary hypertension. Although milrinone and amrinone have been shown to increase effective renal plasma flow and glomerular filtration rate in patients with a stable hemodynamic profile, in clinical practice renal function and urine output usually do not improve without a substantial increase in cardiac output. Like dobutamine, large doses of phosphodiesterase inhibitors may cause hypotension due to excessive peripheral vasodilatation and an inadequate increase in cardiac output, which may be associated with impairment of renal function.

The hemodynamic effects of milrinone have been compared to those of dobutamine during 48 hours of infusion of these agents in patients with chronic heart failure. The magnitude of the increase in cardiac output and stroke volume and of the reduction in mean atrial pressure were similar in response to both agents. However, the magnitude of the reduction in pulmonary capillary wedge pressure in response to milrinone was slightly greater than that in response to dobutamine. The combination of dobutamine, which generates cAMP, and a phosphodiesterase inhibitor, which inhibits degradation of cAMP, produces a greater improvement in hemodynamics and left ventricular performance than either agent alone.[130] Such combination therapy therefore is useful for short-term management of patients with refractory heart failure.

Although phosphodiesterase inhibitors alone or in combination with dobutamine and vasodilators are effective in improving hemodynamics and clinical status during short-term therapy, long-term therapy with phosphodiesterase inhibitors not only does not produce any sustained clinical benefit but also may increase mortality. In the PROMISE trial[131], patients already treated with digoxin, diuretics, and ACE inhibitors were randomized to receive placebo or milrinone; addition of milrinone to triple therapy increased mortality substantially. The risk of mortality increased by 37 percent in patients with severe heart failure. A similar increase in mortality has been observed with the use of other phosphodiesterase inhibitors, such as enoximone.[132] Pimobendan, a predominantly calcium-sensitizing agent with some phosphodiesterase-inhibiting property, has been shown to improve clinical status, exercise tolerance, and left ventricular function during short-term therapy—but at the cost of increased mortality.[133,134] Another vasodilator inotropic agent, flosequinan, has been shown to improve clinical status and exercise tolerance during relatively short-term treatment; but long-term treatment with flosequinan was associated with worsening heart failure and increased mortality.[135,136] Thus any benefits from chronic therapy with this class of medication must be counterbalanced by an apparent substantial increase in mortality rates.

Vesnarinone is another nonglycoside inotropic agent which has been evaluated for long-term management of patients with congestive heart failure. Vesnarinone is a quinoline derivative that inhibits phosphodiesterase isoform III at high doses and increases myocardial contractility through cAMP pathways.[137,138] It also inhibits the inward and outward rectifying potassium currents and increases intracellular sodium by prolonging the opening of sodium channels.[138,139] These effects resemble the properties of type III antiarrhythmia agents and had been expected to provide an advantage over other inotropic agents because of their potential antiarrhythmic effect. Vesnarinone also decreases the levels of cytokines (e.g., tumor necrosis factor and interleukins), which may have a beneficial effect on ventricular remodeling and progression of heart failure. Unfortunately, the initial favorable experience with vernarinone[140] has not been confirmed by the much larger VEST study, which demonstrated an adverse effect on survival without any evidence of clinical improvement.

At present, the use of nonglycoside positive inotropic agents, including β-adrenergic agonists and phosphodiesterase inhibitors, is limited to the treatment of acute exacerbations of chronic refractory heart failure or the maintenance of improved hemodynamics in patients waiting for cardiac transplantation. Although the role of nonglycoside inotropes as a bridge to cardiac transplantation has not been studied prospectively, retrospective studies have reported that these inotropic agents can be used successfully to bridge 45–90 percent of hemodynamically unstable patients to cardiac transplantation.[141–143] Nonparenteral phosphodiesterase inhibitors, particularly enoximone, have been used to wean patients dependent on dobutamine-dopamine infusions. Many patients, such as those weaned from dobutamine-dopamine infusions and maintained on nonparenteral phosphodiesterase inhibitors, survived to undergo cardiac transplantation. The phosphodiesterase inhibitors have also been used in patients with refractory pulmonary hypertension, which is a contraindication for cardiac transplantation.[144] When the reduction in pulmonary hypertension and pulmonary vascular resistance is inadequate with nitroprusside infusion, parenteral and nonparenteral phosphodiesterase inhibitors can often decrease pulmonary artery pressure and pulmonary vascular resistance to an acceptable level for cardiac transplantation. When phosphodiesterase inhibitors or other nonglycoside inotropic agents are used, even in patients waiting for cardiac transplant, it is desirable to add amiodarone, which has been shown to reduce the risk of mortality associated with the use of these inotropic agents. Similarly, patients receiving intermittent dobutamine, dopamine, or phosphodiesterase inhibitors intravenously should be treated with amiodarone concurrently.

Hemodynamic Tailored Therapy for Refractory Heart Failure

Patients with refractory heart failure, particularly those who are being considered for cardiac transplantation, frequently require hemodynamic monitoring and therapy adjusted (tailored) to hemodynamic goals.[145,146] In general, the objective is to maintain systolic blood pressure higher than 85 mmHg, right atrial pressure at 8 mmHg or less, pulmonary capillary wedge pressure at 15 mmHg or less, and the cardiac index at more than 2.5. Unfortunately, in many patients with refractory heart failure these goals cannot be achieved.

Initially, intravenous vasodilators (sodium nitroprusside, nitroglycerin), inotropic agents, and inodilators are used to achieve the desired hemodynamic goals. Sodium nitroprusside is a direct-acting vasodilator with relatively balanced effects on arterial and venous beds, thereby decreasing both arteriolar and venous tone. The hemodynamic effects of sodium nitroprusside are characterized by a substantial decrease in systemic vascular resistance, pulmonary vascular resistance, and pulmonary artery pressure.[29] There is also a significant reduction in right atrial and pulmonary capillary wedge pressure along with an increase in stroke volume and cardiac output. In patients with heart failure, the heart rate usually remains unchanged or may decrease. If the increase in cardiac output is proportional to the decrease in systemic vascular resistance, the mean arterial pressure usually remains unchanged. In clinical practice, however, there is usually some reduction in systolic blood pressure as well as in mean arterial pressure. Indeed, with large doses of sodium nitroprusside the blood pressure may fall substantially owing to marked peripheral vasodilatation, decreased systemic vascular resistance, and inadequately increased cardiac output. The initial dose therefore should be low (5–10, μg/min), and the dose should be increased gradually by 5–10 μg/min every 10–15 minutes; the hemodynamic goals are to maximize the increase in cardiac output and the decrease in pulmonary capillary wedge and right atrial pressures. During dose titration, if there is a substantial reduction in arterial pressure, lower doses should be used to maintain improved hemodynamics.

Nitroglycerin and other nitrates are endothelium-independent vasodilators, although vasodilatation is mediated by the guanosine monophospate–cyclic nitric oxide (GMP-NO) pathway. These agents are predominantly venodilators and cause a substantial reduction in pulmonary capillary wedge, right atrial, and pulmonary artery pressures.[29] Pulmonary vascular resistance also falls in most patients. Nitroglycerin, when given intravenously, increases the compliance of the conduit vessels and improves ventriculoaortic coupling, which facilitates left ventricular ejection. Thus with nitroglycerin, particularly when administered intravenously, there may be an increase in stroke volume and cardiac output. The net hemodynamic effects, however, depend on the relative decrease in left ventricular preload and afterload. It must be appreciated that when pulmonary capillary wedge pressure falls to less than 15 mmHg in patients with chronic left ventricular failure, the cardiac output may not decrease. This lack of decrease in cardiac output associated with a significant reduction in pulmonary capillary wedge pressure is due not only to a concomitant decrease in left ventricular outflow resistance (which increases stroke volume) but to improved left ventricular compliance resulting from ventricular interaction related to decompression of the right ventricle. In clinical practice, nitroglycerin and nitroprusside can be combined to optimize the reduction in pulmonary capillary wedge and right atrial pressure while maintaining cardiac output.

In hypotensive patients with a systolic blood pressure of less than 80–85 mmHg, vasodilators such as sodium nitroprusside or nitroglycerin usually cause a further reduction in arterial pressure and therefore cannot be used initially without concomitant vasopressors, such as norepinephrine, phenylephrine, methoxamine, or large doses of dopamine. Frequently in these patients it is also necessary to use a positive inotropic agent such as dobutamine initially before vasodilator therapy can be instituted. Instead of adding vasodilators such as nitroprusside, addition of a phosphodiesterase inhibitor is likely to produce the same hemodynamic changes. In some patients, however, a vasopressor, an inotropic agent such as dobutamine, an inodilator such as milrinone, and a vasodilator (nitroprusside or nitroglycerin) must be combined to optimize hemodynamic improvements. Addition of diuretics is almost always necessary to decrease right atrial and pulmonary capillary wedge pressures to the desired levels. It is apparent that without hemodynamic monitoring and assessing hemodynamic response of a given therapeutic strategy, hemodynamic tailored therapy is not feasible.

After optimizing the hemodynamic changes with an intravenous vasodilator, inotropic vasopressor, and inodilator therapy, nonparenteral vasodilators such as hydralazine, isosorbide dinitrate, and ACE inhibitors are slowly substituted to maintain the hemodynamic improvement. In many patients the use of nonparenteral phosphodiesterase inhibitors, if available, is helpful for weaning the patient from intravenous therapy and maintaining hemodynamic improvement. The potential clinical problems of such aggressive hemodynamic tailored therapy are hypotension and deterioration of renal function. Thus in addition to hemodynamic monitoring, monitoring renal function and electrolytes is required. The potential pharmacotherapeutic interventions to optimize hemodynamic improvement in patients with refractory heart failure are summarized in Tables 54-2 to 54-5.

Intractable Volume Overload: Therapeutic Approaches

Aggressive diuretic therapy is frequently necessary for the treatment of intractable volume overload.[81,147,148] Refractory congestive heart failure associated with severe right heart failure and volume overload can often be treated by optimizing diuretic therapy. Because bowel wall edema occurs during

Table 54-2. Refractory Heart Failure: Therapeutic Options

Refractory to adequate "triple therapy," but stable
  Evaluate response to combination vasodilator therapy.
  Consider β-blocker therapy (particularly in patients with adequate blood pressure, tachycardia, and evidence of elevated left ventricular diastolic pressure.
  Consider addition of amlodipine in selected patients (particularly in patients with nonischemic cardiomyopathy, hypertension, or unable to tolerate β-blockers).
  Consider low-dose amiodarone in patients with tachycardia, intolerance of β-blockers, or unresponsiveness to β-blocker therapy.

Refractory to adequate "triple therapy," but unstable or refractory to adequate "triple therapy" and β-blocker, amiodarone, or amlodipine
  Hemodynamic monitoring and "tailored therapy."
  Prolonged or intermittent intravenous positive inotropic therapy.

Table 54-3. Tailored Therapy Based on Hemodynamic Profile and Hemodynamic Response to (Intravenous) Therapy

Hemodynamic goals
  Pulmonary capillary wedge pressure (PCWP) $\leq$ 15 mmHg
  Right atrial pressure (RAP) $\leq$ 8 mmHg
  Systemic vascular resistance (SVR) $\leq$ 1200 dynes$\cdot$s$^{-1}\cdot$cm^{-1}
  Systolic blood pressure (SBP) $\geq$ 80 mmHg
  Cardiac index (CI) $\geq$ 2.2 L$\cdot$min$^{-1}\cdot$sq m^{-1}

If PCWP $\uparrow$, RAP $\uparrow$, SVR $\uparrow$, SBP $\uparrow\leftrightarrow$, CI $\downarrow$, initial treatment:
  Increase doses of intravenous sodium nitroprusside (5 μg/min every 10 minutes) until hemodynamic goals are achieved or unacceptable hypotension (SBP $\leq$ 80 mmHg) develops.

With sodium nitroprusside infusion, if PCWP and RAP remain elevated with adequate increase in CI and decrease in SVR:
  Diuretics and/or nitroglycerin (5 μg/min IV initial dose, increased by 5 μg/min every 10 minutes).

With sodium nitroprusside infusion, if CI remains low with adequate decrease in PCWP and RAP:
  Add dobutamine (2.5–10.0 μg$\cdot$kg$^{-1}\cdot$min^{-1}) or milrinone (0.3–1.0 mg/min) and titrate doses of dobutamine and milrinone to avoid hypotension and excessive reduction in SVR.

If PCWP $\uparrow$, RAP $\uparrow$, SVR$\leftrightarrow$ or $\uparrow$, SBP $\leq$ 80 mmHg, CI $\downarrow$:
  Initial treatment is dobutamine.
  If increase in CI is inadequate, add milrinone.
  If BP $\downarrow$, add norepinephrine or phenylephrine.
  If PCWP $\uparrow$ persists, add nitroglycerin and/or diuretics.

Table 54-4. Tailored Therapy for Refractory Heart Failure: Following Intravenous Therapy

1. Maintain the best achievable hemodynamic response with intravenous vasodilators, inotropic agents, and/or vasopressors for 24–48 hours.
2. While on intravenous therapy, restart angiotensin-converting enzyme (ACE) inhibitors (initially low doses, increasing gradually as the intravenous drugs are weaned).
3. Add oral hydralazine and/or isosorbide mononitrate or dinitrate, starting with low doses and increasing as tolerated to maintain optimal hemodynamic responses.
4. Replace intravenous diuretics by equivalent doses of oral diuretics.
5. Maintain digoxin levels at 1.0–2.0 ng/dl if no contraindication.
6. Consider oral amiodarone in patients with atrial fibrillation with rapid ventricular response or with sinus tachycardia (heart rate > 90 bpm).
7. Conduct detailed patient education, including sodium restriction and keeping records of weight changes.
8. Adjust diuretics, ACE inhibitors, and vasodilators on an outpatient basis.
9. Initiate a progressive walking program.
10. Maintain frequent outpatient follow-up to assess changes in clinical status, renal function, and electrolytes.

Table 54-5. Worsening or Recurrent Exacerbation of Heart Failure Despite Tailored Therapy

1. Cardiac transplantation in appropriate patients.
2. When cardiac transplantation is not feasible:
   a. In absence of volume overload: intermittent dobutamine or milrinone infusion, and preferably concomitant amiodarone therapy.
   b. In selected patients with significant mitral and/or tricuspid regurgitation with prolonged P-R interval: DDD pacing with shorter A-V interval.
   c. Noncardiac transplant surgery such as cardiomyoplasty or mitral valve annuloplasty—in selected patients.
   d. In the presence of volume overload:
      (1) Initially aggressive diuretic therapy with sequential nephron blockade (loop diuretics, metolazone, aldosterone antagonists).
      (2) In refractory patients: ultrafiltration, hemodialysis, arteriovenous hemofiltration, peritoneal dialysis in selected patients.

decompensated congestive heart failure with elevated systemic venous pressure, absorption of oral diuretics is impaired. Diuresis can often be restored by intravenous administration of diuretics. Other causes of diuretic resistance during refractory congestive heart failure include diminished renal function, the use of NSAIDs, distal renal tubular hypertrophy with increased sodium and chloride reabsorption, and noncompliance.[147]

The diuretic of choice is a loop diuretic that inhibits chloride reabsorption in the thick ascending loop of the Henle. Sodium reabsorption is concomitantly inhibited. Loop diuretics should be increased until the desired physiologic effects are achieved without compromising renal function. In the presence of impaired renal function, large doses of loop diuretics are necessary and often effective. The use of continuous intravenous furosemide or bumetinide is sometimes more effective than intermittent bolus administration of these drugs.[149,150] The combination of diuretic agents with different modes and different sites of action on the nephron are sometimes necessary to enhance diuresis in patients with intractable peripheral edema and ascites. Thiazide diuretics such as metolazone and intravenous chlorothiazide act at the distal tubal and produce synergistic effects with loop diuretics. Potassium-sparing diuretics, such as spironolactone, triamterene, and amiloride, act in the distal nephron. The addition of potassium-sparing diuretics to the loop diuretics and thiazides not only promotes diuresis but also counteracts the potassium-wasting effect of the loop and thiazide diuretics. If combined sequential nephron blockade with different diuretics is inadequate to achieve the desired physiologic endpoints, diuresis can be sometimes be restored with the addition of low dose captopril or low dose dopamine.[151–154]

Despite the use of combined sequential nephron blockade, diuretic resistance may persist in patients with refractory heart failure. Such persistence may be related to decreased cardiac output, which reduces effective renal plasma flow and therefore the glomerular filtration rate. There is also enhanced reabsorption of sodium and water associated with decreased sodium load to the tubules. In these circumstances, diuresis can be improved only by increasing cardiac output. In some patients, renal function continues to deteriorate with inadequate diuresis despite maintaining arterial pressure and adequate cardiac output. In these patients with so-called cardiorenal syndrome, vasoconstriction of the afferent and efferent renal arterioles might be the pathophysiologic mechanism. No effective treatment is available for such patients, except the use of mechanical means of fluid removal.

Large volumes of excess body water can be rapidly removed by ultrafiltration or hemodialysis or more slowly by continuous arteriovenous hemofiltration with or without dialysis or chronic ambulatory peritoneal dialysis.[155–159] Patients with refractory congestive heart failure and systemic hypotension can undergo ultrafiltration or hemodialysis while the arterial pressure is being supported with vasopressor agents. Mechanical fluid removal, particularly by ultrafiltration, can produce beneficial hemodynamic effects, such as a decrease in right atrial and pulmonary capillary wedge pressure with little or no change in cardiac output or arterial pressure. Ultrafiltration may also promote a sustained autodiuresis and more favorable water balance, which may be related to a decrease in plasma norepinephrine, plasma renin activity, and plasma aldosterone levels. Ultrafiltration usually provides significant relief of congestive symptoms, probably resulting from a reduction in right atrial and pulmonary capillary wedge pressures. Ultrafiltration has been also reported to produce sustained hemodynamic and neurohormonal improvement in patients with congestive heart failure.[155] It should be appreciated, however, that not all patients with refractory heart failure with volume overload respond to mechanical fluid removal. There is also no evidence to indicate that in patients with refractory heart failure ultrafiltration provides any survival benefits.

Dual Chamber Pacing

In patients with chronic congestive heart failure, ventricular dilatation and altered geometry is frequently associated with malfunctioning of the AV valves, producing mitral and tricuspid regurgitation. Mitral and tricuspid regurgitation occur not only during systole but may also be seen at the end of atrial systole: so-called presystolic or diastolic ventriculoatrial regurgitation. In patients with a prolonged P-R interval, diastolic mitral or tricuspid regurgitation can result in shortening of the ventricular filling time, diminished stroke volume, and decreased forward cardiac output. AV sequential (DDD) pacing has been proposed to shorten the P-R interval, decrease AV valve regurgitation, improve ventricular filling, and increase forward cardiac output.[160–164] In a few selected patients, AV sequential pacing with relatively shorter P-R interval has been shown to improve hemodynamics and cardiac performance.[164] However, substantial shortening of the P-R interval may be associated with worse hemodynamics and a reduction in forward stroke volume and cardiac output.[165] Furthermore, in prospective controlled studies in which the P-R interval was varied by programming the DDD pacemaker modes, there was no significant difference in hemodynamic changes and left ventricular function.[166] Presently, therefore, DDD pacing should be considered only for patients with obvious mitral and tricuspid regurgitation and a prolonged P-R interval. Furthermore, the hemodynamic changes and changes in ventricular, systolic, and diastolic function should be evaluated during temporary AV sequential pacing before a permanent pacemaker can be recommended.

Ventricular Tachyarrhythmias and Sudden Death

The incidence of sudden death in patients with heart failure due to systolic dysfunction is approximately 50 percent, and it is presumed that in most patients it results from ventricular tachycardia and fibrillation.[167] It should be appreciated, however, that in about 20–25 percent of patients sudden death syndrome results from advanced AV block or electromechanical dissociation. Pharmacotherapy to prevent recurrence of symptomatic sustained ventricular tachycardia in patients with heart failure primarily consists of the use of amiodarone[168] (Table 54-6).

Table 54-6. Management of Dysrhythmias Contributing to Refractory Heart Failure

Atrial fibrillation or atrial flutter with rapid ventricular response
  Initially amiodarone
  DC cardioversion after adequate anticoagulation
  If successful, long term/low dose amiodarone therapy
Refractory atrial flutter or fibrillation
  Flutter ablation or AV nodal ablation with pacemaker therapy
Sustained recurrent monomorphic ventricular tachycardia
  Without sudden death: initially amiodarone; with suspected bundle branch tachycardia: bundle branch ablation; for refractory ventricular tachycardia: AICD.
  After "sudden death" due to monomorphic or polymorphous ventricular tachycardia: preferably AICD as a bridge to cardiac transplantation, followed by amiodarone therapy.
Unacceptable noniatrogenic bradycardia or advanced AV block.
  Preferably dual chamber rate-responsive pacemaker therapy

Abbreviations: AV, atrioventricular; AICD, automatic, implantable cardioverter defibrillator.

Other class III antiarrhythmic drugs (e.g., sotalol) or type I drugs are either ineffective or cannot be used because of their proarrhythmic and cardiodepressant effects. Nonpharmacologic therapy in these patients consists of use of the automatic implantable cardioverter defibrillator (AICD).[169–172] Uncontrolled prospective studies indicate that AICDs may improve survival in patients with congestive heart failure, sustained symptomatic ventricular tachyarrhythmias, or sudden cardiac death. In patients with severe congestive heart failure (NYHA functional class III or IV) and malignant ventricular arrhythmia AICDs have been reported to be superior to amiodarone in preventing recurrence of ventricular tachycardia and sudden death and therefore have been recommended in such patients as a bridge to a heart transplant.[173] It must be emphasized, however, that no prospective controlled studies have confirmed the potential beneficial effect of AICDs in reducing the incidence of overall mortality or of sudden death in patients with refractory heart failure, and these patients continue to experience high mortality even after device implantation. Therefore such therapy cannot be recommended for all patients; it should be used only in selected patients with a refractory ventricular tachyarrhythmia despite adequate pharmacotherapy with amiodarone.

Patients with advanced heart block or electromechanical dissociation who survive these catastrophic complications should be treated with pacemaker therapy. In addition, these patients frequently require antiarrhythmia therapy with amiodarone because ventricular tachyarrhythmias and bradyarrhythmias often coexist in patients with severe refractory heart failure. In patients with dilated cardiomyopathy who present with ventricular tachycardia with QRS morphology of left bundle branch block pattern, bundle branch block tachycardia should be suspected, particularly in those patients in whom the electrocardiogram reveals the presence of intraventricular conduction defect of left bundle branch type.[174] In these patients, electrophysiologic studies should be considered to identify the mechanism of ventricular tachycardia; and if bundle branch block tachycardia is confirmed, catheter ablation of right bundle branch should be attempted, as it provides a nonpharmacologic cure of ventricular tachycardia.

CONCLUSION

All patients with suspected refractory congestive heart failure should be thoroughly evaluated for the presence of reversible and treatable causes. Frequently, hemodynamic monitoring is necessary to optimize the hemodynamic improvements with the use of a combination of vasodilators, inotropic agents, and inodilators. The goals of treatment of refractory heart failure are primarily palliation of heart failure symptoms, and improvement in the quality of life, although often no survival benefit is expected without cardiac transplantation. Another objective of treatment of refractory heart failure in selected patients is to stabilize hemodynamics and reverse vital organ dysfunction as a bridge to cardiac transplantation. For many patients the complicating factors such as ventricular arrhythmias, atrial fibrillation and flutter, and bradyarrhythmias can be effectively treated and short-term improvement can be expected. There is no simple treatment algorithm that would apply to every patient with refractory congestive heart failure. Each individual patient should be thoroughly investigated in terms of hemodynamic abnormalities, changes in left ventricular function, and evidence of impaired organ perfusion. Therapy should be directed to correct these abnormalities.

REFERENCES

1. Cody RJ, Kubo, SH: Diuretic treatment for the sodium retention of congestive heart failure. Arch Int Med 1994;54:1905–1914.
2. Bayliss J, Norell M, Canea-Anson R et al: Untreated heart failure. Clinical and neuroendocrine effects of introducing diuretics. Br Heart J 1987;57:17–22
3. Ikram H, Chan W, Espinar EA et al: Hemodynamic and hormone responses to acute and chronic furosemide therapy in congestive heart failure. Clin Sci 1980;59:443–449
4. Francis GS, Siegel RM, Goldsmith SR et al: Acute vasoconstrictor response to intravenous furosemide in patients with chronic congestive heart failure. Activation of the neurohumoral axis. Ann Intern Med 1985;103:1–6
5. SOLVD Investigators: Effect of enalapril on survival in patients with reduced left ventricular ejection fractions and congestive heart failure. N Engl J Med 1991;325:293–302
6. CONSENSUS Trial Study Group: Effects of enalapril on mortality in severe congestive heart failure. Results of the Cooperative North Scandinavian Enalapril Survival Study. N Engl J Med 1987;316: 1429–1435
7. SOLVD Investigators: Effect of enalapril on mortality and the development of heart failure in asymptomatic patients with reduced left ventricular ejection fractions. N Engl J Med 1993;327:685–691
8. Cohn JN, Archibald DG, Ziesche S et al: Effects of vasodilator therapy on mortality in chronic congestive heart failure. Results of a Veterans Administration cooperative study. N Engl J Med 1986;314: 1547–1552
9. Cohn JN, Johnson G, Ziesche S et al: A comparison of enalapril with hydralazine-isosorbide dinitrate in the treatment of chronic congestive heart failure. N Engl J Med 1991;325:303–310
10. Uretsky BF, Young JB, Shahidi FE et al: Randomized study assessing the effect of digoxin withdrawal in patients with mild to moderate chronic congestive heart failure. Results of the PROVED trial. J Am Coll Cardiol 1993;22:955–962
11. Packer M, Gheorghiade M, Young JB et al: Withdrawal of digoxin from patients with chronic heart failure treated with angiotensin-converting-enzyme inhibitors (RADIANCE). N Engl J Med 1993;329:1–7
12. Digitalis Investigators Group: Results of the Digitalis Investigators Group trial. Presented at the 45th annual scientific sessions of the American College of Cardiology, Orlando, March 1996
13. Messner-Pellenc P, Ximenes C, Brasileiro CF et al: Cardiopulmonary exercise testing. Determinants of dyspnea due to cardiac or pulmonary limitation. Chest 1994;106:354–360
14. Minotti JR, Dudley G: Pathophysiology of exercise intolerance and the role of exercise training in congestive heart failure. Curr Opin Cardiol 1993;8: 397–403
15. Packer M: The neurohormonal hypothesis. A theory to explain the mechanisms of disease progression in heart failure. J Am Coll Cardiol 1992;20:248–254
16. Chatterjee K, Viquerat CE, Daly P: Neurohormonal abnormalities in heart failure. Heart Failure 1985;1: 69–83
17. Levine B, Kalman J, Mayer L et al: Elevated circulating levels of tumor necrosis factor in severe chronic heart failure. N Engl J Med 1990;323:236–241
18. Dash H, Lipton MJ, Parmley WW, Chaterjee K: Estimation of pulmonary wedge pressure from chest radiograph in patients with chronic congestive cardiomyopathy. Br Heart J 1990;44:322–329
19. Davies SW, Gailey J, Keegan J et al: Reduced pulmonary microvascular permeability in severe chronic left heart failure. Am Heart J 1992;124:137–142
20. Gradman AH, Deedwania PC: Predictors of mortality in patients with heart failure. Cardiol Clin 1994;12: 25–35
21. Pinamonti B, Di Lenarda A, Sinagra G et al: Restrictive left ventricular filling pattern in dilated cardiomyopathy assessed by Doppler echocardiography. Clinical, echocardiographic and hemodynamic correlations and prognostic implications. J Am Coll Cardiol 1993;22:808–815
22. Rockman HA, Juneau C, Chatterjee K, Rouleau JL: Long-term predictors of sudden and low output death in chronic congestive heart failure secondary to coronary artery disease. Am J Cardiol 1989;64: 1344–1348
23. Cohn JN, Levine TB, Olivari MT et al: Plasma norepinephrine as a guide to prognosis in patients with chronic congestive heart failure. N Engl J Med 1984; 311:819–823
24. White M, Rouleau JL, Ruddy RD et al: Decreased coronary sinus oxygen content. A predictor of adverse prognosis in patients with severe congestive heart failure. J Am Coll Cardiol 1991;18:1631–1637
25. Stevenson LW, Tillisch JH, Hamilton M et al: Importance of hemodynamic response to therapy in predicting survival with ejection fraction < 20% secondary to ischemic or nonischemic dilated cardiomyopathy. Am J Cardiol 1990;66:1348–1354

26. Cohn JN, Levine TB, Olivari MT et al: Plasma norepinephrine as a guide to prognosis in patients with chronic congestive heart failure. N Engl J Med 1984; 311:819–823

27. Swedberg K, Eneroth P, Kjekshus J et al: Hormones regulating cardiovascular function in patients with severe congestive heart failure and their relation to mortality. Circulation 1990;82:1730–1736

28. O'Connell JB, Bourge RC, Costanzo-Nordin MR et al: Cardiac transplantation. Recipient selection, donor procurement and medical follow-up. Circulation 1992;86:1061–1079

29. Chatterjee K: Combination therapy in congestive heart failure. pp. 1566–1585. In Messerli FH (ed): Cardiovascular Drug Therapy. WB Saunders, Philadelphia, 1990

30. Elkayam U, Amin J, Mehra A et al: A prospective, randomized, double-blind cross-over study to compare the efficacy and safety of chronic nifedipine therapy with that of isosorbide dinitrate and their combination in the treatment of chronic congestive heart failure. Circulation 1990;82:1954–1961

31. Multicenter Diltiazem Post-Infarction Trial Research Group: The effect of diltiazem on mortality and reinfarction after myocardial infarction. N Engl J Med 1988;319:385–392

32. Schofer J, Hobuss M, Aschenberg W et al: Acute and long-term hemodynamic and neurohumoral response to nisoldipine vs. captopril in patients with heart failure. A randomized double-blind study. Eur Heart J 1990;11:712–721

33. Goldstein RE, Boccuzzi SJ, Cruess D et al: Diltiazem increases late onset congestive heart failure in post-infarction patients with early reduction in ejection fraction. Circulation 1991;83:52–60

34. Elkayam U, Roth A, Hsueh W et al: Neurohumoral consequences of vasodilator therapy with hydralazine and nifedipine in severe congestive heart failure. Am Heart J 1986;111:1130

35. Francis GS: Calcium channel blockers and congestive heart failure. Circulation 1991;83:336

36. O'Connor CM, Belkin RN, Carson PE et al. Effect of amlodipine on mode of death in severe chronic heart failure. The PRAISE trial [abstract]. Circulation, Suppl. I 1995;92:143

37. Cohn JN, Zeische SM, Loss LE et al: Effect of felodipine on short-term exercise and neurohormone and long-term mortality in heart failure. Results of V-HEFT III [abstract]. Circulation, suppl. I 1995;92:143

38. Eichorn EJ: The paradox of β-adrenergic blockade for the management of congestive heart failure. Am J Med 1992;92:527–538

39. Reichenbach DD, Benditt EP: Catecholamines and cardiomyopathy. The pathogenesis and potential importance of myofibrillar degeneration. Hum Pathol 1970;1:125–149

40. Haft JI: Cardiovascular injury induced by sympathetic catecholamines. Prog Cardiovasc Dis 1974;17:73–85

41. Bristow MR, Port JD, Sandoval AB et al: β-Adrenergic receptor pathways in the failing human heart. Heart Failure 1989;5:77–90

42. Kaye DM, Lefkovits J, Jennings GL et al. Adverse consequences of high sympathetic nervous activity in the failing human heart. J Am Coll Cardiol 1995;26:1257–1263

43. Swedberg K, Viquerat C, Rouleau JL et al: Comparison of myocardial catecholamine balance in chronic congestive heart failure and in angina pectoris without failure. Am J Cardiol 1984;54:783

44. Hasking GJ, Esler MD, Jennings GL et al: Norepinephrine spillover to plasma in patients with congestive heart failure. Evidence of increased overall and cardiorenal sympathetic nervous activity. Circulation 1986;73:615

45. Ferguson DW, Berg WJ, Sanders JS: Clinical and hemodynamic correlates of sympathetic nerve activity in normal humans and patients with heart failure. Evidence from direct microneurographic recordings. J Am Coll Cardiol 1990;16:1125–1134

46. Kinugawa T, Dibner-Dunlap ME: Altered vagal and sympathetic control of heart rate in conscious dogs with left ventricular dysfunction and heart failure. Am J Physiol 1995;268:R310–R316

47. Bristow MR, Ginsburg R, Minobe W et al: Decreased catecholamine sensitivity and β-adrenergic receptor density in failing human hearts. N Engl J Med 1982; 307:205–211

48. Fowler MB, Laser JA, Hopkins GL, Minobe W, Bristow MR: Assessment of the β-adrenergic receptor pathway in the intact failing human heart. Progressive receptor down-regulation and subsensitivity to agonist response. Circulation 1986;74:1290–1302

49. Heilbrunn S, Shah P, Bristow M et al: Increased β-receptor density and improved response to catecholamine stimulation during long-term metoprolol therapy in heart failure from dilated cardiomyopathy. Circulation 1989;79:483–490

50. Fowler MB, Bristow MR, Laser JA: Beta-blocker therapy in severe heart failure. Improvement related to beta1-adrenergic receptor up regulation? Circulation, suppl. 2 1984;70:112–116

51. Eichhorn EJ, Bedotto J, Malloy CR et al: Effect of β-adrenergic blockade on myocardial function and energetics in congestive heart failure. Improvements in hemodynamic, contractile, and diastolic performance with bucindolol. Circulation 1989;82:473–483

52. Andersson B, Blomstrom-Lundqvist C, Hedner T, Waagstein F: Exercise hemodynamics and myocardial metabolism during long-term beta-adrenergic blockade in severe heart failure. J Am Coll Cardiol 1991;18:1059–1066

53. Waagstein F, Caidahl K, Wallentin I et al: Long-term β-blockade in dilated cardiomyopathy. Effects of short- and long-term metoprolol treatment followed by withdrawal and re-administration of metoprolol. Circulation 1989;80:551–563

54. Nemanich JW, Veith RC, Abrass JB, Stratton JR: Effects of metoprolol on rest and exercise cardiac function and plasma catecholamines in chronic congestive heart failure secondary to ischemic or idiopathic cardiomyopathy. Am J Cardiol 1990;66:843–848

55. Engelmeier RS, O'Connell JB, Walsh RW et al: Improvement in symptoms and exercise tolerance by metoprolol in patients with dilated cardiomyopathy. A double-blind, randomized, placebo-controlled trial. Circulation 1985;72:536–546

56. Leung WH, Lau CP, Wong CK et al: Improvement in exercise performance and hemodynamics by labetolol

in patients with idiopathic dilated cardiomyopathy. Am Heart J 1990;119:884–890

57. Anderson JL, Lutz JR, Gilbert EM et al: A randomized trial of low-dose beta-blockade therapy for idiopathic dilated cardiomyopathy. Am J Cardiol 1985; 55:471–475

58. Gilbert EM, Anderson JL, Dietchman D et al: Chronic β-blocker-vasodilator therapy improves cardiac function in idiopathic dilated cardiomyopathy. A double-blind, randomized study of bucindolol versus placebo. Am J Med 1990;88:223–229

59. Pollock SG, Lytash J, Tedesco C, Craddock G, Smucker ML: Usefulness of bucindolol in congestive heart failure. Am J Cardiol 1990;66:603–607

60. Woodley SL, Gilbert EM, Anderson JL et al: β-Blockade with bucindolol in heart failure due to ischemic vs. idiopathic dilated cardiomyopathy. Circulation 1991;84:2426–2441

61. Das Gupta P, Broadhurst P, Raftery EB et al: Value of carvedilol in congestive heart failure secondary to coronary artery disease. Am J Cardiol 1990;66: 1118–1123

62. Wisenbaugh T, Katz I, Davis J et al: Long-term (3 month) effects of a new beta blocker (nebivolol) in cardiac performance in patients with dilated cardiomyopathy. J Am Coll Cardiol 1993;21:1094–1100

63. Chatterjee K: Potential use of third-generation β-blockers in heart failure. J Cardiovasc Pharmacol, suppl. 7 1989;14:S22

64. Olsen SL, Gilbert EM, Renlund DG et al: Carvedilol improves left ventricular function and symptoms in chronic heart failure. A double-blind randomized study. J Am Coll Cardiol 1995;25:1225–1231

65. Feldman MD, Gwathmey JK, Phillips P et al: Reversal of the force-frequency relationship in working myocardium from patients with end-stage heart failure. J Appl Cardiol 1988;3:273–283

66. Pieske B, Kretschmann B, Meyer M et al. Alterations in intracellular calcium handling associated with the inverse force-frequency relation in human dilated cardiomyopathy. Circulation 1995;92:1169–1178

67. Yamakawa H, Takeuchi M, Takaoka H et al: Beneficial effect of negative chronotropic action with β-blockade on cardiac energetics in patients with heart failure [abstract]. Circulation, suppl. I 1995;92:394

68. Van der Ent M, Van den H, Reeme WJ et al: Neurohumoral modulation by chronic beta-blockade in moderate to severe heart failure depends on baseline adrenergic activity. A CIBIS study [abstract]. Circulation, suppl. I 1995;92:395

69. Newton GE, Parker JD: β_1 vs non-selective β-blockade in human congestive heart failure. Acute effects on cardiac sympathetic activity [abstract]. Circulation, suppl. I 1995;92:395

70. Henlova MJ, Freudenberger RS, Mannino MM et al: Changes in right ventricular function after beta-blockers in patients with congestive heart failure [abstract]. Circulation, suppl. I 1995;92:395

71. Sharpe N, MacMahon S: Effects of 12 months treatment with carvedilol on left ventricular function and exercise performance in patients with heart failure of ischemic etiology [abstract]. Circulation, suppl. I 1995;92:142

72. Packer M, Bristow MR, Cohn JN et al: Effect of carvedilol on the survival of patients with chronic heart failure [abstract]. Circulation, suppl. I 1995;92: 142

73. Bristow MR, Gilbert EM, Abraham WT et al: Multicenter oral carvedilol heart failure assessment (MOCHA). A six-month dose-response evaluation in class II-IV patients [abstract]. Circulation, suppl. I 1995;92:142

74. Packer M, Colucci WS, Sackner-Bernstein J et al: Prospective randomized evaluation of carvedilol on symptoms and exercise tolerance in chronic heart failure. Results of the PRECISE trial [abstract]. Circulation, suppl. I 1995;92:143

75. Colucci WS, Packer M, Bristow MR et al: Carvedilol inhibits clinical progression with mild heart failure [abstract]. Circulation, suppl. I 1995;92:395

76. Ikram H, Fitzpatrick D: Double-blind trial of chronic oral beta-blockade in congestive cardiomyopathy. Lancet 1981;2:490–493

77. Chadda K, Goldstein S, Byington R, Curb JD: Effect of propranolol after acute myocardial infarction in patients with congestive heart failure. Circulation 1986;73:503–510

78. Kennedy HL, Barker A, Brooks MM et al: Beta-blocker therapy and mortality in the cardiac arrhythmia suppression trial (CAST) [abstract]. Circulation, suppl. I 1992;86:403

79. Waagstein F, Bristow MR, Swedberg K et al: Beneficial effects of metoprolol in idiopathic dilated cardiomyopathy. Lancet 1993;342:1142–1146

80. Lechat P, Jaillon P, Fontaine ML et al: A randomized trial of beta-blockade in heart failure. The cardiac insufficiency bisiprolol study (CIBIS). Circulation 1994;90:1765–1773

81. Chatterjee K, De Marco T: Treatment of symptomatic heart failure. In: Dhalla NS, Beamish RE, Takeda N, Nagano M (eds): The Failing Heart. Lippincott-Raven, Philadelphia, 1995

82. Terce MA, Jessup M: β-Adrenergic blockade in patients with chronic heart failure. Issues and answers. Prim Cardiol 1994;20:33–38

83. Hall SA, Cigarroa CG, Marcoux L et al: Time course of improvement in left ventricular function, mass, and geometry in patients with congestive heart failure treated with beta-adrenergic blockade. J Am Coll Cardiol 1995;25:1154–1161

84. Eichhorn EC, Heesch CM, Risser RC et al: Predictors of systolic and diastolic improvement in patients with dilated cardiomyopathy treated with metoprolol. J Am Coll Cardiol 1995;25:154–162

85. Nademanee K: The amiodarone odyssey. J Am Coll Cardiol 1992;20:1063–1065

86. Nattel S, Talajic M, Fermini B, Roy D: Amiodarone. Pharmacology, clinical actions, and relationship between them. J Cardiovasc Electrophysiol 1992;3: 266–280

87. Nademanee K, Piwonka RW, Singh BN, Hershman JM: Amiodarone and thyroid function. Prog Cardiovasc Dis 1989;31:427–437

88. Shaikh NA, Dounar E, Butany J: Amiodarone—an inhibitor of phospholipase activity. A comparative study of the inhibitory effects of amiodarone, chloroquin, and chlorpromazine. Mol Cell Biochem 1987; 76:163–172

89. Haworth RA, Goknur AB, Berkoff HA: Inhibition of ATP-sensitive potassium channels of adult rate heart

cells by antiarrhythmic drugs. Circulation 1989;65:1157–1160

90. Galli FC, De Marco T, Chatterjee K: Does amiodarone improve survival of patients with refractory heart failure due to dilated cardiomyopathy [abstract]. Clin Res 1994;42:38A

91. Hamer AWR, Arkles LB, Johns JA: Beneficial effects of low dose amiodarone in patients with congestive cardiac failure. A placebo-controlled trial. J Am Coll Cardiol 1989;14:1768–1774

92. Schwartz A, Shen E, Morady F et al: Hemodynamic effects of intravenous amiodarone in patients with depressed left ventricular function and recurrent ventricular tachycardia. Am Heart J 1993;106:848–856

93. Gottlieb SS, Riggio DW, Lauria S et al: High dose oral amiodarone loading exerts important hemodynamic actions in patients with congestive heart failure. J Am Coll Cardiol 1994;23:560–564

94. Massie BM, Fisher SG, Deedwania PC et al: Effect of amiodarone on clinical status and left ventricular function in patients with congestive heart failure. Circulation 1996;93:2128–2134

95. Neri R, Mestroni L, Salvi A, Pandulla C, Camerini F: Ventricular arrhythmias in dilated cardiomyopathy. Efficacy of amiodarone. Am Heart J 1987;113:707–715

96. Nicklas JM, McKenna WJ, Stewart RA et al: Prospective, double-blind, placebo-controlled trial of low-dose amiodarone in patients with severe heart failure and asymptomatic frequent ventricular ectopy. Am Heart J 1991;122:1016–1021

97. Doval HC, Nul DR, Grancelli HO et al: Randomized trial of low-dose amiodarone in severe congestive heart failure. Lancet 1994;344:493–498

98. Singh SN, Fletcher RD, Fisher SG et al: Amiodarone in patients with congestive heart failure and asymptomatic ventricular tachycardia. N Engl J Med 1995;333:77–92

99. Nul DR, Doval HC, Grancelli HO et al: Heart rate is a marker of amiodarone mortality reduction in severe heart failure [abstract]. Circulation, suppl. I 1995;92:666

100. Dristas A, Ciaramella F, Oakley C, Nihoyannopoulos P: Beat-to-beat hemodynamics during atrial fibrillation. Observations in normal and impaired left ventricular function. J Am Coll Cardiol 1994;23:416A

101. Naito M, Daniel D, Michelson EL, Schaffenburg M, Dreifus LS: The hemodynamic consequences of cardiac arrhythmias. Evaluation of the relative roles of abnormal atrioventricular sequencing, irregularity of ventricular rhythm and atrial fibrillation in a canine model. Am Heart J 1983;106:284–291

102. Grogan M, Smith HC, Gersh B, Wood DL: Left ventricular dysfunction due to atrial fibrillation in patients initially believed to have idiopathic dilated cardiomyopathy. Am J Cardiol 1992;69:1570–1573

103. Phillips E, Levine SA: Auricular fibrillation without other evidence of heart disease. A cause of reversible heart failure. Am J Med 1949;7:478–489

104. Tamita M, Spinale FG, Crawford FA, Zile MR: Changes in left ventricular volume, mass and function during the development and regression of supraventricular tachycardia-induced cardiomyopathy. Disparity between recovery of systolic versus diastolic function. Circulation 1991;83:635–644

105. Holinloser SH, Klingenheben T, Singh BN: Amiodarone-associated proarrhythmic effects. A review with special reference to torsade de pointes tachycardia. Ann Intern Med 1994;121:529–533

106. Borowski GD, Garofano CD, Rose LI et al: Effect of long-term amiodarone therapy on thyroid hormone levels and thyroid function. Am J Med 1985;78:443–460

107. Scheinman MM, Morady F, Hess DS, Gonzalez R: Catheter-induced ablation of the atrioventricular junction to control refractory supra-ventricular arrhythmias. JAMA 1982;248:851–855

108. Gallagher JJ, Svenson RH, Kasell JH et al: Catheter technique for closed-chest ablation of the atrioventricular conduction system. N Engl J Med 1982;306:194–200

109. Huang SK, Bharati S, Graham AR et al: Closed-chest catheter desiccation of the atrio-ventricular junction using radiofrequency energy. A new method of catheter ablation. J Am Coll Cardiol 1987;9:349–358

110. Williamson BD, Man KC, Daoud E et al: Radiofrequency catheter modification of atrioventricular conduction to control the ventricular rate during atrial fibrillation. N Engl J Med 1994;331:910–917

111. Jordanes L, Rubben L, Vertongen P: Sudden death and long-term survival after ablation of the atrioventricular junction. Eur JCPE 1993;3:232–237

112. Heinz G, Siostrzonek P, Kreiner G, Gössinger H: Improvement in left ventricular systolic function after successful radiofrequency His bundle ablation for drug refractory, chronic atrial fibrillation and recurrent atrial flutter. Am J Cardiol 1992;69:489–492

113. Fitzpatrick AP, Kourouyan HD, Siu A et al: Quality of life and outcomes after radiofrequency His-bundle catheter ablation and permanent pacemaker implantation. J Am Coll Cardiol 1994;23:350A

114. Packer DL, Bardy GH, Worley SJ et al: Tachycardia-induced cardiomyopathy. A reversible form of left ventricular dysfunction. Am J Cardiol 1986;57:563–570

115. Lemery R, Brugada P, Cheriex E, Wellens HJ: Reversibility of tachycardia-induced left ventricular dysfunction after closed-chest ablation of the atrioventricular junction for atrial fibrillation. Am J Cardiol 1987;60:1406–1408

116. Rosenqvist M, Lee MA, Moulinier L et al: Long-term follow-up of patients after transcatheter direct current ablation of the atrioventricular junction. J Am Coll Cardiol 1990;16:1467–1474

117. Rodriguez LM, Smeets JL, Xie B et al: Improvement in left ventricular function by ablation of atrioventricular conduction in selected patients with lone atrial fibrillation. Am J Cardiol 1993;72:1137–1141

118. Windecker J, Plumb VJ, Epstein AJ, Kay GN: Does AV nodal ablation impair long-term survival compared with medical treatment of atrial fibrillation? J Am Coll Cardiol 1994;23:84A

119. Bendersky R, Chatterjee K, Parmley WW, Brundage BH, Ports TA: Dobutamine in chronic ischemic heart failure. Alterations in left ventricular function and coronary hemodynamics. Am J Cardiol 1981;48:554–558

120. Unverferth DV, Magorien RD, Lewis RP, Leier CV: Long-term benefit of dobutamine in patients with congestive cardiomyopathy. Am Heart J 1980;100:622–630

121. Leier CV, Huss P, Lewis RP, Unverferth DV: Drug-induced conditioning in congestive heart failure. Circulation 1982;65:1382–1387

122. Hodgson JM, Aja M, Sarkin RP: Intermittent ambulatory dobutamine infusions for patients awaiting cardiac transplantation. Am J Cardiol 1984;53:375–376

123. Collins JA, Skidmore MA, Melvin DB, Engel PJ: Home intravenous dobutamine therapy in patients awaiting heart transplantation. J Heart Transplant 1990;9:205–208

124. Dies F: Intermittent dobutamine in ambulatory patients with chronic cardiac failure. Br J Clin Pract, suppl. 1986;45:37–40

125. Xamoterol in Severe Heart Failure Study Group: Xamoterol in severe heart failure. Lancet 1990;336:1

126. Results of the PRIME-II trial. Presented at the 45th scientific sessions of the American College of Cardiology, Orlando, March 1996

127. Rajfer SI, Anton AH, Rossen JD, Goldberg LI: Beneficial hemodynamic effects of oral levodopa in heart failure. Relation to the generation of dopamine. N Engl J Med 1984;310:1357–1362

128. De Marco T, Daly PA, Chatterjee K: Systemic and coronary hemodynamic and neurohormonal effects of levodopa in chronic congestive heart failure. Am J Cardiol 1988;62:1228–1233

129. Chatterjee K: Newer oral inotropic agents. Phosphodiesterase inhibitors. Crit Care Med 1990;18:S34–S38

130. Chatterjee K, Wolfe CL, De Marco T: Non-glycoside inotropes in congestive heart failure. Are they beneficial or harmful? Cardiol Clin 1994;12:63–72

131. Packer M, Carver JR, Rodeheffer RJ et al: Effect of oral milrinone on mortality in severe chronic heart failure. N Engl J Med 1991;325:1468–1475

132. Uretsky BF, Jessup M, Konstam MA et al: Multicenter trial of oral enoximone in patients with moderate to moderately severe congestive heart failure. Lack of benefit compared to placebo. Circulation 1990;82:774–780

133. Katz SD, Kubo SH, Jessup M et al: A multicenter, randomized, double-blind, placebo-controlled trial of pimobendan, a new cardiotonic and vasodilator agent in patients with severe congestive heart failure. Am Heart J 1992;123:95–103

134. Kubo SH, Gollub S, Bourge R et al: Beneficial effects of pimobendan on exercise tolerance quality of life in patients with heart failure. Results of a multicenter trial. Circulation 1992;85:942

135. Packer M, Narahara KA, Elkayam U et al: Double-blind, placebo-controlled study of the efficacy of flosequinan in patients with chronic heart failure. J Am Coll Cardiol 1993;22:65–72

136. Massie BM, Berk MR, Brozena SC et al: Can further benefit be achieved by adding flosequinan to patients with congestive heart failure who remain symptomatic on diuretic, digoxin, and on angiotensin converting enzyme inhibitor? Results of the flosequinan-ACE inhibitor trial (FACET). Circulation 1993;88:442–450

137. Iijima T, Taira N: Membrane current changes responsible for the positive inotropic effect of OPC-8212, a new positive inotropic agent, in single ventricular cells of guinea pig heart. J Pharmacol Exp Ther 1987;240:657–662

138. Lathrop DA, Schwartz A: Evidence for possible increase in sodium channel open time and involvement of Na/Ca exchange by a new positive inotropic drug: OPC-8212. Eur J Pharmacol 1985;117:391–392

139. Feldman AM, Becker LC, LLewllyn MP, Baughman KL: Evaluation of a new inotropic agent, OPC-8212, in patients with dilated cardiomyopathy and heart failure. Am Heart J 1988;116:771–777

140. Feldman AM, Bristow MR, Parmley WW et al: Effects of vesnarinone on morbidity and mortality in patients with heart failure. N Engl J Med 1993;329:149–155

141. Dubois-Rande JL, Loisance D, Duval AM et al: Enoximone, a pharmacologic bridge to transplantation. Br J Clin Pract, suppl. 1988;64:73–79

142. Dreyfus G, Arby B, Jebara V et al: Enoximone as alternative to mechanical support while awaiting cardiac transplantation [letter]. Lancet 1989;1:153

143. Watson DM, Sherry KM, Weston GA: Milrinone. A bridge to transplantation. Anaesthesia 1991;46:285–287

144. Deeb GM, Bolling SF: The role of amrinone in potential heart transplant patients with pulmonary hypertension. J Cardiothorac Anesth, (suppl. 2) 1989;3:33–37

145. Stevenson LW: Tailored therapy before transplantation for treatment of advanced heart failure. Effective use of vasodilators and diuretics. J Heart Lung Transplant 1991;10:468–476

146. De Marco T, Keith F: Bridge to cardiac transplantation. pp. 1–21. In Parmley WW, Chatterjee K (eds): Cardiology. Vol. 3. Lippincott-Raven, Philadelphia, 1994

147. Cody RJ, Pickworth KK: Approaches to diuretic therapy and electrolyte imbalance in congestive heart failure. Cardiol Clin 1994;12:37–50

148. Vasko MR, Broun-Cartwright D, Knochel PA, Nixon JS, Brater DC: Furosemide absorption altered in decompensated congestive heart failure. Ann Intern Med 1985;102:314–318

149. Lahov M, Rege VA, Ra'Anoni P, Theodor E: Intermittent administration of furosemide vs. continuous infusion preceded by a loading dose for congestive heart failure. Chest 1992;102:725–731

150. Van Meyel JJM, Smits P, Dormans T et al: Continuous infusion of furosemide in the treatment of patients with congestive heart failure and diuretic resistance. J Intern Med 1994;235:329–334

151. Motwani JG, Fenwick MK, Morton JJ, Struthers AD: Furosemide-induced natriuresis is augmented by ultra low dose captopril but not by standard doses of captopril in chronic heart failure. Circulation 1992;86:439–445

152. Graziani G, Cantaluppi A, Casati S et al: Dopamine and furosemide in oliguric acute renal failure. Nephron 1984;37:39–42

153. Duke GJ, Bersten AD: Dopamine and renal salvage in the critically ill patients. Anesth Intensive Care 1992;20:277–302

154. De Marco T, Kwasman M, Lau D, Chatterjee K: Dopexamine hydrochloride in chronic congestive heart failure with improved cardiac performance without increased metabolic cost. Am J Cardiol 1988;62:57C–62C

155. Agnostoni P, Marenzi G, Lauri G et al: Sustained improvement in functional capacity after removal of body fluid with isolated ultrafiltration in chronic car-

diac insufficiency. Failure of furosemide to provide the same result. Am J Med 1994;96:191–199

156. Simpson IA, Rae AP, Simpson K et al: Ultrafiltration in the management of refractory congestive heart failure. Br Heart J 1986;55:344–347

157. Akiba T, Taniquchi K, Marumo F, Matsuda O: Clinical significance of renal hemodynamics in severe congestive heart failure. Responsiveness to ultrafiltration therapies. Jpn Circ J 1989;53:191–196

158. Lauer A, Saccaggi A, Ronco C et al: Continuous arteriovenous hemofiltration in the critically ill patient. Clinical use and operational characteristics. Ann Intern Med 1983;99:455–460

159. Cipolla CM, Grazi S, Rimondini A et al: Changes in circulating norepinephrine with hemofiltration in advanced congestive heart failure. Am J Cardiol 1990; 66:987–994

160. Hochleitner M, Hortnagl H, Hortnagl H, Fridrich L, Gschnitzer F: Long-term efficacy of physiologic dual-chamber pacing in the treatment of end-stage idiopathic dilated cardiomyopathy. Am J Cardiol 1992; 70:1320–1325

161. Hochleitner M, Hortnagl H, Ng C-K et al: Usefulness of physiologic dual-chamber pacing in drug-resistant idiopathic dilated cardiomyopathy. Am J Cardiol 1990;66:198–202

162. Kataoka H: Hemodynamic effect of physiological dual chamber pacing in a patient with end-stage dilated cardiomyopathy. A case report. PACE 1991;14: 1330–1335

163. Iskandrian AS: Pacemaker therapy in congestive heart failure. Am J Cardiol 1990;66:223–224

164. Becker SJD, Xiao HB, Sparrow J, Gibson DG: Effects of dual-chamber pacing with short atrioventricular delay in dilated cardiomyopathy. Lancet 1992;340: 1308–1312

165. Nishimura RA, Hayes DL, Holmes DJ, Tajik AJ: Mechanism of hemodynamic improvement by dual-chamber pacing for severe left ventricular dysfunction. An acute Doppler and catheterization hemodynamic study. J Am Coll Cardiol 1995;25:281–288

166. Gold MR, Feliciano Z, Gottlieb SS, Fisher ML: Dual-chamber pacing with a short atrioventricular delay in congestive heart failure. A randomized study. J Am Coll Cardiol 1995;26:967–973

167. Gradman A, Deedwania P, Cody R et al: Predictors of total mortality and sudden death in mild to moderate heart failure. J Am Coll Cardiol 1989;14:564–570

168. Chatterjee K: Amiodarone in chronic heart failure. J Am Coll Cardiol 1989;14:1775–1776

169. Tchou PJ, Kadri N, Anderson J et al: Automatic implantable cardioverter-defibrillators and survival of patients with left ventricular dysfunction and malignant ventricular arrhythmias. Ann Intern Med 1988; 109:529–534

170. Bolling SF, Deeb M, Morady F et al: Automatic internal cardioverter-defibrillator. A bridge to heart transplantation. J Heart Lung Transplant 1991;10: 562–566

171. Jeevanandam V, Bielefeld MR, Auteri JS et al: The implantable defibrillator. An electronic bridge to cardiac transplantation. Circulation, suppl. II 1992;86: 276–279

172. Bardy GH, Hofer B, Johnson G et al: Implantable transvenous cardioverter-defibrillators. Circulation 1993;87:1152–1168

173. Mehta D, Pe E, Gomes JA: Amiodarone versus implantable defibrillator in patients with class III/IV CHF and malignant ventricular arrhythmias [abstract]. Circulation, suppl. I 1995;92:782

174. Tchou P, Tazayeri, M, Denker S et al: Transcatheter electrical ablation of the right bundle branch. A method of treating macroreentrant ventricular tachycardia attributed to bundle branch re-entry. Circulation 1988;78:246

55 Future Directions in the Treatment of Heart Failure*

John R. Teerlink
Barry M. Massie

Our understanding of the pathophysiology of congestive heart failure (CHF) and our ability to treat this syndrome have improved greatly. Indeed, these advances have been closely intertwined, with recognition of the role of the simultaneously adaptive and maladaptive peripheral circulatory and neurohormonal changes stimulating the use of vasodilators and angiotensin-converting enzyme (ACE) inhibitors, and the responses to these agents furthering our knowledge of the underlying pathophysiology. Well designed studies and large trials have demonstrated that ACE inhibitors can prolong survival and prevent the progression of left ventricular dysfunction. The invaluable role of diuretics in symptomatic patients needs no confirmation, and the efficacy of digoxin in reducing symptoms and preventing deterioration in patients with moderate to severe CHF has been substantiated once again by the Digitalis Investigators Group trial (see Chapter 43). The use of these and other currently available agents in the management of CHF has been reviewed,[1] and several guidelines have highlighted the general agreement on most aspects of treatment with these conventional agents.[2-4]

Despite these advances, morbidity and mortality related to CHF remain high and indeed are increasing in absolute numbers.[5,6] The prognosis of patients with CHF remains poor, despite the positive results of recent trials.[7] Therefore interest in new therapeutic agents continues to be high, and novel approaches are sorely needed. The purpose of this chapter is to examine the promise of several currently investigational agents for CHF and to speculate about potential future interventions.

PATHOPHYSIOLOGY OF CHF AND GOALS OF THERAPY

Until fairly recently, symptomatic improvement or stabilization were the primary goals of treatment of CHF, but the demonstration that therapies such as vasodilators and ACE inhibitors reduced mortality rates changed this perspective.[8-10] More recent trials have demonstrated the feasibility of altering the natural history of heart failure; both treatment with ACE inhibitors and β-adrenoreceptor blockers can delay the progression of left ventricular dilatation and dysfunction and so prevent the onset of clinical CHF, thereby improving survival.[11-15] Although intuitively one might expect the beneficial effects regarding symptoms and prognosis to go hand in hand, this does not appear always to be the case. It is now clear that agents that consistently improve exercise tolerance and symptoms may at the same time *increase* mortality, the best example of which was the vasodilator-inotrope flosequinan.[16] The combination of hydralazine and isosorbide dinitrate appears to produce greater improvement in hemodynamics and exercise capacity than ACE inhibitors but to have a lesser benefit for survival.[17] Digoxin may be an example of an agent with the ability to ameliorate clinical status without enhancing survival, and β-block-

* Parts of this chapter have been modified from Massie and Shah,[228] with permission.

ers may improve prognosis with less short-term symptom relief.

On reconsideration, this dichotomy is perhaps not so surprising, as the pathophysiology of CHF is complex and multidimensional. Not only are there hemodynamic derangements resulting from myocardial insufficiency, but there are changes in a plethora of neurohormonal systems, other regulatory and counterregulatory systems, and myocardial energetics. Furthermore, responses at the system, organ, and cellular levels may differ. For instance, an inotropic agent might improve left ventricular performance but produce energetic requirements or cellular responses that are injurious to the remaining myocytes; a diuretic or vasodilator may produce short-term beneficial hemodynamic responses but induce long-term deleterious changes at the organ or cellular level. Appreciating these dichotomies but still not fully understanding their basis leads to the need to define the effect of therapeutic interventions on both symptomatic and mortality/progression endpoints.

POTENTIAL APPROACHES TO THE TREATMENT OF CHF

Table 55-1 lists a number of potential mechanisms by which new or investigational medications may be beneficial in patients with CHF or prevent the progression of left ventricular dysfunction in patients with or without overt CHF. Although medications are currently available in the first three categories, additional approaches continue to be explored. It is the latter three categories that appear to hold the greatest potential. The exciting possibility of "molecular and cellular engineering"[18] still lies in the future, but it is rapidly becoming the foreseeable future and already has captured the imagination and investment of both academia and industry.

Agents That Induce Diuresis

It is with diuretics that currently available medications come closest to meeting the potential clinical needs. With the range of potency provided by thiazides and related agents, loop diuretics, and combinations thereof, most patients can be maintained without excessive fluid retention. The limitations of current diuretics are their variable absorption in severe right-sided failure, the resulting electrolyte imbalances, and their contribution to prerenal azotemia in patients with low cardiac output and hypotension, which is in some cases exacerbated by concomitant ACE inhibitor administration. The first problem can be overcome by intravenous administration, and

Table 55-1. Potential Future Approaches for Treating CHF

Agents that facilitate diuresis
　Natriuretic peptides
　Endopeptidase inhibitors
Agents with positive inotropic activity
　Receptor agonists
　　β-Receptor agonists
　　α-Receptor agonists
　Ion channel modulators
　　Ca^{2+} agonists
　　Na^+ channel agonists
　Modifiers of signal transduction
　　Forskolin
　　Phosphodiesterase inhibitors
　Ca^{2+} sensitizers
Agents with vasodilating activity
　Ca^{2+} antagonists
　Peptide vasodilators
　　Natriuretic peptides
　　Calcitonin gene-related peptide
Neurohormonal antagonists
　Modulators of the sympathetic nervous system
　　β-Blockers
　　Central sympatholytics
　　Dopamine β-hydroxylase inhibitors
　　DA_1 agonists
　Modulators of the renin-angiotensin system
　　Angiotensin II antagonists
　　Renin inhibitors
　Other actions
　　Endothelin antagonists
　　Vasopressin antagonists
　　Stimulants of endothelial-mediated vasodilation
Agents that alter myocardial energetics
　Heart rate depressants
　Modifiers of substrate utilization
Agents that alter gene expression

(From Massie and Shah,[228] with permission.)

the second can be ameliorated by ACE inhibitor or spironolactone therapy; but the third is inherent in the physiology of severe heart failure.

Several approaches are being investigated to improve renal blood flow and natriuresis in CHF patients with impaired renal perfusion. The results with oral dopaminergic agonists, such as levodopa, fenoldepam, and ibopamine, which have at least the theoretic potential to reproduce the renal vasodilation characteristic of low dose intravenous dopamine, have been disappointing,[19,20] although the latter agent continues to be used and investigated as a neurohormonal modulator.[21,22] Of more current interest is the use of atrial natriuretic peptides (ANPs), or inhibitors of neutral endopeptidase, the enzyme responsible for degrading ANP. ANP is a potent vasodilator and natriuretic agent in normal subjects and patients with mild CHF. Tolerance to its actions, however, rather than inadequate endogenous circulating levels (which are typically elevated), appears to be the limiting factor in patients with advanced heart failure.[23,24] The experience thus far with exogenously administered ANP has not been impressive, suggesting that at best it might facilitate aggressive short-term diuresis.[23–26] Brain natriuretic peptide (BNP) has been more promising,[27] though perhaps primarily as a result of its vasodilating properties rather than its ability to stimulate ongoing diuresis in refractory patients. Endopeptidase inhibitors, such as candoxatrilat, have several potential advantages, including the convenience of oral administration and of modulating the levels of endogenously produced natriuretic peptides. They appear to have greater natriuretic activity than would be expected from the changes in plasma ANP levels, suggesting an effect at the tissue level.[23,28–30] Whether endopeptidase inhibitors can act synergistically with other diuretics during long-term therapy in patients with refractory fluid retention, the primary target population for such an agent is uncertain.

Another potential approach that has not yet entered clinical trials is blockade of the potent renal antidiuretic and antinatriuretic actions of adenosine.[31,32] Agents of this class have potent natriuretic and diuretic actions at several tubular sites that persist under conditions of reduced renal blood flow, hypotension, and toxic nephropathy. Of particular interest is that they supplement furosemide activity and produce relatively limited kaliuresis.

Agents with Positive Inotropic Activity

Because impaired cardiac performance is the initial abnormality of systolic heart failure, increasing myocardial contractility is the oldest and most extensively studied pharmacologic approach.[33–35] Figure 55-1 illustrates the many potential avenues for achieving this goal. This complex situation can be simplified into two categories: (1) agents that increase Ca^{2+} release from the sarcoplasmic reticulum (SR) stores, facilitating Ca^{2+} binding to troponin C, which in turn relieves the troponin-tropomyosin inhibition of actin-myosin cross-bridge formation and facilitates sarcomere shortening (sometimes categorized as "upstream" mechanisms); and (2) agents that alter contractile protein sensitivity to Ca^{2+} or the rate of Ca^{2+} reuptake, also with resultant changes in sarcomere shortening and contractility (categorized as "downstream" mechanisms). As can be appreciated from Figure 55-1, not only are there

a number of potential pathways in each category but many agents have multiple actions, sometimes with concordant and sometimes with discordant effects on contractility.

The first category includes (1) agents that directly or indirectly affect ion channels; (2) agents that interact with receptors on the sarcolemmal membrane; and (3) agents that alter signal transduction or second messenger activity. The digitalis glycosides inhibit the sarcolemmal Na^+/K^+-ATPase, increasing intracellular Na^+ concentrations and, by facilitating gradient-dependent Na^+/Ca^{2+} exchange, the Ca^{2+} concentrations, hence stimulating systolic SR Ca^{2+} release.[33,34] Agents that increase flux through Na^+ channels could be expected to have a similar positive inotropic effect.[36,37] Vesnarinone, an agent with relatively modest positive inotropic actions, acts by this mechanism, as well as by weak phosphodiesterase III inhibition.[38] Several investigational compounds have been developed that directly facilitate Ca^{2+} entry through slow Ca^{2+} channels, of which Bay K 8644 is the prototype.[39] Although this compound was not specific to myocyte Ca^{2+} channels and therefore produced undesirable vasoconstriction, other Ca^{2+} promoters have entered clinical investigation.

An important question, based on the overlapping mechanisms of these ion channel modulators, is whether such agents have additive efficacy and at least comparable safety as digoxin. Furthermore, an increase in intracellular Ca^{2+}, by these and other mechanisms, has proarrhythmic potential.[40]

Drugs with receptor-mediated positive inotropic actions have also been extensively investigated.[33,34] β-receptor agonists, such as dobutamine and norepinephrine, are effective and widely used for short-term therapy.[41] Their action is mediated by the adenylate cyclase system and the resultant increase in cyclic adenosine monophosphate (cAMP). cAMP phosphorylates a number of membrane-bound and regulatory proteins, resulting in multiple actions that modulate contractility, including enhancing Ca^{2+} entry through slow calcium channels but also facilitating Ca^{2+} reuptake by the SR and densensitizing contractile proteins to Ca^{2+}. The latter two actions may facilitate diastolic relaxation, but desensitization may have a negative inotropic action and may be a mechanism, in addition to receptor downregulation and desensitization, by which tolerance to the positive inotropic effects of β-adrenoreceptor agonists occurs. Unfortunately, chronic oral therapy with catecholamines (e.g., xamoterol and prenalterol) has not only proved ineffective but also accelerates mortality, at least in part because of increased arrhythmogenesis.[42,43] Intermittent treatment with dobutamine may provide a better balance between efficacy and safety; and chronic intravenous therapy

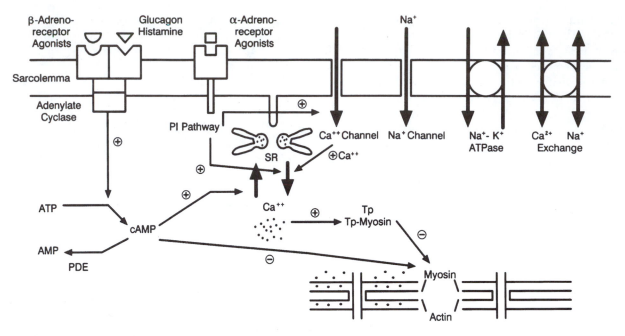

Fig. 55-1. Many of the mechanisms regulating myocardial contractility and some of their important modulators. Ultimately, force development results from actin–myosin cross-bridge formation. In order for it to occur, Ca^{2+} must bind to troponin C, causing a conformational change in the contractile proteins, which permits actin–myosin interaction. Thus any intervention that increases cytosolic Ca^{2+} enhances the contractile force and vice versa. A second mechanism for modulating contractility is to enhance or diminish contractile protein sensitivity to Ca^{2+}. This process is not fully understood, but phosphorylation of troponin I appears to produce this effect. Agents that enhance Ca^{2+} sensitivity include endothelin and a number of investigational drugs (e.g., pimobendan and levosimendan). Agents that increase cyclic adenosine monophosphate (cAMP) decrease Ca^{2+} sensitivity.

Most pharmacologic approaches to modulating contractility affect cytosolic Ca^{2+} concentrations, as small increases in Ca^{2+} concentration are amplified manyfold by facilitating Ca^{2+} release from the sarcoplasmic reticulum (SR). Such approaches include those that are receptor-mediated, alterations in ion channel activity, and phosphodiesterase (PDE) inhibition. β-Adrenoreceptor agonists, as well as such endogenous substances as glucagon and histamine, work through the adenylate cyclase system to increase cAMP, which enhances Ca^{2+} entry through the sarcolemmal slow Ca^{2+} channel. cAMP has additional actions, including enhancing Ca^{2+} reuptake (necessary for relaxation) and densensitizing the contractile proteins (see above). PDE inhibitors produce the same effects by inhibiting the breakdown of cAMP. α-Adrenoreceptors play a less prominent role in regulating myocardial contractility and perhaps a greater role in growth processes. However α-adrenoreceptor stimulation generates inositol triphosphate (IP_3) via the phosphatidyl inositol pathway, and IP_3 facilitates Ca^{2+} entry through slow Ca^{2+} channels and SR Ca^{2+} release.

Of course, most Ca^{2+} channel blockers decrease contractility by decreasing Ca^{2+} entry, and investigation continues into developing Ca^{2+} channel agonists, which would have the opposite effect. Agents that increase Na^+ channel activity also increase Ca^{2+} concentrations by enhancing the activity of the electrogenic Na^+/Ca^{2+} exchanger. Finally, inhibition of the Na^+/K^+-ATPase, which is the primary action of the digitalis glycosides, also increases Ca^{2+} concentrations as a result of the increased Na^+/Ca^{2+} exchange.

may be an option for refractory patients willing to accept the associated risk. Glucagon and histamine also stimulate receptors coupled to adenylate cyclase and produce relatively weak positive inotropic actions; but they have undesirable systemic effects.

α-adrenoreceptor agonists also may enhance contractility, working via the phospholipase C second messenger system, increasing concentrations of inositol trisphosphate, which in turn increases Ca^{2+} entry through slow Ca^{2+} channels and SR Ca^{2+} re-

lease.[44] Oral α-adrenoreceptor agonists have not been investigated for CHF owing to the likely unfavorable balance between peripheral vasoconstriction and positive inotropic activity. However, if more research demonstrates different roles for the various α_1-adrenoreceptor subtypes, specific pharmacologic agents may be developed to not only induce positive inotropy but also modulate these receptors with respect to myocardial hypertrophy and remodeling (see later in the chapter).

The third "upstream" approach to increasing contractility involves modulating the cAMP concentration, the second messenger responsible for β-adrenoreceptor-stimulated positive inotropy. This has been accomplished with forskolin, which stimulates the catalytic subunit of adenylate cyclase, and with inhibitors of myocardial phosphodiesterase III (PDE).[33,34,43,45] The PDE inhibitors are the most extensively studied of the nonglycoside positive inotropic agents. They have potent favorable acute hemodynamic effects, based on a combination of positive inotropic and vasodilating activity, and may not induce short-term tolerance, in distinction to the catecholamines. However, in the dosages evaluated in clinical studies these agents have consistently increased mortality, apparently by inducing ventricular arrhythmias and accelerating the progression of left ventricular dysfunction.[43,46–49]

Our understanding of the "downstream" mechanisms is more primitive, and few pharmacologic agents that modulate them are available. Included in this category are several Ca^{2+} sensitizers, including pimobendan and several newer agents.[50–53] Unfortunately, all of these agents have at least some PDE inhibitor activity, and whether a safe and effective balance between these actions can be obtained is uncertain.[51] In the absence of PDE activity, it is also likely that these agents impair myocardial relaxation and exacerbate the diastolic dysfunction that characterizes most cardiomyopathies. As has been noted,[54] it is also becoming clear that a number of proteins involved in Ca^{2+} transport and the regulation of contractility, including phospholamban, troponin isoforms, myosin light chains, and calmodulin, may be eventual targets for pharmacotherapy or gene therapy.[54,55]

What are the current status and future prospects for positive inotropic therapy? Digoxin remains the only such agent currently available for chronic oral therapy in most countries, and its role in the treatment of heart failure has only recently been definitively clarified by the recently completed Digitalis Investigators Group (DIG) trial and other smaller studies (See Chapter 43). These studies established that digoxin improves symptoms and prevents hospitalizations in patients heart failure due to left ventricular systolic function who are in sinus rhythm. Further, digoxin has neither an adverse nor beneficial effect on survival, confirming the role of digoxin as at least one positive inotropic agent as a valuable adjunctive drug in patients who remain symptomatic on diuretics and ACE inhibitors. An intriguing attribute of digoxin is that it decreases circulating neurohormones and sympathetic nerve activity, so it is difficult to ascribe clinical responses to its positive inotropic actions alone.[56] In contrast to the beneficial effects of digoxin, agents that increase cAMP, by stimulating β-adrenoreceptors or PDE inhibition, increase mortality; and, except during short-term therapy, they produce little clinical benefit.[43] These results raise the crucial question of whether the deleterious effects of cAMP-dependent positive inotropic agents are the result of this particular-mechanism of action or they reflect adverse responses to enhanced contractility. Are they the result of cAMP-induced arrhythmogenesis or possibly desensitization of the contractile apparatus or other injurious responses of nonspecific phosphorylation of proteins? Or do they reflect excessive metabolic demands engendered by inotropic stimulation in energy-depleted myocytes? In any case, it is unlikely that any drug with this predominant mechanism of action will prove useful for long-term therapy, except perhaps for palliation in otherwise refractory patients.

Desite the rather gloomy experience with chronic positive inotropic therapy with agents other than digoxin, investigations have continued with several categories of agents with this mechanism of action. These include drugs that modulate ion channel activity and those that affect the Ca^{2+} sensitivity of the contractile apparatus.[35] Of note is that the agents which have been investigated have usually had multiple actions, including PDE inhibition. Of these, vesnarinone has attracted the most attention. This novel compound appears to activate myocardial Na^+ channels, modulate K^+ currents, inhibit PDE, and, most interestingly, inhibit cytokine production and release.[57] Unfortunately, the early favorable results with vesnarinone were not confirmed in the recently completed 3500 patient VEST trial, which demonstrated 26 percent and 14 percent *increases* in mortality compared to placebo with 60 mg and 30 mg daily doses, respectively. This finding, together with adverse or at best neutral effects of other positive inotropic agents, including the β-adrenoreceptor agonist xamoterol, the PDE inhibitor milrinone, the dopaminergic agonist ibopamine, and the calcium sensitizer pimobendan, have dampened the resurgent interest in positive inotropic drugs. (See Chapter 46).

Agents with Vasodilating Activity

Vasodilating drugs have been responsible for most of the recent successes in the management of heart failure, and hence interest in this class of agent remains high. Figure 55-2 illustrates the numerous potential avenues to achieve vasodilation. Given the heterogeneity of these mechanisms and the dependence of many on nonspecific second messenger systems, it would not be unexpected that they might yield diverse clinical responses. Somewhat arbi-

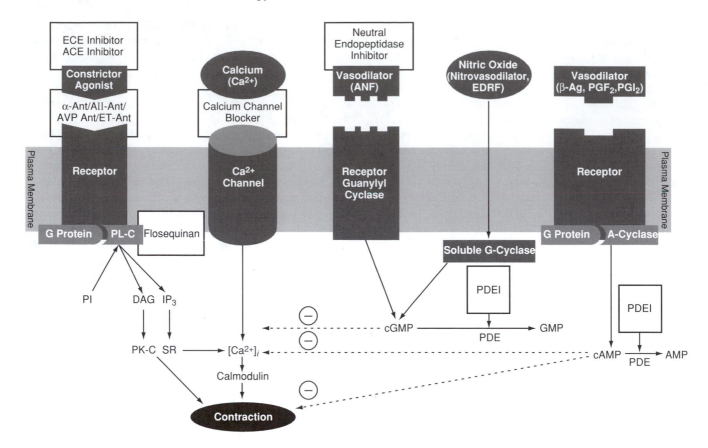

Fig. 55-2. Pathways by which vascular tone is regulated. Some of the drug classes that can cause vasodilation are shown in bold. On the far left, the pathway mediated by the phospholipase C (PL-C)/phosphoinositidyl (PI) pathway is shown. Angiotensin II, α-adrenergic agonists, endothelin, and arginine vasopressin (AVP) all act via this pathway, interacting with their respective surface receptors and activating PL-C via G protein coupling. Downstream, vasoconstriction is enhanced by production of inositidyl triphosphate (IP$_3$) and stimulation of protein kinase C (PK-C), both of which increase cytosolic calcium ([Ca^{2+}]) and enhance vasoconstriction. Vasoconstriction can be decreased with resultant vasodilation via agents that inhibit formation of the agonist, such as the converting enzyme inhibitors for both angiotensin (ACE inhibitor) and probably endothelin (ECE inhibitor), or those that block specific receptors, such as the α-adrenergic antagonists (α-Ant), angiotensin II blockers (AII-Ant), endothelin blockers (ET-Ant), and arginine vasopressin antagonists (AVP-Ant). In addition, agents that act directly on PL-C (e.g., flosequinan) or PK-C can also cause vasodilation.

The second pathway for mediation of vascular tone is directly through the voltage-dependent calcium channels. A wide range of calcium channel blockers have been successfully developed to decrease vasoconstriction.

A third pathway for control of vascular tone is via the guanyl cyclase-mediated increase in cyclic guanosine monophosphate (cGMP), induced by both atrial natriuretic factor (ANF) and activators of endothelium-derived relaxation factors (EDRF) such as nitric oxide (NO), which causes vasodilation by a number of actions, including down-regulation of the calcium channels.

A fourth pathway, represented on the right, induces vasodilation via G protein-coupled stimulation of adenyl cyclase with production of cAMP. β-Adrenergic agonists (β-Ag) and prostaglandins (PG) cause vasodilation by this mechanism. Each of these four pathways is a target for agents that can either inhibit vasoconstriction or promote vasodilation.

trarily, vasodilators have been categorized as neurohormonal agonists or antagonists and direct-acting, with the latter category encompassing agents with undefined mechanisms of action. This section deals with direct-acting agents.

The rationale for vasodilator therapy—to improve

cardiac performance by "unloading" the ventricles—is well accepted. However, it is now clear that although virtually any agent with vasodilating properties can improve some hemodynamic indices of cardiac performance, the effects of these agents on clinical indices and outcomes are variable and sometimes adverse. The list of potent vasodilators that have not proved clinically effective includes hydralazine (administered by itself, without nitrates), prazosin, minoxidil, nifedipine and other Ca^{2+} antagonists (which also have negative inotropic actions), and epoprostenol (a prostacyclin analog),[58-60] as well as other agents for which the negative results have not been published. Other potent vasodilators, such as flosequinan and several PDE inhibitors, have also proved to have adverse effects on survival, although these adverse outcomes may also reflect their positive inotropic actions.[16,43,46,49] Three features characterize the responses to many of these agents. First, they are potent arterial vasodilators, usually producing more marked effects on systemic vascular resistance and cardiac output than on ventricular filling pressures and size. Only in the presence of substantial mitral regurgitation do such arteriolar dilators lower filling pressures.[61] Second, they often increase the heart rate, which may worsen the precarious balance between myocardial energy supply and demand. Third, they often activate neurohormonal mechanisms, such as the sympathetic nervous system and renin-angiotensin system, which appear to play a role in the progression of CHF.[62]

On the other hand, the combination of hydralazine and isosorbide dinitrate improved survival in the V-HeFT I trial and was at least as effective as enalapril for ameliorating symptoms in V-HeFT II.[8,17] This rather unique result in the vasodilator experience has maintained the appeal of this therapeutic approach. It is usually assumed that the combination regimen proved effective where others did not because it satisfied the need for combined arteriolar and venodilatation. This may be the case, although prazosin, flosequinan, and PDE inhibitors also produce venodilation and corresponding hemodynamic changes. Another possibility is that the primary benefit of the combined regimen devolves from the nitrate component, which may have not only a vasodilating effect but also cellular effects that may alter the progression of heart failure while the hydralazine component acts to prevent or reduce nitrate tolerance.[63]

A number of direct-acting vasodilators continue to be investigated and developed. Nitric oxide is an endothelium-derived relaxing factor[64] that is intimately involved in peripheral vascular abnormalities during heart failure. Unfortunately, trials administering inhaled nitric oxide have demonstrated increased left ventricular filling pressures despite reductions in pulmonary vascular resistance,[65,66] suggesting that such therapy may be limited in its applicability. Most other direct-acting vasodilators under investigation are Ca^{2+} antagonists, such as amlodipine and mibefridil (Ro 40–5967),

which are not associated with some of the aforementioned disadvantages such as positive chronotropy, negative inotropy, and significant neurohormonal activation.[67,68] Nonetheless, it is uncertain whether these agents are likely to have important effects on survival and progression of left ventricular dysfunction owing to their unidimensional mechanism of action, which is limited to hemodynamic improvement without affecting other aspects of the pathophysiology of CHF. Indeed, the Prospective Randomized Amlodipine Survival Evaluation (PRAISE) trial failed to find a favorable effect of amlodipine on mortality or severe morbidity in patients with advanced CHF; nor did it demonstrate an adverse effect. Intriguingly, and somewhat paradoxically, there was lower mortality in the subset of patients with nonischemic dilated cardiomyopathy.[69] These results suggest not only that there is a significant difference between the ischemic and nonischemic cardiomyopathies, but that amlodipine may have a role in the treatment of this form of heart failure. A similar effect was not observed in the V-HeFT III trial, which evaluated felodipine.[70] Although this trial was underpowered relative to PRAISE, it suggests that the earlier result may not be related to vasodilation or to Ca^{2+} channel blockade. One possibility is that the potent antioxidant effect of amlodipine might be responsible for this discrepancy.[71,72] A follow-up trial with amlodipine in nonischemic cardiomyopathy is needed to determine if this outcome is reproducible. Such a trial is in progress.

Agents That Alter Neurohormonal Responses

Of course the greatest excitement has come from the introduction of the ACE inhibitors and the delineation of their role in the management of CHF.[73,74] The recognition that these agents, which have rather weak effects on cardiac output in most patients, can produce significant improvements in symptoms and survival brought to the fore the importance of neurohormonal activation[75] and its resultant effects on the pathobiology of the diseased heart and blood vessels. It is now well documented and widely accepted in practice that ACE inhibitors improve symptoms and functional capacity, delay the progression of left ventricular dysfunction, and prolong survival of patients with left ventricular systolic dysfunction, and that they should be administered to all such patients unless contraindicated or not tolerated.[2,73,74] It is likely that angiotensin II blockers and renin inhibitors share at least some of this benefit,[76,77] but the complex interactions between various components of the renin-angiotensin system and other neurohormonal systems make it uncertain as to whether they will be as successful.

The renin-angiotensin system is only one of the many abnormal neurohormonal mechanisms in CHF.[62,78,79] Increased sympathetic nervous system activity, increased circulating levels of endothelin, arginine vasopressin, and the newly discovered adrenomedullin,[80] abnormalities of endothelium-mediated vasodilation (and possibly other endothelium-modulated cellular processes), and resistance to the actions of natriuretic peptides are among other neurohormonal changes that appear to play a role in the pathophysiology of CHF. Each is a possible target for therapy, although paradoxically the success of ACE inhibitors may have dampened the enthusiasm of the industry for developing such agents. The importance of such adjunctive approaches should be readily apparent. The renin-angiotensin system, at least as characterized by its circulating components, is activated relatively late in the natural history of CHF. In the SOLVD trial, measurements of plasma norepinephrine and ANP showed greater differences than plasma renin activity among control subjects, asymptomatic patients with ejection fractions less than 35 percent, and symptomatic CHF patients.[81] The benefit of ACE inhibitor therapy is greatest in patients with more severe symptoms and more severely depressed ejection fractions.[10,12] Even in the refractory patients studied in the CONSENSUS I study, survival improvements were limited to patients with plasma angiotensin II levels above the median, whereas there appeared to be benefit in patients with norepinephrine levels both above and below the median.[82] ACE inhibitors do have indirect effects on the sympathetic nervous system,[83] but they are relatively modest; and changes in plasma norepinephrine are small and inconsistent.

Therefore additional modulation of the sympathetic nervous system has been and remains a prime target for therapy. This concept is not new, of course, and β-adrenoreceptor blockers have been utilized in CHF patients for more than two decades. Their use has grown in acceptance with recognition of the adverse role of neurohormonal activation and with the availability of data from clinical trials.[84–86] The Metoprolol in Dilated Cardiomyopathy (MDC) trial showed strong evidence of delay in the progression of left ventricular dysfunction and the clinical manifestations of deteriorating CHF, but it was inconclusive with regard to mortality.[87] The larger Cardiac Insufficiency Bisoprolol Study (CIBIS) also provided mixed results.[88] In the entire study population, there was no improvement in survival, but when the patients were subdivided by the presence or absence of prior myocardial infarction, mortality was dramatically reduced in the latter group. Again, there was evidence of less deterioration in the bisoprolol-treated patients and extended to patients with and without underlying coronary artery disease. Small controlled studies with bucindolol and carvedilol[89–92] have also provided evidence of benefit, most consistently in the form of improved ejection fraction, reduced heart size, and alleviation of symptoms.[85] More recent results from several carvedilol studies also suggest that this agent improves survival and prevents clinical deterioration in patients with both nonischemic and ischemic CHF.[93,94]

Although this growing experience with β-blockers is encouraging, the ultimate role of these agents remains uncertain. Most of these studies, including those with carvedilol, have only short-term follow-up and few events. The larger MDC and CIBIS studies have not provided definitive evidence of efficacy and do not support a favorable effect on CHF of nonischemic etiology. Important questions remain about the applicability of β-blocker therapy to patients with coronary disease: Should they be used as adjuncts or as substitutes for ACE inhibitors? Are there clinically important differences among agents of this class? New trials should provide some answers. The National Institutes of Health and the Veterans Administration have commenced the β-Blocker Evaluation of Survival Trial (BEST), which should randomize more than 3000 patients to bucindolol or placebo; and a European survival trial with carvedilol is under consideration. Until the answers are known, several speculations seem warranted. First, conventional wisdom to the contrary, β-blockers can be administered safely to patients with clinical CHF, but initiation of therapy in severely symptomatic patients leads to acute deterioration in 10–20 percent. In other words, it is not a form of therapy that is likely to rapidly diffuse into widespread clinical practice. This might be particularly unfortunate because if β-blockers delay the progression of CHF the optimal time to intervene may be early in the natural history, before referral to heart failure specialists. Second, it appears that this mode of therapy has more to offer patients with primary dilated cardiomyopathy than those with ischemic heart disease. Why this might be the case is not clear, but one possibility is that the latter patients are dependent on the compensatory hyperfunction of noninfarcted myocardium. Third, approaches that may modulate the sympathetic nervous system, either by decreasing central sympathetic outflow or decreasing peripheral norepinephrine release, may be advantageous by virtue of blunting rather than blocking catecholamine-mediated responses and by decreasing α-adrenoreceptor-mediated actions, which may have important effects on cell growth and function.

Several agents are being evaluated that have the latter actions. Clonidine and related central α_2-agonists have been used safely but are not well studied in CHF patients.[95] These drugs may have excessive side effects and cause unacceptable hypotension in combination with other hypotensive agents, such as ACE inhibitors and diuretics. However, there are centrally active agents that are more selective for imidazoline I-1 receptors or α_2-receptors, which may down-regulate sympathetic activity with less sedation or less effect on systemic blood pressure.[96,97] These agents are appealing candidates for evaluation in CHF. Another promising approach would be to inhibit dopamine β-hydroxylase, the enzyme responsible for converting dopamine to norepinephrine.[98] Such inhibition should reduce the release of norepinephrine and possibly increase circulating levels of dopamine to the range associated with renal vasodilation. Ibopamine, which is metabolized to epinine, a DA_1 receptor agonist, has produced modest reductions in plasma norepinephrine.[21] However, this agent, which is marketed in several countries, had an adverse effect on survival in a recently terminated European trial.

The endothelin system is emerging as another important element in the pathogenesis of heart failure, as well as many other diseases,[99] and is being targeted by a variety of approaches, analogous to the renin-angiotensin system. Endothelin is the most potent known vasoconstrictor, and current studies in animals[100-102] and humans[103,104] have found evidence for endothelin-induced arterial vasoconstriction mediated by both ET_A and ET_B receptor subtypes. Endothelin concentrations are elevated in patients with heart failure[105-107] and appear to be correlated with disease severity[108]; there also appear to be significant interactions between the endothelin system and the adrenergic and renin-angiotensin systems. These findings suggest that agents that decrease the neurohormonal activation of the endothelin system, either as direct receptor antagonists or endothelin-converting enzyme inhibitors,[109,110] may be beneficial in patients with heart failure. Studies in animal models of heart failure have demonstrated that bosentan, an orally active mixed (ET_A and ET_B) endothelin receptor antagonist,[111] significantly decrease mean arterial pressure, an effect that was additive to treatment with the ACE inhibitor cilazapril.[112] Bosentan has also been shown to ameliorate in vivo norepinephrine-induced hypertrophy in rats,[112] suggesting a potential role for these agents in modifying ventricular remodeling. Other studies in animal models of pulmonary hypertension have demonstrated beneficial effects as well.[114-116] These

preliminary results suggest that endothelin antagonism, either through receptor antagonists or endothelin-converting enzyme inhibitors, may be a useful future therapeutic intervention.

Other neurohormonal systems may also be targets of therapy, even though they do not, at least at first glance, appear as central to the pathophysiology of heart failure as the renin-angiotensin and sympathetic nervous systems. Abnormalities in the parasympathetic nervous system are also important during heart failure and may be related to mortality.[117] Agents that help to restore autonomic balance, such as scopolamine,[118] may have an impact on the high incidence of sudden death in heart failure patients. As mentioned earlier, natriuretic peptides and endopeptidase inhibitors do not appear to be promising candidates for chronic therapy, although research continues in this area. The role of increased vasopressin activity seems too limited for its inhibition to be a prime target,[119] although vasopressin antagonists[120] may be a useful adjunctive therapy.[121-123]

In sum, the interdiction of abnormal neurohormonal mechanisms in CHF is likely to be a successful therapeutic approach, complementary to that already afforded by ACE inhibitors. The optimal agents and the appropriate application of these mechanisms remain to be determined.

Agents That Alter Myocardial Energetics

It is frequently hypothesized that the failing heart is characterized by a perilous balance between myocardial energy availability and demand.[124] This formulation is supported by potential limitations of oxygen supply resulting from changes in the microvasculature, often significant hypertrophy, and the combination of low cardiac output, reduced aortic diastolic pressure, and elevated left ventricular diastolic pressure, which limits coronary reserve. Elevated wall stress and tachycardia combine to increase myocardial energy requirements, and positive inotropic stimulation can exacerbate this problem unless there is a commensurate decrease in other determinants of oxygen consumption. In addition to these factors is the potential for energy wasting during catecholamine stimulation and, possibly, inefficiency of a number of cellular processes, such as Ca^{2+} sequestration and membrane transport in the failing heart.[125]

Although data are limited, there is biochemical evidence to corroborate abnormalities of bioenergetics in the failing heart in both experimental models and some clinical studies.[126,127] This area is important for further investigation, because confirmation and delineation of such abnormalities could point to avenues of therapy. At the current time, a number of therapies have been advocated empirically. One simple tactic is to reduce the sinus rate and hence myocardial energy requirements. Most effective therapies in CHF achieve this aim, but it can also be accomplished with specific pharmacotherapy.[118,128] Whether such an intervention would sufficiently impair cardiac reserve is uncertain, and no clinical data are available.

L-Carnitine and coenzyme Q10 are agents that have been thought to improve fatty acid metabolism. Both have been used and advocated extensively in Asia and parts of Europe, but rigorous clinical trials have not been performed.[129–132] Finally, the failing, or energy-starved, myocardium may utilize energy provided by carbohydrates more easily than that provided by fatty acids. It is possible to shift substrate utilization from fatty acids to glucose with agents that inhibit pyruvate dehydrogenase, such as dichloroacetate or ranolazine.[133,134] The same shift in substrate utilization can be accomplished by administration of glucose and insulin; it also occurs during β-adrenoreceptor blockade. This action may be partly responsible for the improved energy efficiency observed during β-blocker therapy in CHF patients.[135]

Compared to the other approaches of therapeutic intervention in CHF just discussed, the rationale for altering myocardial metabolism is much less clear, and the clinical value of even the empiric therapies now in use is uncertain. Nonetheless, because such agents are likely to complement other treatments and may prevent progressive myocardial dysfunction, further investigation in this area is warranted.

Molecular and Cellular Therapy

As in other areas of medicine and cardiology, advances in molecular and cellular biology are promising to have an important impact on heart failure.[136] Molecular diagnostics, new delivery systems, gene therapy, and other interventions that alter (either upward or downward) the expression of genes or the actions of their protein products are on the horizon.[18] Although wide clinical application of these approaches is unlikely this century, much relevant work is ongoing.

The current techniques available to modify the genetic composition of cells include methods to eliminate expression of a specific gene (knock out the gene, e.g., phospholamban[55]), dramatically increase expression of a gene (over-expression of the gene, e.g., β-adrenergic receptor,[137] c-myc,[138] α_1-receptor[139]), or modulate gene expression (via modulation of transcription factors, e.g., TEF-1[140–142]). These techniques are discussed in detail elsewhere.[143] The possible targets for these interventions are limited only by the determinants of myocardial function, phenotype, or cell cycle control and by the current immature state of knowledge in these fields. The necessary short-term goal is to gain a full enough understanding of the pathophysiology of heart failure on the cellular level to target appropriate genes and cell processes for intervention. These interventions may be viewed as having one or more of three basic goals: (1) increase function of existing myocytes; (2) alter ventricular remodeling; or (3) increase the number of functioning cardiomyocytes.

Potential targets for gene therapy to increase myocardial function are the best understood, given the direct parallel to pharmacologic attempts to discover useful positive inotropic agents. For instance, there are increasing data that the activity and expression of sarcoplasmic Ca^{2+}-ATPase is reduced in CHF.[54] This effect may be mitigated by decreasing the expression of phospholamban, a sarcoplasmic Ca^{2+} reuptake inhibitor, as demonstrated in a mouse model in which the gene for phospholamban had been knocked out.[55] The importance of decreased β-adrenergic receptors during heart failure is well established,[144] and one study demonstrated that mice overexpressing the β_2-adrenergic receptor[137] or the β-adrenergic receptor kinase inhibitor[145] had enhanced cardiac contractility, even in the absence of direct adrenergic stimulation. In addition, these studies have led to the discovery of new molecular targets for traditional pharmacologic therapy. One study[146] demonstrated that co-expression of the third intracellular loop of the α_{1b}-adrenergic receptor, the site that regulates the interaction of the receptor with its G protein, resulted in inhibition of receptor-mediated activation of phospholipase C in a highly specific manner. This result suggests that the receptor–G protein interaction site may be a target for future receptor antagonists. Whether these enhancements in contractility can improve cardiac function in patients with heart failure is unknown at this time,[147] though studies demonstrate the feasibility of molecular approaches to increasing cardiac performance.

Ventricular remodeling is crucial to the pathogenesis of heart failure[148]; and another possible strategy for gene therapy of heart failure is to target either the neurohormonal axis believed to be involved in this process or to directly alter the myocytes or fibroblasts themselves. The renin-angiotensin system plays a central role in the development of heart failure[75] and provides many targets for interventions on the systemic or the local[149,150] level. Angiotensin appears to be involved in the ventricular hypertrophy consequent to myocardial infarction,[151,152] and gene therapy to alter this process could favorably affect ventricular remodeling. Another approach to affect ventricular remodeling and to increase myocardial performance would be to alter the phenotype of the myocytes so they developed "physiologic" versus "pathologic" hypertrophy.[153] Although the approaches discussed above might have this effect through improving ventricular performance, direct interventions to modulate these pathways can be pursued, as the molecular switches that control expression of the various phenotypes are better understood. In addition to changes in myocyte phenotype, there is increasing evidence that the nonmyocyte cells and extracellular matrix[154,155] are important aspects of ventricular remodeling. Cytokines may play an important role in remodeling the myocytes and nonmyocytes,[156] especially tumor necrosis factor α (TNFα), which has been shown to be elevated in patients with heart failure[157,158] and to cause left ventricular dysfunction,[159,160] cardiomyopathy,[161] fibrosis,[162] and cachexia.[163] The role of cytokines in heart failure has received increased interest since the results of the Vesnarinone Study Group heart failure trial[38] and the subsequent studies suggesting that part of the effect of vesnarinone may be due to inhibition of cytokine production.[57] Although the results of the VEST trial have decreased enthusiasm for vesnarinone, other modulators of the cytokine pathways are being actively pursued.

Other cytokine pathways are also potential targets, including transforming growth factor β (TGFβ),[164] interleukin-1 (IL-1), IL-6, and cardiotrophin-1.[165] Specific applications of gene therapy technology to the treatment of heart failure include experiments using plasmid gene transfer,[166] transfected myoblasts,[167] or viral vectors[168] in mice to produce myocardial expression of TGFβ1. This expression has been shown to prolong survival of transplanted myocardium and may represent a future approach to the treatment of heart transplant patients without resort to systemic cytotoxic immunosuppressive agents.[169]

Although considerable attention has been paid to ventricular remodeling, the importance of vascular remodeling[170,171] during heart failure has only recently been appreciated. The peripheral circulation is an essential component in the pathogenesis of heart failure (see Chs. 12 and 14), and the nature and accessibility of endothelial cells make them tempting targets for gene therapy. Gene therapy of the peripheral manifestations of heart failure could address the alterations in the vasculature's response to various neurohormonal agents and its structural characteristics.[172] There are many neurohormonal pathways intricately intertwined in the regulation of vascular tone, including the α- and β-adrenergic, cholinergic, endothelin, vasopressin, and nitric oxide pathways. Elucidation of the nitric oxide pathway[64,173] has led to many studies of heart failure and other pathologic states. Although some studies have shown that basal nitric oxide release is normal[174] or increased[175] in patients with heart failure, this increase may be insufficient to overcome the circulating vasoconstrictors. In addition, many studies in animals[176–178] and patients[179–181] with heart failure have demonstrated decreased stimulated nitric oxide release. The production of nitric oxide is mediated by a number of nitric oxide synthases, all of which are genetically regulated and are potential targets for in situ production and control of vasodilation. Furthermore, the structure of the vascular wall may eventually be controlled through genetic manipulations, most likely as a by-product of work on restenosis after angioplasty.[182]

Myocardial cell loss (both pathologic necrosis and apoptosis) is a major contributing factor to the pathogenesis of heart failure, and the inability of myocytes to proliferate limits the response to myocardial damage. Two main strategies are evolving from studies of the cell cycle to address this decrease in myocyte number: (1) induce the terminally differentiated cardiac myocytes to proliferate; and (2) convert the scar tissue (cardiac fibroblasts) into skeletal or cardiac myocytes. Studies in the cell cycle of skeletal muscle, which is also terminally differentiated, have revealed a set of myogenic transcription factors (the MyoD family) that can induce the skeletal muscle differentiation program.[183] Expression of MyoD in mouse fibroblast cell lines has resulted in conversion to a stable myoblast and subsequently into cells resembling skeletal muscle.[184] Although cardiac myocytes contain basic helix-loop-helix proteins and homeobox genes, they do not express any of the skeletal muscle determination factors such as MyoD, and no cardiac specific determination factors have been isolated to date (though some candidates have been suggested[185,186]). However, if such factors could be isolated, they would represent a potential mechanism through which the remaining cardiac myocytes could be induced to "dedifferentiate" and undergo mitosis, replacing the lost cardiac mass. Another approach is represented by an experiment that demonstrated the in vitro conversion of cardiac fibroblasts into potentially functional skeletal myocytes.[187] This "molecular cardiomyoplasty" would result in converting the cardiac fibroblasts of the scar tissue into skeletal muscle (or cardiac muscle if cardiac-specific myogenic factors are discovered), which could potentially be recruited by the myocardium.

Another possible therapy for the future treatment of heart failure is cardiac myocyte transplantation. Engraftment of transplanted myocytes was first demonstrated using AT-1 cardiomyocytes, a differentiated tumor cell lineage derived from transgenic mice.[188,189] Although these cells did not impair host function, there was no evidence that there were functional connections with the host cardiomyocytes.[190] Other studies attempted the engraftment of skeletal myoblasts using C2C12 myoblasts, which successfully engrafted as fused, multinucleated myotubes that were stable for at least 6 months though still had no evidence of forming functional connections with the host myocardium.[191] One study[192] has demonstrated engraftment of fetal cardiomyocytes in an adult syngeneic mouse using embryonic day 15 cardiomyocytes labeled with a β-galactosidase reporter. These engrafted cells were highly differentiated, binucleated cells with complete sarcomeres, numerous junctional complexes between cells, and abundant mitochondria. More importantly, these cells demonstrated nascent intercalated disks connecting them to the host myocardium,[193] suggesting that there may be functional coupling that allows the engrafted cells to be incorporated into the myocardium. Although these results are encouraging and the electrocardiogram demonstrated no evidence of cardiac arrhythmias, there is no evidence to date that these connections are functional or that these engrafted cells can contribute to myocardial function.

Although ischemic and hypertensive heart disease are the most common causes of heart failure,[194] molecular diagnostic techniques have revealed many genetic abnormalities that can lead to heart failure. These disorders include abnormalities of cardiac energy metabolism and abnormalities of myocardial contractile and structural proteins.[195] Through the use of molecular techniques, specific diagnoses can be made that can lead to important therapeutic interventions, including dietary therapy with appropriate fatty acid and dietary supplements, avoidance of fasting, and specific supportive measures at times of illness. In addition, the increasing knowledge afforded by these investigations of the molecular basis of inherited cardiomyopathies provides targets for future gene therapy and a greater understanding of myocardial function.

As new targets for gene therapy become evident, the problem of delivery systems becomes more important. Much of this technology has been developed to address coronary arterial restenosis after angioplasty, though much of it is probably readily transferable to heart failure therapy. The delivery of these therapies has been described in terms of: (1) direct deposition of therapeutic agents into the tissue through an intravascular delivery system; (2) systemic administration of inactive agents followed by local activation; and (3) systemic administration of agents with specific affinity for the target tissue.[196]

Local delivery via intravascularly administered agents has been shown to transduce perivascular myocytes,[197] although it is not clear as to whether such administration can effect enough cells for clinical benefit. Multiple catheter-based delivery systems, including double-balloon,[198–200] porous balloon,[201–203] iontophoresis,[204] and hydrogel[205] catheters, as well as stents coated with cells, drugs, and genetic vectors, have been developed, but they await more efficient transgenic vectors.

Development of vectors for gene transfer has had to address two main issues: (1) efficiency of gene transfer and subsequent expression; and (2) site specificity. Initial experiments in adult rat myocardium used direct injection of DNA plasmids[206] and were subsequently performed in the canine heart[207]; although these experiments provided useful probes for gene expression, the low efficiency of gene transfer precluded their clinical applicability. Intravenous administration of expression plasmid–cationic liposome complexes has resulted in systemic transgene expression through many tissues and persisted for at least 9 weeks,[208] and newer preparations may increase the efficiency of this method of gene transfer.[209,210] Site specificity with these methods can be either receptor-mediated via liposome target-specific receptors or by using tissue-specific promoter elements. Viruses are a major tool in gene transfer in the laboratory; and with increasing understanding of their molecular biology they have been used in clinical applications.[211–213] Although retroviruses appear to have attractive advantages for gene therapy,[143] their dependence on dividing cells for gene transfer is a limitation for myocytes.[214] Consequently, the ability of adenoviruses to directly transfer DNA into nondividing mammalian cells[215] was exploited by direct injection of adenoviral vectors into the myocardium[216,217] and intravascular injection.[197] At this time, the use of adenoviruses appears to be the most promising vector for gene therapy of heart failure, although other approaches, such as cardiomyocyte transplantation (see above), are also intriguing.

Nonpharmacologic Therapies

The focus of this chapter is on pharmacologic (broadly defined to include gene therapy) approaches to heart failure. Current nonpharmacologic treatments are discussed in detail in Chapter 41. Nonetheless, because some of the latter approaches are underutilized or inadequately evaluated but offer the potential to substantially improve quality of life and outcome, they warrant brief discussion in the current context. Exercise appears to have the best potential for broad applicability. Exercise training and selective respiratory muscle training[218] have been shown to improve exercise performance, left ventricular diastolic filling,[219] hemodynamics, autonomic balance, ventilation, and skeletal muscle oxidative capacity and to alleviate symptoms.[220–222] Other nonpharmacologic treatments address the ventilatory abnormalities of heart failure patients. Continuous positive airway pressure (CPAP) has been shown to have beneficial effects on oxygenation, heart rate variability, and left ventricular afterload in the acute, decompensated setting[223] and, in short-term administration, at baseline.[224,225] Other strategies, such as use of dual-chamber pacing to improve hemodynamics, may be useful in some patients[226,227] though clearly is not of widespread benefit. Perhaps future studies will answer the question as to whether these nonpharmacologic interventions can also have a beneficial effect on survival and which patient populations will benefit most.

CONCLUSION

A great deal of progress has been made with regard to each of the goals of treating CHF: alleviating symptoms and improving functional capacity, preventing progressive left ventricular dysfunction, and prolonging survival. These goals have been partially reached with a relatively limited armamentarium of drugs, but a great deal more remains to be accomplished.

Of the potential therapeutic approaches available, experience and theoretical considerations point toward further development and use of neurohormonal antagonists and away from agents with a primarily narrow hemodynamic mechanism of action, such as direct vasodilation or positive inotropy. After years of controversy, the place of chronic positive inotropic therapy has been clarified by recent trials. Digoxin has at last been proven a valuable agent, although its effect on survival is neutral. However, experience with other positive inotropic agents has been consistently unfavorable, as demonstrated by trials with xamoterol, milrinone, flosequinan, ibopamine, pimobendan, and vesnarinone. Based on these experiences, there appears to be little justification for further investigation of chronic positive inotropic agents, although short-term and intermittent inotropic therapy remains a useful management strategy.

Improving myocardial energetics and altering the pathophysiology of heart failure by interventions at the molecular and cellular level are future approaches that warrant careful attention.

REFERENCES

1. Massie BM: A perspective on the treatment of heart failure. Curr Opin Cardiol 9:255, 1994.
2. Agency for Health Policy and Research: Clinical Practice Guideline 11. Heart Failure. Evaluation and Care of Patients with Left Ventricular Systolic Dysfunction. AHCPR Publication No. 04–0612, 1994
3. Johnstone DE, Abdulla A, Arnold JM et al: Diagnosis and management of heart failure. Canadian Cardiovascular Society. Can J Cardiol 10:613, 1994
4. Williams JF Jr, Bristow MR, Fowler MB et al: Guidelines for the evaluation and management of heart failure. Report of the American College of Cardiology/American Heart Association Task Force on Practice Guidelines (committee on evaluation and management of heart failure). Circulation 92:2764, 1995
5. Massie BM, Shah NB: The heart failure epidemic: magnitude of the problem and potential mitigating approaches. Curr Opin Cardiol 11:221, 1996
6. American Heart Association: Heart and Stroke Facts: 1995 Statistical Supplement. American Heart Association, Dallas, 1995
7. Ho KK, Anderson KM, Kannel WB et al: Survival after the onset of congestive heart failure in Framingham Heart Study subjects. Circulation 88:107, 1993
8. Cohn JN, Archibald DG, Ziesche S et al: Effect of vasodilator therapy on mortality in chronic congestive heart failure. Results of a Veterans Administration Cooperative Study. N Engl J Med 314:1547, 1986
9. CONSENSUS Trial Study Group: Effects of enalapril on mortality in severe congestive heart failure. Results of the Cooperative North Scandinavian Enalapril Survival Study (CONSENSUS). N Engl J Med 316:1429, 1987
10. SOLVD Investigators: Effect of enalapril on survival in patients with reduced left ventricular ejection fractions and congestive heart failure. N Engl J Med 325:293, 1991
11. SOLVD Investigators: Effect of enalapril on mortality and the development of heart failure in asymptomatic patients with reduced left ventricular ejection fractions. N Engl J Med 327:685, 1992
12. Pfeffer MA, Braunwald E, Moye LA et al: Effect of captopril on mortality and morbidity in patients with left ventricular dysfunction after myocardial infarction. Results of the survival and ventricular enlargement trial. The SAVE Investigators. N Engl J Med 327:669, 1992
13. Acute Infraction Ramipril Efficacy (AIRE) Study Investigators: Effect of ramipril on mortality and morbidity of survivors of acute myocardial infarction with clinical evidence of heart failure. The Acute Infarction Ramipril Efficacy (AIRE) Study Investigators. Lancet 342:821, 1993
14. Kober L, Torp-Pedersen C, Carlsen JE, et al: A clinical trial of the angiotensin-converting enzyme inhibitor trandolapril in patients with left ventricular dysfunction after myocardial infarction. N Engl J Med 333:1670, 1995
15. Ambrosioni E, Borghi C, Magnani B: The effect of the angiotensin-converting-enzyme inhibitor zofenopril on mortality and morbidity after anterior myocardial infarction. The Survival of Myocardial Infarction

Long-Term Evaluation (SMILE) study investigators. N Engl J Med 332:80, 1995

16. Packer M, Rouleaou J, Swedberg K et al: Effect of flosequinan on survival in chronic heart failure. Preliminary results of the PROFILE study. Circulation, suppl. 1 88:1, 1993

17. Cohn JN, Johnson G, Ziesche S et al: A comparison of enalapril with hydralazine-isosorbide dinitrate in the treatment of chronic congestive heart failure. N Engl J Med 325:303, 1991

18. Mayer NJ, Rubin SA: The molecular and cellular biology of heart failure. Curr Opin Cardiol 10:238, 1995

19. Van Veldhuisen DJ, Girbes AR, de Graeff PA, Lie KI: Effects of dopaminergic agents on cardiac and renal function in normal man and in patients with congestive heart failure. Int J Cardiol 37:293, 1992

20. Rajfer SI, Davis FR: Role of dopamine receptors and the utility of dopamine agonists in heart failure. Circulation 82:197, 1990

21. Van Veldhuisen DJ, Man in't Veld AJ, Dunselman PH et al: Double-blind placebo-controlled study of ibopamine and digoxin in patients with mild to moderate heart failure. Results of the Dutch ibopamine Multicenter Trial (DIMT). J Am Coll Cardiol 22:1564, 1993

22. Rousseau MF, Konstam MA, Benedict CR et al: Progression of left ventricular dysfunction secondary to coronary artery disease, sustained neurohormonal activation and effects of ibopamine therapy during long-term therapy with angiotensin-converting enzyme inhibitor. Am J Cardiol 73:488, 1994

23. Brandt RR, Wright RS, Redfield MM, Burnett JC Jr: Atrial natriuretic peptide in heart failure. J Am Coll Cardiol 22:86A, 1993

24. Northridge DB, McMurray J, Dargie HJ: Atrial natriuretic factor in chronic heart failure. Herz 16:92, 1991

25. Cody RJ, Atlas SA, Laragh JH et al: Atrial natriuretic factor in normal subjects and heart failure patients. Plasma levels and renal, hormonal, and hemodynamic responses to peptide infusion. J Clin Invest 78:1362, 1986

26. Eiskjaer H, Bagger JP, Danielsen H et al: Attenuated renal excretory response to atrial natriuretic peptide in congestive heart failure in man. Int J Cardiol 33:61, 1991

27. Yoshimura M, Yasue H, Morita E et al: Hemodynamic, renal, and hormonal responses to brain natriuretic peptide infusion in patients with congestive heart failure. Circulation 84:1581, 1991

28. Margulies KB, Burnett JC Jr: Neutral endopeptidase 24.11. A modulator of natriuretic peptides. Semin Nephrol 13:71, 1993

29. Elsner D, Muntze A, Kromer EP, Riegger GA: Effectiveness of endopeptidase inhibition (candoxatril) in congestive heart failure. Am J Cardiol 70:494, 1992

30. Good JM, Peters M, Wilkins M et al: Renal response to candoxatrilat in patients with heart failure. J Am Coll Cardiol 25:1273, 1995

31. Yagil C, Katni G, Yagil Y: The effects of adenosine on transepithelial resistance and sodium uptake in the inner medullary collecting duct. Pflugers Arch 427:225, 1994

32. Kuan CJ, Herzer WA, Jackson EK: Cardiovascular and renal effects of blocking A1 adenosine receptors. J Cardiovasc Pharmacol 21:822, 1993

33. Colucci WS, Wright RF, Braunwald E: New positive inotropic agents in the treatment of congestive heart failure. Mechanisms of action and recent clinical developments. 1. N Engl J Med 314:290, 1986

34. Colucci WS, Wright RF, Braunwald E: New positive inotropic agents in the treatment of congestive heart failure. Mechanisms of action and recent clinical developments. 2. N Engl J Med 314:349, 1986

35. Feldman AM: Classification of positive inotropic agents. J Am Coll Cardiol 22:1223, 1993

36. Schwinger RH, Bohm M, Mittmann C et al: Evidence for a sustained effectiveness of sodium-channel activators in failing human myocardium. J Mol Cell Cardiol 23:461, 1991

37. Hoey A, Amos GJ, Ravens U: Comparison of the action potential prolonging and positive inotropic activity of DPI 201–106 and BDF 9148 in human ventricular myocardium. J Mol Cell Cardiol 26:985, 1994

38. Feldman AM, Bristow MR, Parmley WW et al: Effects of vesnarinone on morbidity and mortality in patients with heart failure. Vesnarinone Study Group. N Engl J Med 329:149, 1993

39. Bechem M, Gross R, Hebisch S, Schramm M: Ca-agonists: a new class of inotropic drugs. Basic Res Cardiol, suppl.1 84:105, 1989

40. Scholz H, Meyer W: Phosphodiesterase-inhibiting properties of newer inotropic agents. Circulation, suppl. III 73:99, 1986

41. Leier CV, Binkley PF: Acute positive inotropic intervention. The catecholamines. Am Heart J 121:1866, 1991

42. Xamoterol in Severe Heart Failure Study Group: Xamoterol in severe heart failure. Lancet 336:1, 1990

43. Packer M: The development of positive inotropic agents for chronic heart failure. How have we gone astray? J Am Coll Cardiol 22:119A, 1993

44. Schmitz W, Kohl C, Neumann J et al: On the mechanism of positive inotropic effects of alpha-adrenoceptor agonists. Basic Res Cardiol, suppl. 1 84:23, 1989

45. DiBianco R: Acute positive inotropic intervention. The phosphodiesterase inhibitors. Am Heart J 121:1871, 1991

46. Packer M, Carver JR, Rodeheffer RJ et al: Effect of oral milrinone on mortality in severe chronic heart failure. The PROMISE Study Research Group. N Engl J Med 325:1468, 1991

47. Lubbe WF, Podzuweit T, Opie LH: Potential arrhythmogenic role of cyclic adenosine monophosphate (AMP) and cytosolic calcium overload. Implications for prophylactic effects of beta-blockers in myocardial infarction and proarrhythmic effects of phosphodiesterase inhibitors. J Am Coll Cardiol 19:1622, 1992

48. Massie BM, Podrid PJ, Hendrix GH et al: Does asymptomatic worsening of arrhythmia predict sudden death in heart failure? Evidence for clinically significant proarrhythmia during milrinone therapy. J Am Coll Cardiol 19:19A, 1992

49. Nony P, Boissel JP, Lievre M et al: Evaluation of the effect of phosphodiesterase inhibitors on mortality in chronic heart failure patients. A meta-analysis. Eur J Clin Pharmacol 46:191, 1994

50. Kubo SH: Inotropic agents with calcium-sensitizing properties. Clinical and hemodynamic effects of pimobendan. Coron Artery Dis 5:119, 1994

51. Hagemeijer F: Calcium sensitization with pimobendan. Pharmacology, haemodynamic improvement, and sudden death in patients with chronic congestive heart failure. Eur Heart J 14:551, 1993

52. Pagel PS, Harkin CP, Hettrick DA, Warltier DC: Levosimendan (OR–1259), a myofilament calcium sensitizer, enhances myocardial contractility but does not alter isovolumic relaxation in conscious and anesthetized dogs. Anesthesiology 81:974, 1994

53. Sundberg S, Lilleberg J, Nieminen MS, Lehtonen L: Hemodynamic and neurohumoral effects of levosimendan, a new calcium sensitizer, at rest and during exercise in healthy men. Am J Cardiol 75:1061, 1995

54. Figueredo VM, Camacho SA: Basic mechanisms of myocardial dysfunction. Cellular pathophysiology of heart failure. Curr Opin Cardiol 10:246, 1995

55. Luo W, Grupp IL, Harrer J et al: Targeted ablation of the phospholamban gene is associated with markedly enhanced myocardial contractility and loss of beta-agonist stimulation. Circ Res 75:401, 1994

56. Ferguson DW: Digitalis and neurohormonal abnormalities in heart failure and implications for therapy. Am J Cardiol 69:24G, 1992

57. Matsumori A, Shioi T, Yamada T et al: Vesnarinone, a new inotropic agent, inhibits cytokine production by stimulated human blood from patients with heart failure. Circulation 89:955, 1994

58. Packer M: Long-term strategies in the management of heart failure. Looking beyond ventricular function and symptoms. Am J Cardiol 69:150G, 1992

59. Elkayam U, Shotan A, Mehra A, Ostrzega E: Calcium channel blockers in heart failure. J Am Coll Cardiol 22:139A, 1993

60. Packer M: Pathophysiological mechanisms underlying the adverse effects of calcium channel-blocking drugs in patients with chronic heart failure. Circulation, suppl. IV 80:59, 1989

61. Haeusslein EA, Greenberg BH, Massie BM: Does the magnitude of mitral regurgitation determine hemodynamic response to vasodilation in chronic congestive heart failure? Chest 100:1312, 1991

62. Packer M: The neurohormonal hypothesis. A theory to explain the mechanism of disease progression in heart failure. J Am Coll Cardiol 20:248, 1992

63. Bauer JA, Fung HL: Concurrent hydralazine administration prevents nitroglycerin-induced hemodynamic tolerance in experimental heart failure. Circulation 84:35, 1991

64. Palmer RM, Ferrige AG, Moncada S: Nitric oxide release accounts for the biological activity of endothelium-derived relaxing factor. Nature 327:524, 1987

65. Loh E, Stamler JS, Hare JM et al: Cardiovascular effects of inhaled nitric oxide in patients with left ventricular dysfunction. Circulation 90:2780, 1994

66. Semigran MJ, Cockrill BA, Kacmarek R et al: Hemodynamic effects of inhaled nitric oxide in heart failure. J Am Coll Cardiol 24:982, 1994

67. Packer M, Nicod P, Khandheria BR et al: Randomized, multicenter, double-blind, placebo-controlled evaluation of amlodipine in patients with mild-to-moderate heart failure. J Am Coll Cardiol 17:274A, 1991

68. Veniant M, Clozel JP, Hess P, Wolfgang R: Ro 40–5967, in contrast to diltiazem, does not reduce left ventricular contractility in rats with chronic myocardial infarction. J Cardiovasc Pharmacol 17:277, 1991

69. Packer M, O'Connor CM, Ghali JK, et al: Effect of amlodipine on morbidity and mortality in severe chronic heart failure. N Engl J Med, 1996 (in press)

70. Cohn JN, Ziesche SM, Loss LE et al: Effect of felodipine on short-term exercise and neurohormone and long-term mortality in heart failure: Results of V-HeFT III. Circulation 95:1, 1995

71. Kramsch DM, Sharma RC: Limits of lipid-lowering therapy. The benefits of amlodipine as an anti-atherosclerotic agent. J Hum Hypertens, suppl. 1 9:S3, 1995

72. Lupo E, Locher R, Weisser B, Vetter W: In vitro antioxidant activity of calcium antagonists against LDL oxidation compared with alpha-tocopherol. Biochem Biophys Res Commun 203:1803, 1994

73. Massie BM, Amidon T: Angiotensin converting enzyme inhibitor therapy for congestive heart failure. p. 380. In Hosenpud JD, Greenberg BH (eds): Congestive Heart Failure. Springer-Verlag, New York, 1993

74. Teerlink JR: The evolving role of angiotensin-converting enzyme inhibition in heart failure. Expanding the protective envelope. J Cardiovasc Pharmacol, suppl. 3 24:S32, 1994

75. Teerlink JR: Neurohumoral mechanisms in heart failure. A central role for the renin-angiotensin system. J Cardiovasc Pharmacol, suppl. 2 27:1, 1996

76. Cody RJ: The clinical potential of renin inhibitors and angiotensin antagonists. Drugs 47:586, 1994

77. Gottlieb SS, Dickstein K, Fleck E et al: Hemodynamic and neurohormonal effects of the angiotensin II antagonist losartan in patients with congestive heart failure. Circulation 88:1602, 1993

78. Benedict CR: Neurohumoral aspects of heart failure. Cardiol Clin 12:9, 1994

79. Francis GS, Chu C: Compensatory and maladaptive responses to cardiac dysfunction. Curr Opin Cardiol 9:280, 1994

80. Jougasaki M, Wei C-M, McKinley LJ, Burnett JC Jr: Elevation of circulating and ventricular adrenomedullin in human congestive heart failure. Circulation 92:286, 1995

81. Francis GS, Benedict C, Johnstone DE et al: Comparison of neuroendocrine activation in patients with left ventricular dysfunction with and without congestive heart failure. A substudy of the Studies of Left Ventricular Dysfunction (SOLVD). Circulation 82:1724, 1990

82. Swedberg K, Eneroth P, Kjekshus J, Wilhelmsen L: Hormones regulating cardiovascular function in patients with severe congestive heart failure and their relation to mortality. CONSENSUS Trial Study Group. Circulation 82:1730, 1990

83. Gilbert EM, Sandoval A, Larrabee P et al: Lisinopril lowers cardiac adrenergic drive and increases beta-receptor density in the failing human heart. Circulation 88:472, 1993

84. Eichhorn EJ: Do beta-blockers have a role in patients with congestive heart failure? Cardiol Clin 12:133, 1994

85. Gottlieb SS: Beta-blockers for heart failure. Where are we now? Curr Opin Cardiol 9:295, 1994

86. Doughty RN, MacMahon S, Sharpe N: Beta-blockers in heart failure. Promising or proved? J Am Coll Cardiol 23:814, 1994

87. Waagstein F, Bristow MR, Swedberg K et al: Beneficial effects of metroprolol in idiopathic dilated cardiomyopathy. Metroprolol in Dilated Cardiomyopathy (MDC) Trial Study Group. Lancet 342:1441, 1993

88. CIBIS Investigators and Committees: A randomized trial of beta-blockade in heart failure. The Cardiac

Insufficiency Bisoprolol Study (CIBIS). Circulation 90:1765, 1994

89. Metra M, Nardi M, Giubbini R, Dei Cas L: Effects of short- and long-term carvedilol administration on rest and exercise hemodynamic variables, exercise capacity and clinical condition in patients with idiopathic dilated cardiomyopathy. J Am Coll Cardiol 24:1678, 1994

90. Bristow MR, O'Connell JB, Gilberg EM et al: Dose-response of chronic beta-blocker treatment in heart failure from either idiopathic dilated or ischemic cardiomyopathy. Bucindolol investigators. Circulation 89:1632, 1994

91. Olsen SL, Gilbert EM, Renlund DG et al: Carvedilol improves left ventricular function and symptoms in chronic heart failure. A double-blind randomized study. J Am Coll Cardiol 25:1225, 1995

92. Australia-New Zealand Heart Failure Research Collaborative Group: Effects of carvedilol, a vasodilator-beta-blocker, in patients with congestive heart failure due to ischemic heart disease. Circulation 92:212, 1995

93. Packer M, Bristow MR, Cohn JN, et al: The effect of carvedilol on morbidity and mortality in patients with chronic heart failure. N Engl J Med 334:1349, 1996

94. Colucci WS, Packer M, Bristow MR et al: Carvedilol inhibits clinical progression in patients with mild heart failure. Circulation, suppl. I 92:395, 1995

95. Manmontri A, MacLeod SM: Centrally acting sympatholytic agents in the treatment of congestive heart failure. A review of the literature. Drugs 40:169, 1990

96. Ernsberger P, Damon TH, Graff LM et al: Moxonidine, a centrally acting antihypertensive agent, is a selective ligand for I1-imidazoline sites. J Pharmacol Exp Ther 264:172, 1993

97. Noyer M, De Laveley F, Vauquelin G et al: Mivazerol, a novel compound with high specificity for alpha 2 adrenergic receptors. Binding studies on different human and rate membrane preparations. Neurochem Int 24:221, 1994

98. Brooks DP, Fredrickson TA, Koster PF, Ruffolo RR Jr: Effect of the dopamine beta-hydroxylase inhibitor, SK&F 102698, on blood pressure in the 1-kidney, 1-clip hypertensive dog. Pharmacology 43:90, 1991

99. Levin ER: Endothelins. N Engl J Med 333:356, 1995

100. Harrison VJ, Randriantsoa A, Schoeffter P: Heterogeneity of endothelin-sarafotoxin receptors mediating contraction of pig coronary artery. Br J Pharmacol 105:511, 1992

101. Clozel M, Gray GA, Breu V et al: The endothelin ET_B receptor mediates both vasodilation and vasoconstriction in vivo. Biochem Biophys Res Commun 186:867, 1992

102. Teerlink JR, Breu V, Sprecher U et al: Potent vasoconstriction mediated by endothelin ET_B receptors in canine coronary arteries. Circ Res 74:105, 1994

103. Seo B, Oemar BS, Siebenmann R et al: Both ET_A and ET_B receptors cause vasoconstriction of human resistance and capacitance vessels in vivo. Circulation 92:357, 1995

104. Haynes WG, Strachan FE, Webb DJ: Endothelin ET_A and ET_B receptors cause vasoconstriction of human resistance and capacitance vessels in vivo. Circulation 92:357, 1995

105. Cody RJ, Haas GJ, Binkley PF et al: Plasma endothelin correlates with the extent of pulmonary hypertension in patients with chronic congestive heart failure. Circulation 85:504, 1992

106. Steward DJ, Cernacek P, Costello KB, Rouleau JL: Elevated endothelin-1 in heart failure and loss of normal response to postural change. Circulation 85:510, 1992

107. McMurray JJ, Ray SG, Abdullah I et al: Plasma endothelin in chronic heart failure. Circulation 85:1374, 1992

108. Wei CM, Lerman A, Rodeheffer RJ et al: Endothelin in human congestive heart failure. Circulation 89:1580, 1994

109. Shimada K, Masushita Y, Wakabayashi K et al: Cloning and functional expression of human endothelin-converting enzyme cDNA. Biochem Biophys Res Commun 207:807, 1995

110. Tsurumi Y, Fujie K, Nishikawa M et al: Biological and pharmacological properties of highly selective new endothelin converting enzyme inhibitor WS79089B isolated from Streptosporangium roseum No. 79089. J Antibiot (Tokyo) 48:169, 1995

111. Clozel M, Breu V, Burri K et al: Pathophysiological role of endothelin revealed by the first orally active endothelin receptor antagonist. Nature 365:759, 1993

112. Teerlink JR, Löffler BM, Hess P et al: Role of endothelin in the maintenance of blood pressure in conscious rats with chronic heart failure. Acute effects of the endothelin receptor antagonist Ro 47-0203 (bosentan). Circulation 90:2510, 1994

113. Kaddoura S, Firth JD, Boheler KR, Sugden PH, Poole-Wilson PA: Endothelin-1 is involved in norepinephrine-induced ventricular hypertrophy in vivo. Acute effects of bosentan, an orally active, mixed endothelin ET_A and ET_B receptor antagonist. Circulation 93:2068, 1996

114. Eddahibi S, Raffestin B, Clozel M et al: Protection from pulmonary hypertension with an orally active endothelin receptor antagonist in hypoxic rats. Am J Physiol 268:H828, 1995

115. Okada M, Yamashita C, Okada M, Okada K: Endothelin receptor antagonists in a beagle model of pulmonary hypertension. Contribution to possible potential therapy? J Am Coll Cardiol 25:1213, 1995

116. Oparil S, Chen SJ, Meng QC et al: Endothelin-A receptor antagonist prevents acute hypoxia-induced pulmonary hypertension in the rat. Am J Physiol 268:L95, 1995

117. Eckberg DL, Drabinsky M, Braunwald E: Defective cardiac parasympathetic control in patients with heart disease. N Engl J Med 285:877, 1971

118. La Rovere MT, Mortara A, Pantaleo P et al: Scopolamine improves autonomic balance in advanced congestive heart failure. Circulation 90:838, 1994

119. Riegger AJ: Role of neuroendocrine mechanisms in the pathogenesis of heart failure. Basic Res Cardiol, suppl. 3 86:125, 1991

120. Yamamura Y, Ogawa H, Chihara T et al: OPC–21268, an orally effective, nonpeptide vasopressin V1 receptor antagonist. Science 252:572, 1991

121. Mulinari RA, Gavras I, Wang YX et al: Effects of a vasopressin antagonist with combined antipressor and antiantidiuretic activities in rats with left ventricular dysfunction. Circulation 81:308, 1990

122. Raya TE, Gay RG, Goldman S: Selective vasopressin inhibition in rats with heart failure decreases af-

terload and results in venodilatation. J Pharmacol Exp Ther 255:1015, 1990

123. Naitoh M, Suzuki H, Murakami M et al: Effects of oral AV receptor antagonists OPC–21268 and OPC–31260 on congestive heart failure in conscious dogs. Am J Physiol 267:H2245, 1994

124. Katz AM: Cardiomyopathy of overload. A major determinant of prognosis in congestive heart failure. N Engl J Med 322:100, 1990

125. Takaoka H, Takeuchi M, Odake M et al: Depressed contractile state and increased myocardial consumption for non-mechanical work in patients with heart failure due to old myocardial infarction. Cardiovasc Res 28:1251, 1994

126. McDonald KM, Yoshiyama M, Francis GS et al: Myocardial bioenergetic abnormalities in a canine model of left ventricular dysfunction. J Am Coll Cardiol 23:786, 1994

127. Neubauer S, Krahe T, Schindler R et al: ^{31}P magnetic resonance spectroscopy in dilated cardiomyopathy and coronary artery disease. Altered cardiac high-energy phosphate metabolism in heart failure. Circulation 86:1810, 1992

128. Koenig W, Stauch M, Sund M et al: Hemodynamic effects of alinidine (ST 567) at rest and during exercise in patients with chronic congestive heart failure. Am Heart J 119:1348, 1990

129. Regitz V, Shug AL, Fleck E: Defective myocardial carnitine metabolism in congestive heart failure secondary to dilated cardiomyopathy and to coronary, hypertensive and valvular heart diseases. Am J Cardiol 65:755, 1990

130. Kobayashi A, Masumura Y, Yamazaki N: L-Carnitine treatment for congestive heart failure—experimental and clinical study. Jpn Circ J 56:86, 1992

131. Mortensen SA, Vadhanavikit S, Muratsu K, Folkers K: Coenzyme Q10. Clinical benefits which biochemical correlates suggesting a scientific breakthrough in the management of chronic heart failure. Int J Tissue React 12:155, 1990

132. Sanbe A, Tanonaka K, Niwano Y, Takeo S: Improvement of cardiac function and myocardial energy metabolism of rats with chronic heart failure by long-term coenzyme Q10 treatment. J Pharmacol Exp Ther 269:51, 1994

133. Bersin RM, Wolfe C, Kwasman M et al: Improved hemodynamic function and mechanical efficiency in congestive heart failure with sodium dichloroacetate. J Am Coll Cardiol 23:1617, 1994

134. Clarke B, Spedding M, Patmore L, McCormack JG: Protective effects of ranolazine in guinea-pig hearts during low-flow ischaemia and their association with increases in active pyruvate dehydrogenase. Br J Pharmacol 109:748, 1993

135. Eichhorn EJ, Bedotto JB, Malloy CR et al: Effect of beta-adrenergic blockade on myocardial function and energetics on congestive heart failure. Improvements in hemodynamic, contractile, and diastolic performance with bucindolol. Circulation 82:473, 1990

136. Nabel EG: Gene therapy for cardiovascular disease. Circulation 91:541, 1995

137. Milano CA, Allen LF, Rockman HA et al: Enhanced myocardial function in transgenic mice overexpressing the beta 2-adrenergic receptor. Science 264:582, 1994

138. Jackson T, Allard MF, Screenan CM et al: The *c-myc* proto-oncogene regulates cardiac development in transgenic mice. Mol Cell Biol 10:3709, 1990

139. Milano CA, Dolber PC, Rockman HA et al: Myocardial expression of a constitutively active alpha$_{1B}$-adrenergic receptor in transgenic mice induces cardiac hypertrophy. Proc Natl Acad Sci USA 91:10109, 1994

140. Kariya K, Karns LR, Simpson PC: An enhancer core element mediates stimulation of the rat beta-myosin heavy chain promoter by an alpha 1-adrenergic agonist and activated beta-protein kinase C in hypertrophy of cardiac myocytes. J Biol Chem 269:3775, 1994

141. Kariya K, Farrance IK, Simpson PC: Transcriptional enhancer factor-1 in cardiac myocytes interacts with an alpha 1-adrenergic- and beta-protein kinase C-inducible element in the rat beta-myosin heavy chain promoter. J Biol Chem 268:26658, 1993

142. Chen Z, Friedrich GA, Soriano P: Transcriptional enhancer factor 1 disruption by a retroviral gene trap leads to heart defects and embryonic lethality in mice. Genes Dev 8:2293, 1994

143. Mulligan RC: The basic science of gene therapy. Science 260:926, 1993

144. Bristow MR, Ginsburg R, Minobe W et al: Decreased catcholamine sensitivity and beta-adrenergic-receptor density in failing human hearts. N Engl J Med 307:205, 1982

145. Koch WJ, Rockman HA, Samama P et al: Cardiac function in mice overexpressing the beta-adrenergic receptor kinase or a beta ARK inhibitor. Science 268:1350, 1995

146. Luttrell LM, Ostrowski J, Cotecchia S et al: Antagonism of catecholamine receptor signaling by expression of cytoplasmic domains of the receptors. Science 259:1453, 1993

147. Williams RS: Boosting cardiac contractility with genes. N Engl J Med 332:817, 1995

148. Pfeffer MA, Braunwald E: Ventricular remodeling after myocardial infarction. Experimental observations and clinical implications. Circulation 81:1161, 1990

149. Hirsch AT, Talsness CE, Schunkert H et al: Tissue-specific activation of cardiac angiotensin converting enzyme in experimental heart failure. Circ Res 69:475, 1991

150. Lindpaintner K, Ganten D: The cardiac renin-angiotensin system. An appraisal of present experimental and clinical evidence. Circ Res 68:905, 1991

151. Sadoshima J, Izumo S: Molecular characterization of angiotensin II-induced hypertrophy of cardiac myocytes and hyperplasia of cardiac fibroblasts. Critical role of the AT1 receptor subtype. Circ Res 73:413, 1993

152. Sadoshima J, Izumo S: Signal transduction pathways of angiotensin II-induced *c-fos* gene expression in cardiac myocytes in vitro. Roles of phospholipid-derived second messengers. Circ Res 73:424, 1993

153. Scheuer J, Malhotra A, Hirsch C et al: Physiologic cardiac hypertrophy corrects contractile protein abnormalities associated with pathologic hypertrophy in rats. J Clin Invest 70:1300, 1982

154. Marijianoswki MM, Teeling P, Mann J, Becker AE: Dilated cardiomyopathy is associated with an increase in the type I/type III collagen ratio. A quantitative assessment. J Am Coll Cardiol 25:1263, 1995

155. Klappacher G, Franzen P, Haab D et al: Measuring extracellular matrix turnover in the serum of patients with idiopathic or ischemic dilated cardiomy-

opathy and impact on diagnosis and prognosis. Am J Cardiol 75:913, 1995

156. Mann DL, Young JB: Basic mechanisms in congestive heart failure. Recognizing the role of proinflammatory cytokines. Chest 105:897, 1994

157. Levine B, Kalman J, Mayer L et al: Elevated circulating levels of tumor necrosis factor in severe chronic heart failure. N Engl J Med 323:236, 1990

158. McMurray J, Abdullah I, Dargie HJ, Shapiro D: Increased concentrations of tumour necrosis factor in "cachectic" patients with severe chronic heart failure. Br Heart J 66:356, 1991

159. Gulick T, Chung MK, Pieper SJ et al: Interleukin 1 and tumor necrosis factor inhibit cardiac myocyte beta-adrenergic responsiveness. Proc Natl Acad Sci USA 86:6753, 1989

160. Yokoyama T, Vaca L, Rossen RD et al: Cellular basis for the negative inotropic effects of tumor necrosis factor-alpha in the adult mamalian heart. J Clin Invest 92:2303, 1993

161. Hegewisch S, Weh HJ, Hossfeld DK: TNF-induced cardiomyopathy. Lancet 335:294, 1990

162. Castagnoli C, Stella M, Berthod C et al: TNF production and hypertrophic scarring. Cell Immunol 147:51, 1993

163. Oliff A, Defeo-Jones D, Boyer M et al: Tumors secreting human TNF/cachectin induce cachexia in mice. Cell 50:555, 1987

164. Border WA, Noble NA: Transforming growth factor beta in tissue fibrosis. N Engl J Med 331:1286, 1994

165. Pennica D, King KL, Shaw KJ et al: Expression cloning of cardiotrophin 1, a cytokine that induces cardiac myocyte hypertrophy. Proc Natl Acad Sci USA 92:1142, 1995

166. Qin L, Chavin KD, Ding Y et al: Gene transfer for transplantation. Prolongation of allograft survival with transforming growth factor-beta 1. Ann Surg 220:508, 1994

167. Koh GY, Kim SJ, Klug MG et al: Targeted expression of transforming growth factor-beta 1 in intracardiac grafts promotes vascular endothelial cell DNA synthesis. J Clin Invest 95:114, 1995

168. Qin L, Chavin KD, Ding Y et al: Multiple vectors effectively achieve gene transfer in a murine cardiac transplantation model. Immunosuppression with TGF-beta 1 or vIL-10. Transplantation 59:809, 1995

169. Costanzo MR, Franco KL: New frontiers in heart transplantation. Clinical applications of basic research and new surgical approaches. Cardiol Clin 13:101, 1995

170. Weber KT, Anversa P, Armstrong PW et al: Remodeling and reparation of the cardiovascular system. J Am Coll Cardiol 20:3, 1992

171. Gibbons GH, Dzau VJ: The emerging concept of vascular remodeling. N Engl J Med 330:1431, 1994

172. Giannattasio C, Failla M, Stella ML et al: Alterations of radial artery compliance in patients with heart failure. Am J Cardiol 76:381, 1995

173. Furchgott RF, Zawadzski JV: The obligatory role of endothelial cells in the relaxation of arterial smooth muscle by acetylcholine. Nature 288:373, 1980

174. Kubo SH, Rector TS, Bank AJ et al: Lack of contribution of nitric oxide to basal vasomotor tone in heart failure. Am J Cardiol 74:1133, 1994

175. Winlaw DS, Smythe GA, Keogh AM et al: Increased nitric oxide production in heart failure. Lancet 344:373, 1994

176. Kaiser L, Spickard RC, Olivier NB: Heart failure depresses endothelium-dependent responses in canine femoral artery. Am J Physiol 256:H926, 1989

177. Ontkean M, Gay R, Greenberg B: Diminished endothelium-derived relaxing factor activity in an experimental model of chronic heart failure. Circ Res 69:1088, 1991

178. Teerlink JR, Clozel M, Fischli W, Clozel JP: Temporal evolution of endothelial dysfunction in a rat model of chronic heart failure. J Am Coll Cardiol 22:615, 1993

179. Treasure CB, Vita JA, Cox DA et al: Endothelium-dependent dilation of the coronary microvasculature is impaired in dilated cardiomyopathy. Circulation 81:772, 1990

180. Kubo SH, Rector TS, Bank AJ et al: Endothelium-dependent vasodilation is attenuated in patients with heart failure. Circulation 84:1589, 1991

181. Katz SD, Biasucci L, Sabba C et al: Impaired endothelium-mediated vasodilation in the peripheral vasculature of patients with congestive heart failure. J Am Coll Cardiol 19:918, 1992

182. Epstein SE, Speir E, Unger EF et al: The basis of molecular strategies for treating coronary restenosis after angioplasty. J Am Coll Cardiol 23:1278, 1994

183. Weintraub H, Davis R, Tapscott S et al: The myoD gene family. Nodal point during specification of the muscle cell lineage. Science 251:761, 1991

184. Davis RL, Weintraub H, Lassar AB: Expression of a single transfected cDNA converts fibroblasts to myoblasts. Cell 51:987, 1987

185. Daud AI, Lanson NA Jr, Claycomb WC, Field LJ: Identification of SV40 large T-antigen-associated proteins in cardiomyocytes from transgenic mice. Am J Physiol 264:H1693, 1993

186. Grepin C, Robitaille L, Antakly T, Nemer M: Inhibition of transcription factor GATA–4 expression blocks in vitro cardiac muscle differentiation. Mol Cell Biol 15:4095, 1995

187. Tam SK, Gu W, Nadal-Ginard B: Molecular cardiomyoplasty. Potential cardiac gene therapy for chronic heart failure. J Thorac Cardiovasc Surg 109:918, 1995

188. Field LJ: Atrial natriuretic factor-SV40 T antigen transgenes produce tumors and cardiac arrhythmias in mice. Science 239:1029, 1988

189. Steinhelper ME, Lanson NA Jr, Dresdner KP et al: Proliferation in vivo and in culture of differentiated adult atrial cardiomyocytes from transgenic mice. Am J Physiol 259:H1826, 1990

190. Koh GY, Soonpaa MH, Klug MG, Field LJ: Long-term survival of AT-1 cardiomyocyte grafts in syngeneic myocardium. Am J Physiol 264:H1727, 1993

191. Koh GY, Klug MG, Soonpaa MH, Field LJ: Differentiation and long-term survival of C2C12 myoblast grafts in heart. J Clin Invest 92:1548, 1993

192. Soonpaa MH, Koh GY, Klug MG, Field LJ: Formation of nascent intercalated disks between grafted fetal cardiomyocytes and host myocardium. Science 264:98, 1994

193. Nowak R: New cell transplants may mend a broken heart. Science 264:31, 1994

194. Teerlink JR, Goldhaber SZ, Pfeffer MA: An overview of contemporary etiologies of congestive heart failure. Am Heart J 121:1852, 1991

195. Kelly DP, Strauss AW: Inherited cardiomyopathies. N Engl J Med 330:913, 1994

196. Riessen R, Isner JM: Prospects for site-specific deliv-

ery of pharmacologic and molecular therapies. J Am Coll Cardiol 23:1234, 1994

197. Barr E, Carroll J, Kalynych AM et al: Efficient catheter-mediated gene transfer into the heart using replication-defective adenovirus. Gene Ther 1:51, 1994

198. Goldman B, Blanke H, Wolinsky H: Influence of pressure on permeability of normal and diseased muscular arteries to horseradish peroxidase. A new catheter approach. Atherosclerosis 65:215, 1987

199. Jorgensen B, Tonnesen KH, Bulow J et al: Femoral artery recanalisation with percutaneous angioplasty and segmentally enclosed plasminogen activator. Lancet 1:1106, 1989

200. Nabel EG, Plautz G, Nabel GJ: Site-specific gene expression in vivo by direct gene transfer into the arterial wall. Science 249:1285, 1990

201. Wolinsky H, Thung SN: Use of a perforated balloon catheter to deliver concentrated heparin into the wall of the normal canine artery. J Am Coll Cardiol 15:475, 1990

202. Flugelman MY, Jaklitsch MT, Newman KD et al: Low level in vivo gene transfer into the arterial wall through a perforated balloon catheter. Circulation 85:1110, 1992

203. Chapman GD, Lim CS, Gammon RS et al: Gene transfer into coronary arteries of intact animals with a percutaneous balloon catheter. Circ Res 71:27, 1992

204. Fernandez-Ortiz A, Meyer BJ, Mailhac A et al: A new approach for local intravascular drug delivery. Iontophoretic balloon. Circulation 89:1518, 1994

205. Riessen R, Rahimizadeh H, Blessing E et al: Arterial gene transfer using pure DNA applied directly to a hydrogel-coated angioplasty balloon. Hum Gene Ther 4:749, 1993

206. Lin H, Parmacek MS, Morle G et al: Expression of recombinant genes in myocardium in vivo after direct injection of DNA. Circulation 82:2217, 1990

207. Von Harsdorf R, Schott RJ, Shen YT et al: Gene injection into canine myocardium as a useful model for studying gene expression in the heart of large mammals. Circ Res 72:688, 1993

208. Zhu N, Liggitt D, Liu Y, Debs R: Systemic gene expression after intravenous DNA delivery into adult mice. Science 261:209, 1993

209. Felgner JH, Kumar R, Sridhar CN et al: Enhanced gene delivery and mechanism studies with a novel series of cationic lipid formulations. J Biol Chem 269:2550, 1994

210. San H, Yang ZY, Pompili VJ et al: Safety and short-term toxicity of a novel cationic lipid formulation for human gene therapy. Hum Gene Ther 4:781, 1993

211. Zabner J, Couture LA, Gregory RJ et al: Adenovirus-mediated gene transfer transiently corrects the chloride transport defect in nasal epithelia of patients with cystic fibrosis. Cell 75:207, 1993

212. Crystal RG, McElvaney NG, Rosenfeld MA et al: Administration of an adenovirus containing the human CFTR cDNA to the respiratory tract of individuals with cystic fibrosis. Nat Genet 8:42, 1994

213. Wilson JM, Engelhardt JF, Grossman M et al: Gene therapy of cystic fibrosis lung disease using E1 deleted adenoviruses. A phase I trial. Hum Gene Ther 5:501, 1994

214. Miller DG, Adam MA, Miller AD: Gene transfer by retrovirus vectors occurs only in cells that are actively replicating at the time of infection. Mol Cell Biol 10:4239, 1990

215. Brody SL, Crystal RG: Adenovirus-mediated in vivo gene transfer. Ann NY Acad Sci 716:90, 1994

216. Guzman RJ, Lemarchand P, Crystal RG et al: Efficient gene transfer into myocardium by direct injection of adenovirus vectors. Circ Res 73:1202, 1993

217. Kass-Eisler A, Falck-Pedersen E, Alvira M et al: Quantitative determination of adenovirus-mediated gene delivery to rat cardiac myocytes in vitro and in vivo. Proc Natl Acad Sci USA 90:11498, 1993

218. Mancini DM, Henson D, LaManca J et al: Benefit of selective respiratory muscle training on exercise capacity in patients with chronic congestive heart failure. Circulation 91:320, 1995

219. Belardinelli R, Georgiou D, Cianci G et al: Exercise training improves left ventricular diastolic filling in patients with dilated cardiomyopathy. Clinical and prognostic implications. Circulation 91:2775, 1995

220. Coats AJ, Adamopoulos S, Radaelli A et al: Controlled trial of physical training in chronic heart failure. Exercise performance, hemodynamics, ventilation, and autonomic function. Circulation 85:2119, 1992

221. Minotti JR, Massie BM: Exercise training in heart failure patients. Does reversing the peripheral abnormalities protect the heart? Circulation 85:2323, 1992

222. McKelvie RS, Teo KK, McCartney N et al: Effects of exercise training in patients with congestive heart failure. A critical review. J Am Coll Cardiol 25:789, 1995

223. Bersten AD, Holt AW, Vedig AE et al: Treatment of severe cardiogenic pulmonary edema with continuous positive airway pressure delivered by face mask. N Engl J Med 325:1825, 1991

224. Naughton MT, Rahman MA, Hara K et al: Effect of continuous positive airway pressure on intrathoracic and left ventricular transmural pressures in patients with congestive heart failure. Circulation 91:1725, 1995

225. Butler GC, Naughton MT, Rahman MA et al: Continuous positive airway pressure increases heart rate variability in congestive heart failure. J Am Coll Cardiol 25:672, 1995

226. Linde C, Gadler F, Edner M et al: Results of atrioventricular synchronous pacing with optimized delay in patients with severe congestive heart failure. Am J Cardiol 75:919, 1995

227. Nishimura RA, Hayes DL, Holmes DR Jr, Tajik AJ: Mechanism of hemodynamic improvement by dual-chamber pacing for severe left ventricular dysfunction. An acute Doppler and catheterization hemodynamic study. J Am Coll Cardiol 25:281, 1995

228. Massie BM, Shah NB: Future approaches to pharmacologic therapy for congestive heart failure. Curr Opin Cardiol 10:229, 1995

Index

Page numbers followed by *f* indicate figures; those followed by *t* indicate tables.